# SKANDALAKIS'

# *Surgical Anatomy*

*The Embryologic and Anatomic*
*Basis of Modern Surgery*

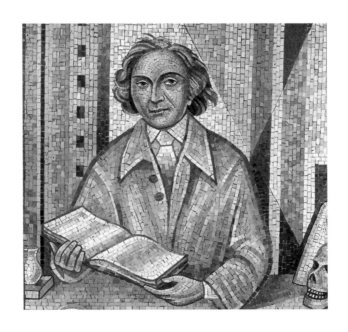

# PMP

## PASCHALIDIS MEDICAL PUBLICATIONS

**Front Page:** John Hunter (1728-1793) finalized the progression of surgery from a technical mode of treatment to a true science based on physiology and pathology. This representation is part of a mosaic mural of the history of medicine at Emory University School of Medicine in Atlanta, Georgia.

*SKANDALAKIS'*

# *Surgical Anatomy*

## *The Embryologic and Anatomic Basis of Modern Surgery*

# II

*Editor in Chief*
## JOHN E. SKANDALAKIS

*Associate Editors*

**GENE L. COLBORN • THOMAS A. WEIDMAN • ROGER S. FOSTER, Jr.**
**ANDREW N. KINGSNORTH • LEE J. SKANDALAKIS**
**PANAJIOTIS N. SKANDALAKIS • PETROS MIRILAS**

*P M P*
**PASCHALIDIS MEDICAL PUBLICATIONS**

PMP (Paschalidis Medical Publications, Ltd.).
14th, Tetrapoleos str., Athens, 115 27, Greece
Tel.: 003-210-7789125, 003-210-7793012, Fax: 003-210-7759421,
e-mail:
orders: Paschalidis@Medical-Books.gr
© information: GP@Medical-Books.gr, CP@Medical-Books.gr

ISBN:    960-399-074-4

**SURGICAL ANATOMY: The Embryologic and Anatomic Basis of Modern Surgery – 2 Volumes**

## EDITOR IN CHIEF

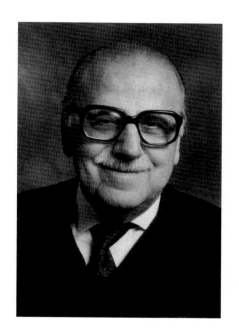

**John E. Skandalakis**
(1920- )

# Contributors

**John A. Androulakis, MD, FACS**
Professor and Chairman of Surgery
University of Patras Medical School
Greece

**Robert A. Badalament, MD, FACS**
Rochester Urology, P.C.
Rochester Hills, Michigan

**Gene D. Branum, MD, FACS**
Harrisonburg Surgical Associates
Harrisonburg, Virginia

**Grant W. Carlson, MD, FACS**
Wadley Glenn Professor of Surgery
Professor of Surgery/Oncology/Plastics
Emory University School of Medicine
Atlanta, Georgia

**Gene L. Colborn, MS, PhD**
Clinical Professor of Surgical Anatomy and Technique
Emory University School of Medicine, Atlanta, Georgia
Director (Emeritus), Center for Clinical Anatomy
Professor Emeritus, Department of Cellular Biology and Anatomy
Professor Emeritus, Department of Surgery
Medical College of Georgia, Augusta, Georgia
Chairman of Anatomy (Retired), Ross University, School of Medicine
Commonwealth of Dominica, West Indies
Professor and Director of Clinical Anatomy
American University of the Caribbean School of Medicine
St. Maarten, Netherlands Antilles

**John M. DelGaudio, MD, FACS**
Assistant Professor of Otolaryngology - Head and Neck Surgery
Emory University School of Medicine
Atlanta, Georgia

**Roger S. Foster, Jr., MD, FACS**
Professor Emeritus, Surgery
University of Vermont, Burlington, Vermont
Wadley Glenn Professor of Surgery (Retired)
Emory University School of Medicine, Atlanta, Georgia

**Niall T. M. Galloway, MD, FRCS**
Associate Professor, Department of Urology
Emory University School of Medicine
Medical Director, Emory Continence Center
Atlanta, Georgia

**George F. Hatch III, MD**
Resident, Department of Orthopedic Surgery
Emory University School of Medicine
Atlanta, Georgia

**Kathryn F. Hatch, MD**
Resident, Department of Surgery
University of Utah
Salt Lake City, Utah

**Ian N. Jacobs, MD, FAAP**
Assistant Professor of Otolaryngology
University of Pennsylvania School of Medicine
Philadelphia, Pennsylvania

**Andrew N. Kingsnorth, BSc (Hons), MBBS, MS, FRCS, FACS**
Professor of Surgery
Derriford Hospital, Postgraduate Medical School
University of Plymouth
Devon, U.K.

**Richard C. Lauer, MD, FACP**
Attending Physician
Piedmont Hospital
Atlanta, Georgia

**Dorothea Liebermann-Meffert, MD, Professor Dr, FACS**
Professor of Surgery, Surgical Clinic and Policlinic r.d. Isar
Technical University
Munich, Germany

**David A. McClusky III, MD**
Resident, Department of Surgery
Emory University School of Medicine
Atlanta, Georgia

**Petros Mirilas, MD, MSurg**
Clinical Associate Professor of Surgical Anatomy and Technique
Emory University School of Medicine, Atlanta, Georgia
Lecturer in Anatomy, Department of Anatomy-Embryology
University of Crete Medical School
Heraklion, Crete, Greece

**Thomas S. Parrott, MD, FAAP, FACS†**
Assistant Professor of Urology
Emory University School of Medicine
Atlanta, Georgia

**Dimitry Rabkin, FAAP, FACS**
Attending Otolaryngologist
Lenox Hill Hospital
Manhattan Eye, Ear & Throat Hospital
New York, New York

**Daniel D. Richardson, MD, FACS**
Clinical Associate Professor of Surgical Anatomy and Technique
Emory University School of Medicine
Atlanta, Georgia
Attending Physician, Highlands-Cashier Hospital
Highlands, North Carolina

**Robert M. Rogers, Jr., MD, FACOG**
Attending Gynecologist
Reading Hospital and Medical Center
Reading, Pennsylvania

**William M. Scaljon, MD, FACS**
Clinical Associate Professor of Surgical Anatomy and Technique
Emory University School of Medicine
Atlanta, Georgia
Chief, Section of Urology
Piedmont Hospital
Atlanta, Georgia

**Ahmed Shafik, MD, PhD**
Professor and Chairman, Department of Surgery and
    Experimental Research
Faculty of Medicine, Cairo University
Cairo, Egypt

**John E. Skandalakis, MD, PhD, FACS**
Chris Carlos Distinguished Professor of Surgical Anatomy
    and Technique
Director, Centers for Surgical Anatomy and Technique
Professor of Surgery
Emory University School of Medicine, Atlanta, Georgia
Senior Attending Surgeon (Retired)
Piedmont Hospital, Atlanta, Georgia
Clinical Professor of Surgery
Medical College of Georgia, Augusta, Georgia, and
Mercer University School of Medicine, Macon, Georgia

**Lee J. Skandalakis, MD, FACS**
Clinical Professor of Surgical Anatomy and Technique
Emory University School of Medicine, Atlanta, Georgia
Attending Surgeon and Director of Surgical Education
Piedmont Hospital, Atlanta, Georgia

**Panajiotis N. Skandalakis, MD, MS**
Clinical Professor of Surgical Anatomy and Technique
Emory University School of Medicine
Atlanta, Georgia
Assistant Professor of Surgery
University of Athens School of Medicine
Athens, Greece

**C. Daniel Smith, MD, FACS**
Clinical Associate Professor of Surgical Anatomy and Technique
Associate Professor of Surgery/General
Chief, General and Gastrointestinal Surgery
Emory University School of Medicine
Atlanta, Georgia

**Panagiotis Symbas, MD, FACS**
Professor of Cardiothoracic Surgery
Emory University School of Medicine
Director of Cardiothoracic Surgery
Grady Memorial Hospital
Atlanta, Georgia

**Thomas A. Weidman, PhD[†]**
Associate Professor of Anatomy (Retired)
Department of Cellular Biology and Anatomy
Medical College of Georgia, Augusta, Georgia

**Odysseas Zoras, MD**
Associate Professor of Surgery
University of Crete Medical School
Heraklion, Crete, Greece

---

[†]Deceased

*TO*

*Dr. William McClatchey,*
*Thanks, William, for your early*
*discovery of my prostate cancer.*

*Dr. Sam Ambrose,*
*Thank you, brother Sam,*
*for keeping me alive.*

*The late Dr. John Akin,*
*With profound gratitude for supporting me*
*to become Chief Resident at Piedmont Hospital.*

*The late Dr. Stephen W. Gray,*
*Heartfelt gratitude to my former*
*friend, teacher, and mentor.*

*JOHN E. SKANDALAKIS*

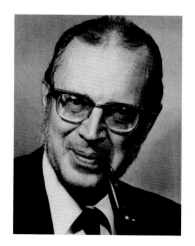

*The late Stephen W. Gray*
*(1915-1996)*

# *Foreword*

It is indeed both a pleasure and a privilege to have been asked to write the Foreword to this book of which Dr. John E. Skandalakis is the editor in chief. Known to most people simply as "Dr. Skan," he has been my teacher and academic scholar/idol, and this book is another of his many works of art. I first met this unique, seriously infectious personality in Chicago at an American College of Surgeons meeting in the late 1970s. Still but a lowly surgical resident at Johns Hopkins, I was working my way through the poster exhibits when I came upon a marvelous spread of posters on surgical anatomy. The subject matter belied the reputation of the author – Skandalakis – who even to a 3rd-year resident in General Surgery was well known as an embryologist. Of course, I stopped and started to devour the posters. As I began to read, I felt a warm, gentle hand on my shoulder, and a deeply-accented voice asked my name. Quite surprised, I turned to encounter the owner of the hand and the voice only to find a face that actually appeared interested in me  – truly interested in me and my obvious interest in the posters. Little was I to know that this would be the start of a friendship for several decades to come and a chance for me to acquire both a mentor in the science of surgical anatomy as well as (eventually) an adopted father (having lost my own father in 1983).

These past two decades have further proven the worth of this initial encounter with this learned American anatomist of Greek birth. Although now into his 9th decade, Dr. Skan remains a pupil of anatomy and continues to lead and teach us – his disciples. Rarely will the surgical world find a scientist so devoted to any one calling. Dr. Skan has been a surgical embryologist/anatomist now for 50+ years and is (not even arguably) the preeminent surgical anatomist of our time. His numerous books, articles, reviews, and book chapters reflect a singular study of surgical anatomy of many different regions – from rostral to caudal, anterior to posterior, dorsal to ventral, ulnar to radial, volar to palmar. One need only read any of his works to realize his clarity of both thought and word and the ease by which we as the readers are guided through the material – and it becomes interesting, enthralling, captivating, and often for the first time clear and understandable. For instance, read just the chapters in this book on the peritoneum/omentum or the liver and you will immediately appreciate my point.

In Dr. Skan's Preface he writes of his half century of experience teaching surgery and surgical anatomy. It is the magic of his clarity of presentation combined with his 50 years of hands-on operative experience with surgical anatomy that has allowed Dr. Skan to recognize and select the salient points of embryology and anatomy within this book; and that is its attraction for both the initiate and seasoned surgeon alike. Dr. Skan continues to remind us of the importance of an understanding of embryology, not just in our dealings with anomalies in pediatric surgery, but also in our trials and tribulations of finding the non-typically oriented parathyroid glands, or appreciating the vagaries of the blood vessels to the liver and gallbladder, or in preventing injuries to anomalous extrahepatic bile ducts during a laparoscopic cholecystectomy. In addition, the advent of laparoscopic surgery demands a new look at anatomy from a smaller, different, but more magnified laparoscopic purview – and while the anatomy itself does not change, our view does.

One of the unique approaches Dr. Skandalakis uses so effectively is to trace the history of some aspects of anatomic thought. This approach not only allows us to see the development of our understanding of anatomy, but also allows the insightful reader to merge the history of anatomic knowledge with the current concept of physiology; one will recognize how each field has driven the other to advance.

To try to put this book in perspective, let me tell you a bit about Dr. Skan, the man. Born in Greece, Dr. Skan became interested in anatomy early on, possibly under the aura and influence of the past Greek masters of his nationality, his heritage, and his geographic region. To further his studies, he came to the United States in 1951. In Atlanta, the academic environment and Dr. Skan's mentors allowed him to flourish, a privilege and freedom he has never forgotten. He has taken this opportunity very seriously as his obligation, giving back of his time, effort, and devotion to further the study and understanding of anatomy. Moreover, this **Greek American** became actively ensconced in the Atlanta scene by his own volition, not just in the medical or academic world, but also in the social and religious communities. Dr. Skan is known in Atlanta as a skilled, eminent surgeon, the consummate educator, a social philanthropist, and a loving, devoted father of a family itself prominent in the community. He is supported by his delightful and equally respected wife of 50 years – Mimi.

Even now at 83 years young, his clarity of thought and word in this book continue to guide us through the vagaries as well as the constancies of anatomy. Through his devotion and discipline, he has established and run the Thalia and Michael Carlos Center for Surgical Anatomy and Technique and the Alfred A. Davis Research Center for Surgical Anatomy at Emory University School of Medicine. From these centers and this man have been born many surgical anatomists destined to keep alive his words, devotion, and love of anatomy. This book is the Current Bible for the Surgical Anatomist and will undoubtedly remain so for many years to come. Thank you, Dr. Skan.

*Your friend and adopted son,*

**Michael G. Sarr, M.D.**
*Professor of Surgery*
*Chair, Division of General and Gastroenterologic Surgery*
*Mayo Clinic*
*Rochester, Minnesota*

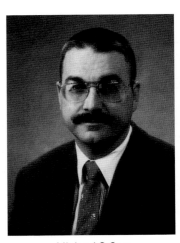

*Michael G.Sarr*
*(1950- )*

# *Preface*

*In writing for this book the lives of Alexander the king, and of Caesar, the conqueror of Pompey, I have before me such an abundance of materials that I shall make no other preface but to beg my readers not to complain of me if I do not relate all their celebrated exploits or even any one in full detail, but in most instances abridge the story.*

*Plutarch[1] (A.D. 46-120)*

*You will have to blame me for my boldness – I do not hesitate to confess it myself – when you remember with what presumption I formerly always strove for more, as long as the benevolent opinion of me held by the Governors, the excessive expectations of my pupils concerning the mediocre gifts I may possess, as well as the fire of my yet unimpaired youth, stimulated me to activity and perhaps also to an ambition of which I do not feel ashamed.*

*Hermann Boerhaave: Oration of 1729[2]*

This book derives from the half century of my experience – teaching surgery and surgical anatomy and technique at the Emory University School of Medicine, and practicing general surgery at Piedmont Hospital, both located in Atlanta, Georgia – and from the extensive and varied experiences of my associate editors and contributors in their specialized fields of endeavor. My hope is that we have articulated our collection of anatomic pearls to form a precious possession on paper for the student, the resident, and the practicing surgeon.

I selected the photographs of men and women who have contributed to their fields, and I regret that we could not include more. I take full responsibility for any omissions or if insufficient importance has been ascribed to someone's work. I, solely, am accountable for any errors in this book.

Our historical tables are by no means complete; our objective is only to stimulate the reader to go back and learn about the glory of yesterday.

Brief facts of embryogenesis are included because embryology leads the student to a more thorough understanding of the human anatomy. We present applied, surgically oriented anatomy emphasizing both surgical applications and ways to avoid anatomic complications. We approach the study of anatomic entities -- to paraphrase Treves -- upon the circumstances of practice. To be more specific, we present the anatomic entities with which the surgeon should be very familiar. Because minimally invasive and robotic surgery is definitely the surgery of today and tomorrow, the modern surgeon must now know this other type of anatomy, the "non-touch, non-see" anatomy. In other words, the surgeon must know the anatomy VERY WELL.

This book would never have come to fruition without contributions from numerous sources. I'd like to express my most profound appreciation to my associate editors and contributors who accepted the invitation to create this book with me. It is my admiration for them and their work that made me seek them out; and they acceded to my demands with grace and tolerance. The editorial comments of Dr. Roger S. Foster, Jr., are an invaluable addition to the text. Dr. Gary Bernstein, my former student and associate,

1. Plutarch. Selected Lives and Essays (trans. Loomis LR), vol. 2. Roslyn, NY: Walter J. Black, 1951.
2. Lindeboom GA. Herman Boerhaave: The Man and his Work. London: Methuen, 1968.

reviewed several chapters, and I'm grateful for the improvements his insights provided. It was a pleasure for me to have a very promising young resident, Dr. David A. McClusky III, as an assistant in researching facts for the history tables.

I'm very much indebted to my two editorial assistants, Phyllis H. Bazinet and Carol R. Froman, for their excellent work in preparing this material for publication. My grateful thanks also go to my secretary, Cynthia Painter, for her faithful service.

Eric Grafman's superb illustrations are found in almost every chapter of this book. His talent and skills, along with those of his associates Susan Brust, Robin Jensen, Barbara Cousins, Paul Chason, Andrew Matlock, and Mary Beth Clough add immeasurably to the book's usefulness.

At all phases of this endeavor, Paschalidis Medical Publications has provided important professional support. I truly appreciate it. As an aid to the reader, our publisher has added color to most of the illustrations that were originally black and white. I'm deeply grateful to Dr. John Louis-Ugbo for the significant refinements that resulted from his painstaking attention to detail in reviewing the illustrations.

In most cases the designation "Modified from ..." in the figure legend refers to the addition of color. In some cases the illustration itself was modified (with permission), and in some cases the term "Modified from ..." refers to both of the preceding.

The last thought I must share with the reader is that I mourn the passing of one of the associate editors of this book, Dr. Thomas A. Weidman, who was an excellent embryologist and a valued colleague. And I miss my former student and colleague, the late Dr. Thomas S. Parrott, who served as co-author of several chapters and who was an excellent pediatric urologist.

*John E. Skandalakis, MD, PhD, FACS*

# Contents

# Chapter 16

# Small Intestine

John A. Androulakis, Lee J. Skandalakis,
Andrew N. Kingsnorth, Gene L. Colborn,
Thomas A. Weidman, Daniel D. Richardson,
John E. Skandalakis, Panajiotis N. Skandalakis

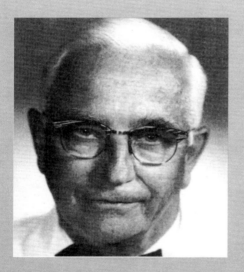

Owen H. Wangensteen (1898-1981), one of the
patriarchs of surgery in the United States.

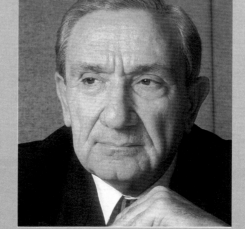

John Androulakis (1934--), Professor and
Chairman, Department of Surgery, University of
Patras Medical School, Greece; excellent inside
and outside the operating room.

*I hav finally kum to the konklusion, that a good reliable sett ov bowels
iz wurth more tu a man, than enny quantity ov brains.*

**Josh Billings**[1]

## HISTORY

The anatomic and surgical history of the small intestine is found in Table 16-1.

## EMBRYOGENESIS

### Normal Development

The distal foregut and the proximal midgut are responsible for the genesis of the three parts of the small bowel (duodenum, jejunum, and ileum). The approximate junction of the distal foregut and proximal midgut lies just distal to the ampulla of Vater in the adult. The demarcation of the small bowel into three parts takes place by the start of the third week of embryonic life.

The position of the duodenum posterior to the superior mesenteric artery is the result of the normal development and rotation of the embryonic gut. According to O'Rahilly and Müller,[3] duodenal rotation is unlikely, and the extended peritoneal cavity is responsible for the duodenal mesenteric attachment. The same authors believe that the duodenum's largely retroperitoneal position is the result of an increase in mesenchyme around the duodenum.

Early in the second month of gestation, the intestines, which elongate faster than the abdominal cavity expands, push a loop out into the umbilical cord (Fig. 16-1). This is the "midgut" of the embryologist, not the "midgut" of the surgeon. The herniated segment extends from approximately the distal one-third of the duodenum through the proximal one-third of the transverse colon. It is supplied by branches of the superior mesenteric artery. The axis of this herniation is the superior mesenteric artery. This artery, together with the celiac axis and the inferior mesenteric artery, is a remnant of the arterial side of the primitive vitelline circulation to the yolk sac. Originally paired and segmentally arranged, the pairs of arteries fuse, and their number is reduced to three by the sixth week of development. At this stage, the superior mesenteric artery continues past the intestine to supply the vitelline stalk, which occasionally persists as Meckel's diverticulum.

Rotation of the intestinal loop counterclockwise through 90° brings the future duodenum and proximal small intestine to the right of the future colon. The axis of this rotation is the superior mesenteric artery. The intestines continue to elongate in the umbilical cord. In the tenth week, they rather suddenly return to the abdomen. The cranial limb of the intestinal loop returns first, so that the duodenum passes behind the superior mesenteric artery. The caudal limb, which will form the distal ileum and the entire colon, returns later, bringing the transverse colon in front of the artery and the duodenum by a further 180° counterclockwise rotation (Fig. 16-2A & B).

In the final adult relations, the third part of the duodenum lies in the angle formed by the superior mesenteric artery and the aorta, having passed under the artery. It is this relationship that may lead to duodenal compression by the artery.

Movement of the contents of the duodenum is rarely impeded by the superior mesenteric artery early in life. A few cases in infants are known, but the condition cannot qualify as a frank congenital defect. A predisposition to vascular compression may exist in some individuals and not in others, but it is improbable that it can be recognized. Changes in habitus, posture, and diet later in life seem to be more important than anatomic configuration at birth. Burrington and Wayne[4] documented the influence of these extrinsic factors in adolescence.

As early as the beginning of the fifth week, the duodenal epithelium begins to proliferate, especially along the right wall near the origin of the hepatic diverticulum. By the end of the fifth week, only a few luminal clefts remain in the multilayered epithelium.[5] The lumen is restored by the eighth week, and the epithelium is a single layer of cells by the tenth week.

**TABLE 16-1. Anatomic and Surgical History of the Small Intestine**

| | | |
|---|---|---|
| Sushruta | 6th century B.C. | Wrote oldest known descriptions of bowel surgery. Described using a cautery over the swelling of strangulated hernias. Used the mandibles of black ants to clamp the edges of bowel wounds together. |
| Hippocrates (460-370 B.C.) | | Argued against surgical treatment of the abdomen. Provided a detailed description of intestinal obstruction: "In ileus, the belly becomes hard, there are no motions; the whole abdomen is painful, there are fever and thirst and sometimes the patient is so tormented that he vomits bile." |
| Praxagoras | 350 B.C. | Advocated opening the abdomen as a last resort to relieve "iliac passion" making an incision over the swelling of a strangulated hernia, freeing the intestine and establishing an artificial anus |
| Herophilus (334-280 B.C.) | | Referred to the "beginning of the intestines, prior to the beginning of the loops" as the "dodekadactilon" |
| Rufus of Ephesus (98-117 A.D.) | | Noted that a sphincter regulated the flow of gastric contents into the duodenum |
| Aretaeus the Cappadocian (81-138 A.D.) | | Described in detail ileus secondary to incarcerated hernia |
| Galen (131-201) | | In performing several abdominal procedures as surgeon to the Roman gladiators, he observed and described the anatomy of the small intestine |
| Fabricius d'Aqua-pendente | 12th century | As reported by Duverger, he described a procedure of intestinal repair involving end-to-end anastomosis |
| Roger of Palermo | Early 13th century | Wrote, "...if a part of the tender intestine is wounded, it is better to leave the treatment to God than to man, since Death will follow it very soon." Used the entrails of animals to protect eviscerated bowel until it could be replaced within the abdominal cavity. |
| Lanfranc | 13th century | Used animal tracheas to connect divided segments of bowel |
| Rolandus | ca. 1400 | Wrote a surgical text in which a picture depicts a physician preparing a patient with an eviscerated intestine using the open abdomen of a cat |
| Benedetti | 1497 | Claimed that the duodenum served as a "gate" controlling stomach-to-jejunal passage |
| Paracelsus (1491-1541) and Fabricius Hildanus (1560-1624) | | Each observed spontaneous fistulas due to penetrating bowel injury |
| Sanctus | 16th century | Treated intestinal obstructions by giving patients metallic mercury (up to three pounds) and using the weight of the mercury to try to open the intestines |
| Vesalius | 1543 | Studied the relationship between the duodenum and the extrahepatic biliary tract |
| Franco | 1556 | Described his experience in surgically treating strangulated inguinal hernia. He made an incision over the swelling, divided the constricting band, inserted a goose-quill-sized cannula, and returned the bowel to the peritoneum. |
| Sydenham (1624-1689) | | Managed intestinal obstruction using opium. He also recommended rest and horseback rides as therapy. |
| Kerckring | 1670 | Described the intestinal valvulae conniventes |
| Peyer | 1677 | Noted the presence of lymphoid follicles in the small intestine |
| Bidloo | 1685 | Provided a description of the duodenal papillae, the hepatopancreatic ampulla, and the junction of the pancreatic and common bile ducts |
| Nuck | 1692 | Reported his experiences helping a young surgeon treat volvulus, using his finger to draw out and treat a strangulated hernia |
| Mery | 1701 | Removed several feet of gangrenous bowel and established an artificial anus in a woman suffering from a strangulated hernia |
| Vater | 1720 | Described the duodenal papilla now commonly called the papilla of Vater |

**TABLE 16-1 (cont'd). Anatomic and Surgical History of the Small Intestine**

| | | |
|---|---|---|
| Le Peyronie | 1723 | Removed gangrenous bowel from a man with intestinal obstruction. Brought two loops out into the wound to serve as an artificial anus, placing traction on a suture placed in the mesentery between the two loops to quickly heal the fistula. |
| Ramdohr | 1727 | Removed two feet of gangrenous small bowel and invaginated the proximal end of the bowel into the lumen of the distal segment, securing the connection with a few sutures |
| Duverger | 1747 | Excised several inches of gangrenous bowel while suturing the two ends together over a piece of dog trachea that was passed 21 days later |
| Velse | 1751 | According to von Haller, he repaired an intestinal intussusception by removing the bowel, placing it in tepid milk until it returned to normal, and replacing it inside the abdomen |
| Mensching | 1756 | Used repeated intestinal puncture to treat obstructed bowels |
| Pott | 1771 | Inverted his patients to treat intestinal strangulation, arguing, "The nearer the posture approaches to what is commonly called standing on the head, the better, as it causes the whole packet of small intestines to hang, as it were, but the strangulated portion, and may thereby disengage it" |
| Meckel | 1781-1833 | Described diverticulum iliei verum, also known as Meckel's diverticulum |
| Cooper | 1804 | Inverted patients, suspending them over the shoulders of a strong attendant, to treat strangulated hernias. Also used isinglass (ichthyocolla) and suture in experiments connecting divided canine intestines. |
| Travers | 1812 | While experimenting with suture techniques, he noted that wounds closed with sutures that passed through all layers of the bowel wall healed well |
| Jobert | 1824 | Performed end-to-side anastomoses in dogs and cats using continuous wax suture |
| Lembert | 1826 | Developed a suture technique employing interrupted sutures that passed through the entire bowel wall except for the mucous membrane |
| d'Etiolles | 1826 | Used electrical stimulation of the abdominal wall to treat intestinal obstructions |
| Amussat | 1839 | Presented an autointoxication theory of intestinal obstruction, based on the assumption that it was caused by enteric toxin. Essentially the theory was used as a means for justifying the continued usage of emetics, laxatives, and bloodletting to treat obstructions. |
| Nélaton | 1839-1840 | Fixed a distended loop of bowel, proximal to the obstruction, in the wound using sutures penetrating the lumen and incising the exposed bowel (enterostomy). Although his first patient died, he was successful in 1849 and in 1852. |
| Duchenne | 1855 | Reported several successful instances where he treated intestinal obstruction with faradic current (electrodes placed in the rectum, abdomen, and sometimes the stomach) |
| Pfluger | 1857 | Observed that splanchnic nerve stimulation inhibited small intestinal movement |
| Ludwig | 1861 | Observed what he called "Pendelbwegungan" or the motion made by the bowel between peristaltic contractions |
| Auerbach and Meissner | 1862 | Published a study describing the intrinsic nerve plexus of the small intestine |
| Kussmaul | 1869 | Used gastric lavage to treat intestinal obstructions |
| Hutchinson | 1871 | Performed a successful operation for the reduction of intussusception in an infant. He published a review on the subject in 1874. |
| H.O. Thomas | 1879 | Enthusiastically followed Sydenham's opium recommendations, adding more to the recommended dosages. He thought that abdominal operations were not only unsuccessful but dangerous. |
| Billroth | 1881 1885 | Anastomosed parts of the small bowel to circumvent intestinal obstructions Invented the Billroth II procedure |
| Halsted | 1887 | Altered Lembert's suture technique, passing the needle through the submucosa but not into the bowel lumen |
| Witzel | 1891 | Published a description of an oblique enterostomy over a catheter |
| J.B. Murphy | 1892 | Used a button he devised to simplify intestinal anastomosis (Murphy's button) |

## TABLE 16-1 *(cont'd)*. Anatomic and Surgical History of the Small Intestine

| | | |
|---|---|---|
| Jourdain | 1895 | Performed what may have been the first mobilization of the duodenum |
| Mall | 1896 | Caused an acute intestinal obstruction by reversing a piece of bowel in order to prove that intestinal anatomy ensured that peristalsis moves only in the aboral direction |
| Schlatter | 1897 | Anastomosed the lower esophagus to the upper small intestine after performing a total gastrectomy |
| Bayliss and Starling | 1899 | Discovered that peristalsis was due to a reflex of the intrinsic nerve plexus |
| Treves | 1899 | After winning the 1883 Jacksonian Prize of the Royal College of Surgeons for a thesis regarding the benefits of operative management of intestinal obstruction, he wrote in 1899: "It is less dangerous to leap from the Clifton Suspension Bridge than to suffer from acute intestinal obstruction and decline operation." His work stimulated a movement toward the modern era of surgical management of intestinal obstruction. |
| MacCormac | 1899-1902 | As consulting surgeon during the Boer War he claimed, ". . . in this war, a man wounded in the abdomen dies if he is operated upon and remains alive if he is left in peace." This "MacCormac's Aphorism" was widely adopted. |
| Kocher | 1903 | Developed his classical method of duodenal mobilization (Kocher's maneuver) |
| Schwartz | 1911 | Used x-ray films to determine areas of intestinal distention |
| Hartwell and Hoguet | 1912 | Proved that subcutaneous injections of saline prolonged the life of dogs with (artificially produced) bowel obstruction. Their findings helped debunk the theory of autointoxication. |
| Richards | 1915 | Recorded his World War I experience with five cases of laparotomy. Two of his patients survived resections of 2-4 feet of bowel. |
| Dragstedt | 1918 | Proved that experimental animals could survive a total duodenectomy |
| Kloiber | 1919 | Published a paper emphasizing the usefulness of x-rays in discerning the level of intestinal obstruction |
| Ryle | 1920s | Introduced methods of passing tubes into the stomach for decompression |
| Gamble | 1925 | Used prolific fluid resuscitation in patients undergoing abdominal surgery |
| Monrad | 1926 | Treated intussusception using manipulative taxis through the abdominal wall after anesthetizing his patients |
| Hipsley | 1926 | Recommended using hydrostatic pressure from water in a rectal tube to treat intussusception |
| Olsson and Pallin | 1926-1927 | Used a column of barium passed through a rectal tube to treat intussusception |
| Wangensteen | 1932 | Advanced methods of intestinal decompression to treat intestinal obstruction (reducing mortality from 60-80% to 20%) while advocating excessive saline infusion for patients with a high obstruction. He changed the initial stage of a three-stage decompression from a proximal cutaneous jejunostomy to a more distal cutaneous jejunostomy; the other two stages (enterolysis and stoma closure) went unchanged. |
| Miller and Abbot | 1934 | Invented a tube to be passed into the intestine for decompression |
| Segi | 1935 | Discovered concentration of basal-granulated cells in intestinal villi of fetus (thesis published in 1936). Structure termed "Segi's cap" in 1980. |
| Klass | 1950 | Diagnosed mesenteric ischemia before infarction. Performed embolectomy without intestinal resection (patient died of acute heart failure). |
| Shaw & Rutledge | 1957 | Reported successful superior mesenteric vein embolectomy without bowel resection |
| Ende | 1958 | First description of nonocclusive mesenteric ischemia |
| Skandalakis et al. | 1962 | Collective review of cases of smooth muscle tumors of the small intestine as reported in the world literature |
| Aylett | 1963 | Performed ileorectal anastomosis with proximal loop ileostomy |
| Root | 1965 | Used a peritoneal tap to diagnose peritoneal insult (>200 leukocytes/mL) |
| Kock | 1970 | Developed continent abdominal ileostomy pouches |

**TABLE 16-1 *(cont'd)*. Anatomic and Surgical History of the Small Intestine**

| | | |
|---|---|---|
| Ghanem et al. | 1970 | Observed increased peritoneal leukocytes after intestinal arterial supply was cut off in dogs and cats |
| Boley et al. | 1971 | Edited first textbook on mesenteric ischemia |
| Guseinov | 1975 | Studied embryology of lymphatic capillaries in small bowel |
| Vantrappen et al. | 1977 | Published first description of human small bowel interdigestive motor complex |
| Traverso & Longmire | 1978 | Reported pylorus-sparing pancreaticoduodenectomy |
| Bookstein | 1982 | Used angiography to diagnose and treat small bowel bleeding |
| Saini et al. | 1986 | Described percutaneous drainage of diverticular abscesses |
| Gauderer & Stellato | 1986 | Performed gastrostomy without celiotomy or sutures |
| McKee et al. | 1994 | Evaluated diagnostic procedures for diverticular disease (CT scan, contrast enema, ultrasonography) |
| Zielke et al. Yacoe et al. | 1994 1997 | |

*History table compiled by David A. McClusky III and John E. Skandalakis.*

**References:**

Boley SJ, Sammartano RJ, Brandt LJ. Historical perspective. In: Longo WE, Peterson GJ, Jacobs DL. Intestinal Ischemia Disorders. St. Louis: Quality Medical, 1999. pp. 1-16.

Ellis H. The history of small-intestinal surgery. In: Wastell C, Nyhus LM, Donahue PE (eds). Surgery of the Esophagus, Stomach, and Small Intestine (5th ed). Boston: Little, Brown, 1990, pp. 774-782.

Ghanem E, Goodale RL, Spanos P, Tsung MS, Wangensteen OH. Value of leukocyte counts in the recognition of mesenteric infarction and strangulation of shorter intestinal lengths: an experimental study. Surgery 68(4):635-645, 1970.

Khubchandani IT. Evolution of surgical management of ulcerative colitis. Dis Colon Rectum 1989;32:911-917.

Nelson RL. Introduction and history. In: Nelson RL, Nyhus LM (eds.) Surgery of the Small Intestine. Norwalk, CT.: Appleton and Lange, 1987, pp. 3-12.

Peters JH. Historical review of pancreaticoduodenectomy. Am J Surg 1991:161:219-225.

Rachmilewitz D (ed). V International Symposium on Inflammatory Bowel Diseases. Boston: Kluwer, 1997.

Richardson DD, Gray SW, Skandalakis JE. The history of the small bowel. J Med Assoc Ga 1991;80:439-443.

Skandalakis JE, Gray SW, Shepard D, Bourne GH. Smooth Muscle Tumors of the Alimentary Canal: Leiomyomas and Leiomyosarcomas, a Review of 2525 Cases. Springfield, IL: Charles C. Thomas, 1962.

Wangensteen OH, Wangensteen SD. The Rise of Surgery: From Empiric Craft to Scientific Discipline. Minneapolis: University of Minnesota Press, 1978, pp. 106-141.

The first part of the duodenum retains both dorsal and ventral mesentery. However, during the rotation, the duodenal loop is fixed in the retroperitoneal space. Therefore, the dorsal mesentery of the rest of the duodenum disappears. The "disappearing" dorsal duodenal mesentery remains as an avascular plane of loose connective tissue (the fascia of Treitz) (Fig. 16-3). It is not related to the ligament of Treitz.

A duodenal mesentery is very rare; the authors of this chapter have seen only two cases in 40 years in both the operating room and the anatomy laboratory. This plane is entered into when the Kocher maneuver is performed to lift the second part of the duodenum to the left, thereby exposing the retroduodenal and retropancreatic regions.

As to the maturation of the duodenum, at first there is a single layer of endodermal cells surrounded by un-differentiated mesenchyme cells. By the end of the fourth week, the duodenal mucosa begins to proliferate, especially along the right wall near the origin of the hepatic diverticulum, which arises from the ventral wall during this stage. By the sixth week, only a few luminal clefts remain in the epithelium. By the tenth week, the lumen is completely restored and has become almost entirely single-layered.

Around the turn of the 19th century, it was believed that diverticula, duplications, and atresia resulted from a failure of recanalization of the epithelial plug.[6] It now appears that the occlusion is the incidental result of epithelial proliferation, rather than a definite, necessary stage in foregut development. It is probable that some intramural duplications and small diverticula may be the result of persistence of tissue spaces that failed to coalesce with the main portion of the lumina.[7]

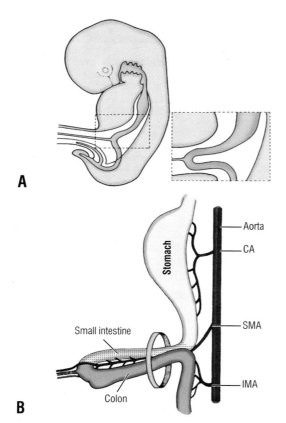

**FIG. 16-1.** Development of the small intestine. **A.** Elongation and herniation of the midgut into the umbilical cord early in the fifth week. *(Inset)* Late fifth week. **B.** Primary rotation of the herniated gut around the superior mesenteric artery. Prearterial limb *stippled. CA,* celiac axis; *SMA,* superior mesenteric artery; *IMA,* inferior mesenteric artery. (Modified from Gray SW, Akin JT Jr, Milsap JH Jr, Skandalakis JE. Vascular compression of the duodenum. (Part 1) Contemp Surg 9:37, 1976; with permission.)

The foregut will differentiate into the pharynx, esophagus, and stomach. The transverse septum, into which the liver cords of endoderm will grow, forms the anterior cranial boundary of the foregut and the open midgut. Posteriorly, the dorsal pancreatic primordium will develop. These structures define the future duodenum.

During the third and fourth weeks, the embryo grows rapidly, but the yolk sac and open midgut do not. By the fifth week, the foregut is as large as the opening of the midgut, which may then be called the *yolk stalk,* the *vitelline duct,* or the *omphalomesenteric duct.* At this time, a ventral swelling of the midgut just caudal to the yolk stalk marks the site of the cecum, and hence, the boundary between the small and large intestine.

Elongation of the midgut, especially of the portion between the yolk stalk and the duodenum, proceeds faster than elongation of the whole body of the embryo. The result

of this growth differential is a series of movements that ends with the adult position of the intestines in the abdomen. These movements occur in three well-defined stages that will be described only briefly here. For further details, consult Estrada[8] and Skandalakis and Gray.[9]

### *Stage 1: Herniation*

The midportion of the growing intestine buckles ventrally and protrudes into the coelom of the body stalk in the fifth week (Fig. 16-1A). The apex of the protrusion is marked by the yolk stalk. Its axis is marked by the superior mesenteric artery, which represents part of the primitive blood supply to the yolk sac. This loop of intestine undergoes a counterclockwise twist of 90°, so that the "prearterial" (cranial) limb lies to the right of the postarterial (caudal) limb (Fig. 16-1B). The caudal limb remains nearly straight, while the cranial limb grows rapidly and is thrown into coils.

### *Stage 2: Return (Reduction)*

The intestines return to the abdomen rather suddenly during the tenth week. The cranial limb enters first, to the right of the superior mesenteric artery (Fig. 16-2A & B). The caudal loop enters later: the left colon first; the transverse colon in front of the superior mesenteric artery; and lastly, the cecum with the terminal ileum.

### *Stage 3: Fixation*

From the fourth month until well after birth, the growth of the colon is completed. The mesenteries of the ascending and descending portions become obliterated by fusion with the peritoneum of the body wall. The transverse mesocolon fuses with the posterior leaf of the omental bursa.

Slovis et al.[10] reported on 19 patients with incomplete intestinal rotation, six (32%) of whom had normal cecal position and abnormal duodenojejunal junction. Among these six patients midgut volvulus was present in three, and obstructing duodenal bands were present in one. Postnatal fixation of the duodenojejunal junction was accomplished over a ten-month to two-year period in two of the six patients.

Intestinal villi begin to appear in the distal duodenum and the proximal ileum in the eighth week. The whole intestine is provided with villi by the end of the fourth month (the villi of the colon will disappear after birth). Brunner's glands appear in the third and fourth months, and may be capable of secretion by the end of the fifth month.[11] The striate border of the epithelial cells is visible by the third month.

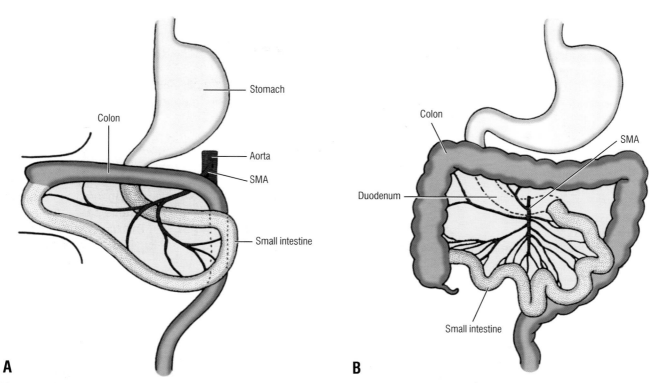

**FIG. 16-2. A.** Return of the intestines to the abdomen in the tenth week. The prearterial *(stippled)* limb returns first, passing behind the superior mesenteric artery. **B.** Final position of the intestines attained shortly after birth. *SMA,* superior mesenteric artery. (Modified from Gray SW, Akin JT Jr, Milsap JH Jr, Skandalakis JE. Vascular compression of the duodenum. (Part 1). Contemp Surg 9:37, 1976; with permission.)

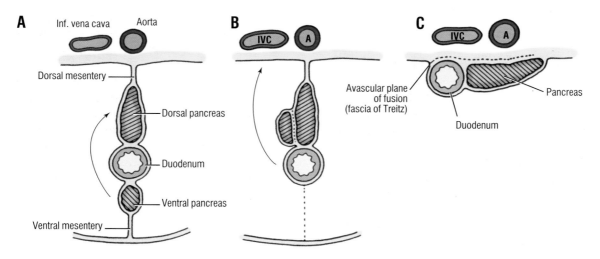

**FIG. 16-3.** Diagram of the rotation of pancreas and duodenum. **A.** Primitive relation of dorsal and ventral pancreatic primordia. **B.** Disappearance of ventral mesentery and rotation of ventral pancreas. **C.** Final retroperitoneal position of duodenum and pancreas. The plane of fusion of the mesoduodenum is the avascular fascia of Treitz. (Modified from Gray SW, Colborn GL, Pemberton LB, Skandalakis LJ, Skandalakis JE. The duodenum. Part 1: History, embryogenesis, and histologic and physiologic features. Am Surg 55(4):257-261, 1989; with permission.)

Circular muscle appears in the duodenum late in the fifth week; longitudinal muscle is visible in the third month. Before the longitudinal muscle appears, neuroblasts of the myenteric plexus follow the vagus nerve down the surface of the circular muscle. By the eighth week, all but the distal colon is innervated. The nerve supply is completely in place by the twelfth week.

## Congenital Anomalies

### Duodenum

#### Stenoses and Atresias

Stenosis of the duodenum is often associated with an anular pancreas or with aberrant pancreatic tissue in the duodenal wall. Stenosis may also result from a perforated diaphragmatic atresia (see type III below). The aperture may be so small that functional atresia develops later in life.[12]

We quote from Ladd and Madura[13]:

> Duodenal anomalies are rare in adults. Duodenal webs are best managed by transduodenal excision and duodenoplasty. Annular pancreas is generally best treated by duodenal bypass to the distal duodenum or the jejunum. Annulus division can be carried out if the annulus is extramural, without duodenal stenosis, and if access to the pancreaticobiliary sphincters is necessary.

Atresias may be divided into three types (Fig. 16-4).[9]

In *type A,* a membrane composed of mucosa and submucosa closes the duodenal lumen. There may be a secondary perforation. This is the most frequent type. Because it bulges downward under proximal pressure, the diaphragm usually appears to be more distal than is actually the case.

In *type B,* the proximal and distal ends are blind. They are joined by a fibrous band lying in the edge of the mesentery.

In *type C,* the proximal and distal blind ends have no connection with each other, and the mesentery between them is absent. This type is rare.

In all three types, the proximal segment is dilated and the distal segment is completely unexpanded. Seventy-five percent of intestinal stenoses and 40 percent of intestinal atresias are found in the duodenum.

Vecchia et al.[14] reported that the major causes of morbidity and mortality in patients with intestinal atresia were cardiac anomalies (with duodenal atresia) and ultrashort bowel syndrome (<40 cm), which requires long-term total parenteral nutrition and which can be complicated by liver disease with jejunoileal atresia. They advised that long-term outcomes may be improved by the use of growth factors to enhance adaptation and advances in small bowel transplantation.

Duodenectomy-duodenoplasty for chronic intestinal pseudo-obstruction (megaduodenum) is recommended by Loire et al.[15]

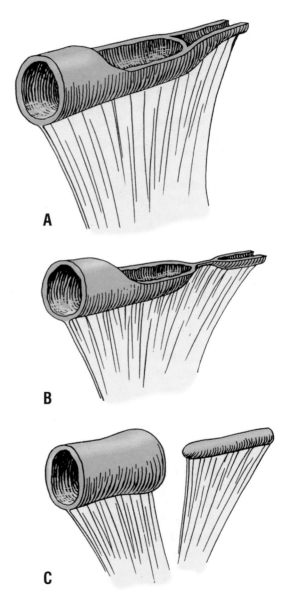

**A**

**B**

**C**

FIG. 16-4. Types of intestinal atresia. **A.** The lumen is closed by a mucosal and submucosal diaphragm. **B.** The atretic segment is a solid fibrous cord. **C.** There is complete absence of a segment of intestine and its mesentery. Note the dilatation of the intestine proximal to the atresia. (Modified from Colborn GL, Gray SW, Pemberton LB, Skandalakis LJ, Skandalakis JE. The duodenum. Part 3: Pathology. Am Surg 55(7):469-473, 1989; with permission.)

## Duodenal Diverticula

Most duodenal diverticula are found on the concave (pancreatic) wall of the second and third portions of the duodenum. They are usually solitary; however, they may be multiple. Duodenal diverticula are often asymptomatic.

Large symptomatic diverticula should be excised and closed with inversion of the sac. A long T-tube and duodenostomy are recommended for safe dissection of diverticula near the duodenal papilla. Neill and Thompson[16] studied complications of duodenal diverticula.

Vassilakis et al.[17] reported that Roux-en-Y choleduodenojejunostomy and duodenojejunostomy give satisfactory results for the treatment of complicated duodenal diverticulum.

Chiu et al.[18] evaluated a large series of small bowel diverticula and concluded the following:

> Duodenal diverticulum was the most common small bowel diverticulum. Abdominal pain and gastrointestinal bleeding were the most common clinical presentations. The small bowel diverticula, except for Meckel's diverticulum, did not need to be treated if there were no significant symptoms.

## *Jejunoileum*

### Atresias and Stenoses

Congenital intestinal atresia is a major cause of intestinal obstruction in infants. As in the duodenum (see above), jejunoileal atresia occurs in three types (Fig. 16-4).

In *type A,* obstruction is produced by a diaphragm or a membrane of mucosa and submucosa. It may be complete or may have perforations.

In *type B,* two blind ends of the intestine are connected by a fibrous cord lying on the edge of the intact mesentery.

In *type C,* two blind ends of the intestine are not connected with each other, and the mesentery between the ends is absent.

In all except perforated membranes of type A, the proximal segment is greatly dilated and the distal segment is completely unexpanded. If there are multiple atresias, the dilation is proximal to the first one only. Stenoses and all types of atresias are more common in the duodenum than in the ileum and the jejunum.

Matsumoto et al.[19] reported on jejunoileal atresia in identical twins, attributing most such cases to environmental influences during gestation. The authors of this chapter have reservations about accepting this etiology for an extremely rare anomaly.

Treatment comprises the excision of the atretic or stenotic segment and anastomosis of the ends. End-to-end anastomosis is rendered difficult by the disparity in size between the dilated proximal segment and the unexpanded distal segment. A side-to-side anastomosis or a Mikulicz exteriorization of the ends, dilation of the distal segment, and subsequent return of the intestines to the abdomen are the procedures of choice. For duodenal atresias, a retrocolic, isoperistaltic, two-layered duodenojejunostomy should be done whenever possible.[20] Stenoses should be treated similarly.

### Intestinal Duplications

Long intestinal duplications (Fig. 16-5) are the result of a failure of the endoderm to separate from the overlying notochord during the eighteenth to twenty-first day of gestation. Subsequent embryonic growth results in a band of endodermal cells attached to the normal gut at the caudal end and to the notochord at the cranial end. The band of endodermal cells will differentiate into a tubular gutlike structure on the mesenteric side of the normal gut. The notochordal attachment usually fails to persist, but one or more anomalous vertebrae are usually present to indicate the site of the abnormal attachment.

The resulting entities may be cystic duplications or long tubular duplications in the mesentery parallel to the normal intestine. They frequently contain gastric or pancreatic mucosa, usually at the proximal end. Communication with the normal intestine is usually at the distal end only.

Cystic duplications and short parallel duplications should be resected entirely, together with the normal intestine served by the same blood vessels (Fig. 16-6A). Longer duplications, and hence, the adjacent intestine, may be preserved by creating a fistula at the distal end of the duplication (Fig. 16-6B), or by extirpation of the common wall (Fig. 16-6C), if there is no ulceration present.

### Meckel's Diverticulum

A remnant of the proximal portion of the yolk stalk (base of the vitelline stalk) is responsible for the formation of Meckel's diverticulum. It may be connected to the umbilicus by a fibrous cord that may be patent (ileo-umbilical fistula). Persistence of that portion of the duct between the umbilicus and the ileum results in the diverticulum of Meckel.

Persistence is a misleading term. If the duct fails to degenerate, it not only persists, but usually grows to keep pace with the ileum to which it is attached. Rarely, the entire abdominal portion of the vitelline duct survives as an omphaloileal fistula. Even more rarely, an umbilical sinus or an umbilical polyp may represent the undegenerated distal end of the tract, or an abdominal cyst may indicate disappearance of all but the midportion of the vitelline duct. Much more frequently, a short portion of the ileal end persists and develops into a blindly ending diverticulum of the ileum.

Why epithelial cells of the yolk sac in certain individuals

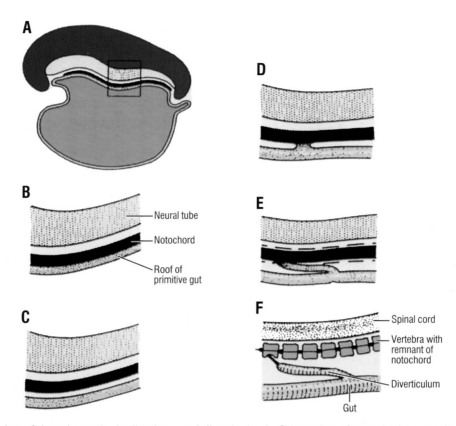

FIG. 16-5. The formation of dorsal enteric duplications and diverticula. **A.** Orientation of neural tube notochord and primitive gut. **B.** Before the fourth week the notochord is attached to the underlying endoderm forming the roof of the primitive gut. **C.** Separation during the fourth week is normally complete. **D, E.** Incomplete separation and differences in growth of notochord and endoderm result in a band of endoderm cells pulled from the roof of the gut. **F.** The band of cells forms a tubular structure similar to and parallel with the normal gut. Note the deformed vertebra. (Modified from Skandalakis JE, Gray SW, Rowe JS Jr. Anatomical Complications in General Surgery. New York: McGraw-Hill, 1983; with permission.)

continue to flourish and differentiate instead of following the usual pattern of ceasing to divide during the fifth week of embryonic life is a mystery. Sorokin and Padykula[21] reported that rat embryo yolk sac will survive in tissue culture and that regression is not intrinsic to the endoderm. This suggests that it is the mesodermal component which governs epithelial development.

Werner et al.[22] reported that Meckel's diverticulum is the most common congenital anomaly of the gastrointestinal tract and its complications are hemorrhage (due to acid secretion by ectopic gastric mucosa), inflammation (similar to acute appendicitis), and intestinal obstruction (due to intussusception, volvulus, or adhesive bands).

Additional information about Meckel's diverticulum will be found later in this chapter in the anatomy section.

### Small Bowel Diverticulosis

A prevalence of small bowel diverticulosis of 0.3-2.5% was cited by de Lange et al.[23]

## SURGICAL ANATOMY OF THE DUODENUM

## Topography and Relations

### *Relations of the Duodenum*

**First Part (Superior):** 5 cm long. The proximal half is mobile; the distal half is fixed.

The duodenum passes upward from the pylorus to the neck of the gallbladder (Fig. 16-7). It is related (1) posteriorly to the common bile duct, portal vein, inferior vena cava, and gastroduodenal artery; (2) anteriorly to the quadrate lobe of the liver; (3) superiorly to the epiploic foramen; and (4) inferiorly to the head of the pancreas.

The initial 2.5 cm is freely movable and is covered by the same two layers of peritoneum that invest the stomach. The

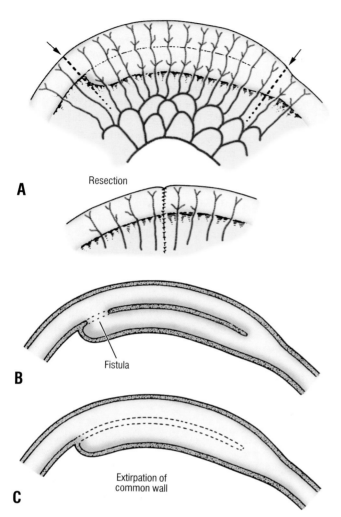

**A**

Resection

**B**

Fistula

**C**

Extirpation of
common wall

**FIG. 16-6.** Intestinal duplication. **A.** Blood supply to duplications and normal intestine. Resection *(at arrows)* removes both normal and duplicated segment. **B.** Resection may be avoided by the creation of a fistula at the blind end of the duplication. **C.** Extirpation of the common wall between normal and duplicated segments may be feasible. (Modified from Skandalakis JE, Gray SW, Rowe JS Jr. Anatomical Complications in General Surgery. New York: McGraw-Hill, 1983; with permission.)

hepatoduodenal portion of the lesser omentum attaches to the superior border of the duodenum; the greater omentum attaches to its inferior border. The distal 2.5 cm is covered with peritoneum only on the anterior surface of the organ, so that the posterior surface is in intimate contact with the bile duct, the portal vein, and the gastroduodenal artery. The duodenum is separated from the inferior vena cava by a small amount of connective tissue.

**Second Part (Descending):** 7.5 cm long. It extends from the neck of the gallbladder to the upper border of L4.

This part of the duodenum is crossed by the transverse colon and the mesocolon and consists, therefore, of a supramesocolic portion and an inframesocolic portion. The parts above and below the attachment of the transverse colon are covered with visceral peritoneum. The first and second parts of the duodenum join behind the costal margin a little above and medial to the tip of the ninth costal cartilage and on the right side of the first lumbar vertebra.

The second part of the duodenum forms an acute angle with the first part, and descends from the neck of the gallbladder anterior to the hilum of the right kidney, the right ureter, the right renal vessels, the psoas major, and the edge of the inferior vena cava. It is related anteriorly to the right lobe of the liver, the transverse colon, and the jejunum. At about the midpoint of the second part of the duodenum, the pancreaticobiliary tract opens into its concave posteromedial side. The right side is related to the ascending colon and the right colic flexure.

**Third Part (Horizontal or Inferior):** 10 cm long. It extends from the right side of L3 or L4 to the left side of the aorta.

The third part of the duodenum begins about 5 cm from the midline, to the right of the lower end of the third lumbar vertebra, at about the level of the subcostal plane. The third, or transverse, part passes to the left, anterior to the ureter, the right gonadal vessels, the psoas muscle, the inferior vena cava, the lumbar vertebral column, and the aorta. It ends to the left of the third lumbar vertebra.

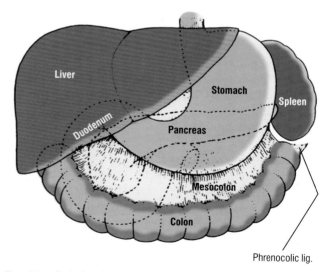

**FIG. 16-7.** Anterior view of the relationships of the duodenum and pancreas. (Modified from Skandalakis JE, Skandalakis LJ, Colborn GL, Pemberton LB, Gray SW. The duodenum. Part 2: Surgical anatomy. Am Surg 55(5):291-298, 1989; with permission.)

This inframesocolic portion of the duodenum is covered anteriorly by the peritoneum. It is crossed anteriorly by the superior mesenteric vessels and, near its termination, by the root of the mesentery of the small intestine. The third part is related superiorly to the head and uncinate process of the pancreas. The inferior pancreaticoduodenal artery lies in a groove at the interface of the pancreas and the duodenum. Anteriorly and inferiorly, this part of the duodenum is related to the small bowel, primarily to the jejunum.

**Fourth Part (Ascending):** 2.5 cm long. It extends from the left side of the aorta to the left upper border of L2.

The fourth, or ascending, part of the duodenum is directed obliquely upward. It ends at the duodenojejunal junction to the left and at the level of the second lumbar vertebra at the root of the transverse mesocolon. This junction occurs at about 4 cm below and medial to the tip of the ninth costal cartilage. The fourth part is related posteriorly to the left sympathetic trunk, the psoas muscle, and the left renal and gonadal vessels. Its termination is very close to the terminal part of the inferior mesenteric vein, to the left ureter, and to the left kidney. The upper end of the root of the mesentery also attaches here. The duodenojejunal junction is suspended by the ligament of Treitz, a remnant of the dorsal mesentery, which extends from the duodenojejunal flexure to the right crus of the diaphragm.

## Pancreaticobiliary Structures

The fourth (intramural) portion of the common bile duct passes obliquely through the wall of the second part of the duodenum with the main pancreatic duct (Wirsung). Other associated structures are the major and minor papillae, the ampulla of Vater (if present), and the sphincteric mechanism of Boyden. Taken together, they form what Dowdy called the "Vaterian system."[24] This term expresses the anatomic and surgical unity of these structures, but has no functional significance.

The terminal portion of the common bile duct passes through the duodenal wall; it is about 1.5 cm in length, and narrows from 1.0 cm extramurally to 0.54 cm at the papilla. The main pancreatic duct enters the duodenum caudal to the bile duct, also decreasing in diameter. The ducts usually lie side by side, with a common adventitia for several millimeters. The septum between them becomes reduced to a mucosal membrane before actual confluence is reached.

### Major Duodenal Papilla

There is confusion in the literature regarding the true definitions of the terms papilla of Vater and ampulla of Vater. The papilla of Vater, which should be called the major duodenal papilla, is a nipplelike formation and pro-

jection of the duodenal mucosa through which the distal end of the ampulla of Vater passes into the duodenum. The ampulla of Vater (hepatopancreatic), with its several formations, is the union of the pancreaticobiliary ducts.

The major papilla is on the posteromedial wall of the second (descending) portion of the duodenum to the right of the second or third lumbar vertebra. In older patients, it may lie at a slightly lower level. The distance from the pylorus varies from 7 to 10 cm, with extremes of 1.5 to 12 cm. The distance is decreased in the presence of inflammation of the cap or the postbulbar region of the duodenum.

Viewed from the mucosal surface, the papilla (Fig. 16-8) may be hard to locate because of the mucosal folds; sometimes it is completely overlaid by a transverse fold of duodenal mucosa. Its oval or slitlike orifice lies at its tip, the posterior end of which projects downward, and raises a longitudinal fold, known as the plica longitudinalis. The orifice is frequently filled by villuslike projections called valvules, or valvulae. Occasionally, a diverticulum lying near the papilla can cause difficulty for the surgeon or the endoscopist.

### Ampulla (of Vater)

The ampulla is a dilatation of the common pancreatico-

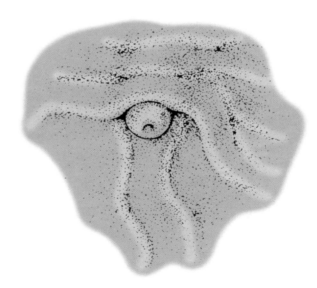

**FIG. 16-8.** The T arrangement of duodenal mucosal folds indicating the site of the major duodenal papilla. In some cases, a mucosal fold may cover the orifice of the papilla. The major papilla is rarely as obvious as this illustration. No such arrangement marks the site of the minor papilla. (Originally, in 1775, a plate by Santorini, and reproduced in 1932 by Livingston. Modified from Skandalakis JE, Skandalakis LJ, Colborn GL, Pemberton LB, Gray SW. The duodenum. Part 2: Surgical anatomy. Am Surg 55(5):291-298, 1989; with permission.)

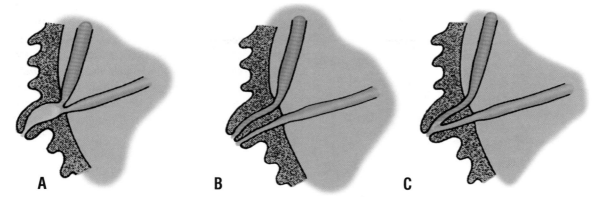

FIG. 16-9. Diagram of the variations in the relation of the common bile duct and main pancreatic duct at the duodenal papilla. **A.** Minimal absorption of the ducts into the duodenal wall during embryonic development; an ampulla is present. **B.** Maximum absorption of the ducts into the duodenum. There are separate orifices on the papilla; no ampulla is present. **C.** Partial absorption of the common channel; no true ampulla is present. (Modified from Skandalakis JE, Skandalakis LJ, Colborn GL, Pemberton LB, Gray SW. The duodenum. Part 2: Surgical anatomy. Am Surg 55(5):291-298, 1989; with permission.)

biliary channel within the papilla and below the junction of the two ducts (Fig. 16-9A). If a septum is present as far as the duodenal orifice, the ampulla is said to be absent (Fig. 16-9B). Michels[25] collected the findings of 25 investigators in 2500 specimens and concluded that an ampulla was present in 63 percent of cases. By definition, an ampulla was said to be present if the edge of the septum between the two ducts fell short of the tip of the papilla. Actual measurements of the distance between the septal edge and the papillary tip range from 1 to 14 mm, with 75 percent being 5 mm or less.[26]

Purists would require a dilatation of the common channel before they would apply the term ampulla. Where the common channel is less than 5 mm long, there is little or no dilatation.[27] In such specimens, the presence of a true ampulla becomes a matter of opinion (Fig. 16-9C). We agree with Michels[25] that the following classification is the most useful:

- **Type 1.** The pancreatic duct opens into the common bile duct at a variable distance from the opening in the major duodenal papilla. The common channel may or may not be dilated (85 percent).
- **Type 2.** The pancreatic and bile ducts open close to one another but separately on the major duodenal papilla (5 percent).
- **Type 3.** The pancreatic and bile ducts open into the duodenum at separate points (9 percent).

A true dilated ampulla is present in about 75 percent of individuals of type 1, and is absent in types 2 and 3.

The variations in the distance between the pancreaticobiliary junction and the duodenal lumen result from developmental processes.[28] In the embryo, the main pancreatic duct arises as a branch of the common bile duct, which in turn arises from the duodenum. Growth of the duodenum absorbs the proximal bile duct up to its junction with the pancreatic duct. When the resorption is minimal, there is a long ampulla, and the junction of the ducts is high in the duodenal wall (type 1), or even extramural. With increased resorption of the terminal bile duct, the junction lies closer to the duodenal orifice and the ampulla is shortened. The maximum resorption results in separate orifices for the main pancreatic duct and the common bile duct (type 3).

### Sphincter of Boyden

A complex of several sphincters, composed of circular or spiral smooth muscle fibers, is found around the intramural part of the common bile duct, the main pancreatic duct, and the ampulla, if present. This sphincteric complex is called the sphincter of Boyden.[29] The muscle fibers have an embryonic origin separate from that of the duodenal muscularis and are functionally separate from it (Fig. 16-10).

Like the papilla of Vater, another example of a misnamed anatomic entity is the sphincter of Oddi at the duodenal end of the pancreatic and common bile ducts. By priority of description, it should have been named for Francis Glisson.[30] In 1654 he described anular fibers around the entire intramural portion of the bile duct, and believed that they guarded the opening against the reflux of the contents of the duodenum. Glisson's account of his work is found in Boyden.[31]

### Minor Duodenal Papilla

The minor papilla, through which the accessory pancreatic duct (Santorini) opens, is about 2 cm cranial and slightly anterior to the major papilla. It is smaller and less

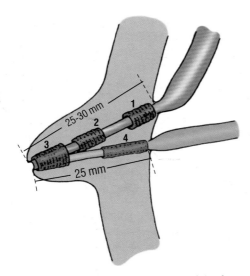

FIG. 16-10. Diagrammatic representation of the four sphincters making up the sphincter of Boyden. **1.** Superior choledochal sphincter. **2.** Inferior (submucosal) choledochal sphincter. **3.** Sphincter ampullae (papillae). **4.** Pancreatic sphincter. The measurements are those of White.[179] (Modified from Skandalakis JE, Skandalakis LJ, Colborn GL, Pemberton LB, Gray SW. The duodenum. Part 2: Surgical anatomy. Am Surg 55(5):291-298, 1989; with permission.)

easily identified than the major papilla. The most useful landmark is the gastroduodenal artery, behind which lies the accessory duct and the minor papilla. Duodenal dissection for gastrectomy should end proximal to the artery. The minor papilla may contain no duct or only a microscopic, tortuous channel. A true sphincter (of Helly) is rarely present. In about 10 percent[32] of individuals, the duct of Santorini is the only duct draining most of the pancreas. Accidental ligation of this duct, together with the gastroduodenal artery, would result in catastrophic pancreatitis.

### Duodenal "Sphincters"

The debates concerning the so-called duodenal sphincters remind the authors of the controversy surrounding the gastroesophageal sphincters in regard to their anatomic or physiologic existence and their relation to duodenal pathology. The authors' knowledge about duodenal sphincters was obtained from the excellent book by DiDio and Anderson, *The "Sphincters" of the Digestive System*.[33] In addition to the well-known gastroduodenal pyloric sphincter, the duodenum has the following controversial sphincters:

- The first duodenal sphincter is said to be located at the distal end of the duodenal bulb and is perhaps related to, if not responsible for, segmental achalasia and "megabulb."

- The sphincter of Villemin is proximal to the ampulla of Vater.[34,35]
- If the so-called "Ochsner muscle" exists, it is probably located below the ampulla of Vater, according to Ochsner, who presented his findings in two publications in 1906.[36] In 1907, Boothby expressed doubt as to the existence of the sphincter.[37] A sphincter just proximal to the duodenojejunal flexure was also described by both Ochsner and Villemin.

In the introduction to his book about Antonio Scarpa, Monti stated: "Like the poet, and perhaps even more so, the scientist is the product of the period in which [he] lives."[38] It may be that the period in which Ochsner, Boothby, and Villemin lived stimulated them to perform their investigative work. The authors of this chapter agree with DiDio and Anderson that the descriptions of the sphincteric component are vague and that their clinical significance is nonexistent.

## Vascular Supply

### Arteries

The blood supply of the duodenum is confusing due to the diverse possibilities of origin, distribution, and individual variations (Fig. 16-11, Fig. 16-12, Fig. 16-13). This is especially true of the blood supply of the first portion of the duodenum. In his fine presentation about the stomach and the duodenum, Griffith[39] warned surgeons to be very cautious, because of these variations of the main arteries. Akkinis[40] stated that there is no collateral circulation beyond the terminal arcades of the small bowel. Do we have the same phenomenon in the first portion of the duodenum? What about the anemic spot of Mayo that corresponds to the distribution of the supraduodenal artery? Does it exist? Do the variations of the above-named arteries represent, as Griffith states, an underlying factor in necrosis and leakage? The authors of this chapter do not want to take a position on these questions. Our only advice is to use good surgical technique when surgery is definitely required, and not take an overenthusiastic approach when dealing with benign disease.

The first part of the duodenum is supplied by the supraduodenal artery (Fig. 16-11) and the posterior superior pancreaticoduodenal branch of the gastroduodenal artery (retroduodenal artery as described by Edwards, Michels, and Wilkie), which is a branch of the common hepatic artery. In many individuals, the upper part of the first 1 cm is also supplied by branches of the right gastric artery. In some individuals, one may see separate small branches to the superior and posterior aspects of the first part of the

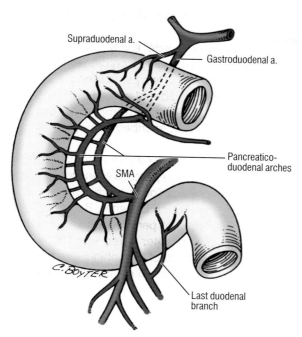

FIG. **16-11.** Major arterial supply to the duodenum. (Modified from Skandalakis JE, Skandalakis LJ, Colborn GL, Pemberton LB, Gray SW. The duodenum. Part 2: Surgical anatomy. Am Surg 55(5):291-298, 1989; with permission.)

rately, or in various combinations. It is preferable, therefore, that the term retroduodenal not be used as a synonym for the posterior superior pancreaticoduodenal branch, the principal role of which is to supply the second part of the duodenum and pancreatic head. *Nomina Anatomica* (6th ed)[41] also acknowledges the separate identity of the supraduodenal, retroduodenal, and posterior superior pancreaticoduodenal arteries; the supraduodenal artery is frequently absent, however.

After giving origin to the supraduodenal, retroduodenal, and posterior superior pancreaticoduodenal branches, the gastroduodenal artery descends between the first part of the duodenum and the head of the pancreas. It terminates by dividing into the right gastroepiploic and anterior superior pancreaticoduodenal arteries, both supplying twigs to this part of the duodenum.

The remaining three parts of the duodenum are supplied by an anterior and a posterior arcade. From the arcades spring pancreatic and duodenal branches. Those supplying the duodenum are called arteriae rectae; they may be embedded in the substance of the pancreas. Four arteries contribute to the pancreaticoduodenal vascular arcades:

1. The anterior superior pancreaticoduodenal arteries, commonly two in number, arise from the gastroduodenal artery on the ventral surface of the pancreas.
2. The posterior superior pancreaticoduodenal (retroduodenal) artery usually crosses in front of the common bile

duodenum; they can be properly called supraduodenal and retroduodenal, respectively. Each may arise separately,

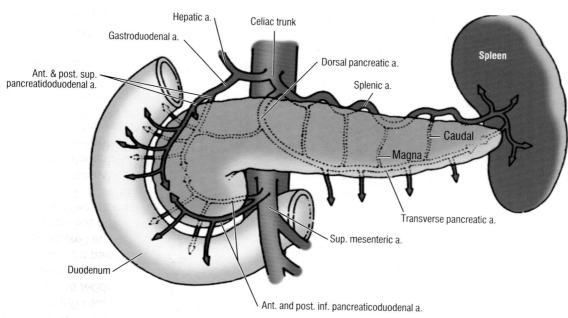

FIG. **16-12.** Anterior view of arterial supply of the duodenum and pancreas. (Modified from Skandalakis JE, Skandalakis LJ, Colborn GL, Pemberton LB, Gray SW. The duodenum. Part 2: Surgical anatomy. Am Surg 55(5):291-298, 1989; with permission.)

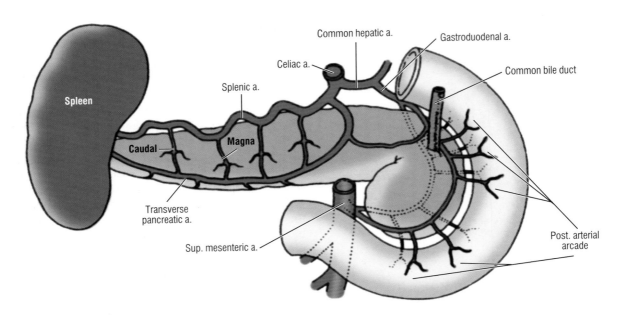

FIG. 16-13. Posterior view of arterial supply of duodenum and pancreas. (Modified from Skandalakis JE, Skandalakis LJ, Colborn GL, Pemberton LB, Gray SW. The duodenum. Part 2: Surgical anatomy. Am Surg 55(5):291-298, 1989; with permission.)

duct. The artery then spirals to the right and posterior to the duct, descending deep to the head of the pancreas. Several of the retroduodenal artery branches anastomose inferiorly with rami from the posterior branch of the inferior pancreaticoduodenal artery.

3 & 4. Anterior inferior and posterior inferior pancreaticoduodenal arteries arise from the superior mesenteric artery or its first jejunal branch, either separately or from a common stem. Blood reaches the concave surface of the duodenum by the vasa recta from the pancreaticoduodenal arcades. At first supplying the muscularis externa, they form a large plexus in the submucosa, from which arteries pierce the muscularis mucosae and form a second rich plexus just beneath the epithelium of the villi. The surgeon should be sure to ligate only one of the two arcades, the superior or the inferior only.

Lately, Hentati et al.[42] proposed a new classification of the arterial supply of the duodenal bulb (Fig. 16-14, Fig. 16-15, Fig. 16-16), as follows:

*The two arterial pedicles (infra- and supraduodenal) reach the bulb on its posterior aspect; each pedicle is made up of two sorts of blood currents (right and left); the posterior aspect of the bulb seems to be the most vascularized one, explaining, apart from bleeding from gastroduodenal [artery] erosion, the hemorrhagic character of ulcers of the posterior aspect of the bulb. The predominance of the left-hand currents explains the possible ischemia of the duodenal bulb and/ or rupture of the duodenal stump after their interruption.*

## Veins

Veins of the lower first part of the duodenum and the pylorus usually open into the right gastroepiploic veins (Fig. 16-17); they are the subpyloric veins. The upper first part of the duodenum is drained by suprapyloric veins, which open into the portal vein or the posterior superior pancreaticoduodenal vein. Anastomoses between subpyloric and suprapyloric veins pass around the duodenum. One of these has been said to mark the site of the pylorus (prepyloric vein of Mayo).[43] It is not a constant indicator of the location of the pylorus.

The venous arcades draining the duodenum follow the arterial arcades and tend to lie superficial to them. The anterior superior vein drains into the right gastroepiploic vein while the posterior superior vein usually passes behind the common bile duct to enter the portal vein. The inferior veins can enter the superior mesenteric (Fig. 16-18), the inferior mesenteric, the splenic, or the first jejunal vein. The veins may terminate separately or by a common stem.

## Lymphatics

The duodenum is richly supplied with lymphatics (Fig. 16-19). They originate as blind-ending vessels (lacteals) in

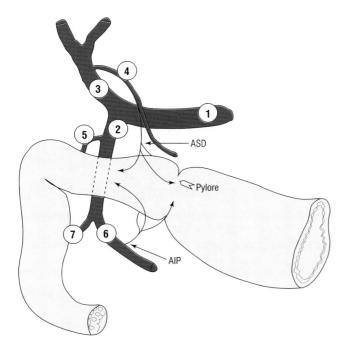

FIG. 16-14. General layout of the vessels on the anterior aspect of the duodenal bulb (classic concept). **1,** common hepatic a.; **2,** gastroduodenal a.; **3,** hepatic a.; **4,** right gastric a.; **5,** posterior duodenopancreatic a.; **6,** right gastroepiploic a.; **7,** anterior superior duodenopancreatic a.; ASD, supraduodenal a.; AIP, intrapyloric a.; pylore, pylorus. (Modified from Hentati N, Fournier HD, Papon X, Aube Ch, Vialle R, Mercier Ph. Arterial supply of the duodenal bulb: an anatomoclinical study. Surg Radiol Anat 1999;21:159-64; with permission.)

each villus of the mucosa. These vessels form a plexus in the lamina propria and, piercing the muscularis mucosae, form a second submucosal plexus. Still another lymphatic plexus lies between the circular and longitudinal layers of the muscularis. Collecting trunks pass over the anterior and posterior duodenal wall toward the lesser curvature to enter the anterior and posterior pancreaticoduodenal lymph nodes.

The anterior extramural collecting ducts drain to nodes anterior to the pancreas. The posterior ducts pass to nodes posterior to the head of the pancreas. These follow the veins and arteries to nodes related to the superior mesenteric artery.

At the turn of the 20th century, Bartels[44] presented evidence that the valves of the lymphatic vessels connecting the duodenal wall with the head of the pancreas are arranged so that normal lymph flow is from pancreas to duodenum, and not the reverse. This theory has not been confirmed recently. Although the lymphatics of the pancreas have received some attention, those of the duodenum have received very little.

## Innervation

Within the duodenal wall are the two well-known neural plexuses of the gastrointestinal tract, each of which is composed of groups of neurons interconnected by networks of fibers. One plexus (of Meissner) is in the submucosa; another plexus (of Auerbach) is in the connective tissue between the circular and longitudinal layers of muscularis externa. Some of the neuronal cell bodies and processes in the plexuses are assumed to be postganglionic parasympathetic. Several studies indicate that many are related (1) to circuitry for processing information received from various types of sensory receptors, (2) to synaptic complexes for directing neural outflow, and (3) to interconnecting neurons.[45]

Preganglionic parasympathetic fibers in the plexuses are carried initially by the vagus nerves. Postganglionic sympathetic fibers arise from cell bodies located in the celiac and superior mesenteric ganglia, in sympathetic chain ganglia ranging from T-6 to T-12, or scattered along

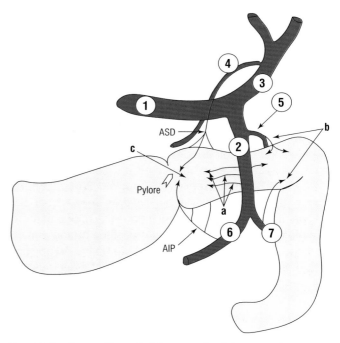

FIG. 16-15. General layout of the vessels of the posterior aspect of the bulb (classic concept). **1,** common hepatic a.; **2,** gastroduodenal a.; **3,** hepatic a.; **4,** right gastric a.; **5,** posterior duodenopancreatic a.; **6,** right gastroepiploic a.; **7,** anterior superior duodenopancreatic a.; ASD, supraduodenal a.; AIP, intrapyloric a.; pylore, pylorus; **a,** retroduodenal aa.; **b,** accessory duodenal aa.; **c,** poorly vascularized area. (Modified from Hentati N, Fournier HD, Papon X, Aube Ch, Vialle R, Mercier Ph. Arterial supply of the duodenal bulb: an anatomoclinical study. Surg Radiol Anat 1999;21:159-64; with permission.)

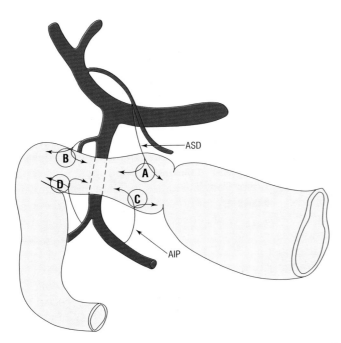

**Fig. 16-16.** General layout of the vessels of the bulb (concept of Hentati et al.). **A,** left supraduodenal current; **B,** right supra-duodenal current; **C,** left intraduodenal current; **D,** right intra-duodenal current; ASD, supraduodenal a.; AIP, intrapyloric a. (Modified from Hentati N, Fournier HD, Papon X, Aube Ch, Vialle R, Mercier Ph. Arterial supply of the duodenal bulb: an anatomo-clinical study. Surg Radiol Anat 1999;21:159-64; with permission.)

the course of the splanchnic nerves. The extrinsic nerve supply to the duodenum probably includes contributions which leave the anterior hepatic plexus close to the origin of the right gastric artery. In six out of 100 specimens examined by Skandalakis et al.,[46] nerves from the hepatic division of the anterior vagal trunk gave rise to one or more branches that innervated the first part of the duodenum. In most specimens, some branches could be traced upward toward the gastric incisura. The vagaries of the vagus are well known.[47,48]

## SURGICAL ANATOMY OF THE JEJUNUM AND THE ILEUM

### Topography and Anatomy

#### Length of the Jejunoileum

For all practical purposes, 60 percent of the length of

the GI tract is composed of jejunoileum,[49] which performs 90 percent of the absorption.[50,51]

The beginning and the end of the jejunum and ileum are topographically related to peritoneal pockets or fossae which are usually very shallow. Occasionally, when they are very deep, they may be the cause of internal herniation. At the beginning of the jejunum there are paraduodenal fossae; at the end, ileocecal fossae; in the center, there is non-fusion of the intestinal root.

Touloukian and Smith,[52] in an autopsy study of children, reported that total intestinal length ranged from 142 ± 22 cm for preterm infants 19 to 27 gestational weeks to 304 ± 44 cm for preterm infants more than 35 gestational weeks. The same authors reported that the average length of jejunoileum was 248 ± 40 cm for preterm infants more than 35 gestational weeks.

The length of the alimentary tract in humans is surprisingly difficult to measure. In the older literature, reviewed by Bryant,[53] the length of the jejunum and ileum in cadavers was reported to be from 10 to 40 feet. Based upon his own studies, Bryant recorded an average length of 20.5 feet (624.8 cm). From his tables, an average of 20 to 22 feet has been widely quoted in textbooks up to the present.

That the "normal" length of 20 to 22 feet bears no relation to the jejunoileum in the living patient was apparent in 1924 when Reis and Schembra[54] measured the jejunoileum in living dogs and remeasured it at various intervals after death. In the first 10 minutes, it elongated 23 to 25 percent. Four hours after death, the increase in length reached 135 percent. This occurs because tonus of the longitudinal muscle is lost much faster than that of the circular muscle.

Blankenhorn and associates[55] intubated eight patients and from their measurements determined the average length of the duodenum to be about 22 cm (8.5 inches); jejunoileum, 258 cm (8.5 ft); and colon, 110 cm (3 ft, 7 inches). The overall nose-to-anus length of the gastrointestinal tract averaged 452 cm (14 ft, 10 inches). There is some evidence that intestinal length is greater in obese individuals.[56]

A 1995 study by Nightingale and Lennard-Jones[57] found that the normal adult human small intestinal length, measured surgically or at autopsy from the duodenojejunal flexure, ranges from 275 to 850 cm. According to Nordgren et al.,[58] in patients with Crohn's disease the small bowel was significantly shorter than in patients with ulcerative colitis and in a control population.

The surgeon is more concerned with the length of intestine remaining after a resection than with the amount resected. In the older literature there are lists of operations in which 4-5 m or more of intestine were removed, with survival of the patient.[59] Undoubtedly, the resected seg-

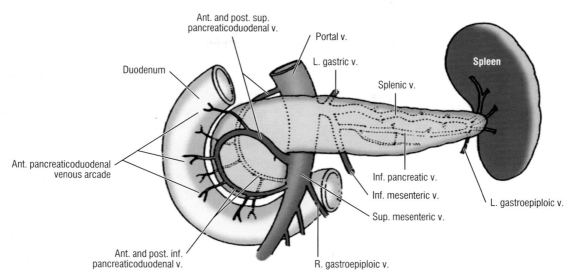

**FIG. 16-17.** The venous drainage of the duodenum and pancreas: anterior view. (Modified from Skandalakis JE, Skandalakis LJ, Colborn GL, Pemberton LB, Gray SW. The duodenum. Part 2: Surgical anatomy. Am Surg 55(5):291-298, 1989; with permission.)

ment was measured only after the resection was completed and the abdomen closed; elongation of the specimen was by then well under way. Accurate measurements should be made before the intestine is removed and with the least manipulation possible. We cannot explain why the older measurements are still widely accepted.

Weser[60,61] studied the functional capacity of the jejunoileum. He reported that 50 percent resection can be tolerated well by the patient, but 75 percent resection will produce severe malabsorption syndrome. Winawer and Zamchek[62] believed that patient survival is possible with the duodenum in situ following resection of approximately 50 cm of the jejunoileum. Wilmore[63] stated that 15 cm of je-

junum or ileum with the ileocecal valve in situ can be tolerated, but 40 cm of small bowel is needed if the ileocecal valve is resected. Total parenteral nutrition is an extremely useful treatment with short bowel syndrome in infants as well as in adults.

Thompson[64] reported the surgical aspects of the short-bowel syndrome. He stated that:

- Ostomy formation is often prudent at the time of initial resection
- Factors influencing restoration of intestinal continuity must be considered (Table 16-2)
- Prophylactic cholecystectomy is often advisable to avoid cholelithiasis

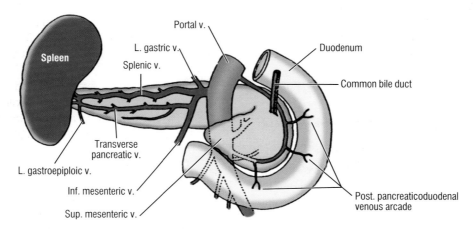

**FIG. 16-18.** The venous drainage of the duodenum and pancreas and formation of the hepatic portal vein: posterior view. (Modified from Skandalakis JE, Skandalakis LJ, Colborn GL, Pemberton LB, Gray SW. The duodenum. Part 2: Surgical anatomy. Am Surg 55(5):291-298, 1989; with permission.)

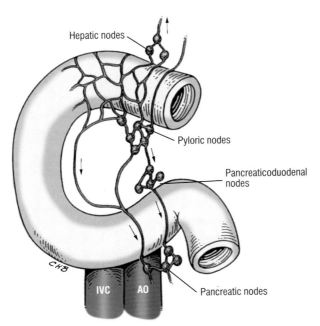

**FIG. 16-19.** Diagrammatic presentation of duodenal lymphatics. (Modified from Skandalakis JE, Skandalakis LJ, Colborn GL, Pemberton LB, Gray SW. The duodenum. Part 2: Surgical anatomy. Am Surg 55(5):291-298, 1989; with permission.)

- Surgical therapy includes procedures to slow intestinal transit
- Intestinal transplantation may be the most promising therapy

In a more recent publication, the same author stated the following[65]:

> The outcome of short bowel syndrome is influenced by several factors including intestinal disease, remnant length and location, the other digestive organs, and intestinal adaptation...Patients with short bowel syndrome resulting from inflammatory disease appear to have a better nutritional prognosis after the first year. While they are more likely to have had multiple resections and develop short bowel syndrome with longer remnant length, inflammatory disease itself is an important prognostic factor. This may be related to resolution of inflammatory disease or a greater adaptive response.

Dyke and Vinocur[66] noted that "pneumatosis cystoides intestinalis has been encountered in a large number of infants with necrotizing enterocolitis and short gut syndrome and in children who are immunosuppressed following liver transplantation."

In resecting a segment of the proximal part of the jejunoileum, remove at least 10 cm of healthy small bowel on each side of the lesion, as well as a V-like mesenteric excision. In performing a resection of the terminal ileum, surgery by right colectomy is the appropriate procedure, due to the anatomic lymphatic pathway.

## Differential Characteristics of the Jejunum and Ileum

There is no good way to identify an isolated loop of small intestine with absolute certainty without following it in one direction to the duodenojejunal junction, or in the other direction to the ileocecal junction. Table 16-3 may be consulted as an additional, but not very satisfactory, guide for distinguishing the jejunum from the ileum. It is our opinion that the clearest distinction between the jejunum and the ileum is based upon the differences between the topographic features of the blood supply to these two regions of the bowel.

Remember that each typical segment of jejunum characteristically has one or two arterial arcades in the mesentery. These arcades join parallel jejunal arteries, with parallel, long vasa recta arising from the arcades, then pass to the intestinal wall. Such vasa recta have a length of approximately 4 cm. A typical segment of the ileum often has three or more arterial arcades in the mesentery, with great numbers of relatively short vasa recta (approximately 1.5 cm in length) passing to the ileal wall. The great number of short vasa recta is related, presumably, to the large role in absorption played by the ileum. Similarly, the increase in the quantity of fat seen in the mesentery of some individuals correlates with the relative significance of the absorption of fatty elements in the ileum, in comparison with that in the jejunum.

Theoretically, the preceding information is correct; in a virgin peritoneal cavity in a thin patient, these facts may as-

## TABLE 16-2. Factors Influencing Decision to Restore Intestinal Continuity

Factors for restoring intestinal continuity
 Absorptive capacity increased
 Intestinal transit time prolonged
 Effects of short-chain fatty acids enhanced
 Intestinal stoma avoided
Factors against restoring intestinal continuity
 Secretory diarrhea from bile acids
 Perianal complications increased
 Dietary restrictions
 Incidence of nephrolithiasis increased

*Source:* Thompson JS. Surgical aspects of the short-bowel syndrome. Am J Surg 1995;170:532-536; with permission.

**TABLE 16-3. Some Differences Between Jejunum and Ileum**

| Jejunum | Ileum |
|---|---|
| Wall thicker | Wall thinner |
| Lumen larger | Lumen smaller |
| Fat on mesentery | Fat on ileum and mesentery |
| Prominent plicae circulates | Less prominent plicae |
| Single line of arterial arcades | Several lines of arterial arcades |
| Aggregate lymph nodules (Peyer's patches) sparse | Aggregate lymph nodules frequent |

*Source:* Skandalakis JE, Gray SW, Rowe JS Jr. Anatomical Complications in General Surgery. New York: McGraw-Hill, 1983; with permission.

sist in identification. However, in patients with fatty mesentery, even translumination with a sterile lighting device does not help. Our final recommendation is to use the ligament of Treitz and the ileocecal junction to distinguish the jejunum from the ileum.

## *Vascular Supply*

### Arteries

The superior mesenteric artery arises from the aorta below the origin of the celiac trunk. In about one percent of individuals, there is a combined celiacomesenteric trunk.[67] The celiac, superior, and inferior mesenteric arteries are the remnants of the paired vitelline arteries of the embryo. The superior mesenteric artery continues beyond the ileal border to supply the Meckel's diverticulum (if one is present).

The basic patterns of the intestinal arteries have been described by Noer and colleagues,[68] Michels and associates,[67] and others. On average, the left side of the superior mesenteric artery gives origin to five intestinal arteries above the origin of the ileocolic artery, and 11 arteries below that level. Eight more arteries arise from the ileal branch of the ileocolic artery.[67] A few centimeters from the border of the intestine, these intestinal vessels branch to form a series of arterial arcades connecting the intestinal arteries with one another (Fig. 16-20). Proximally, in the jejunum, one to three arcades are present; distally, in the ileum, there is an increased number of arcades.

The vascular arches form the primary anastomoses of the arterial supply. A complete channel may exist from the posteroinferior pancreaticoduodenal artery, which is parallel to the intestine and joins the marginal artery (of Drummond) of the colon. In some individuals, the pathway is incomplete, usually at the end of the ileum.[67] From the arches of the arcades, numerous arteries (the vasa recta)

arise, then pass (without cross-communication) to enter the intestinal wall. They may bifurcate to supply each side, or they may pass singly to alternate sides of the intestine (Fig. 16-21).

The vasa recta branch beneath the serosa without anastomosing, before piercing the muscularis externa. There is no collateral circulation between the vasa recta or their branches at the surface of the intestines. This configuration provides the best supply of oxygenated blood to the mesenteric side of the intestine, and the poorest supply to the antimesenteric border.

If we accept that there is no collateral circulation beyond the terminal arcades (in other words, no communication between the vasa recta and/or within the intramural network), then the blood supply of the antimesenteric border of the small bowel is probably relatively poor. Therefore, during surgery, the bowel ought to be opened halfway between the mesenteric and the antimesenteric border. We have made incisions many times at the antimesenteric border, and have had no complications.

Within the intestinal wall, the arteries form a large plexus in the submucosa. From this plexus, short vessels reach the lamina propria to supply a network of capillaries around the intestinal crypts, while longer arteries supply the cores of the intestinal villi (Fig. 16-22). Thus, there are two regions

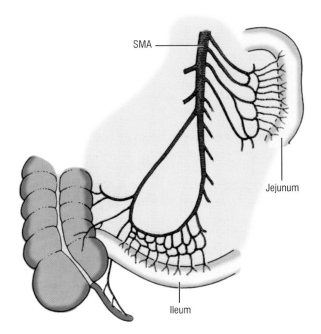

**FIG. 16-20.** The blood supply of the jejunum and ileum. The arcades of the superior mesenteric artery increase in complexity distally. (Modified from Skandalakis JE, Gray SW, Rowe JS Jr. Anatomical Complications in General Surgery. New York: McGraw-Hill, 1983; with permission.)

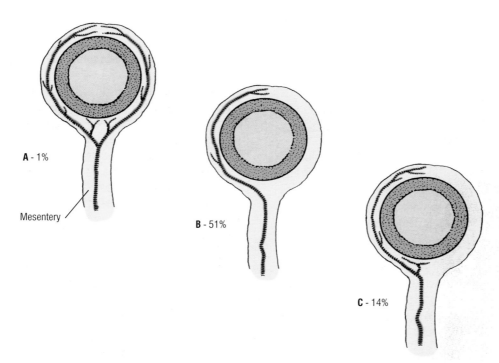

**A** - 1%

Mesentery

**B** - 51%

**C** - 14%

**FIG. 16-21. A.** The vasa recta may divide into two short vessels to the mesenteric side of the intestine and two long vessels supplying the rest of the intestinal wall. **B.** More frequently, a single long vessel supplies one side of the intestine, alternating with a vessel supplying the other side. **C.** A single long and short vessel serving one side only. The remaining 34 percent are various combinations of paired or single long or short vessels. (Modified from Skandalakis JE, Gray SW, Rowe JS Jr. Anatomical Complications in General Surgery. New York: McGraw-Hill, 1983; with permission. Data from Michels NA, Siddharth P, Kornblith PL, Parke WW. The variant blood supply to the small and large intestines: Its import in regional resections. J Int Coll Surg 1963;39:127.)

of anastomoses of intestinal arteries: the extramural arches between intestinal arteries, and the intramural submucosal plexus.

### Veins

One or more small veins originate near the tip of each intestinal villus and travel outward, receiving contributions from a plexus of veins around the intestinal glands. They enter the submucosal plexus, which is drained through the muscular layer by larger veins traveling with the arteries in the mesentery, to reach the superior mesenteric vein. These intestinal veins are interconnected by venous arcades that are similar to, but less complex than, the accompanying arterial arcades. The superior mesenteric vein belongs to the portal system, which drains the intestinal blood into the liver.

### Lymphatics

Lymphatic vessels (lacteals) arise in the cores of the intestinal villi. They form plexuses at the base of the villi, the base of the crypts, in the muscularis mucosa, in the submucosa, and between the circular and longitudinal layers of the muscularis externa. This series of plexuses is drained by large lymphatics that travel in the mesentery with the arteries and veins. The lymph flows to nodes residing between the leaves of the mesentery. Over 200 small mesenteric nodes lie near the vasa recta and along the intestinal arteries. Drainage from the mesenteric nodes is finally to the large, superior mesenteric lymph nodes at the root of the mesentery. Efferent vessels from these and the celiac nodes form the intestinal lymphatic trunk. This trunk passes beneath the left renal artery and ends in the left lumbar lymphatic trunk (70 percent) or in the cisterna chyli (25 percent).

In summary, the pathways of small bowel lymphatics are as follows:
- *Intramural:* Lacteals → mucosal vessels → submucosal plexus → subserosal plexus
- *Extramural:* Vasa recta → lymph nodes along the mesenteric vessels → lymph nodes along the superior mesenteric artery and celiac artery → cisterna chyli

### *Innervation*

The innervation of the jejunum and the ileum is by the

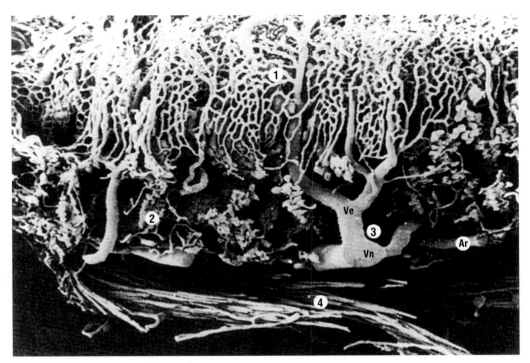

**FIG. 16-22.** A cast of the blood vascular system of the jejunal wall. **1.** Capillaries of villi. **2.** Capillaries of intestinal crypts. **3.** Submucosa with venules (Ve), veins (Vn), and arteries (Ar). **4.** Vessels of the muscularis. Scanning electron microscope ×180. (From Kessel RG, Kardon RH. Tissues and Organs: A Text-Atlas of Scanning Electron Microscopy. San Francisco: Freeman, 1979; with permission.)

autonomic system. Pain secondary to small bowel pathology is referred to the 9th, 10th, and 11th thoracic nerves, and usually is periumbilical.

## *Dimensions of the Mesentery*

Shackleford[69] stated that the length of the mesentery of the small intestine, measured between the attachment to the intestine and the root of the mesentery, usually does not exceed 20 to 25 cm. This length will permit a loop of intestine to slide down into an inguinal hernia, especially if the mesentery is slightly relaxed at its extraperitoneal attachment. Similarly, it is usually long enough to permit the surgeon to bring a loop up to form an esophagojejunostomy.

There is considerable variation in the breadth of the small bowel mesentery and that of the sigmoid mesentery. In patients with volvulus and intestinal knots, the breadth of the affected mesentery is greater than that found in healthy patients[70] (Fig. 16-23). It has not yet been determined whether there are any ethnic differences in these dimensions and their variations. The topographic anatomy and relation of the mesenteric root of the small bowel on its oblique pathway from the left upper quadrant to the right

lower quadrant is as follows:
1. The proximal end of the mesenteric root is found at the left side of L2, which is the most likely location of the duodenojejunal junction.
2. The uncinate process of the pancreas is characteristically located (when it is present) between the aorta and the superior mesenteric artery.
3. The mesentery crosses in front of the third, or horizontal, part of the duodenum.
4. It descends obliquely downward to the right, in front of the inferior vena cava.
5. The mesentery attaches to the lateral border of the right common iliac vessels.
6. It passes in front of the psoas major muscle, crossing the right ureter and the right gonadal vessels.
7. The mesentery root terminates at the ileocecal junction; there it contains the ileocolic vessels, in front of the upper end of the right sacroiliac joint.

In extremely rare cases, the mesentery of the small bowel is not totally fixed in the retroperitoneal space. Such a defect can permit an intestinal loop to enter, and can produce intestinal obstruction.[71]

To prepare a long loop of jejunum for anastomosis, the following steps can be used, after securing the duo-

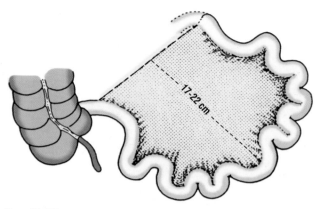

FIG. 16-23. The breadth of the mesentery. It is usually long enough to reach the internal inguinal ring. (Modified from Skandalakis JE, Gray SW, Rowe JS Jr. Anatomical Complications in General Surgery. New York: McGraw-Hill, 1983; data from Vaez-Zadeh K, Dutz W. Ileosigmoid knotting. Ann Surg 172:1027, 1970; with permission.)

denojejunal junction and drawing the proximal jejunum out of the abdomen:[72]

1. The peritoneum is incised and the selected loop is isolated and inspected. Fat and lymph nodes are removed to within 1-2 cm from the wall of the intestine.
2. The jejunal vessels are skeletonized of connective tissue, nerve fibers, and lymphatic vessels. The arteries and veins are freed to their bifurcations to form the anastomotic arcades.
3. The exposed blood vessels are again covered with peritoneum. The anatomy of the jejunal arteries and their arcades is examined to determine the feasibility of dividing the necessary number of arteries (usually 3 or 4) required for mobilization of a loop of adequate length.
4. The root of the mesentery is divided as necessary to gain length, if required.

Wind et al.[73] presented the anatomic basis of mesenteric elongation and the use of the ileum for tension-free ileo-anal anastomosis. We advise interested surgeons to put this article in their collections, and we present verbatim results along with four anatomic drawings (Fig. 16-24, Fig. 16-25, Fig. 16-26, Fig. 16-27):

*Twenty-two fresh cadavers had an ileal J-shaped reservoir of 18 cm fashioned from the last loop of small intestinal loop after section of the root of the mesentery. The gains in length so obtained were measured after section of the ileocolic artery at its origin (group A) or section between the two vascular arches of the last small intestinal group (group B); the superior mesenteric vessels were then injected with colored resin. The gain in length obtained by these two methods was iden-*

*tical (2.3 ± 1.1 cm for group A as against 2.18 ± 0.9 cm for group B), but only if the section of the ileocolic artery was accompanied by section of the mesenteric peritoneum up to the vascular arch formed by the anastomosis between the terminal branch of the superior mesenteric artery and the ileocolic artery. The constancy of this anastomosis always allowed section of the ileocolic artery while preserving good vascular distribution to the entirety of the reservoir. Section between the two arches was difficult when the distance separating them was small.*

## Anatomy of the Ileocecal Valve

For almost 400 years after its first description by Bauhin in 1579,[74] the ileocecal valve was considered to be a slitlike valve with two major lips. As early as 1914, Rutherford noticed the differences between the valve of the cadaver and that of the living patient. With the development of new methods (such as colonoscopy and photography through a cecostomy) for studying the ileocecal area in living patients, it was demonstrated that the "valve" in most patients resembles the cervix protruding into the vagina or the pyloric opening into the duodenum.[74]

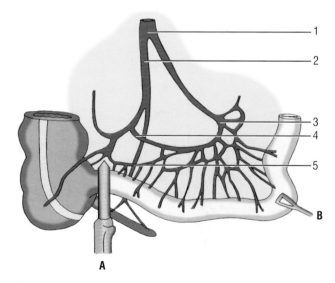

FIG. 16-24. Ileocecal region. The staple applicator **(A)** shows section of the last loop flush with the ileocecal valve. The forceps **(B)** is located at the site of the future apex of the J-shaped reservoir. 1. superior mesenteric artery. 2. ileocolic artery. 3. terminal ileal branch of superior mesenteric artery. 4. ileal branch of ileocolic artery. 5. recurrent ileal artery. (Modification from Wind P, Chevallier JM, Sauvanet A, Delmas V, Cugnenc PH. Anatomic basis of mesenteric elongation for ileo-anal anastomosis with J-shaped reservoir: comparison of two techniques of vascular selection. Surg Radiol Anat 1996;18:11-16; with permission.)

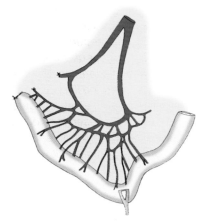

**FIG. 16-25.** Appearance of terminal loop of small intestine after section. The recurrent ileal artery has been sectioned at its origin and the ileocecal artery has been divided below the origin of the ileal branch. (Modified from Wind P, Chevallier JM, Sauvanet A, Delmas V, Cugnenc PH. Anatomic basis of mesenteric elongation for ileo-anal anastomosis with J-shaped reservoir: comparison of two techniques of vascular selection. Surg Radiol Anat 1996;18:11-16; with permission.)

The slitlike orifice of the ileocecal valve appears to be a postmortem artifact. Ulin and colleagues[75] illustrated the changes in appearance of the valve, from a "papilla" to a bilabial valve, that take place within the first hour after death (Fig. 16-28). The closing mechanism of the papilla is formed by two rings of thickened circular muscle, one at the base of the papilla and one at the free end.

### *Terminal Ileum and Appendiceal Abscess*

An appendiceal abscess may be palpated by abdominal examination when it is located posteriorly or anteriorly to the terminal ileal loop. The abscess located anteriorly is occasionally referred to as an abscess behind the right rectus abdominis muscle.

### *Anatomy of Meckel's Diverticulum*

#### Surgical Anatomy

When present, Meckel's diverticulum arises from the antimesenteric surface of the ileum about 40 cm from the ileocecal valve in infants, and almost 50 cm in adults. It may be less than 15 cm (4% of cases) or as much as 167 cm from the valve (Fig. 16-29).[20] Not less than 5 feet (about 2 meters) of ileum should be inspected to be sure that the diverticulum has not been overlooked.

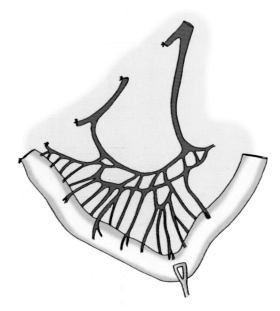

**FIG. 16-26.** For elongation of the mesenteric axis, the ileocolic artery has been sectioned at its origin from the superior mesenteric artery. (Modified from Wind P, Chevallier JM, Sauvanet A, Delmas V, Cugnenc PH. Anatomic basis of mesenteric elongation for ileo-anal anastomosis with J-shaped reservoir: comparison of two techniques of vascular selection. Surg Radiol Anat 1996;18:11-16; with permission.)

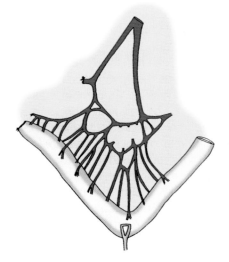

**FIG. 16-27.** For elongation of the mesenteric axis, some vascular connections between the primary arch and the second-order arch have been sectioned. (Modified from Wind P, Chevallier JM, Sauvanet A, Delmas V, Cugnenc PH. Anatomic basis of mesenteric elongation for ileo-anal anastomosis with J-shaped reservoir: comparison of two techniques of vascular selection. Surg Radiol Anat 1996;18:11-16; with permission.)

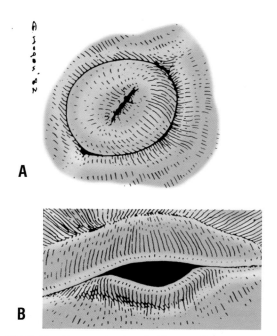

**FIG. 16-28.** The ileocecal valve. **A.** The papillary appearance of the valve in the living patient. **B.** The bilabial appearance of the valve in the cadaver. (Modified from Skandalakis JE, Gray SW, Rowe JS Jr. Anatomical Complications in General Surgery. New York: McGraw-Hill, 1983; with permission.)

The diverticulum may be as short as 1 cm or as long as 26 cm: 75 percent will be from 1 to 5 cm; the rest will be longer.[9] In spite of these wide variations, there are limits to the possible size and position of vitelline duct remnants. Their length is not measured in meters. They do not arise from the colon, the duodenum, or even from the jejunum (for rare exceptions, see Benson[76]). Although they may appear to do so, vitelline duct remnants cannot arise from the mesenteric side of the ileum. Remember: very long diverticula, those beyond the boundaries of the ileum, and diverticula on the mesenteric side are not Meckelian in origin.

Three major types of Meckel's diverticulum are shown in Figure 16-30. The usual condition (Fig. 16-30A) is a blind diverticulum with a free and mobile tip (74 percent). In most of the remainder (24 percent), the tip is attached to the anterior body wall at the umbilicus (Fig. 16-30B). In a few cases (2 percent), the structure is patent to the outside (omphalo-ileal fistula), a solid cord, or a cystic remnant (Fig. 16-30C).

The mucosa of the diverticulum is largely ileal; gastric, pancreatic, or duodenal mucosa may also be present. Gastric mucosa was present in 80 percent of specimens examined by Stewart and Storey.[77] Far from being merely an embryologic curiosity, ectopic gastric mucosa with parietal cells leads to ileal ulceration, and is an important con-

duit of pathology of the diverticulum to the adjacent ileum.

Remember that the independent blood supply of Meckel's diverticulum originates from an intestinal arcade.

Meckel's diverticulum is discovered only incidentally during surgery (2 to 4.5 percent of individuals) or at autopsy (1.1 to 2.5 percent of individuals, unless the organ is diseased).[9] It is widely stated to be more frequent in males than in females, but this is true only in the presence of disease. Incidentally-found Meckel's diverticula are equally distributed between the sexes (Fig. 16-31).[78]

**Pathology**

Obstruction produced by Meckel's diverticulum is a complication, rather than a disease of the diverticulum. Since the pathologic findings originate with the diverticulum, Androulakis et al.[78] categorized obstruction under Meckel's diverticulum disease.

Ulceration accounts for about 40 percent of Meckel's diverticulum disease. It is produced by secretions from ectopic gastric mucosa in the diverticulum. Ulceration acts on unprotected ileal mucosa in the diverticulum or in the ileum distal to it. Bright red or brick red rectal bleeding secondary to ulceration is painless and episodic.[79] In 90 percent of cases of bleeding associated with a Meckel's diverticulum, Tc-99m pertechnetate (nuclear scan with technetium pertechnetate) confirms the clinical diagnosis by demonstrating the ectopic gastric mucosa in the diverticulum.[79]

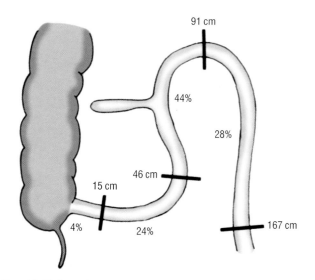

**FIG. 16-29.** Location on the ileum and frequency of occurrence of Meckel's diverticulum. (Modified from Skandalakis JE, Gray SW (Eds). Embryology for Surgeons, 2nd Ed. Baltimore: Williams & Wilkins, 1994; data from Jay GD III, Margulis RR, McGraw AB, Northrip RR. Meckel's diverticulum: a survey of one hundred and three cases. Arch Surg 61:158-169, 1950; with permission.)

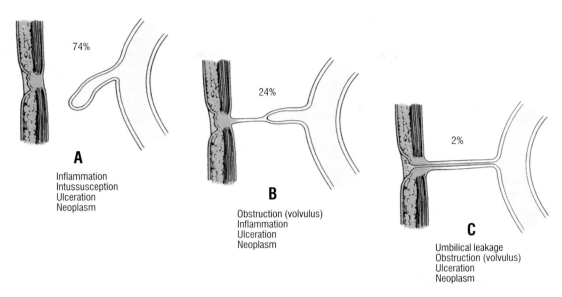

FIG. 16-30. Major types of Meckel's diverticulum. **A.** Diverticulum with free end not attached to body wall. **B.** Diverticulum connected with the anterior body wall by a fibrous cord. **C.** Fistula opening through the umbilicus. (Modified from Skandalakis JE, Gray SW, Rowe JS Jr. Anatomical Complications in General Surgery. New York: McGraw-Hill, 1983; with permission.)

Lichtstein and Herskowitz[80] reported on a 91-year-old male with massive lower gastrointestinal bleeding secondary to Meckel's diverticulum with ectopic gastric mucosa.

Obstruction and intussusception together account for about 32 percent of Meckel's diverticulum disease. Obstruction can be caused by volvulus. A diverticulum attached to the abdominal wall can also cause obstruction by incarceration of an intestinal loop. The diverticulum is the leading point of intussusception. According to Oldham and Wesley,[79] five to ten percent of patients with symptomatic diverticular disease present with the clinical picture of intussusception.

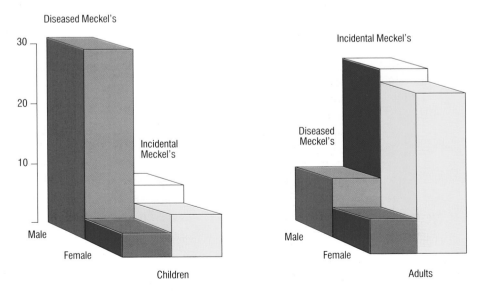

FIG. 16-31. Difference in age and sex distribution of diseased (symptomatic) and incidental (asymptomatic) Meckel's diverticulum among 53 children and 71 adults. A sex difference is apparent only in children with diseased Meckel's diverticulum. Scale indicates the number of cases. (Modified from Skandalakis JE, Gray SW, Rowe JS Jr. Anatomical Complications in General Surgery. New York: McGraw-Hill, 1983; with permission.)

Appendicitis-like inflammation, often from the presence of a foreign body and narrow base, accounts for 17 percent of Meckel's diverticulum disease.[79]

Neoplasms are found in about 6 percent of Meckel's diverticulum disease. In order of frequency, these neoplasms are leiomyomas, leiomyosarcomas (malignant gastrointestinal stromal tumors), carcinoid tumors, and adenocarcinomas. Lin et al.[81] reported a case of gastric adenocarcinoma of Meckel's diverticulum which completely obstructed the sigmoid colon. Carcinoid tumors may be the most common neoplastic lesions of the diverticulum.[82]

Umbilical symptoms (umbilical leakage from an omphaloileal fistula, weeping from an umbilical polyp, or infection of an umbilical sinus) account for the remaining 5 percent of Meckel's diverticulum disease.[9]

The symptomatology of Meckel's diverticulum disease is the clinical picture of acute appendicitis, or symptoms produced by the accompanying pathology (rectal bleeding, intestinal obstruction, etc.).

### Incidental Meckel's Diverticulum

It is our opinion that an asymptomatic Meckel's diverticulum should always be excised if found during an exploratory laparotomy. The only question is the type of excision: a wide V-wedge excision with intact mesenteric borders, or a minimal segmental bowel resection. We prefer the latter if the general condition of the patient permits, and if the surgeon is not absolutely sure about any possible pathology involving the diverticulum.

We quote Yahchouchy et al.[83] on the prophylactic removal of a incidentally discovered Meckel's diverticulum, "The risk of complications of a Meckel's diverticulum has not been found to decrease with age. So the benefits of incidental diverticulectomy outweighed its attending morbidity and mortality."

# HISTOLOGY AND PHYSIOLOGY OF THE SMALL INTESTINE

## Histology of the Duodenum

The duodenal wall, from inside to outside, consists of a mucous membrane, a submucosa, a muscularis externa, and an external serosa. The mucosa is thrown up into large crescentic folds (plica circulares, or valves of Kerckring) that project into the intestinal lumen transverse to its long axis. These folds are absent in the proximal 2.5 to 5 cm of the duodenum. The folds are very large and close together just distal to the entrance of the common bile and pancreatic ducts. The duodenal mucosa is characterized by a columnar epithelium on a lamina propria of loose connective tissue, bounded by a thin layer of smooth muscle, the muscularis mucosae. Leaf-shaped villi of mucosa project into the intestinal lumen.

The epithelial surface of the villi contains columnar absorptive intestinal cells capped with microvilli and a glycoprotein surface coat; there are also goblet cells, Paneth cells, argentaffin cells, and a variety of endocrine polypeptide-secreting cells, not all of which are yet understood. The absorptive cells are the most numerous and have the greatest rate of replacement.

Between the villi projecting from the surface into the lumen are openings of simple tubular glands (crypts of Lieberkühn) extending into the lamina propria. Beneath the muscularis mucosa, the submucosa is filled with the coiled tubular glands of Brunner that pierce the muscularis mucosa and open into the bottoms of the crypts. These glands, which are characteristic of the duodenal portion of the small intestine, become less frequent, and finally disappear, in its dis-

### Editorial Comment

*The management of an incidental finding of a Meckel's diverticulum is controversial. In my opinion it is not always appropriate to excise an asymptomatic Meckel's diverticulum. The decision is based in part on patient age and in part on the appearance of the diverticulum. Development of pathology related to a Meckel's diverticulum is rare in adults and thus I do not believe excision of an incidental normal-appearing diverticulum is appropriate. In pediatric patients, particularly under the age of two years, resection should be considered in the following situations: heterotopic gastric mucosa is suspected because there is a palpable thickening at the base of the diverticulum; there is an unusually long diverticulum with a narrow opening that might become obstructed. Diverticulectomy may be considered if there is an attachment of the diverticulum to the umbilicus, but, even here, resection may not be necessary when there is only a band. (RSF Jr)*

tal segment. Their secretion is alkaline, probably to neutralize the acid gastric secretion of the stomach. The submucosa is bounded by the muscularis externa, having a deep layer of circular smooth muscle and a superficial layer of longitudinal smooth muscle. These two layers form the contractile basis of peristalsis.

The duodenum, together with the pylorus of the stomach, controls the passage of food to the jejunum and the ileum. The anatomic basis for this action rests on the structure of the proximal duodenum.

At the gastroduodenal junction, the continuity of the circular musculature is interrupted by a ring-shaped septum of connective tissue derived from the submucosa. Proximal to this ring, the circular muscle layer is thickened to form the pyloric sphincter of the stomach. Distal to the ring, there is an abrupt decrease in the thickness of the circular muscle that forms the relatively thin-walled duodenum. At its distal end, the pylorus ("os pylorus") is surrounded by a duodenal fornix. This arrangement must be kept in mind when performing pyloromyotomy.

The longitudinal external muscle layer, without a change in thickness, is also interrupted at the gastroduodenal junction (except on the side of the lesser curvature, where some peripheral muscle fibers are continuous with fibers of the duodenal musculature). This arrangement may serve to carry peristaltic contractions across the interruption at the connective tissue septum.[84]

Internally, the appearance of the submucosal glands of Brunner marks the gastroduodenal junction. This may not correspond with the muscular junction. In human beings, the submucosal glands may extend a few centimeters into the pylorus. Occasionally, antral gastric mucosa may prolapse through the pylorus, producing a radiological finding but not a true clinical syndrome.

Where the common bile duct and the main pancreatic duct pass through the wall of the duodenum to open into its lumen, there is an absence of Brunner's glands. The duodenojejunal junction also is marked internally by the disappearance of Brunner's glands, and externally by the attachment of the suspensory ligament of Treitz. There is no line of demarcation at this junction.

The suspensory muscle (or, ligament) of Treitz is a fibromuscular band that arises from the right crus of the diaphragm and inserts on the upper surface of the duodenojejunal flexure. It passes posterior to the pancreas and the splenic vein, and anterior to the left renal vein. It may surround the celiac artery or course to its left as the ligament passes toward the terminal region of the duodenum. At its origin, the band contains striated muscle fibers continuous with those of the right crus of the respiratory diaphragm. Near its insertion, the suspensory band contains smooth muscle fibers continuous with those of the longitudinal duo-

denal muscularis. According to O'Rahilly and Müller,[3] the suspensory duodenal muscle, which develops at the beginning of the third trimester, descends from the vicinity of the celiac axis and small intestine down to the duodenojejunal flexure.

The suspensory ligament usually inserts on the duodenal flexure and the third and fourth portions of the duodenum (Fig. 16-32A); it may insert on the flexure only (Fig. 16-32B), or on the third and fourth portions only (Fig. 16-32C). There can also be multiple attachments (Fig. 16-32D). In almost one-fifth of cadavers, the ligament is absent, apparently without associated symptoms.[85]

The proximal half of the first part of the duodenum is completely covered by peritoneum, but all the other parts are located retroperitoneally. The second and third parts are overlapped by the head of the pancreas, so that there is a pancreatic bare area of the duodenum not covered by peritoneum. A second bare area exists on the anterior surface of the second part of the duodenum, where the trans-

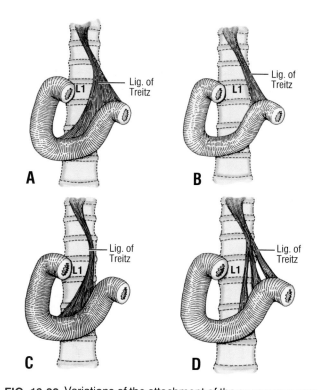

**FIG. 16-32.** Variations of the attachment of the suspensory muscle (ligament) of Treitz. **A.** Attachments to the flexure and the third and fourth portions of the duodenum. This is the most common type. **B.** Attachment to the duodenojejunal flexure. **C.** Attachments to the third and fourth portions only. **D.** Multiple separated attachments of the suspensory ligament. (Modified from Skandalakis JE, Skandalakis LJ, Colborn GL, Pemberton LB, Gray SW. The duodenum. Part 2: Surgical anatomy. Am Surg 55(5):291-298, 1989; with permission.)

verse colon is attached (Fig. 16-33). With pancreatic cancer or pancreatitis, the pancreas and mesocolon, with its middle colic artery, become firmly fixed. The anatomic entities responsible for duodenal fixation are the pylorus, the superior mesenteric vessels, the ligament of Treitz, and, of course, the peritoneum.

## Physiologic Characteristics of the Duodenum

Although the duodenum's control over gastric emptying was known, or at least suspected, in antiquity, the action of the duodenum on the pylorus is far more complex than Rufus of Ephesus could have imagined. Nerve reflexes acting from the duodenum to the pylorus are partly through the extrinsic nerves. Some go via prevertebral sympathetic ganglia, and return through inhibitory sympathetic nerve fibers to the stomach. In addition to extrinsic nerves, the enteric nervous system within the wall of the gastrointestinal tract is now recognized as an independent integrative system with structural and functional properties akin to those of the central nervous system. Thus, the enteric nervous system plays a major role in coordinating and programming gastrointestinal functions within the walls of the duodenum and the stomach.[45]

We quote from Nemeth et al.[86] on the embryology of peristalsis:

> [N]eurone density of myenteric plexus is significantly higher in the mesenteric border of the small bowel compared with antimesenteric border in premature infants. The marked morphological differences observed in neurone density in the small bowel of premature infants may contribute to immature small bowel activity.

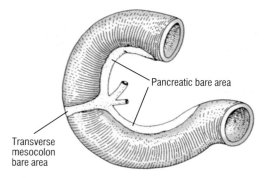

FIG. 16-33. Bare areas of the duodenum. The pancreas is in intimate contact with the duodenum along the concave surface. The attachment of the transverse mesocolon produces an additional bare area. (Modified from Skandalakis JE, Skandalakis LJ, Colborn GL, Pemberton LB, Gray SW. The duodenum. Part 2: Surgical anatomy. Am Surg 55(5):291-298, 1989; with permission.)

In addition to the neural mechanisms, there is a humoral effect on the stomach from the duodenum. It appears to respond chiefly to fat in the gastric chyme. The two feedback systems (neural and humoral) work together to inhibit gastric emptying when the duodenum is full or the chyme contains excess acid, protein, or fat. Emptying of the stomach depends upon the amount of chyme to be processed.

## Histology of the Jejunum and the Ileum

The intestinal wall (Fig. 16-34) is composed of a serosa of visceral peritoneum, longitudinal and circular muscle, a submucosa of connective tissue, and a mucosa of connective tissue, smooth muscle, and epithelium. The plicae circulares of the small intestine are most obvious in the jejunum. The villi of the jejunum are the most distinctly long, tongue-shaped, or fingerlike projections. The villi of the ileum are shorter and shaped more bluntly, disappearing gradually as the ileocecal valve is approached.

Almost a century ago, Halsted pointed out the importance of the submucosal connective tissue in holding sutures.[87] One should remember that when butchers make beef or pork sausage, it is from this layer of the intestine that casings are made; "catgut" sutures also used to be made from this layer. Fear of perforating the mucosa with a stitch makes seromuscular sutures seem to be safer, but the integrity of an anastomosis is greater if the submucosa is included.[88-91]

The serosa surrounds the jejunum and ileum completely, except at the mesenteric border. Together with the muscular coat, the serosa is the well-known stroma for the application of seromuscular sutures during surgical procedures. The muscular coat, which is formed by the inner circular and outer longitudinal layers, should be considered, at least surgically, as one layer. The muscular coat is responsible for intestinal motility. It contains the myenteric plexus of Auerbach, as well as ganglia for non-myelinated nerve fibers. The submucosa is the home of the very rich network of neuronal elements of Meissner's plexus, as well as arteries, veins, and lymphatics. It also hosts the Peyer's patches of isolated and confluent masses of lymphatic nodules in the antimesenteric side of the ileum.

## Physiologic Characteristics of the Jejunum and the Ileum

The multitude of villi and their innumerable microvilli vastly increase the surface area of the mucosa of the small intestine that is responsible for absorption and secretion.

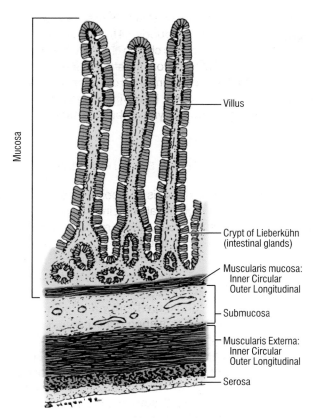

Mucosa

Villus

Crypt of Lieberkühn
(intestinal glands)

Muscularis mucosa:
Inner Circular
Outer Longitudinal

Submucosa

Muscularis Externa:
Inner Circular
Outer Longitudinal

Serosa

FIG. 16-34. Section through the wall of the small intestine. The submucosa should be included in stitches forming an anastomosis. (Modified from Skandalakis JE, Gray SW, Rowe JS Jr. Anatomical Complications in General Surgery. New York: McGraw-Hill, 1983; with permission.)

Intestinal absorptive cells, goblet exocrine cells, and Paneth cells are found in the villi. T-cells and APUD (amine precursor uptake and decarboxylation) cells also are found there. According to Guyton,[92] the small intestine absorbs almost all the ingested fluid (about 1.5 liters per day), plus all the fluid from gastrointestinal secretions (approximately 7 liters). The large bowel absorbs only 1.5 liters. The substances absorbed by the small bowel include water, ions, and nutrients (carbohydrates, proteins, and fats).

The small bowel makes the following nonimmunologic contributions:[92,93]

- Degradation of harmful toxins by enteric proteolytic enzymes, lysozymes, and hydrochloric acid
- Inhibition of bacteria by mucin, as well as protection of the enteric epithelium
- Removal of microbes and parasites by peristaltic activity
- Dilution and exclusion of antigens by rapid turnover of the epithelium, minimizing violation of the epithelial surface

- Competition for inhibition taking place between the pathologic and the endogenous bacteria

The histologic and functional integrity of the small bowel mucosa is maintained by the genesis of cells that replace the old dying cells. The rapid turnover of the epithelium of the mucosa of the small bowel (in comparison with the slow turnover of that in the large bowel) makes neoplasia of the small bowel unusual. Townsend et al.,[94] reporting on growth factors and intestinal neoplasms, wrote that, despite the huge surface area of the small intestines, the interactions of the factors responsible for growth and differentiation are less frequently deranged than in the large bowel. Sarr[95] speculates that the following factors may explain why the small bowel has fewer benign and malignant neoplasia in comparison with the stomach and large bowel:

- Mucosal cells are replaced rapidly
- Small bowel chyme has a high liquid content and is, therefore, less "irritating"
- Contents move rapidly through the small bowel, minimizing exposure to carcinogens
- Alkaline pH and decreased bacterial concentration minimize the formation of carcinogens from bile and ingested precarcinogens
- High activity of the enzyme benzopyrene hydroxylase in the small intestinal mucosa results in detoxification of carcinogens
- The small intestine offers humoral and cellular immune surveillance (secretory IgA, abundant immunocompetent lymphoid tissue)

Sarr[95] believes that depressed overall immune surveillance by the small intestine may support the genesis of neoplasia in immunocompromised individuals.

## SURGERY OF THE SMALL INTESTINE

## Decalogue of Good and Safe Intestinal Surgery

1. Start by carefully exploring the peritoneal cavity and examining the intraperitoneal organs for primary, secondary, or metastatic disease from the tumor in question, or for metastasis from other tumors, especially melanoma.
2. Inspect and gently palpate the tumor to be resected.
3. Perform good mobilization (both proximal and distal) of the area in question, to avoid tension and to perform an anastomosis without tension.

4. Be extremely careful of the blood supply. Angiography prior to surgery gives the surgeon information about the vascular topography of the duodenum. In a mesentery with a lot of adipose tissue, pulsation of vessels in the mesentery may not be obvious, but gentle palpation can reveal vessels. Very minimal bleeding at the edges is a good sign.

5. Form larger proximal and distal stomata by oblique placement of the noncrushing clamps.

6. After the resection, a good, tension-free apposition of the distal and proximal stomata with serosa-to-serosa approximation is essential.

7. Prepare both stomata for anastomosis by cleaning fat and adhesions approximately 0.5-1.0 cm from the cut edge (especially in the mesenteric border, where leaks always occur).

8. Include the submucosa with the seromuscular layer to better ensure the integrity of the intestinal anastomosis.

9. Avoid hematomata on the anastomotic side.

10. Check anastomotic patency with the thumb and index finger.

## Neoplasms of the Small Intestine

The small bowel from the gastroduodenal junction to the ileocecal junction is the home of rare benign and malignant tumors. Because of the differences in anatomic topography of the duodenum and the jejunum/ileum, surgical techniques differ according to the location of the tumor.

The classification and distribution of small bowel neoplasms can be appreciated by study of Table 16-4, Table 16-5, and Table 16-6. Blanchard et al.[96] reviewed benign and malignant smooth muscle tumors, and their results are shown in Figure 16-35 and Figure 16-36. According to Sarr,[95] the malignant tumors of the small bowel are adenocarcinoma (30-50 percent), leiomyosarcoma (10-20 percent), lymphoma (10-15 percent), and carcinoid tumors (13 percent). Again according to Sarr, adenocarcinoma occurs in the duodenum in 40 percent of cases, in the jejunum in 40 percent, and in the ileum in 20 percent.

Several authors[96,97] strongly advise that leiomyoma of the gastrointestinal tract be treated as a malignant tumor, due to the difficulty of diagnosis by frozen or permanent section. This enigmatic presentation dictates radical surgery, even though it may actually be a benign disease. A similar situation exists with sessile villous adenoma. Because of the possibility of malignancy, it should be treated not by enterotomy and excision, but by segmental resection.

Polyps and polyposis present a similar scenario. Sarr[95] states that 30 percent of these harbor adenocarcinoma;

therefore, radical surgery is the appropriate response. However, since it is not within the scope of this book to present detailed pathologic descriptions of the many lesions that can involve the small bowel, we end the listing of them at this point.

Wängberg et al.[98] studied 64 patients with disseminated midgut carcinoids and concluded that an active surgical approach must be recommended to patients with midgut carcinoid syndrome. Figures 16-37 and 16-38 summarize their treatment program and results.

In commenting on the above paper, Farley[99] noted that aggressive surgical therapy with improved adjuvant therapy of carcinoid malignancies provides hope for patients with hepatic involvement of midgut carcinoid.

Kirshbom et al.[100] stated that metastatic carcinoids of

### TABLE 16-4. Pathology of Primary Small Bowel Tumors by Cell of Origin

| Cell of Origin | Benign | Malignant |
|---|---|---|
| Epithelium | Adenoma | Adenocarcinoma |
| Connective tissue | Fibroma | Fibrosarcoma |
| Smooth muscle | Leiomyoma | Leiomyosarcoma |
| Fat | Lipoma | Liposarcoma |
| Vascular endothelium | Hemangioma | Angiosarcoma |
| Lymphatics | Lymphangioma | Lymphangiosarcoma |
| Lymphoid tissue | Pseudolymphoma | Lymphoma |
| Nerve | Neurofibroma | Neurofibrosarcoma |
|  | Ganglioneuroma | GAN tumor |
| Argentaffin cell | – | Carcinoid |
| Mixed | Hamartoma |  |

*Source:* Coit DG. Cancer of the small intestine. In: DeVita VT Jr, Hellman S, Rosenberg SA (eds). Cancer: Principles & Practice of Oncology, 5th Ed. Philadelphia: Lippincott-Raven, 1997; with permission.

**TABLE 16-5. Distribution of Malignant Tumors of the Small Bowel by Site in 27 Series**

| Tumor | Duodenum | Jejunum | Ileum | Total | |
|---|---|---|---|---|---|
| Adenocarcinoma | 634 | 454 | 301 | 1389 | (44%) |
| Carcinoid | 60 | 92 | 781 | 933 | (29%) |
| Lymphoma | 34 | 183 | 276 | 493 | (15%) |
| Sarcoma | 61 | 159 | 148 | 368 | (12%) |
| Total | 789 (25%) | 888 (28%) | 1506 (47%) | 3183 | (100%) |

*Source:* Coit DG. Cancer of the small intestine. In: DeVita VT Jr, Hellman S, Rosenberg SA (eds). Cancer: Principles & Practice of Oncology, 5th Ed. Philadelphia: Lippincott-Raven, 1997; with permission.

**TABLE 16-6. Distribution of Benign Tumors of the Small Bowel by Site in 13 Series**

| Tumor | Duodenum | Jejunum | Ileum | Total | |
|---|---|---|---|---|---|
| Leiomyoma | 24 | 64 | 47 | 135 | (37%) |
| Polyp, adenoma | 34 | 17 | 17 | 68 | (19%) |
| Lipoma | 11 | 13 | 30 | 54 | (15%) |
| Hemangioma | 1 | 10 | 26 | 37 | (10%) |
| Fibroma | 4 | 7 | 12 | 23 | (6%) |
| Other | 27 | 8 | 13 | 48 | (13%) |
| Total | 101 (27%) | 119 (33%) | 145 (40%) | 365 | (100%) |

*Source:* Coit DG. Cancer of the small intestine. In: DeVita VT Jr, Hellman S, Rosenberg SA (eds). Cancer: Principles & Practice of Oncology, 5th Ed. Philadelphia: Lippincott-Raven, 1997; with permission.

unknown origin behave like midgut carcinoids with respect to hormone production, indolence, and survival.

Surgery of the duodenum can be summarized as follows:

1. With malignancy in the first, third, and fourth part of the duodenum, a segmental resection may be advisable, depending on many other factors.

2. With malignancy of the second part, Whipple resection with regional lymphadenectomy is the procedure of choice. We feel that periampullary carcinoma should be treated radically; occasionally, depending on the age and general condition of the patient, local excision will be performed instead.

3. We agree with the conclusion of Rose et al.,[101] and Lil-

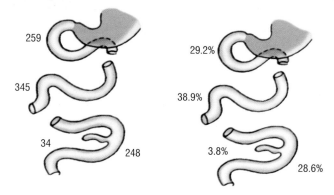

FIG. 16-35. Incidence of leiomyomas in the small intestine. n = 886 cases, plus 166 not specified. (Modified from Blanchard DK, Budde JM, Hatch GF III, Wertheimer-Hatch L, Hatch KF, Davis GB, Foster RS Jr, Skandalakis JE. Tumors of the small intestine. World J Surg 24:421-429, 2000; with permission.)

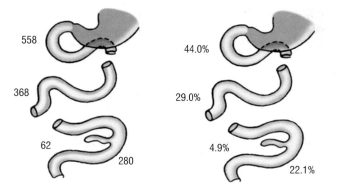

FIG. 16-36. Incidence of leiomyosarcomas in the small intestine. n =1268 cases, plus 387 not specified. (Modified from Blanchard DK, Budde JM, Hatch GF III, Wertheimer-Hatch L, Hatch KF, Davis GB, Foster RS Jr, Skandalakis JE. Tumors of the small intestine. World J Surg 24:421-429, 2000; with permission.)

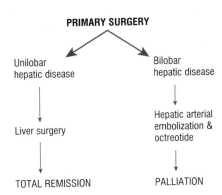

PRIMARY SURGERY

**FIG. 16-37.** Treatment program aiming at aggressive tumor reduction in patients with the midgut carcinoid syndrome using surgery and hepatic artery embolization. All interventional procedures were performed under octreotide protection. (From Wängberg B, Westberg G, Tylén U, Tisell L-E, Jansson S, Nilsson O, Johansson V, Scherstén T, Ahlman H. Survival of patients with disseminated midgut carcinoid tumors after aggressive tumor reduction. World J Surg 1996;20:892; with permission.)

lemoe's concurrence,[102] that duodenal carcinoma is biologically comparable to pancreatic and gastric cancer. Therefore, the procedure of choice is pancreatoduodenectomy.

4. According to Farnell and colleagues,[103] "Pancreaticoduodenectomy is appropriate for villous tumors containing cancer and may be considered an alternative for select patients with benign villous tumors of the duodenum. If local excision is performed, regular postoperative endoscopic surveillance is mandatory."

Bleeding, perforation, and obstruction are the complications of small bowel neoplasia. The peculiar anatomy of the lymphatics of the small bowel, together with the above complications, lessens the possibility of a cure if the tumor is malignant.

The mesentery should be inspected for lymph nodes. An excisional biopsy of any enlarged lymph nodes or perhaps two to three suspect lymph nodes should be performed. Careful incision of the overlying peritoneum and excision of the lymph nodes in toto should follow a report of malignancy in the lymph nodes. What appears to be a discolored lymph node may actually be an accessory or ectopic spleen, rather than a lymph node.

## Surgical Applications to the Duodenum

### First Part of the Duodenum

The relative paucity of collateral pathways in the arterial supply to the first part of the duodenum should cause the

surgeon to exercise all possible care in operative procedures in this area. Here, solidly based anatomic knowledge, skillful technique, and conservative skeletonization will produce good results with surgical procedures.

### Second Part of the Duodenum

The duodenum is one of the most difficult areas to approach when operating, because of the fixation of the duodenum and the pancreas, the common blood supply for both organs (superior and inferior pancreaticoduodenal arcades), and the opening of the common bile duct and pancreatic ducts. With malignant disease, a pancreaticoduodenectomy should be performed. In the presence of benign disease, a more conservative approach, such as segmental resection, is the preferred treatment. Edwards et al.[104] describe two cases in which pancreaticoduodenectomy with en bloc colectomy were attempted as curative procedures for primary malignancies of the duodenum.

### Third Part of the Duodenum

The proximal one-third of this part of the duodenum is difficult to deal with because of its relationship posterosuperiorly to the head of the pancreas and the uncinate process. The third part is related posteroinferiorly to the inferior mesenteric artery, which arises from the aorta just behind the duodenum. The surgeon should remember that the third part is crossed ventrally by the superior mesenteric vessels in the vertical plane. The horizontal plane is crossed by the transverse mesocolon, with its marginal

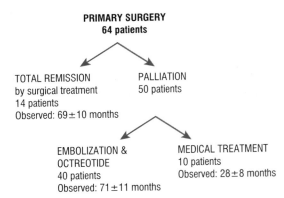

**FIG. 16-38.** Flow chart of 64 patients with the midgut carcinoid syndrome according to the treatment program in Fig. 16-37. Observation time is given as the mean ± SEM (standard error of mean). (From Wängberg B, Westberg G, Tylén U, Tisell L-E, Jansson S, Nilsson O, Johansson V, Scherstén T, Ahlman H. Survival of patients with disseminated midgut carcinoid tumors after aggressive tumor reduction. World J Surg 1996;20:892; with permission.)

artery and the middle colic artery. The surgeon should proceed slowly with the uncinate process, which is closely related to the superior mesenteric vessels. Many small vessels originate from the inferior pancreaticoduodenal arcades. Other small twigs from the superior mesenteric artery are commonly present.

## *Fourth Part of the Duodenum*

The fourth portion of the duodenum is related to two anatomic entities of importance: the ligament of Treitz above, and the inferior mesenteric vein, which is to the left of the paraduodenal fossae. The surgeon should use the fourth portion to begin the exploration of the distal duodenum (third and fourth portions). Remember that mobilization of the right colon and transection of the ligament of Treitz are necessary for good exposure of the distal duodenum. The blood supply here originates from the divisions of the intestinal branches of the superior mesenteric artery, and is similar to that of the rest of the small bowel. The arteries of the fourth part of the duodenum have little or no collateral circulation, and the blood supply is "least efficient" in the "antimesenteric" border (the duodenum loses its mesentery in development but, embryologically, the middle of the anterior wall, which is covered by peritoneum, should be considered its "antimesenteric" border).

## *Bleeding Duodenal Ulcer*

A duodenal ulcer is a peptic ulceration that is located on the posterior wall of the duodenal bulb. When bleeding occurs, it is the gastroduodenal artery that has been eroded, and in most cases the erosion is close to the springing of the transverse pancreatic artery. Turnage[105] advised three-point ligation of these vessels to prevent future bleeding.

Remember, in 10 percent[32] of the cases there is only one pancreatic duct: the duct of Santorini. The gastroduodenal artery passes "behind" the duodenum and in front of the duct of Santorini. A very deep suture to stop the bleeding can ligate, with catastrophic results, the only pancreatic duct that is present. (See additional information about the accessory pancreatic duct in the section "Surgical Notes to Remember" in this chapter.)

## *Vascular Compression of the Duodenum*

### Anatomy of Vascular Compression

A consequence of the erect posture of humans is that the superior mesenteric artery leaves the aorta at a more acute angle than it does in quadrupeds. Through this vascular angle passes the third or fourth part of the duodenum, held in place by the suspensory muscle of Treitz. The posterior limb of the angle is formed by the vertebrae and the paravertebral muscles, as well as by the aorta. The anterior limb is formed by the superior mesenteric artery; the middle and right colic arteries (the superior mesentery artery's first two branches in the transverse mesocolon) sometimes join in. The most narrow part of the angle, above the duodenum, contains the uncinate process and the left renal vein. The relation of the third portion of the duodenum to the superior mesenteric artery, middle colic artery, aorta, and mesentery is shown in sagittal section in Fig. 16-39. An anterior view of the duodenum, superior mesenteric artery, middle colic artery, and vertebral column is shown in Fig. 16-40.

The position of the duodenum beneath the superior mesenteric artery is the result of normal intestinal rotation. Vascular compression syndrome was first described by Rokitansky[106] in 1861. Compression in patients with malrotation and grossly altered vascular relationships[107] or duodenal compression by anomalous hepatic portal veins[108] are not considered here.

### Anatomic Variations of Vascular Compression

Three anatomic variations are important in vascular compression:

1. Variations in the length and attachment of the suspensory muscle
2. Variations in the level at which the duodenum crosses the vertebral column
3. Variations in the level of the origin of the superior mesenteric artery

The duodenum usually crosses the vertebral column at the level of the third lumbar vertebra,[109] but it may cross at a lower level, especially in women. In a few patients, the crossing may be as high as the second lumbar vertebra. Either the third or the fourth part of the duodenum may lie over the vertebral column.

A lower crossing might seem to allow more room for the duodenum. However, the lumbar curve of the spine reaches its most anterior position at the fourth lumbar vertebra; therefore, the space between the limbs of the angle does not increase. This lumbar curvature is usually more pronounced in females than in males.

The suspensory muscle of the duodenum (ligament of Treitz) connects the right crus of the diaphragm with the duodenojejunal flexure. Variations in insertion are shown in Fig. 16-32; the type shown in Fig. 16-32A is the most common. Multiple separate divisions are not unusual; occurrences of three and four divisions have been reported.[110]

The duodenum may be pulled higher into the vascular angle if the suspensory muscle is short. Since only

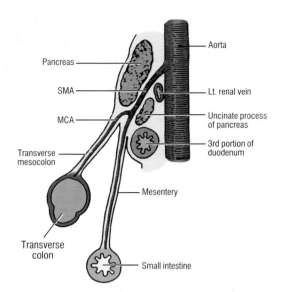

FIG. 16-39. Diagrammatic sagittal section through the neck of the pancreas showing the relation of the third portion of the duodenum to the superior mesenteric artery (SMA), middle colic artery (MCA), aorta, and mesentery. (Modified from Akin JT Jr, Gray SW, Skandalakis JE. Vascular compression of the duodenum: presentation of ten cases and review of the literature. Surgery 79(5):515-522, 1976; with permission.)

the flexure may be raised, the angulation of the fourth part is increased, while the third part remains at the usual level.

According to Cauldwell and Anson,[111] in 75 percent of individuals, the superior mesenteric artery arises from the aorta at a level between the upper one-third of the first lumbar vertebra and the disc between the first and second lumbar vertebrae. The artery frequently produces a groove on the anterior surface of the duodenum. Figure 16-39 shows the course of the superior mesenteric artery and its relations to posterior entities.

Compression is occasionally produced by the middle colic artery, which arises from the superior mesenteric artery at the inferior border of the pancreas. This branch lies in the transverse mesocolon and crosses the third part of the duodenum.

The normal angle made by the superior mesenteric artery and the aorta has been measured in cadavers by Derrick and Fadhli[112] and Byers and Mansberger, as reported by Mansberger et al.,[113] and in living patients by Hearn.[114] Of six cases reported by Hearn, five showed radiologic evidence of superior mesenteric artery compression, and the diagnosis was confirmed by surgery in four. The measurements reported in these studies are shown in Table 16-7; it is apparent that the angle is less than normal in two patients in the study by Hearn.

## Symptoms

The chief symptoms of vascular compression of the duodenum are vomiting and epigastric pain after meals. Weight loss commencing after the onset of symptoms is frequent, since the patient regurgitates food or becomes afraid to eat.[110]

## Treatment

Section or lysis of the suspensory ligament (ligament of Treitz) is the procedure of choice. Occasionally, duodenojejunostomy may be necessary.

REMEMBER: Vascular compression of the duodenum, while not rare, can be considered a matter of degree. While many individuals with marked compression are easily diagnosed, many other patients with equally real but less severe compression escape diagnosis and live in discomfort, more or less palliated by medical regimens.

### Exposures of the Duodenum

Exposure of the duodenum can be necessary in a search for traumatic injury, for pancreatic procedures, for exploration of the distal common bile duct, for section of the suspensory ligament to relieve duodenal compression, or to reduce a redundant proximal loop of a gastrojejunostomy above the transverse mesocolon.[115] The following maneuvers will provide the needed exposures:

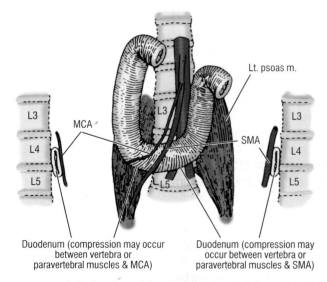

FIG. 16-40. Anterior view of the duodenum, superior mesenteric artery (SMA), middle colic artery (MCA), and vertebral column. (Modified from Akin JT Jr, Gray SW, Skandalakis JE. Vascular compression of the duodenum: presentation of ten cases and review of the literature. Surgery 79(5):515-522, 1976; with permission.)

**TABLE 16-7. Aortomesenteric angles**

| | No. | Average angle (degrees) | Range (degrees) |
|---|---|---|---|
| *Cadavers:* | | | |
| Derrick and Fadhli (1965)[a] | 64 | 41.25 | 20 to 70 |
| Mansberger et al. (1968)[b] | 31 | 30 | 18 to 60 |
| *Living subjects* [Hearn (1966)][c]: | | | |
| Normal arteriograms | 5 | 56 | 45 to 65 |
| Patients with superior mesenteric artery syndrome | 2* | 11 | 10 to 12 |

*One following body cast, one following 30 lb. weight loss (dieting).

a. Derrick JR, Fadhli HA: Surgical anatomy of the superior mesenteric artery. Am Surg 31:545, 1965.

b. Hearn JB: Duodenal ileus with special reference to superior mesenteric artery compression. Radiology 86:305, 1966.

c. Mansberger AR, Hearn JB, Byers RM, et al.: Vascular compression of the duodenum: Emphasis on accurate diagnosis. Am J Surg 115: 89, 1968.

*Source:* Akin JT, Gray SW, Skandalakis JE. Vascular compression of the duodenum: Presentation of ten cases and review of the literature. Surgery 1976; 79:515-22; with permission.

1. Mobilization of the second and proximal third portions of the duodenum is obtained by incising the parietal peritoneum along the descending duodenum (second portion), and by retracting the duodenum medially with the head of the pancreas (the "Kocher maneuver"). Madden states that this procedure should bear the name of Jourdain, who described it in 1895.[116] This maneuver permits examination of the posterior wall of the duodenum, as well as exploration of the retroduodenal and pancreatic portions of the common bile duct.

2. Exposure of the third portion of the duodenum, proximal to the superior mesenteric vessels, can be obtained by an incision through the transverse mesocolon, an incision through the gastrocolic omentum, or reflection of the right half of the colon.[117]

3. Exposure of the duodenum distal to the superior mesenteric vessels can be accomplished by incision through the gastrocolic omentum and further reflection of the right colon. In addition, division of the parietal fold just inferior to the paraduodenal fossa will permit visualization of the distal duodenum. Further mobilization of the duodenum can be obtained by transection of the ligament of Treitz.[85] In dividing the mesocolon, the surgeon must watch for the right colic, the middle colic, and the marginal vessels. The gastroepiploic arteries lie near the greater curvature of the stomach, within the gastrocolic ligament, and must also be handled appropriately.

## Surgical Notes to Remember

(See table "Anatomic Complications of Some Gastric, Duodenal, and Pancreatic Procedures" in stomach chapter).

- Duodenectomy alone is impossible because of the fixation of the head of the pancreas to the duodenal loop; pancreaticoduodenectomy is the only practical procedure. However, pancreas-sparing duodenectomy or duodenum-sparing pancreatectomy for benign diseases are new procedures currently being tried, but not used by the majority of surgeons.

- Do not ligate both the superior and the inferior pancreaticoduodenal arteries. Ligation of both can cause necrosis of the head of the pancreas and of a great part of the duodenum.

- The accessory pancreatic duct (of Santorini) passes deep to the gastrointestinal artery. For safety, ligate the artery away from the anterior medial duodenal wall where the papilla is located. Such a maneuver avoids injury to or ligation of the duct. The well-known phrase "water under the bridge" applies to the relation of the ureter and the uterine artery, as well as to the relation of the accessory pancreatic duct and the gastroduodenal artery. Keep in mind that in 10 percent[32] of cases, the duct of Santorini is the only duct draining the pancreas. Therefore, ligation of the gastroduodenal artery with accidental inclusion of the duct will be catastrophic.

- With the Kocher maneuver, the surgeon reconstructs the primitive mesoduodenum and achieves mobilization of the duodenum. This is useful for some surgical procedures.

- Do not skeletonize more than 2 cm of the first part of the duodenum. If more than 2 cm of skeletonization is done, a duodenostomy may be necessary to avoid blowout of the stump secondary to poor blood supply.

- The suspensory ligament can be transected with impunity. It should be ligated before being sectioned, so that bleeding from small vessels contained within it can be avoided. Failure to completely sever the suspensory muscle (which is possible if the insertion is multiple) will, of course, fail to relieve the symptoms of vascular compression of the duodenum (Fig. 16-41).

- With a large, penetrating, posterior duodenal or pyloric ulcer, the surgeon should remember the following:
  - The proximal duodenum shortens because of the inflammatory process (duodenal shortening)
  - The anatomic topography of the distal common bile duct, the opening of the duct of Santorini, and the ampulla of Vater are distorted
  - Leaving the ulcer in situ is a wise decision
  - The following two procedures are extremely useful:
    ▶ Careful palpation for, or visualization of, the location

of the ampulla of Vater

▶ Common bile duct exploration, with insertion of a catheter into the common bile duct and the duodenum

- Chang et al.[118] advise partial and complete circular duodenectomy as well as highly selective vagotomy for the treatment of duodenal ulcer with obstruction.
- Katkhouda et al.[119] stated that a perforated duodenal ulcer may be repaired laparoscopically.
- In the majority of cases, the common bile duct is located to the right of the gastroduodenal artery at the posterior wall of the first portion of the duodenum. In many cases, the artery crosses the supraduodenal portion of the common bile duct anteriorly or posteriorly. This phenomenon may also be observed with the posterior superior pancreaticoduodenal artery, which crosses the common bile duct ventrally, to the right, and then dorsally.
- According to Nassoura et al.,[120] the vast majority of penetrating duodenal injuries should be treated by primary repair or resection and anastomosis. Degiannis[121] recommended the addition of pyloric exclusion to the operative management of penetrating duodenal injuries.
- A retrospective study by Allen et al.[122] of 22,163 cases of blunt trauma identified 35 (0.2%) cases of blunt duodenal injury. Despite modern diagnostic techniques (CT scan, diagnostic peritoneal lavage), diagnosis was delayed (more than 6 hours) in seven (20%) of these 35. Delayed diagnosis was associated with an increase in abdominal complications.
- Chou et al.[123] concluded after reviewing 309 CT examinations that CT imaging is a reliable method for localizing the duodenojejunal junction because the inferior mesenteric vein can be clearly demonstrated. They identified the junction in 224 examinations.
- Bouvier et al.[124] stated that duodenojejunal junction tumors may be excised in a single block if the superior mesenteric artery is not involved with the tumor.

## Surgical Applications to the Jejunum and Ileum

### Diagnostic Procedures for the Jejunum and Ileum

Morphology, topography, functional problems, and pathology may be visualized by several methods, such as:
- Barium swallow
- Barium enema (if the ileocecal valve permits entrance of the barium into the terminal ileum)
- Selective superior mesenteric artery arteriography
- Phlebography

- Enteroscopy
- Tc-99m pertechnetate (nuclear scan with technetium pertechnetate)

Peck et al.[125] advised use of computed tomography for detection of the cause of intestinal obstruction and the presence of strangulation.

### Resection of the Jejunum and the Ileum

#### Pathologic Indications for Resection

Jejunal or ileal resection may be done in response to several pathologic entities of the small bowel. To name a few:
- Internal hernia, intussusception
- Intestinal obstruction secondary to Crohn's disease, mesenteric cysts, lymphangioma or other causes[126]
- Mesenteric thrombosis of arterial or venous type, with infarction (ischemia)
- Benign or malignant tumors
- Intestinal injury secondary to bleeding or penetrating abdominal trauma; traumatic perforation
- Adhesions
- Obstruction by food, foreign bodies, or gallstones
- Volvulus with bowel necrosis
- Meckel's diverticulum

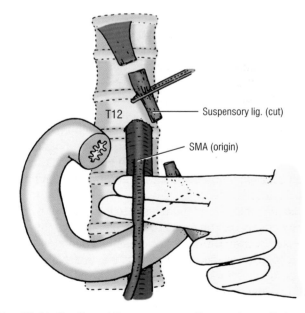

FIG. 16-41. Section of the suspensory ligament usually lowers the duodenum two fingerbreadths below the origin of the superior mesenteric artery (SMA). (Modified from Akin JT Jr., Milsap JH Jr., Gray SW, Skandalakis JE. Pictorial presentation of the vascular compression of the duodenum. III. Contemp Surg 1977;10:52-6. Used with permission.)

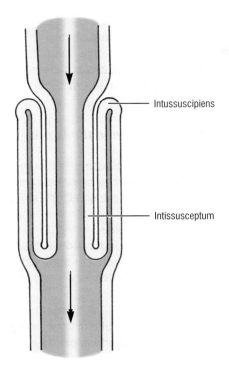

**FIG. 16-42.** Diagram of the anatomy of an intestinal intussusception. Such a formation can enlarge distally until the leading edge reaches the anus. (Modified from Skandalakis JE, Gray SW, Rowe JS Jr. Anatomical Complications in General Surgery. New York: McGraw-Hill, 1983; with permission.)

- Duplication of the intestine
- Atresias and stenoses of the intestine

Bemelman and colleagues[127] favored laparoscopic ileocolic resection for Crohn's disease over open surgery, based on early hospital discharge and improved cosmetic results.

Here we will consider only intussusception, mesenteric cysts, and mesenteric ischemia.

**INTUSSUSCEPTION.** An intussusception is created when a proximal segment of intestine (the intussusceptum) invaginates into the portion of the intestine immediately distal to it (the intussuscipiens) (Fig. 16-42). Intussusceptions are named for their location; the most frequent are ileocolic. They tend to increase in length, frequently appearing at the anus. Figure 16-43 shows the location and extent of 120 intussusceptions in infants and children.[128]

Meckel's diverticulum is the most common identifiable cause of intussusception in children. Other known causes are intestinal polyps, duplications, atresias, and tumors of the intestine, but 85 percent of our cases of intussusceptions in children could not be assigned to any cause (Fig. 16-44). A seasonal cycle, with more admissions in the spring and the summer, has been observed in children.[128]

The Centers for Disease Control and Prevention[129] in Atlanta reported preliminary findings of an increased risk of intussusception among healthy infants who were recipients of the rotavirus vaccine. Perhaps this is another etiologic factor for the genesis of intussusception.

Zapas et al.[130] presented ileocecal duplication (cyst), which was the focal point for ileocolic intussusception. The treatment was bowel resection and primary anastomosis.

Oldham and Wesley[79] presented a table (Table 16-8) of predisposing factors for the development of intussusception.

In adults, our "two-thirds rule" can be applied[131]: Two-thirds of adult intussusceptions are from known causes. Of these, two-thirds are due to neoplasms. Of those caused by neoplasms, two-thirds of the neoplasms will be malignant.

The first stage of intussusception is edema of the intussusceptum, owing to lymphatic obstruction. Venous obstruction occurs next, followed by infarction and gangrene. The final stage is necrosis and perforation. Very rarely, the intussusception sloughs, and anastomosis with the normal proximal portion produces a spontaneous cure.

Oldham and Wesley[79] stated that ultrasound examination is a very reliable tool, demonstrating intussusception as a mass, with a double lumen resembling a "bull's eye." They added that an air contrast enema or a barium enema

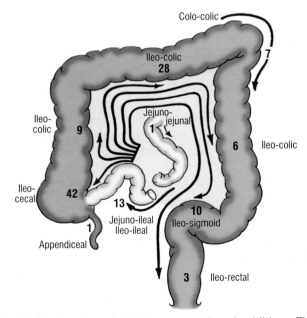

**FIG. 16-43.** Location of 120 intussusceptions in children. The head of the arrow indicates the position of the advancing head of the intussusception. (Modified from Lionakis B, Gray SW, Skandalakis JE, Akin JT Jr. Intussusception in infants and children. South Med J 1960:53:1226; with permission.)

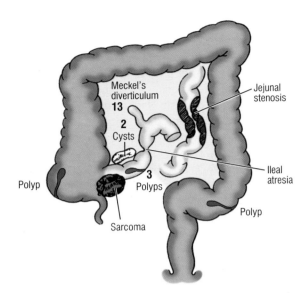

FIG. 16-44. Cause of intussusception in 23 cases, 14.5% of total cases. The remaining 136 cases had no evident anatomic cause. (Modified from Lionakis B, Gray SW, Skandalakis JE, Akin JT Jr. Intussusception in infants and children. South Med J 1960: 53:1226; with permission.)

serves both diagnostic and therapeutic purposes.

As previously noted, reduction of the intussusception can be spontaneous, or it may be achieved by a barium enema, an air enema, or with operation. With operation, reduction can be attempted, or resection with anastomosis of the healthy ends may be necessary. We believe that reduction by enema should be attempted in children. Wang et al.[132] reported that pneumatic reduction, with air and fluoroscopic guidance, afforded them a 97 percent success rate for reduction without surgery.

If the reduction is successful, the patient should be watched for 48 hours for possible recurrence. If the enema is unsuccessful or the intussusception recurs, operation should be undertaken at once. For children, we recommend reduction with resection if necessary; for adults, we recommend resection without reduction.

**MESENTERIC CYSTS.** Mesenteric cysts are fluid-filled chambers lined by cuboidal or columnar epithelium or without lining. No smooth muscle is present. Blood vessels infrequently adhere to the wall of the cyst.[133] The fluid inside may be clear if located in the mesentery of the distal small bowel or colon, or chylous if in the mesentery of the proximal small bowel.[133] Baird et al.[134] presented a case of mesenteric cyst containing milk of calcium.

Mesenteric cysts are uncommon. Since 1507, only 820 cases of mesenteric cysts have been reported.[135] From 1900 to 1926 at the Massachusetts General Hospital only six cases of mesenteric cyst were recorded.[136] There were only seven cases at the Mayo Clinic in more than one million patients.[137] At Saint Joseph's Infirmary, Atlanta, Skandalakis[138] found only two cases of mesenteric cyst in 67,000 admissions between 1922 and 1955. Mesenteric cysts occur in about 1 in 100,000 general hospital admissions and in 1 in 4000 to 34,000 pediatric admissions.[133]

Mesenteric cysts may be malignant or benign. They may be unilocular or multilocular, single or multiple.[139] The home of mesenteric cysts in most cases is the mesentery of the small bowel (60%) or of the colon (40%)[140] (Fig. 16-45). Mourad et al.[141] presented a cyst localized in the hepatogastric mesentery and made reference to two similar cases from the literature. Chung et al.[142] reported on several cysts located in the mesentery of the small bowel (5 cases), the base of the mesentery with retroperitoneal extension (4 cases), transverse mesocolon (4 cases), and gastrocolic ligament (2 cases).

Confusion exists in the literature regarding mesenteric, omental, and retroperitoneal masses; between benign or malignant cystic neoplasms and cysts; and between solid and cystic neoplasms. We do not propose to resolve this issue, other than to point out that benign mesenteric cystic neoplasms and mesenteric cysts are usually assumed to be terms referring to the same pathologic entities, and we do not disagree with that view. For a more detailed presentation of the classification of mesenteric cysts, see Table 16-9.

The incidence may be highest in the fourth decade of life and lowest in the first and sixth.[143] Takiff et al.[144] stated that cysts are more common in middle-aged adults and

| TABLE 16-8. Predisposing Factors to the Development of Intussusception | |
|---|---|
| **Anatomic Lead Points** | **Bleeding Disorders*** |
| Meckel's diverticulum | Henoch-Schönlein purpura |
| Polyp | Hemophilia |
| Hypertrophied Peyer patch | Leukemia |
| Appendix | **Trauma*** |
| Duplication or enteric cyst | Blunt abdominal trauma |
| Lymphoma | Major retroperitoneal operative |
| Other neoplasm | procedures |
| Ectopic pancreas | **Other** |
| **Associated Infections** | Cystic fibrosis |
| Adenovirus | |
| Rotavirus | |
| Others | |

*These factors are more likely to be associated with small bowel-to-small bowel intussusception than with ileocolic intussusception.

*Source:* Oldham KT, Coran AG, Wesley JR. Pediatric abdomen. In: Greenfield LJ, ed. Surgery: Scientific Principles and Practice, 2nd Ed. Philadelphia: Lippincot-Raven, 1997; with permission.

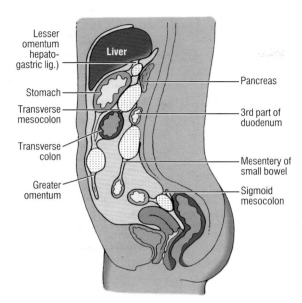

Fig. 16-45. Topographic anatomy showing 5 omental and mesenteric cysts *(dotted)*. (Modified from Skandalakis JE, Gray SW [eds]. Embryology for Surgeons, 2nd Ed. Baltimore: Williams & Wilkins, 1994; with permission.)

more common in women. However, they may occur in either sex and at any age. There is a case in the literature of a cyst in a neonate[142] and one in a 72 year old.[138]

Cystic tumors of the mesentery are rare. They are typically benign. Cystic lymphangiomas are the most common type of benign tumor and are lined by endothelium. Their gross structure is often indistinguishable from that of mesenteric cysts. Knol and Eckhauser[133] stated that despite the fact that the incidence of malignant change is low the cystic wall should be examined for "rough, friable, papillary projections that suggest malignancy."

How these cysts arise is a matter of speculation. Orobitg et al.[145] reported a case of mesenteric cyst of lymphatic origin. Lee et al.[146] presented a cyst of mullerian origin that was located between the liver and right adnexa. Mullerian cysts of the mesentery and retroperitoneum are extremely rare and may be of urogenital origin.

Some published hypotheses (Table 16-10) suggest that mesenteric cysts may arise from degeneration of lymph nodes,[147,148] or result from congenital malformation of lymphatic vessels,[149] developmental anomalies,[137] and trauma.[150] Guthrie and Wakefield[151] suggested that mesenteric cysts originate from true diverticula of the small intestine that grow into the mesentery and become pinched off. Gross and Ladd[152] described mesenteric cysts as "[m]isplaced bits of lymphatic tissue which proliferate and ...accumulate fluid because they do not possess communications which allow them to drain properly into the re-

mainder of the lymphatic system." Beahrs et al.[153] stated: "It is felt that chylous cysts do not have a common mode of origin but may come from several sources."

The severity of symptoms correlates with cyst size.[133] Cysts may be asymptomatic or may present with abdominal pain, fever, vomitting, diarrhea or constipation, ascites, and abdominal mass. Mohanty et al.[154] described a case of mesenteric cyst that presented as an inguinal hernia, and these authors found four more such cases from the English literature. Chung et al.[142] reported that several

---

### TABLE 16-9. Classification

I. Embryonal cysts
   A. Arising from embryonic remnants and sequestrated tissue
      1. Serous
      2. Chylous
      3. Sanguineous
      4. Dermoid
   B. Arising by sequestration from the bowel
      1. Including Meckel's diverticulum
   C. Of urogenital origin
II. Pseudocysts
   A. Of infective origin
      1. Hydatids
      2. Cystic degeneration of tuberculous nodes
   B. Cystic malignant disease
III. Embryonic and developmental cysts
   A. Enteric
   B. Urogenital
   C. Lymphoid
   D. Dermoid
   E. Embryonic defects in early formation of lymphatic vessels, lymph nodes, etc.
IV. Traumatic or acquired cysts (cyst wall composed of fibrous tissue without a lining membrane)
   A. Those caused by injury
      1. Hemorrhage causing sanguineous cysts
      2. Rupture of lacteals
      3. Extravasation of chyle into surrounding tissue
V. Neoplastic cysts
   A. Benign cysts
      1. Hyperplastic lymph of vessels resolving in lymphangiomata
   B. Malignant cysts
      1. Lymphangioendothelioma
VI. Infective and degenerative cysts
   A. Mycotic
   B. Parasitic
   C. Tuberculous
   D. Cystic degeneration of lymph nodes and other tissue

Classification from Caropreso P. Mesenteric cysts: a review. Arch Surg 1974; 108:242-246. After Ford JR. Mesenteric cyst: review of the literature with report of an unusual case. Am J Surg 1960;99:878-883; with permission.

cases presented as appendicitis. Namasivayam et al.[155] reported on a mesenteric cyst producing volvulus of the proximal small bowel.

Ultrasonography,[156] and CT and MR imaging, together with history and physical examination, is used to diagnose mesenteric cysts.[133]

Treatment is surgical: (1) resection and primary anastomosis, if the cyst is unduly adherent to the intestine, (2) dissection and enucleation, or (3) marsupialization. The treatment of choice is dissection and enucleation; if this is not possible, resection with anastomosis of the remaining ends may be done. Tuttle et al.[157] advised simple enucleation as the treatment of choice for all types of mesenteric cysts.

The first step is to study the cyst through the open abdomen and to make the differential diagnosis between a true mesenteric cyst and an enteric cyst. Then one must try to locate and displace all the important vessels of the mesentery. If this can be done, the dissection is easy. If this is not possible we must think of resection. We cannot agree with Parsons[158] that marsupialization is an obsolete procedure. When indicated, it is a necessary evil and "the way of necessity."

In summarizing the operative aspects of mesenteric cysts, one should emphasize the following:
- Always have in mind the blood supply of the intestine
- Carefully close the opened mesentery
- Avoid rough or ragged areas on bowel or mesentery
    Several reports[159-161] indicate that laparoscopic surgery for mesenteric cysts can be successful.

**MESENTERIC ISCHEMIA.** Mesenteric ischemia, the acute type, is a real surgical emergency. Divino et al.[162] urged that aggressive treatment be immediately instituted when mesenteric vein thrombosis is suspected. We quote Skandalakis et al.[163]:

> Mesenteric venous thrombosis appears to be a distinct clinical entity among the group of conditions generally referred to as mesenteric vascular occlusions. In contrast to catastrophic arterial occlusions, mesenteric venous thrombosis follows a different course. The latter is much nore amenable to surgery, and because of the more insidious onset of symptoms, earlier recognition of this entity offers an opportunity for early and adequate treatment in a large percentage of cases.

According to Hassan and Raufman,[164] the following eight conditions are associated with mesenteric venous thrombosis:
- previous abdominal surgery
- blunt abdominal trauma
- hypercoagulable states

- oral contraceptive use
- inflammation
- portal hypertension
- decompression disease, sickle-cell anemia, hypoperfusion syndrome
- paroxysmal nocturnal hemoglobulinuria, volvulus, intussusception

Hassan and Raufman found that previous abdominal surgery and hypercoagulable states are the most common of the above conditions. Gewertz,[165] in an invited critique of the paper of Mansour,[166] wisely stated the following:

> The morbidity and mortality of acute mesenteric ischemia has remained high despite heightened sensitivity to the diagnosis. Since the duration of the ischemic episode is the most important determinant of outcome, an aggressive diagnostic and treatment protocol must be maintained. While this stance may precipitate many negative angiographic studies, such an approach is the only opportunity to save in these critically ill patients.

### Non-Pathologic Reasons for Resection
Intestinal resection can be performed for inherent dis-

**TABLE 16-10. Theories on the Etiology of Mesenteric Cysts**

| Name | Theory |
|---|---|
| Rokitansky | Degeneration of lymph nodes |
| Carson | Degeneration of lymph nodes |
| Hill | Congenital malformation of the lymphatic vessels |
| Godel | Neoplasia in the presence of lymph vessel hyperplasia |
| Handfield-Jones | Developmental anomalies |
| Arzella | Developmental anomalies |
| Lee | Traumatic origin |
| Ewing | Traumatic origin |
| Guthrie-Wakefield | Embryologic origin from true diverticula of the small intestine which grew into the mesentery and became pinched off |
| Gross-Ladd | "Misplaced bits of lymphatic tissue which proliferate and they accumulate fluid because they do not possess communications which allow them to drain properly into the remainder of the lymphatic system" |
| Beahrs et al. | "It is felt that chylous cysts do not have a common mode of origin but may come from several sources" |

*Source:* Skandalakis JE. Mesenteric cyst: a report of three cases. J Med Assoc Ga 44(2):75-80, 1955; with permission.

ease of the segment resected, or to obtain a normal segment for use elsewhere in the body. Healthy intestinal segments have been used in the gastrointestinal tract in the following ways, both in experimental animals[167] and in human patients:[168,169]

- as jejunal loops for stomach reconstruction
- as intestinal transplant for chronic short gut syndrome following surgical intervention for necrotizing enterocolitis[170]
- as graft material for treatment of desmoid tumors in patients with familial adenomatous polyposis[171]
- as intestinal loops for esophageal reconstruction
- as segments of intestine for biliary tract surgery
- as surgical treatment of postgastrectomy syndrome
- as mucosal grafts of jejunum for large duodenal defects[172]

Similar use of the intestine has been successful in such urologic procedures as:
- Ileal graft to enlarge the bladder
- Ileal loop to reimplant a ureter into the bladder
- Ureteroileosigmoidostomy
- Ileal pouch formation and ileoanal anastomosis

In addition, the small intestine has been used for:
- Vaginal reconstruction
- Reinforcement of vascular grafts
- Revascularization of the breast
- Strictureplasty for obstructing small bowel Crohn's disease[173]

Some of these techniques have been abandoned, but several are still being used today very successfully. Few organs are more easily exposed and mobilized than are loops of small intestine. Size reductions of adult cadaveric small bowels can provide suitable grafts for pediatric transplantation.[174] Adhesions from previous surgery are the chief obstacles to good mobilization.

# ANATOMIC COMPLICATIONS OF INTESTINAL RESECTION

Dhar and Kirsner[175] reported the possible consequences of ileal resection as follows:
- Diarrhea and steatorrhea
- Bacterial overgrowth
- Nutritional deficiencies
- Cholelithiasis
- Hyperoxaluria and nephrolithiasis
- Gastric hypersecretion

## Vascular Injury

Table 16-11 summarizes some of the anatomic complications of resection. The most serious vascular injury by far in resecting the small intestine is that to the superior mesenteric artery. This must be repaired at once. Injury to the mesentery and one or more of the intestinal arteries will require ligation. It will also increase the length of a devitalized segment of intestine and hence, the length of the resection needed.

Any line of resection must be placed where it minimizes injury to the blood supply. Clamps should be placed such that there is at least 1 cm free on either side of the line of transection. Preserve as many vascular arches and vasa recta as possible (Fig. 16-46).

Hematomas at the anastomotic site will cause ischemia, necrosis, and perforation. Hematomas are most common at the junction of the mesentery with the anastomotic site. Here, mesenteric vessels can be occluded, producing local ischemia.

## Organ Injury

The only organ at risk, of course, should be the intestine being resected. The abdominal cavity should be well packed before any enterotomy or enterostomy to avoid contamination and future infection with resulting intraperitoneal or abdominal wall abscesses. The surgeon must exercise judgment as to how much intestine is to be resected. There is no excuse for resecting too little; if in doubt, the surgeon should remove the segment in question.

Leakage at the suture line is the result of poor technique and will be followed by a fistula or general peritonitis. The possibility of leakage can be reduced by careful closure of the mesentery at the suture line to avoid damaging blood vessels, use of a nasogastric tube to avoid distention, and avoidance of tension on the anastomosis.

An inadequate stoma will result in stasis of intestinal contents, and possible obstruction. A slightly oblique line of resection will help enlarge the anastomotic opening and will preserve the blood supply to the antimesenteric border. The proper angle is shown in Fig. 16-47. Surgeons must use their judgment in cutting adhesions. They should ligate both distal and proximal ends of adhesion bands to prevent possible bleeding. Simple adhesions are usually avascular; no ligation is needed.

**TABLE 16-11. Summary of Anatomic Complications of Small Intestine Resections**

| Procedure | Vascular Injury | Organ Injury | Inadequate Procedure |
|---|---|---|---|
| Intestinal resection | Ischemia at antimesenteric border from injury to vasa recta, at mesenteric border from hematoma at junction of mesentery and anastomotic site, from injury to intestinal arteries and arcades supplying intestinal segment to be preserved | Peritoneal soiling, adhesions from raw surfaces, tension on anastomosis | Too short a segment resected, leakage of anastomosis at suture line, inadequate stoma, failure to look for possible additional distal obstructions, side-to-side anastomosis with long stump of proximal limb |

*Source:* Skandalakis JE, Gray SW, Rowe JS Jr. Anatomical Complications in General Surgery. New York: McGraw-Hill, 1983; with permission.

Surgeons should make every effort to avoid producing raw surfaces during dissection. In very rare cases, raw surfaces should be repaired with 3-0 Vicryl. But the pathobiology of adhesion formation is foreign-body reaction, and sutures serve as the nidus for such reactions. An end-to-end anastomosis is the preferred method for intestinal resection. If a side-to-side anastomosis is to be used, the opening should be carried as close to the blind ends as possible to avoid blowout of the stumps or the blind stump syndrome (Fig. 16-47).

Tension and torsion at the anastomosis must be avoided. The surgeon must be sure that any tension or torsion has not been merely transferred to a more distal or prox-imal site. The resection of an intestinal obstruction does not preclude the presence of another obstruction distal to the anastomosis. This is of great importance in surgery for intestinal atresias in infancy.[152]

Complications related to needle catheter jejunostomy were studied by Myers et al.[176] These complications are detailed in Table 16-12. North and Nava[177] report that it is possible to introduce air into the portal vein during a needle catheter jejunostomy.

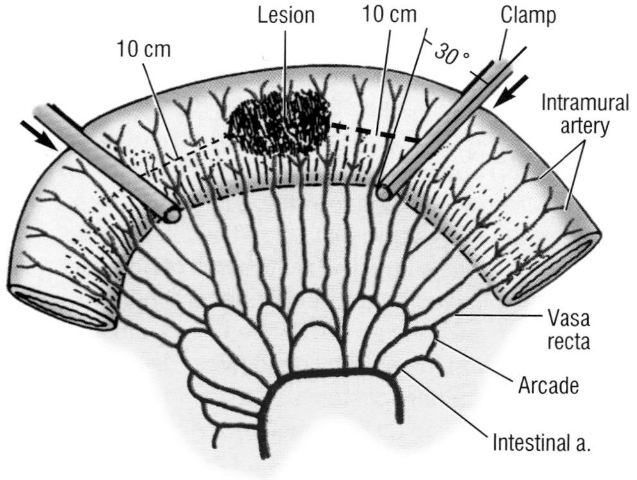

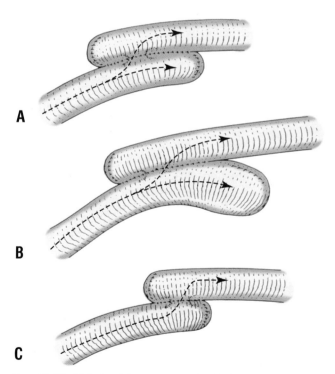

FIG. 16-46. Recommended position of noncrushing clamps for segmental resection of intestine. The 30° angle from a vertical transection preserves as much of the antimesenteric blood supply as possible *(arrows)* and slightly increases the functional diameter of the anastomosis. (Modified from Skandalakis JE, Skandalakis PN, Skandalakis LJ. Surgical Anatomy and Technique: A Pocket Manual, 2nd Ed. New York: Springer, 2000; with permission.)

FIG. 16-47. Side-to-side anastomosis. **A.** Stoma too proximal. **B.** Dilated stump of proximal loop resulting in the blind stump syndrome. **C.** Proper location of the stoma at the distal end of proximal loop. (Modified from Skandalakis JE, Gray SW, Rowe JS Jr. Anatomical Complications in General Surgery. New York: McGraw-Hill, 1983; with permission.)

**TABLE 16-12. Complications Related to Needle Catheter Jejunostomy in 2022 Consecutive Applications**

| Category | Complication | Reoperation | Death | Avoidable Complication | Avoidable Reoperation |
|---|---|---|---|---|---|
| Abdominal wall infection | 3 | 3 | 0 | 2 | 2 |
| Bowel necrosis | 3 | 3 | 2 | 2 | 2 |
| Pneumatosis intestinalis | 3 | 2 | 0 | 0 | 0 |
| Bowel obstruction | 3 | 3 | 1 | 1 | 1 |
| Fistula | 1 | 0 | 0 | 0 | 0 |
| Intra-abdominal infection | 3 | 3 | 0 | 1 | 1 |
| Central line sepsis | 1 | 0 | 0 | 1 | 0 |
| Subcutaneous abscess | 2 | 0 | 0 | 0 | 0 |
| Dislodgment | 10 | 3 | 0 | 10 | 4 |
| Occlusion | 5 | 1 | 0 | 5 | 2 |
| Total | 34 | 18 | 3 | 22 | 10* |

*Two repeat operations involved 2 complications.

*Source:* Myers JG, Page CP, Stewart RM, Schwesinger WH, Sirinek KR, Aust JB. Complications of needle catheter jejunostomy in 2,022 consecutive applications. Am J Surg 1995;170:547-551; with permission.

Nussbaumer et al.[178] reported traumatic perforation of the small bowel as the rare complication of inguinal hernia.

# REFERENCES

1. Billings J. Josh Billings: hiz sayings, with comic illustrations. New York: Carleton, 1865, chapter 29.

2. Androulakis J, Colborn GL, Skandalakis PN, Skandalakis LJ, Skandalakis JE. Embryologic and anatomic basis of duodenal surgery. Surg Clin North Am 80(1):171-199, 2000.

3. O'Rahilly R, Müller F. Human Embryology & Teratology, 2nd ed. New York: Wiley-Liss, 1996, p. 229.

4. Burrington JD, Wayne ER. Obstruction of the duodenum by the superior mesenteric artery - does it exist in children? J Pediatr Surg 1974;9:733.

5. Moutsouris C. The "solid stage" and congenital intestinal atresia. J Pediatr Surg 1966;1:446.

6. Bremer JL. Diverticula and duplications of the intestinal tract. Arch Pathol 1944;38:133-140.

7. Bremer JL. Congenital Anomalies of Viscera. Cambridge MA: Harvard University Press, 1957.

8. Estrada RL. Anomalies of Intestinal Rotation and Fixation. Springfield IL: Thomas, 1958.

9. Skandalakis JE, Gray SW. Embryology for Surgeons. 2nd ed. Baltimore: Williams & Wilkins, 1994.

10. Slovis TL, Klein MD, Watts FB Jr. Incomplete rotation of the intestine with a normal cecal position. Surgery 1980;87:325-30.

11. Nagakawa T. Histogenetic and cytological studies on the duodenal mucous membrane in human foetuses. Arch Histol 1959;16:495.

12. Hudson CN. Congenital diaphragm of the duodenum causing intestinal obstruction in an adult. Br J Surg 1961;49:234.

13. Ladd AP, Madura JA. Congenital duodenal anomalies in the adult. Arch Surg 2001;136:576-584.

14. Vecchia LKD, Grosfeld JL, West KW, Rescorla FJ, Scherer LR, Engum SA. Intestinal atresia and stenosis. A 25-year experience with 277 cases. Arch Surg 133:490-496, 1998.

15. Loire J, Gouillat C, Partensky C. [Megaduodenum in chronic intestinal pseudo-obstruction: management by duodenectomy-duodenoplasty]. Gastroenterol Clin Biol 2000;24:21-25.

16. Neill SA, Thompson NW. The complications of duodenal diverticula and their management. Surg Gynecol Obstet 1965;120: 1251-1258.

17. Vassilakis JS, Tzovaras G, Chrysos E, Mouzas I, Manousos O, Xynos E. Roux-Y choledochojejunostomy and duodenojejunostomy for the complicated duodenal diverticulum. Am J Surg 1997;174:45-48.

18. Chiu EJ, Shyr YM, Su CH, Wu CW, Lui WY. Diverticular disease of the small bowel. Hepatogastroenterology 2000;47:181-184.

19. Matsumoto Y, Komatsu K, Tabata T. Jejuno-ileal atresia in identical twins: report of a case. Surg Today 2000;438-440.

20. Jay GD III, Margulis RR, McGraw AB, Northrip RR. Meckel's diverticulum: A survey of one hundred and three cases. Arch Surg 1950;61:158.

21. Sorokin SP, Padykula HA. Differentiation of the rat's yolk sac in organ culture. Amer J Anat 1964;114:457.

22. Werner AM, Zunzunegui RG, Williams JT, White JJ, Solis MM. Complications of Meckel's diverticulum: Case reports and literature review. Contemp Surg 1998;53:382-85.

23. de Lange DW, Cluysenaer OJ, Verberne GH, van de Wiel A. [Diverticulosis of the small bowel]. Neder Tijd Geneeskunde 2000; 144:946-949.

24. Dowdy GS Jr. The Biliary Tract. Philadelphia: Lea & Febiger, 1969, p. 174.

25. Michels NA. Blood Supply and Anatomy of the Upper Abdominal Organs. Philadelphia: JB Lippincott, 1955.

26. Reinhoff WF Jr, Pickrell KL. Pancreatitis: An anatomic study of pancreatic and extrahepatic biliary systems. Arch Surg 1945;51: 205.

27. Dardinski VJ. The anatomy of the major duodenal papilla of man, with special reference to its musculature. J Anat 1935;69:469.

28. Schwegle RA Jr, Boyden EA. The development of the pars intestinalis of the common bile duct in the human fetus, with special reference to the origin of the ampulla of Vater and the sphincter of

Oddi. Anat Rec 1937;67:441.

29. Jones SA. Sphincteroplasty (not sphincterotomy) in the treatment of biliary tract disease. Surg Clin North Am 1973;28:1123.

30. Glisson F. Anatomia Hepatis (2nd ed). London: Hagae, 1654.

31. Boyden EA. The pars intestinalis of the common bile duct, as viewed by the older anatomists (Vesalius, Glisson, Bianchi, Vater, Haller, Santorini, etc.). Anat Rec 1936;66:217.

32. Silen W. Surgical anatomy of the pancreas. Surg Clin North Am 44:1253, 1964.

33. DiDio LJA, Anderson MC. The "Sphincters" of the Digestive System. Baltimore: Williams & Wilkins, 1968.

34. Villemin F. A propos de la limite inférieure du duodénum chez l'homme adulte. Le rétrécissement et la valvule duodénojéjunaux: leur signification anatomique. 17th Internat Congress of Med, London, August 12, 1913, Section Anat Embryol 1914;2: 131-5.

35. Villemin F. Recherches d'anatomie comparée sur le duodénum de l'homme et des mammiferes. Sa signification morphologique et functionnelle. Arch Morphol Génél Exp 1922;3:1-142.

36. Ochsner AJ. Constriction of the duodenum below the entrance of the common duct and its relation to disease. Ann Surg 1906;43: 80-88.

37. Boothby WM. The so-called "Ochsner muscle" of the duodenum. Boston Med Surg J 1907;157:80-81.

38. Monti A. Antonio Scarpa. Loria FL (trans). New York: Vigo Press, 1957.

39. Griffith CA. Anatomy. In: Nyhus LM, Wastell C (eds). Surgery of the Stomach and Duodenum (4th ed). Boston: Little, Brown and Company, 1986, p. 74.

40. Akkinis AJ. (No title given as cited in McGregor AL, Du Plessis DJ. A Synopsis of Surgical Anatomy, 10th ed. Baltimore: Williams & Wilkins, 1969.) J Anat (Paris) 1930;64:200.

41. International Anatomical Nomenclature Committee. Nomina Anatomica (6th ed). Edinburgh: Churchill Livingstone, 1989.

42. Hentati N, Fournier HD, Papon X, Aube Ch, Vialle R, Mercier Ph. Arterial supply of the duodenal bulb: an anatomoclinical study. Surg Radiol Anat 1999;21:159-64.

43. Mayo WJ. The contributions of surgery to a better understanding of gastric and duodenal ulcer. Ann Surg 1907;45:810.

44. Bartels P. Uber die Lymphage faesse des Pankreas, III. Die regionaeren Drusen des Pankreas beim Menschen. Archiv Anat Entwicklungsgesch 1907;35:267.

45. Wood JD. Physiology of the enteric nervous system. In: Johnson LR (ed). Physiology of the Gastrointestinal Tract. New York: Raven Press, 1987.

46. Skandalakis JE, Gray SW, Soria RE, Sorg JL, Rowe JS. Distribution of the vagus nerve to the stomach. Am Surg 1980;46:130-139.

47. Skandalakis JE, Rowe JS, Gray SW, Androulakis JA. Identification of vagal structures at the esophageal hiatus. Surgery 1974;75:233-237.

48. Skandalakis LJ, Donahue PE, Skandalakis JE. The vagus nerve and its vagaries. Surg Clin North Am 1993;73:769-784.

49. Warwick R, Williams PL (eds). Gray's Anatomy (35th British ed). Philadelphia: WB Saunders, 1973.

50. Ross RK, Hartnett NM, Bernstein L. Epidemiology of adenocarcinoma of small intestine: Is bile a small bowel carcinogen? Br J Cancer 1991;63:143.

51. Schier J. Diagnostic and therapeutic aspects of tumors of the small bowel. Int Surg 1972;57:789.

52. Touloukian RF, Smith GJW. Normal intestinal length in preterm infants. J Pediatr Surg 1983;18:720.

53. Bryant J. Observations upon the growth and length of the human intestine. Am J Med Sci 1924;167:499.

54. Reis van der V, Schembra FW. Länge und Lage des Verdauungsrohres beim Lebenden. Z Ges Exp Med 1924;43:94.

55. Blankenhorn DH, Hirsch J, Ahrens EH Jr. Transintestinal intubation: Technique for measurement of gut length and physiologic sampling at known loci. Proc Soc Exp Biol Med 1955;88: 356.

56. Backman L, Hallberg D. Small-intestinal length. Acta Chir Scand 1974;140:57.

57. Nightingale JM, Lennard-Jones JE. Adult patients with a short bowel due to Crohn's disease often start with a short normal bowel. Eur J Gastroenterol Hepatol 1995;7:989-991.

58. Nordgren S, McPheeters G, Svaninger G, Oresland T, Hulten L. Small bowel length in inflammatory bowel disease. Int J Colorectal Dis 1997;12:230-234.

59. Flint JM. The effect of extensive resections of the small intestine. Johns Hopkins Hosp Bull 1912;23:127.

60. Weser E. Management of patients after small bowel resection. Gastroenterology 1976;71:146.

61. Weser E. Nutritional aspects of malabsorption: Short gut syndrome. Am J Med 1979;67:1014.

62. Winawer SJ, Zamchek N. Pathophysiology of small intestinal resection in man. In: Glass GBJ (ed). Progress in Gastroenterology, Vol. 1. New York: Grune and Stratton, 1968, p. 339.

63. Wilmore DW. Factors correlating with a successful outcome following extensive intestinal resection in newborn infants. J Pediatr 1972;80:88.

64. Thompson JS. Surgical aspects of the short-bowel syndrome. Am J Surg 1995;170:532-536.

65. Thompson JS. Inflammatory disease and outcome of short bowel syndrome. Am J Surg 2000;180:551-555.

66. Dyke VR, Vinocur CD. Pneumatosis cystoides intestinalis in children. Contemp Surg 2001;57:83-86.

67. Michels NA, Siddharth P, Kornblith PL, Parke WW. The variant blood supply to the small and large intestines: Its import in regional resections. J Int Coll Surg 1963;39:127.

68. Noer RJ, Derr JW, Johnston CG. The circulation of the small intestine: An evaluation of its revascularizing potential. Ann Surg 1949;130:608.

69. Shackleford RT. Surgery of the Alimentary Tract. Philadelphia: WB Saunders, 1955.

70. Vaez-Zadeh K, Dutz W. Ileosigmoid knotting. Ann Surg 1970: 172:1027.

71. Skandalakis JE, Gray SW, Harlaftis M, Collier HS. Hernia into the fossa of Waldeyer: Three cases of right paraduodenal hernia with emphasis on surgical anatomy. In Honour of Thomas Doxiadis. Athens, Greece: Hospital Evangelismos, 1976.

72. Wong J. Small-intestinal interpositions for esophageal replacement. In: Nelson RL, Nyhus LM (eds). Surgery of the Small Intestine. Norwalk, CT: Appleton & Lange, 1987.

73. Wind P, Chevallier JM, Sauvanet A, Delmas V, Cugnenc L. Anatomic basis of mesenteric elongation for ileo-anal anastomosis with J-shaped reservoir: comparison of two techniques of vascular section. Surg Radiol Anat 1996;18:11-16.

74. Rosenberg JC, DiDio LJA. Anatomic and clinical aspects of the junction of the ileum with the large intestine. Dis Colon Rectum 1970;13:220.

75. Ulin AW, Shoemaker WC, Deutsch J. The ileocecal valve and papilla. Arch Intern Med 1956;97:409.

76. Benson CD. Discussion. McRoberts JW. Meckel's diverticulum. Arch Surg 1948;56:718.

77. Stewart JH, Storey CF. Meckel's diverticulum: A study of 141 cases. South Med J 1962;55:16.

78. Androulakis JA, Gray SW, Lionakis B, Skandalakis JE. The sex ratio of Meckel's diverticulum. Am Surg 1969;35:455.

79. Oldham KT, Wesley JR. The pediatric abdomen. In: Greenfield LJ (ed). Surgery: Scientific Principles and Practice. Philadelphia: JB Lippincott, 1993, pp. 1832-82.

80. Lichtstein DM, Herskowitz B. Massive gastrointestinal bleeding from Meckel's diverticulum in a 91-year-old man. South Med J 1998;91:753-54.

81. Lin PH, Koffron AJ, Heilizer TJ, Theodoropoulus P, Pasikhov D, Lujan HJ. Gastric adenocarcinoma of Meckel's diverticulum as a cause of colonic obstruction. Am Surg 2000;66:627-630.

82. Singhabhandhu B, Gray SW, Krieger H, Gerstmann KE, Skandalakis JE. Carcinoid tumor of Meckel's diverticulum: Report of a case and review of literature. J Med Assoc Ga 1973;62:84-9.

83. Yahchouchy EK, Marano AF, Etienne JCF, Fingerhut AL. Meckel's diverticulum. J Am Coll Surg 2001;192:658-661.

84. Torgerson J. Muscular build and movements of stomach and duodenal bulb: especially with regard to problem of segmental divisions of stomach in light of comparative anatomy and embryology. Acta Radiol 1942;45(Suppl):1.

85. Cocke WM, Meyer KK. Retroperitoneal duodenal rupture. Proposed mechanism, review of literature and report of a case. Am J Surg 1964;108:834.

86. Nemeth L, Fourcade L, Puri P. Marked morphological differences in the myenteric plexus between the mesenteric and antimesenteric sides of small bowel in premature infants. J Ped Surg 2000;35:748-752.

87. Burket WC (ed). Surgical Papers by William Stewart Halsted, vol 1. Baltimore: John Hopkins Press, 1952.

88. Burket WC. The surgical significance of the anatomical layers of the gastro-intestinal tract. J Int Coll Surg 1944;7:462.

89. Lord MG, Broughton AC, Williams HTG. A morphologic study on the effect of suturing the submucosa of the large intestine. Surg Gynecol Obstet 1978;146:211.

90. Poth EJ, Gold D. Intestinal anastomosis — A unique technic. Am J Surg 1968;116:643.

91. Trimpi HD, Khubchandani IT, Sheets JA, Stasik JJ Jr. Advances in intestinal anastomosis: Experimental study and an analysis of 984 patients. Dis Colon Rectum 1977;20:107.

92. Guyton AC. Textbook of Medical Physiology (7th ed). Philadelphia: WB Saunders, 1986.

93. Koltun WA, Pappas TN. Anatomy and physiology of the small intestine. In: Greenfield LJ (ed). Surgery: Scientific Principles and Practice. Philadelphia: JB Lippincott, 1993.

94. Townsend CM Jr, Beauchamp RD, Singh P, Thompson JC. Growth factors and intestinal neoplasms. Am J Surg 1988;155: 526-536.

95. Sarr MG. Small intestinal neoplasms. In: Greenfield LJ (ed). Surgery: Scientific Principles and Practice. Philadelphia: JB Lippincott, 1993.

96. Blanchard DK, Budde JM, Hatch GF III, Wertheimer-Hatch L, Hatch KF, Davis GB, Foster RS Jr, Skandalakis JE. Tumors of the small intestine. World J Surg 24:421-429, 2000

97. Skandalakis JE, Gray SW, Skandalakis LJ. Metastasis of malignant smooth muscle tumors of the gastrointestinal tract: Pattern and process. J Med Assoc Ga 1991;80:701-709.

98. Wängberg B, Westberg G, Tylén U, Tisell L-E, Jansson S, Nilsson O, Johansson V, Scherstén T, Ahlman H. Survival of patients with disseminated midgut carcinoid tumors after aggressive tumor reduction. World J Surg 1996;20:892.

99. Farley DR. Invited Commentary. In: Wängberg B, Westberg G, Tylén U, Tisell L-E, Jansson S, Nilsson O, Johansson V, Scherstén T, Ahlman H. Survival of patients with disseminated midgut carcinoid tumors after aggressive tumor reduction. World J Surg 1996;20:892.

100. Kirshbom PM, Kherani AR, Onaitis MW, Feldman JM, Tyler DS. Carcinoids of unknown origin: comparative analysis with foregut, midgut, and hindgut carcinoids. Surgery 1998;124:1063-70.

101. Rose DM, Hochwald SN, Klimstra DS, Brennan MF. Primary duodenal adenocarcinoma: a ten-year experience with 79 patients. J Am Coll Surg 1996;183:89-96.

102. Lillemoe KD. Primary duodenal adenocarcinoma: role for aggressive resection. (Editorial). J Am Coll Surg 1996;183:155-156.

103. Farnell MB, Sakorafas GH, Sarr MG, Rowland CM, Tsiotos GG, Farley DR, Nagorney DM. Villous tumors of the duodenum: reappraisal of local vs. extended resection. J Gastrointest Surg 2000;4:13-21.

104. Edwards MJ, Nakagawa K, McMasters KM. En bloc pancreaticoduodenectomy and colectomy for duodenal neoplasms. South Med J 1997;90:733-735.

105. Turnage RH. Acute gastrointestinal hemorrhage. In Greenfield LJ, ed. Surgery: Scientific Principles and Practice, 2nd Ed. Philadelphia: Lippincott-Raven, 1997, p. 1164.

106. Rokitansky C. Lehrbuch der pathologischen Anatomie (first edition). Vienna: W. Braumüller, 1861.

107. Buchanan EP. Congenital duodenal obstruction from anomalous mesenteric vessels. Am J Surg 1935;30:499.

108. Braun P, Collin PP, Ducharme JC. Preduodenal portal vein: A significant entity. Report of two cases and review of the literature. Can J Surg 1974;17:316.

109. Fawcett E, Blotchford JV. Observation on the line at which the lower border of the third portion of the duodenum crosses the vertebral column. J Anat Physiol 1903;38:435.

110. Akin JT, Gray SW, Skandalakis JE. Vascular compression of the duodenum: Presentation of ten cases and review of the literature. Surgery 1976;79:515-22.

111. Cauldwell EW, Anson BJ. The visceral branches of the abdominal aorta; topographic relationships. Am J Anat 1943; 73:27.

112. Derrick JR, Fadhli HA. Surgical anatomy of the superior mesenteric artery. Am Surg 1965;31:545.

113. Mansberger AR Jr, Hearn JB, Byers RM, Fleisig N, Bruxton RW. Vascular compression of the duodenum. Emphasis on accurate diagnosis. Am J Surg 1968;115:89.

114. Hearn JB. Duodenal ileus with special reference to superior mesenteric artery compression. Radiology 1966;86:305.

115. Lahey FH. A method of dealing with the proximal jejunal loop in posterior polya anastomosis. Surg Gynecol Obstet 1933;57:227-303.

116. Madden JL. Excision of duodenal diverticula. In: Madden JL, ed. Atlas of Technics in Surgery. Vol. 1, 2nd ed. New York; Appleton-Century-Crofts, 1964.

117. Cattell RB, Braasch JW. A technique for the exposure of the third

and fourth portions of the duodenum. Surg Gynecol Obstet 1960;111:379-83.

118. Chang TM, Chen TH, Shih CM, Gueng MK, Tsou SS. Partial or complete circular duodenectomy with highly selective vagotomy for severe obstructing duodenal ulcer disease. Arch Surg 1998;133:998-1001.

119. Katkhouda N, Mavor E, Mason RJ, Campos GMR, Soroushyari A, Berne TV. Laparoscopic repair of perforated duodenal ulcers: Outcome and efficacy in 30 consecutive patients. Arch Surg 1999; 134:845-50.

120. Nassoura ZE, Ivatury RR, Simon RJ, Kihtir T, Stahl WM. A prospective reappraisal of primary repair of penetrating duodenal injuries. Am Surg 1994;60:35.

121. Degiannis E, Krawczykowski D, Velmahos GC, Levy RD, Souter I, Saadia R. Pyloric exclusion in severe penetrating injuries of the duodenum. World J Surg 1993;17:751-4.

122. Allen GS, Moore FA, Cox CS Jr., Mehall JR, Duke JH. Delayed diagnosis of blunt duodenal injury: an avoidable complication. J Am Coll Surg 1998;187:393-99.

123. Chou CK, Chang JM, Tsai TC, Mak CW, How CC. CT of the duodenojejunal junction. Abdom Imaging 1995;20:425-30.

124. Bouvier S, Le Borgne J, Lehur PA, Smaili M, Moussu P. [Excision of the duodenojejunal angle for tumor: from simple excision to locoregional excision]. [French] J Chir 1997;134:122-27.

125. Peck JJ, Milleson T, Phelan J. The role of computed tomography with contrast and small bowel follow-through in management of small bowel obstruction. Am J Surg 1999;177:375-78.

126. Troum S, Solis MM. Mesenteric lymphangioma causing bowel obstruction in a child. South Med J 89(8):808-809, 1996.

127. Bemelman WA, Slors JF, Dunker MS, van Hogezand RA, van Deventer SJ, Ringers J, Griffioen G, Gouma DJ. Laparoscopic-assisted vs open ileocolic resection for Crohn's disease: a comparative study. Surg Endosc 2000;14:721-725.

128. Lionakis BS, Gray SW, Skandalakis JE, Akin JT Jr. Intussusception in infants and children. South Med J 1960:53:1226.

129. Centers for Disease Control and Prevention. Intussusception among recipients of rotavirus vaccine — United States, 1998-1999. JAMA 1999;282:520-21.

130. Zapas JL, Selby DM, Sato TT. Ileocecal duplication cyst: An unusual cause of childhood intussusception. Contemp Surg 1998; 53:339-41.

131. Harlaftis N, Skandalakis JE, Droulias C, Gray SW, Akin JT Jr. The pattern of intussusceptions in adults. J Med Assoc Ga 1977; 66:534.

132. Wang G, Liu XG, Zitsman JL. Nonfluoroscopic reduction of intussusception by air enema. World J Surg 1995:19:435-438.

133. Knol JA, Eckhauser FE. Inguinal anatomy and abdominal wall hernias. In: Greefield LJ, Mulholland MW, Oldham KT, Zelenock GB, Lillemoe KD (eds.). Surgery: Scientific Principles and Practice. Philadelphia: Lippincott-Raven, 1997.

134. Baird D, Radvany MG, Shanley DJ, Fitzharris GA. Mesenteric cyst with milk of calcium. Abdom Imaging 1994;19:347-48.

135. Liew SC, Glenn DC, Storey DW. Mesenteric cyst. Aust NZ J Surg 1994;64:741-44.

136. Slocum MA. Surgical treatment of chylous mesenteric cyst by marsupialization. Am J Surg 1938;41:464-473.

137. Beahrs OH, Judd ES. Chylangiomas of the abdomen. Proc Staff Meet Mayo Clin 1937;22:297-304.

138. Skandalakis JE. Mesenteric cyst: a report of three cases. J Med Assoc Ga 44(2):75-80, 1955.

139. Ellis H. Lesions of the mesentery, omentum, and retroperitoneum. In: Maingot H. Abdominal Operations. 6th ed, Vol 2, New York: Appleton-Century-Crofts, 1974, p.1469.

140. Kurtz RJ, Heimann TM, Beck AR, et al. Mesenteric and retroperitoneal cysts. Ann Surg 1986;203:109.

141. Mourad M, Desrousseaux B, Atat I, Abizeid G, Ampe J. [Cystic formations of the mesentery: appropos a case report of a pseudocyst of the lesser omentum]. Acta Chir Belgica 1991;91: 145-49.

142. Chung MA, Brandt ML, St.-Vil D, Yazbeck S. Mesenteric cysts in children. J Pediatr Surg 1991;26:1306-8.

143. Brown RB, Shaul JF. Mesenteric cyst complicated by intestinal obstruction. US Armed Forces Med J 1950;1:437-42.

144. Takiff H, Calabria R, Yin L, et al. Mesenteric cysts and intra-abdominal cystic lymphangiomas. Arch Surg 1985;120:1266.

145. Orobitg FJ, Vazquez L, De Franceschini AB, Ramos-Ruiz E. Mesenteric cyst of lymphatic origin: a radiopathological correlation and case report. Puerto Rico Health Sciences J 1994;13: 171-74.

146. Lee J, Song SY, Park CS, Kim B. Mullerian cysts of the mesentery and retroperitoneum: a case report and literature review. Pathol Int 1998;48:902-6.

147. Rokitansky quoted by Slocum MA. Surgical treatment of chylous mesenteric cyst by marsupialization. Am J Surg 1938;41: 464-473.

148. Carson quoted by Beahrs OH, Judd ES Jr, Dockerty MB. Chylous cysts of the abdomen. Surg Clin North Am Aug 1950: 1081-96.

149. Hill LG. Lymphagioma of the abdomen. Lancet 1930;2:897-98.

150. Lee FC. Large retroperitoneal chylous cyst: report of a case, with experiments on lymphatic permeability. Arch Surg 1942;44:61-71.

151. Guthrie RF, Wakefield EG. Mesenteric cysts. Proc Staff Meet Mayo Clin 1943;18:52-58.

152. Gross RE. The Surgery of Infancy and Childhood. Philadelphia: WB Saunders, 1953.

153. Beahrs OH, Judd ES Jr, Dockerty MB. Chylous cysts of the abdomen. Surg Clin North Am, Aug 1950;1981-1996.

154. Mohanty SK, Bal RK, Maudar KK. Mesenteric cyst: an unusual presentation. J Pediatr Surg 1998;33:792-93.

155. Namasivayam J, Ziervogel MA, Hollman AS. Case report: volvulus of a mesenteric cyst — an unusual complication diagnosed by CT. Clin Radiol 1992;46:211-12.

156. Ling JH, Chou YH, Tiu CM, Yeh TJ, Wei CF. [Sonographic appearances of mesenteric cysts: report of 2 cases]. Chin Med J 1991; 47:213-17.

157. Tuttle AE, Jones DB, Buchman TG. Mesenteric cyst in a 96-year-old woman: case report. Contemp Surg 1998;53:343-46.

158. Parsons OE. Cystic lymphangioma of mesentery. Ann Surg 1936; 103:595-604.

159. Rosado R, Flores B, Medina P, Ramirez D, Silic J. Laparoscopic resection of a mesenteric cyst: presentation of a new case. J Laparoendosc Surg 1996;6:353-55.

160. Shimura H, Ueda J, Ogawa Y, Ichimiya H, Tanaka M. Total excision of mesenteric cysts by laparoscopic surgery: report of two cases. Surg Laparosc Endosc 1997;7:173-76.

161. Brentano L, Faccini P, de Castro Oderich GS. Laparoscopic resection of a mesenteric cyst. Surg Laparosc Endosc 1998; 8:402-3.

162. Divino CM, Park IS, Angel LP, Ellozy S, Spiegel R, Kim U. A retrospective study of diagnosis and management of mesenteric vein thrombosis. Am J Surg 2001;181:20-23.

163. Skandalakis JE, Acosta FV, Veatch JW. Venous mesenteric thrombosis. J Med Assoc Ga 1958;47:222-228.

164. Hassan HA, Raufman J-P. Mesenteric venous thrombosis. South Med J 1999;92:558-62.

165. Gewertz BL. Invited critique. Arch Surg 1999;134:331.

166. Mansour MA. Management of acute mesenteric ischemia. Arch Surg 1999;134:328-30.

167. Hammer JM, Seay PH, Hill EJ, Prust FW, Campbell RB. Intestinal segments as internal pedicle grafts. Arch Surg 1955; 71:625.

168. Gentil F, Shahbender S. The use of segments of small intestine in surgery. Surg Gynecol Obstet 1959;109:417.

169. Winchester DP, Dorsey JM. Intestinal segments and pouches in gastrointestinal surgery. Surg Gynecol Obstet 1971;132:131.

170. Vennarecci G, Kato T, Misiakos EP, Neto AB, Verzaro R, Pinna A, Nery J, Khan F, Thompson JF, Tzakis AG. Intestinal transplantation for short gut syndrome attributable to necrotizing enterocolitis. Pediatrics 2000;105:E25.

171. Chatzipetrou MA, Tzakis AG, Pinna AD, Kato T, Misiakos EP, Tsaroucha AK, Weppler D, Ruiz P, Berho M, Fishbein T, Conn HO, Ricordi C. Intestinal transplantation for the treatment of desmoid tumors associated with familial adenomatous polyposis. Surgery 2001;129:277-281.

172. DeShazo CV, Snyder WH, Daugherty CG, Crenshaw CA. Mucosal pedical graft of jejunum for large gastroduodenal defects. Am J Surg 1972;124:671.

173. Dietz DW, Laureti S, Strong SA, Hull TL, Church J, Remzi FH, Lavery IC, Fazio VW. Safety and longterm efficacy of strictureplasty in 314 patients with obstructing small bowel Crohn's disease. J Am Coll Surg 2001;192:330-338.

174. Delrivière L, Muiesan P, Marshall M, Davenport M, Dhawan A, Kane P, Karani J, Rela M, Heaton N. Size reduction of small bowels from adult cadaveric donors to alleviate the scarcity of pediatric size-matched organs: an anatomical and feasibility study. Transplantation 2000;69:1392-1396.

175. Dhar GJ, Kirsner JB. Consequences of ileal resection. In: Nelson RL, Nyhus LM (eds). Surgery of the Small Intestine. Norwalk, CT: Appleton & Lange, 1987.

176. Myers JG, Page CP, Stewart RM, Schwesinger WH, Sirinek KR, Aust JB. Complications of needle catheter jejunostomy in 2,022 consecutive applications. Am J Surg 1995;170:547-551.

177. North JH, Nava HR. Pneumatosis intestinalis and portal venous air associated with needle catheter jejunostomy. Am Surg 1995;61:1045-1048.

178. Nussbaumer P, Weber D, Hollinger A. [Traumatic perforation of the small intestine - a rare complication of inguinal hernia]. Schweiz Rundsch Med Prax 2000;89:934-936.

179. White TT. Surgical anatomy of the pancreas. In Carey LC, ed. The Pancreas. St. Louis: CV Mosby Co, 1973, p. 12.

# Chapter *17*

# *Appendix*

Lee J. Skandalakis, Gene L. Colborn,
Thomas A. Weidman, John E. Skandalakis,
Panajiotis N. Skandalakis

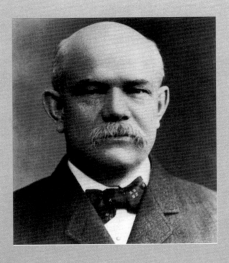

**Reginald Heber Fitz (1843-1913),** professor of pathologic anatomy at Harvard University, recognized appendicitis as a pathologic and clinical entity.

*Photo:* Meade RH. An Introduction to the History of General Surgery. Philadelphia: Saunders, 1968; with permission.

*"It is the duty of every physician to be mindful that, for all practical purposes, perityphlitis, perityphlitic tumor, and perityphlitic abscess mean inflammation of the vermiform appendix."*

**Reginald Fitz (1886)**[1]

*"What we wish to accomplish in the treatment of appendicitis is, not to save half of our cases, nor four cases out of five, but all of them."*

**C. McBurney (1889)**[2]

*"There is only one logical treatment of the disease, namely, the excision of the diseased organ as soon as the diagnosis is made."*

**A. Worcester (1892)**[3]

*"It is interesting and humiliating that a small organ which in Man performs no useful function can so frequently give rise to problems which, if not promptly and correctly treated, may have fatal complications, and of which we still do not fully know the cause."*

**Basil Morson (1972)**[4]

## HISTORY OF THE APPENDIX

The anatomic and surgical history of the appendix is shown in Table 17-1.

## EMBRYOGENESIS

### Normal Development

The appendix is the terminal portion of the embryonic cecum. The appendix becomes distinguishable by its failure to enlarge as fast as the proximal cecum. This difference in growth rate continues into postnatal life. At birth, the diameter of the colon is 4.5 times that of the appendix; at maturity, it is 8.5 times larger.[5]

The appendix is visible at about the eighth week of gestation. At first, it projects from the apex of the cecum. As the cecum grows, the origin of the appendix shifts medially toward the ileocecal valve (Fig. 17-1C). The taeniae of the longitudinal muscle coat of the colon originate from the base of the appendix, showing the same displacement.

The medial shift of the adult appendix fails to occur in 5-15% of individuals.[6] In these cases, the appendix is funnel-shaped (Fig. 17-1A). If the appendix is of normal shape, it is still located symmetrically on the cecal apex (Fig. 17-1B).

Wakeley[7] believed that asymmetric positioning of the appendix is due to faster relative growth of the right and anterior cecal walls in childhood. The symmetric position is the normal mature condition.

Maisel[8] argued that there is a rotation of the right colon and cecum about their own long axis. Thus, the retrocecal appendix is the juvenile condition. The authors of this chapter do not find this argument convincing.

Until the 12th week, the appendix is circular in cross-section. After this time, it appears as lobed. Villi are found in the fourth and fifth months, disappearing before birth. A few lymph nodules appear in the wall of the appendix by the seventh month. They increase up to puberty, after which they gradually decrease. Obliteration of the lumen is common in elderly patients.

### Congenital Anomalies

Because of its seemingly vestigial nature, one would expect to find great variability of the appendix, but this is not the case. Appendiceal variations are few, and are all rare. Although in humans the appendix appears to be vestigial as a digestive organ, it emerges as a fully developed and functional lymphoid organ.

#### *Absence of the Appendix*

Both Morgagni (in 1719)[9] and Hunter (in 1762)[10] reported on the absence of the appendix. Few cases of ab-

## TABLE 17-1. Anatomic and Surgical History of the Appendix

| | | |
|---|---|---|
| Leonardo da Vinci | 1492 | Showed appendix in drawings and called it "orecchio" (little ear); published in the 18th century |
| Berengario da Carpi | 1521 | First person to describe the appendix |
| Andreas Vesalius | 1543 | Showed the appendix in a drawing but did not describe it in the text |
| Jean Fernel | 1544 | Early description of appendicitis |
| Von Hilden | 1652 | Early description of appendicitis |
| Lorenz Heister | 1711 | Unequivocal description of perforated appendix with abscess formation |
| Giovanni Battista Morgagni | 1719 | First detailed anatomic description of appendix |
| Claudius Amyand | 1736 | Performed the first appendectomy? or Tait, 1980? or Krönlein, 1884? |
| Mestivier | 1759 | Described perforation of the appendix by a pin; considered perforation the cause of the abscess; the second unequivocal case identifying appendix as site of disease |
| John Hunter | 1767 | Described gangrenous appendix at autopsy |
| John Parkinson | 1812 | Described autopsy findings of 5-year-old child with perforated appendix containing a fecalith |
| Louyer-Villemay | 1824 | Described fatal gangrenous appendix in two young men; first clinical history of acute suppurative appendicitis |
| Francois Melier | 1827 | Presented six autopsy descriptions of appendicitis and suggested that perhaps surgical removal of the appendix was in order |
| Goldbeck | 1830 | Described acute suppurative appendicitis but said cause was irritation of cecum; first use of term "perityphlitis" |
| Guillaume Dupuytren | 1835 | Ascribed RLQ abscesses to pericecal origin without mention of appendix |
| Stokes | 1838 | Used large doses of opium to treat intraabdominal inflammations |
| Thomas Addison and Richard Bright | 1839 | Described symptomatology of appendicitis; stated that appendix was the cause of many or most of the inflammatory processes of the right iliac fossa |
| A. Grisolle | 1839 | Advocated drainage of abdominal abscesses following watchful waiting until fluctuation |
| Volz | 1846 | Identified the appendix as the origin of RLQ inflammatory process |
| Henry Hancock | 1848 | Recommended earlier operation for drainage of abscesses |
| Willard Parker | 1867 | Recognized obstructive origin of appendicitis; reported four cases of abscess secondary to perforated appendix; advised surgical drainage after the 5th day of the disease, but did not advise operation before perforation |
| Lawson Tait | 1880 | Removed a gangrenous appendix; in 1890 abandoned appendectomy |
| Abraham Groves | 1883 | Removed an inflamed appendix; not published until 1934 |
| Mikulicz | 1884 | Removed the appendix but patient did not survive |
| Krönlein | 1884 | Perhaps, rather than Amyand in 1736, was first to perform appendectomy |
| Charter-Symonds | 1885 | Extraperitoneal removal of fecalith |
| Reginald Heber Fitz | 1886 | Advocated early surgical removal of acute appendix; first used term "appendicitis" |
| R.J. Hall | 1886 | Successfully removed perforated appendix within an irreducible inguinal hernia with pelvic abscess |
| John Homans | 1886 | Operated on an 11-year-old boy, draining the abscess with good recovery |
| Thomas G. Morton | 1887 | Successful operative removal of perforated appendix with draining of abscess |
| Edward R. Cutler | 1887 | Performed one of the first "clean" unruptured appendectomies; reported in 1889 |
| Henry Sands | 1888 | Removed two fecaliths and closed the perforation of the appendix |
| Charles McBurney | 1889<br>June, 1894 | Described abdominal point tenderness (McBurney's point)<br>Presented "gridiron incision" (McBurney's incision) to Chicago Medical Society (CMS) |
| Lewis L. McArthur | July, 1894 | Published his vertical midline incision technique, which was postponed from presentation at June meeting of CMS |

## TABLE 17-1 (cont'd). Anatomic and Surgical History of the Appendix

| | | |
|---|---|---|
| G.R. Fowler | 1894 to 1895 | Advocated "cuffing" of appendiceal stump |
| R.H.M. Dawbarn | 1895 | Advocated invagination of appendiceal stump to prevent postoperative fistula |
| William Henry Battle | 1897 | Advocated a vertical incision through the lateral edge of the right rectus sheath; others also advocated it, and incision sometimes is referred to as Battle-Jalaguier-Kammerer incision |
| A.C. Bernays | 1898 | Reported 71 consecutive appendectomies without mortality |
| Harrington, Weir, and Fowler | 1899 | Described medial extension of gridiron incision by dividing lateral portion of rectus sheath (Fowler-Weir extension) |
| A.J. Ochsner | 1902 | Advocated nonoperative treatment to localize spreading peritonitis |
| John B. Murphy | 1904 | Reported 2000 appendectomies without death |
| H.A. Kelly | 1905 | Advocated against "ligating, amputating, and burying the little stump" |
| A. E. Rockey, G. G. Davis | 1905 1906 | Each advocated transverse skin incision (later called Rockey-Davis incision) |
| P. Masson | 1921 | Described neuromas of the appendix; studied relationship between neuroendocrine cells and origin of carcinoid tumors |
| Arthur Rendle Short | 1925 | Investigated appendicitis as "a disease of Western civilization," low-fiber diet |
| LeGrand Guerry | 1926 | Cited 2,959 personal cases of appendectomy |
| A.J.E. Cave | 1936 | Described appendiceal duplications and abnormalities |
| D.C. Collins | 1951 1955 1963 | Described agenesis of the appendix Study of 50,000 human appendix specimens Study of 71,000 human appendix specimens |
| Skandalakis et al. | 1962 | Collective review of cases of smooth muscle tumors of the colon and appendix as reported in the world literature |
| O'Neill | 1966 | Described use of appendix as fallopian tube |
| E. Higa et al. | 1973 | Described proliferative epithelial tumors of appendiceal mucosa |
| de Kok | 1977 | Laparoscope-aided appendectomy with mini-laparotomy |
| A.P. Dhillon, L. Papadaki, J. Rode | 1982 to 1983 | Studied subepithelial neuroendocrine cells; immunoreactivity for serotonin |
| Semm | 1983 | Laparoscopic appendectomy |

History table compiled by David A. McClusky III and John E. Skandalakis.

**References:**

de Kok HJ. A new technique for resecting the non-inflamed not-adhesive appendix through a mini-laparotomy with the aid of the laparoscope. Arch Chir Neerl 1977;29:195-98.

Moore FD. The gastrointestinal tract and the acute abdomen. In: Warren R. (ed) Surgery. Philadelphia: WB Saunders, 1963.

O'Neill JJ. The use of the vermiform appendix as a fallopian tube. Am J Obstet Gynecol 1966;95:219-21.

Skandalakis JE, Gray SW, Shepard D, Bourne GH. Smooth Muscle Tumors of the Alimentary Canal: Leiomyomas and Leiomyosarcomas, a Review of 2525 Cases. Springfield, IL: Charles C. Thomas, 1962.

Skandalakis JE, Gray SW. Embryology for Surgeons (2nd ed). Baltimore: Williams & Wilkins, 1994.

Williams GR. Presidential address: A history of appendicitis. Ann Surg 1983;197:495-506.

Williams RS. Appendicitis: historical milestones and current challenges. Med J Aust 1992;157:784-87.

Williams RA, Myers P. Pathology of the Appendix and Its Surgical Treatment. New York: Chapman & Hall Medical, 1994.

sent appendix or both absent appendix and cecum have been reported. Collins found 4 cases in 71,000 specimens examined,[11] and reported only 46 cases in the literature (by 1931).[12]

An absent appendix may have failed to form in the eighth week. Alternatively, it may have developed at the same rate as the cecum, and thus be present, but lacking demarcation from the rest of the cecum. The latter is probably the case where there are more than four haustra in the cecum.[13] According to Williams,[14] the possibility of appendiceal autoamputation, intussusception, or volvulus[15] suggests that any diagnosis of agenesis should be preceded by inspection of the bowel and abdominal cavity for a mummified appendix.

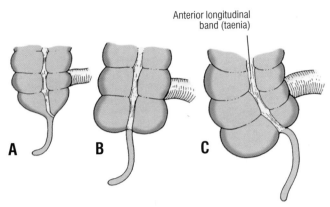

Anterior longitudinal
band (taenia)

**A**  **B**  **C**

FIG. 17-1. Three types of cecum and appendix. **A** and **B.** Infantile forms. When present in the adult, they represent mild developmental arrest. **C.** Mature and most common form. (Modified from Skandalakis JE, Gray SW, Rowe JS Jr. Anatomical Complications in General Surgery. New York: McGraw-Hill, 1983; with permission.)

Chevre et al.,[16] who encountered a case of appendiceal agenesis, cautioned that the diagnosis not be made without thorough exploration of the ileocecal and retrocecal areas.

## Ectopic Appendix

Fawcitt found an appendix in the thorax, in association with malrotation and diaphragmatic defect.[17] Babcock reported the removal of an appendix in the lumbar area.[18] Abramson presented a case of an appendix which was located within the posterior cecal wall, and which did not have a serous coat.[19]

## Left-Sided Appendix

There are four conditions that can result in a left-sided appendix. In order of frequency, they are: (1) situs inversus viscerum, (2) nonrotation of the intestines, (3) "wandering" cecum with a long mesentery, and (4) an excessively long appendix crossing the midline. Nisolle et al.[20] described a case of left-sided appendicitis in which the extremity of a dilated right appendix was located in the left lower quadrant (LLQ) along the lateral pelvic wall.

Smith and colleagues stated that there were 40 cases of appendicitis and malrotation with the appendix in the left lower quadrant reported by 1933, and 97 cases of appendicitis and situs inversus reported by 1949.[21] Collins found 40 cases of LLQ appendix and 17 cases of situs inversus (11 with dextrocardia) in his series of 71,000.[11] Altogether, some 200 cases of left-sided appendix are in the literature.

Situs inversus can be predicted by noting the position of the patient's heart. Nonrotation, however, may not be recognized if there are no radiographic films available. Further, it should be noted that in about one-half of patients with situs inversus, the pain of appendicitis is felt in the right lower quadrant (RLQ).

If the cecum and appendix are not in the right iliac fossa, the right paravertebral gutter and the right subhepatic space should be searched. If the cecum still cannot be found, the incision should be closed. A midline incision should be made that will give access to both the left and right lower quadrants.

## Duplication of the Appendix

Waugh[22] described three types of duplication of the appendix:

- Double-barreled appendix, with a common muscularis and often a distal communication between the lumina (this type of tubular duplication is also found elsewhere in the large and small intestine)
- "Bird-type" paired appendix. Structures are symmetrically placed on either side of the ileocecal valve (this condition occurs in conjunction with other severe defects, and may be a mild form of hindgut twinning)
- Taenia coli-type duplication. A normal appendix develops at the usual site, and an additional small appendix forms on a taenia. This may represent a continued development of the transitory cecal protuberance observed from the sixth to the seventh week of development.

Appendiceal duplications as classified by Cave[23] and Wallbridge[24] are shown in Figures 17-2A-E. Kjossev and Losanoff[25] found a second appendix at the splenic flexure (Fig. 17-2D), which they considered to be a new subtype of the Cave-Wallbridge Type B anomaly.

Duplication is rare; Collins found only two cases of true congenital double appendix and one case of post-inflammatory pseudo-duplication in 71,000 specimens.[11] Arda et al.,[26] reporting in 1992, expanded case reports to around 100. A triplicated appendix with other anomalies was reported by Tinckler;[27] a horseshoe appendix having a patent continuous lumen with two separate openings into the cecum and a fan-shaped mesoappendix was discovered during surgery by Mesko et al.[28]

Lin et al.[29] urged surgeons to routinely check for appendiceal duplication at surgery, especially when clinical signs of appendicitis occur with visualization of a normal appendix at laparotomy. We agree that this is very wise advice.

## Congenital Appendiceal Diverticula

Although the appendix is subject to diverticulum formation like the rest of the intestine, there have been few re-

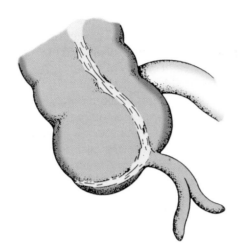

**A**

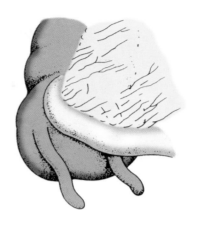

**B**

**C**

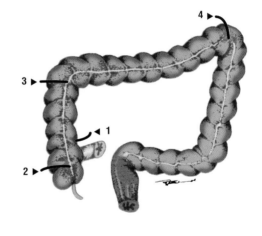

**D**

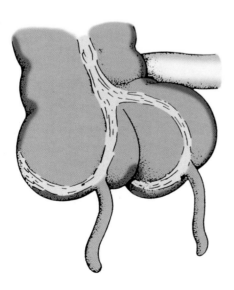

**E**

Fig. 17-2. Duplication classification system of Cave and Wall-bridge. **A.** Wallbridge type A anomaly. Single cecum and a partial duplication of the appendix with a single base. Varying degrees of appendiceal duplication are possible. **B.** Wallbridge type B1 anomaly. Two completely separate appendices arise from a single cecum and are disposed on either side of the ileocecal valve. **C.** Wallbridge type B2 anomaly. The second appendix is usually found arising from the taenia coli of the wall of the cecum. **D.** Figure shows type B1 (1) and B2 (2) anomalies; 3 represents duplication from the hepatic flexure; 4 represents duplication from the splenic flexure. **E.** Wallbridge type C anomaly. Double cecum, each with its own appendix. (**A, B, C, E** Modified from Williams RA. Development, structure and function of the appendix. In: Williams RA, Myers P. Pathology of the Appendix and Its Surgical Treatment. New York: Chapman & Hall Medical, 1994, pp. 9-30, with permission). (**D** Modified from Kjossev KT, Losanoff JE. Duplicated vermiform appendix. Br J Surg 1996;83:1259, with permission.)

nerves. Anteriorly it is related to the abdominal wall, the greater omentum, or coils of ileum. In the cadaver, the apex of the cecum is usually found slightly to the medial side of the middle of the right inguinal ligament.

In living individuals the position of the cecum varies with posture, respiration, abdominal muscle tone, and state of intestinal distention. When an individual is standing upright, the cecum and appendix often hang over the pelvic brim. From the apex of the cecum (the only relatively fixed point) the appendix can project in any direction and the tip can become attached to almost any abdominal organ except the spleen (Fig. 17-4).

There is little doubt that the terminology used to describe the position of the appendix is a major source of confusion to those who would attempt to apply the descriptions in the literature to the reality of the operating room. Sir Frederick Treves derived a schema for appendiceal positions based on the hands of a clock (Fig. 17-5).[37]

The exact meaning of "retrocecal" is disturbingly unclear in a report by Wakeley in 1933,[7] in which he reviewed 10,000 postmortem cases and described five typical locations of the appendix. In order of frequency they are (1) retrocecal-

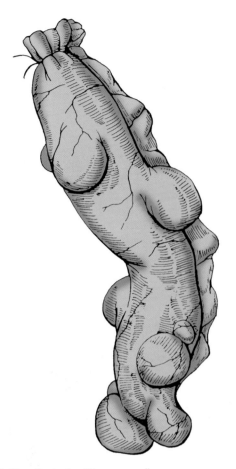

**FIG. 17-3.** Diverticulosis of the appendix.

ports of the formation of true congenital appendiceal diverticula (Fig. 17-3).[30-33] Favara[31] found an association between genetic abnormalities and congenital diverticula.

### *Heterotopic Mucosa in the Appendix*

Gastric mucosa, pancreatic tissue,[34] and esophageal mucosa[35] have been reported in the appendix. Haque et al.[36] found heterotopic bone associated with mucin-producing tumors of the appendix.

## SURGICAL ANATOMY

## Topography, Position, and Relations

The appendix arises from the cecum, which is related posteriorly to the iliopsoas muscle and the lumbar plexus of

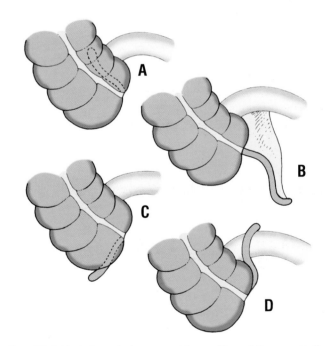

**FIG. 17-4.** Variations in topographic position of the appendix. From its base at the cecum, the appendix may extend **(A)** upward, retrocecal and retrocolic; **(B)** downward, pelvic; **(C)** downward to the right, subcecal; or **(D)** upward to the left, ileocecal (may pass anterior or posterior to the ileum). (Modified from Skandalakis JE, Gray SW, Rowe JS Jr. Anatomical Complications in General Surgery. New York: McGraw-Hill, 1983; with permission.)

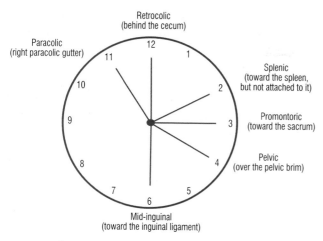

FIG. 17-5. Graphic illustration of appendiceal position. (Adapted from Decker GAG, Du Plessis DJ. Lee McGregor's Synopsis of Surgical Anatomy (12th ed). Bristol: Wright, 1986; with permission.)

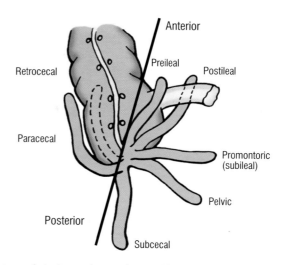

FIG. 17-6. Anterior and posterior positions of the appendiceal tip. (From O'Connor CE, Reed WP. In vivo location of the human vermiform appendix. Clin Anat 1994; 7:139-142; with permission.)

retrocolic, free or fixed; (2) pelvic or descending; (3) subcecal, passing downward and to the right; (4) ileocecal, passing upward and to the left anterior to the ileum; and (5) ileocecal, posterior to the ileum. If the position of the appendix is "retrocecal" or "retrocolic," does this indicate whether the organ is intraperitoneal or extraperitoneal? Such a difference is no small matter.

Most series concurred with Wakeley's findings regarding the two most common locations, but Buschard and Kjaeldgaard[38] compiled significant variations from reports of many surgeons (Table 17-2).

O'Connor and Reed[39] studied the location of the appendix in 129 patients undergoing abdominal procedures; these authors also had their own terminology of anatomic location of the appendix (Fig. 17-6). A summary of the findings of these workers is presented in Table 17-3. They stated that the retrocecal position of the appendix was indeed the most common, although it occurred in only 28-33% of instances.

O'Connor and Reed's findings included the observation that only 10% of the 21.5% rate of retrocecal appendices reported by Collins[12] were mobile, but more than 40% of the Danish patients (out of a total of 56.7%) reported by

### TABLE 17-2. Survey of the Position of the Appendix, in Per Cent, in Various Materials

| | | | Position, % | | | | | |
|---|---|---|---|---|---|---|---|---|
| | | | Anterior | | Posterior | | | |
| Material | Country | No. | Pelvic | Ileocecal | Retrocecal | Subcecal | Anterior | Posterior |
| Collins | USA | 4,680 | 78.5 | | 20.2 | 1.3 | 78.5 | 21.5 |
| Peterson | Finland | 373 | 42.2 | 26.8 | 31.0 | — | 69.0 | 31.0 |
| Maisel | South Africa | 300 | 58.0 | 10.2 | 26.7 | 5.0 | 68.2 | 31.7 |
| Shah & Shah autopsy | India | 186 | 34.9 | 28.0 | 30.1 | 7.0 | 62.9 | 37.1 |
| Liertz | Germany | 2,092 | 42.1 | 13.9 | 35.0 | 9.0 | 56.0 | 44.0 |
| B & K | CSSR | 93 | 44.1 | 11.8 | 44.1 | 0.0 | 55.9 | 44.1 |
| Waas | Ceylon | 266 | 24.1 | 28.6 | 35.3 | 12.0 | 52.7 | 47.3 |
| Solanke | Nigeria | 125 | 31.2 | 29.2 | 38.4 | 11.2 | 50.4 | 49.6 |
| B & K | Denmark | 141 | 33.4 | 7.8 | 56.7 | 2.1 | 41.2 | 58.8 |
| Shah & Shah operation | India | 405 | 8.2 | 26.9 | 61.2 | 3.7 | 35.1 | 64.9 |
| Wakeley | Great Britain | 10,000 | 31.0 | 1.4 | 65.3 | 2.3 | 32.4 | 67.6 |

*Source:* Buschard K, Kjaeldgaard A. Investigation and analysis of the position, fixation, length, and embryology of the vermiform appendix. Acta Chir Scand 1973;139:293-298.

### TABLE 17-3. Distribution of Locations of the Vermiform Appendix

| Position[a,b] | Nonappendicitis | Appendicitis[c] | Total | Percentage[d] | |
|---|---|---|---|---|---|
| Preileal | 1 | 5 | 6 | 4 | (5%) |
| Postileal | 7 | 3 | 10 | 8 | (7%) |
| Subileal | 11 | 8 | 19 | 15 | (15%) |
| Pelvic | 14 | 11 | 25 | 19 | (19%) |
| Subcecal | 9 | 5 | 14 | 11 | (13%) |
| Paracecal | 4 | 9 | 13 | 10 | (13%) |
| Retrocecal | 18 | 24 | 42 | 33 | (28%) |
| Totals | 64 | 65 | 129 | 100 | (100%) |

[a]Anterior positions 1-5: 56%.
[b]Posterior positions 6-7: 44%.
[c]Distribution of positions analyzed by Pearsons Chi-square (P >0.2).
[d]Percentages in parentheses include the 27 excluded cases.

*Source:* O'Connor CE, Reed WP. *In vivo* location of the human vermiform appendix. Clin Anat 1994;7:139-142.

Buschard and Kjaelgaard[38] had mobile retrocecal appendices. Whether the appendix is "fixed" or "unfixed," it would seem fairly reasonable to think that the truly major factor in appendectomy has to do with its intraperitoneal or extraperitoneal position.

Puylaert[40] classified the orientation of the appendix as medial (35%), caudal (30%), retrocecal/retroperitoneal (25%), and lateral (10%).

Ajmani and Ajmani[41] studied appendiceal arteries and the position of the appendix in natives of India. The most common position of the appendix was retrocecal/ retrocolic (58%); the pelvic position accounted for 23%. The other positions, in descending order of occurrence, were: postileal, 10%; subcecal, 5%; paracecal, 2%; and preileal, 2% (Table 17-4). The same authors reported an average appendiceal length of 9.5 cm in males and 8.7 cm in females.

Wakeley,[7] who focused on Great Britain, reported that only 1.4% of appendices were ileocecal. Solanke,[42] in Nigeria, found 19.2% in this position. Buschard and Kjaeldgaard,[38] using measurements made in Denmark and the former Czechoslovakia (see Table 17-2), concluded that

the pelvic position represented immaturity of cecal development and that the retrocecal position represented complete maturity. This theory concurs with those of Wakeley[7] and DeGaris.[43]

The appendix can possibly change its position in living subjects when not held in place by adhesions. Buschard and Kjaeldgaard[38] sought evidence of such change, but observed none. Although it has often been suggested,[11,44] no consistent correlation between position of appendix and frequency of appendicitis has been confirmed. In a retrospective review of operative reports and in an analysis of 94 appendectomies, Shen and colleagues[45] found that the retrocecal position of the appendix did not alter the clinical course of appendicitis.

## Appendiceal Wall

The appendiceal wall is similar to the wall of the colon. It is formed by
- The serosa
- A muscular layer composed of the longitudinal and cir-

### TABLE 17-4. Showing Various Positions of Appendix and their Percentage

| Classification Sex | Retrocecal and Retrocolic | | Pelvic | | Postilial | | Subcecal | | Preilial | | Paracecal | |
|---|---|---|---|---|---|---|---|---|---|---|---|---|
| | M | F | M | F | M | F | M | F | M | F | M | F |
| No. of cases | 52 | 6 | 15 | 8 | 9 | 1 | 5 | nil | 2 | nil | 2 | nil |
| Total | 58 | | 23 | | 10 | | 5 | | 2 | | 2 | |
| Total in % | 58% | | 23% | | 10% | | 5% | | 2% | | 2% | |

*Source:* Ajmani ML, Ajmani K. The position, length and arterial supply of vermiform appendix. Anat Anz (Jena) 1983;153:369-74.

cular layers. At the appendiceal base, the longitudinal muscle produces a thickening that is related to all cecal taeniae

- The submucosa, which contains many lymphoid islands
- The mucosa

According to Owen and Nemanic,[46] columnar epithelial cells and attenuated antigen-transporting membrane or M cells cover the mucosa. Ferguson[47] stated that even though the association between columnar epithelial cells and lymphocytes within the epithelial layer of the gut and other organs is well known, much work remains to establish the real role of interactions between lymphocytes and the enteric mucosa.

Brunagel et al.[48] described an appendicocutaneous fistula which occurred as a complication of abdominal draining.

## Mesentery of the Appendix

Hollinshead[49] proposed that "since the appendix is a part of the cecum and the latter has no true mesentery, the appendix does not either; however, there is usually a peritoneal fold enclosing the artery to the appendix which is commonly referred to as the mesenteriole or mesentery of the appendix."

The mesentery of the appendix is embryologically derived from the posterior side of the mesentery of the terminal ileum. The mesentery attaches to the cecum as well as to the proximal appendix. It contains the appendicular artery. The mesentery frequently appears to be too short for the appendix, which may be sharply bent on itself.

## Morphology of the Appendix

The posteromedial side of the cecum gives origin to the vermiform appendix about 1.7 cm from the end of the ileum. Variations have been found in the diameter of the appendix at its base at the cecum: Hollinshead[49] found an average of 0.6 cm, Anson and McVay[50] reported an average of 0.8 cm, and Maingot[51] found a range of 0.5-1.5 cm.

The average appendiceal length as reported by a number of authors is shown in Table 17-5. Apparent differences in dimension seem to exist in varying populations, but no correlation exists between the length of the appendix and its position.[38]

## Vascular Supply

### *Arteries* (Figs. 17-7, 17-8) *and Veins*

The appendicular artery arises from the ileocolic artery, an ileal branch, or from a cecal artery. Although the ap-

pendicular artery is usually singular (Fig. 17-7A, B), Michels[52] found two appendicular arteries in 10 of 132 specimens examined (Fig. 17-7C). A much higher frequency of duplication among Indian subjects was reported by Shah and Shah.[44] In 30% of their subjects, there were two arteries. In addition to the typical appendicular artery, the base of the appendix may be supplied by a small branch of the anterior or posterior cecal artery.

Solanke,[53] in his study of Nigerians, found variation in the pattern of arterial blood supply to the appendix. Eighty of the 100 cadavers received, in addition to blood from the main appendicular artery, supply from one or more accessory appendicular arteries. He also noted a high frequency of arterial anastomoses, which could serve as alternate routes for circulation in the event of occlusion of the main appendicular artery.

Van Damme[54] stated that the appendicular branch of the ileocolic artery can be doubled in 5% of cases. In agreement with Van Damme, Bertelli et al.[55] consider the cecoappendicular branches of the ileocolic artery to be terminal branches.

Ajmani and Ajmani,[41] in their study of Indian subjects, stated that the main appendicular artery springs from the ileocecal artery. In 39% of their cadavers, the accessory appendicular arteries arose from various vessels (Fig. 17-8, Table 17-6).

The appendicular vein and artery are enveloped by the mesentery of the appendix. The appendicular vein joins cecal veins to become the ileocolic vein, which is a tributary of the right colic vein.[56]

### *Lymphatic Drainage*

Lymphatic drainage from the ileocecal region is through a chain of nodes on the appendicular, ileocolic, and superior mesenteric arteries through which the lymph passes to reach the celiac lymph nodes and the cisterna chyli (Figs. 17-9, 17-10). A secondary drainage (which

---

### Editorial Comment

*Knowledge of lymphatic drainage and the regional nodes is important in the management of the rare malignancies of the appendix. A formal right hemicolectomy should be performed for primary adenocarcinomas of the appendix and for carcinoid tumors greater than 2 cm or carcinoid tumors less than 2 cm with extension of the tumor into the mesoappendix. (RSF Jr)*

## TABLE 17-5. Average Dimensions of the Appendix from Various Sources

| Authors | Year | Length, cm |
|---|---|---|
| Ferguson | 1891 | 11.5 |
| Kelynack | 1893 | 9.0 |
| Bryant | 1893 | 8.25 |
| Monks & Blake | 1902 | 7.9 |
| Kelly & Hurdon | 1905 | 9.1 |
| Deaver | 1913 | 8.9 |
| MacPhail | 1917 | 9.9 |
| Lewis | 1918 | 8.3 |
| Robinson | 1923 | 9.2 |
| Royster | 1927 | 7.5 |
| Henke & Lubarsch | 1929 | 9.5 |
| Hafferl | 1953 | 9.0 |
| Hollinshead | 1956 | 8.5 |
| Goss | 1959 | 8.3 |
| Solanke | 1970 | 9.6 |
| Anson & McVay | 1971 | 6-12 (range) |
| Warwick & Williams | 1973 | 9.0 |
| Buschard & Kjaeldgaard | 1973 | 9.12 (operation) (CSSR)<br>9.75 (operation) (Denmark)<br>9.96 (autopsy) (Denmark) |
| Ajmani & Ajmani | 1983 | 8.7 (female)<br>9.5 (male) |
| Puylaert | 1990 | 9.0 |
| Williams & Myers | 1994 | 9.0 |

**Based on data from the following:**
Ajmani ML, Ajmani K. The position, length and arterial supply of vermiform appendix. Anat Anz (Jena) 1983;153:369-374.
Buschard K, Kjaeldgaard A. Investigation and analysis of the position, fixation, length, and embryology of the vermiform appendix. Acta Chir Scand 1973;139:293-298.
Puylaert JBCM. Ultrasound of Appendicitis. New York: Springer-Verlag, 1990.
Solanke TF. The position, length and content of the vermiform appendix in Nigerians. Br J Surg 1970;57:100-102.
Williams RA, Myers P. Pathology of the Appendix and Its Surgical Treatment. New York: Chapman & Hall Medical, 1994.

passes anterior to the pancreas) to subpyloric nodes was described by Braithwaite.[57] It should be remembered that lymph nodules in the wall of the appendix are not connected with the lymphatic drainage of the organ. The lymphocytes formed in the nodules pass into the lumen of the appendix.

### Innervation

Sympathetic innervation of the appendix originates from the celiac and superior mesenteric ganglia. Parasympathetic innervation originates from the vagus nerve. Sensory innervation for pain is carried by the eighth thoracic spinal nerve, or perhaps by the 10th and 11th thoracic nerves.

## HISTOLOGY

Though the thick appendiceal wall has the same four layers as the colon (serosa or adventitia, muscularis externa, submucosa, and mucosa), it differs by having the following characteristics: its outer layer of longitudinal smooth muscle is complete, and the mucosa and submucosa have multiple lymph nodules.

The histology of the appendix has been considered

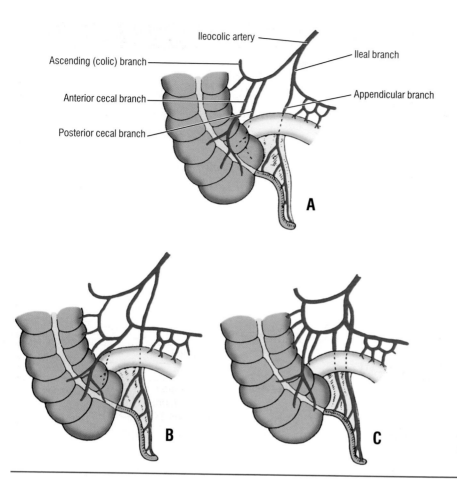

Fig. 17-7. Blood supply to the appendix. **A** and **B.** Usual type with a single appendicular artery. **C.** Paired appendicular arteries. (Modified from Skandalakis JE, Gray SW, Rowe JS Jr. Anatomical Complications in General Surgery. New York: McGraw-Hill, 1983; after Solanke TF. The blood supply of the vermiform appendix in Nigerians. J Anat 1968;102:353-361; with permission.)

previously in this chapter under the heading "Appendiceal Wall."

## PHYSIOLOGY

The physiologic action of this vestigial organ in human beings is not known. Due to the presence of numerous lymphatic follicles however, it is generally accepted that the appendix performs immune functions. But this does not mean that a normal appendix should not be removed in an exploratory (diagnostic) laparotomy. The reason is very simple: there is the possibility of future acute appendicitis with or without gangrene, perforation, and localized or generalized peritonitis.

### Editorial Comment

*Two anatomically distinct systems of innervation are responsible for the different pain patterns of appendicitis. Distension of stretch of the sympathetic fibers of the visceral peritoneum of the appendix causes moderately severe periumbilical pain which may be either cramping or steady. The sympathetic nerve fibers that transmit signals of pain when distended are not sensitive to inflammation. In contrast, inflammation of the parietal peritoneum causes pain. The parietal peritoneum is innervated by the thoracic somatic sensory nerves. When the inflamed appendix lies in the anterior position, it causes the classic findings, initially a hyperesthesia and then a localized pain and tenderness at the site of the inflammation. (RSF Jr)*

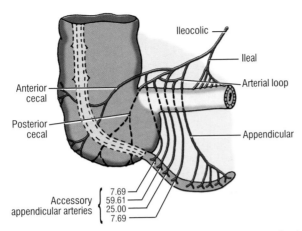

**Fig. 17-8.** Variations in the origin of the accessory appendicular arteries. (Modified from Ajmani ML, Ajmani K. The position, length and arterial supply of vermiform appendix. Anat Anz 1983; 153:369-374; with permission.)

## SURGICAL ANATOMY OF APPENDECTOMY

### Exposure and Mobilization

The incision for appendectomy (Fig. 17-11) is usually made over McBurney's point.[58] It is made at right angles to a line between the anterior superior iliac spine and the umbilicus at two-thirds the distance from the umbilicus. One-third of the incision should be above the line; two-thirds should be below.[59]

The surgeon must not expect to find the appendix exactly at McBurney's point. Using roentgenography, DeGaris[43] found the base of the appendix to be near McBurney's point in 7 of 30 patients; it was displaced in 23 (Fig. 17-11). Karim et al.[60] described 70% of appendices visualized in 51 subjects as lying inferior to the interspinous line. In a study of 275 double-contrast barium enemas,

Ramsden and colleagues[61] found only 35% of appendiceal bases lying within 5 cm of McBurney's point; 15% were more than 10 cm away.

### Identification

The cecum should be identified first. The cecum can be distinguished from the transverse colon by the absence of attachments of the greater omentum. If the cecum cannot be located, malrotation of the intestines or an undescended cecum should be considered (see "Topography, Position, and Relations").

Once the cecum has been identified, one of the taeniae coli should be traced downward to the base of the appendix. The base always arises from the cecum at the convergence of the taeniae, even though the tip of the appendix is very mobile. It may be necessary to incise the posterior peritoneum lateral to the cecum to expose a deeply buried retrocecal appendix.

Congenital absence of the appendix is too rare to be entertained seriously. However, apparent absence of the appendix can be the result of intussusception. With intus-

| TABLE 17-6. Showing Origin of Accessory Appendicular Arteries | | | | | | | | |
|---|---|---|---|---|---|---|---|---|
| **Origin** | **Posterior Cecal** | | **Ileocecal** | | **Anterior Cecal** | | **Arterial Loop** | |
| **Sex** | M | F | M | F | M | F | M | F |
| No. of cases | 22 | 5 | 6 | 2 | 1 | 1 | 2 | nil |
| Total (39) | 27 | | 8 | | 2 | | 2 | |
| Total in percentage | 69.23% | | 20.5% | | 5.12% | | 5.12% | |

*Source:* Ajmani ML, Ajmani K. The position, length and arterial supply of vermiform appendix. Anat Anz (Jena) 1983; 153:369-74.

susception, there should be an obvious dimple at the normal site of the appendix. The wise surgeon will always inspect the abdomen for signs of previous operation.

## Surgical Applications

- The convergence of the taeniae coli at the appendiceal base will help the surgeon find a hidden appendix.
- Right psoas muscle test: The forced extension of the right thigh produces increased pain in the RLQ of the abdomen when the inflamed appendix and its short mesentery rest on the peritoneum which covers the right major psoas muscle.
- Right obturator muscle test: Flexion and lateral rotation of the right thigh produces increased pain in the RLQ and right pelvic area when the inflamed appendix is

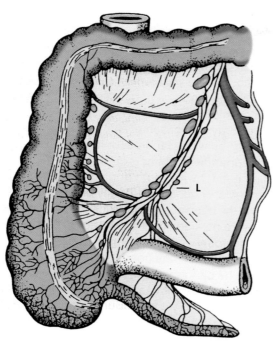

FIG. 17-9. Anterior view of the external lymphatic drainage of the appendix with the position of the lower ileocolic lymph nodes indicated (L). (Modified from Williams RA. Development, structure and function of the appendix. In: Williams RA, Myers P. Pathology of the Appendix and Its Surgical Treatment. New York: Chapman & Hall Medical, 1994, pp. 9-30; with permission.)

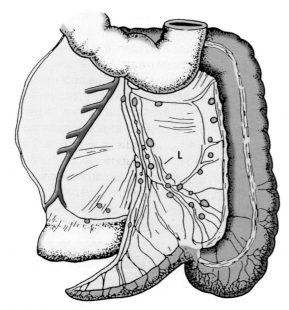

FIG. 17-10. Posterior view of the external lymphatic drainage of the appendix and cecum with the position of the lower ileocolic lymph nodes indicated (L). (Modified from Williams RA. Development, structure and function of the appendix. In: Williams RA, Myers P. Pathology of the Appendix and Its Surgical Treatment. New York: Chapman & Hall Medical, 1994, pp. 9-30; with permission.)

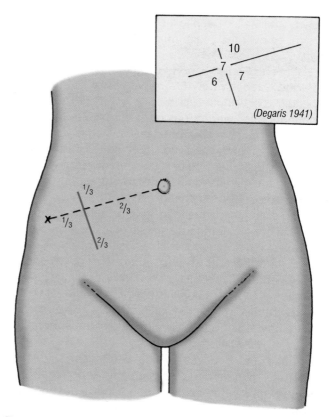

FIG. 17-11. Incision for appendectomy (blue line) in relation to McBurney's point. Inset: Actual location of 30 appendices in 30 patients. (Modified from Skandalakis JE, Gray SW, Rowe JS Jr. Anatomical Complications in General Surgery. New York: McGraw-Hill, 1983; redrawn from DuPlessis DJ. A Synopsis of Surgical Anatomy, 11th Ed. Bristol, England: Wright and Sons, 1975; with permission. Inset: Redrawn from DeGaris CF. Topography and development of the cecum and appendix. Ann Surg 113:540, 1941; with permission.)

closely related to the obturator internus muscle.

- Each position of the appendix produces and mimics a different clinical picture:
  - *Retrocecal appendix:* RLQ or right flank pain with ureteric irritation
  - *Pelvic appendix:* Pelvic pain with urinary symptoms; rule out pelvic inflammatory disease
  - *Subhepatic appendix:* Due to cecal malrotation; presents gallbladder symptoms
  - *Upper or lower midline appendix:* Epigastric or hypogastric pain
  - *Situs inversus:* When present, pain is located at the LLQ
- If the diagnosis of acute appendicitis in children is not certain, we advise emergency surgery for females and close follow-up for males. Diagnostic aids, such as an emergency Gastrografin enema, are of occasional help. Delay in making the appropriate diagnosis is a major factor in the occurrence of perforation, according to Berry and Malt.[62] Despite the fact that mortality has been reduced over the years, morbidity is high with delayed diagnosis and surgery.
- Guidry and Poole[63] reported that the appendix was in a "hidden" location in 15% of patients with simple appendicitis or without appendicitis, compared with 68% of patients with gangrenous or perforative appendicitis. The same authors concluded that anatomic variations in the location of the appendix may be responsible for a late diagnosis, causing delayed appendectomy.
- Stevenson[64] advised elective appendectomy with the clinical diagnosis of appendiceal colic.
- Wong et al.[65] recommended Tc-99m IgG scintigraphy as a definitive test for the diagnosis of acute appendicitis. This test did not produce false-positive results. Chen et al.[66] reported that abdominal sonography to detect acute appendicitis has a sensitivity of 99.3%, an accuracy of 91.6%, a positive predictive value of 90.5%, and a negative predictive value of 97.0%. Chen and colleagues advise routine sonography of the abdomen in patients with clinical appendicitis.
- Crombe et al.,[67] in a study similar to that of Chen et al., likewise recommended systematic abdominal ultrasonography when acute appendicitis is suspected in adults.
- Buckley et al.[68] advocate laparoscopic appendectomy because of the reduction in complications and shorter hospital stay. Reiertsen et al.[69] found laparoscopic appendectomy "at least as good" as open appendectomy. Williams et al.[70] reported that laparoscopic appendectomy resulted in less parenteral analgesia and made earlier hospital discharge possible, but at a significantly higher expense. Ortega and colleagues[71] mentioned the

same benefits, but coupled with increased operative time. In the majority of cases retroperitoneal dissection is not required. O'Connor and Reed[39] observed that the appendix was most commonly retrocecal in position, but this accounted for only 33% of cases. This fact, they believed, may encourage greater use of laparoscopic appendectomy.

The study by Hansen et al.[72] found no difference in morbidity between laparoscopic and open cases of acute appendicitis. Minné et al.[73] stated that for the routine patient with acute appendicitis, laparoscopic appendectomy does not offer any proven benefits compared to the open approach. Mutter et al.[74] reported that there were no significant advantages of laparoscopic appendectomy over open appendectomy for male patients, and recommended that laparoscopic appendectomy be performed only in men with atypical symptomatology and in obese patients. In contrast, Cox et al.[75] stated that there were significant advantages for men in terms of a more rapid recovery compared to open appendectomy, and no significant disadvantages.

- Appendicitis in pregnancy is a diagnostic problem. Baer et al.[76] emphasized the displacement of the appendix by the gravid uterus and the corresponding relocation of the pain (Fig. 17-12).
- Serour et al.[77] reported 3 cases of acute appendicitis following blunt abdominal trauma, and after an extensive review of the world literature found posttraumatic appendicitis to be a real entity to take into consideration.
- Ohno et. al.[78] presented the first report of appendiceal intussusception secondary to tubulovillous adenoma arising from the appendix.
- Nycum et al.[79] reported a case of asymptomatic intussusception of the appendix secondary to endometriosis. Collins,[11] after studying 71,000 human appendiceal specimens over the course of 40 years, reported the incidence of all causes of intussusception to be 0.1%.
- Hoeksema and Gusz[80] used colonoscopy to diagnose appendiceal intussusception, which was treated by laparoscopic appendectomy.
- Lessin et al.[81] stated that in clinically equivocal cases of appendicitis, ultrasonography is a good diagnostic modality.
- Scineaux et al.[82] recommended transvaginal ultrasonography as a diagnostic tool for patients with recurrent pelvic pain. They relied on this modality to diagnose appendicitis in a woman with chronic endometriosis.
- In contrast, a study by Lee et al.[83] disputes the value of ultrasound and CT as a diagnostic tool, and recommends selective use of diagnostic laparoscopy. We quote:

*Migratory pain, physical examination, and initial leukocytosis remain reliable and accurate in diagnos-*

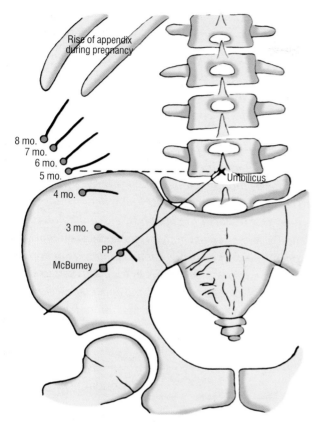

**FIG. 17-12.** Changes in position and direction of appendix during pregnancy. PP = postpartum. (Modified from Baer JL, Arens RA. Appendicitis in pregnancy. JAMA 1932;98:1359; with permission.)

*ing acute appendicitis. Neither CT nor US improves the diagnostic accuracy or the negative appendectomy rate; in fact, they may delay surgical consultation and appendectomy. In atypical cases, one should consider the selective use of diagnostic laparoscopy instead.*

- Benign and malignant neoplasms of the appendix are very rare, and according to Lyss,[84] occur in 1.08% to 1.3% of all appendiceal specimens. The most common

neoplastic processes are carcinoids, mucoceles, and rarely, epithelial and nonepithelial tumors.

- In a review of the world literature from 1875 to 1996, Hatch et al.[85] found only 23 leiomyomas and 5 leiomyosarcomas of the appendix. They strongly advised a right colectomy if the tumor shows two or more mitotic figures in every ten high-power fields.
- Krisher et al.[86] reported significantly increased rates of postoperative intra-abdominal abscess in children with perforated appendicitis when laparoscopic appendectomy was compared with open surgery in a tertiary care facility.

## ANATOMIC COMPLICATIONS OF APPENDECTOMY (Table 17-7)

### Vascular Injury

Hematoma of the mesentery of the appendix or of the ileocecal mesentery can occur as a result of appendectomy. Intraluminal bleeding is also possible. The right iliac vessels may be injured, especially with a downward-projecting "pelvic" appendix.

Hemoperitoneum can occur secondary to improper ligation of the mesentery of the appendix. McGraw[87] recommended ligation of individual branches of the appendicular artery in the mesoappendix. Kazarian et al.[88] found 6 cases of intraperitoneal hemorrhage among 539 operations for appendicitis.

### Organ Injury

The cecum, the terminal ileum, or any loop of intestine can be injured by excessive traction or rough handling. Difficult pelvic appendectomy can also cause injury to the right ureter, right uterine tube, or ovary.

A fecal fistula can form secondary to inadequate ligation or failure to invert the appendiceal stump. The fistula may

**TABLE 17-7. Summary of Anatomical Complications of Appendectomy**

| Procedure | Vascular Injury | Organ Injury | Inadequate Procedures |
|---|---|---|---|
| Appendectomy | Hematoma of the mesentery, hemoperitoneum, intraluminal bleeding, right iliac artery and vein | Perforation of cecum or intestinal loop, of right ureter, of right uterine tube or ovary | Unnecessary delay in locating appendix, failure to remove tip of appendix, remaining stump too long (appendicitis may recur) |

*Source:* Skandalakis JE, Gray SW, Rowe JS Jr. Anatomical Complications in General Surgery. New York: McGraw-Hill, 1983; with permission.

## Editorial Comment

*Adequate visualization should prevent injury to other structures. Adequate visualization may be impossible with delayed diagnosis when a patient with localized perforation of the appendix presents several days after the initiation of the process. The inflammatory mass at this stage may range from a phlegmon to a pus-filled abscess cavity. The initial treatment should usually be nonoperative. Phlegmons will usually resolve with antibiotics. True abscesses may require either surgical drainage or image-guided drainage. If surgical drainage is undertaken, appendectomy should not usually be attempted. An exception can be made when the appendix is readily visible within the abscess cavity. It is usually more prudent to carry out a delayed appendectomy after resolution of the inflammation in order to prevent damage to adjacent structures and/or spilling the contents of the abscess into the peritoneal cavity.*

*Fecal fistulas are annoying but are not usually dangerous complications of an appendectomy. They have occurred with both the inversion and noninversion techniques. A fecal fistula occurring after inversion technique may, perhaps, be due to necrosis from a purse-string suture tied too tightly or perhaps due to cecal injury. Fecal fistulas from noninverted appendiceal stump may be due to slippage of too loose a ligature or necrosis from too tight a ligature. Most fistulas will close spontaneously unless there is a retained foreign body, a distal colon obstruction, or retention of a mucous producing remnant of the appendix. Selection of inversion or noninversion technique appears to be dictated more by tradition than scientific data. With careful technique, the appendiceal stump can be managed either by simple ligation or by ligation and inversion. (RSF Jr)*

occur when preoperative perforation or severe inflammation is located at the base of the appendix or in the wall of the cecum; notwithstanding, many surgeons do not invert the stump. Kazarian et al.[88] reported an occurrence rate of fecal fistula of 0-1.4%.

## Nerve Injury

### Motor Nerves

With the use of a vertical incision, there is always the possibility of injury to the 10th, 11th, or 12th thoracic nerves, or occasionally, the iliohypogastric nerve. Such an injury will result in some degree of late muscle atrophy of the lower part of the internal oblique and transversus abdominis muscles, as well as the rectus abdominis, and the possible (but rare) development of inguinal hernia. It is always good practice to avoid damaging nerves whenever possible.

### Sensory Nerves

Division of lateral and anterior cutaneous branches of the intercostal nerves may produce transitory numbness around the incision. This will disappear in 2 to 3 months.

## Inadequate Procedure

Sound knowledge of the embryology and anatomy of the intestines is necessary to avoid inadequate procedures. Such information reduces the time a surgeon spends trying to locate and identify the appendix. This embryologic/anatomic knowledge can prevent mismanagement of acute appendicitis in an undescended cecum.

Examples of inadequate procedure are an uninverted long appendiceal stump that may be subject to recurring acute appendicitis, and a long inverted stump that may produce a radiographic filling defect that simulates a tumor. When surgeons leave an appendiceal tip in situ because of local severe inflammatory process, they do so of necessity, but realizing that complications may follow later.

The advice of Lin and colleagues[29] (which we presented earlier in the chapter) to routinely check for appendiceal duplication at surgery is another version of the sage advice that to be forewarned is to be forearmed.

Price et al.[89] advocated interval appendectomy as a critical component of the complete management of appendiceal abscess, and presented two cases in which initial drainage did not obviate the need for later extirpation.

Katkhouda et al.,[90] citing results from a minimally invasive surgical service and a general service, found significantly reduced rates of intra-abdominal abscess for perforated appendicitis in the former.

# REFERENCES

1. Fitz R. N Y Med J 1886;47:508
2. McBurney C. N Y Med J 1889;i:679
3. Worcester A. Ann Gyn Pediatr 1892;v:49
4. Morson DP, Dawson IMP. Gastrointestinal Pathology. London: Blackwell Scientific Publications, 1972, p 397.
5. Collins DC. The length and position of the vermiform appendix: a study of 4,680 specimens. Ann Surg 1932; 96:1044-48.
6. May EA. Chronic appendicitis: its roentgen diagnosis. J Med Soc NJ 1937; 34:91.
7. Wakeley CPG. The position of the vermiform appendix as ascertained by an analysis of 10,000 cases. J Anat 1933; 67:277.
8. Maisel H. The position of the human vermiform appendix in fetal and adult age groups. Anat Rec 1960; 136:385.
9. Morgagni JB. The seats and causes of disease investigated by anatomy. Alexander LB (trans). New York: Hafner Publishing, 1960.
10. Hunter W. Medical commentaries. London, 1762.
11. Collins DC. 71,000 human appendix specimens: a final report, summarizing forty years' study. Am J Proctol 1963; 14:365-81.
12. Collins DC. The chronic inflammatory and obliterative reactions of the vermiform appendix. Thesis. Post-Graduate School, University of Minnesota, June 1932.
13. Schridde H. Über den angeborenen Mangel des Processus vermiformis. Virchows Arch (Pathol Anat) 1904; 177:150.
14. Williams RA. Development, structure and function of the appendix. In: Williams RA, Myers P. Pathology of the Appendix and Its Surgical Treatment. New York: Chapman & Hall Medical, 1994, pp. 9-30.
15. Fenoglio-Preiser CM, Lantz PE, Listrom MB. Gastrointestinal Pathology: An Anthology and Text. New York: Raven Press, 1989.
16. Chevre F, Gillet M, Vuilleumier H. Agenesis of the vermiform appendix. Surg Laparosc Endosc Percutan Tech 2000; 10:110-112.
17. Fawcitt R. Appendix situated within thorax. Br J Radiol 1948; 21:523-5.
18. Babcock WW. Lumbar appendicitis and lumbar appendectomy. Surg Gynecol Obstet 1946; 82:414-6.
19. Abramson DJ. Vermiform appendix located within the cecal wall. Dis Colon Rectum 1983; 26:386-9.
20. Nisolle JF, Bodart E, de Caniere L, Bahati M, Michel L, Trigaux JP. [Acute left-side appendicitis: diagnostic contribution of tomodensitometry.] Arch Pediatr 1996;3:47-50.
21. Smith DE, Jacquet JM, Virgilio RW. Left upper quadrant appendicitis. Arch Surg 1974; 109:443.
22. Waugh TR. Appendix vermiformis duplex. Arch Surg 1941; 42:311-320.
23. Cave AJE. Appendix vermiformis duplex. J Anat 1936;70:283-292.
24. Wallbridge PH. Double appendix. Br J Surg 1963;50:346-347.
25. Kjossev KT, Losanoff JE. Duplicated vermiform appendix. Br J Surg 1996;83:1259.
26. Arda IS, Şenocak ME, Hiçsönmez A. Duplication of the vermiform appendix: case report and review of the literature. Paed Surg Int 1992;7:221-222.
27. Tinckler LF. Triple appendix vermiformis: a unique case. Br J Surg 1968;55:79-81.
28. Mesko TW, Lugo R, Breitholz T. Horseshoe anomaly of the appendix: a previously undescribed entity. Surgery 1989;106:563-566.
29. Lin BC, Chen RJ, Fang JF, Lo TH, Kuo TT. Duplication of the vermiform appendix. Eur J Surg 1996;162:589-591.
30. Royster HA. Appendicitis. New York: Appleton, 1927.
31. Favara BE. Multiple congenital diverticula of the vermiform appendix. Am J Clin Pathol 1968; 49:60-64.
32. Balsano NA, Reynolds BM. Ruptured true congenital diverticulum of vermiform appendix without associated appendicitis. NY State J Med 1971; 71:2877-78.
33. Wetzig NR. Diverticulosis of the vermiform appendix. Med J Aust 1986; 145:464-5.
34. Budd DC, Fouty WJ. Familial retrocecal appendicitis. Am J Surg 1977; 133:670-1.
35. Droga BW, Levine S, Baber JJ. Heterotopic gastric and esophageal tissue in the vermiform appendix. Am J Clin Pathol 1963; 40:190.
36. Haque S, Eisen RN, West AB. Heterotopic bone formation in the gastrointestinal tract. Arch Pathol Lab Med 1996;120:666-670.
37. Treves F. Lectures on the anatomy of the intestinal canal and peritoneum in man. Br Med J 1885; 1:527-30.
38. Buschard K, Kjaeldgaard A. Investigation and analysis of the position, fixation, length, and embryology of the vermiform appendix. Acta Chir Scand 1973;139:293-298.
39. O'Connor CE, Reed WP. In vivo location of the human vermiform appendix. Clin Anat 1994; 7:139-142.
40. Puylaert JBCM. Ultrasound of Appendicitis. New York: Springer-Verlag, 1990.
41. Ajmani ML, Ajmani K. The position, length and arterial supply of vermiform appendix. Anat Anz (Jena) 1983; 153:369-74.
42. Solanke TF. The position, length and content of the vermiform appendix in Nigerians. Br J Surg 1970; 57:100-2.
43. DeGaris CF. Topography and development of the cecum and appendix. Ann Surg 1941; 113:540-48.
44. Shah MA, Shah M. The position of the vermiform appendix. Indian Med Gaz 1945; 80:494-5.
45. Shen GK, Wong R, Daller J, Melcer S, Tsen A, Awtrey S, Rappaport W. Does the retrocecal position of the vermiform appendix alter the clinical course of acute appendicitis? Arch Surg 1991; 26:569-70.
46. Owen RL, Nemanic P. Antigen processing structures of the mammalian intestinal tract. Scanning Electron Microsc 1978;II: 367-78.
47. Ferguson A. The immune system and mucosal transformation - historical perspective. Digestion 1990;46(Suppl 2):255-61.
48. Brunagel G, Decker P, Hirner A. [Delayed appendico-cutaneous fistula: a rare complication of simple abdominal drainage.] Zentralbl Chir 1996;121:67-69.
49. Hollinshead WH. Anatomy for Surgeons. New York: Hoeber-Harper, 1956.
50. Anson BJ, McVay CB. Surgical Anatomy (5th ed). Philadelphia: Saunders, 1971.
51. Maingot R. Abdominal Operations (6th ed). New York: Appleton-Century-Crofts, 1974.
52. Michels NA. The variant blood supply to the small and large intestines. J Int Coll Surg 1963; 39:127.
53. Solanke TF. The blood supply of the vermiform appendix in Nigerians. J Anat 1968;102:353-361.
54. Van Damme JPJ. Behavioral anatomy of the abdominal arteries.

Surg Clin North Am 1993;73:699-725.

55. Bertelli L, Lorenzini L, Bertelli E. The arterial vascularization of the large intestine: anatomical and radiological study. Surg Radiol Anat 1996;18(Suppl I):S1-S59.

56. Kelly HA, Hurdon E. The Vermiform Appendix and Its Diseases. Philadelphia: Saunders, 1905.

57. Braithwaite LR. The flow of lymph from the ileocecal angle and its possible bearing on the cause of duodenal and gastric ulcer. Br J Surg 1923; 11:7.

58. McBurney C. Experiences with early operative interference in cases of disease of the vermiform appendix. NY Med J 1889, 50:676.

59. Du Plessis DJ. A Synopsis of Surgical Anatomy (11th ed). Bristol: Wright and Sons, 1975.

60. Karim OM, Boothroyd AE, Wyllie JH. McBurney's point - fact or fiction? Ann R Coll Surg Engl 1990; 72:304-8.

61. Ramsden WH, Mannion RA, Simpkins KC, deDombal FT. Is the appendix where you think it is — and if not does it matter? Clin Radiol 1993; 47:100-3.

62. Berry J Jr., Malt RA. Appendicitis near its centenary. Ann Surg 1984; 200:567-75.

63. Guidry SP, Poole GV. The anatomy of appendicitis. Am Surg 1994;60:68-71.

64. Stevenson RJ. Chronic right-lower-quadrant abdominal pain: is there a role for elective appendectomy? J Pediatr Surg 1999;34:950-54.

65. Wong DW, Vasinrapee P, Spieth ME, Cook RE, Ansari AN, Jones M Jr, Mandal A. Rapid detection of acute appendicitis with Tc-99m-labeled intact polyvalent human immune globulin. J Am Coll Surg 185:534-543, 1997.

66. Chen SC, Chen KM, Wang SM, Chang KJ. Abdominal sonography screening of clinically diagnosed or suspected appendicitis before surgery. World J Surg 1998;22:449-452.

67. Crombe A, Weber F, Gruner L, Martins A, Fouque P, Barth X. [Abdominopelvic ultrasonography in suspected acute appendicitis: prospective study in adults]. Ann Chir 2000;125:57-61.

68. Buckley RC, Hall TJ, Muakkassa FF, Anglin B, Rhodes RS, Scott-Conner CEH. Laparaoscopic appendectomy: is it worth it? Am Surg 1994; 60:30-4.

69. Reiertsen O, Trondsen E, Bakka A, Andersen OK, Larsen S, Rosseland AR. Prospective nonrandomized study of conventional versus laparoscopic appendectomy. World J Surg 1994; 18:411-6.

70. Williams MD, Miller D, Graves ED, Walsh C, Luterman A. Laparoscopic appendectomy, is it worth it? South Med J 1994; 87:592-8.

71. Ortega AE, Hunter JG, Peters JH, Swanstrom LL, Schirmer B, and the Laparoscopic Appendectomy Study Group. A prospective, randomized comparison of laparoscopic appendectomy with open appendectomy. Am J Surg 1995; 169:208-213.

72. Hansen JB, Smithers BM, Schache D, Wall DR, Miller BJ, Menzies BL. Laparoscopic vesus open appendectomy: prospective randomized trial. World J Surg 20:17-21, 1996.

73. Minné L, Varner D, Burnell A, Ratzer E, Jeffrey Clark, Haun W. Laparoscopic vs open appendectomy: prospective randomized study of outcomes. Arch Surg 132:708-712, 1997.

74. Mutter D, Vix M, Bui A, Evrard S, Tassetti V, Breton JF, Marescaux J. Laparoscopy not recommended for routine appendectomy in men: results of a prospective randomized study. Surgery 120:71-74, 1996.

75. Cox MR, McCall JL, Toouli J, Padbury RTA, Wilson TG, Wattchow DA, Langcake M. Prospective randomized comparison of open versus laparoscopic appendectomy in men. World J Surg 20:263-266, 1996.

76. Baer JL, Reis RA, Arens RA. Appendicitis in pregnancy. JAMA 1932; 98:1359.

77. Serour F, Efrati Y, Klin B, Shikar S, Weinberg M, Vinograd I. Acute appendicitis following abdominal trauma. Arch Surg 131: 130-785-786, 1996.

78. Ohno M, Nakamura T, Hori H, Tabuchi Y, Kuroda Y. Appendiceal intussusception induced by tubulovillous adenoma with carcinoma in situ: report of a case. Surg Today 2000;30:441-444.

79. Nycum LR, Moss H, Adams JQ, Macri CI. Asymptomatic intussusception of the appendix due to endometriosis. So Med J 1999;92(5):524-25.

80. Hoeksema MA, Gusz JR. Appendiceal intussusception. J Am Coll Surg 2001;192:538.

81. Lessin MS, Chan M, Catallozzi M, Gilchrist BF, Richards C, Manera L, Wallach MT, Luks FI. Selective use of ultrasonography for acute appendicitis in children. Am J Surg 1999;177:193-96.

82. Scineaux TL, Sills ES, Perloe M, Daly JP. Transvaginal ultrasonographic identification of appendicitis in a setting of chronic pelvic pain and endometriosis. South Med J 2001;94:73-74.

83. Lee SL, Walsh AJ, Ho HS. Computed tomography and ultrasonography do not improve and may delay the diagnosis and treatment of acute appendicitis. Arch Surg 136:556-562, 2001.

84. Lyss AP. Appendiceal malignancies. Semin Oncol 15:129, 1988.

85. Hatch KF, Blanchard DK, Hatch GF III, Wertheimer-Hatch L, Davis GB, Foster RS Jr, Skandalakis JE. Smooth muscle (stromal) tumors of the appendix and colon. World J Surg 2000;24:430-436.

86. Krisher SL, Browne A, Dibbins A, Thacz N, Curci M. Intra-abdominal abscess after laparoscopic appendectomy for perforated appendicitis. Arch Surg 2001;136:438-441.

87. McGraw AB. Factors contributing to low mortality from appendectomy for acute appendicitis: ten year study. Arch Surg 1949;58:171.

88. Kazarian KK, Roeder WJ, Mersheimer WL. Decreasing mortality and increasing morbidity from acute appendicitis. Am J Surg 1970; 119:681.

89. Price MR, Haase GM, Sartorelli KH, Meagher DP Jr. Recurrent appendicitis after initial conservative management of appendiceal abscesses. J Pediatr Surg 1996;31:291-294.

90. Katkhouda N, Friedlander MH, Grant SW, Achanta KK, Essani R, Paik P, Velmahos G, Campos G, Mason R, Mavor E. Intra-abdominal abscess rate after laparoscopic appendectomy. Am J Surg 2000;180:456-461.

# Chapter *18*

# *Large Intestine and Anorectum*

JOHN E. SKANDALAKIS, ANDREW N. KINGSNORTH,
GENE L. COLBORN, THOMAS A. WEIDMAN,
PANAJIOTIS N. SKANDALAKIS, LEE J. SKANDALAKIS

*Followed by a Special Section Written by* AHMED SHAFIK

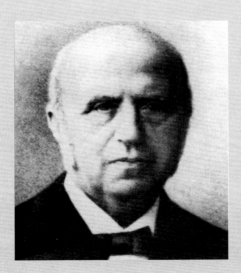

**Harald Hirschsprung (1830-1916)** published his classic work about congenital megacolon (Hirschsprung's disease) in 1889.

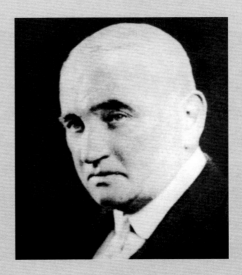

**W. Ernest Miles (1869-1947)** developed the combined abdominoperineal resection in 1926.

*For surgical practice, behavioral anatomy is more important than variational anatomy. It has been possible, indeed, to define rules and behavioral explanations that allow us to understand and thus memorize easily the overwhelming number of variations in the abdominal blood supply. Variational anatomy is like the wiring diagram of a television set, whereas behavioral anatomy is its remote controller.*

*Van Damme*[1]

*If it looks like a clover, the trouble is over,
If it looks like a dahlia, it's surely a failure.*

*(Description by* **Ferguson and Parks**[2] *of the margins of the wound after hemorrhoidectomy)*

The large intestine is formed by the following anatomic entities:
- Ileocecal valve
- Appendix
- Cecum
- Ascending colon
- Hepatic flexure
- Transverse colon
- Splenic flexure
- Descending colon
- Sigmoid colon
- Anorectum

In this book, the appendix has been presented in the preceding chapter.

Following our presentations on the above list of topics is a special section written by Professor Ahmed Shafik. Dr. Shafik, who is chairman of the Department of Surgery and Experimental Research at the medical school of Cairo University, Egypt, is such an original thinker in regard to the large intestine and anorectum that we invited him to share his unique perspective with our readers. We are grateful to him for interpreting his research and offering his philosophy to us, and we are honored to provide his excellent work on the large intestine and anorectum to our readers. We encourage careful thought about Dr. Shafik's innovative ideas.

Note: Some writers use the word "colon" to mean the collectivity of four anatomic entities: ascending, transverse, descending, and sigmoid colons. Occasionally we will employ the word "colon" or "colonic" in that manner to mean "large intestine" (e.g. "colonic" wall for "large intestinal" wall).

## HISTORY

The anatomic and surgical history of the large intestine and anorectum is shown in Table 18-1.

## EMBRYOGENESIS

### Normal Development

During herniation of the intestines into the umbilical cord (Fig. 18-1), a slight local enlargement of the portion posterior to the superior mesenteric artery marks the site of the future cecum. Growth and differentiation of this postarterial limb lags behind that of the proximal prearterial limb when the intestines return to the abdomen.

Goblet cells and epithelial cells with a striate border may be found in the colon by the eleventh week. During the third month, villi and glands appear. The villi reach their maximum development in the fourth month and gradually shorten and disappear with the enlargement of the colon in the seventh and eighth months.

Langman and Rowland[3] reported that the estimated total number of lymphoid follicles in the large intestine is between 12,761 and 18,432. The average follicular density is 18.4 per $cm^2$ in the cecum, 15.0 per $cm^2$ in the colon, and 25.4 per $cm^2$ in the rectum. Previously reported numbers were very low; perhaps these new numbers will remind the physician about the diagnosis of lymphoid hyperplasia.

| T A B L E | | 18-1. Anatomic and Surgical History of the Large Intestine |
|---|---|---|
| Hippocrates | ca. 400 B.C. | Treated hemorrhoids with white-hot iron or by burning them off; treated fistulas by use of seton |
| Aristotle (384-322 B.C.) | | Used the word "colon"; noted that congenital malformations occurred more often in boys than girls |
| Soranos of Ephesus (A.D. 98-138) | | Performed digital rupture of membranes of the anal canal of newborns |
| Galen (121-201 A.D.) | | Named the rectum "apefthismenon" |
| Paul of Aegina (625-690 A.D.) | | Collected lost works of Heliodorus, Leonidas, and Antyllus, and presented first description of a surgical technique for anal atresia |
| Albertus Magnus (1193-1280) | | Works indicate that anal atresia was well known during Middle Ages |
| John Arderne | 1367 | Wrote paper that contained the basis of anorectal surgery |
| Antonius Benivenius (1513-1572) | | Studied recto-anal agenesis in autopsy; reported recto-anal agenesis with vaginal fistula |
| Tobias Cneulinus | ca. 1580 | Unsuccessful perineal operation for recto-anal agenesis because the rectum could not be identified |
| Fabricius Hildanus | 1593 | Successfully opened anal agenesis by incision, introduction of rectal speculum, dilatation of the opening, and application of lead carbonate and meninge-dye |
| J.S. von Grafenberg | 1609 | Reported the first case of anal agenesis with urethral fistula; reported isolated rectal atresia without anal atresia |
| G.T. Dürr | 1668 | Described anus copertus with perineal fistula; incised the anal membrane and the obstructed anus, curing the child |
| Hendrik van Roonhuysen | 1676 | Ruptured anal stenosis with a knife and successfully maintained the opening with salves and instruments |
| Physician to King Louis XIV | 1686 | Conceived of and performed fistulotomy on the king |
| Frederik Ruysch (1638-1731) | ca. 1700 | Reported spontaneous rupture of anal atresia in a 5-day-old child (who died soon thereafter) |
| Saviard | 1702 | In a child with no trace of an anus, he inserted a lancet, and entered the blind rectal pouch. Meconium was released and the child survived. |
| Littré | 1710 | Successfully treated imperforate anus by opening colon in left lower quadrant of abdomen |
| Heister | 1718 | Operated – using a trocar – on two children whose rectum ended at the level of upper sacrum; both died |
| Barbout | 1739 to 1775 | Reported two cases of recto-anal agenesis with recto-cloacal fistula |
| Percivall Pott | 1765 | British doctor whose writings pointed up the advances Britons had made in colorectal diseases and surgery |
| Pillore | 1776 | Performed cecostomy for cancer of the lower bowel |
| Petit | 1781 | Incising for recto-anal agenesis, a tumor, but no rectum, was found. After incision of the tumor, meconium discharged. Patient died. |
| Benjamin Bell | 1787 | Successfully treated 2 cases of recto-anal agenesis; newly formed orifices tended to shrink from scar tissue |
| Duret | 1793 | Successfully treated imperforate anus by opening left lower quadrant of colon |
| Latta | 1795 | Successfully treated recto-anal agenesis, but dilatation therapy was required for nine full months |
| Callisen | 1798 | Suggested extraperitoneal colostomy at the lumbar area for imperforate anus |
| Meckel | 1817 | Studied embryology of the normal colon |
| Lisfranc (1790-1847) | | Operated on colonic tumors |

| T A B L E | | 18-1 *(cont'd)*. Anatomic and Surgical History of the Large |
|---|---|---|
| Frederick Salmon<br><br>William Allingham | 1835 | Salmon was founder and chief surgeon of St. Mark's Hospital in London, which was the pinnacle of knowledge and treatment of colon and rectal diseases<br>At this hospital William Allingham wrote the first textbook devoted entirely to anorectal disease; it describes hemorrhoid treatment by excision and ligature |
| Amussat | 1835<br>1839 | Described surgery for imperforate anus.<br>Adopted Callisen's procedure. |
| G.M. Bushe | 1837 | Wrote first American proctology book that later acquired international acclaim |
| Nélaton | 1839 | Exposed, fixed, and incised distended loop of bowel proximal to obstruction |
| Miller | 1857 | First successful operation for recto-anal agenesis with bladder fistula |
| J.H. Bigelow | 1858 | Wrote that at the present state of the art of surgery, children with rectal or anal atresia should die without operation |
| W.H. Bodenhamer | 1860 | First to produce a clear classification of rectal and anal malformations |
| Teale (1801-1868) | | Favored exploratory surgery for bowel obstruction |
| Mason | 1873 | Reported 80 cases of colostomy for obstruction with 32.5% mortality |
| Wilks | 1875 | Described ulcerative colitis |
| Hutchinson | 1878 | "...exploratory operations for the relief of abdominal obstruction, the cause of which cannot be diagnosed, are not warrantable." Stated that by the time a surgeon is called, "the stage at which abdominal taxis is most hopeful has passed." |
| J.W. Matthews | 1878 | American physician began teaching in America the principals of anorectal surgery he had learned at St. Mark's Hospital, London |
| Edmund Andrews & E.W. Andrews | 1878 | Co-authored one of the first textbooks on anorectal surgery |
| Billroth | 1879 | Performed sigmoid resection and exteriorization of the proximal bowel as permanent colostomy |
| Kraske & Kocher | ca. 1880 | Perfected the sacral approach to rectal tumors |
| Parker | 1883 | Urged extension of protracted palliative management of intestinal obstruction |
| Reybard | 1884 | Reported survival after resection and anastomosis for cancer of the colon |
| Greves | 1885 | Advocated operative intervention for intestinal obstruction |
| Bryant | 1885 | Reverted to the intraperitoneal maneuvers of Pillore and Duret |
| Tait (1845-1899) | | Remarked that accurate diagnosis could only be made by exploration, "which is better performed before than after death" |
| H.O. Thomas | 1885 | Published monograph against surgical intervention for intestinal obstruction, "The Collegian of 1666 and the Collegians of 1885." Stated that cases of acute intestinal obstruction "belonged to the department of medicine, the surgeon was a mere assistant... An operation may be required in a few hours or it may not be required for weeks." |
| Mikulicz | 1886 | Reverting from his formerly more aggressive surgical approach, decided that laparotomy often offered no hopeful prospect for relief of acute intestinal obstruction |
| Hirschsprung | 1886 | Described autopsies of two infants who died from congenital megacolon (Hirschsprung's disease) |
| Fitz & Senn | 1888 | Advised 48-72 hours observation before patient diagnosed with intestinal obstruction was turned over to the surgeon |
| Retterer | 1890 | Studied urorectal septum and cloaca |
| Bloch & Paul | 1892<br>to 1895 | Development of "obstructive resection," in which portion of bowel with tumor is brought outside abdominal cavity; 1-2 days later, it is divided by cautery, forming a "loop" or "double-barreled" colostomy |
| Mall | 1898<br>1899 | Studied the development and position of the human intestine.<br>Observed the extraembryonic growth of the intestines and their return to the abdomen. |
| J.W. Matthews | 1899 | Became one of founders of American Proctologic Society. Later called "the Father of Proctology." |

## TABLE 18-1 *(cont'd)*. Anatomic and Surgical History of the Large

| | | |
|---|---|---|
| Mikulicz | 1905 | Perfected and popularized obstructive resection |
| W.E. Miles | 1908 | British surgeon who described combined abdominoperineal resection for rectal cancer |
| Chilaiditi | 1910 | Described hepatic flexure between liver and diaphragm |
| Morton | 1912 | Offered a description of congenital absence of the colon using segmental arterial ligation in dogs |
| Johnson | 1913 | Studied development of colonic mucosa |
| Dott | 1923 | Developed a classification of abnormalities of intestinal rotation based on embryologic observations |
| Henri Hartmann | 1923 | Described treatment for obstructing carcinoma of the distal colon |
| Miles | 1926 | Developed combined abdominoperineal resection |
| Rankin | 1930 | Improved the double-barreled colostomy |
| Cuthbert Dukes | 1932 | Originated classification for carcinoma of the rectum |
| Ladd & Gross | 1934 | Created a new classification of anorectal anomalies that was the standard for many years |
| Kirschner | 1934 | German doctor demonstrated a combined synchronous approach to the abdominoperineal resection |
| Gilchrist | 1938, 1952 | Published studies of retrograde lymphatic spread in regard to gastrointestinal carcinoma |
| Swenson | 1950 | Designed operation for anal sphincter-preserving removal of aganglionic segments of colon |
| Stephens | 1953 | Recognized that the puborectalis muscle is the most critical to continence |
| Scott | 1959 | Investigated autonomic supply of the rectum and anorectum |
| Duthie & Gairns | 1960 | Investigated sensory innervation of the lower anal canal |
| Skandalakis et al. | 1962 | Collective review of cases of smooth muscle tumors of the colon, appendix, and rectum as reported in the world literature |
| Painter & Burkitt | 1971 | Studied relationship of low-residue diet to diverticulosis |
| Stephens & Smith | 1984 | Classified anorectal anomalies as high, intermediate, low cloacal, and rare |
| Peña | 1990 | Recommended posterior sagittal anorectoplasty |

*History table compiled by David A. McClusky III and John E. Skandalakis.*

**References**

Estrada RL. Anomalies of Intestinal Rotation and Fixation. Springfield IL: Charles C. Thomas, 1958.

Kevorkian J. The Story of Dissection. New York: Philosophical Library, 1959.

Muldoon JP. History of colorectal surgery. In: Mazier WP, Levien DH, Luchtefeld MA, Senagore AJ (eds). Surgery of the Colon, Rectum, and Anus. Philadelphia: WB Saunders, 1995.

Schärli AF. Malformations of the anus and rectum and their treatment in medical history. Prog Pediatr Surg 11:141-172, 1978.

Skandalakis JE, Gray SW, Shepard D, Bourne GH. Smooth Muscle Tumors of the Alimentary Canal: Leiomyomas and Leiomyosarcomas, a Review of 2525 Cases. Springfield IL: Charles C. Thomas, 1962.

Skandalakis JE, Gray SW. Embryology for Surgeons (2nd ed). Baltimore: Williams & Wilkins, 1994.

Wangensteen OH, Wangensteen SD. The Rise of Surgery. Minneapolis: University of Minnesota Press, 1978.

Warren R. Surgery. Philadelphia: WB Saunders, 1963.

The circular layer of muscularis externa appears caudally in the ninth week and spreads cranially. Ganglion cells of the myenteric plexus of Auerbach reach the colon in the seventh week, and innervation appears to be complete by the twelfth week.[4] The first longitudinal muscle fibers are present at the anal canal in the tenth week. Above the sigmoid colon, the longitudinal fibers extend cranially only along the mesenteric border of the colon, reaching the cecum in the eleventh week. By the fourth month, the entire colon is covered, but growth of the muscle coat does not keep up with increasing colon diameter. By the fourth month, the longitudinal muscle coat becomes separated into three bands, the taeniae coli. Meconium gradually fills the colon and the lower ileum until birth.

REMEMBER: The colon is produced by both the midgut and

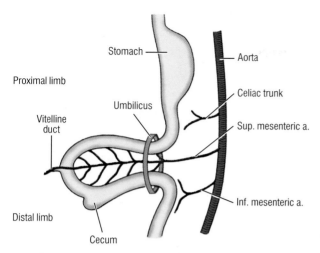

**FIG. 18-1.** Diagram of the growth of the embryonic midgut into the umbilical cord. Fifth week of gestation. The distal limb shows a swelling at the site of the cecum. The three great arteries supplying the stomach and intestines are remnants of the earlier vitelline arteries. (Modified from Skandalakis JE, Gray SW, Rowe JS Jr. Anatomical Complications in General Surgery. New York: McGraw-Hill, 1983; with permission.)

the hindgut. The midgut is responsible for the genesis of the cecum, the ascending colon, and the proximal 2/3 of the transverse colon. The hindgut is responsible for the remainder of the colon, the rectum, and the proximal part of the anus. To be more specific, the distal 1/3 of the transverse colon, the descending colon, the sigmoid colon, the rectum and the proximal part of the anal canal develop from the hindgut.

The distal part of the surgical anal canal is not related embryologically to the hindgut. It most likely originates from the anal pit, which is of ectodermal origin. As O'Rahilly and Müller[5] wrote, "the anal canal is probably derived from the cloaca." To be more anatomically correct but still speculative about the embryology of the anorectum, we present the following information by Rowe et al.[6] about the cloacal region.

*In the fifth week, the embryonic cloaca is an endodermal sac receiving the hindgut dorsally and the allantoic stalk ventrally. The cloaca (Fig. 18-2A, B) is separated from the outside by a thin cloacal membrane (proctodeum), which occupies the embryo's ventral surface between the tail and the body stalk. During the sixth week, a septum of mesoderm divides the cloaca into a ventral urogenital sinus and a dorsal rectum (Fig. 18-2C) . This mesodermic septum fuses with the cloacal membrane in the seventh week to form the perineal body. The cloacal membrane is divided into a larger, ventral urogenital membrane and a*

*smaller, dorsal anal membrane. Externally, the anal membrane becomes slightly depressed, forming the anal dimple.*

*By the eighth week, the anal membrane ruptures, leaving no trace of itself (Fig. 18-2D). The pectinate line in the adult is often considered to be at the level of the anal membrane, but little evidence exists to either support or contradict this view. Whatever the exact line of demarcation, the rectum and the upper anal canal are endodermal and are supplied by the inferior mesenteric artery, while the lower anal canal is ectodermal and is supplied by branches of the internal iliac artery.*

*On either side of the anal membrane, the somatic mesoderm forms a pair of anal tubercles. These tubercles fuse dorsally into a horseshoe-shaped structure. By the tenth week, the ventral tips of the horseshoe fuse with the perineal body. Striated muscle in this horseshoe-shaped structure will later become the superficial portion of the external anal sphincter. The anal sphincter will form at the normal location even if the rectum should end blindly or should open at another site.*

The superior mesenteric artery (SMA) and the inferior mesenteric artery (IMA) provide the blood supply of the entire colon. In the surgical anal canal, the branches of the internal pudendal artery participate.

## Congenital Anomalies of the Colon

### Stenoses and Atresias

Stenoses and atresias occur in the same pattern as those of the small intestine (see "Stenoses and Atresias" in the small intestine chapter). They are less common in the large intestine, with an incidence ranging from 4.6 percent[7] to 11.7 percent[8] of all intestinal atresias. More type I (diaphragmatic) atresias occur in the ascending and sigmoid colons, and more type III (complete segmental) atresias occur in the transverse colon.[9] Treatment is the same as that for atresias of the small intestine.

Dalla Vecchia et al.[10] reported 277 cases of intestinal atresia and stenosis, detailing the treatment and results. The obstruction was duodenal in 138 (50%) [79 (57%) female, 59 (43%) male], jejunoileal in 128 (46%) [61 (48%) female, 67 (52%) male], and colonic in 21 (8%) [8 (38%) female, 13 (62%) male]. Patients with colon atresia were managed with initial ostomy and delayed anastomosis in 18 of 21 patients (86%) and resection with primary anastomosis in 3 (14%).

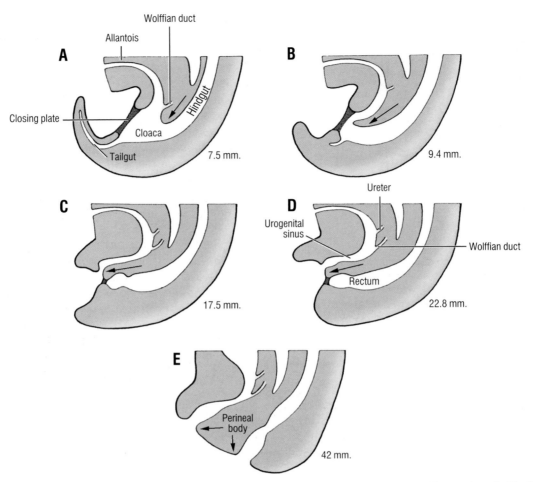

FIG. 18-2. Diagram of stages in development of the anus and rectum from the fifth to tenth weeks of gestation. **A,** Closing plate (proctodeum separates the cloaca from the outside). Urorectal septum *(arrow)* grows downward to divide the cloaca. **B,** Cloaca almost separated into dorsal rectum and ventral urogenital sinus. Tailgut is vanishing. **C,** Fusion of urorectal septum with closing plate to form the perineal body. **D,** Closing plates rupture. **E,** Division into rectum and urogenital sinus by the perineal body is complete. (Modified from Skandalakis JE, Gray SW. Embryology for Surgeons (2nd ed). Baltimore: Williams & Wilkins, 1994; with permission.)

We quote from Lambrecht and Kluth[11] on hereditary multiple atresias of the gastrointestinal tract:

*Hereditary multiple atresias have several unique features: (1) the abdominal x-ray shows signs of gastric or duodenal atresia combined with typical large rounded or oval homogeneous calcifications in the abdominal cavity, (2) intraoperatively widespread atresias (exclusively type I and II) extending mostly from the stomach to rectum are found, (3) cystic dilatation of the bile ducts can be present in cases with both complete pyloric and duodenal or proximal jejunal atresia, (4) the pathogenesis is still speculative; a combined immunodeficiency should be excluded, and (5) a fatal outcome is the rule.*

## Congenital Aganglionic Megacolon (Hirschsprung's Disease)

Aganglionic megacolon is the result of an absence of ganglion cells in a distal segment of colon. Neurenteric ganglion cells normally originate in the neural crest, enter the cranial end of the esophagus, and then follow vagus nerve fibers caudally until the entire gut is innervated. Why the migrating cells sometimes stop short of the rectum is unknown.

As seen in Fig. 18-3, only 4%[12] of the aganglionic segments of the colon are found proximal to the splenic flexure. It is interesting to note that the neural crest cells forming these intestinal ganglia follow the vagus with a

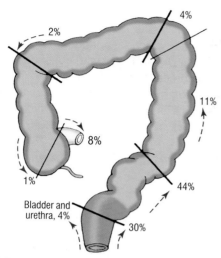

**FIG. 18-3.** Relative frequency of aganglionic segments by length of segment affected. Most cases involve the rectum and sigmoid colon only. (Modified from Skandalakis JE, Gray SW. Embryology for Surgeons (2nd ed). Baltimore: Williams & Wilkins, 1994; with permission.)

low failure rate to the end of that nerve's distribution, i.e., approximately up to the splenic flexure. The remainder of the colon and rectum receive their parasympathetic innervation via the second, third, and fourth sacral nerves which have a more or less diffuse pathway to the colon themselves. Perhaps they do not serve as effectively as a "guide" or "transporter" of the neural crest cells for their migration into the hindgut derivative. Postganglionic fibers from proximal normal ganglia, as well as preganglionic parasympathetic fibers, are usually present. The aganglionic segment usually extends into the sigmoid colon, but the whole of the large intestine and even part of the small intestine can be affected (Fig. 18-3).[13]

The greatly dilated proximal segment is normal; the narrowed distal segment is without ganglia (Fig. 18-4). The line of resection must be within the area in which ganglion cells are present. Because aganglionosis (Fig. 18-5) is not the only cause of megacolon, a biopsy is necessary to demonstrate the absence of ganglion cells in the narrowed segment and their presence in the dilated segment.

Remember to differentiate between congenital megacolon and massive fecal impaction. Because massive fecal impaction may lead to megarectum causing abdominal compartment syndrome and colorectal obstruction, perforation, or necrosis, Lohlun et al.[14] recommend prompt manual disimpaction or appropriate operative treatment.

Wulkan and Georgeson[15] recommend primary laparo-

scopic endorectal pull-through surgery as a safe and effective procedure for Hirschsprung's disease in infants and children.

### Colonic Malposition

There are several types of malposition. In Chilaiditi syndrome, the hepatic flexure is situated between the liver and the diaphragm due to anomalies of the hepatic ligaments. We quote from Balthazar:[16]

> Positional anomalies of the colon may be explained by an arrest in the normal development of the distal midgut. Aberrations involving the incipient stages of rotation lead to severe malpositions, while those involving the latter stages to milder forms... There is a high incidence of associated failure of fixation resulting in mobile colons that can be demonstrated radiographically. In addition, the great majority of colonic malrotations demonstrate rotational abnormalities involving the proximal intestinal tract. Their clinical implication is related to the presence of other incidental congenital anomalies or to complications derived from faulty mesenteric fixations such as peritoneal bands, adhesions, kinking, or intestinal volvulus.

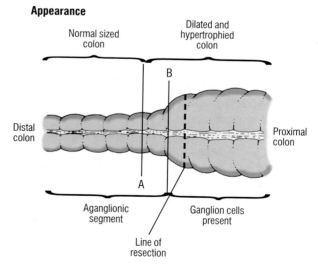

**FIG. 18-4.** Gross appearance and biopsy findings in aganglionic megacolon. On gross examination the normal colon is thought to end at *A,* but biopsy findings reveal that the aganglionic segment extends to *B.* Resection must be through the dilated proximal portion in which ganglion cells are present. (Modified from Skandalakis JE, Gray SW, Rowe JS Jr. Anatomical Complications in General Surgery. New York: McGraw-Hill, 1983; with permission.)

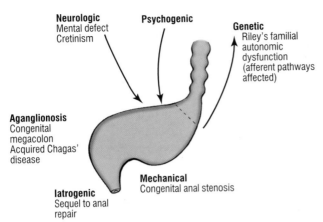

FIG. 18-5. Possible causes of megacolon which must be considered in diagnosis. (Modified from Skandalakis JE, Gray SW. Embryology for Surgeons (2nd ed). Baltimore: Williams & Wilkins, 1994; with permission.)

DePrima et al.[17] reported reversed intestinal rotation due to abnormal rotation and fixation.

Retropsoas positioned bowel (colonic positioning posterior or posterolateral to the psoas muscle at a level below the lower kidney pole) may occur in the ascending or descending colon. Prassopoulos et al.[18] advised that this condition be considered when performing percutaneous diskectomy or other interventional procedures in the posterior retroperitoneum.

## Congenital Short Colon

Congenital short colon is total or partial replacement of the colon by a pouch, as well as associated anorectal malformation and colourinary fistula. A case of congenital short colon with imperforate anus was reported by Herman et al.[19] An excellent paper about congenital short colon by Wakhlu et al.[20] advised that the initial procedure be a window colostomy, followed by pouch excision/ coloplasty and pull-through by a combined abdominal and posterior sagittal approach when the baby is 6 months old.

## Congenital Anomalies of the Anorectum

Multiple classifications of anorectal anomalies exist; none is perfect. We present a highly diagrammatic review of these anomalies with the hope that the student of embryology will be able to visualize these enigmatic malformations topographicoanatomically (Table 18-2 and Figs. 18-6 through 18-11).

While most anorectal malformations are diagnosed at birth, a significant number of mild lesions may not be recognized until later. Kim et al.[21] recommend that older infants and children with cardiac, genitourinary, or VACTERL (vertebral, anal, cardiac, tracheosophageal, esophageal, renal, limb) anomalies who present with constipation be evaluated for low anorectal malformations.

Connaughton et al.[22] presented a case of rectal duplication cyst with a large perineal hernia which presented as recurrent perineal abscesses.

## Imperforate Anus and Related Anomalies

Immediate relief of the acute colonic obstruction is provided by colostomy, after which further repair can be planned. Remember that the first operation has the greatest chance for a successful outcome. The best procedure may be less than perfectly successful if it follows an earlier, inadequate attempt at repair.

The procedures following colostomy vary with the specific anatomy of the defect to be treated. They are outside the field of general surgery.

Another anomaly is the posteriorly situated retroperitoneal colon (see Descending Colon, Surgical Considerations).

### TABLE 18-2. Anatomic Classification of Anorectal Malformations

| Female | Male |
|---|---|
| High | High |
|   Anorectal agenesis |   Anorectal agenesis |
|     With rectovaginal fistula |     With rectoprostatic urethral fistula[a] |
|     Without fistula |     Without fistula |
|   Rectal atresia |   Rectal atresia |
| Intermediate | Intermediate |
|   Rectovestibular fistula |   Rectobulbar urethral fistula |
|   Rectovaginal fistula |   Anal agenesis without fistula |
|   Anal agenesis without fistula | |
| Low | Low |
|   Anovestibular fistula[a] |   Anocutaneous fistula[a] |
|   Anocutaneous fistula[a,b] |   Anal stenosis[a,c] |
|   Anal stenosis[c] | |
| Cloacal malformations[d] | |
| Rare malformations | Rare malformations |

[a]Relatively common lesion.
[b]Includes fistulae occurring at the posterior junction of the labia minora often called "fourchette fistulae" or "vulvar fistulae."
[c]Previously called "covered anus."
[d]Previously called "rectocloacal fistulae." Entry of the rectal fistula into the cloaca may be high or intermediate, depending on the length of the cloacal canal.

*Source:* Skandalakis JE, Gray SW (eds). Embryology for Surgeons, 2nd Ed. Baltimore: Williams & Wilkins, 1994; with permission.

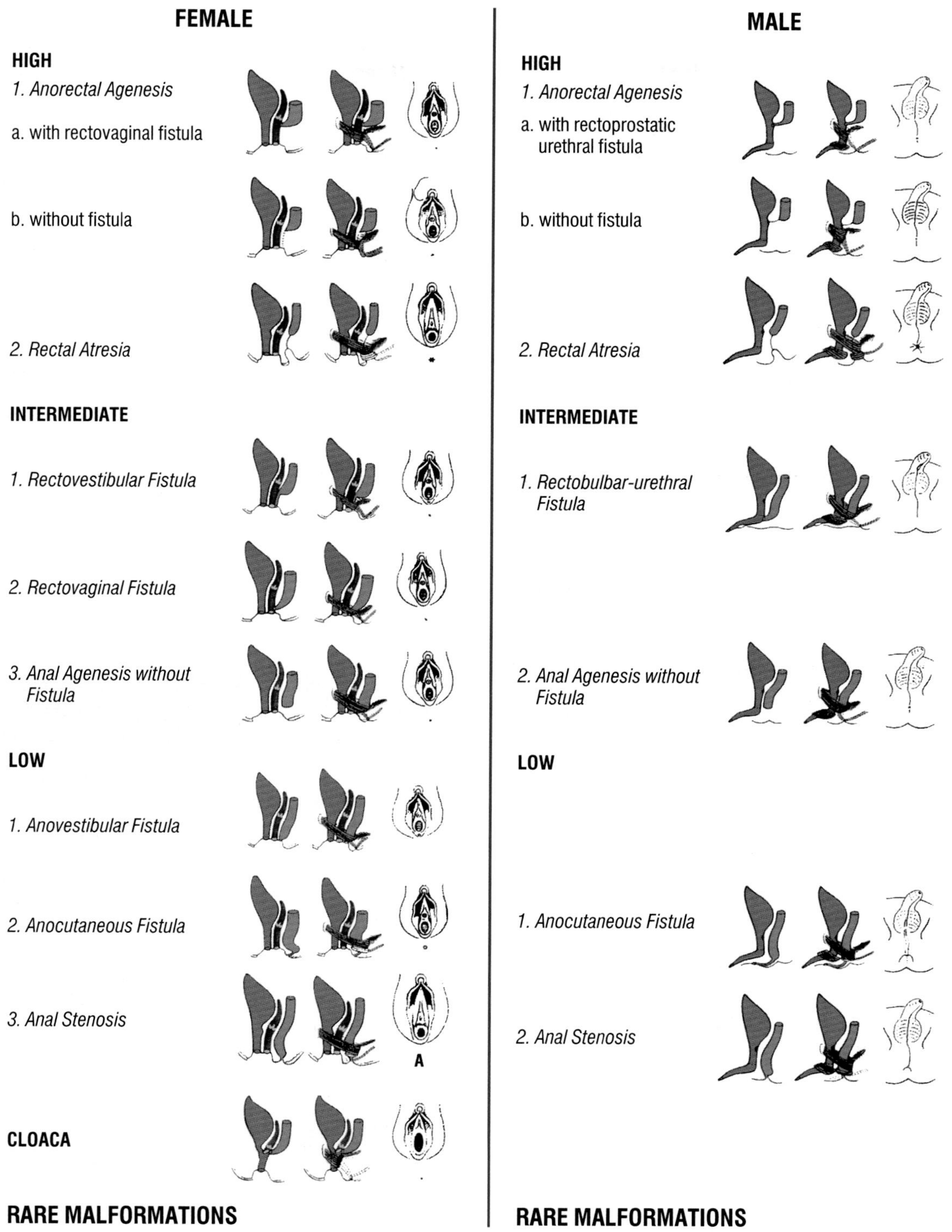

## FEMALE

**HIGH**

1. Anorectal Agenesis

a. with rectovaginal fistula

b. without fistula

2. Rectal Atresia

**INTERMEDIATE**

1. Rectovestibular Fistula

2. Rectovaginal Fistula

3. Anal Agenesis without Fistula

**LOW**

1. Anovestibular Fistula

2. Anocutaneous Fistula

3. Anal Stenosis

A

**CLOACA**

**RARE MALFORMATIONS**

## MALE

**HIGH**

1. Anorectal Agenesis

a. with rectoprostatic urethral fistula

b. without fistula

2. Rectal Atresia

**INTERMEDIATE**

1. Rectobulbar-urethral Fistula

2. Anal Agenesis without Fistula

**LOW**

1. Anocutaneous Fistula

2. Anal Stenosis

**RARE MALFORMATIONS**

FIG. 18-6. Classification of anorectal malformations. (Modified from Raffensperger JG (ed). Swenson's Pediatric Surgery (5th ed). Norwalk CT: Appleton & Lange, 1990; with permission. Prepared by Kascot Media, Inc., for the Department of Surgery, Children's Memorial Hospital, Chicago IL.)

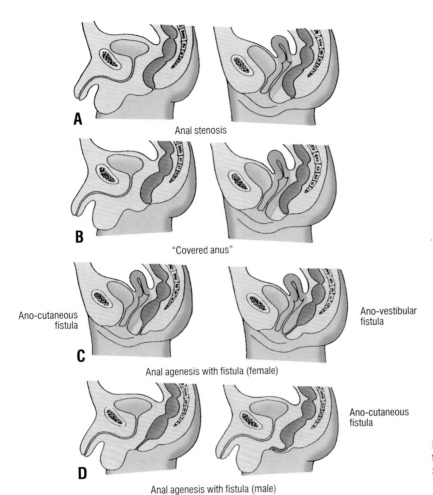

A

Anal stenosis

B

"Covered anus"

Ano-cutaneous fistula

C

Anal agenesis with fistula (female)

Ano-vestibular fistula

Ano-cutaneous fistula

D

Anal agenesis with fistula (male)

**FIG. 18-7.** Types of anal ("low") defects. (Modified from Skandalakis JE, Gray SW. Embryology for Surgeons (2nd ed). Baltimore: Williams & Wilkins, 1994; with permission.)

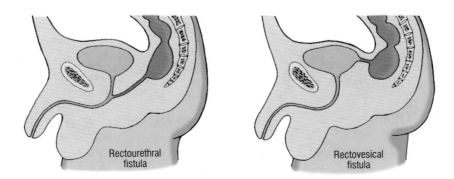

Rectourethral fistula

Rectovesical fistula

Anorectal agenesis with fistula (male)

**FIG. 18-8.** Types of anorectal ("high") defects. (Modified from Skandalakis JE, Gray SW. Embryology for Surgeons (2nd ed). Baltimore: Williams & Wilkins, 1994; with permission.)

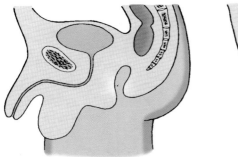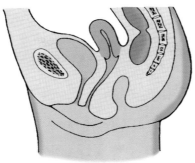

**FIG. 18-9.** High rectal atresia. These forms do not arise from abnormal partition of the cloaca; they are related to other intestinal atresias. (Modified from Skandalakis JE, Gray SW. Embryology for Surgeons (2nd ed). Baltimore: Williams & Wilkins, 1994; with permission.)

Susuki et al.[23] presented two cases of nonrotation in adults. The authors of this chapter are in agreement with Susuki et al. that the anomaly is more common in infants, but we have seen several cases in adults in the lab of the Emory Medical School as well as on barium enemas with x-rays at Piedmont Hospital.

### *Idiopathic Anal Incontinence*

Peveretos et al.[24] reported 3 cases of idiopathic anal incontinence. They supported the theory that the etiology is secondary to degeneration of the nerves supplying the pelvic floor muscles resulting in partial or total disappearance of the double right angle between the anal canal and the rectum which is essential for anal continence.

We quote from Skandalakis and Gray[13] on cloacal exstrophy, the most severe of the ventral wall defects, as well as the most rare:

*Superficially, the anomaly resembles exstrophy of the bladder, but the defect is larger...The lateral portion of the exposed mucosa represents the posterior wall of the bladder, but the central portion is intestinal epithelium. Superiorly, just below the umbilicus, the ileum opens to the surface and usually is prolapsed. On the exposed intestinal mucosa, one or occasionally two vermiform appendices open. At the inferior end of the mucosal surface, a segment of colon, which usually ends blindly, opens. The ureters open low on*

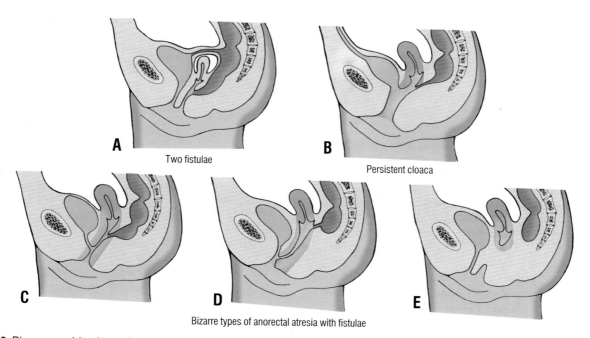

A — Two fistulae

B — Persistent cloaca

C      D      E

Bizarre types of anorectal atresia with fistulae

**FIG. 18-10.** Bizarre combinations of developmental arrests, atresias, and fistulas. All are rare. **A,** Rare. **B,** Cloaca. **C,** Cloaca. **D,** Rare. **E,** Rare. (Modified from Skandalakis JE, Gray SW. Embryology for Surgeons (2nd ed). Baltimore: Williams & Wilkins, 1994; with permission.)

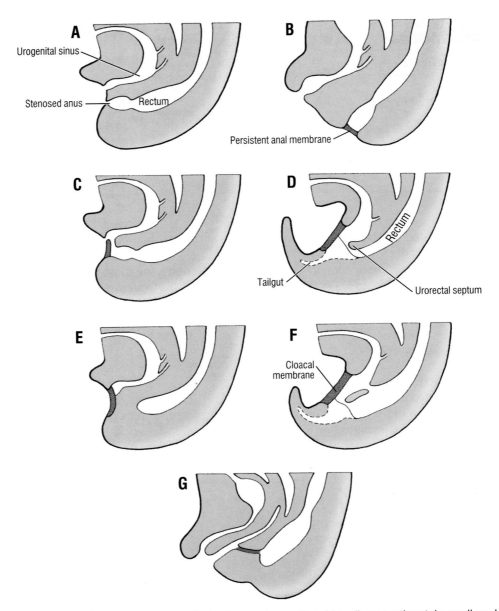

FIG. 18-11. Embryogenesis of anal and anorectal defects. **A,** Anal stenosis resulting from disproportionately small anal portion of the cloacal membrane. **B,** Membranous atresia from persistent anal closing plate. **C,** Covered anus. The perineal body has not fused with the persistent cloacal plate, and a perineal fistula is present. **D** and **E,** Anorectal agenesis with and without arrested descent of the urorectal septum. **F,** Anal agenesis with failure of midline fusion of the folds forming the urorectal septum, leaving two fistulous openings. **G,** Anal agenesis with rectovaginal fistula. (Modified from Skandalakis JE, Gray SW. Embryology for Surgeons (2nd ed). Baltimore: Williams & Wilkins, 1994; with permission.)

*the lateral bladder mucosa, and in males there may be two penes or hemipenes. Females may have müllerian duct orifices on the bladder mucosa, or two vaginae may end blindly. Exomphalos may extend the defect cranially, and the pubic bones are separated, as in exstrophy of the bladder. Spina bifida, myelomeningocele, and a single umbilical artery are common...*

*Exstrophy of the cloaca arises from the failure of secondary mesoderm from the primitive streak to cover the infraumbilical wall. It differs from exstrophy of the bladder in that midline rupture has occurred earlier (about the fifth week), before the fusion of the genital tubercles (hence the double penis) and before the descent of the urorectal septum, which separates the cloaca into*

**TABLE 18-3. Germ Layer Origin of Developmental Cysts**

| | Epidermoid | Dermoid | Enterogenous | Teratomatous |
|---|---|---|---|---|
| **Tissue of origin** | Ectoderm | Ectoderm | Endoderm | All three layers |
| **Histologic characteristics** | Stratified squamous | Stratified squamous with skin appendages (sweat glands, sebaceous glands, hair follicles) | Columnar or cuboidal lining; may have secretory function | Varying degrees of differentiation between cysts and cell layers of single cyst |
| **General state** | Benign* | Benign* | Benign | Benign or malignant |

*Malignant variants are rare.

*Source:* Goldberg SM, Gordon PH, Nivatvongs S. Essentials of Anorectal Surgery. Philadelphia: JB Lippincott, 1980; with permission.

bladder and rectum. *As the individual cloaca is exposed, its central portion is the posterior wall of the gut, while its lateral portions receive the ureters and differentiate into bladder mucosa.*

### Retrorectal Lesions

According to Gordon,[25] retrorectal lesions may be congenital, inflammatory, neurogenic, osseous, or miscellaneous. More than half of all presacral lesions are congenital, and approximately two-thirds of these are of developmental origin. Table 18-3 describes the formation of these benign or malignant developmental cysts from an embryologic and histologic point of view.

## SURGICAL ANATOMY OF THE COLON

### Topographic Anatomy and Relations

The large intestine extends from the terminal ileum to the anus. To be more embryologically and anatomically correct, it extends to the pectinate (dentate) line, in other words, to the proximal 2 cm of the anal canal. The classic divisions of the colon are the cecum, the colon proper, the rectum, and the anal canal. The first 6 cm of the large intestine just below the ileocecal valve, the ascending colon, and the hepatic flexure form a surgical unit, the right colon (right colectomy). The distal transverse colon, splenic flexure, and descending and sigmoid colons constitute the left colon (left colectomy).

### Length and Diameter of the Large Intestine

Textbooks of anatomy offer no agreement about the length of the segments of the large intestine. We have used the lengths and diameters from several studies to present averages for Figure 18-12. Estimates of the length of the large bowel average about 1.3-1.8 m. According to *Gray's Anatomy* (37th ed.),[26] the length from the end of the distal ileum to the anus is about 1.5 m. Goligher[27] estimated the length of the colon to be 4½ ft (1.25 m).

Saunders et al.[28] reported intraoperative measurements of colonic anatomy in 118 patients, reporting a mean total colonic length of 114. 1 cm (range 68-159 cm). A free sigmoid loop was not present in 20 patients (17%) because of adhesions. Ten patients (8%) had a descending mesocolon of 10 cm or more, and 11 patients (9%) had an ascending mesocolon of 10 cm or more. Twenty-four patients (20%) had mobile splenic flexures. The mid-transverse colon reached the symphysis pubis in 34 patients (29%).

The caliber of the large bowel is greater close to the cecum; it gradually gets smaller toward the rectum, then dilates again at the rectal ampulla just above the surgical anal canal. A sigmoid colon loop is occasionally as wide as a loop of terminal ileum.

Sadahiro et al.,[29] in a study of Japanese patients, reported that the transverse colon was the largest in length and surface area of the 6 segments of large intestine. They also reported that the length of the entire colon tended to become longer with age. Is this, perhaps, one of the etiologic factors for the phenomenon of geriatric constipation? Sadahiro and colleagues also found the diameters of the descending colon, sigmoid colon, and rectum to be larger in males. However, the length of the entire intestine was shorter, and the surface area was smaller, in males than in females.

A discussion of the colonic wall is presented in this chapter in the section on histology.

### Vascular Supply

The large intestine is supplied by the superior and infe-

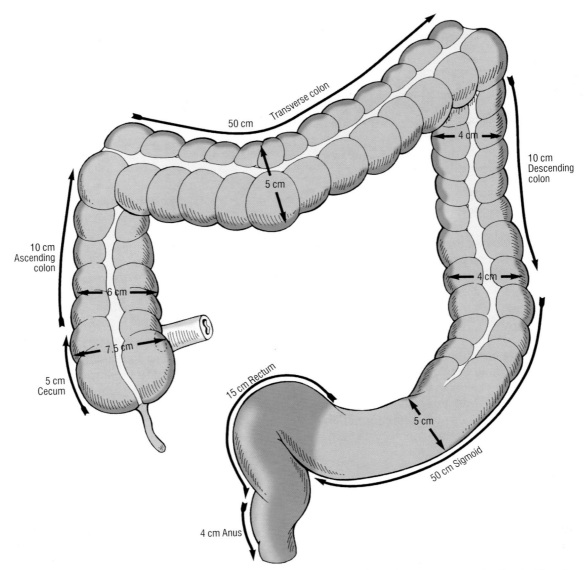

**FIG. 18-12.** Average lengths and diameters of the segments of the large intestine (based on an average of estimated lengths presented by studies of many researchers.)

rior mesenteric arteries and branches of the internal iliac (hypogastric) artery; it is drained by the superior and inferior mesenteric veins and tributaries to the internal iliac vein.

## Arterial Supply

### Superior Mesenteric Artery

The cecum and the ascending colon receive blood from two arterial branches of the superior mesenteric artery: the ileocolic and right colic arteries (Figs. 18-13, 18-14). These arteries form arcades from which vasa recta pass to the medial colonic wall. As the vasa recta reach the

surface of the colon, they divide into short and long branches. The short branches serve the medial or mesenteric side of the colon; the long branches serve the lateral and antimesenteric side. The long branches send twigs into the epiploic appendages (Fig. 18-15).

The transverse colon is similarly supplied by the middle colic artery from the superior mesenteric artery. Steward and Rankin[30] found the splenic flexure supplied by the middle colic artery in 37 percent of their specimens. In the remainder, the flexure and the left portion of the transverse colon were supplied by the left colic artery, a branch of the inferior mesenteric artery.

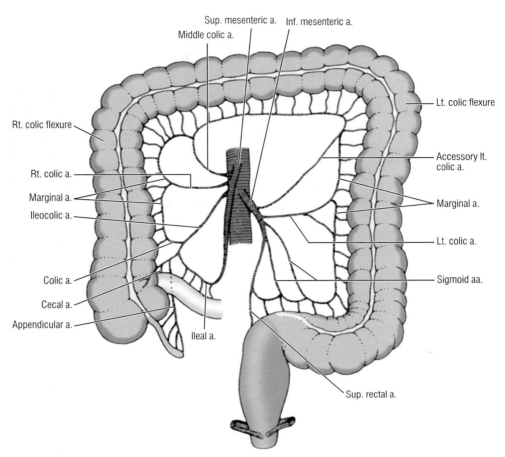

FIG. 18-13. Schema of the arterial blood supply to the large intestine. There are many variations of this basic pattern. (Modified from Skandalakis JE, Gray SW, Rowe JS Jr. Anatomical Complications in General Surgery. New York: McGraw-Hill, 1983; with permission.)

## Inferior Mesenteric Artery

The inferior mesenteric artery (Fig. 18-16) arises from the aorta opposite the lower portion of the 3rd lumbar vertebra, at or near the lower margin of the transverse segment of the duodenum. The origin tends to become lower with age.[31] The length of the artery prior to its first branch varies from 1.5 cm to 9.0 cm.[32]

The branches of the inferior mesenteric artery (Figs. 18-13 and 18-17C, D, E) are the left colic artery, with its ascending and descending branches for the descending colon, 1 to 9 sigmoid arteries for the sigmoid colon, and the superior rectal (hemorrhoidal) artery for the rectum. An accessory middle colic artery is present in about 38 percent of subjects. The left colic artery may reach the splenic flexure (86 percent of cases) or may join the marginal artery short of the flexure (14 percent of cases).

In the anatomy of the colon vasculature, the ascending branch of the left colic artery is the primary supplying vessel (96.91%).[33] According to Furst et al.,[34] an intact left colic artery, including its collaterals at the splenic flexure, will supply sufficient blood to the proximal ascending colon after central ligation of the middle and right colic artery. By including the ascending colon in their alternative colon interposition procedure, they were able to obtain a sufficient graft length without mobilization of the left flexure.

Is the splenic flexure vulnerable to ischemic injury due to a compromised blood flow, as Griffiths[35] stated? Van Damme and Bonte,[36] without supporting or denying the dogma of Griffiths, stated that the splenic flexure has 3 types of arcades: paracolic, anastomotic in the mesentery, and possibly a small intermesenteric arcade or a left accessory colic vessel close to the duodenojejunal flexure.

Dworkin and Allen-Mersh[37] found that the "significant blood flow reduction after ligation of the inferior and distal mesenteric arteries supports the hypothesis that anastomotic leakage after restorative rectal excision may result from ischemia associated with inadequate blood flow in the marginal artery-dependent sigmoid colon. Improvement in inadequate intraoperative colonic perfusion

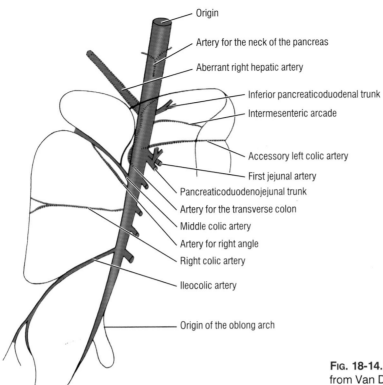

**FIG. 18-14.** The collaterals of the superior mesenteric artery. (Modified from Van Damme JP, Bonte J. Vascular Anatomy in Abdominal Surgery. New York: Thieme Verlag, 1990; with permission.)

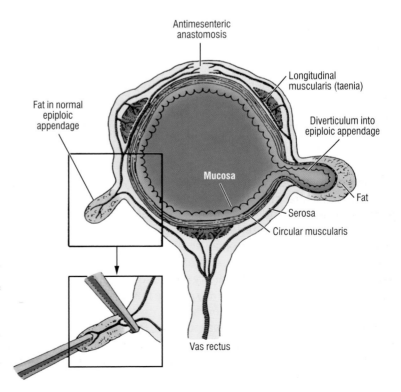

**FIG. 18-15.** Diagram of the transverse colon showing long and short branches of the vasa recta. On the left is a normal epiploic appendage; on the right, a diverticulum extending into an epiploic appendage. *Inset:* Effect of too much traction on an epiploic appendage resulting in injury to one of the long branches of vasa recta followed by antimesenteric ischemia. (Modified from Skandalakis JE, Gray SW, Rowe JS Jr. Anatomical Complications in General Surgery. New York: McGraw-Hill, 1983; with permission.)

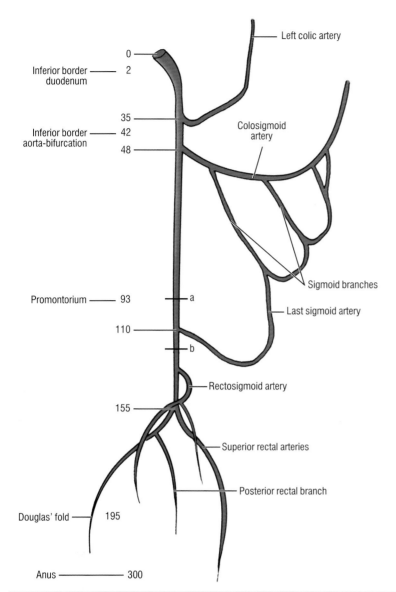

Fig. 18-16. The inferior mesenteric artery and its branches; origin distance in millimeters. If the inferior mesenteric artery is divided at "a", above the last full anastomosis, collateral circulation toward the rectum is still possible. Division at "b" would interrupt the collateral circulation. (Modified from Van Damme JP, Bonte J. Vascular Anatomy in Abdominal Surgery. New York: Thieme Verlag, 1990; with permission.)

from increased collateral circulation is unlikely to develop in the marginal-artery dependent colon during the first five postoperative days."

Adachi et al.[38] stated that poor bowel function after low anterior resection is associated with high ligation of the inferior mesenteric artery and injury to the pelvic autonomic nerve, and urged less aggressive surgery. Poor bowel function after sigmoid colectomy was correlated with length of the resected colon.

Remember the long and short vasa recta (Fig. 18-18). The long vasa recta branches bifurcate and anastomose at the antimesenteric border of the bowel after encircling it. The short ones, branches of the marginal artery, are responsible for the mesocolic two-thirds of the colonic circumference.

### Marginal Artery (of Drummond)

The marginal artery (Fig. 18-17A, B, C) is composed of a series of anastomosing arcades between branches of the ileocolic, right colic, middle colic, left colic, and sigmoidal arteries. These form a single, looping vessel. The marginal artery courses roughly parallel with the mesenteric border of the large intestine, from 1 cm to 8 cm from the intestinal wall. It may or may not terminate at the superior rectal artery (Fig. 18-17C).

The blood supply to the colon is adequate, but without

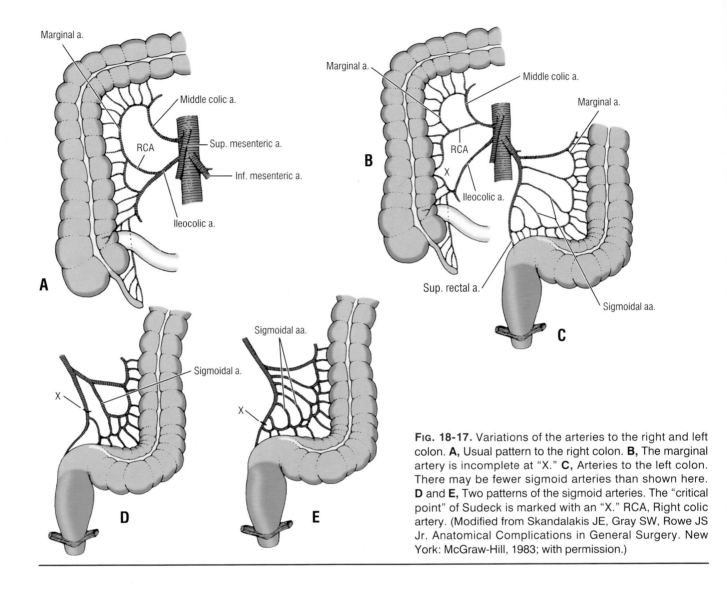

**FIG. 18-17.** Variations of the arteries to the right and left colon. **A,** Usual pattern to the right colon. **B,** The marginal artery is incomplete at "X." **C,** Arteries to the left colon. There may be fewer sigmoid arteries than shown here. **D** and **E,** Two patterns of the sigmoid arteries. The "critical point" of Sudeck is marked with an "X." RCA, Right colic artery. (Modified from Skandalakis JE, Gray SW, Rowe JS Jr. Anatomical Complications in General Surgery. New York: McGraw-Hill, 1983; with permission.)

much margin of safety. Anastomosis between the right colic and ileocolic arteries is absent in 5 percent of subjects (Fig. 18-17B).[30]

Griffiths[35] described a point of circulation weakness at the splenic flexure. In 200 subjects, Michels and colleagues[32] found good anastomosis of arteries in this area in 61 percent, poor anastomosis in 32 percent, and no anastomosis in 7 percent.

Haigh and Temple[39] presented a case of a dilated marginal artery (Fig. 18-19B) providing collateral blood supply from the middle colic artery to the ileocolonic artery to compensate for the occlusion of the superior mesenteric artery secondary to chronic volvulus of the small intestine. The authors advise 1) complete knowledge of mesenteric collateral circulation; 2) relocation and repositioning of the small bowel, if necessary, prior to closing the abdomen; and 3) delineating the dilated marginal artery before performing a resection.

### Critical Point of Sudeck

The critical point of Sudeck is no longer considered to be as "critical" as was once thought. Its location is unimportant in present-day abdominal and abdominoperineal resections. We present it here only for historical reasons.

Sudeck[40] described a point on the superior rectal artery at which ligation of the artery would not devascularize a long rectosigmoid stump. This point is just above the origin of the last sigmoid artery; its position varies with the number of such arteries (Fig. 18-17D, E). In about 50 percent of individuals, the marginal artery continues downward to join the superior rectal artery. Sudeck's point would be just proximal to that junction.

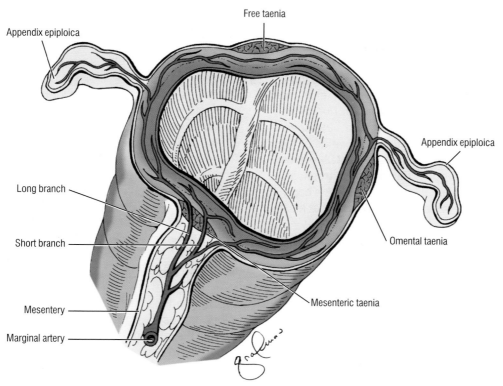

FIG. 18-18. The terminal arterial supply to the colon and its relation to the taenia coli and appendices epiploicae.

The significance of Sudeck's point depends on the surgical procedure to be performed. In 1907, Sudeck was interested in perineal excision of the rectum, the procedure of choice at the beginning of the century. Ligation of the superior rectal artery was necessary for mobilization of the rectum.

In some cases of left colectomy in which a long sigmoid stump is left, it may be difficult to bring the transverse colon

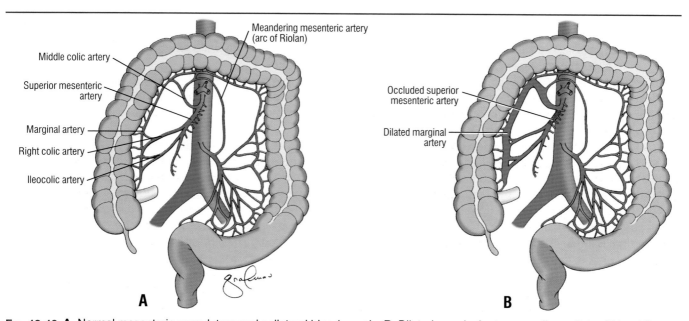

FIG. 18-19. **A,** Normal mesenteric vasculature and collateral blood supply. **B,** Dilated marginal artery supplies collateral blood flow to small bowel in case of superior mesenteric artery occlusion.

down to the stump because of a short transverse mesocolon. This problem could be solved by ligation of the superior rectal artery above Sudeck's point.

The concept of Sudeck's critical point fails to recognize two other sources of blood to the rectum. One is the intramural network of arteries in the submucosal layer of the wall. The other is from the middle and inferior rectal arteries, especially the latter. Goligher[41] stated: "Experience with sphincter-saving resections for carcinomas of the upper rectum and lower sigmoid shows that after division of the inferior mesenteric/superior hemorrhoidal trunk, the middle and inferior hemorrhoidal [rectal] arteries are capable of nourishing a distal rectal stump up to a point at least 8 to 10 cm above the peritoneal reflection."

According to Michels et al.,[32] in addition to the three pairs of rectal (hemorrhoidal) arteries, other sources of collateral blood supply to the rectum and sigmoid might include:

- branches of the inferior vesical artery
- arteries supplying the levator ani muscle
- the middle sacral artery
- the posterior retroperitoneal arterial plexus uniting the parietal and visceral circulation

The inferior rectal artery is responsible for the arterial blood supply of the distal 2 cm of the anal canal.

We strongly advise the reader to consult the excellent works of Van Damme[1] and Bertelli et al.[42]

## Venous Drainage

Veins of the colon (Fig. 18-20) follow the arteries. On the right (the cecum, ascending colon, and right transverse colon), the veins join to form the superior mesenteric vein. Veins of the hepatic flexure and the right portion of the transverse colon enter the gastroepiploic vein or the anterior superior pancreaticoduodenal vein. Voiglio et al.[43] studied and defined the gastrocolic vein and reported two cases of avulsion secondary to abdominal trauma. It is present in 70% of patients, it is short (less than 25 mm), and its calibre ranges from 3 mm to 10 mm. It is located at the anterior surface of the head of the pancreas and beneath the root of the transverse mesocolon as a confluence between the right gastroepiploic and right upper colic veins. The above authors emphasize the surgical importance of this vein during surgery of the pancreas, in portal hypertension, and in abdominal trauma. Drainage from the left portion of the transverse colon enters the superior mesenteric vein. The superior rectal vein drains the descending and sigmoid colons; it passes upward to form the inferior mesenteric vein.

The rectum is drained by the superior rectal veins (Fig. 18-21), which enter the inferior mesenteric vein. This drainage is to the portal system. The middle and inferior rectal veins enter the internal iliac vein and thus drain into the systemic circulation.

REMEMBER:

- The inferior rectal vein is mainly responsible for the venous return of the distal 2 cm of the anal canal.
- Anastomoses occur between the superior rectal vein (portal) and the middle and inferior rectal veins (systemic). These constitute a potential portosystemic shunt.
- Because lower intestinal venous malformations may cause significant chronic and acute gastric hemorrhage, Fishman et al.[44] recommend colectomy with mucosectomy and endorectal pull-through before the development of large transfusion requirements.

## Lymphatic Drainage

Lymph nodes of the large intestine have been divided into four groups (Fig. 18-22): epicolic (under the serosa of the wall of the intestine); paracolic (on the marginal artery); intermediate (along the large arteries [superior and inferior mesenteric arteries]); and principal (at the root of the superior and inferior mesenteric arteries). This last group includes mesenteric root nodes (which also receive lymph from the small intestine), aortic nodes, and left lumbar nodes. The number of nodes of the large intestine is shown in Table 18-4.

Although lymph flow follows the arteries, there are cross-connections at the level of the arcades that are parallel with the intestine. In addition, communication between the lymphatics of the transverse colon and those of the stomach, and between lymphatics of the ascending and descending colon and the body wall have been described in the medical literature.

Wide resection of the colon should include the entire segment supplied by a major artery. This will also remove most, but not all, the lymphatic drainage of the segment (Figs. 18-23, 18-24).

Yada et al.[45] analyzed the vascular anatomy and lymph node metastases in carcinoma of the colon:

*Because the ileocecal artery always arises from the superior mesenteric artery and lymph node metastases of cecum cancer were limited to nodes along the ileocolic artery, cecum cancer can be cured by ileocecal resection. The right colic artery has various origins, and ascending colon cancer shows various patterns of lymph node metastases. Therefore a right hemicolectomy should be performed for ascending colon cancer. The middle colic artery forks into right and left branches, and each branch has different branching variations. If the right colic and middle colic arteries*

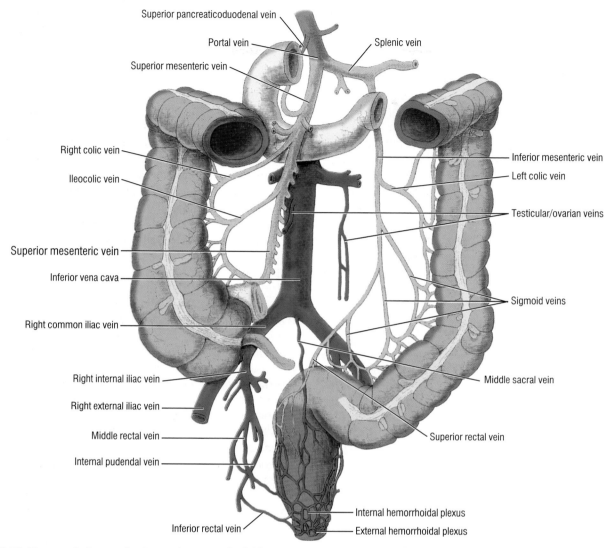

**FIG. 18-20.** Venous drainage of colon and rectum. *Dark blue,* systemic venous drainage. *Light blue,* portal venous drainage. (Modified from Gordon PH, Nivatvongs S (eds). Principles and Practice of Surgery for the Colon, Rectum, and Anus. St. Louis, MO: Quality Medical Publishing, 1992; with permission.)

*have a common trunk, a right hemicolectomy should be performed for transverse colon cancer on the right side. If the left branch of the middle colic artery has an independent replaced origin, lymph node dissection should be modified according to the variant origin. If the left colic artery and the first sigmoidal artery have a common trunk, the lymph nodes along the common trunk should be removed for sigmoid colon cancer and for descending colon cancer. Of the patients with sigmoid colon cancer, 6.3% also had lymph node metastases along the superior rectal artery. Given that the lymph nodes along the superior rectal artery are skeletonized, sigmoid colon cancer can be also cured by partial sigmoidectomy.*

REMEMBER:
- The lymphatic vessels of the distal 2 cm of the anal canal drain to the inguinal nodes.

## Innervation

### *Intrinsic Innervation*

From the esophagus to the anus, the digestive tract is supplied with two intramural nerve networks. The myenteric plexus (Auerbach) (Fig. 18-25) controls motility, and the submucosal plexus (Meissner) controls secretion. Vagal and sympathetic fibers synapse with these intra-

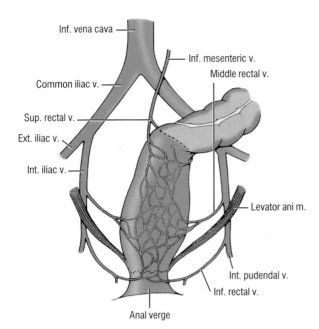

**FIG. 18-21.** Detailed diagram of the venous drainage of the rectum and anus. The superior rectal vein drains to the portal system, and the middle and inferior rectal veins drain to the systemic veins. The venous plexus between the veins forms a potential portacaval shunt. (Modified from Skandalakis JE, Gray SW, Rowe JS Jr. Anatomical Complications in General Surgery. New York: McGraw-Hill, 1983; with permission.)

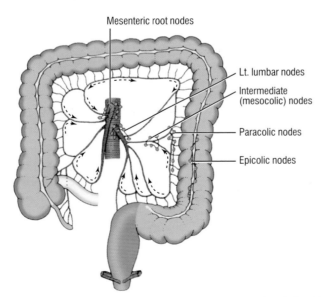

**FIG. 18-22.** The lymphatics of the large intestine follow the arteries and drain to the principal nodes at the root of the mesentery. The path is by way of epicolic, paracolic, and mesocolic lymph nodes. (Modified from Skandalakis JE, Gray SW, Rowe JS Jr. Anatomical Complications in General Surgery. New York: McGraw-Hill, 1983; with permission.)

mural ganglion cells. Innervation of the gastrointestinal system is now considered to have its own intrinsic set of nerves known as the *intramural plexus* or the *intestinal enteric nervous system*.[46] The number of neurons this system comprises is estimated to be 100 million, equal to that of the whole neuronal population of the spinal cord. Postganglionic sympathetic and parasympathetic neurons synapse on neurons of both myenteric and submucosal plexuses. Postganglionic sympathetic fibers also synapse directly on the epithelial cells.

The neurons of the two plexuses, generally regarded as postganglionic parasympathetic fibers, form a reticulum of neurons with widespread synapses; and within these plexuses there are also interneurons. Some sensory neurons with receptors in the epithelium are now known to collateralize into both plexuses and then continue on so that some follow parasympathetic fibers back to the brain or sacral segments of the spinal cord and sympathetic fibers back to the T1-L2,3 spinal cord segments. However, in addition to those sensory fibers, others have been identified which synapse in the collateral (prevertebral) (sympathetic) ganglia.

## Sympathetic Innervation

The sympathetic supply to the right colon originates from the lower six thoracic segments of the spinal cord. Preganglionic fibers pass through the sympathetic chain ganglia, then pass as thoracic splanchnic nerves to synapse in the celiac, aortic, and superior mesenteric plexuses. From the plexuses, postganglionic fibers pass with the arteries in the mesentery to the small intestine and the right colon.

On the left, preganglionic fibers arise from the first two (or three) lumbar segments of the cord, then travel as lumbar splanchnic nerves to the aortic plexus and the inferior mesenteric plexus. From ganglia in this diffuse plexus, postganglionic fibers follow branches of the inferior mesenteric artery to the left colon and the upper rectum.

| **TABLE 18-4. Numbers of Lymph Nodes in the Mesentery of the Large Intestine by Regions** | |
|---|---|
| **Nodes** | **Average number** |
| Ileocolic | 29 |
| Right colic | 11.1 |
| Midcolic | 22.4 |
| Left colic | 25.2 |
| Sigmoid and rectal | 32.8 |

*Source:* Skandalakis JE, Gray SW, Rowe JS Jr. Anatomical Complications in General Surgery. New York: McGraw-Hill, 1983; with permission.

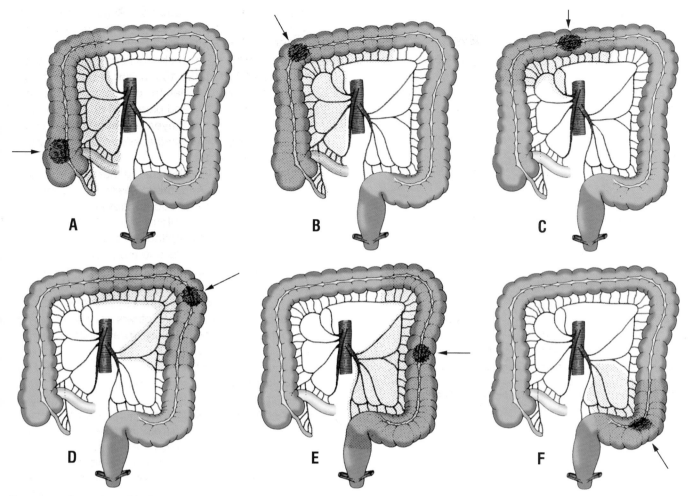

**FIG. 18-23.** Resection of the large intestine should include the entire area served by a major artery as well as the lesion itself. Most of the lymphatic drainage will be included. Areas of resection (stippled) for lesions in various segments of the large bowel are shown in **A-F.** An arrow indicates the site of the lesion. (Modified from Skandalakis JE, Gray SW, Rowe JS Jr. Anatomical Complications in General Surgery. New York: McGraw-Hill, 1983; with permission.)

## *Parasympathetic Innervation*

Vagal fibers from the posterior trunk pass as the celiac division to and through the celiac ganglion without synapse. From the ganglion, preganglionic fibers pass on the superior mesenteric artery to the small intestine and the right colon, where they synapse with ganglion cells of the intramural plexuses.

The left colon receives parasympathetic fibers from pelvic splanchnic nerves, which arise from the 2nd, 3rd, and 4th sacral nerves. These fibers follow the course of the presacral nerve to reach the inferior mesenteric plexus. From this plexus, the preganglionic fibers follow the branches of the inferior mesenteric artery to the left colon and the upper rectum.

REMEMBER:

- The proximal 2 cm of the anal canal is innervated by visceral autonomic fibers.
- The distal 2 cm of the anal canal is innervated by somatic rectal nerves.

## Detailed Anatomy of Colonic Segments

### *Cecum and Ileocecal Valve*

The cecum lies in the right iliac fossa; in about 60 percent of living, erect individuals, it lies partly in the true pelvis. Anson and McVay[47] distinguished six types and several subtypes of peritoneal reflections of the cecum. In

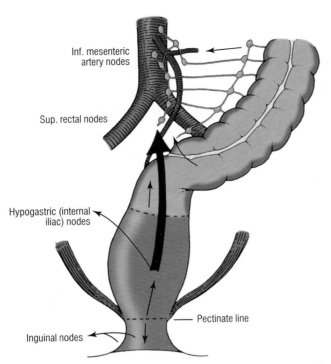

**FIG. 18-24.** Lymphatic drainage of the sigmoid colon, rectum, and anus. Above the pectinate line, drainage is to inferior mesenteric nodes. Below the line, drainage is to the inguinal nodes. (Modified from Skandalakis JE, Gray SW, Rowe JS Jr. Anatomical Complications in General Surgery. New York: McGraw-Hill, 1983; with permission.)

of cases. At the other extreme, the cecum was wholly unattached in 24 percent of cases. Among the latter group are cases of true "mobile cecum," in which the cecum and the lower part of the ascending colon are unattached. Pavlov and Pétrov[48] stated that the cecum was mobile more often in females than in males by a factor of 20 percent.

Because the cecum is located at the right iliac fossa, it is related to the right iliacus muscle posteriorly. In most cases, it is covered 90 to 100 percent by peritoneum. The cecum usually is not fixed by the posterior peritoneum which covers the right iliac fossa. The relations and variations of the cecum at the iliac fossa are shown in Figures 18-26 and 18-27.

A fold of peritoneum from the mesentery of the terminal ileum may cross the ileum to attach to the lower colon and the cecum. This is the superior ileocecal fold (Fig. 18-28); the anterior cecal artery lies within it. This fold, the mesentery, and the ileum may form a superior ileocecal fossa. Inferior to the terminal ileum, an inferior ileocecal fold may lie anterior to the mesentery of the appendix. Between them is the inferior ileocecal fossa (paracecal herniation). Both the superior and inferior ileocecal folds are inconstant, and the associated fossae can be shallow or absent. Some types of cecal attachment to the body wall may form a retrocecal fossa. In 78 cadavers dissected by Skandalakis,[49] 12 had a fixed terminal ileum and 1 had a common ileocecal mesentery.

Four types of human cecum were postulated by Treves[50] in a developmental model (he referred to them as the "first" through "fourth" types).
- First (Infantile): During the neonatal period, the cecum

their series, almost the entire posterior surface of the cecum was attached to the posterior abdominal wall in 19.6 percent

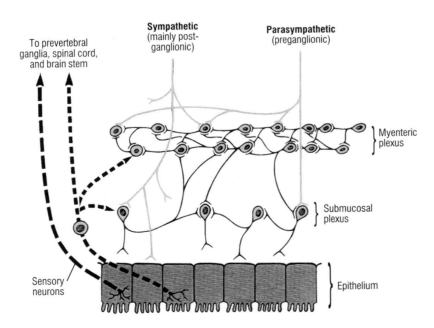

**FIG. 18-25.** Neural control of the gut wall, showing 1) the myenteric and submucosal plexuses; 2) extrinsic control of these plexuses by the sympathetic and parasympathetic nervous systems; and 3) sensory fibers passing from the luminal epithelium and gut wall to the enteric plexuses and from there to the prevertebral ganglia, spinal cord, and brain stem. (Modified from Guyton AC, Hall JE. Textbook of Medical Physiology, 9th ed. Philadelphia: WB Saunders, 1996; with permission.)

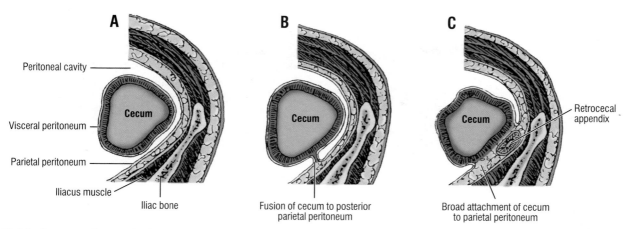

**FIG. 18-26.** Cross sections at the level of the cecum and the iliac fossa showing variations in the degree of fusion of the cecum to the peritoneum. **A,** The cecum is unattached at this level and quite free to move about. **B,** The cecum is held by a narrow mesenteric fold, permitting moderate mobility. **C,** Cecum with a retrocecal appendix is bound down to the iliac peritoneum over an extensive area. (Modified from McVay CB. Anson & McVay Surgical Anatomy, 6th ed. Philadelphia: WB Saunders, 1984; with permission.)

grows to a conical formation. The appendix hangs from its apex. The 3 taeniae are present, beginning at the appendiceal base. This form persists in approximately 2 percent of the population.

- Second (Childhood): The cecum becomes quadrate by forming saccules medial and lateral to the anterior taeniae. The appendix hangs from the area between the saccules and not from the apex. This form persists in about 3 percent of the population.
- Third (Adult): A new apex is formed by rapid growth of the right lateral saccule. The old apex is pushed to the left lateral area toward the ileocecal valve. The appendix hangs between the anterior and posterolateral taeniae. This form occurs in roughly 90 percent of the population.
- Fourth (Geriatric): There is atrophy of the left saccule and enlargement of the right saccule. The apex and the appendix are now close to the ileocecal valve. The fourth form, actually a progression of the third form, is found in approximately 4 percent of the population.

Pavlov and Pétrov,[48] after studying the ceca of 126 subjects, classified them as follows: infantile type (which they named "infundibular"), 13%; adult type (which they called "ampullary"), 78%; "intermediate" type, 9%.

The cecum and ascending colon are related posteriorly to the following anatomic entities, which should be protected during mobilization of the right colon:

- psoas major muscle
- nerves (lateral femoral cutaneous, femoral, genitofemoral)
- gonadal arteries and veins
- ureter

Sappey[51] attributes the discovery of the ileocecal valve to C. Varolius, based on the following lines which were published by Varolius in 1573:

> *Where the ileum joins the colon, there is a certain membrane which protrudes into the cavity of the latter. Of this membrane, which is the very end of the ileum extending to this junction, I who am the inventor, name it operculum of the ileum.*

DiDio and Anderson[52] used the term ileal pylorus, which is anatomically correct, rather than the term ileocecal valve. They stated that the ileum opens into the transitional zone between the cecum and the ascending colon, thereby asserting that the name "ileocecal valve" does not have any anatomic meaning. However, for the sake of convenience, we will continue to call this anatomic entity the "ileocecal valve."

The cadaveric valve is formed by two parallel transverse folds (labia, lips, or flaps) which project within the colon and form a transverse slit of 1-1.5 cm. At each end, the folds are united and form the frenulum. For all practical purposes, the protrusion of the small bowel into the colon is formed by the circular muscle of the terminal ileum which is covered by the mucosa.

In living subjects, the ileocecal valve has a papillary shape with a conoid ileal projection or intrusion into the cecum.

Kumar and Phillips[53] stated that the superior and the inferior ileocecal ligaments are responsible for the competence of the ileocecal valve.

The purpose of the ileocecal valve is not definitely known. Bogers and Van Marck[54] stated that "the ileocecal junction remains a controversial region of the gut." They

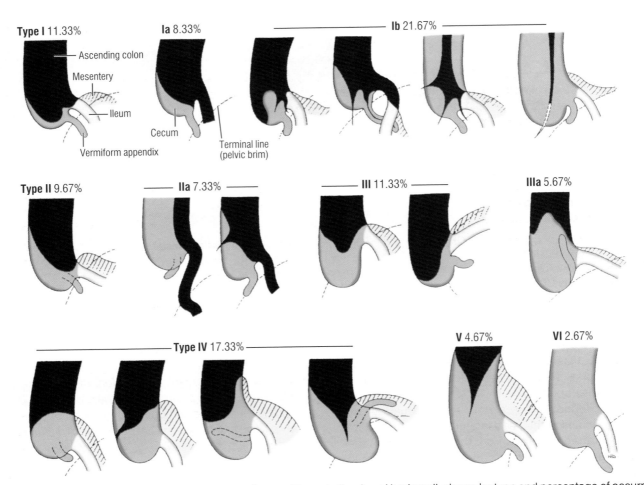

FIG. 18-27. Attachment of the cecum, ascending colon, and ileum to the dorsal body wall, shown by type and percentage of occurrence (areas of fixation shown in *black*), based on 300 laboratory specimens. **Types I and I-a,** Almost complete dorsal fixation of the cecum. **Type I-b,** Examples of retrocecal recess (spaces occurring as offsets of the cecal fossa) arranged in order of descending fixation. **Types II and II-a,** Fixation is chiefly medial (in **II-a,** with continuing attachment of the terminal ileum). **Types III, III-a, and IV,** Cecum free of dorsal attachment, in varying degree. In several cases, the proximal segment of the ascending colon also found without posterior parietal attachment. **Type V,** Nonfixation of the cecum, with continuing mobility of the greater part of the ascending colon. **Type VI,** Complete absence of dorsal attachment. (Modified from McVay CB. Anson & McVay Surgical Anatomy, 6th ed. Philadelphia: WB Saunders, 1984; with permission.)

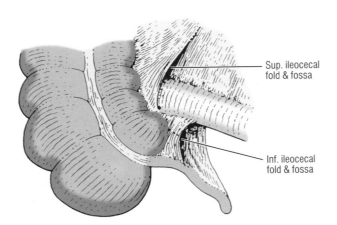

FIG. 18-28. Superior and inferior ileocecal folds forming fossae. (Modified from Skandalakis JE, Gray SW, Rowe JS Jr. Anatomical Complications in General Surgery. New York: McGraw-Hill, 1983; with permission.)

wrote in a review in 1993, "Based on the available data from the literature, evidence is accumulating for a sphincteric function."

The definition of the ileocecal valve differs with various specialties. Anatomists define it as a bilabial type with a horizontal slit, formed by the upper and lower lips which are united medially and laterally to form the frenula. Endoscopists consider it a papillary type, which is like a uterine cervix, a round or conical projection with a starlike orifice, but without the frenula. To radiologists,[55] the ileocecal valve appears as a round or oval protuberance, which usually arises from the posteromedial wall of the cecum. It is composed of superior and inferior lips which, at the corners of fusion, taper to form a part of the cecal wall.

Identification of the ileocecal region can be aided by a CT scan. In a study by Silverman et al.,[56] the region was identified using CT scan in 18 of 25 patients (72 percent) without pathology.

### Arterial Supply, Venous Drainage

The ileocolic artery (Fig. 18-29), which arises from the right side of the superior mesenteric artery, is the chief blood supply of the cecum. This artery divides into two branches before approaching the cecal wall. The colic branch anastomoses with the right colic artery. The ileal branch anastomoses with the terminal intestinal branch of the superior mesenteric artery. Close to its bifurcation, the ileocolic artery gives off two more branches: the anterior and the posterior cecal arteries.

The ileocolic vein is a tributary of the superior mesenteric vein.

### Lymphatics

The lymphatic vessels of the cecum (Figs. 18-30, 18-31) drain to lymph nodes along the anterior network of the ileocolic arteries. There are two groups of lymph nodes. The ileocolic lymph nodes are found along the ileocolic artery. The cecal lymph nodes are located in the vicinity of the anterior and posterior cecal arteries.

### Innervation

The sympathetic innervation of the cecum arises from the celiac and superior mesenteric ganglia. The parasympathetic innervation of the cecum comes from the vagus nerve.

### Surgical Considerations

- Volvulus of the cecum is an extremely rare phenomenon. The term "cecal volvulus" is frequently misused. The correct terminology is "volvulus of the right colon." Cecal volvulus in a 2 month-old boy was reported by Khope and Rao.[57] Laparoscopic cecopexy for intermittent cecal volvulus was reported by Shoop and Sackier.[58] Frank et al.[59] reported the first description of the CT diagnosis of cecal volvulus, emphasizing the significance of the "whirl sign." Moore et al.[60] reported a case with synchronous cecal and sigmoid volvulus, an extremely unusual phenomenon. Theuer and Cheadle[61] reported a similar case.

- The wall of the cecum is thin in comparison with the wall of the other colonic segments. The best and most secure part of the wall for cecotomy, cecorrhaphy, anastomosis with other viscera, and cecopexy is the taeniae (especially the anterior one, which is most approachable).

- Ileocecal intussusception can be idiopathic or secondary to benign or malignant tumors of the terminal ileum and of the ileocecal area generally. Idiopathic intussusception is a disease of the neonatal period; it may be secondary to the hypertrophy of the patches of Peyer. VanderKolk et al.[62] studied cecal-colic adult intussusception and recommended surgical reduction; colectomy was recommended only if the bowel is gangrenous. However, the authors of this chapter believe that cecopexy is a wise choice when the bowel wall is healthy.

- Cecal diverticulitis is rare. It is always solitary, in contrast to that of the left colon, where the diverticula are multiple. Efforts must be made to save the ileocecal valve if possible when operating in the ileocecal area. Two such cases with acute diverticulitis among 7 cases of benign lesions of the right colon were reported by Lear et al.[63] The following material is taken from that paper.

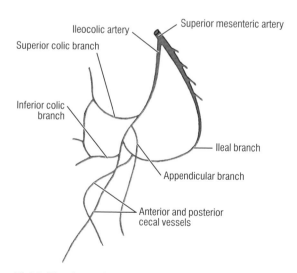

**FIG. 18-29.** The branches of the ileocolic artery. The ileocolic artery can be traced as a stem until it ends in two cecal branches. The other branches are direct collaterals of the main stem. (Modified from Van Damme JP, Bonte J. Vascular Anatomy in Abdominal Surgery. New York: Thieme Verlag, 1990; with permission.)

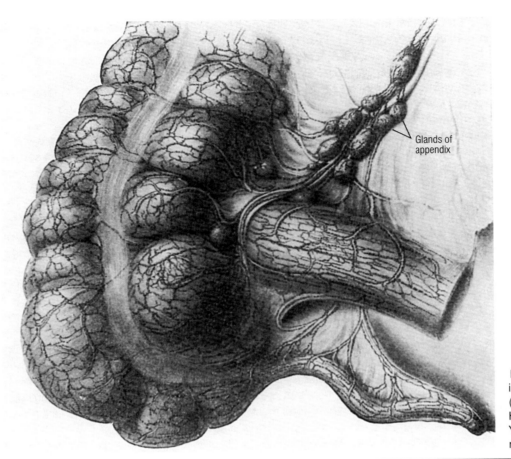

Glands of appendix

**Fig. 18-30.** The lymphatics of the ileocecal region, ventral view. (From Schaeffer JP (ed). Morris' Human Anatomy (11th ed). New York: Blakiston, 1953; with permission.)

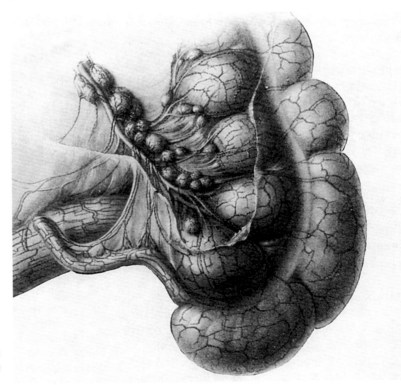

**Fig. 18-31.** The lymphatics of the ileocecal region, dorsal view. (From Schaeffer JP (ed). Morris' Human Anatomy (11th ed). New York: Blakiston, 1953; with permission.)

Many benign conditions occur in the right colon, and the differential diagnosis of these lesions is frequently difficult. This report concerns seven patients seen at Piedmont Hospital in the past six years, whose ultimate diagnoses illustrate several of the many benign conditions which may occur in the right colon. Patients with acute appendicitis have not been included in this report, nor have those with neoplasms which are frequently malignant such as carcinoid and polyps.

Astler et al.[64] divided benign lesions of the right colon into four groups as follows:

1. *Benign neoplasms (benign variants of carcinoids, hemangiomas, lymphangiomas, lipomas, fibromas, adenomas, etc.)*
2. *Inflammatory and parasitic conditions (regional enteritis, mucocele of appendix, ameboma, tuberculoma, actinomycosis, etc.)*
3. *Anatomic and congenital abnormalities (diverticula, hypertrophic mucosal folds, inverted appendiceal stump, etc.)*
4. *Physiologic defects (hypertrophied ileocecal valve, fecalith, prolapsed ileal mucosa, etc.)*

The grouping is not exclusive, and a lesion may fall into more than one class. A benign neoplasm such as a lipoma may involve the ileocecal valve, and this may become ulcerated and produce a nonspecific inflammatory mass. Table 18-5 shows pre- and postoperative diagnoses.

- The appendix, colon, anorectum, and surgical anal canal follow the pathologic destiny of other parts of the alimentary tract, developing cancers of epithelial and nonepithelial origin. Two studies by Hatch et al.[65,66] of stromal tumors of the appendix, colon, anorectum, and anal canal (leiomyomas and leiomyosarcomas) are recommended to the interested student.
- Isolated cecal infarction should be included in the differential diagnosis of acute right lower quadrant pain.[67]
- Nelson[68] stated that surgeons routinely divide the col-

orectum into anatomic subsites when treating colorectal cancer. He finds that the best classification is as follows:

1. *Proximal colon: cecum, transverse colon, descending colon*
2. *Distal colon: sigmoid, rectosigmoid, rectum (above anal canal)*
3. *Anal canal*

Justification for these three divisions is embryologic (midgut-hindgut).

- Poon and Chu[69] reported the following:

   Most inflammatory cecal masses are caused by benign pathology, and ileocecal resection is the procedure of choice. We do not recommend routine right hemicolectomy, as it requires conversion to a midline incision and is associated with a longer operation time, higher morbidity rate, and longer hospital stay. However, careful intraoperative assessment and, in particular, examination of the resected specimens is essential to exclude an underlying malignancy that would require right hemicolectomy.

- The competence of the ileocecal valve depends on the presence and action of the sphincteric mechanism in this area, which is the result of the formation of the sphincter of the valve (the valve itself is a thickening of the circular muscle). In most cases, a retrograde state exists.
- With total colonic obstruction, if the ileocecal valve is competent, the colon proximal to the obstruction is dilated. This type of valve –which does not permit the colonic contents to enter the ileum, but permits ileal contents to enter the colon– will produce a closed, looplike formation with increased tension. With an incompetent ileocecal valve, the closed-loop phenomenon does not exist: the small bowel receives the colonic contents and becomes distended, and nausea and vomiting follow.
- Mann et al. presented a case of right thigh abscess secondary to perforated adenocarcinoma of the cecum.[70] The pathway of the cecal contents most likely followed

**TABLE 18-5.**

| Patient No. | Age | Sex | Preoperative Diagnosis | Postoperative Diagnosis |
|---|---|---|---|---|
| 1 | 51 | F | Probable carcinoma of cecum | Lipoma of valve |
| 2 | 49 | F | Appendiceal abscess | Inflammation of cecum |
| 3 | 38 | F | Probable carcinoma of cecum | Non-specific inflammation |
| 4 | 50 | M | Possible carcinoma of cecum | Mucosal fold |
| 5 | 47 | F | Possible carcinoma | Diverticulum |
| 6 | 46 | F | Volvulus | Diverticulum |
| 7 | 59 | F | Probable carcinoma of cecum | Constriction ring |

*Source:* Astler VB, Miller EB, Snyder RS, McIntyre CH, Lillie RH. Benign surgical lesions of the cecum. Arch Surg 1963;86:435; with permission.

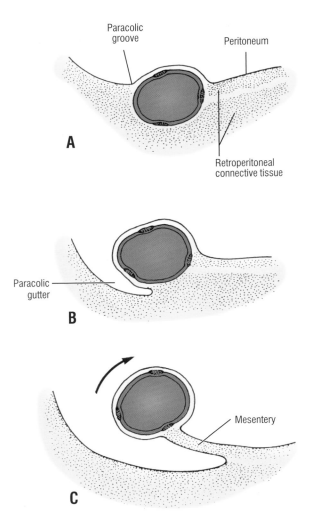

**FIG. 18-32.** Degrees of attachment of the right colon to the abdominal wall. **A,** Normal retroperitoneal location of the colon. **B,** Paracolic gutter. **C,** Mobile colon with mesentery. (Modified from Skandalakis JE, Gray SW, Rowe JS Jr. Anatomical Complications in General Surgery. New York: McGraw-Hill, 1983; with permission.)

the anatomy of the iliopsoas fascia which may be continuous with the fascia lata of the thigh.[71]

### Ascending Colon

Normally the ascending limb of the right colon is fused to the posterior body wall and covered anteriorly by the peritoneum (Fig. 18-32). There are variations of incomplete fusion, ranging from a deep lateral paracolic groove to the persistence of an entire ascending mesocolon. A mesocolon long enough to permit volvulus occurs in approximately 11 percent of cases.[72] In cadavers, the ascending colon may be mobile in approximately 37 percent of

cases.[48] A mobile cecum, together with a mobile right colon, may be present; this is the justification for volvulus of the right colon.

The older literature[50] reported a much higher incidence of right mesocolon from autopsy specimens. Symington[73] observed that laxity of the parietal peritoneum in the unembalmed body will permit the colon to be pulled anteriorly to produce a pseudomesentery. This cannot be done in the embalmed cadaver. To what extent this colonic mobility can occur in the living patient is not known.

Where the mesocolon is present, the cecum and proximal ascending colon are unusually mobile. It is this condition that is termed mobile cecum (Fig. 18-33); it can result in volvulus of the cecum and the right colon. In a study of 87 cadavers,[49] the cecum alone was mobile in 55. In 6 of these, enough of the right colon was mobile so that volvulus could have occurred.

Two conditions must be present for right colon volvulus to occur:[74] (1) an abnormally mobile segment of colon, and (2) a fixed point around which the mobile segment can twist. The first condition is often present in many individuals (Table 18-6). The second can be provided by the normal attachments of the colon or by postoperative adhesions.

Rogers and Harford[75] reported on five patients with mobile cecum syndrome. In all these patients, the cecum and ascending colon were not attached to the lateral peritoneum for 15-18 cm. According to these authors, cecopexy is the procedure of choice to reduce the colonic mobility.

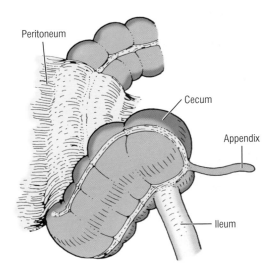

**FIG. 18-33.** Mobile cecum, distal ileum, and proximal right colon. This configuration is subject to volvulus. (Modified from Skandalakis JE, Gray SW, Rowe JS Jr. Anatomical Complications in General Surgery. New York: McGraw-Hill, 1983; with permission.)

**TABLE 18-6. Percent Frequency of Persistent Right and Left Mesocolon**

| Source | Right | Left |
|---|---|---|
| Adults (Treves, 1885) | 26 | 36 |
| Infants (Smith, 1911) | 30.75 | 37.1 |
| Adults (Harvey, 1918) | 13 | – |
| Adults (Hendrick, 1964) | 11.2 | – |
| Adults (Skandalakis, 1949) | 36.9 | – |

*Source:* Skandalakis JE, Gray SW, Rowe JS Jr. Anatomical Complications in General Surgery. New York: McGraw-Hill, 1983; with permission.

In a study by Wright and Max[76] of 12 patients with cecal volvulus, 2 who were treated by simple detorsion without fixation did not experience recurrence. Nevertheless, the authors of this chapter strongly advise fication, with or without cecostomy.

Ballantyne et al.[77] reported 137 cases of colonic volvulus between 1960 and 1980 at the Mayo Clinic: 52 percent were cecal; 3 percent were transverse; 2 percent were at the splenic flexure; 43 percent were sigmoid. Mortalities with cecal volvulus involving the cecum, transverse colon, and splenic flexure were 17 percent; with sigmoid volvulus, 11 percent.

Rabinovici et al.[78] reviewed 568 cases of cecal volvulus. The mean age of the patients was 53 years. The female/ male ratio was 1.4:1. There was gangrenous cecum in 20 percent of the cases. These authors emphasized that cecostomy had more complications in comparison with other techniques. They advised that with a necrotic cecum, resection should be done; with a viable cecum, detorsion and cecopexy is the procedure of choice. They also advised that cecostomy should be abandoned. Other authors disagree, however. For cecal volvulus with a viable colon, Jones and Fazio[79] recommended detorsion, cecopexy, and tube cecostomy as a combined procedure.

Benacci and Wolff[80] of the Mayo Clinic stated the indications for catheter cecostomy as follows:

• Colonic pseudo-obstruction
• Distal colonic obstruction
• Cecal perforation
• Cecal volvulus
• Preanastomotic decompression
• Miscellaneous usage

These authors conclude that good selection of patients, good cecostomy technique, and good postoperative care will provide good results.

Marinella[81] reported colonic pseudo-obstruction complicated by cecal perforation in a patient with Parkinson's disease.

Decreased mobility of the colon can result from abnormal connective tissue bands that pass across the ascending colon beneath the peritoneum. If the band is broad, covering most of the colon, it is designated as Jackson's membrane or veil (Fig. 18-34). It may or may not be vascularized. The origin of this membrane is not known with certainty, but probably results from improper fixation of the bowel in embryologic development. Indeed, the gradation from normal to abnormal is so subtle that its incidence cannot be stated. Such bands and membranes can constrict the colon, reduce its mobility, and provide a basis for volvulus.

**Arterial Supply, Venous Drainage**

The right colic artery participates in the blood supply of the ascending colon. It is usually said to be a branch of the superior mesenteric artery, and anastomoses with the colic branch of the ileocolic artery. Variations of the right colic artery are frequent, however.

According to Van Damme,[1] the vascularization of the ascending colon is through a paracolic arcade supplied by

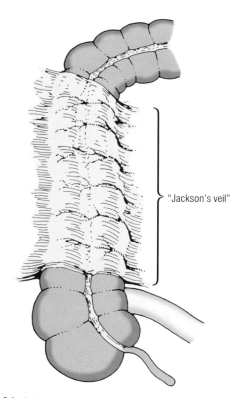

"Jackson's veil"

FIG. 18-34. "Jackson's veil" may contain many small blood vessels from the second lumbar or renal arteries. The extent of the "veil" is variable. (Modified from Skandalakis JE, Gray SW, Rowe JS Jr. Anatomical Complications in General Surgery. New York: McGraw-Hill, 1983; with permission.)

the ileocolic and middle colic arteries, with the potential reinforcement of two right colic arteries. Van Damme stated that the ileocolic artery is the most consistent branch leaving the right side of the superior mesenteric artery. The ileocolic artery is also an important landmark for the interpretation of arteriograms.

Bertelli et al.[42] found the number of right colic arteries to be variable. In most cases, there are two or three.

The right colic vein, a tributary of the superior mesenteric vein, provides the venous return for the ascending colon.

### Lymphatics

The lymphatic drainage is to the right colic nodes, which are located along the network of the right colic artery and the marginal artery of Drummond. According to Woodburne and Burkel,[82] the total number of lymph nodes of the ascending colon and cecum averages 75.

### Innervation

The sympathetic innervation of the ascending colon comes from the celiac and superior mesenteric ganglia. The parasympathetic innervation of the ascending colon arises from the vagus nerve. Cell bodies of sensory fibers from this part of the bowel are located in dorsal root ganglia of the eighth and ninth spinal nerves; therefore, pain is referred to the paraumbilical region of the abdominal wall.

### Surgical Considerations
- The ascending colon can be mobilized by incision of the right lateral peritoneal reflection.
- Dangers from incision are: bleeding from the gonadal vessels, injury to the right ureter, and injury to the duodenum.

### *Hepatic Flexure, Transverse Colon, Splenic Flexure, and Transverse Mesocolon*

The hepatic flexure is located under the 9th and 10th costal cartilages in the vicinity of the midaxillary line between the anterior surface of the lower half of the right kidney and the inferior surface of the right hepatic lobe. The gallbladder is located anteriorly, and the duodenum is located posteriorly.

Occasionally, there is a peritoneal fold between the hepatic flexure and the gallbladder (cystocolic ligament). Also, occasionally, there is another peritoneal fold which starts from the hepatogastric or hepatoduodenal ligament and ends at the right part of the hepatic flexure (hepatocolic ligament). A similar, but rare, peritoneal fold starts from the right lobe of the liver and extends over the entire hepatic flexure. For all practical purposes, this is a wide hepatocolic ligament.

The transverse colon begins where the colon turns sharply to the left (the hepatic flexure), just beneath the inferior surface of the right lobe of the liver. It ends at a sharp upward and then downward bend (the splenic flexure) related to the posterolateral surface of the spleen. The tail of the pancreas is above. The anterior surface of the left kidney lies medially.

The transverse colon, unlike the ascending and descending colon, has a mesentery which has fused secondarily with the posterior wall of the omental bursa (Fig. 18-35). At the beginning of the mesentery, there may be additional bands of peritoneum, the hepatocolic and cystocolic ligaments. These are adhesion bands, not persistent remnants of the ventral mesentery. At the splenic flexure, the colon is supported by the phrenocolic ligament, a part of the left side of the transverse mesocolon.

Between the hepatic and splenic flexures, the transverse colon hangs in a U- or V-shaped curve. It may lie above the umbilicus, but is often lower, even extending into the true pelvis. The transverse colon varies with individuals and with body position.

The transverse mesocolon is formed by a double peritoneal fold which extends upward and attaches to the an-

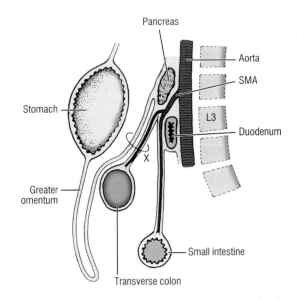

**FIG. 18-35.** Diagrammatic sagittal section showing the developmental relation of the transverse colon and its mesentery to the omentum. The two are fused at "X" to form the transverse mesocolon containing the middle colic artery. SMA, Superior mesenteric artery. (Modified from Skandalakis JE, Gray SW, Rowe JS Jr. Anatomical Complications in General Surgery. New York: McGraw-Hill, 1983; with permission.)

terior pancreatic border, suspending the transverse colon from the pancreas. It ranges in length from 3 to 12 cm. The transverse mesocolon contains the middle colic artery and vein, and lymph nodes as well as nerves. Occasionally, the superior fold of the transverse mesocolon is fixed by adhesions to the posterior wall of the stomach. Gastric ulcers and benign or malignant tumors may be firmly fixed to the mesocolon and despite all efforts to preserve integrity, the middle colic artery may be injured when the stomach wall is separated from mesocolon.

The transverse mesocolon and transverse colon provide the barrier between the supracolic and infracolic compartments of the peritoneal cavity; they are responsible for supracolic or infracolic collections of fluid.

The splenic flexure has an acute angle. It is located higher than the hepatic flexure, at the level of the 8th interspace in the midaxillary line. This high position is due not only to the small left hepatic lobe, but also to the multiple splenic ligaments and other ligaments in its vicinity (see the chapter on the spleen). The splenic flexure is related posteriorly to the left kidney and anteriorly to the left costal arch and occasionally to the stomach.

Charnsangavej and colleagues reviewed CT studies of the mesocolon in health[83] and disease,[84] and reported the following:

> The mesocolon of the cecum and ascending colon can be identified by following the ileocolic vessels at the root of the mesentery and the marginal vessels along the mesocolic side of the colon, whereas the IMV [inferior mesenteric vein] and the marginal vessels of the descending colon serve as landmarks for the descending mesocolon. These vessels ...can be readily identified on CT scans. The transverse mesocolon and the sigmoid mesocolon are less constant because they are more mobile, but the vessels in them can also be traced on CT scans. The middle colic vessels that originate from the marginal vessels of the transverse colon and run toward the pancreas to drain into the SMV (superior mesenteric vein] serve as landmarks for the transverse mesocolon; the marginal vessels of the descending colon and the sigmoid colon and the superior hemorrhoidal vessels form the IMV and serve as landmarks for the sigmoid mesocolon.

The anatomy of the colon and mesocolon is well defined and can be recognized by following the vascular anatomy and by understanding the relationship between the colon and mesocolon and its attachment to retroperitoneal structures, particularly to the pancreas. Common pathologic conditions in the mesocolon result from the spread of disease either from the colon or the pancreas.

The pathway for the spread of disease may be seen along the mesocolon via the lymphatic vessels in the mesocolon and involvement of mesocolic vessels.

### Arterial Supply, Venous Drainage

In the "typical" arrangement, the right colic artery (Fig. 18-36) bifurcates into ascending and descending branches. The ascending branch anastomoses with the right branch of the middle colic artery. The descending branch anastomoses with the ileocolic artery. The left colic artery (Fig. 18-36) also bifurcates; its ascending branch anastomoses with the left branch of the middle colic artery, and its descending branch anastomoses with the first branch of the sigmoid artery.

The main blood supply of the transverse colon is the middle colic artery (Fig. 18-36), but the ascending branch of the left colic artery contributes circulation for the distal part of the transverse colon. Anatomically, the entrance of the middle colic artery into the antimesenteric border of the transverse colon is very close to the pancreatic neck. If adhesions of benign or malignant origin are present in this area, this is another point of danger.

The middle colic artery bifurcates from 3 cm to 11 cm from the colonic wall, and may be absent in 5-8 percent of individuals. In most cases, the middle colic artery originates from the superior mesenteric artery. It can arise as a stem from which the inferior pancreaticoduodenal artery, right hepatic artery, jejunal artery, or other branches take origin. It may be absent.[85]

Van Damme[1] stated that the middle colic artery is not a single artery, but a complex system of different vessels. He described the "composed system of the middle colic artery" as follows:

> The middle colic artery is not a single vessel. Five different vessels can be discerned (Fig. 18-36) behaving as arteries or as branches: (1) the middle colic artery (46% of specimens), dividing into a branch for the right angle and one for the transverse colon; (2) the artery for the right angle of the colon (32%); (3) the artery for the transverse colon (12%); (4) the accessory artery for the transverse colon (3%); and (5) the accessory left colic artery (7%).

Bertelli et al.[42] noted a middle colic artery in more than 95% of their subjects.

The venous return is formed by right and left networks. The right network drains into the right gastroepiploic vein or the superior mesenteric vein. The left network drains into the inferior mesenteric vein.

### Lymphatics

The lymphatics of the transverse colon can be sub-

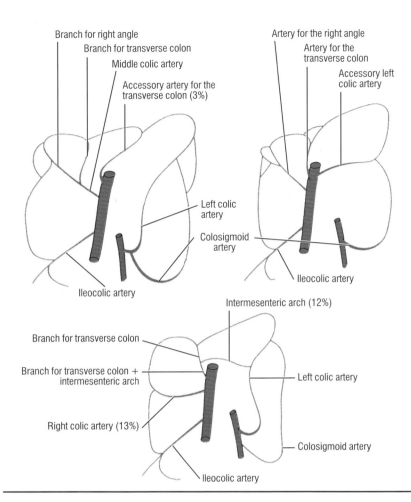

**FIG. 18-36.** Nomenclature of the colic arteries. Only colic vessels arising directly from the superior mesenteric artery deserve the name of arteria colica. The right colic artery is an exceptional vessel (13%). The middle colic is not a single vessel but a complex system of five different vessels that behave as arteries or as branches: (1) middle colic artery dividing into a branch for the right angle and one for the transverse colon; (2) artery for the right angle of the colon; (3) artery for the transverse colon; (4) accessory artery for the transverse colon; (5) accessory left colic artery. (Modified from Van Damme JP, Bonte J. Vascular Anatomy in Abdominal Surgery. New York: Thieme Verlag, 1990; with permission.)

divided into two networks: the right serves the proximal two-thirds, and the left serves the distal one-third.

In the right network, the lymphatic vessels follow the right and middle colic arteries to the lymph nodes of the superior mesenteric artery, and then to the aortic nodes, and finally reach the intestinal lymphatic trunk.

In the left network, some of the lymphatic vessels follow the middle colic artery, while most accompany the left colic artery to the lymph nodes of the inferior mesenteric artery and lumbar lymph nodes.

REMEMBER:
- Lymphatic drainage of the proximal transverse colon including the hepatic flexure usually drains into the middle colic or right colic system; rarely it drains into the ileocolic system.
- The middle transverse colon is served by the middle colic system.
- Lymphatic drainage of the distal transverse colon including the splenic flexure drains to the middle colic and

left colic systems.
- Retrograde systems may be present.

**Innervation**

The innervation of the transverse colon is by the autonomic system. Postganglionic sympathetic fibers arise from the superior mesenteric ganglia. Preganglionic parasympathetic fibers from the vagi supply two-thirds or somewhat more of the transverse colon. The remainder arise by way of the pelvic splanchnic parasympathetic outflow from the intermediolateral cell column at levels S2, S3, and S4. Postganglionic cell bodies are present within the terminal ganglia of the wall of the colon.

**Surgical Considerations**
- Mobilization of the hepatic flexure can be accomplished by: (a) incision of the upper right lateral peritoneal reflection (as is done for mobilization of the ascending colon), (b) placement of the colon in a medial position.

- Mobilization of the right colon (cecum, ascending colon, hepatic flexure) can be combined with duodenal mobilization by kocherization (see the duodenum chapter).
- The retroperitoneal anatomic entities with which the hepatic flexure is related are the right kidney and the ureter, and the descending part of the duodenum and the gonadal vessels.
- The right gonadal vein is more vulnerable than the right gonadal artery. This is because the entrance of the vein to the inferior vena cava is higher, and the origin of the artery is lower. Both vessels are very close together just above the right iliac fossa. They travel downward together.
- The anterior relations with the gallbladder can be seen very well by the orthodox or laparoscopic approach.
- Separation of the posterior gastric wall from the transverse mesocolon requires great care.
- It is also essential to separate the transverse mesocolon very carefully from the pancreas at the neck of the pancreas.
- The left mesocolon is less vascular than the right. These avascular areas should be used in surgery for posterior gastrojejunostomy, Roux-en-Y, and other procedures. Remember that the "arc of Riolan" may be present in the more cranial part of the mesocolon. This is an artery of respectable size interconnecting the inferior mesenteric or left colic arteries with the superior mesenteric or middle colic arteries. Hollinshead[86] states that Griffiths reported the incidence of the arc of Riolan to be 10%.
- The posterior area of the splenic flexure is usually not covered by peritoneum and is fixed to the posterior abdominal wall. Occasionally, it is covered completely by peritoneum and its mesocolon is fixed to the distal body and tail of the pancreas.
- The splenocolic ligament, a remnant of the left end of the transverse mesocolon, is a peritoneal bridge between the splenic flexure and the lower spleen. The left gastroepipolic artery and some aberrant inferior polar vessels may be in the vicinity. Incise the ligament between clamps and ligate. Should excessive traction be applied to this ligament, tearing of the splenic pole can result, with profuse bleeding.
- The phrenocolic ligament, between the splenic flexure and the diaphragm at the level of the 10th rib at the mid-axillary line, forms a hammock in which the spleen rests. The ligament should be incised for mobilization of the splenic flexure.
- Mesenteric cysts of the small or large bowel are uncommon, but may be benign or malignant; thus the surgeon should be alert to them. Horiuchi et al.[87] state that retroperitoneoscopic resection of such cysts has a lower risk of traumatizing the bowel than laparoscopic intra-abdominal excision, with a further advantage of not com-

pressing other intra-abdominal organs. Forty percent of all mesenteric cysts occur in the colon. A complete discussion of mesenteric cysts can be found in the chapter on the small intestine.

## *Descending Colon*

The descending colon is related to the following anatomic entities: the quadratus lumborum muscle, left adrenal gland, left kidney and left ureter, left gonadal vessels, and the iliohypogastric and ilioinguinal nerves.

Like the ascending colon, the left or descending colon is covered anteriorly and on its medial and lateral sides by peritoneum. It normally has no mesentery. During the last decade, several authors, such as Dixon et al.[88] have investigated the superficial or deep retroperitoneal topographical anatomy of the descending colon with the use of CT scans and MRIs. Hadar and Gadoth,[89] Sherman et al.,[90] Hopper et al.,[91] Helms et al.,[92] and Prassopoulos et al.[93] investigated the retroperitoneal relations between the descending colon and the left kidney. Because the goal of these articles is to avoid anatomic complications and injury to the left kidney during percutaneous renal and vertebral procedures when the descending colon is too deep, they should have presented more details of the anatomy of the descending colon.

LeRoy et al.[94] stated that a descending colon that is located more posteriorly than expected may be injured if too posterior an approach is used. According to Dixon et al.,[88] in rare cases, the descending colon (which is situated within the retroperitoneal fat) passes between the psoas major and the quadratus lumborum muscles in a posterolateral location, which makes it possible for the bowel to be injured during posterior percutaneous procedures. LeRoy et al.,[94] Helms et al.[92] and Bonaldi et al.[95] emphasized the possibility of puncturing the descending colon.

According to Dixon et al.,[88] there are several explanations for these variations. in topography and location of the descending colon. These include: obesity, variations of the architecture and topography of the psoas major muscle, and the more posterior location of the colon in women. The authors of this chapter emphasize that these variations are not of congenital origin and we concur with Dixon et al. that they constitute anatomic variations.

When the left or descending colon has a mesentery, it is rarely long enough to permit a volvulus to occur. The surgical unit of the left colon consists of the splenic flexure and the descending and sigmoid colons.

### Arterial Supply, Venous Drainage

The descending colon is supplied by the left colic

artery. The inferior mesenteric vein provides venous drainage. This then passes into the portal vein. The route may be via the splenic vein, the superior mesenteric vein, or venous flow may pass directly into the origin of the portal vein at the junction of the two previous veins. These pathways occur with nearly equal frequency.

According to Grant and Basmajian,[96] "a large branch ...not rarely connects the stem of the superior mesenteric artery with the left colic artery on the posterior abdominal wall." This branch is the arc of Riolan.

Van Damme[1] reported the following observations on the arterial supply of the left colon:

> *The left colic artery... has a long S-like course and ends at the splenic flexure. Its behavior is influenced by the presence of an accessory left colic artery or branch (14% of specimens) from the middle colic artery group, yet they arise from a completely different area. If this accessory left colic vessel is present, the normal left colic artery is absent (12%), atrophic, or displaced. In the absence of the left colic artery, both the colosigmoid artery and the paracolic arcade are usually reinforced by an accessory vessel... The left colic artery gives rise to the colosigmoid (38%) and sigmoid (4%) vessels and seldom to an intermesenteric arcade. We reintroduced the name "colosigmoid artery"[97] because this vessel plays a key role in the supply of the descending and sigmoid colons. It arises close to the angle between the left colic and the inferior mesenteric artery from one of these constituents and points to the colosigmoid transition area. Sigmoid branches arise from the colosigmoid, the left colic, the inferior mesenteric, or the superior rectal arteries. The last sigmoid artery is a troublesome heritage from the discussion about the critical point of Sudeck.[40] It deserves no special attention.*

Bertelli et al.[42] agree with several authors that the left colic artery is the only true colic artery.

### Lymphatics

The lymphatic drainage is to nodes of the superior mesenteric artery.

### Innervation

The autonomic system is responsible for the innervation of the descending colon. Preganglionic and postganglionic sympathetic fibers are carried by lumbar splanchnic branches of the sympathetic chain, the preganglionic fibers synapsing in inferior mesenteric ganglia. Preganglionic parasympathetic fibers are carried by the pelvic splanchnic nerves from the ventral primary rami of S2, S3, and S4; these fibers synapse in intramural (terminal) parasympathetic ganglia in the rich intermuscular and submucosal plexuses.

### Surgical Considerations

- Mobilization of the descending colon is accomplished by incising the peritoneal reflection at the left gutter along the "white line of Toldt." During mobilization, the most vulnerable anatomic entities are the left ureter and the left gonadal vessels.
- Remember that the inferior mesenteric vein may also lie, often well-concealed, behind the mesentery of the descending colon, if a mesentery is present.

## *Sigmoid Colon*

At the level of the iliac crest, the descending colon becomes the sigmoid colon and acquires a mesentery. The sigmoid colon is described as having two portions: (1) the iliac portion, which is fixed and located at the left iliac fossa; and (2) the pelvic portion, which is mobile. This entity is called "sigmoid" because of its "S" shape in many people. For all practical purposes, the sigmoid colon begins at the iliac crest and ends at the 3rd sacral vertebra. The iliac part is the downward continuation of the descending colon. It does not have a mesentery, and it ends at the pelvic brim, where the pelvic colon and its mesentery (pelvic mesocolon) start.

The mobile, omega-shaped (Ω) pelvic colon begins at the medial border of the psoas major muscle. It has a mesentery (the pelvic mesocolon) that is fixed to the posterior pelvic wall, its fixation being like the capital Greek letter lambda (Λ). The pelvic colon terminates at the rectosigmoid junction, which is located at the area of the 3rd sacral vertebra. At this point, its mesentery ceases. The middle of the base of the lambda is located at the point where the left ureter crosses the pelvic brim –at the intersigmoid mesenteric recess– just lateral and posterior to the fossa in which the left ovary rests. The left leg of the lambda is attached to the pelvic brim. The right leg travels medially and downward to the 3rd sacral vertebra. The superior rectal vessels are within the mesentery of the sigmoid colon.

Shafik[98] suggested that the rectosigmoid junction acts as a functional sphincter: opening reflexively upon sigmoid contraction (rectosigmoid inhibitory reflex) and allowing feces to pass to the rectum, and closing upon rectal contraction (rectosigmoid excitatory reflex) and preventing stool reflux into the sigmoid.

### Arterial Supply, Venous Drainage

The sigmoid branches of the inferior mesenteric artery supply the sigmoid colon. There can be a left colic-sigmoid branch of the left colic artery that supplies the proximal sigmoid. The inferior mesenteric vein drains the area.

### Lymphatics

The course of the lymphatics of the descending colon

is as follows: the lymphatic vessels drain to nodes along the left colic artery, then to inferior mesenteric artery nodes, then to left lumbar nodes or left aortic nodes.

### Innervation

Autonomic nerves, as described for the descending colon, innervate the sigmoid colon. Pain fibers for the sigmoid colon and the descending colon pass upward via lumbar splanchnic nerves and the sympathetic chain to the upper 1 or 2 lumbar segments of the spinal cord (the site to which pain may be referred from the descending colon). Their path is via white communicating rami, connecting the sympathetic chains to the spinal nerves at those levels.

### Surgical Considerations

- During mobilization of the ileal and pelvic parts of the sigmoid colon, it is necessary to protect the left ureter and the left gonadal vessels (just as with the descending colon).
- The inferior mesenteric vein can be ligated with impunity. If possible, ligate it close to its termination or to its entrance to the splenic or superior mesenteric vein.
- Transection of the colon 3-4 cm below the tumor is adequate for rectosigmoid tumors because the lymphatic flow in most cases is not retrograde. Most, if not all, involved lymph nodes are 2 cm or less below the tumor.
- The promontory of the sacrum is perhaps a landmark for the termination of the sigmoid colon. Remember that in rare cases there are tongues of short mesentery for both the proximal rectum and the terminal sigmoid colon.
- The inferior mesenteric artery also can be ligated with impunity if normal anastomoses are present between the right colic artery (if present), middle colic artery, and the marginal artery interconnecting them with the left colic artery.
- The attachment of the mesosigmoid to the body wall shows much variation.[99] In most individuals, the attachment starts in the left iliac fossa and extends diagonally downward and to the right. In others, the attachment is sinuous (shaped like a C, S, or inverted U). According to Vaez-Zadeh and Dutz,[100] the average length of the attachment in 140 autopsies was 7.9 cm (Fig. 18-37A). These authors found the breadth of the mesentery ranging from an average of 5.6 cm in 100 autopsies in New York to 15.2 cm in 40 autopsies in Iran. Whether this difference is genetic or dietary is not clear. The left ureter passes through the base of the sigmoid mesocolon through the intersigmoid recess (Fig. 18-37B).

## SURGICAL ANATOMY OF THE RECTUM AND ANAL CANAL

The junction between the sigmoid colon and the rectum has been variously described:

- A point opposite the left sacroiliac joint
- Level of the 3rd sacral vertebra
- Level at which the sigmoid mesentery disappears
- Level at which sacculations and epiploic appendages disappear and taeniae broaden to form a complete muscle layer (long transition)

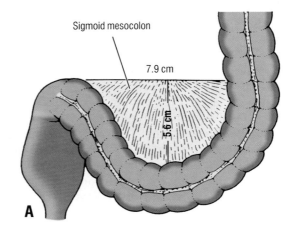

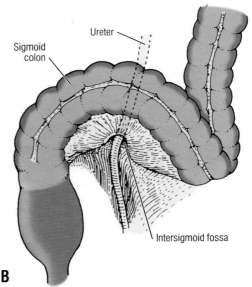

FIG. 18-37. Sigmoid mesocolon. **A,** Average measurements. **B,** The relation of the base of the sigmoid mesocolon to the left ureter. (Modified from Skandalakis JE, Gray SW, Rowe JS Jr. Anatomical Complications in General Surgery. New York: McGraw-Hill, 1983. Data in **A** from Vaez-Zadeh K, Dutz W. Ileosigmoid knotting. Ann Surg 1970;172:1027; with permission.)

- Level at which the superior rectal artery divides into right and left branches
- Construction with anterior angulation (proctoscopy)
- Level of superior rectal fold (inconstant)
- Transition between rugose mucosa of colon and smooth mucosa of rectum (cadaver)

These levels are neither consistent with each other nor constant from one individual to another. Some are useful to the surgeon, some to the anatomist, and some to the proctoscopist. The reader need not be discouraged. There is, fortunately, no compelling surgical reason for establishing a definite boundary between the sigmoid colon and the rectum.

The lower boundary of the rectum is no more agreed upon than the upper boundary. Part of the disagreement between the surgeon and the anatomist lies in differences between the living patient and the cadaver, but much of it is due to a terminology rich in both synonyms and ambiguities.

Some anatomy textbooks describe the anal canal as the region lying distal to the pectinate (dentate) line, while to the surgeon, all the region distal to the insertion of the levator ani muscles is the anal canal. The surgical anal canal (the anorectum of Harkins) includes the anatomic anal canal and the distal 2 cm of the rectum above the pectinate line. In addition to the changes in anatomy and physiology at the pectinate line, pathology unique to the distal 4 cm of the intestinal tract (2 cm above and 2 cm below the line) distinguishes a unit, the "surgical anal canal" (Table 18-7).[6]

## Peritoneal Reflections

The entire upper one-third of the rectum is covered by peritoneum (Fig. 18-38). As the rectum passes deeper into the pelvis, more and more fat is interposed between the rectal musculature and the peritoneum. The mesorectum, which suspends the rectum from the posterior body wall, comes off more laterally, leaving bare progressively more of the posterior rectal wall. The peritoneum finally leaves the rectum and passes anteriorly and superiorly over the posterior vaginal fornix and the uterus in females or over the superior ends of the seminal vesicles and the bladder in males. This creates a depression, the rectouterine or rectovesical pouch; with infection, this may become filled with pus.

In summary, the relations of the rectum are as follows:
- Male (extraperitoneal)
  - Anterior: prostate, seminal vesicles, ductus (vas) deferens, ureters, urinary bladder
  - Posterior: sacrum and fascia of Waldeyer, coccyx and its muscles, levator ani, median sacral vessels, roots of the sacral nerve plexus
- Female
  a. Extraperitoneal
  - Anterior: posterior vaginal wall
  - Lateral: intestinal loops
  b. Intraperitoneal
  - Anterior: posterior vaginal wall, upper uterus, uterine (fallopian) tubes, ovaries
  - Lateral: pelvic wall
  - Posterior: as in the male

Some authors like to divide the anorectum into 3 parts. This division also is acceptable if the student of rectal surgery remembers that the upper one-third is surrounded by peritoneum, the middle one-third is covered only anteriorly by peritoneum (being located nearly retroperitoneally) and the lower one-third is extraperitoneal (retroperitoneal).

**TABLE 18-7. The Pectinate Line and Changes in the Surgical Anal Canal**

|  | Below the Pectinate Line | Above the Pectinate Line |
|---|---|---|
| Embryonic origin | Ectoderm | Endoderm |
| Anatomy |  |  |
|   Lining | Stratified squamous | Simple columnar |
|   Arterial supply | Inferior rectal artery | Superior rectal artery |
|   Venous drainage | Systemic, by way of inferior rectal vein | Portal, by way of superior rectal vein |
|   Lymphatic drainage | To inguinal nodes | To pelvic and lumbar nodes |
|   Nerve supply | Inferior rectal nerves (somatic) | Autonomic fibers (visceral) |
| Physiology | Excellent sensation | Sensation quickly diminishes |
| Pathology |  |  |
|   Cancer | Squamous cell carcinoma | Adenocarcinoma |
|   Varices | External hemorrhoids | Internal hemorrhoids |

*Source:* Skandalakis JE, Gray SW, Rowe JS Jr. Anatomical Complications in General Surgery. New York: McGraw-Hill, 1983; with permission.

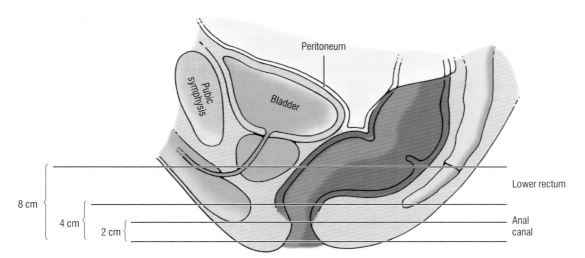

**FIG. 18-38.** The line of peritoneal reflection on the rectum; lateral view in the male. More of the rectum is covered anteriorly than posteriorly. The measurements of the anal canal and lower rectum from the anal verge are approximate. (Modified from Skandalakis JE, Gray SW, Rowe JS Jr. Anatomical Complications in General Surgery. New York: McGraw-Hill, 1983; with permission.)

## Pelvic Diaphragm and Continence

The floor of the pelvis is the pelvic diaphragm, through which the rectum passes. The diaphragm is composed of two paired muscles, the levator ani and the coccygeus (Fig. 18-39). The levator ani may be considered to be made up of three muscles: the iliococcygeus, the pubococcygeus, and the puborectalis. The puborectalis is essential to maintaining rectal continence, and is considered by some authors to be part of the external sphincter and not a part of levator ani. The visible, intrapelvic border of the levator hiatus is formed by the medial borders of the pubococcygeus, not the puborectalis. The puborectalis is attached to the lower back surface of the symphysis pubis and the superior layer of the deep perineal pouch (urogenital diaphragm). Fibers from each side of the muscle pass posteriorly and then join posterior to the rectum, forming a well-defined sling (Fig. 18-39).

The puborectalis with the superficial and deep parts of the external sphincter and the proximal part of the internal sphincter form the so-called anorectal ring. This ring can be palpated; and since cutting through it will produce incontinence, it must be identified and protected during surgical procedures. The details of the external sphincter will be discussed with the morphology of the anal canal (see "Anal Canal").

REMEMBER:
- The anal verge is the junction of skin around the anal opening and the anal mucosa.

- The dentate or pectinate line is located 2 cm above the anal verge and represents the junction between the anal transition zone below and the anal nonkeratinizing squamous mucosa.
- In the upper end of the surgical anal canal (which is located 4 cm from the anal verge and 2 cm from the dentate line) is the palpable anorectal ring. This is the level of the sling provided by the puborectalis.

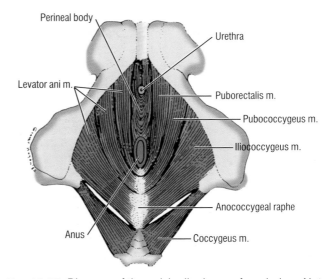

**FIG. 18-39.** Diagram of the pelvic diaphragm from below. Note that the levator ani is composed of three muscles: puborectalis, pubococcygeus, and iliococcygeus. (Modified from Skandalakis JE, Gray SW, Rowe JS Jr. Anatomical Complications in General Surgery. New York: McGraw-Hill, 1983; with permission.)

- The divisions of the anorectum can be remembered as 4 and its multiples. The surgical anal canal is 4 cm long; the rectum, 12 cm long; the total anorectum is approximately 16 cm.
- Fibrofatty tissue covers the surgical anal canal anteriorly, laterally, and posteriorly. The distal 8 cm of the anorectum is mostly (or partially) retroperitoneal; posteriorly it is related to the sacrum and coccyx.
- The posterior rectal wall is related to two fasciae: a thin one close to the rectal wall, and a thick one (the fascia of Waldeyer) covering the anterior aspects of the sacrococcygeal area.
- Only the thin fascia should be removed with the rectum. Removal of the sacral fascia will produce venous bleeding which is extremely difficult to control.
- Careful cleaning of the distal 8 cm of the anorectum will produce enough length for a sphincter-saving procedure.
- Anorectal anastomosis after good mobilization of the distal 8 cm of the anorectum can be safely done at the dentate line (endo-anal anastomosis).
- Some anatomic guidelines vary depending on the peritoneal reflection, sex of the patient, peculiarity of pelvic anatomy, and weight of the patient.
- The rectal mucosa has no role in the act of defecation.
- Today's acceptable "save" rule is a resection line of 2.5-3 cm distal to the lower margin of the tumor mass.
- The surgeon should always remember the magic number 4 for the segmental anatomy of the anorectum, as well as an empiric 2.5-3 cm margin below the tumor as the line of resection. Frozen specimen of the distal end, appropriately marked, is essential. If the tumor is located 2-3 cm above the dentate line, abdominoperineal resection is the procedure of choice. Discussion with the patient prior to surgery about the possibility of permanent colostomy is imperative.
- During a low anterior resection, the length of the rectum after good mobilization may be increased by 4 cm to 5 cm.

## Fascial Relations and Tissue Spaces

The parietal fascia of the pelvic basin is continuous with the transversalis fascia of the abdominal cavity. In the pelvis this fascia would include that which covers the obturator internus laterally and the piriformis posterolaterally. It also includes the fascial layers of the pelvic diaphragm; that is, the fascia of the levator ani (Fig. 18-40) and coccygeus muscles.

Six potential spaces around the rectum (Fig. 18-41) are recognized by Shafik.[101] They are important because they may become sites of infection. The fascial layers that bound these spaces help limit the spread both of infection and of neoplastic disease, although all are potentially confluent with one another.

### Subcutaneous Space

The subcutaneous space corresponds to the perianal space of Milligan and associates.[102] It is bounded above by the lowest muscular loop of the external sphincter, below by the perianal skin, and medially by the epithelium of the anal verge. It is filled with fat and by fibers of the corrugator ani cutis. The subcutaneous space is in communication above with the central space and laterally with the ischioanal (ischiorectal) space. Medially, the medial central septum separates it from the submucous space. The subcutaneous space is often considered to be a part of the ischioanal space.

### Central Space

The central space is considered by Shafik[101] to be the main perianal space; it is in communication with each of the others. It surrounds the anal canal and is bounded by the termination of the longitudinal muscles above and the lowest muscular loop of the external sphincter below. Within it lie the tendon fibers of the longitudinal muscles.

### Intersphincteric Spaces

The intersphincteric spaces are four upward extensions of the central space. They are the fascial planes between the longitudinal intersphincteric muscles that form the upper boundary of the central space. Proceeding from lateral to medial, the first and third spaces open into the ischioanal space, the second space opens into the pelvirectal space, and the most medial space communicates with the submucous space. These "spaces" are potential pathways of infection and are potential spaces only.

### Ischioanal (Ischiorectal) Fossa

The ischioanal (ischiorectal) fossa is a pyramidal space on either side of the anal canal and lower rectum, posterior to the base of the urogenital diaphragm. Its base is at the perianal skin; its medial wall is the external anal sphincter and levator; its lateral wall is the internal obturator fascia; and its apex is where the levator muscles join the obturator internus muscle. The two spaces communicate posteriorly through the *retrosphincteric space*.[103]

The lower portion of the ischioanal (ischiorectal) space has been termed the *perianal space* by Milligan.[104] Laterally it

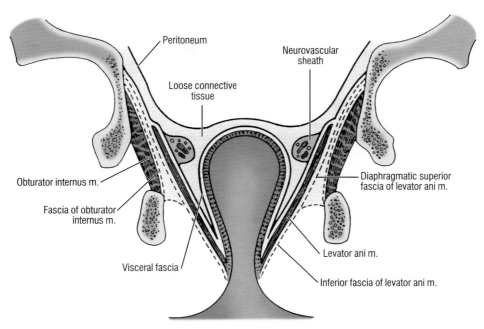

**FIG. 18-40.** Diagram of some of the fasciae of the pelvis seen in coronal section. (Modified from Skandalakis JE, Gray SW, Rowe JS Jr. *Anatomical Complications in General Surgery.* New York: McGraw-Hill, 1983; with permission.)

communicates with the gluteal fat and the subcutaneous space. It is usually considered a part of the ischioanal fossa.

## Pelvirectal Spaces

The pelvirectal spaces lie above the levators and are bounded superiorly by the pelvic peritoneum, laterally by the pubococcygeus muscle, and medially by the rectum. The spaces are filled with fibroadipose tissue. The fibrous elements of the tissue, known as the lateral ligaments of the rectum, are part of the pelvic fascia and connect the parietal pelvic fascia with the walls of the rectum and pelvis. These ligaments form a triangle, with its base on the side wall of the pelvis and the apex joining the rectum. The lateral ligaments conduct the middle rectal vessels and nerves.

The lateral pelvirectal spaces on either side of the rectum communicate behind the rectum, in front of the sacrum, and above the levators. This communication is separated from the rectal wall by the fascia propria of the rectum and from the sacrum by a thickened parietal pelvic fascia called the *fascia of Waldeyer*. The middle sacral vessels lie within this fascia, which is often considered to be a separate space (the rectorectal or presacral space).

The extraperitoneal anterior part of the rectum is covered with a bilaminar fascial layer *(Denonvilliers' fascia)* that extends from the anterior peritoneal reflection above to the perineal body below. Posterolaterally, this connective tissue septum is continuous with connective tissue of the sacrogenital or uterosacral folds and the lateral pillar of the rectum. This bilaminar fascial layer, also called the rectovaginal or rectovesical septum, separates the rectum from the prostate and seminal vesicles in males or from the vagina in females. This fascia forms a barrier to the spread of cancer or infection either anteriorly or posteriorly.

## Submucous Space

The submucous space of Shafik[105] lies beneath the anal mucosa and the internal sphincter. It is the most distal portion of the submucosa of the digestive tract. While it is certainly a possible pathway for infection, it does not contribute to the longitudinal spread of cancer.[106] The authors of this chapter consider it a definite and rather stout layer of the enteric wall; however, it can be considered a space.

A mucosal ligament described by Parks[107] as connecting the anal mucosa and the internal sphincter would form the lower limit of the submucous space. The presence of such a ligament has not been confirmed by Shafik[105] or by Goligher.[41]

## Retrorectal Space

The retrorectal space, according to Jackman et al.,[108]

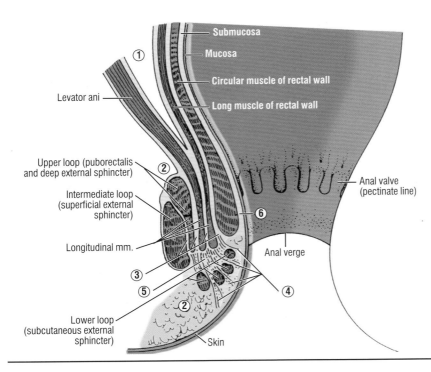

FIG. 18-41. The spaces of the anus and rectum. 1. Pelvirectal space. 2, Ischioanal (ischiorectal) space. 3, Intersphincteric spaces. 4, Subcutaneous space. 5, Central space. 6, Submucous space. (Modified from Skandalakis JE, Gray SW, Rowe JS Jr. Anatomical Complications in General Surgery. New York: McGraw-Hill, 1983; with permission.)

has the following boundaries:

- Anterior: Fascia propria of the posterior rectal wall
- Posterior: Presacral fascia
- Lateral: Iliac vessels, ureters, lateral rectal ligaments
- Superior: Peritoneum
- Inferior: Retrosacral fascia

## Mesorectum

In *Embryology for Surgeons*,[13] which was co-written by the senior author of this chapter the mesorectum was neither mentioned nor discussed. *Gray's Anatomy*[26] refers to the "dorsal mesorectum...which does not form a true mesentery, however, but... a woven fibroelar sheet with patterned variations in thickness and fibre orientation." The rectum is said to differ from the sigmoid colon by having "no sacculations, appendices epiploicae or mesentery"[26] (emphasis ours).

Heald and colleagues[109] have published multiple excellent articles providing a complete education about the mesorectum. Heald[110] defines the mesorectum as "the integral visceral mesentery surrounding the rectum ...covered by a layer of visceral fascia providing a relatively bloodless plane, the so-called 'holy plane' (Fig. 18-42A & B). The dorsal mesentery is embryologically responsible for the genesis of the mesorectum.

In the lab, the senior author of this chapter has found this 'holy plane,' and he agrees with Heald about its sev-

eral relations. Posteriorly, the plane is located between the visceral fascia which surrounds the mesorectum and the parietal presacral fascia (fascia of Waldeyer). In the male, Denonvilliers' fascia (Fig. 18-43) constitutes the anterior surface of the mesorectum, which is fused with the posterior surface of the fascia of Denonvilliers'. Inferiorly, the mesorectum and the fascia of Waldeyer condense to form the rectosacral ligament in the vicinity of S4.

The senior author of this chapter is sure that the readers of the beautiful publications of Heald would have no objections to renaming the 'holy plane,' the Plane of Heald.

We quote from Konerding et al.:[111]

*The perirectal tissue gives rise to the rectal fascia or adventitia, also known as mesorectum. The connective tissue space between rectal and parietal pelvic fascia can be dissected as a plane free of vessels and nerves. Surgical dissection along this plane with complete mesorectum excision results in reliable excision of all relevant lymphatic pathways with extensive preservation of continence and sexual function.*

Enker et al.[112] presented four surgical planes for anatomic dissection of the rectum for the following oncologic surgeries (see the section "Anorectal Cancer Surgery" later in this chapter for details):

- Total mesorectal excision
- Total mesorectal excision with autonomic nerve preservation
- Mesorectal excision

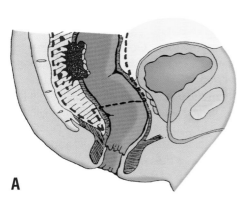
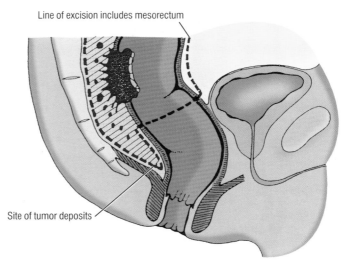

**A**               **B**

Line of excision includes mesorectum

Site of tumor deposits

FIG. **18-42.** The "holy plane." **A,** Diagrammatic representation. **B,** Suggested plane of excision shown by dashed line. (**A,** Modified from Heald RJ. The "holy plane" of rectal surgery. J R Soc Med 1988;81:503-508. **B,** Modified from Heald RJ, Husband EM, Ryall RDH. The mesorectum in rectal cancer surgery - the clue to pelvic recurrence? Br J Surg 1982;69:613-616; with permission.)

• Extrafascial excision of the rectum

After low anterior resection with total mesorectal excision, Law et al.[113] recommend routine creation of a stoma for males and selective use of diversion for females for the avoidance of lower anastomotic leakage.

Total or partial mesorectal excision for rectal carcinoma has been advocated by several authors.[114-119] Maurer et al.[120] stated that continence-preserving surgery on patients with rectal carcinoma may be performed in over 80% of patients by partial or total removal of the mesorectum with positive results.

## Arterial Supply, Venous Drainage

The following is a detailed presentation of the blood supply of the anorectum. Some of this material has already been presented in less detailed form in other sections of "Surgical Anatomy of the Colon"; because it is a complicated topic, some repetition is worthwhile.

The arteries of the rectum and anal canal are the unpaired superior rectal artery, the paired middle and inferior rectal arteries (Fig. 18-44), and the median sacral arteries. The superior rectal (hemorrhoidal) artery arises from the inferior mesenteric artery and descends to the posterior wall of the upper rectum. Supplying the posterior wall, it divides and sends right and left branches to the lateral walls of the middle portion of the rectum down to the pectinate (dentate) line.

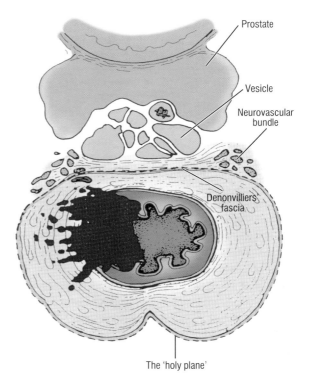

Prostate

Vesicle

Neurovascular bundle

Denonvilliers' fascia

The 'holy plane'

FIG. **18-43.** Schematic representation of the relationships of the mesorectum to the anatomic structures in the male. The neurovascular bundle contains the nerves responsible for erection and ejaculation, and aspects of bladder function. (Modified from Heald RJ, Moran BJ. Embryology and anatomy of the rectum. Semin Surg Oncol 1998;15:66-71; with permission.)

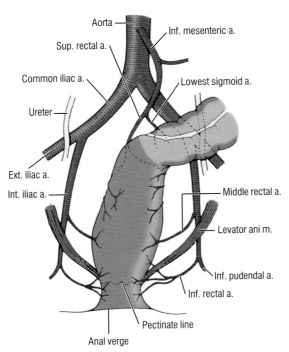

Aorta

Inf. mesenteric a.

Sup. rectal a.

Common iliac a.

Lowest sigmoid a.

Ureter

Ext. iliac a.

Int. iliac a.

Middle rectal a.

Levator ani m.

Inf. pudendal a.

Inf. rectal a.

Pectinate line

Anal verge

FIG. 18-44. Diagram of the arterial supply to the rectum and anus. The median sacral artery supplying a few small branches to the posterior wall of the rectum is not shown. (Modified from Skandalakis JE, Gray SW, Rowe JS Jr. Anatomical Complications in General Surgery. New York: McGraw-Hill, 1983; with permission.)

Many surgeons are under the impression that the *middle rectal (hemorrhoidal) arteries* are always present in the lateral rectal stalks. Some authors[30,121] have found these arteries to be inconstant; Michels[122] found them to be constant, but varying in number and in origin. All originated (directly, or often indirectly) from the internal iliac artery. The number varied from three to nine and the diameter from 1.0 mm to 2.5 mm. In 58 percent of subjects, there was a grossly visible anastomosis between the middle and superior rectal arteries.

Boxall et al.[123] found that the vessel in the lateral ligaments of the rectum, called the *middle rectal artery* by surgeons, was actually an "accessory" middle rectal artery that is present in about 25 percent of individuals. The main trunk of the middle rectal artery was inferior to the rectal stalk and could be endangered when the rectum is separated from the seminal vesicle, prostate, or vagina. In 12 cadavers, the arteries entered the rectal wall with the levator ani muscle; in 9 it was 2-4 cm higher. These findings may explain why some surgeons feel that the lateral ligaments may be cut with impunity.

In our experience, the middle rectal artery is usually absent in the female. It is probably replaced by the uterine artery. In the male, the chief beneficiaries of the artery are the rectal musculature and the prostate gland. Last[124] agrees.

Vogel and Klosterhalfen[125] reported that the middle rectal artery supplies the rectum accessorily and stated that this is the reason for suture leaks at the dorsocaudal area of the profunda. However, Goligher[126] reported that the rectum and anus can survive divisions of the superior and middle rectal arteries.

The *inferior rectal (hemorrhoidal) arteries* arise from the internal pudendal arteries and proceed ventrally and medially to supply the anal canal distal to the pectinate line.

The median sacral artery arises just above the bifurcation of the aorta and descends beneath the peritoneum on the anterior surface of the lower lumbar vertebrae, the sacrum, and the coccyx. It sends several very small branches to the posterior wall of the rectum.

Venous drainage of the rectum and anal canal is discussed in "Vascular Supply" of the large intestine.

## Lymphatics

Lymph channels of the rectum and anal canal form two extramural plexuses, one above and one below the pectinate line (see Fig. 18-24). The upper plexus drains through posterior rectal nodes to a chain of nodes along the superior rectal artery to the pelvic nodes. Some drainage follows the middle and inferior rectal arteries to hypogastric nodes. Below the pectinate line, the plexus drains to the inguinal nodes.

There is considerable disagreement about connections between the two plexuses across the pectinate line, but if such connections exist, they are small. Regardless of this, drainage above the pectinate line from any part of the rectum is upward to the pelvic nodes; drainage below the line is to inguinal nodes. The importance of this line is that 85 percent of pathology is located in this area. External drainage to inguinal nodes appears to be limited to lesions involving the skin of the anal or perianal region.[41]

The watershed of the extramural lymphatic vessels is at the pectinate line (Fig. 18-44). The watershed for the intramural lymphatics is higher, at the level of the middle rectal valve (Fig. 18-45). These two landmarks may be kept in mind by the mnemonic "two, four, eight," meaning:

2 cm = anal verge to pectinate line

4 cm = surgical anal canal (above and below the pectinate line)

8 cm = anal verge to middle rectal valve

The anatomy of metastasis of malignant tumors of the colon and rectum is perhaps as follows (Fig. 18-46):

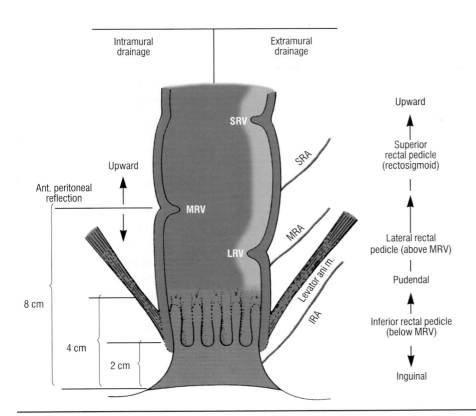

FIG. 18-45. Diagram of lymph drainage of the anus and rectum. The watershed for extramural drainage is at the pectinate line. The watershed for intramural drainage is at the level of the middle rectal valve, about 8 cm above the anal verge. IRA, Inferior rectal artery. MRA, Middle rectal artery. SRA, Superior rectal artery. LRV, Lower rectal valve. MRV, Middle rectal valve. SRV, Superior rectal valve. (Modified from Skandalakis JE, Gray SW, Rowe JS Jr. *Anatomical Complications in General Surgery.* New York: McGraw-Hill, 1983; with permission.)

1. *Intramural stage.* Cancer begins in the epithelium of the colon wall. Longitudinal spread in the submucosa is not common and, when present, extends only a few centimeters.[106] Until the tumor has penetrated the mucosa and submucosa and involved the muscular and serosal layers, no metastasis occurs.

2. *Direct extension.* The pericolic fat is usually the first of the neighboring structures to be involved.

3. *Venous drainage.* Metastasis to the liver and lungs by way of the inferior mesenteric vein and the portal veins is an obvious pathway. A second pathway is from pelvic veins to the vertebral veins.[127] This explains metastases to the vertebral column.

We quote from Koch et al.[128]:

> *Metastatic disease in colorectal cancer results from hematogenic dissemination of tumor cells...The significantly higher detection rate in mesenteric venous blood emphasizes the importance of the filter function of the liver for circulating tumor cells in the portal venous blood. Tumor cell detection in central and peripheral venous blood, however, shows that this filtering process is limited and indicates early systemic hematogenic tumor cell dissemination in colorectal cancer.*

4. *Additional pathways by which cancer spreads.* Cancer spreads: (a) by lymphatics from nearby epicolic to paracolic to intermediate to principal lymph nodes; (b) by means of the peritoneal cavity with implants on the serosal surfaces of other viscera. Ueno et al.[129] stated that indirect cancer involvement of the extrarectal autonomic nerves and/or the surrounding tissue occurred in direct proportion to the extent of cancer spread to the mesorectum. Nerve plexus involvement had an unfavorable prognosis.

Lateral lymphatic spread is uncommon and is limited to lesions less than 4 cm from the pectinate line. Lesions above this level spread upward along the superior rectal/inferior mesenteric artery system.[130] The fact that recurrence of tumors of the lower one-third of the rectum is much higher than that of tumors of the upper two-thirds suggests that lateral spread may be more frequent than has been suspected.[131]

Downward spread of lesions of the rectum is similarly rare, probably only about 2 percent.[132] A margin of 2-3 cm distal to the tumor should be allowed in anterior resection.

Williams and Beart[133] stated that despite the fact that the Dukes 1932 system is considered the gold standard and is still used because of its simplicity and accuracy, the following should be considered predictors of survival and will play a role in the equation of staging: the number of

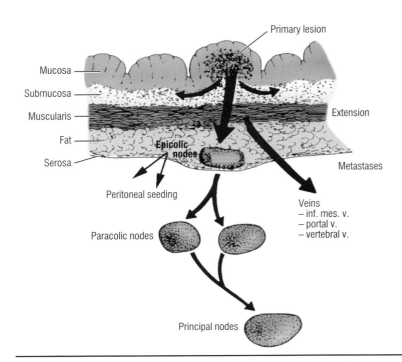

**FIG. 18-46.** Spread from a primary carcinoma of the colonic epithelium. Spread may be by extension in the submucosa, or by peritoneal seeding from extension into the subserous fat. More commonly, metastases travel through lymphatics to principal lymph nodes at the root of the mesentery, or by veins to the portal system. Thickness of arrows indicates the frequency with which spread occurs. (Modified from Skandalakis JE, Gray SW, Rowe JS Jr. Anatomical Complications in General Surgery. New York: McGraw-Hill, 1983; with permission.)

positive lymph nodes, the depth of invasion, nucleopathology, flow cytometric characteristics, histological grade, and vascular or lymphatic invasion. The same authors recommend the use of the TNM (tumor, nodes, metastasis) system.

Granfield et al.[134] reported that routine CT of the abdomen and pelvis will show the distribution of regional lymph node metastases in carcinoma of the left side of the colon, rectum, and anus.

### *Lymphatic Drainage to Adjacent Organs*

Madden and McVeigh[135] emphasized the importance of lymphatic communication between tumors of the colon at the splenic flexure and lymph nodes in the hilum of the spleen. To perform an adequate resection including the lymphatic drainage, they recommended removing en bloc the distal one-half of the transverse colon, the flexure, the whole of the descending and the proximal sigmoid colon with the mesentery, the distal one-half of the greater omentum, the proximal two-thirds of the gastrocolic ligament, the spleen, and the tail of the pancreas.

Block and Enquist[136] found a large number of lymphatic channels passing from the lower one-third of the rectum to the posterior vaginal wall, the cul-de-sac, broad ligaments, and lateral cervical (cardinal) ligaments. For this reason, they recommended that resection for carcinoma of the lower two-thirds of the rectum in women include the rectum, the cul-de-sac, the uterus, tubes, ovaries, and posterior vaginal wall, the lateral cervical and broad ligaments, the levator ani muscles, and the ischioanal (ischiorectal) fat in continuity.

## Innervation

The possible autonomic innervation of the anorectum is as follows. The internal rectal sphincter's motor innervation is supplied by sympathetic fibers that cause contraction. The pelvic splanchnic nerve (parasympathetic) and the hypogastric nerve (sympathetic) supply the lower rectal wall. Together these two nerves serve to form the rectal plexus. The levator ani muscles are controlled by the third and the fourth sacral nerves.

Davies[137] reported the following about the innervation of the rectum, bladder, and internal genitalia in anorectal dysgenesis in the male.

*Using a posterior sagittal approach to expose retroperitoneal viscera and nerves, the anatomy of the pelvic autonomic nerve plexus was studied in normal and abnormal male cadaver specimens. This plexus is found on the anterolateral surface of the lower rectum surrounded by endopelvic fascia. The autonomic nerves that supply the plexus reach it from posterior, lateral to the midline by passing over the surface of the rectum. The nerves of this plexus are distributed with the termi-*

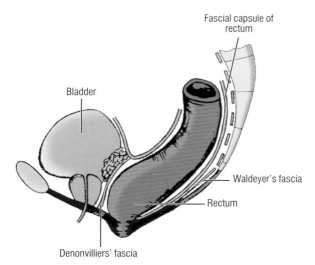

**FIG. 18-47.** The dissection planes in front and behind the normal rectum. (Modified from Davies MRQ. Anatomy of the nerve supply of the rectum, bladder, and internal genitalia in anorectal dysgenesis in the male. J Pediatr Surg 32:536-541, 1997; with permission.)

*nal branches of the internal iliac arteries, mainly with the vessels of the inferior vesical plexus. The rectum receives its autonomic nerves with its arterial blood supply, the superior rectal artery. The nerves of the pelvic plexus supply the genitourinary viscera that lie anterior to the rectum and in front of the fascia of Denonvilliers. The named fascial layers of the pelvis play a major role in determining the anatomic plane of these structures. In anorectal agenesis the plexus becomes a more midline structure. Because the pelvic fascia is often deficient in these cases these nerves lie vulnerable to inappropriate midline dissection (Figs. 18-47 through 18-49).*

Motor innervation of the internal rectal sphincter is supplied by sympathetic fibers that cause contraction and by parasympathetic fibers that inhibit contraction. The parasympathetic fibers are carried by pelvic splanchnic nerves which also convey the afferent nerve fibers that mediate the sensation of rectal distention. The external rectal sphincter is innervated by the inferior rectal branch of the internal pudendal nerve and by the perineal branch of the fourth sacral nerve.

The pelvic splanchnic nerves (parasympathetic and sensory) and the hypogastric nerve (sympathetic) supply the lower rectal wall. These two sources together form the rectal plexus. The levator ani muscles are supplied by the nerve to the levator ani, usually a branch from S4, with variant contributions from S3 and S5.

The inferior rectal branches of the internal pudendal nerve follow the inferior rectal arteries and supply the sensory innervation of the perianal skin.[138]

Remember that the pudendal nerve innervates the external sphincter and possibly the puborectalis muscle. The sympathetic nerves have no influence on the muscular wall of the rectum. Evacuation is accomplished by the pelvic splanchnic nerves; continence is maintained by the pudendal and the pelvic splanchnic nerves.

Since the pelvic parasympathetic nerves are responsible for erection and the sympathetic nerves of the hypogastric plexus are responsible for ejaculation, the surgeon should be familiar with the pathway of these nerves and dissect the posterior rectal wall from the sacrum, the prostate, and the lateral pelvic wall as close to the posterior rectal wall as possible.

The topographic anatomy of the nervi erigentes was studied by Stelzner et al.,[139] who reported that the nerves are located along the diaphragmatic part of the urethra before entering the cavernous bodies. During procto-colectomy, in order to preserve sexual function, these au-

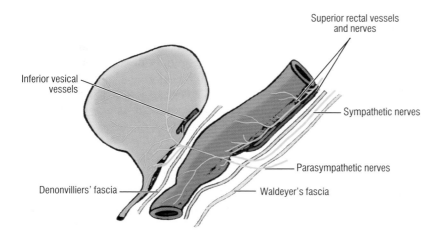

**FIG. 18-48.** The anatomy of the pelvic nerve plexus in the presence of a normal rectum and anal canal. (Modified from Davies MRQ. Anatomy of the nerve supply of the rectum, bladder, and internal genitalia in anorectal dysgenesis in the male. J Pediatr Surg 32:536-541, 1997; with permission.)

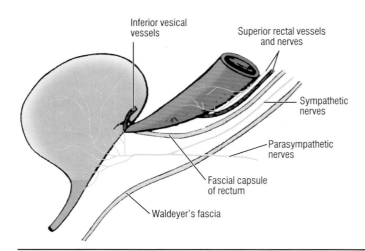

**FIG. 18-49.** The anatomy of the pelvic nerve plexus in anorectal agenesis with a rectovesical fistula. (Modified from Davies MRQ. Anatomy of the nerve supply of the rectum, bladder, and internal genitalia in anorectal dysgenesis in the male. J Pediatr Surg 32:536-541, 1997; with permission.)

thors advised leaving a piece of the rectal muscle that covers the diaphragmatic part of the urethra.

Williams and Slack[140] studied the sexual function of males and females after rectosigmoid and rectum excision by examining the specimens for the presence of nerve tissue. Their results suggest that as the amount of nerve tissue in the specimen increases, impaired sexual activity increases.

For a conceptual picture of the "flow" of pelvic autonomic nerves which cannot be seen during mobilization of the rectosigmoid, and to help surgeons avoid inadvertent injury to these nerves, we recommend reading a brief review by Pearl et al.[141] of the structure and function of these nerves.

### *Defecation and Continence*

Distention of the rectum is the initial stimulus for defecation. Distention (Fig. 18-50A), with a rise in pressure, acting on mural receptors, produces reflex contraction of the rectal musculature. At the same time, the internal sphincter relaxes. This portion of the process is mediated by the intrinsic nerves only, with no contribution from extrinsic nerves.

The external (voluntary) sphincter (Figs. 18-50, 18-51) is normally in a state of contraction by a reflex from muscle spindles by means of the sacral spinal cord. Continence is obtained by a second reflex from the distended rectal wall to the sacral cord increasing contraction of the external sphincter and relaxing the rectal wall, reducing the urge to defecate. This reflex can be reinforced by voluntary effort if defecation is inhibited.

If defecation is to proceed, facilitating impulses arise from the cerebrum, pass to the sacral cord, then to the external sphincter to relax it[142] (Fig. 18-50B). Contraction of

the longitudinal muscles, together with peristalsis starting in the sigmoid colon, results in extrusion of the stool. The process is aided by voluntary straining (Valsalva maneuver).

Gunterberg et al.[143] stated that damage to the parasympathetic nerves can almost completely abolish activity of the internal sphincter. Speakman et al.[144] speculated that incontinence in some patients is from as yet unidentified defects in the innervation of the internal anal sphincter.

Is damage to the puborectalis during vaginal delivery the most significant cause of incontinence? Sunderland[145] and Henry et al.[146] support this concept. But recent studies indicate that a great proportion of incontinence is from other types of injuries during delivery. Fornell and her colleagues[147] reported a high incidence of fecal incontinence after anal sphincter rupture at childbirth.

## Surgical Considerations

- Digital examination of the anus and lower rectum is essential. No patient should leave the office without rectal examination. In the male both lobes of the prostate gland should be palpated, as well as the right and left seminal vesicles and the retrorectal or presacral space, the ischioanal space, and the cystorectal space. The sphincteric mechanism should be evaluated. In the female palpate the cervix, posterior uterine wall, space of Douglas, ischioanal space, and retrorectal space. Try to palpate both ovaries and both tubes.
- In the female, the cul-de-sac (space of Douglas) is lower in comparison to the male; a pelvic abscess formation can be drained by aspiration or incision of the postvaginal vault. In the male, the only way to drain such an abscess is through the posterior rectal wall after per-

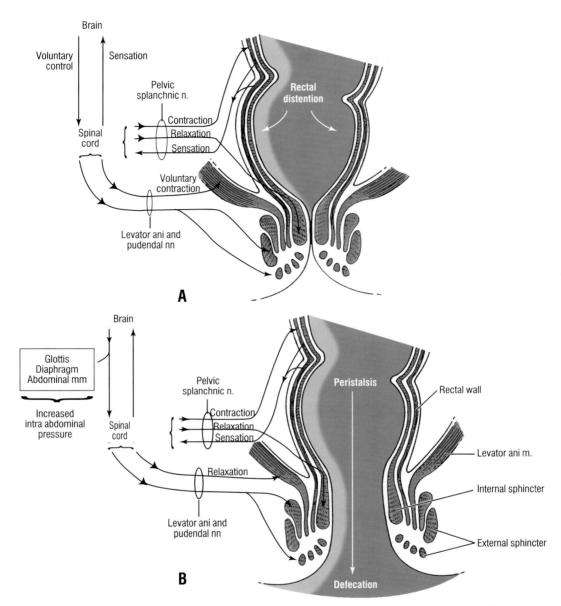

**FIG. 18-50.** Neural pathways involved in defecation. **A,** Rectal distension initiates relaxation of the internal sphincter and effective voluntary closure by the external sphincter. **B,** Defecation with relaxation of both sphincters, contraction of muscles in the rectal wall, and increased intraabdominal pressure. (Modified from Skandalakis JE, Gray SW, Rowe JS Jr. Anatomical Complications in General Surgery. New York: McGraw-Hill, 1983; with permission.)

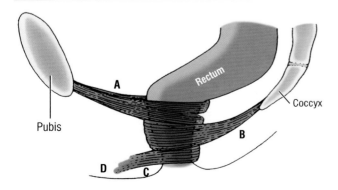

**FIG. 18-51.** The three loops of the external anal sphincter: subcutaneous **(C)**, superficial **(B)**, and deep **(A)**. Continence depends on the preservation of at least one of the three. Some subcutaneous muscle fibers encircle the anus; some attach to the perianal skin anteriorly at **D**. (Modified from Skandalakis JE, Gray SW, Rowe JS Jr. Anatomical Complications in General Surgery. New York: McGraw-Hill, 1983; with permission.)

forming a careful digital examination to find a better location for the incision or insertion of the trocar.

- Chifflet[148] observed that there is no fascial barrier between rectum and vagina in women as there is in men between the rectum and the prostate (Denonvilliers' fascia). Two of the authors of this chapter (GLC and JES) have routinely noted the presence of the septum in dissections of female cadavers, however. Transverse or vertical breaks in the rectovaginal septum often presage the occurence of enteroceles and rectoceles in women. Surgical correction of these problems is often performed by repair of the septum or the insertion of a prosthetic mesh to replace its function. Watson et al.[149] advised operative repair of the rectovaginal septum (transperineal with Marlex mesh) in patients with large rectoceles.

- Merad et al.[150] stated that "prophylactic drainage of the pelvic space does not improve outcome or influence the severity of complications." Ross et al.[151] advised mesorectal excision and radiotherapy for patients with local recurrence of rectal cancer if these tumors are identified with endorectal ultrasound or pathology.

- The superior rectal artery (which is the downward continuation of the inferior mesenteric artery) can be ligated with impunity and must be ligated during rectosigmoid resections. The needs of this area for arterial blood will be taken care of by the middle and inferior rectal arteries.

- The controversy regarding ligation of the middle rectal artery continues. We quote from Siddharth and Ravo:[152]

    *The superior rectal artery is the main blood supply of the rectum. Its branching on the rectum is varied, but it has a rich anastomosis with the other rectal arteries, namely, the middle rectal and inferior rectal arteries. Sudeck's point is not critical. The middle rectal artery varies in number and origin and is not essential provided the inferior rectal artery is intact.*

    At a 1986 meeting of the American Association of Clinical Anatomists attended by the senior author of this chapter (JES), the position of the Mayo Clinic (as represented by Oliver Beahrs) was that ligation of the middle rectal artery is not necessary. The Vanderbilt surgeons (represented by H. William Scott, Jr.) disagreed. Anatomically Beahrs was right when he expressed his belief that the middle rectal artery is, for all practical purposes, a prostatic small artery. However Scott, also, was correct when he advised ligation to avoid a possible hematoma.

    Our advice is to ligate all tissues on the superior surface of the levator ani at its insertion to the rectal wall; among them should be the middle rectal artery.

- Remember that a presacral plexus of veins is located under the endopelvic fascia that covers the sacral periosteum; this is the No. 1 danger zone during low anterior resection. Do not remove the fascia. Work close to the posterior rectal wall. If bleeding occurs use thumbtacks, bone wax, Oxycel (oxidized cellulose), or apply pressure with a surgical pad and lap packs. Leave the endopelvic fascia in situ and *always* dissect close to the posterior rectal wall. This is the correct plane for avoiding anatomic complications. Another source of bleeding is the median sacral artery. This can be controlled without too much difficulty.

- The lateral ligaments of the rectum should be divided using Hemoclips, which work better than suture ligations. These poorly defined anatomic entities are controversial. Are they related to the middle rectal artery or to the nerves of the rectum? From a surgical standpoint it makes no difference whether the ligaments are posterolateral, the middle rectal artery is anterolateral, and the nerves are closer to the ligaments. All these perirectal components should be divided between hemoclips.

- To avoid impotence, protect the nerves of the right and left pelvic plexuses. The parasympathetic fibers responsible for erection arise as the nervi erigens (pelvic splanchnic nerves) from the second, third and fourth sacral ventral primary rami. To avoid anatomic complications of neurologic origin, dissection close to the posterior rectal wall is mandatory.

- During the perineal part of abdominoperineal resection, remember the location of the following anatomic entities (which are located within the anal triangle) from below upward. There are two surgical zones: the posterior (safe) and the anterior (dangerous).
  - *Posterior:* Cut the strong rectococcygeal fascia (anococcygeal ligament) close to and anterior to the coccyx. Cut the puborectalis muscle close to the anorectal wall using an anterior incision.
  - *Anterior:* The transverse perineal muscle should be identified and used as a landmark. Always dissect posterior to the muscle to avoid urethral injury. A Foley catheter prior to surgery is essential.

  Protect the pudendal nerve by dissecting close to the anorectal wall. Between the surgical anal canal and the prostate in the male or vagina in the female is the perineal body in the general surgeon's terms, or the area called the perineum by the gynecologist. The anatomic landmarks in this area are the superficial transverse perineal muscle and the urogenital diaphragm. The membranous urethra penetrates the muscle and is protected only by not extending any anterior dissection. The fascia of Denonvilliers will be found by posterior traction and downward pushing of the specimen. The prostate will be found in this area; protect it.

  Laterally, of course, ligate the inferior rectal vessels at the medial wall of the ischioanal fossa.

Remember the double fascia of Denonvilliers, the rectovesical or rectovaginal septum. Infiltration of the rectovesical septum by prostatic or rectal carcinoma is well known. Since the anterior leaflet of the fascia is related to the prostate and the posterior leaflet is related to the rectum, ideally the surgeon should explore the space (of Proust) between. But as Healey and Hodge[153] stated in their beautiful book *Surgical Anatomy,* "it is not always easy to find the passage between 'wind and water.'"

- Remember that external hemorrhoids are covered by skin; internal hemorrhoids are covered by anal mucosa.
- Anal fissure is a longitudinal crack from the anal verge very near the dentate line. In both males and females it is most common at the posterior anal wall. An anterior anal fissure may be present in females; it may be single or multiple.

Characteristically the fissure has two pockets: one close to the dentate line (anal crypt) and one (subcutaneous pocket) at the anal verge.

Therefore, the fissure is anatomically associated with the subcutaneous ring of the external sphincter.

- Anal fistulas (Figs. 18-52 through 18-54) extend from an anal crypt in the vicinity of the dentate line (internal or primary opening) to a possible pathway along the lymphatics to the skin, forming the external or secondary opening. Remember Goodsall's rule on location and pathway of fistula tracts (Fig. 18-54): A posterior external opening has a curved pathway to the internal primary opening in the midline and posteriorly; an anterior external opening has a straight pathway to an opposite internal opening.
- With ischioanal (ischiorectal) abscess, early draining with skin incision as close to the anus as possible is mandatory to avoid supralevator space inflammatory process and external fistula far away from the anus.

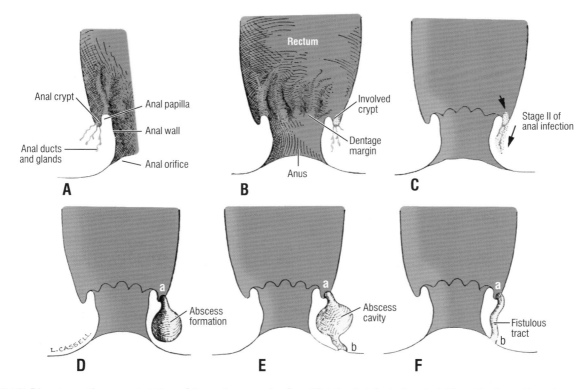

FIG. 18-52. Diagrammatic representation of the pathogenesis of anal fistula. **A,** Infected material from the bowel invades one or more of the anal crypts and the tiny vestigial anal glands. This "primary" process is at the dentate line. **B** and **C,** The infection spreads to the perianal and perirectal tissue indirectly by way of the lymphatics or directly by breaks in the continuity of the gland duct structure. **D,** Abscess formation. **E,** The abscess spontaneously ruptures or is incised on the perianal skin surface, and the fistulous tract is complete. The skin opening (at "b") is a "secondary" opening. If the abscess had drained into the rectum (at "a"), the secondary opening would have been at that point. **F,** Collapse of the abscess leaves the commonly seen narrow fistulous tract. *Editor's note: For instructional purposes, Nesselrod divides anal infection into 3 stages. Stage I is entry of infectious material into anal crypts that funnel the material into anal ducts and glands. In Stage II the perianal tissues, and possibly perirectal tissues, are invaded by infection. Stage III consists of manifestations of infection, including abscess and fistula.* (Modified from Nesselrod JP. Proctology in General Practice. Philadelphia: WB Saunders, 1950; with permission.)

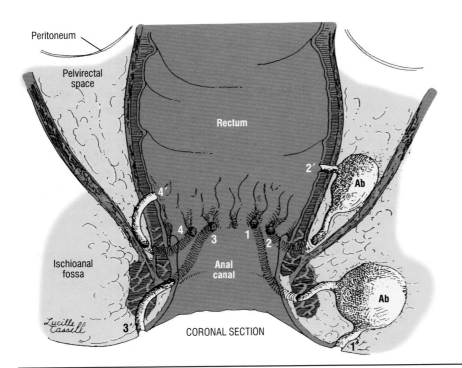

**FIG. 18-53.** Common locations of anal abscesses and fistulous openings. The ischioanal (ischiorectal) fossae (infralevator spaces) are much more commonly involved than the pelvirectal (supralevator) spaces. From the latter an abscess may extend through the intervening pelvic diaphragm to the lower ischioanal space. A supralevator abscess may drain spontaneously into the rectum, as at *2′*. Subsequent shrinkage of the abscess leads to a chronic fistulous process similar to the tract from *4* to *4′*. Occasionally an abscess will drain through its primary opening, and is then a sinus. An ordinary anal fistula is *3* to *3′*; *1, 2, 3* and *4* are primary openings; *1′, 2′, 3′* and *4′* are secondary openings. Ab, Abscess. (Modified from Nesselrod JP. Proctology in General Practice. Philadelphia: WB Saunder, 1950; with permission.)

## HISTOLOGY OF THE COLONIC WALL

The layers of the wall of the large intestine are essentially similar to those of the wall of the small intestine. The chief differences are: (1) the absence of mucosal villi; (2) the longitudinal muscularis externa in three discrete bands (taeniae) rather than in a continuous cylinder; (3) the presence of epiploic appendices (appendages); and (4) the presence of haustra or sacculations.

The colonic wall has 5 layers:
- serosa
- muscularis externa
- submucosa
- muscularis mucosa
- mucosa

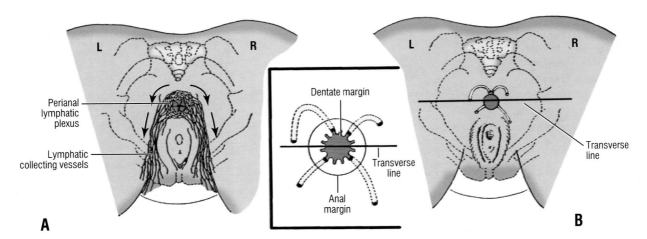

**FIG. 18-54.** Perianal lymphatic drainage and Goodsall's rule. **A,** Direction of perianal lymphatic plexus. **B,** Goodsall's rule: Fistulas with an external (secondary) opening situated posterior to an imaginary line passing transversely through the center of the anus usually have the internal (primary) opening in the midline and posteriorly, so that the tract is curved. When the external (secondary) opening is anterior to the transverse line, the internal (primary) opening is immediately opposite; hence the tract is straight. (Modified from Nesselrod JP. Anal, perianal, perineal and sacrococcygeal sinuses. Am J Surg 1942;56:154-165; with permission.)

Serosa is the visceral peritoneum that covers the colon, abdominal pelvic viscera, and the mesenteries; it does not cover the posterior attachments of the colon. The appendix, cecum, and transverse and sigmoid colons are covered totally by peritoneum.

The muscularis externa layer is composed of the inner circular and outer longitudinal layers, between which lies the myenteric plexus (of Auerbach). The outer layer is not as complete as the inner; it is responsible for the formation of the taeniae coli. Both layers form a network of smooth muscle.

The submucosa is areolar tissue containing veins, lymphatics, the terminal portion of small arteries, and the submucosal plexus (of Meissner).

The muscularis mucosa is a thin network of circular and longitudinal smooth muscle, fixed and interwoven together.

The mucosa is formed by a simple columnar epithelium containing goblet cells.

Dieulafoy's lesion (cirsoid aneurysm) may cause massive lower gastrointestinal bleeding from a minute submucosal arteriole that bleeds through a punctate erosion in an otherwise normal mucosa. Dieulafoy's lesions of the colon, rectum, and anal canal have been reported.[154]

The colon is characterized by three longitudinal muscular bands, the taeniae coli. Between these bands, the longitudinal muscle layer is highly attenuated, reduced to a thickness of less than half that of the circular coat. The bands begin their divergence from one another at the base of the appendix and, as a result, provide a useful guide to the position of the appendix. The taenia libera or free taenia (see Fig. 18-18) is located on the ventral surface of the cecum and the ascending and descending colons. The taenia omentalis (omental taenia) is found posterolaterally. Posteromedially, at the attachment of the mesocolon, is the taenia mesocolica (mesenteric taenia).

Between the taeniae are saccular formations, the haustra, which are characteristic of the colon. The haustra have an enigmatic origin. It is presumed that the length of the taeniae is less than that of the bowel itself, resulting in the formation of the haustra. Indeed, if the taeniae are cut, the colon increases in length.

The taeniae coli are about 1 cm wide. They are most completely developed in the right colon. In the rectum, their architecture changes to broad bands. These are located anteriorly and posteriorly in the rectal wall, and occasionally completely cover the rectosigmoid area and the rectum. Distally, on the rectal ampulla, some anterior longitudinal fibers leave the bowel as the rectourethralis muscle to insert upon the perineal body.

The epiploic appendages (appendices epiploica) (see Fig. 18-18) are another characteristic of the external surface of the colon. They are sessile or pedunculated adipose masses enveloped by the serosa of the colon. They are absent from the rectum. The epiploic appendages can become infarcted or gangrenous, thereby producing severe epigastric or left abdominal pain. These fat-filled pouches can also serve to conceal true diverticula from the wall of the bowel.

The appendages are small pouches of peritoneum that arise from the external surface of the colon. They range from 3 cm to as much as 15 cm in length, depending on the obesity of the patient. The epiploic appendices arise in two rows, chiefly from the lateral and medial intertaenial areas of the transverse and descending colons. They may be present anywhere from the cecum to the proximal rectum.

The surgeon is interested in the epiploic appendages because they may be the sites of diverticula (see Fig. 18-15). Fat may conceal the presence of the diverticulum on inspection, but fecoliths in the diverticula are frequently palpable.[41] The appendices are also subject to infarction and torsion; both produce symptoms of an acute abdomen. Goligher[41] warned that epiploic appendages should be ligated without traction (see Fig. 18-15). This prevents unintentional pulling of a loop of a long colic artery into the appendiceal neck, and its accidental inclusion in the ligation.

Occasionally the epiploic appendix becomes inflamed secondary to venous thrombosis or torsion, producing a clinical picture similar to diverticulitis; but primary epiploic appendagitis (PEA) is rarely diagnosed. Rao et al.[155] reported significant potential to accurately differentiate PEA from diverticulitis and appendicitis at CT scanning if the correct CT techniques are used and radiologists become aware of the CT features of PEA.

Kuganeswaran and Fisher[156] reported a giant sigmoid diverticulum of 33 cm, the largest recorded in the literature.

REMEMBER:
- The large bowel epithelium is columnar, without any villi. Characteristically, the flat mucosa of the large bowel is penetrated by tubular glands, forming the crypts of Lieberkühn which open into its lumen. Mucus-secreting goblet cells and some endocrine cells are found within the epithelium of the crypts.
- Welton[157] proposed that the "human colonic microvascular endothelial cell in culture is a legitimate model for the study of the human colon in the normal and diseased states."
- The muscularis externa of the colonic wall is formed by smooth muscles (longitudinal and circular). These are responsible for peristaltic contraction.
- The arrangement of the muscular network of the colonic wall from mucosa to serosa is as follows: the muscularis

mucosa just below the colonic epithelium is formed by an inner circular and outer longitudinal layer which are heavily fixed and interwoven together.

- The circular layer surrounds the colonic wall; the longitudinal layer covers the circular layer (responsible for formation of the taeniae).

## HISTOLOGY OF THE RECTUM

The upper rectum contains one to four crescentic plicae, the rectal folds or valves of Houston. Typically there are three folds: left superior, right middle, and left inferior. They are encountered by the sigmoidoscope at 4-7 cm, 8-10 cm, and 10-12 cm from the anal verge.

These folds contain mucosa, submucosa, and some muscle. Their positions are marked by a groove on the outer wall, and they do not disappear on rectal distention.

Gordon and Nivatvongs[158] state that the Houston valves do not contain all the layers of the rectal wall and biopsy of the valves has minimal risk of perforation.

## HISTOLOGY OF THE ANAL CANAL

### Musculature of the Wall of the Anal Canal

Two layers of smooth muscle surround the anal canal. The innermost layer is formed by a greatly thickened circular coat which is continuous with the circular muscularis externa of the colon. This is the internal sphincter of the anal canal (see Fig. 18-41). The second smooth muscle layer is composed of longitudinal fibers continuous with the fibers of the taeniae coli.

The downward continuation of the longitudinal muscle is the so- called *conjoined longitudinal coat* which forms fibers that penetrate both internal and external sphincters and extends to the perianal connective tissue and perhaps to the skin and the anal mucosa. Therefore, the conjoined longitudinal coat is considered the anchor of the surgical anal canal. However, the anatomy of the perianal area is still very controversial. O'Kelly et al.[159] stated that in the anal canal both the conjoined longitudinal coat and the internal anal sphincter are specialized sphincteric smooth muscle which relax under the influence of beta-adrenoceptor stimulation.

Shafik[101] would divide the longitudinal muscle fibers into three layers that lie between the internal and external sphincters. These layers, the medial, intermediate, and lateral longitudinal muscles, are separated by fibrous connective tissue septa that join to form a "central tendon." Fibers from this pierce the external sphincter to form the corrugator cutis ani.

The longitudinal muscle fibers prevent separation of the sphincteric elements from each other and also permit a telescopic movement between internal and external sphincters. We witness this in the operating room when the external sphincter rolls back and the internal sphincter rolls forward. Goligher[41] suggested that this is why, in the past, surgeons performing sphincterotomy sometimes thought they were cutting the external sphincter but were, in reality, cutting the internal sphincter. They were unknowingly performing the correct operation.

Delancey et al.[160] performed cadaveric evaluation of the length of the internal and external anal sphincters. The internal sphincter, located between the anal mucosa and the external sphincter, extends more than a centimeter above the cranial margin of the external sphincter. This region is damaged in fourth-degree obstetric lacerations.

Haas and Fox,[161] emphasizing the importance of the perianal connective tissue, state that the anus is anchored by fibers of the conjoined longitudinal coat which bundle the internal and external sphincters, penetrate the perianal fat, reach the pelvic wall and the lower levator fascia, and end at the perianal skin. This peculiar complicated network acts in an antagonistic action to the muscles of the anal canal which are able to overcome such action and close the anus.

The same authors suggest that stretching (transecting the sphincters) may cause loss of elasticity or mobility in the sphincteric anal apparatus with some impairment of function. Maybe so, but we have our doubts; therefore we agree with the anatomy described by Haas and Fox, but we perhaps disagree with the possible pathology.

We quote from Sangwan and Solla[162]:

> *The internal anal sphincter, the smooth muscle component of the anal sphincter complex, has an ambiguous role in maintaining anal continence. Despite its significant contribution to resting anal canal pressures, even total division of the internal anal sphincter in surgery for anal fistulas may fail to compromise continence in otherwise healthy subjects. However, recently reported abnormalities of the innervation and reflex response of the internal anal sphincter in patients with fecal incontinence indicate its significance in maintaining continence. The advent of sphincter-saving surgery and restorative proctocolectomy has re-emphasized the major contribution of the internal anal sphincter to resting pressure and its significance in preventing fecal leakage. The variable*

*effect of rectal excision on rectoanal inhibitory reflex has led to a reappraisal of the significance of this reflex in discrimination of rectal contents and its impact on anal continence. Electromyographic, manometric, and ultrasonographic evaluation of the internal anal sphincter has provided new insights into its pathophysiology.*

Unlike the longitudinal and circular muscles of the anal canal which are smooth and arise from splanchnic mesoderm, the external sphincter is striated muscle and arises from somatic mesoderm.

The external sphincter is often described as having three separate fiber bundles or loops (see Fig. 18-51): subcutaneous, superficial, and deep. Although in normal individuals these bundles are continuous and show no gross or histologic evidence of separation, it is useful to consider the three parts separately. Shafik[163] believes that the three loops together form an efficient anal closure. Any single one of the loops is capable of maintaining continence to solid stools, but not to fluid or gas. The subcutaneous portion surrounds the outlet of the anus, attaching to the perianal skin anteriorly. Some fibers completely encircle the anus.

The superficial portion surrounds the anus and continues within the anococcygeal ligament, which attaches posteriorly to the coccyx. This creates the small triangular space of Minor behind the anus. It is worth noting that the contraction of this part of the sphincteric mechanism pulls the anus posteriorly toward the coccyx, perhaps serving to augment the posterior angulation of the anal canal and thus enhancing the action of the puborectalis. Anteriorly, some fibers insert into the transverse perineal muscles at the perineal body, creating a potential space toward which anterior midline fistulas may point.

The deep portion, like the subcutaneous portion, surrounds the canal, with no obvious anterior or posterior attachments. In Shafik's view, the deep portion and the puborectalis muscle are a single unit.[164]

The degree to which these portions, together with their anterior and posterior attachments, are separated from one another has been a source of controversy. We agree that no real separation exists between deep and superficial portions of the sphincter, although an intersphincteric groove is palpable. We question, however, some of the anterior and posterior attachments described by Oh and Kark.[165] Our view is shown in Figure 18-55.

## Lining of the Surgical Anal Canal

There are three histologic regions of the anal canal. The

*cutaneous zone,* up to the anal verge (anocutaneous line), is covered by pigmented skin that has hair follicles and sebaceous glands. Above the anal verge is the *transitional zone,* which consists of modified skin that has sebaceous glands without hair. It extends to the pectinate line defined by the free edges of the anal valves. Above the line begins the *true mucosa of the anal canal* (Fig. 18-56).

The pectinate line is formed by the margins of the anal valves, small mucosal pockets between the 5-10 vertical folds of the mucosa known as the *anal columns of Morgagni.* These columns extend upward from the pectinate line to the upper end of the surgical anal canal, at the level of the puborectalis sling. They are formed by underlying parallel bundles of the muscularis mucosae. Hollinshead[166] noted that the actual junction of stratified squamous and columnar epithelia is usually just above the pectinate line; hence the *mucocutaneous line* is not precisely equivalent to the pectinate line.

The pectinate line is the most important landmark in the anal canal. It marks the transition between the visceral area above and the somatic area below. The arterial supply, the venous and lymphatic drainage, the nerve supply, and the character of the lining all change at or very near the pectinate line (see Table 18-7).

In spite of all the changes that occur at the pectinate line, pathology, unique to a region 2 cm above and 2 cm below the line, makes a unit of the "surgical anal canal."[6]

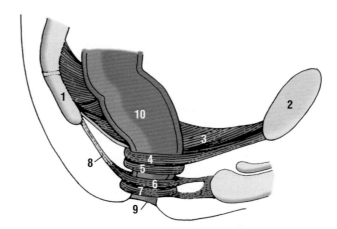

FIG. **18-55.** Diagram of the extrinsic muscles of the surgical anal canal. 1, Coccyx. 2, Pubis. 3, Levator ani muscle. 4, Puborectalis muscle. 5, Deep external sphincter. 6, Superficial external sphincter. 7, Subcutaneous external sphincter. 8, Anococcygeal ligament. 9, Anal verge. 10, Rectum. (Modified from Skandalakis JE, Gray SW, Rowe JS Jr. Anatomical Complications in General Surgery. New York: McGraw-Hill, 1983; with permission.)

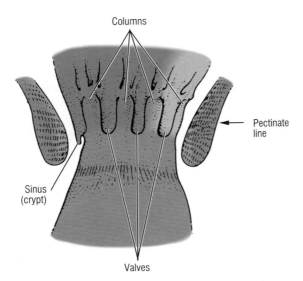

Columns

Pectinate line

Sinus (crypt)

Valves

**Fig. 18-56.** The interior of the anal canal showing the rectal columns, anal valves, and anal sinuses (crypts). They form the pectinate line. (Modified from Skandalakis JE, Gray SW, Rowe JS Jr. Anatomical Complications in General Surgery. New York: McGraw-Hill, 1983; with permission.)

## HISTOLOGY OF THE ANAL GLANDS AND ANAL PAPILLAE

The pockets formed by the anal valves are termed *anal sinuses or crypts* (Fig. 18-56). In 4-8 of these, especially those on the posterior rectal wall, ducts lead downward and outward, reaching the intersphincteric longitudinal muscle and occasionally penetrating the internal sphincter. Such anal ducts are present in about three-fourths of fetuses[121] and in about one-half of adults.[167] When present, these ducts appear to be vestigial structures; most lack mucus-secreting gland cells.[121] Anal ducts may become infected and provide pathways for anal fistulas. We quote from Klosterhalfen et al.:[168] "[A]nal sinuses and anal intramuscular glands are separate anatomic entities... For idiopathic, chronic anal diseases anal sinuses have little surgical significance. Anal intramuscular glands should be the anatomic correlate of anal fistulas."

Where the margins of the anal valves join the anal column, some individuals have small projections, the anal papillae. Usually they cause no symptoms. In a few patients, one or more of these may become hypertrophied and, when large enough, may prolapse.[169,170] Schutte and Tolentino[171] found papillae in 13 percent of newborns and 46 percent of adults. Most were at the apices of the anal column. They varied from 2 mm or less

to a "fibrous polyp" 2 cm in length.

The surgical anal canal is lined by squamous epithelium along the 2 cm below the dentate line and by columnar epithelium above the dentate line. The anal transitional zone has a length 0.5 cm to 2 cm; it is located just above the anal valves. The peculiar innervation of the anal canal is shown in Figure 18-57.

## PHYSIOLOGY

Colonic motility is enigmatic. Each segment, part, or region functions in a seemingly independent manner. Practically speaking, the right colon accepts the ileal contents. Multiple phenomena take place: mixing, stirring, kneading, some absorption, and propulsion. These phenomena are manifestations of colonic contraction.

The left colon is a storage reservoir, with further propulsion activities directed toward the anorectum.

Colonic and anorectal function are altered after posterior rectopexy. Mollen and colleagues[172] reported that total and segmental transit times doubled, while the effects on anorectal function were not statistically significant. Division of the lateral ligaments did not significantly influence postoperative functional outcome.

## SURGERY OF THE COLON

### Abdominoperitoneal Resection

The abdominal phase of an abdominoperineal resection is an extended left colectomy with a presacral dissection to mobilize the rectum, which will be removed in the perineal phase.

The left colon should be mobilized down to the rectovesical or rectouterine fossa by medial and lateral incision of the peritoneal ligaments of the sigmoid colon. The left ureter and left gonadal vessels are visualized; the inferior mesenteric artery and its downward continuation as the superior rectal artery are identified, the duodenum is pushed upward, and the surgeon is ready to enter the pre-sacral area by bloody presacral dissection.

Potential bleeding may occur from the presacral veins which lie beneath the endopelvic fascia. The fascia should not be removed. Use clips for hemostasis; warm packs

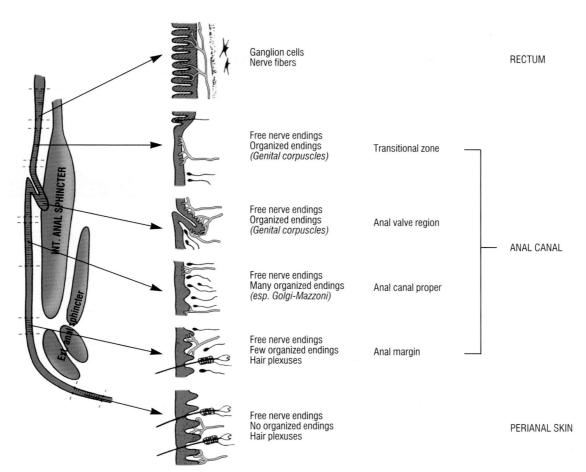

FIG. 18-57. A diagrammatic representation of the innervation of the anal canal and perianal skin. The nerve endings characteristic of the transitional zone and the anal valve region are shown. (Modified from Keighley MRB, Williams NS. Surgery of the Anus, Rectum and Colon. Philadelphia: Saunders, 1993; with permission.)

with Gelfoam will reduce bleeding.

Use long scissors for the perirectal tissues and the fascia of Waldeyer which bridges the sacrum and coccyx to the lower rectum. Blunt dissection with the surgeon's hand may be used to complete the procedure. Remember the complicated anatomy of the mesorectum.

The tip of the prostate, with Denonvilliers' fascia, or the tip of the uterine cervix as well as the tip of the coccyx may now be palpated; the hypogastric nerve and hypogastric (pelvic) plexus must be preserved to avoid problems with ejaculation or a neurogenic bladder.

We quote from Havenga et al.[173]:

*Between the rectum and the sacrum a retrorectal space can be developed, lined anteriorly by the visceral leaf and posteriorly by the parietal leaf of the pelvic fascia. The hypogastric nerve runs anterior to the visceral fascia, from the sacral promontory in a laterocaudad direction. The splanchnic sacral nerves originate from the sacral foramina, posterior to the parietal fascia, and run caudad, laterally and anteriorly. After piercing the parietal layer of the pelvic fascia, approximately 4 cm from the midline, the sacral nerves run between a double layer of the visceral part of the pelvic fascia. The relationship between the hypogastric nerves, the splanchnic nerves and the pelvic fascia was comparable in all six specimens examined.*

The perineal phase of the abdominoperineal resection encounters the following structures: pudendal vessels (which should be ligated), levator sling (which should be excised widely), and membranous urethra of the male (in which a Foley catheter has been placed prior to surgery). Use sharp dissection to separate the prostate from the lower rectum. The perineum should be partially or completely closed; a suction drain is advisable.

**TABLE 18-8. Malignant Retrorectal Tumors**

|  | Total (%) |
|---|---|
| **Congenital** | |
| Chordoma | 140 (50.7) |
| Teratocarcinoma | 12 (4.3) |
| **Neurogenic** | |
| Neurofibrosarcoma | 12 (4.3) |
| Neuroblastoma | 9 (3.3) |
| Ependymoma | 7 (2.5) |
| **Osseous** | |
| Osteosarcoma | 7 (2.5) |
| Ewing's tumor | 6 (2.2) |
| Chondrosarcoma | 9 (3.3) |
| Myeloma | 6 (2.2) |
| **Miscellaneous** | |
| Metastatic carcinoma | 21 (7.6) |
| Liposarcoma | 3 (1.1) |
| Hemangiosarcoma | 6 (2.2) |
| Fibrosarcoma | 5 (1.8) |
| Leiomyosarcoma | 9 (3.3) |
| Unknown origin | 9 (3.3) |
| Lymphoma | 8 (2.9) |
| Pericytoma | 4 (1.4) |
| Carcinoid | 1 (0.4) |
| Other | 2 (0.7) |
| **Total** | 276 (100) |

*Source:* Modified from Gorski T, Khubchandani IT, Stasik JJ, Riether R. Retrorectal carcinoid tumor. South Med J 1999; 92:417-420; with permission.

Gorski et al.,[174] in a review of the literature, reported 276 cases of retrorectal malignancy. Table 18-8 indicates the tumor types.

## Surgery of Colonic Trauma

Brasel et al.[175] stated that "simple suture or resection and anastomosis at the time of initial exploration is the dominant management method for penetrating colonic trauma."

Curran and Borzotta,[176] after evaluating 5,400 cases of colon injury, advised primary repair of colon injury, but in selected cases advised colostomy.

## Colon Resection: Open Method

Specific knowledge of normal and abnormal anatomy is mandatory for the uncomplicated resection of part or all of the large bowel. The surgeon must be familiar with the

### Editorial Comment

*In the past most surgeons did not do primary repairs for colon injuries. As indicated above this policy has changed as numerous retrospective and prospective studies have demonstrated that the majority of patients with colon trauma are candidates for primary repair. Conditions that would lead to avoidance of primary repair in a minority of patients include: extensive contamination, a long interval from injury to treatment, protracted shock, multiple other injuries, and left colon injuries that are extensive enough to require resection. (RSF Jr)*

peritoneal attachments, the blood supply, and the lymphatic pathways in this area where cancer is so common. Lack of knowledge of the peritoneal reflections and the mesenteries will produce technical problems in the operating room, such as poor mobilization or tension at the anastomosis, with postoperative leakage and peritonitis. Inadequate knowledge of the blood supply and its variations can be catastrophic. Ignorance of the pathways and patterns of lymphatic distribution may result in a fatal disseminated disease. Therefore, a brief summary with emphasis on specific anatomy and some of the anatomic entities involved with techniques of colon surgery is necessary.

We agree with the statement of McDaniel et al.[177]:

*The distribution of regional lymph node metastases in carcinomas of the cecum, ascending colon, and transverse colon follows the vascular distribution in the ileocolic mesentery, ascending mesocolon, and transverse mesocolon. The location of these metastatic nodes can be recognized on CT scans when the anatomy of the vessels in the ileocolic mesentery and mesocolon is well understood. This knowledge is important in the preoperative staging of carcinomas of the colon for curative surgery and in the early detection of recurrent nodal disease after curative surgery.*

Lane et al.[178] advised the following procedures for cecal diverticulitis:

- If solitary diverticulum is present, only diverticulectomy
- With multiple diverticuli and cecal phlegmon or if neoplastic disease cannot be ruled out, right hemicolectomy is recommended even if the colon is not prepared

McDonald et al.[179] reported that the size the colonic polyp plus the presence of high-grade dysplasia are key factors to be considered in formulating a treatment plan.

Opinions vary on the value of total mesorectal excision (TME). Lopez-Kostner et al.[180] reported that total mesorectal excision is not necessary for cancers of the upper rectum. Heald et al.[181] concluded that "precise total mesorectal excision from above appears oncologically superior to abdominoperineal resection." Havenga et al.[182] stated that TME and extended lymphadenectomy gives better recurrence and survival results than conventional surgery in the treatment of primary rectal cancer.

Very rarely colonic adenocarcinoma may arise without a gross mucosal lesion. Such a case was presented by Wimmer et al.[183] when the tumor developed in the underlying submucosa with negative colonoscopy.

Hayashi et al.[184] reported the no-touch isolation technique without surgical manipulation may be useful in preventing cancer cells from being shed into the portal vein during resection of colorectal cancer.

## Anatomy of Exposure and Mobilization

Condon and Lamphier[185] suggested the concept of three layers of structures in the abdominal cavity. The first layer is the digestive tube with its nerves and vessels. The second layer contains the kidneys, adrenals, ureter, aorta, and inferior vena cava. The third layer is the transversalis fascia lining the parietal muscles.

Figure 18-23 shows the extent of colectomy recommended for cancer at various sites in the colon. A standard right colectomy is essentially a midline resection; it includes a few centimeters of the terminal ileum, the cecum, the right colon, and the proximal half of the transverse colon. These are the segments served by the ileocolic, right colic, and right branches of the middle colic arteries (Fig. 18-23B). Following mobilization of the right colon, expose the kidney, ureter, spermatic vessels, inferior vena cava, aorta, iliac vessels, duodenum, pancreas, and retroperitoneal muscles.[186]

There are four reasons for choosing the standard right colectomy rather than a lesser resection:
(1) the lymphatic drainage makes a lesser resection inadequate
(2) the proximal colon is more difficult to use for anastomosis because it is not completely covered by peritoneum and may have attached fat or membranous veils
(3) the ileum has a good blood supply and is less subject to suture-line necrosis than is the colon
(4) the operation is easier, since the hepatic flexure is easy to mobilize

An exception may be made for benign tumors. In these cases, as much of the terminal ileum as possible should be preserved to prevent diarrhea resulting from a lack of resorption of bile salts.

Koea et al.[187] reported that extended resection by right colectomy and en bloc duodenectomy or by en bloc pancreaticoduodenectomy for localized primary colon carcinoma invading the pancreas or duodenum are safe procedures associated with prolonged survival time.

In left colectomy, the lowest sigmoid artery may be too short for adequate sigmoid resection. Dixon[188] suggested a method to overcome this problem (Fig. 18-58): the last sigmoid artery, together with a small portion of the proximal stump, may be sectioned to permit an anastomosis free from tension. The sigmoid artery and the problem of the short transverse mesocolon should be evaluated before resection is started.

Mobilization of the left colon for a successful pull-through operation was discussed by Barnes.[189]

Sharma and Klaasen[190] reported that the procedure of choice for elderly patients with colonic carcinoma adherent to the duodenum is duodenal seromyectomy.

## Editorial Comment

*In studies done in the 1950s Rupert Turnbull and Edwin Fisher identified colon cancer cells in the portal vein blood of patients undergoing colon resections for cancer. It was also known that intraluminal tumor fragments could be incorporated into the anastomosis and lead to suture line recurrence. On the basis of these observations, many years ago Turnbull advocated a no-touch technique of colon resection: prior to mobilization of the colon at the site of the tumor the bowel lumen was isolated by encircling the bowel proximally and distally, and the arterial and venous supply was also ligated prior to the mobilization of the tumor-containing colon. Turnbull reported very good results with his no-touch technique, but others have reported similar results when the vascular supply was ligated after mobilization of the colon. Most surgeons find it technically more difficult to ligate the vessels before the colon is mobilized, and vascular isolation prior to mobilization is not performed by the majority. The biologic significance of the cancer cells detectable in the portal vein blood is unclear. Isolating the bowel lumen by encirclement is easily accomplished and is probably appropriate. (RSF Jr)*

Eisen et al.[191] made the following recommendations about intussusception in adults:

- Colectomy should be performed without reduction of intussusception because malignant tumor is often the cause of intussusception in adults
- Small bowel intussusception should be reduced only if there is benign disease or if resection is likely to result in short bowel syndrome

Total proctocolectomy with pouch ileoanal anastomosis is used to treat patients with ulcerative colitis and familial polyposis. Michelassi and Hurst[192] reported that the procedure allows patients to live without a permanent stoma and experience a high degree of continence and an acceptable number of daily bowel movements.

## Colostomy

Below we list several types of colostomy; some are included entirely for historical interest. The procedures in *italics* are those that are currently being performed, and here we will describe only those. End colostomies with Hartmann's pouch or mucous fistula have limited application, but ReMine and Dozois[193] and Bell[194] have reaffirmed their usefulness.

1. Cecostomy
   a. Cecal exteriorization
   b. *Tube cecostomy*
2. *Loop colostomy*
3. Double-barreled colostomy (Bloch-Paul-Mikulicz)
4. Tube and marsupialization colostomy
5. Interrupted colostomy
   a. *End colostomy with Hartmann's pouch*
   b. *End colostomy with mucous fistula*

We quote from Bardoel et al.[195] on their cadaveric studies:

*[T]he rectus abdominis muscle is ideally suited for the construction of a stoma sphincter. The muscle is located in the appropriate anatomical location for stoma creation; it has a long vascular pedicle; and the preserved, segmental intercostal innervation pattern allows the muscle to be tailored and mobilized so as to completely wrap a fecal stoma without significant muscle denervation.*

They plan future "functional" studies to see if the rectus abdominis muscle can be successfully trained to become fatigue-resistant.

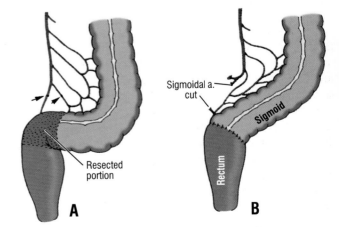

FIG. 18-58. **A,** Following resection of the sigmoid colon, the last sigmoid artery may be too short to permit the required anastomosis. **B,** The last sigmoid artery together with a small portion of the proximal stump may be sectioned to permit an anastomosis free from tension. (Modified from Skandalakis JE, Gray SW, Rowe JS Jr. Anatomical Complications in General Surgery. New York: McGraw-Hill, 1983; with permission.)

## Tube Cecostomy

A double purse-string absorbable suture at the anterior taenia is the first step in a tube cecostomy (Fig. 18-59A). The cecum must be fixed to the abdominal wall without leaving a dead space between the stoma and the wall. Removal of the appendix is desirable. The appendiceal stump may be used to insert the Foley catheter before closing it. A three-way, large Foley catheter can be used for irrigation and suction as well as for injection of antibiotics when necessary.

Although cecostomy is less popular than it once was, we have used the procedure successfully several times for decompression and for suture-line protection. With a short transverse mesocolon in an obese patient, cecostomy is the ideal operation.

Tschmelitsch et al.[196] compared loop colostomy/ ileostomy (C/I) and tube cecostomy (TC) in patients who had undergone low anterior resections for rectal cancer. They reported that the rate of anastomotic leaks, fecal peritonitis, reoperation for anastomotic leak/fistulas, permanent colostomies, and postoperative mortality was not significantly different between the groups, and concluded, "a C/I for protection of the anastomosis did not improve outcome significantly as compared with a TC. With a properly fashioned TC and adequate postoperative management a second operation (for colostomy closure) can be avoided and the overall hospital stay is significantly reduced."

## Loop Colostomy

A loop colostomy (Fig. 18-59B) is feasible only in the transverse or sigmoid colon because a mesentery is required. If the transverse mesocolon is short, mobilization of the hepatic and splenic flexures will provide a more mobile loop.

At the hepatic flexure, the colon is attached to the second part of the duodenum and the lower pole of the right kidney. There is no right phrenocolic ligament. At the splenic flexure, the colon is attached to the lower pole of the left kidney and to the diaphragm by the phrenocolic ligament. Careful division of the ligament is important to avoid injury to the spleen.

With obstruction of the left colon, the transverse colon is dilated; unless adhesions hold it in the pelvis, the transverse colon is high. Identification of dilated intestine can be a problem. The presence of taeniae distinguishes the colon from the small intestine, but with dilatation, the taeniae tend to become less visible. The left colon has many more epiploic appendages than does the transverse colon. Trans-

illuminate the mesocolon if possible. The middle colic and marginal arteries should be identified and preserved. Keep in mind that the blood supply of the colon is not as rich as that of the small intestine.

Sigmoid loop colostomy is, for practical purposes, left colon colostomy. The stoma should be located at the junction of the descending and sigmoid colons so that the peritoneal fixation of the descending colon will protect the proximal stoma from prolapse.

Sakai et al.[197] stated that transverse colostomy and loop ileostomy are equally safe procedures for temporary fecal diversion, and recommend further comparative study of these procedures for patient satisfaction and quality of life.

## End Colostomy

In end colostomy (Fig 18-59C), the stoma should be in the most proximal sigmoid loop, very close to the distal end of the descending colon. Externally, the stoma should be in the left lower quadrant somewhere between the umbilicus and the left anterior superior iliac spine. A site which is the mirror image of McBurney's point is usually ideal. The considerations are: (1) mechanical, for optimum placement of the colostomy bag, and (2) anatomic, for closure of the left paracolic gutter to avoid obstructing the small intestine.

The proximal cut end of the sigmoid colon should be brought 5 to 8 cm above the surface of the skin and observed for color. The colostomy should be loose enough to permit the insertion of one finger. Be sure to close the space between the superficial fascia and the aponeuroses of the external oblique muscle and the anterior rectus sheath. If this space is not closed, it will become the site of a postoperative hernia.

The distal rectal stump can be closed to form Hartmann's pouch,[198] or it may be brought to the surface to form a "mucous" fistula. With modern knowledge of colon anatomy and with good colonic preparation, Hartmann's procedure is performed less frequently today. ReMine and Dozois[193] defended the use of this procedure, pointing out its safety and good long-term survival as well as its advantage in permitting subsequent restoration of bowel continuity, especially if the resection is above the line of peritoneal reflection. Another advocate of the Hartmann procedure was Bell,[194] who performed a typical Hartmann procedure or used a distal mucous fistula.

However Belmonte et al.[199] reported that colostomy closure after Hartmann's procedure is associated with significant length of hospitalization and morbidity, and leaves one third of patients with permanent stomas.

Rosoff[200] introduced the question of the value of the

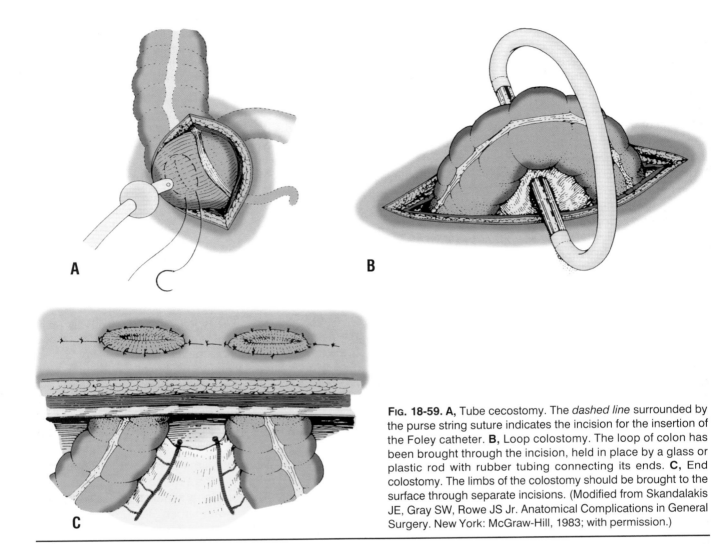

**FIG. 18-59. A,** Tube cecostomy. The *dashed line* surrounded by the purse string suture indicates the incision for the insertion of the Foley catheter. **B,** Loop colostomy. The loop of colon has been brought through the incision, held in place by a glass or plastic rod with rubber tubing connecting its ends. **C,** End colostomy. The limbs of the colostomy should be brought to the surface through separate incisions. (Modified from Skandalakis JE, Gray SW, Rowe JS Jr. Anatomical Complications in General Surgery. New York: McGraw-Hill, 1983; with permission.)

critical point of Sudeck (see "Critical Point of Sudeck" earlier in this chapter). Ligation of the inferior mesenteric or superior rectal artery almost never results in necrosis of the left colon.[35,41]

The surgeon should perform the colostomy he or she judges to be best. The critical point of Sudeck may be ignored; however, the surgeon must observe the color, bleeding, and arterial pulsation in the segment to be anastomosed or to be brought outside. No one need be critical if the surgeon chooses to do a loop colostomy or an end colostomy with a pouch or mucous fistula.

## Laparoscopic Colectomy

Liu et al.[201] concluded that laparoscopic intestinal surgery is both feasible and safe in selected patients with inflammatory bowel disease. Technical advances have enabled laparoscopic lower anterior resection to transect the lower rectum in the same way as is done with laparotomy.[202] Reissman et al.[203] concluded that the feasibility of laparoscopic and laparoscopy-assisted colorectal surgery has been well established. Leung et al.[204] stated that the immediate and medium-term results of laparoscopy-assisted resection of rectosigmoid carcinoma are promising.

There is controversy as to the safety of laparoscopic colectomy for malignancy. Bouvet et al.[205] advocate laparoscopic colectomy for carcinoma of the colon, as a sound oncologic procedure.

Targarona et al.[206] reported that laparoscopy can help disseminate aggressive tumors and therefore should be reserved for diagnostic and staging procedures or for treatment of low-grade malignant tumors.

Tomita et al.[207] considered laparoscopic surgery for treatment of colorectal cancer, including indications and contraindications. They stated that more research on surgery for colorectal carcinoma, as well as advances in laparoscopic technology, will be needed for future successful application of laparoscopic surgery to the treatment of colorectal carcinoma.

Stocchi and Nelson[208] recommended worldwide trials for laparoscopic colectomy to treat carcinoma of the colon. We agree.

We quote the wise counsel of Marubashi et al.[209]:

*[W]hile laparoscopy-assisted colectomy (LAC) is a safe and minimally invasive form of surgery from which faster recovery can be expected, it should only be performed in carefully selected patients with advanced colorectal carcinomas because most of the major complications associated with LAC using current devices and techniques may be prevented by performing traditional open surgery.*

The authors of this chapter consider laparoscopic procedures for the colon to be evolutionary. Therapeutic laparoscopic resection of carcinoma of the colon should be restricted to prospective and randomized trials until there is enough hard data to indicate its safety.

## The Colon as a Reconstructive Entity

Bussi et al.[210] advised that pharyngocoloplasty after total pharyngolaryngoesophagectomy for carcinoma of the hypopharyngoesophageal junction is a reliable treatment option when gastric pull-up is considered risky or is contraindicated.

## SURGERY OF THE ANORECTUM

## Cloacal Exstrophy

Soffer et al.[211] reported on the surgical treatment of cloacal exstrophy:

*During neonatal repair, a colostomy should be formed incorporating all pieces of colon, no matter how small. With time, most patients will be able to form solid stool, and a pull-through should be undertaken if that ability exists. Decisions regarding genitourinary reconstruction should be made only after the gastrointestinal plan is established to achieve the optimal use of available bowel.*

Howell et al.[212] and Ricketts et al.[213] advised the following about the surgery and treatment of exstrophy of the cloaca:

1. Preservation of the entire hindgut, including the terminal colon
2. End colostomy using the tailgut
3. Primary closure of omphalocele, if possible at once or in stages
4. Reapproximation of the bladder halves
5. Closure of the exstrophic bladder
6. Bladder augmentation at a later stage, using either bowel or stomach
7. Conversion to female gender
8. Staged abdominoperineal pull-through of the fecal stoma, or conversion to a continent ileostomy, depending on the anatomy and available bowel

## Anatomic Guidelines

No anorectal procedure should be undertaken without digital and sigmoidoscopic examination. The following is the anatomy as encountered by the examiner's finger or as seen in the sigmoidoscope. Digital examination should always precede sigmoidoscopy. It relaxes the sphincters and reveals any obstruction that might be injured by the sigmoidoscope.

The anal verge (Fig. 18-60) separates the pigmented perianal skin from the pink transition zone. The verge is the reference line for the position of all other structures encountered.

When the gloved and lubricated index finger is inserted so that the distal interphalangeal joint is at the anal verge (Fig. 18-61A), the subcutaneous portion of the external (voluntary) sphincter is felt as a tight ring around the distal half of the distal phalanx. The fingertip should detect the pectinate line of anal valves that lies about 2 cm above the anal verge. The anal columns (Morgagni) above valves also may be felt. External hemorrhoids, polyps, and hypertrophied anal papillae in this region are readily detected.

Further insertion of the finger to the level of the middle interphalangeal joint (Fig. 18-61B) brings the first joint to the anorectal ring formed by the deep component of the external sphincter, the puborectalis loop, and the upper margin of the internal sphincter. The ring is felt posteriorly and laterally, but not anteriorly.

Still further penetration of the finger to the level of the metacarpophalangeal joint (Fig. 18-61C) allows the distal phalanx to enter the rectum. The left lower rectal fold may often be touched. At this point the pelvirectal space lies lateral and the rectovesical or rectovaginal space lies anterior. Further anterior to the rectum one can palpate the prostate gland in men and the upper vagina and cervix in women.

The sigmoidoscope should be inserted, aimed at the patient's umbilicus (Fig. 18-62A). At 4 cm from the anal verge, the tip will be at the anorectal ring. With the obturator removed (Fig. 18-62B), the left lower rectal fold should be visible. At about 8 cm from the verge, the middle rectal fold may be seen. This is the level of the peritoneal reflection. The superior rectal fold is reached at 10 to 12 cm, and beyond this, passage of the instrument is easy.

The rectum, despite its name (which means "straight"), is not straight. The perineal flexure is a posterior bend just above the anorectal ring. Beyond this is the sacral flexure as the rectum follows the curve of the sacrum anteriorly. Lateral flexure to the left occurs at the first and third (inferior and superior) rectal folds and to the right at the middle rectal fold. The most dangerous area is between the middle and superior rectal folds, just above the peritoneal reflection. This is the area in which perforation by the sigmoidoscope may occur.

Saunders et al.[214] investigated the thesis that colonoscopy is a more difficult procedure in Western than Oriental patients by comparing anatomic findings at laparotomy of 115 Western (Caucasian) and 114 Oriental patients:

*Sigmoid adhesions were found more frequently in Western (17%) compared to Oriental (8%) patients, P = 0.047. A descending mesocolon of ≥10 cm occurred in 10 (8%) Western patients but only 1 (0.9%) Oriental patient, P = 0.01. The splenic flexure was more frequently mobile in Western patients (20%) compared to Oriental (9%) patients, P = 0.016. In 29% of Western patients the mid-transverse colon reached the symphysis pubis, or lower when pulled downward, in contrast to 10% of Oriental patients, P <0.001. There was no significant difference in total colonic length comparing Western (median = 114 cm, range 68-159 cm) to Oriental (median = 111 cm, range 78-161 cm) patients. Western patients have a higher incidence of sigmoid colon adhesions and increased colonic mobility when compared to Orientals.*

## Anorectal Fistulas

Most anal fistulas are complications of anorectal abscesses, and most such abscesses arise in the anal glands that open into the base of the anal valves. Incision and drain-

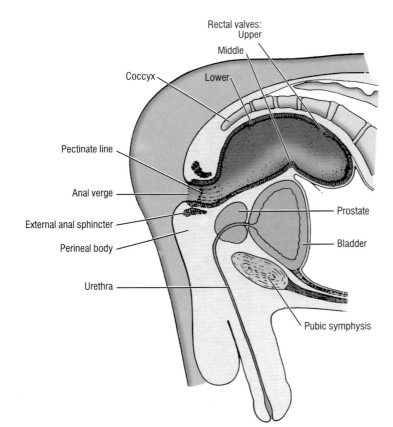

**FIG. 18-60.** Diagram of anorectal landmarks for sigmoidoscopic examination. Patient in knee-chest or knee-elbow position. (Modified from Skandalakis JE, Gray SW, Rowe JS Jr. Anatomical Complications in General Surgery. New York: McGraw-Hill, 1983; with permission.)

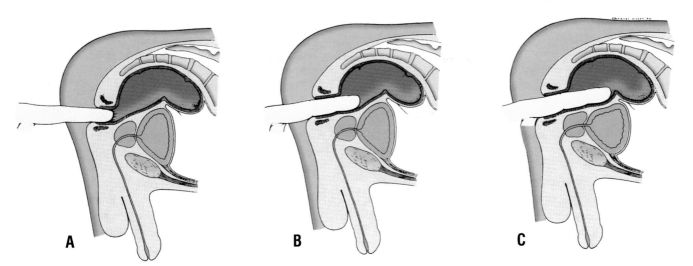

FIG. **18-61.** Digital examination. **A,** Distal interphalangeal joint at the anal verge. Hemorrhoids can be detected at this stage. **B,** Middle interphalangeal joint at the anal verge. **C,** Metacarpophalangeal joint at the anal verge. The tip of the finger is at or just above the inferior rectal valve. (Modified from Skandalakis JE, Gray SW, Rowe JS Jr. Anatomical Complications in General Surgery. New York: McGraw-Hill, 1983; with permission.)

age of an abscess predisposes to fistula formation.[107,215,216]

Conservative treatment is called for here. Fistulectomy (radical removal of the fistula) with extensive section of the sphincters will produce incontinence. Fistulectomy is safe only where preservation of the anal ring can be ensured; otherwise fistulotomy is the procedure of choice.

## Anorectal Abscesses

With anorectal abscesses, early drainage by a long, radial incision is the correct technique to avoid recurrence. An excellent presentation by Nomikos[217] advised accurate anatomic localization of anorectal abscesses.

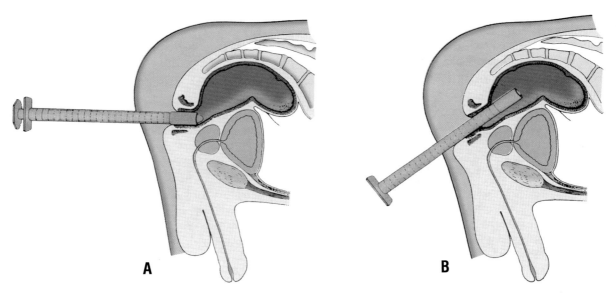

FIG. **18-62.** Sigmoidscopic examination. **A,** The instrument is directed toward the umbilicus. The tip is just past the anorectal ring. **B,** With obturator removed, the instrument is passed by direct observation. The tip shown here is almost up to the middle rectal valve. (Modified from Skandalakis JE, Gray SW, Rowe JS Jr. Anatomical Complications in General Surgery. New York: McGraw-Hill, 1983; with permission.)

## Anal Fissure

An anal fissure, which has a boatlike shape, is a painful ulcer in the anal canal, and may be superficial or deep. In children it is usually secondary to constipation; in adults it is most likely idiopathic (except in cases of preexisting disease such as Crohn's disease, AIDS, or anal tuberculosis, or predisposing factors such as anal intercourse) or iatrogenic.

The accepted treatment is partial internal sphincterotomy (lateral or midline) or pharmacologic sphincterotomy (topical application of glyceryl trinitrate or intrasphincteric injection of botulinum toxin). A superficial vertical mucosal tear secondary to severe and tight spasm of the anal sphincters may be treated by four finger dilatation and very rarely by lateral internal sphincterotomy. Argov and Levandovsky[218] state that open lateral sphincterotomy performed in an ambulatory setting is the gold standard treatment for chronic anal fissure due to the very high long-term success rate and negligible occurrence of complications. Fecal or flatus incontinence is reported with lateral sphincterotomy; according to Sharp[219] the incidence is 0-35%.

REMEMBER: Rule out epidermoid carcinoma as well as venereal diseases prior to any dilatation.

## Pilonidal Disease

Pilonidal disease produces a cyst or sinus with hair. While it may be of congenital origin, it is most likely that this enigmatic condition is acquired. The treatment is also controversial. If abscessed, incise and drain. Incision and curettage is favored by da Silva[220] with regard to morbidity, healing, recurrence, and cure. If a persistent sinus remains, then excision of the sinus in toto, leaving the wound open, is perhaps the procedure of choice.

Malignant degeneration of pilonidal cysts was reported by Davis and colleagues.[221]

## Hemorrhoids

Hemorrhoids may be internal or external.
Good knowledge of technique and surgical anatomy is essential when treating hemorrhoids.

## Rectal Prolapse

Rectal prolapse (Fig. 18-63) is a pathologic entity in which some or all layers of the rectum protrude mucosal side out from the surgical anal canal.

There are several approaches and procedures which may be employed:
- Perineal approach with amputation of the sigmoid colon and rectosigmoid anastomosis
- Thiersch perineal approach
- Rectopexy by abdominal approach or low anterior resection. Herold and Bruch[222] reported good results with laparoscopic retropexy in patients with rectal prolapse and morphologic outlet constipation.
- Rectal sling of Ripstein. Schultz et al.[223] reported low mortality and recurrence, but high complication rate, with Ripstein rectopexy. Increased constipation occurred with improved continence in some patients, especially those with internal rectal intussusception.
- Ivalon sponge wrap of Wells
- Transanal excision. Transanal excision for low rectal cancer in early stage disease (carcinoma in situ and T1 lesion) with favorable histology was reported safe and effective by Blair and Ellenhorn.[224]

Agachan et al.[225] advised perineal rectosigmoidectomy with levatoroplasty for the treatment of rectal prolapse.

Pikarsky and colleagues[226] stated that the outcome of surgery is similar in cases of primary or recurrent prolapse, with the same surgical options valid in both scenarios. They reported an overall success rate of 85.2 percent.

For further information and techniques, please consult *Modern Hernia Repair*.[227]

## Anorectal Cancer Surgery

We quote from the beautiful anatomical presentation of Enker et al.[112]:

*In the posterior visceral compartment of the pelvis, four anatomic layers determine which surgical planes are available for sharp dissection within the pelvis. These layers are 1) the visceral layer of the pelvic fascia; 2) the parietal layer(s) of the pelvic fascia; 3) the medial layer of the internal iliac vascular adventitia; and 4) the lateral layers of the internal iliac vascular adventitia and the obturator spaces. The bilateral paravesical spaces may also provide ventral access to the deep pelvis in rare instances.*

*The circumstances defining the use of each of the planes include:*
- *Primary rectal cancers without extension to the visceral layer of the pelvic fascia.*
- *Primary rectal cancers with extension to the visceral layer of the pelvic fascia.*
- *Primary rectal cancers with extension beyond the*

*visceral layer of the pelvic fascia, but resectable with negative (uninvolved) margins. Examples include 1) attachment to or invasion of the so-called lateral ligament (which actually contains no ligamentous tissue), 2) localized involvement of the middle rectal artery or the internal iliac vessels, and 3) middle rectal or internal iliac node involvement.*

- *Recurrent rectal cancer due to previously unresected internal iliac or mid-rectal artery node involvement.*
- *Obturator space involvement by either primary or recurrent disease, or by nodal disease presenting as a resectable mass.*
- *Direct spread to the levator ani by a laterally located, low-lying rectal cancer.*

*Under these differing circumstances, the knowledge and use of these planes can make a difference between successful resection of a primary or recurrent rectal cancer and a negative outcome, such as uninvolved circumferential margins or the death of the patient due to unresectable pelvic disease.*

Approaches and procedures include:
- Anterior resection if margin distal to the tumor is 5 cm
- Abdominoperineal rectal excision
- Sphincter-saving resection
- Transsacral

The surgical treatment of anorectal cancer is controversial; most controversial are the sphincter-saving procedures. As Dehni and colleagues[228] wisely stated, "Conservation of the sphincter mechanism should never compromise the oncologic outcome of surgery and the method

of neorectum construction must provide acceptable function for patients."

Several factors influence the choice of procedure:
- Anatomic location of tumors (above or below dentate line)
- Pathology (epithelial or nonepithelial)
- Invasion
- Fixation
- Involvement of other anatomic entities related to the anorectum such as parts of the urogenital system (including lymph nodes)
- Age and general condition of patient
- Distal metastasis

Read and Kodner[229] reported that restoration of intestinal continuity following proctectomy for cancer is now possible due to better understanding of the spread of rectal cancer as well as of pelvic physiology. Occasionally a diverting loop ileostomy may be necessary. Di Matteo et al.[230] reported better anal sphincteric continence with high or low colorectal anastomosis than with coloanal anastomosis. Madoff et al.[231] reported that sphincter replacement by electrically stimulated skeletal muscle neosphincter and artificial anal sphincter provide a continent option for patients with end-stage fecal incontinence and those requiring abdominoperineal resection.

Locally excised T1 rectal cancer with negative surgical margins should receive adjuvant chemoradiation.[232] Adequate shielding of the anal sphincter during chemoradiation is essential when a sphincter-preserving procedure is performed for low rectal cancer.[233]

This is the era of the sentinel lymph node in cancer surgery not only in the breast, but also in other anatomic

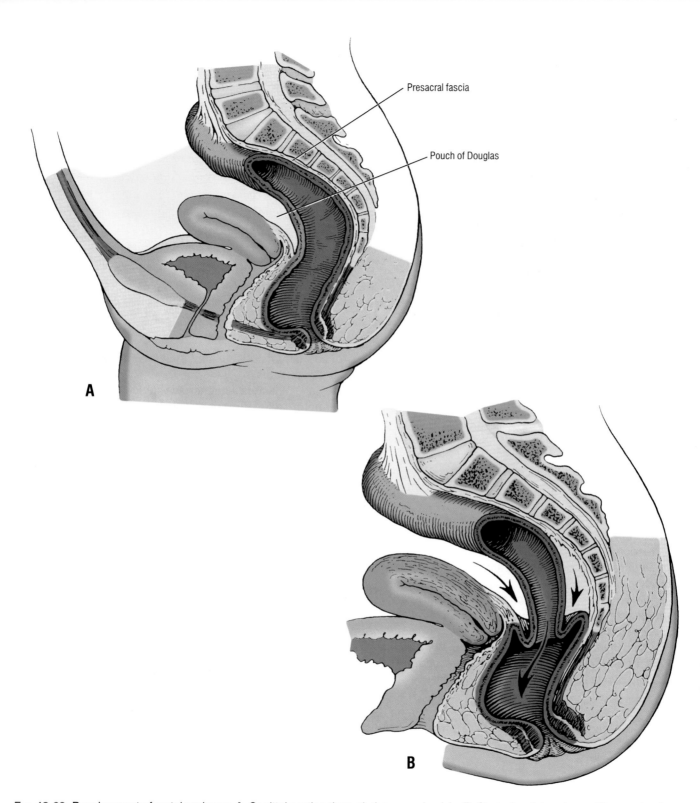

Presacral fascia

Pouch of Douglas

**A**

**B**

FIG. 18-63. Development of rectal prolapse. **A,** Sagittal section through the normal pelvis. **B,** Start of rectal prolapse. The proximal segment (intussusceptum) is telescoping into the distal segment (intussuscipiens). **C,** Intussusceptum at the pectinate line. **D,** Intussusceptum protrudes through the anus. (Modified from Skandalakis LJ, Gadacz TR, Mansberger AR Jr, Mitchell WE Jr, Colborn GL, Skandalakis JE. Modern Hernia Repair. New York: Parthenon, 1996; with permission.)

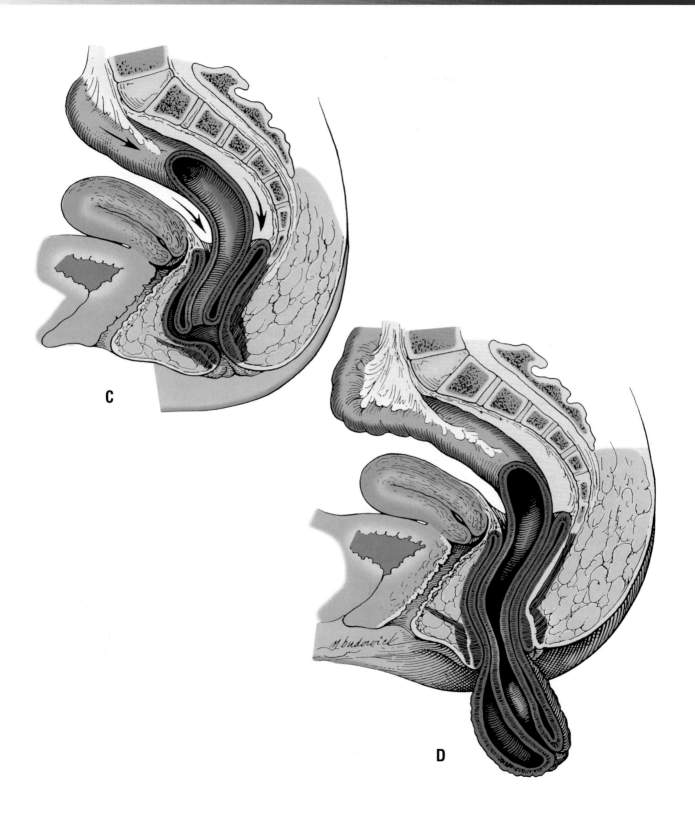

C

D

entities such as the colorectum.[234] Saha et al.[235] reported that sentinel lymph node mapping can easily be performed in colorectal cancer patients, with an accuracy rate of more than 95%.

## ANATOMIC COMPLICATIONS OF THE COLON

### Colon Resection

#### *Anastomotic Complications*

Schrock and colleagues[236] investigated leakage in 1,703 colonic anastomoses. Disruption of the anastomosis occurred in 4.5 percent. The mortality among patients with leakage was 36.8 percent in enterocolic anastomoses, 36.8 percent in left colocolostomies, and 26.5 percent in left colorectal anastomoses. The incidence of anastomotic dehiscence increased with the age of the patient, anemia, prior radiation therapy, infection, hypotension, intraoperative transfusion, and carcinoma at the line of resection. Anastomotic dehiscence occurred in 1.7 percent of colonic anastomoses performed under ideal circumstances and in 6.7 percent of anastomoses performed with one or more unfavorable conditions present. Neither the experience of the surgeon nor the details of the technique showed significant differences.

One- or two-layered anastomosis, omental wrapping, proximal colostomy, preoperative cleansing, and antibiotics all reduce leakage, but they do not eliminate it entirely. Welch et al.[237] stated: "It could be assumed that if barium enemas were given almost immediately after every colonic anastomosis, 100 percent of them would show some leakage." While we consider this view too pessimistic, we recognize that leakage of colonic anastomoses is a much more frequent problem than leakage of small intestinal anastomoses. Tocchi et al.[238] reported that omentoplasty by means of intact omentum reduced the severity of anastomotic leakage following rectal resection, although the incidence of anastomotic disruption was not affected by the use of omentoplasty. Moran and Heald[239] stated that with optimum technique and the use of a combination of linear and circular staplers, leakage is a problem largely confined to anastomoses within 6 cm of the anal verge.

Vogel and Klosterhalfen[125] stated that the dorsocaudal sector of the rectal ampulla is an area of the rectum defi-

cient in blood supply. This is due to the separation of the inferior and superior rectal arteries by the pelvic diaphragm.

Patricio et al.[240] reported that in patients older than 50, the hypogastric (internal iliac) arteries provide less blood to the anorectum. These authors hypothesize that a deficient blood supply is one of several factors responsible for leakage at a colorectal anastomosis. Because the inferior mesenteric artery is ligated, this hypothesis is very sound.

Jansen et al.[241] reported an ingenious method to close the anastomosis. Two ring magnets were used to produce end-to-end approximation of the layers of the gut wall. Following healing of the resection, the magnets pass out of the body. The report covered 21 patients in whom the magnetic anastomosis was employed. In two (9.5 percent), dehiscence took place.

In spite of the fact that leakage cannot be entirely prevented, principles of good technique must be observed:
- Anastomose only healthy colon
- Avoid tension on the anastomosis
- Ensure a good blood supply at the cut ends of both bowels. Good color, bleeding at the cut edge, and pulsation of mesenteric vessels are indicators of a good blood supply.
- Avoid intramural hematoma. If a hematoma appears to be spreading, do not hesitate to resect more colon. Good hemostasis is absolutely mandatory; ligate all vessels.
- Clean fat, epiploic appendices, and mesentery from both proximal and distal edges of the anastomosis. Clean not more than 1 to 1.5 cm.
- Preserve an adequate lumen
- Close mesenteric gaps if possible. If they cannot be closed, open them as wide as possible.
- Avoid sepsis by good preparation of the colon prior to surgery. Careful selection of appropriate antibiotics is mandatory before and after surgery.
- If there is doubt about the anastomosis, perform a proximal colostomy. This is a life-saving procedure.

In addition to postoperative leakage, colon anastomoses are subject to bleeding and hematoma formation as well as ischemia, necrosis, and fistula formation.

Early obstruction at the anastomotic site can result from edema or excessive inversion; late obstruction can be caused by recurrent carcinoma. Hernia through a mesenteric defect is a possible complication. Mesenteric defects should be closed or enlarged to avoid the possibility of strangulated transmesenteric hernia.

Remember:
- The circular muscle is probably the strongest stroma of the intestinal wall.

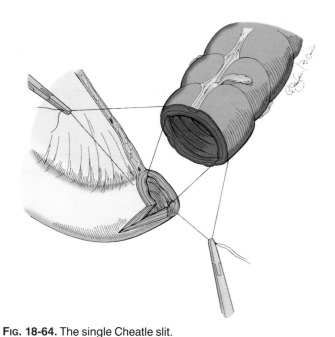

FIG. **18-64.** The single Cheatle slit.

- The single Cheatle slit (Fig. 18-64) is made by incising longitudinally the antimesenteric border of the narrow intestinal segment.
- The double Cheatle slit (Fig. 18-65) is made by incising both antimesenteric borders of the proximal and distal segments. The more mobile bowel end is rotated approximately 180°. The end of the Cheatle incision is sutured to the cutting edge (rim) of the bowel. The same technique is used to approximate the remaining Cheatle incision.

## *Vascular Injury*

Several vessels are subject to injury with consequent hemorrhage.
- In right colectomy: the superior mesenteric artery, superior mesenteric vein, branches of the middle colic vein extending to the first part of the duodenum, and marginal artery
- In left colectomy: the left gastroepiploic artery, left splenic polar artery, vessels of the renocolic ligament that may connect Gerota's fascia of the kidney, left gonadal vein, marginal artery, and middle colic artery
- In low anterior resection: most of the vessels endangered by left colectomy (left iliac vein, veins of the left pelvic wall, and presacral venous plexus which is beneath the endopelvic fascia)

In addition, hematomas, abscesses, or fistulas are possible.

## *Organ Injury*

### Ureters

Graham and Goligher[242] reviewed 1,605 patients, 14 of whom suffered ureteric injury (one bilateral) during rectal excision. A higher frequency was reported by Andersson and Bergdahl,[243] who found 30 ureteric injuries among 801 patients. The two sides are almost equally affected. Injuries occur either at the level of ligation of the inferior mesenteric vessels or, more often, just above the level of the lateral rectal ligaments. Graham and Goligher[242] observed that the left ureter lies 1.25-5 cm or more lateral to the inferior mesenteric artery. Where the ureter is close to the artery, it can inadvertently be hooked with the vessel and ligated. This must be avoided by pushing the left ureter laterally and backward following incision of the left lateral peritoneum.

If the tumor is not adherent, the ureter can be retracted blindly from the lateral ligament. However, the only reliable method for sparing the ureter is by exposing it from the brim of the pelvis almost to the bladder. If the ureter is infiltrated by the tumor, it will, of course, have to be resected.

The ureter may survive ligation or crushing injury if the ligation or clamp is removed at once. If the ureter does not appear normal, the injured portion must be resected. Where resection has occurred, the choice is between end-to-end anastomosis of the ureter or reimplantation of the ureter into the bladder. The latter procedure is the easier of the two.[244]

### Duodenum, Liver, Pancreas, and Spleen

In right colectomy, mobilization of the hepatic flexure and the right transverse mesocolon may accidentally in-

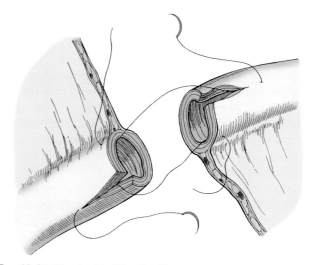

FIG. **18-65.** The double Cheatle slit.

jure the duodenum, liver, or pancreas. In left colectomy, the duodenum, spleen, and tail of the pancreas may be injured during mobilization of the splenic flexure and the left transverse colon.

### Prostate, Seminal Vesicle, Vagina, Bladder, and Rectum

The prostate, seminal vesicle, vagina, and bladder can be injured during low left colon resections. In 11 of 801 patients reviewed by Andersson and Bergdahl,[243] trauma to the bladder appeared following operation. Voiding dysfunction was described by Kirkegaard and associates[245] in 20 patients who underwent low anterior resection of midrectal carcinoma. These conditions were the result of autonomic nerve injury, and did not arise from direct trauma to the bladder.

Autonomic nerve preservation in association with total mesorectal excision for cancer of the rectum minimizes sexual and urinary dysfunction, according to Havenga et al.[246]

We quote Mancini et al.[247]:

> Traditional rectal cancer surgery has been burdened with a high rate of sexual and urinary dysfunctions due to intraoperative injury or the cutting of the sympathetic and/or parasympathetic nerves...The parasympathetic nerve trunks were those most often damaged because of perineural tumor spreading. Partial to complete sexual impotence was observed in 44% of the patients and surprisingly, preoperative dysfunctions were detected by means of the multidisciplinary approach in one third of these patients. Therefore, only 30.5% of the patients presented with strictly postoperative sexual impotency, above all, those who had undergone high-dose preoperative chemoradiation for T3 or T4 middle to low rectal cancer.

### *Inadequate Procedure*

A leaking anastomosis is the most obvious sign of an inadequate procedure, but, as we have seen, it is unrealistic to expect every anastomosis to be free from leakage. Goligher and colleagues[248] reported radiological leakage in 51 percent of low and high anterior resections. Chassin[249] had only two patients with clinical leakage in 62 anastomoses. Many radiological leaks do not present with clinical symptoms.

Other evidence of inadequate procedure includes:

- Obstruction resulting from turning in too much tissue at the anastomosis
- Improper preparation of the ends to be anastomosed
- Failure to close (or open widely) a mesenteric defect

- Excessive tension on the anastomosis from a short transverse mesocolon
- Poor lymphadenectomy with future recurrence

The following are several anatomic points to be remembered to ensure performance of a complete lymphadenectomy (and, therefore, adequate cancer surgery):

*Right Colectomy*
- Ligate the ileocolic artery at its point of origin from the superior mesenteric artery, or as high as possible. Preserve ileal branches.
- If an extended right colectomy is necessary, ligate the middle colic artery in the above fashion.

*Left Colectomy*
- High ligation of the inferior mesenteric artery must be carried out. To accomplish this, elevate the third part of the duodenum, which is notorious for covering the origin of the inferior mesenteric artery from the aorta.
- Perform high ligation of the inferior mesenteric vein employing slight, gentle elevation of the pancreas, in order to explore the entrance of this vein into the splenic vein.
- Avoid traction of the spleen (see surgical anatomy section of the spleen chapter for details).

## Cecostomy

Anatomic complications of cecostomy include:
- Intraperitoneal abscess secondary to leakage at the stoma; poor purse-string suture is a contributing factor
- Abdominal wall abscess resulting from failure to completely fix the cecum to the abdominal wall
- Poor or nonfunctioning cecostomy due to a Foley catheter that is too small, has blockage, or its catheter tip in the cecum is located poorly, especially when the appendiceal stump is used

## Colostomy

Most of the anatomic complications of colostomy result from inadequate procedures. Many sources of error are possible.

Among a series of 181 consecutive colostomies,[250] one patient died, and 50 suffered complications. Of the 50 complications, 12 resulted from an opening that was too tight; 24 resulted from an opening that was too loose. An excessively tight opening leads to edema, ischemia, and stenosis; an excessively loose opening leads to prolapse, redundant mucosa, peristomal hernia, retraction, evisceration, and small intestinal obstruction. Wound infection and tumor recurrence each occurred in 3 patients.

In 100 of the patients in Hines and Harris' series,[250] the colostomy was subsequently closed. There was 1 death; 17 patients had complications. Incisional hernia occurred in 7 patients, obstruction in 4, and infection in 2. A much higher rate (43.5 percent) of complications at closure has been reported by Varnell and Pemberton.[251] The Hartmann procedure had significantly more complications than did loop colostomy. Nearly two-thirds of the complications were the result of infection.

In a series reported by Stothert and colleagues,[252] 41 patients underwent emergency colonic stoma formation. Six patients died and 19 had major or minor complications. Among the major complications were intraabdominal abscesses, peristomal abscesses, necrosis of the stoma, and peristomal hernia. The researchers advised using better technique to avoid complications.

Establishment of an end colostomy requires a good blood supply to the distal stump. If the end of the colon is ischemic, the tightness of the stoma will be irrelevant. If the terminal blood supply is good, strangulation from an abdominal aperture that is too small or is stenosed by skin may produce ischemia and necrosis in spite of a well-prepared colonic end.

Remember that retraction of a colostomy is due to peristaltic contractions trying to move feces from the obstructed colon. These contractions can be powerful.

We quote Kasperk et al.[253]:

> *Parastomal herniation is a very frequent complication in enterostomy. The therapeutic strategy consists of three approaches: local fascial repair, relocation of the stoma, and a variety of more elaborate procedures, many of which also involve the use of nonabsorbable meshes. Despite this multitude of available techniques, recurrence rates are high, and longterm complications, especially after mesh implantation, are frequent.*

## Abdominoperineal Resection

The complications of abdominoperineal resection can be summarized as: (1) vascular injury, (2) organ injury, and (3) nerve injury.

Presacral veins, the left iliac vein, the middle rectal artery (if present), and inferior hemorrhoidal vessels are subject to injury.

Trauma to the left ureter, duodenum, urinary bladder, or male urethra must be avoided. Other complications of abdominoperineal resection are inadequate reconstruction of the peritoneal floor, small bowel obstruction, colostomy complications, rupture of the rectum, and contamination.

Injury to the sympathetic or parasympathetic nerves may result in bladder dysfunction, failure of ejaculation, and severance of the nervi erigentes with impotence and retention of urine.[41] The surgeon should remember that the nervi erigentes penetrate the fascia of Waldeyer; the fascia of Waldeyer should be divided at the tip of the coccyx. Nakai et al.[254] reported that unilateral sacrifice of sacral nerves results in little bladder or anorectal dysfunction.

The ureter (and the lateral ligaments of the rectum) must be traced deep into the pelvis by careful dissection without elevation. Division of the colon and formation of the colostomy can then be done. The pelvic peritoneum should be closed to avoid herniation and obstruction of the small bowel.

According to Porter et al.,[255] 62% of inadvertent rectal perforations during abdominoperineal resection take place during the perineal part of surgery. The authors advised special care.

## Iatrogenic Perforations with Barium Enema or Colonoscopy

Gedebou et al.[256] stated that in iatrogenic colon perforations due to barium enema or colonoscopy without significant contamination, either primary repair or resection and anastomosis can be performed with acceptable morbidity.

# ANATOMIC COMPLICATIONS OF THE ANORECTUM

## Anorectal Fistulas

Among 133 patients in the series of Adams and Kovalcik,[216] there were 80 fistulectomies, with 1 patient in whom section of the sphincter was necessary. The other 53 patients had fistulotomy. Complications occurred in 14 patients: recurrence in 5, spinal headache in 3, postoperative bleeding in 2, and temporary rectal incontinence in 1. Other complications are stenosis and stricture. Avoid complete division of the external sphincter. Avoid complete anterior division of the external sphincter in females.

Church et al.[257] reported that hemorrhage from presacral veins, perforation of the rectum, damage to the pelvic autonomic nerves, and inadequate clearance of rectal cancer are major complications of rectal surgery.

## Anorectal Abscesses

Fistulas may form due to poor drainage of abscesses. Initial fistulotomy reduces the number of recurrences requiring surgery. Knoefel et al.[258] state that the risk of developing incontinence increases with recurrent anorectal disease, not with careful fistulotomy.

## Anal Fissure

Fecal incontinence in elderly patients may occur secondary to dilatation or sphincterotomy.

## Hemorrhoids

We quote Liberman and Thorson[259]:

*Anal stenosis may be anatomic (stricture) or functional (muscular). Anal stricture is most often a preventable complication. It is most commonly seen after overzealous surgical hemorrhoidectomy. A well-performed hemorrhoidectomy is the best way to avoid anal stricture. Symptomatic mild functional stenosis and stricture may be managed conservatively with diet, fiber supplements, and stool softeners. A program of gradual manual or mechanical dilation may be required. Sphincterotomy and various techniques of anoplasty have been used successfully in the treatment of symptomatic moderate to severe functional anal stenosis and stricture, respectively.*

Anal or distal rectal strictures can occur secondary to nonepithelialization of the mucosa of the surgical anal canal and distal rectum when the mucosa is removed in toto. Anal fissure is a rare complication of hemorrhoids. Incontinence is very rare.

Timaran et al.[260] reported a case of unexpected anal adenocarcinoma in a hemorrhoidectomy specimen, but they advised that the rarity of this finding does not support routine histopathological examination.

## Rectal Prolapse

The complications of the surgical treatment of rectal prolapse depend on the procedure chosen by the surgeon:

- Anastomotic complications
  - Leakage
  - Disruption of anastomosis
  - Obstruction
- Vascular injury. The following vessels should be protected to prevent bleeding:
  - Left gastrohepatic artery and vein
  - Left splenic polar artery
  - Renocolic vessels
  - Left gonadal vein
  - Marginal artery
  - Middle colic artery
  - Vein of the left pelvic wall
  - Presacral venous plexus
  - Superior, middle, and inferior rectal veins
- Organ injury
  - Ureters
  - Spleen
  - Prostate
  - Seminal vesicles
  - Vagina
  - Urinary bladder
- Nerve injury
  - Autonomic nerve injury with bladder dysfunction and impotence
- Inadequate procedures
  - Failure to close mesenteric defect

## Anorectal Cancer Surgery

Complications of anorectal cancer surgery may include impotence, anastomotic leak with local abscess formation or generalized peritonitis, bleeding of venous origin, or urinary retention.

Bissett and Hill[261] present the following complications which may occur during rectal mobilization for carcinoma:

- Ureteric injury
- Rectal perforation
- Hemorrhage
- Injury to the autonomic nerves
- Recurrence of cancer in the pelvis

Ho et al.[262] stated that transanally introduced stapling technique which involves anal manipulation may result in postoperative anal sphincter defects and impaired anal pressures.

*AHMED SHAFIK: THE LARGE INTESTINE AND ANORECTUM*

*As promised earlier in this chapter, we present here some selected topics on the large intestine and extensive research on the anorectum by Dr. Ahmed Shafik.*

*Dr. Shafik wishes to acknowledge his great appreciation to Margot Yehia and Waltraut Reichelt for their invaluable assistance in preparing this material.*

# *Large Intestine*

## RIGHT COLON FLEXURE SYNDROME

The right colon flexure syndrome, which was described by Shafik,[263] presented with right-sided abdominal pain, distension and constipation. At operation a triangular web (Fig. 18-66) with an underlying narrow segment at the hepatic colonic flexure was found responsible for colonic obstruction. The stenotic segment had complete longitudinal muscle coverage due to fusion of the 3 taenia coli. Colo-colic anastomosis relieves the symptoms. The condition seems to have a developmental origin.

## RECTOSIGMOID JUNCTION

The physioanatomic aspects of the rectosigmoid junction (RSJ) are rarely considered in the literature. Herein is a concise review of the surgical anatomy and related physiology of the RSJ.

### Sigmoidorectal Junction Sphincter and Reflex

A recent study has recognized the presence of a high pressure zone in the RSJ at rest.[98] It exists between two lower pressure zones: the sigmoid colon above and the rectum below. The segment of the colon at the RSJ seems to act as a physiologic sphincter preventing feces from crossing automatically from the sigmoid colon to the rectum during a cycle of mass colonic contraction.

Upon colonic contraction, the colonic contents travel downward through the descending colon to the sigmoid colon. The factors preventing the colonic contents from continuing directly to the rectum during colonic contraction are believed to be:
- The S-curve of the sigmoid colon
- A flap-valve action induced by the angle that links the sigmoid with the rectum
- The high pressure zone at the RSJ

During the time of fecal collection in the sigmoid colon, the pressures in the RSJ and rectum showed no significant change against the resting state suggesting that the rectum and RSJ did not exhibit mechanical activity. This state was maintained until the fecal mass attained a certain vol-

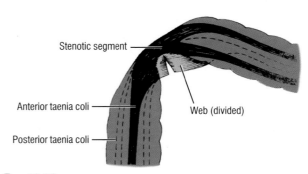

**FIG. 18-66.** Operative findings at the hepatic flexure. Web is divided to demonstrate the stenotic segment. (Modified from Shafik A. Right colon flexure syndrome. Report of two cases. Coloproctology 1981;3:105-106; with permission.)

ume, at which point the sigmoid colon contracts and the RSJ relaxes, dispelling the sigmoid contents to the rectum.[98] A reflex relationship exists between the sigmoid colon and the RSJ which is mediated through what Shafik calls: "sigmoidorectal junction inhibitory reflex."[98] The reflex functions to relax the RSJ upon sigmoid contraction, thereby allowing the sigmoid contents to cross into the rectum. It seems to also regulate the process of sigmoid stool delivery to the rectum: it does not relax until the colonic mass reaches a certain volume that would initiate sigmoid contraction.

Studies have demonstrated that the RSJ pressure increases upon rectal contraction. This reflex relationship, which Shafik termed "sigmoidorectal junction excitatory reflex,"[98] closes the RSJ upon rectal contraction, resulting in the rectal contents being dispelled distally. This in turn prevents reflux of rectal contents back to the sigmoid colon. The sigmoido-rectal junction excitatory reflex seems to function only upon rectal contraction leading to RSJ closure.

Thus, a physiologic sphincter appears to exist at the RSJ. Researchers failed to detect such a sphincter anatomically. The same state of affairs is found with respect to the lower esophageal sphincter: it exists functionally but not anatomically.

## Functional Activity of Sigmoid Colon and Rectum During Fecal Storage in the Sigmoid

Another study[264] revealed that slow sigmoid colon distension did not effect the increase of sigmoid pressure, indicating that the sigmoid colon adapts as it receives new material from the colon. This adaptation continued with increasing balloon distension of the sigmoid, until, at a certain volume, the sigmoid colon contracted and pushed the balloon to the rectum (Fig. 18-67). It seems that the stretch receptors in the sigmoid colon wall, which initiate sigmoid contraction, are not stimulated before a certain level of distension is reached.

This is in contrast to rapid sigmoid distension which effected sigmoid contraction with approximately half the volume required for sigmoid contraction by the slow distension test (Fig. 18-68). There might be 2 types of stretch receptors in the sigmoid wall: one responding to slow distension and the other to rapid distension. Under normal physiologic conditions, the sigmoid receives the feces from the colon and stores them until a volume has accumulated which is big enough to stimulate the stretch receptors and initiate sigmoid colon contraction which would push the

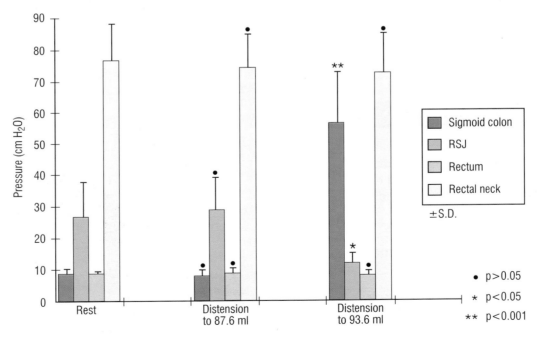

**FIG. 18-67.** Pressure response of the sigmoid colon, rectosigmoid junction (RSJ), rectum, and rectal neck (anal canal) to slow-rate balloon distension of the sigmoid colon. (Modified from Shafik A. Functional activity of the sigmoid colon and rectum. A study during fecal storage in the sigmoid. Coloproctology 1997;19:236-241; with permission.)

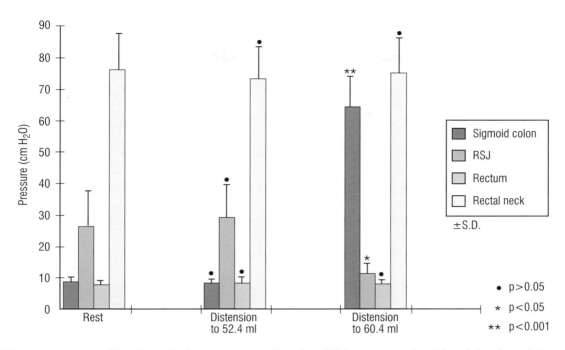

**FIG. 18-68.** Pressure response of the sigmoid colon, rectosigmoid junction (RSJ), rectum, and rectal neck (anal canal) to rapid-rate balloon distension of the sigmoid colon. (Modified from Shafik A. Functional activity of the sigmoid colon and rectum. A study during fecal storage in the sigmoid. Coloproctology 1997;19:236-241; with permission.)

stools to the rectum. Shafik speculates that rapid sigmoid distension occurs in pathologic conditions, such as diarrhea, and triggers sigmoid contraction with smaller amounts of fecal material than normal.

## Hypertonic Rectosigmoid Junction Syndrome

The presence of a new clinicopathological entity causing constipation which Shafik termed the 'hypertonic rectosigmoid junction'[265] could be demonstrated in 6 women and 2 men (mean age 44.2 ± 10.3 years) who complained of chronic constipation. They had normal bowel habits before that time. Intestinal transit was delayed with accumulation of pellets in the sigmoid colon. Defecography and electromyography of the external anal sphincter and levator ani muscle were normal. The resting pressure was normal in the sigmoid colon, rectum, and rectal neck, but elevated in the rectosigmoid sphincter (RSS). The sigmoidorectal inhibitory and excitatory reflexes were absent. Histologic findings in biopsies from the sigmoid colon and rectum were normal, but from the RSS were aganglionic (Fig. 18-69). RSS "achalasia" was diagnosed. Endoscopic dilatation of the RSS effected improvement of 5 patients. The remaining 3 patients underwent sigmoidomyotomy (Fig. 18-70A, B).

The 8 patients are now 9 to 38 months without recurrence of the constipation. RSS achalasia constitutes a clinicopathologic entity which should be considered in the etiology of constipation.

## Electrorectogram and Rectosigmoid Pacemaker

The electrical activity of the rectal detrusor was studied experimentally and in humans both intrarectally and transcutaneously.[266-268] Pacesetter potentials (PPs) or slow wave activity was recorded in the rectum. PPs start in an area that corresponds anatomically to the RSJ. The PPs propagate distally in a caudad direction with the same frequency and velocity in the individual subject.

Action potentials (APs) followed or were superimposed on the PPs. They were accompanied simultaneously with increased rectal pressure, which denotes rectal contraction. They occurred less frequently than the PPs, and their frequency was inconsistent in each individual subject. The frequency and amplitude of PPs and APs increased with increasing rectal distension until the rectal balloon was dispelled. The occurrence of APs in relation with PPs was usually random. This points to irregular or nonrhythmic

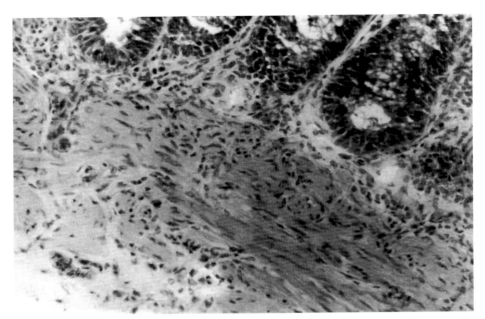

**FIG. 18-69.** Photomicrograph of a biopsy from the rectosigmoid sphincter showing aganglionosis. Hematoxylin eosin x 1000. (From Shafik A. The hypertonic rectosigmoid junction: description of a new clinicopathologic entity causing constipation. Surg Laparosc Endosc 1997;7:116-120; with permission.)

segmental rectal contraction. However, once they occurred they were conducted distally in a regular fashion like PPs. After rectal myotomy, the orderly distal propagation of APs disappeared because myotomy had interrupted their pathway. The APs cause a contractile sweep along the rectum. Yet, this contractile activity induces a rectal pressure increase which is too small to be perceived as rectal sensation.

The aforementioned findings would suggest that the RSJ is the site of a pacemaker.[266-268] It triggers the PPs

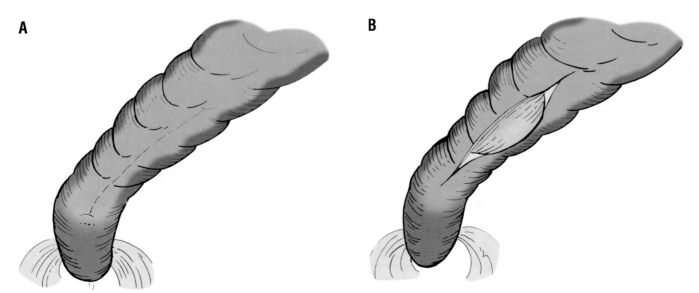

**FIG. 18-70.** Technique of sigmoidomyotomy. **A,** Muscle coat of the rectosigmoid junction is incised down to the mucosa. **B,** Mucosa bulges throughout the length of the incision. (Modified from Shafik A. The hypertonic rectosigmoid junction: description of a new clinicopathologic entity causing constipation. Surg Laparosc Endosc 1997;7:116-120; with permission.)

which are propagated distally along the rectum. The PPs seem to initiate the APs which are accompanied with episodes of rectal pressure elevation representing contractile activity. This postulates that rectal contractions result from APs and not from PPs. The PPs seem to pace the rectal contractile activity in terms of direction and frequency.

### Rectosigmoid Pacemaker Evidence

It seems that there are specialized receptors at the RSJ that trigger rectal detrusor contraction on stimulation by distension of the RSJ. These receptors act as a 'pacemaker' regulating the stool delivery from the sigmoid colon through the rectum to the rectal neck.[269,270] The concept of a 'recto-sigmoid pacemaker' is evidenced[269-271] by: (a) rectal detrusor contraction on RSJ distension, (b) propagation of the rectal electric waves from the RSJ proximodistally, (c) absence of rectal detrusor response to distension of the anesthetized RSJ, (d) absence of detrusor contraction on distension of the colon in anterior resection operation for rectal cancer, and (e) reproducibility. The mechanism of action of the rectosigmoid pacemaker in rectal motility needs to be discussed.

### Rectosigmoid Pacemaker and Rectal Motility

When the sigmoid colon contracts, it delivers its stool contents to the rectum. As the stools pass across the RSJ, they stimulate the rectosigmoid pacemaker leading to rectal detrusor contraction.[98,264] A contraction wave seems to start at the RSJ and to spread into the rectal detrusor, serving a dual action: a) it closes the RSJ, and b) it amputates the fecal column delivered by the sigmoid colon. The upper part remains in the sigmoid colon, while the lower part is delivered to the rectal neck by a wave of 'mass-squeeze' contraction of the rectal detrusor[98,272,273] (Fig. 18-71). The contraction wave travels caudad across the rectal detrusor pushing the fecal column into the rectal neck.

After the rectum evacuates its contents, it relaxes. The fecal portion that remained in the sigmoid colon is then delivered to the rectum, stimulating the recto-sigmoid pacemaker into evoking another rectal contraction wave that evacuates the rectum. The process of rectosigmoid pacemaker stimulation is repeated until the sigmoid reservoir becomes empty.[98,272,273] The stimulus to sigmoid colon contraction is unknown. Relaxation, following the contraction of the rectal detrusor, seems to trigger sigmoid contraction to deliver further stools into the rectum.

If, after the rectal contraction wave has been initiated, evacuation is inopportune, the external anal sphincter is voluntarily contracted, hence preventing internal sphincter relaxation and reflexively aborting rectal detrusor contraction; this occurs through the voluntary inhibition reflex.[163] The rectum relaxes and accommodates for the new contents. It is under these conditions that stools can be palpated in the rectum on digital examination, though under normal physiologic conditions the rectum is empty. When conditions are favorable, the loaded rectum is emptied either by straining with resulting mechanical compression of the detrusor or by a rectal contraction wave initiated when the RSJ is stimulated by another fecal mass delivered from the sigmoid colon to the rectum.

### Artificial Pacemaker

The role of an artificial pacemaker in initiating rectal contractions was assessed both experimentally and in humans.

#### Experimental

An artificial pacemaker was applied to the rectum of 18 mongrel dogs aiming at assessing its effectiveness in inducing rectal contraction.[271] The pacemaker consisted of a hooked needle, a metal plate, a battery, and a tele-

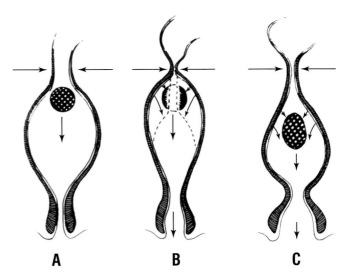

**FIG. 18-71.** "Mass-squeeze" contraction of the rectal detrusor. **A,** Stool distends the rectum. **B,** Rectosigmoid junction closed by means of the rectosigmoid junction excitatory reflex. **C,** Rectal contractile wave travels caudad pushing the fecal column to the rectal neck. (Modified from Shafik A. Study of the rectal detrusor motility in normal and constipated subjects. Proc 2nd Int Mtg Coloproct, Ivrea/Italy 1992:78-90; with permission.)

grapher's key. The needle was hooked into the dog's rectal muscle coat at the RSJ and the metal piece was applied to the skin. Upon electric pulsing of the pacemaker, the rectal pressure showed significant increase while the rectal neck pressure was significantly decreased. Electric pacing succeeded in expelling the balloon in all the dogs.

### Human

In 46 patients, the effectiveness of an artificial pacemaker in the treatment of chronic idiopathic constipation was studied: 26 had chronic idiopathic constipation and 20 were normal controls.[274] The results demonstrated the effectiveness of the artificial pacemaker in inducing rectal contraction in both the normal controls and constipated subjects. This is evident from the significant rectal pressure increase as well as from balloon expulsion upon electric pulsing of the pacemaker.

### Relationship Between Electrosigmoidogram and Electrorectogram

In the sigmoid colon, slow waves or PPs were monophasic with a large negative deflection, while the rectal PPs were triphasic with a small positive, large negative, and another small positive deflection[275] (Figs. 18-72, 18-73). The frequency and amplitude of the PPs in the rectum were significantly higher than those of the sigmoid colon. The fact that shape, frequency, amplitude, and velocity of conduction of the electric waves differed in the electrosigmoidogram (ESG) from those in the electrorectogram (ERG) suggests that the rectal electromechanical activity is not a continuation of the sigmoid colon activity and seems to be initiated in the rectum.[275] This agrees with previous studies which have shown that the rectal motility may be regulated by a "pacemaker"

at the rectosigmoid junction.[266,269] The increased intrasigmoid and rectal pressures associated with APs indicate that they possess contractile activity that continued to increase with increasing balloon distension until, at a certain volume, the balloon is dispelled outside the sigmoid colon or rectum.

### Motility of Sigmoid Colon and Rectum

The sigmoid colon receives the stools from the colon by a mass action.[276] The new contents distend the sigmoid colon and augment its electromechanical activity.[275] The latter increases with growing accumulation of sigmoid contents until the stools are expelled to the rectum. The movements of the sigmoid colon appear to be of the "mass type." Shafik's study showed that the proximal contraction of the sigmoid colon and its relaxation distal to the simulated stool occurred synchronously in one comprehensive mass action and not segmentally.[264,275] This mechanism pushes the contents of the sigmoid colon en masse to the rectum. The results showed also that the distension of the sigmoid colon did not affect the electromechanical activity of the rectum. Therefore, the mass action of the sigmoid colon is independent from the rectal mass action.

### Tube and Marsupialization Colostomy

The technique for tube and marsupialization colostomy consists of creating a small opening into the colon (1-2 cm in length) and suturing its edges to the abdominal wall.[277] The procedure is referred to as a tube colostomy when a tube is put into the colostomy (Fig. 18-74), and a marsupialization colostomy (Fig. 18-75) when no tube is used. The technique is especially indicated in seriously ill patients

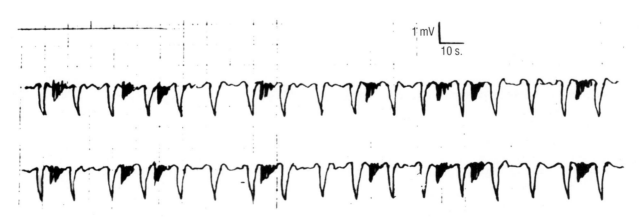

**FIG. 18-72.** Electrorectogram showing triphasic pacesetter potentials followed randomly by action potentials. (From Shafik A. Electrosigmoidogram, electrorectogram and their relation. Front Biosci 1997;2:12-16 Pub Med No. 9294095; with permission.)

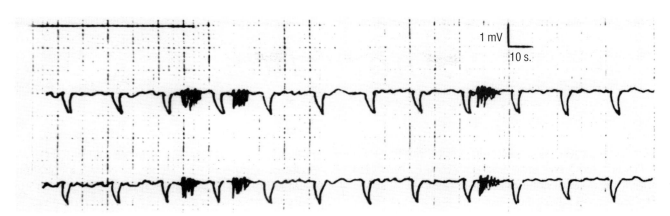

**FIG. 18-73.** Electrosigmoidogram showing monophasic pacesetter potentials followed randomly by action potentials. (From Shafik A. Electrosigmoidogram, electrorectogram and their relation. Front Biosci 1997;2:12-16 Pub Med No. 9294095; with permission.)

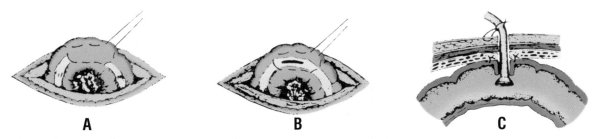

**A**                    **B**                    **C**

**FIG. 18-74.** "Tube colostomy." **A,** Purse-string suture applied to the colon. **B,** Incision into the colon. **C,** Tube introduced into the bowel lumen. (Modified from Shafik A. "Tube" and "marsupialization" colostomy: a simplified technique for colostomy. Am J Proct 1982;33:12-16; with permission.)

with colonic obstruction.

"Tube" colostomy is a deflating colostomy whereas "marsupialization" colostomy is both deflating and defunctioning. Both colostomies have advantages over the formal colostomies. The operations are easily and rapidly performed in any part of the colon, and do not require colonic mobilization or exteriorization. They are performed under local anesthesia, and preserve colonic length. They require a small parietal opening, thus avoiding colostomy prolapse or hernia. Tube colostomy closes spontaneously and marsupialization colostomy requires simple closure.

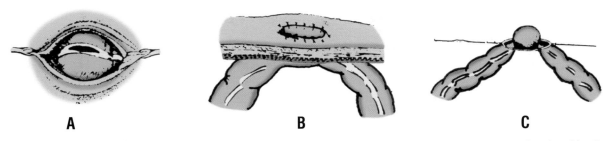

**A**                    **B**                    **C**

**FIG. 18-75.** "Marsupialization colostomy." **A,** Incision into the colon. **B,** Edges of the colonic opening sutured to the skin. **C,** A wide colonic opening showing eversion of posterior colonic wall forming a spur. (Modified from Shafik A. "Tube" and "marsupialization" colostomy: a simplified technique for colostomy. Am J Proct 1982;33:12-16; with permission.)

# *Anorectum*

Intense research by Shafik and others into the anorectal region has been provoked both by unsatisfactory results from diverse clinical procedures and by some key references in the medical literature that are still taken for granted, even though they date back about 400 years to the time of Vesalius (1514-1564).[278] As a result of research in recent years, ample new anatomic and physiologic data have become available which have shed brighter light on the anatomy and function of the anorectal region.

Some of the new data are consistent with our classical knowledge; some negate older observations and conclusions. The majority of findings are intriguing additions to our perception of the physioanatomic relationships of this area. They have had a direct bearing on the adaptation of the basic concepts of the anorectal region. The newer concepts have taken a significant place in our understanding of the etiologies of hitherto unresolved rectal pathologies, including some that had been earlier considered idiopathic.

The findings obtained by intensive investigations into the embryologic aspects of the anorectum, in particular, have provided missing links which have contributed in large measure to our understanding of the functions, the interdependence of the different elements contained in the area, and the disorders that affect them. Hence, by drawing from and applying modern knowledge and understanding, modern surgery stands an incomparably better chance of improving the results of treatment.

## EMBRYOLOGY

Embryologic investigations have supplied the essential bits of mosaic which are necessary for the understanding of the principles governing the anorectum through its development from the hindgut. Studies have conclusively revealed that the rectum extends down to the perineal skin and constitutes one single embryologic, anatomic, and functional unit, together with its neck (the anal canal). The anal canal consequently exists neither as an embryologic entity, nor as an anatomically separate entity, but only as the epithelium that lines the terminal part of the hindgut and forms an opening for the course of the hindgut to the exterior. Failure to comprehend these facts has contributed to the controversy about the embryologic bases of the different congenital anomalies of the area.

## Anatomic Evidence Related to the Anal Musculature

The anal musculature consists of two components: visceral and somatic, which are separated by the intersphincteric space.

### *Visceral Component*

The visceral component of the anal musculature comprises the internal sphincter and the longitudinal muscle, both of which are formed of smooth muscle bundles and are autonomically innervated. Contrary to the views of some investigators[41,279] who hold that these muscles belong to the anal canal, all evidence suggests that they are part of the rectum. Accordingly, the internal sphincter is the downward extension of the circular muscle coat of the rectum which is thickened at the rectal neck inlet, and proceeds down to the perineal skin, from which it is separated by the subcutaneous space[101] (Fig. 18-76A). The longitudinal muscle is but a continuation of the rectal longitudinal muscle coat. It stretches along the rectal neck to stop short of the lower end of the internal sphincter, where it contributes to the central tendon which inserts into the perineal skin by multiple tendinous fibers (Fig. 18-76B).

### *Somatic Component*

The somatic component of the anal musculature consists of striated muscles which include parts of the levator ani, including the puborectalis, and the external sphincter. The somatic component forms the levator tunnel (Fig. 18-77) which embraces the lower end of the hindgut. It develops in the perineum independently of the visceral component.[280] It functions under voluntary control, and serves to control the involuntary visceral component.

The two components, visceral and somatic, although

separate anatomically, have been found to be functionally interrelated so that the voluntary component acts through the involuntary, and vice versa. Thus, the "voluntary inhibition reflex" action of the external sphincter is effected through the involuntary internal sphincter.[163] Furthermore, the suspensory sling of the levator ani (somatic) and the longitudinal muscle (visceral) act jointly to open the rectal neck at defecation.[281] For these reasons, the somatic component is an integral part of the hindgut visceral component.

## Intersphincteric Space

The intersphincteric space is an embryologically developed space which acts to separate the visceral and somatic components of the hindgut, and is occupied by areolar tissue. It lies between the longitudinal muscle and the suspensory sling of the levator ani muscle; it extends along the lower part of the hindgut to the subcutaneous space, and is continuous above with the pelvirectal space.[101] Through the intersphincteric space, the lower part of the

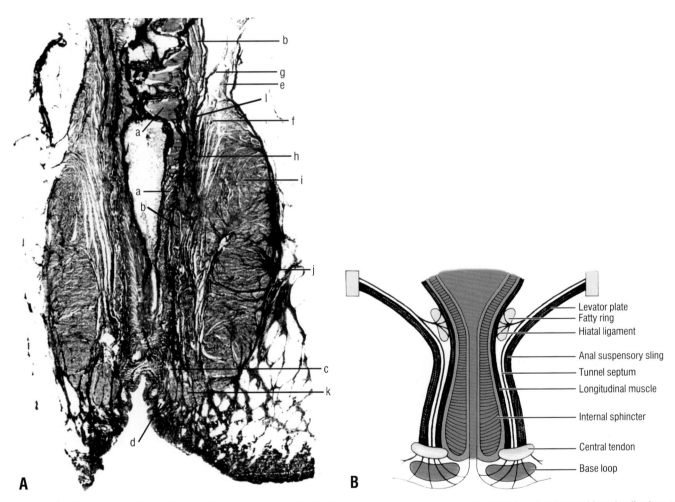

**A**  **B**

FIG. 18-76. Coronal sections of the rectal muscle coats. **A,** Cadaveric specimen demonstrates that the circular and longitudinal rectal muscle coats extend down to the perineal skin, and that the longitudinal muscle inserts into the perineal skin after base loop penetration. Verhoeff-van Gieson × 7. a, Rectal circular muscle coat and internal sphincter. b, Rectal longitudinal muscle coat. c, Central tendon. d, Rectal longitudinal muscle insertion in perineal skin. e, Levator plate. f, Suspensory sling. g, Fascia covering levator plate. h, Tunnel septum. i, Top loop of external sphincter (conjoined deep external sphincter and puborectalis). j and k, Intermediate and base loops of external sphincter. l, Hiatal ligament. **B,** Diagrammatic coronal section of the muscle coats. (**A,** From Shafik A. A new concept of the anatomy of the anal sphincter mechanism and the physiology of defecation. II. Anatomy of the levator ani muscle with special reference to puborectalis. Invest Urol 1975;13:175-182; with permission. **B,** Modified from Shafik A. A new concept of the anatomy of the anal sphincter mechanism and the physiology of defecation. V. The rectal neck: Anatomy and function. Chir Gastroenterol 1977:11:319; with permission.)

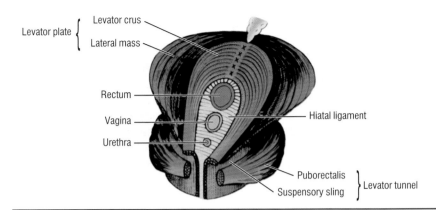

FIG. 18-77. The levator tunnel. (Modified from Shafik A. A new concept of the anatomy of the anal sphincter mechanism and the physiology of defecation. VIII. Levator hiatus and tunnel. Anatomy and function. Dis Colon Rectum 1979;22: 539; with permission.)

rectum, including its visceral component, can be mobilized from within the levator tunnel (somatic component) for removal of otherwise inaccessible rectal lesions, with preservation of the voluntary somatic component[282] (Fig. 18-78).

## Embryologic Evidence

The rectum develops from the hindgut (Fig. 18-79A, B, C), which extends down to the perineal skin as can be deduced from the extension of its circular and longitudinal muscle coats to this level. The blind end of the hindgut, reaching the perineal skin, is invaginated by the proctodeal dimple (Fig. 18-79D). The invagination is effected by

the ectoderm only, without muscular elements.[282] In the course of invagination, an anorectal sinus forms, but is usually obliterated (Fig. 18-79E, F); and the proctodeal skin is remodeled[282,283] (Fig. 18-79G). It seems that the hindgut is guided to its normal location in the perineum by tracking through the levator tunnel (Fig. 18-79B, C).

The stimulus to proctodeal dimpling has not been identified. It may be triggered either by the fixation of longitudinal hindgut fibers to the perineal skin or in the course of formation of the levator tunnel.[282] The latter possibility seems more likely, because proctodeal dimpling occurs also without the hindgut having entered the tunnel or being fixed to the perineal skin. The formation of the levator tunnel may therefore stimulate not only normal hindgut migration to the perineum, but also proctodeal dimpling. As

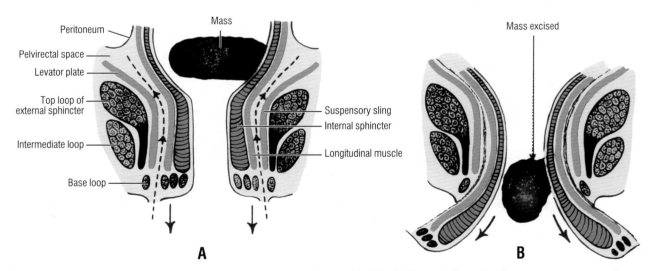

FIG. 18-78. The technique of rectal mobilization for local removal of a rectal lesion. A, Plane of dissection between suspensory sling and longitudinal muscle. B, Rectal neck and lower rectum proper mobilized and pulled down outside anal wound. (Modified from Shafik A. A new concept of the anatomy of the anal sphincter mechanism and the physiology of defecation. XII. Anorectal mobilization. A new surgical access to rectal lesions. Preliminary report. Am J Surg 1981;142:625-635; with permission.)

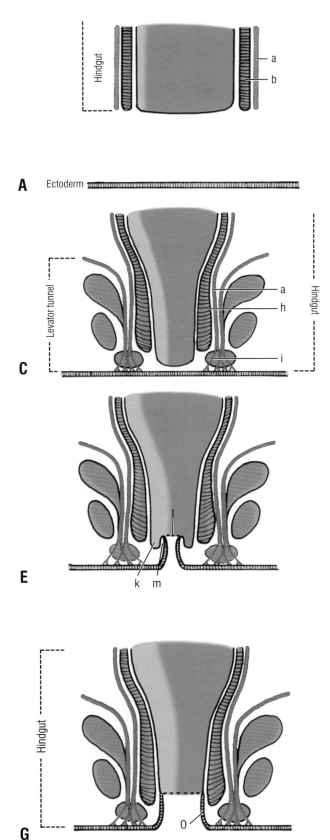

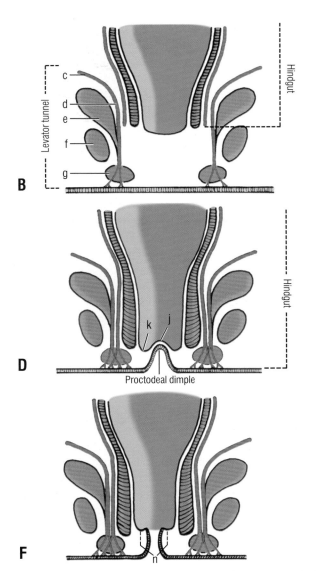

**Fig. 18-79.** The embryologic development of the lower end of the hindgut. **A,** Hindgut migrating toward perineal skin. **B,** Levator tunnel formation. Hindgut migrates through and is guided by levator tunnel to the perineal skin. **C,** Hindgut reaches and is fixed to perineal skin by its longitudinal muscle coat. **D,** Proctodeal dimple invaginates hindgut lower end with resultant anorectal sinus formation. **E,** Rectal membrane rupture with a resulting hindgut opening to the exterior and paraanal space formation. **F,** Anorectal sinus obliteration with persistence of paraanal space. **G,** Rectal neck remodeling resulting in paraanal space obliteration. a, Hindgut longitudinal muscle coat. b, Hindgut circular muscle coat. c, Levator plate. d, Suspensory sling. e, Top loop of external sphincter (conjoined deep external sphincter and puborectalis). f,g, Intermediate and base loops of external sphincter. h, Internal sphincter (hindgut circular muscle coat). i, Hindgut longitudinal muscle attachment to perineal skin. j, Hindgut membrane (rectal membrane). k, Anorectal sinus. l, Pectinate line. m, Paraanal space. n, Obliterated anorectal sinus. o, Skin lining hindgut. (Modified from Shafik A. A new concept of the anatomy of the anal sphincter mechanism and the physiology of defecation. X. Anorectal sinus and band: anatomic nature and surgical significance. Dis Colon Rectum 1980;23:170; with permission.)

an embryologic result of this process, proctodeum-hindgut intussusception achieves both rupture of the rectal membrane (Fig. 18-79E) to open the hindgut to the exterior, and fusion of the lining of the endodermal hindgut with the perineal ectoderm within the lower end of the hindgut at the pectinate line.

## Vascular Supply

The hindgut artery is the inferior mesenteric artery. Its continuation, beyond the last sigmoid branch, is the superior rectal artery which normally accompanies the hindgut to its termination at the perineal skin. In postnatal life, however, the artery normally ends approximately at the pectinate line – probably because invagination of the hindgut by the proctodeum involves its lower part during the obliteration of the anorectal sinus. The hindgut below this level acquires blood supply from the inferior rectal branch of the internal pudendal artery.

## Rectal Neck

The rectum is the terminal part of the hindgut, between the third sacral vertebra and the perineal skin. Its lower segment, which can be termed "rectal neck" (Fig. 18-80) due to the narrowing imposed on it by the surrounding sphincters, extends downward from the level of the levator plate to the perineal skin, whereas the part above is the "rectum proper." The rectal neck therefore represents that portion of the bowel usually referred to as the "anal canal."[282] The only role the proctodeum has in the rectal neck is as the lining of its terminal end, which develops in

the course of fusion of the hindgut mucosa with the perineal skin, as described above.

This simulates the case of the gastric columnar mucosa: although it normally extends upward into the distal 3 cm of the esophagus to fuse with its squamous epithelium,[284] this columnar-lined esophageal segment is neither considered a separate entity of the esophagus nor given a separate name. The junction of the rectum proper with its neck is the "rectal neck inlet" (Fig. 18-80), whereas the rectal neck opening to the exterior is the "rectal neck outlet." The skin lining the lower rectal neck is the "intrarectal skin," while the skin surrounding the rectal neck outlet is the "perirectal skin".

## Structural-Functional Adaptation of the Rectal Neck

The rectal neck has undergone certain anatomic changes in adaptation to its function as a regulator of the mechanisms of continence and defecation.[285] Thus, the presence of the rectal angle induced by the puborectalis sling and levator plate (Fig. 18-81), at the junction of the rectum proper with its neck, seems to play a role in rectal continence. The thickening of the rectal circular muscle coat around the rectal neck to form the internal sphincter keeps the rectal neck closed involuntarily. Also the longitudinal muscle attachments to the perineal skin, after penetrating the base loop, are of functional significance: they fix the rectum to the perineal skin in such a way that the longitudinal muscle, on contraction at stool, not only shortens and opens up the rectal neck, but also stretches open and pulls up the base loop to unseal the rectal neck outlet.[105,281] The intrarectal skin lining is functionally important in that the rich somatic ectodermal innervation supplies the lower

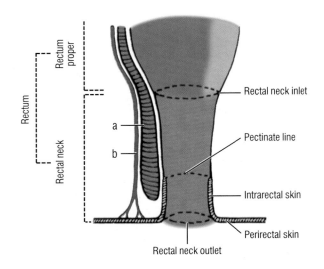

**FIG. 18-80.** The new anatomic features of the rectum. a, Internal rectal sphincter. b, Longitudinal rectal muscle. (Courtesy of Prof. Ahmed Shafik, MD.)

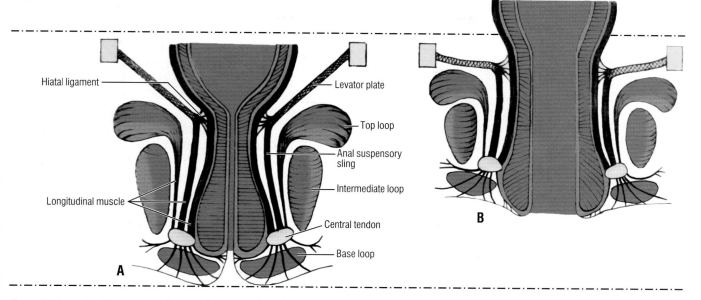

FIG. 18-81. Defecation mechanism. **A,** At rest. **B,** At defecation. Observe opening of both rectal neck inlet and outlet as well as opening and shortening of rectal neck. (Modified from Shafik A. A new concept of the anatomy of the anal sphincter mechanism and the physiology of defecation. V. The rectal neck: Anatomy and function. Chir Gastroenterol 1977;11:319; with permission.)

rectal neck with sensitivity to stimuli, and thus constitutes an essential component in the mechanisms of continence and defecation.

Furthermore, the rectal neck sphincter apparatus is arranged to keep each involuntary muscle under the control of a voluntary one.[163] Hence, the external sphincter voluntarily opposes the involuntary action both of the internal sphincter and the longitudinal muscle. In order to resist the desire to pass stool or flatus, external sphincter contraction inhibits the reflex internal sphincter relaxation on detrusor contraction; this is called the "voluntary inhibition reflex" action.[163] At the same time, base loop contraction stretches tight, and inhibits contraction of, the longitudinal muscle which passes through the base loop substance.[163] More information on this subject follows under "Mechanism of Continence."

# Congenital Rectal Anomalies

## *A New Concept of Genesis*

The conclusion that the hindgut migrates to the perineal skin, guided by the levator tunnel, to be invaginated and perforated by the proctodeal dimple could explain the different congenital rectal anomalies.[283,285] The rectum may develop completely, enter the levator tunnel and reach the perineal skin, but not be invaginated by the proctodeum (Fig. 18-

82A, B); or it may be invaginated without rupture of the rectal membrane (Fig. 18-82C, D). In both conditions, the end of the hindgut may remain blind or result in a fistula in the perineum or genitourinary tract (Fig. 18-82B, D). Failure of rectal neck remodeling could result in rectal neck stenosis (Fig. 18-82E). The hindgut might fail to enter the levator tunnel because of delayed formation of, or poor development of, the levator tunnel and hence not be guided to its normal location in the perineum. In such cases then, the end of the hindgut lies above the levator tunnel and either remains blind (Fig. 18-82F) or seeks a way to the exterior by development of a fistular connection to the genitourinary tract (Fig. 18-82G).

## *Anorectal Sinus and Band*

The proctodeal dimple, by invaginating the lower end of the hindgut (Fig. 18-79A, B) as it approaches the perineal skin, pushes up and tightly stretches the rectal membrane which separates the hindgut from the proctodeum; meanwhile it enfolds the lower end of the hindgut mucosa[285] (Fig. 18-79C, D). Invagination continues until the rectal membrane ultimately ruptures, leaving the anal valves to mark its site (Fig. 18-79E, F).

Two spaces result from proctodeal "invagination" of the hindgut: (1) an outer space which can be termed the "anorectal sinus," and (2) an inner space which can be

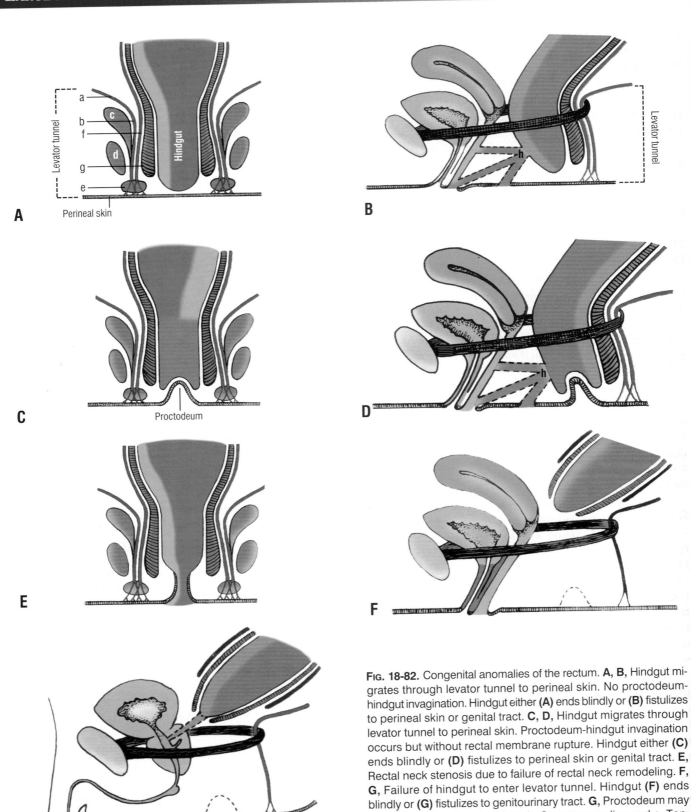

**FIG. 18-82.** Congenital anomalies of the rectum. **A, B,** Hindgut migrates through levator tunnel to perineal skin. No proctodeum-hindgut invagination. Hindgut either **(A)** ends blindly or **(B)** fistulizes to perineal skin or genital tract. **C, D,** Hindgut migrates through levator tunnel to perineal skin. Proctodeum-hindgut invagination occurs but without rectal membrane rupture. Hindgut either **(C)** ends blindly or **(D)** fistulizes to perineal skin or genital tract. **E,** Rectal neck stenosis due to failure of rectal neck remodeling. **F, G,** Failure of hindgut to enter levator tunnel. Hindgut **(F)** ends blindly or **(G)** fistulizes to genitourinary tract. **G,** Proctodeum may dimple or not. a, Levator plate. b, Suspensory sling. c,d,e, Top, intermediate, and base loops of external sphincter. f, Longitudinal rectal muscle. g, Internal rectal sphincter. h, Fistula. (Courtesy of Prof. Ahmed Shafik, MD.)

called the "paraanal space"[283,285] (Fig. 18-79E). The anorectal sinus represents the enfolded part of the hindgut mucosa and seems to include the structures which investigators refer to as the anal glands.

### Histopathology of the Anorectal Sinus and Band and Epithelial Debris

The anorectal sinus (Fig. 18-83) is a diverticulum-like process which extends downward to a variable extent in the lower rectal neck submucosa from the level of the anal valves.[285] The sinus may be deep and narrow and extend along the internal sphincter, or it may be small and shallow. Deep sinuses are commonly found in deceased neonates and children, and are complete circumferentially around the lower rectal neck.[285] In adult specimens the anorectal sinus is shallow and divided longitudinally into 4 to 9 compartments. It is lined by columnar epithelium in some areas, and stratified columnar in others.

The anorectal band (Fig. 18-84) is a fibroepithelial tube which lies in the submucosa of the rectal neck below the anal valves.[285] Histologically, it consists of collagen fibers impregnated with islands of epithelial cells. Clumps of epithelial cells found scattered in the lower rectal neck submucosa constitute epithelial debris[285] (Fig. 18-85). These clumps are composed of round, oval, or columnar cells and are arranged in masses, sheets, or in the form of pseudoacini. The cells have been found to occur at the site of the absent anorectal sinus, and probably represent remnants of the sinus.

### Fate and Anomalies of the Anorectal Sinus

Normally the anorectal sinus is obliterated. The process of obliteration simply represents the completion of the embryonic fusion of the proctodeum with the hindgut. Sinus obliteration leads to the formation of the anorectal band (Fig. 18-79F) which normally disappears.[285] This is followed by rectal neck remodeling in such a way that the proctodeal wall recedes laterally to come into alignment with the rectal wall, with the obliteration of the paraanal space and widening of the lower rectal neck (Fig. 18-79G).

The sinus has been found divided into 4 to 9 compartments, however, indicating irregularity in the process of closure.[285] This is consistent with Shafik's findings that the anorectal sinus may persist or be only partially obliterated and form epithelium-lined structures in the submucosa of the lower rectal neck. On the other hand, obliteration of the sinus may be complete, yet leave the anorectal band or epithelial debris that marks the position of the anorectal sinus[285] (Fig. 18-79F). Failure of rectal neck remodeling, with persistence of the paraanal space, results in narrowing of the lower rectal neck (Fig. 18-79E).

### *Role of the Anorectal Sinus, Anorectal Band, and Epithelial Debris in the Genesis of Rectal Pathology*

Persistence of the anorectal sinus or its epithelial elements, as represented in the anorectal band or epithelial debris, could explain the pathogenesis of some idiopathic rectal neck lesions such as perirectal abscess and fistula, chronic fissure, pruritus ani, hemorrhoids, cysts, and rectal neck adenocarcinoma.[285]

### *Perirectal Suppurations and Fistulas*

A study of the pathology of perirectal fistula[286,287] revealed a significantly higher rectal neck pressure (128 cm

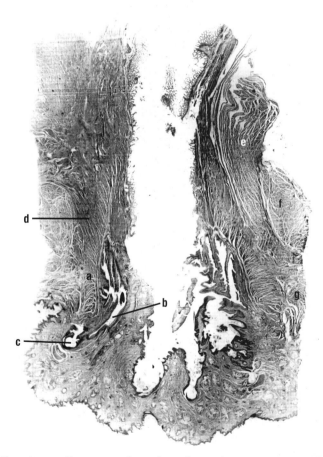

**FIG. 18-83.** Paracoronal section of rectal neck showing an anorectal sinus extending down to the central space (hematoxylin and eosin; magnification × 8). a, Internal sphincter. b, Anorectal sinus extending down to (c) central space. d, Longitudinal muscles. e, f, g, Top, intermediate, and base loops of external sphincter. (Courtesy of Prof. Ahmed Shafik, MD.)

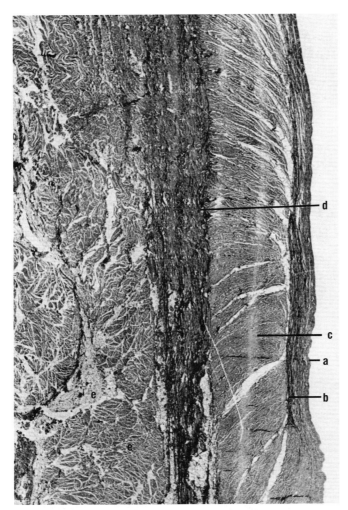

FIG. 18-84. Coronal section of rectal neck showing anorectal band in anal submucosa (Verhoeff-van Gieson; magnification × 27). a, Anal lining. b, Anorectal band. c, Internal sphincter. d, Longitudinal muscle. e, External sphincter. (Courtesy of Prof. Ahmed Shafik, MD.)

H$_2$O) than normal (78 cm H$_2$O). Epithelial cells were detected in the vicinity of the fistular track in 90% of the cases studied. These cells were arranged in acini or masses (Fig. 18-86). Multiple intraepithelial microabscesses were detected in these masses. Presumably, these epithelial cells are but the epithelial debris of the anorectal sinus. Chronic perirectal suppuration is believed to be due to the epithelial debris which maintains the infective process.[287] The cure of perirectal suppuration of a nonchronic form would be related to absence of epithelial debris, or its destruction in the course of infection. The cause of fistular recurrence following properly performed operations could be due to the infection of other islands of epithelial debris.[287] The rectal neck pressure becomes normal after correction of the fistula.

## Perianal Spaces and Anorectal Suppuration

Studies by Shafik[101] have identified 6 perianal spaces: subcutaneous, central, intersphincteric, ischiorectal (ischioanal), submucosal, and pelvirectal (Fig. 18-87). Infection was found to start as a central abscess in the central space, which, if neglected, spread to the above mentioned spaces, and led to central, intersphincteric, ischiorectal, and pelvirectal abscess and fistula formation[286] (Fig. 18-88).

Fistula cauterization was performed with a cautery probe. By destroying the epithelial debris, this treatment alternative achieves satisfactory results.[288]

## Role of the Anorectal Sinus in Chronic Anal Fissure

Assessment of pathologic changes in chronic fissure[289] resulted in identification of epithelial cells in the

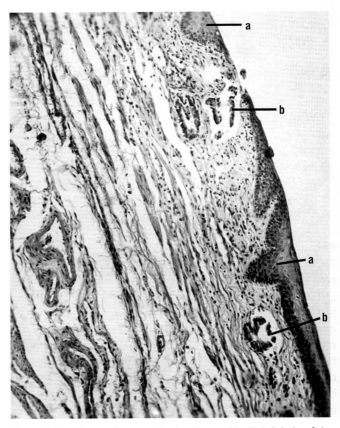

FIG. 18-85. Photomicrograph showing epithelial debris of the anorectal sinus in the anal submucosa (hematoxylin and eosin; magnification × 110). a, Anal lining. b, Epithelial debris. (Courtesy of Prof. Ahmed Shafik, MD.)

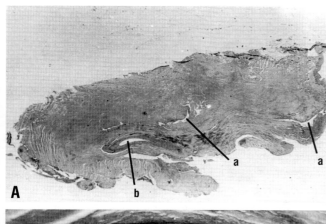

A

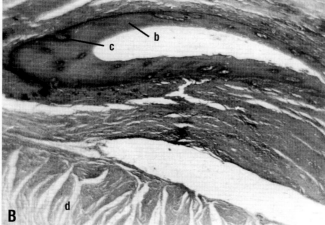

B

**FIG. 18-86.** Photomicrograph showing epithelial debris in the vicinity of the fistulous track. The cells are arranged in masses lined by hyperplastic nonkeratinized stratified squamous epithelium which contains multiple microabscesses (hematoxylin and eosin). **A,** Magnification × 5. **B,** Magnification × 60. a, Fistulous track. b, Squamous epithelial mass. c, Microabscess. d, Rectal muscle bundles. (Courtesy of Prof. Ahmed Shafik, MD.)

Epithelial cells act as multiple sites (sequestra) for harboring the infection and are responsible for fissure chronicity. Where epithelial debris could not be detected in the fissure, the death of the epithelial cells over the course of infection was assumed –which would explain the spontaneous cure of some fissures.[289]

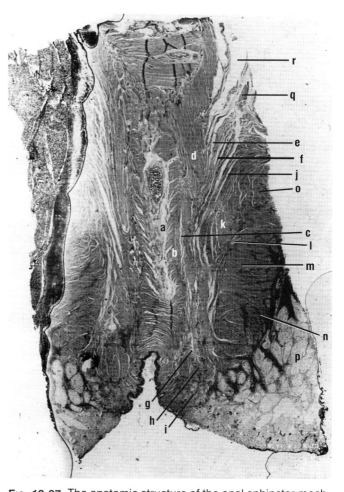

**FIG. 18-87.** The anatomic structure of the anal sphincter mechanism and the perianal spaces. Paracoronal section of rectal neck (hematoxylin and eosin; magnification × 19). a, Submucous space. b, Internal sphincter. c, e, j, l, Intersphincteric space. d, Medial layer of longitudinal muscle. f, Intermediate layer of longitudinal muscle, anal suspensory sling. g, Central space and central tendon. h, Base loop of external sphincter. i, Subcutaneous space containing corrugator cutis. k, Lateral layer of longitudinal muscle. m, Intermediate loop of external sphincter. n, External anal septum. o, Top loop of external sphincter. p, Ischiorectal (ischioanal) space. q, Levator plate. r, Pelvirectal space. (From Shafik A. A new concept of the anatomy of the anal sphincter mechanism and the physiology of defecation. IV. Anatomy of perineal spaces. Invest Urol 1976;13:424; with permission.)

floor of the fissure, superficial to the internal sphincter. The cells were round, oval, or columnar, and were arranged in clumps or in the form of pseudoacini (Fig. 18-89). It is believed that these epithelial cells are just anorectal sinus remnants that exist in the rectal neck submucosa either as epithelial debris or an anorectal band.[289] In a few cases, the anorectal sinus was detected in the floor of the fissure (Fig. 18-90), whereas in others no epithelial cells could be found, as occurs in heavily infected fissures. The mean maximal rectal neck pressure was significantly above normal (124 cm H_2O).

The mechanism of fissure formation (Fig. 18-91) includes disruption of the lower rectal neck lining and the resulting exposure of the epithelial cells or the anorectal sinus to repeated infection in the floor of the wound.[289]

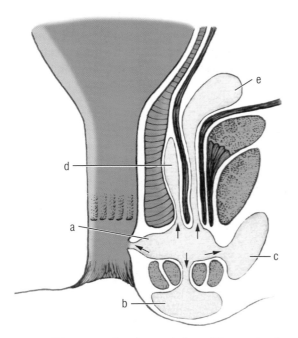

**FIG. 18-88.** Diagrammatic representation of the mode of spread of central space infection and the resultant anorectal abscess. a, Central abscess. b, Subcutaneous abscess. c, Ischiorectal (ischioanal) abscess. d, Intersphincteric abscess. e, Pelvirectal abscess. (Courtesy of Prof. Ahmed Shafik, MD.)

The presence of high pressure in the rectal neck predisposes it to trauma by feces, due to the partial stenosis of the rectal neck. The stenosis can be induced either by the constricting effect of the anorectal band or failure of rectal neck remodeling.[285,289] Evidence of partial stenosis is provided both by the significant high rectal neck pressure and the necessity of straining at stool, even with soft and bulky stools. The location of the fissure exclusively in the lower, and not in the upper rectal neck, is due to the anorectal sinus remnants contained therein; whereas, on the other hand, the posterior and (rarely seen) anterior median fissure is ascribed to the existence of 2 weak areas opposite the intermediate and base loop ellipses of the external sphincter[289] (Fig. 18-92). Tears are more frequent posteriorly because the posterior rectal neck wall is less supported than the anterior wall.

Treatment of chronic fissure is directed at ablation of epithelial debris in the fissure. Both internal sphincterotomy and anal dilatation aim at sectioning the rigid, fibrous, tube-shaped anorectal band ("anorectal bandotomy"),[290] and provide the expansion of the rectal neck on defecation that prevents the repeated trauma from fecal material. These procedures do not eradicate the epithelial remnants in the fissure floor, however; fissure excision does remove these remnants.[289]

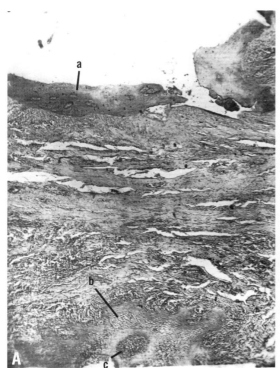

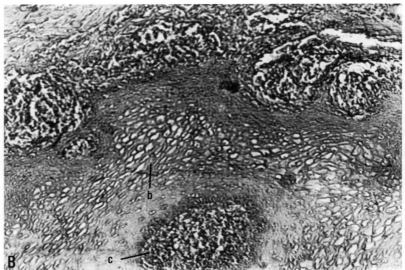

**FIG. 18-89.** Photomicrographs showing the epithelial debris in the floor of a chronic anal fissure. (Hematoxylin-eosin stain). **A,** Magnification × 40. **B,** Magnification × 150, reduced 17 percent. a, Squamous epithelium at the edge of the fissure. b, Epithelial cells. c, Inflammatory cells. (Courtesy of Prof. Ahmed Shafik, MD.)

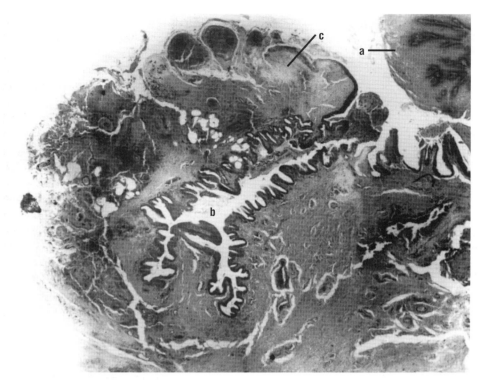

**FIG. 18-90.** Chronic anal fissure showing an anorectal sinus at its floor. a, Squamous epithelium. b, Anorectal sinus. c, Granulations of the fissure. (Hematoxylin-eosin stain; magnification × 18.5, reduced 13 percent). (Courtesy of Prof. Ahmed Shafik, MD.)

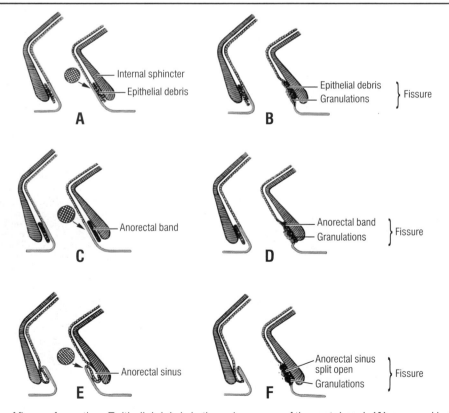

**FIG. 18-91.** Mechanism of fissure formation. Epithelial debris in the submucosa of the rectal neck **(A)** exposed in the wound floor due to anal lining disruption **(B)**. Anorectal band in the submucosa of the rectal neck **(C)** exposed in the wound floor due to anal lining traumatization **(D)**. Anorectal sinus in the submucosa of the rectal neck **(E)** exposed in the wound floor due to anal lining traumatization **(F)**. (Courtesy of Prof. Ahmed Shafik, MD.)

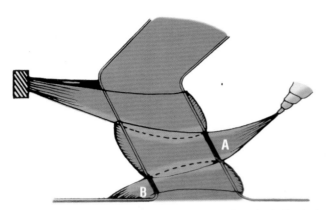

FIG. 18-92. The two weak areas in the rectal neck. A, Posterior area corresponds to the intermediate loop ellipse. B, Anterior area corresponds to the base loop ellipse. (Courtesy of Prof. Ahmed Shafik, MD.)

### Role of the Anorectal Sinus in Hemorrhoids

In the presence of hemorrhoids, the mean rectal neck pressure is significantly higher than normal, 118 cm $H_2O$ ± 24 (s) versus 76 cm $H_2O$ ± 18 (s).[290] There is, however, no significant difference in the rectal neck pressures between large and small hemorrhoids. Fibrous bands (Fig. 18-93) were detected in the lower rectal neck submucosa of all studied hemorrhoid patients, but in only 1 of the control subjects.[290] The bands may extend from the bottom of an incompletely obliterated anorectal sinus. The hemorrhoid neck overhangs the top end of the fibrous band. Evidence suggests that this fibrous band is the anorectal band, an embryonic vestige.[290]

The invariable detection of fibrous bands (anorectal bands) with hemorrhoids postulates a relationship. High rectal neck pressure indicates a degree of stenosis which commonly accompanies the anorectal band.[285] The presence of the fibrous band and the accompanying stenosis of the lower rectal neck hinder full rectal neck expansion at defecation, with a resulting partial obstruction to the descending fecal mass (Fig. 18-94). An excessive straining effort is necessary to achieve dilatation sufficient for evacuation. This would explain the cause of straining, even with soft and bulky stools, which precedes and accompanies hemorrhoid formation. The fecal mass, passing through the stenosed lower rectal neck, repeatedly traumatizes the mucosa at the upper end of the anorectal band, which would slacken and ultimately prolapse[290] (Fig. 18-94).

The 25% incidence of hemorrhoids in our population above 45 years corresponds with the 20% incidence of persisting anorectal bands in a series of normal cadaveric

specimens.[285] This suggests an individual susceptibility to hemorrhoids related to the presence of the anorectal band. It appears that the constricting nature of the anorectal band not only leads to mucosal prolapse and hemorrhoid formation, but is also responsible for the higher fissure incidence in patients with hemorrhoids, in comparison to patients without hemorrhoids.[290] Moreover, the constricting effect of the anorectal band could explain the manifestations in the syndrome of "urethral discharge, constipation, and hemorrhoids."[291] In this syndrome, the hemorrhoid patient experiences urethral discharge only when he is constipated. The discharge results from the squeezing effect of the descending hard fecal mass on the prostate, seminal vesicles, and vasal ampullae which are compressed, consequent to lower rectal neck congestion induced by hemorrhoids. In these patients, the anorectal band seems not only to cause hemorrhoid formation, but also to augment the squeezing effect of the hard feces.[291]

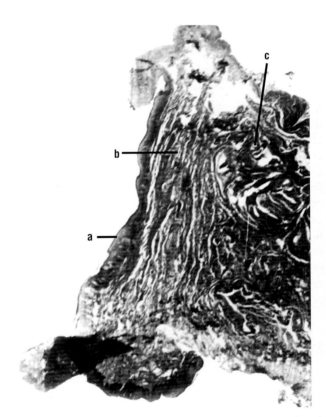

FIG. 18-93. Photomicrograph of biopsy from the lower rectal neck of hemorrhoid patient, showing a fibrous tissue band extending in the submucosa from the level of pectinate line downward. (Verhoeff-van Gieson stain, magnification × 13). a, Squamous epithelium. b, Fibrous band. c, Internal sphincter. (Courtesy of Prof. Ahmed Shafik, MD.)

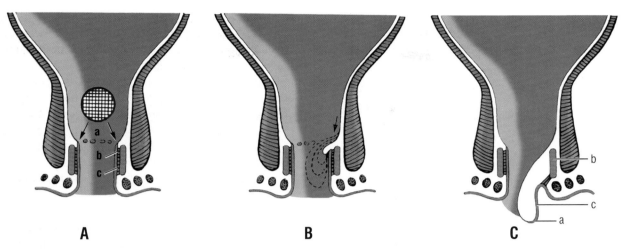

**A**                    **B**                    **C**

FIG. 18-94. Mechanism of hemorrhoid formation. **A,** Descending fecal mass partially obstructed at lower rectal neck with extra straining due to forcing of the fecal mass through the stenosed rectal neck with resultant mucosal slackening. **B,** Gradual mucosal prolapse. Prolapsing mucosa overhangs top end of anorectal band. *Arrow* points to loose mucosa, which glides to share in hemorrhoid formation. Pectinate line is in its place. **C,** Firm attachment of the cutaneous lining of the rectal neck (c) to the anorectal band (b) is loosened by the hemorrhoid mass. The cutaneous lining is dragged downward, displacing the pectinate line (a) outside the rectal neck orifice. a, Pectinate line. b, Anorectal band. c, Cutaneous lining of rectal neck. (**A, B,** Modified from Shafik A, Mohi-el-Din M. A new concept of the anatomy of the anal sphincter mechanism and the physiology of defaecation. XXII. The pathogenesis of hemorrhoids and their treatment by anorectal bandotomy. J Clin Gastroent 1984;6:129-137; with permission; **C,** Courtesy of Prof. Ahmed Shafik, MD.)

Shafik's studies have shown that hemorrhoids are a "disease" in which the rectal masses represent a "manifestation," but not the cause.[285,290] Both the high rectal neck pressure and hemorrhoid masses are attributable to lower rectal neck stenosis due to the constricting action of the anorectal band and the failure of rectal neck remodeling with a resulting mucosal prolapse and venous congestion.[290] In light of these findings, a new technique has been devised for treatment of hemorrhoids consisting of 2 main steps:[292] (1) anorectal bandotomy (Fig. 18-95) involving division of the anorectal band and (2) ligation of the hemorrhoid mass at its base (Fig. 18-96). The achieved results are satisfactory. Preoperative high rectal neck pressures normalized postoperatively.[292] The procedure is easy, and prevents the otherwise not infrequent recurrence by dealing directly with the primary etiologic factor.

### Role of the Anorectal Sinus in Pruritus Ani

The cause of pruritus ani was unknown in more than 50% of the cases until the detection of epithelial cells in the dermis of the lower rectal neck offered new possibilities regarding its etiology.[293] The cells were oval and arranged in sheets, showed acinar arrangements of columnar cells, or were arranged in sheets of squamous epithelium (Fig. 18-97). They were swollen and vacuolated, with the nucleus displaced and edematous. Lymphocytic aggregations

were found in close proximity to the ectopic epithelial cells. Occasionally the pruritic areas were found heavily infected, and epithelial debris could not be detected.

Epidermal hyperplasia, prickle cell hydrops, dermal edema, and lymphocytic aggregations, as well as absence of leucocytes, are changes which are characteristic of dermatitis due to "sterile" irritation. The irritant factor seems to exist locally, because pruritus affects no other parts of the body. The local sterile irritative changes are probably produced by the epithelial elements, which are believed to be anorectal sinus remnants.[293] These changes are initiated by the antigenic action of either the epithelial cells or their secretions, as evidenced by epidermal hydropic degeneration, as well as by edema and infiltration of the dermis with plasma cells and lymphocytes.[293] Where epithelial debris could not be identified it was assumed that it was destroyed by infection. Pruritus ani seems to be an "autoimmune reaction" resulting from cell antigenicity induced by buried "epithelial remnants" which probably originate in the anorectal sinus.

The treatment of pruritus ani aims at destruction of the epithelial debris in the submucosa of the lower rectal neck as the primary cause of pruritus ani. Injection of a 5% solution of phenol in almond oil into the submucosa of the lower rectal neck under short duration general anesthesia achieves a cure.[294] Relapse, if any, might be ascribed to incomplete epithelial debris destruction, as a result either of

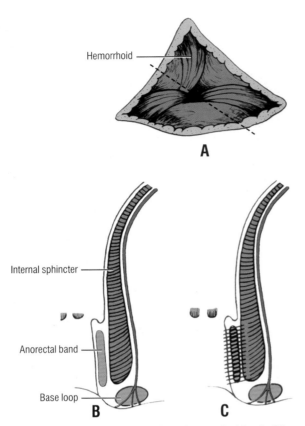

**FIG. 18-95.** Anorectal bandotomy of the hemorrhoids. **A,** Site. **B,** Anorectal band in lower rectal neck. **C,** Shaded area showing the extent of division. (Courtesy of Prof. Ahmed Shafik, MD.)

insufficient dosage or improper placement of the solution; it is easily cured with a second injection.

## SURGICAL ANATOMY AND PHYSIOLOGY

### Anatomy of Anal Sphincters and Pelvic Floor

#### *Smooth Musculature*

In the past our conventional textbooks described the anatomic concept of this area with the classical information: *The internal anal sphincter starts at the anorectal junction by thickening of the rectal circular muscle coat (Fig. 18-98). The sphincter is up to 5 mm thick. It has a rounded lower border which lies in the lowest part of the external anal sphincter. The sphincter consists of smooth muscle bundles which run obliquely at the proximal and distal ends of the muscle and horizontally in its middle part.*

*At the anorectal junction, the rectal longitudinal muscle coat fuses with inferiorly directed fibers of the pubococcygeus to form a conjoined longitudinal muscle layer (Fig. 18-98). Strands from this muscle layer penetrate the internal anal sphincter and the lower part of the external anal sphincter; some fibers reach the ischiorectal (ischioanal) fossa, the perianal skin and the mucous membrane of the intersphincteric groove. Puckering of the perianal skin was ascribed to some of these fibroelastic strands, while other investigators attributed it to the corrugator cutis ani muscle which is considered part of the panniculus carnosus.*

This picture differed after Shafik's studies[105,282] revealed that the longitudinal anal muscle consists of 3 layers: medial, intermediate, and lateral (see Figs. 18-76, 18-81, 18-87), each having a different origin and being separated from the other by a fascial septum. The medial layer is a continu-

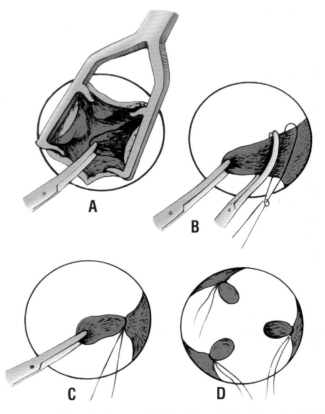

**FIG. 18-96.** Steps in hemorrhoid ligation. **A,** Tip of hemorrhoid mass is seized in an artery forceps. **B,** Curved forceps applied to hemorrhoid pedicle and a ligature placed proximal to it. **C** and **D,** Ligatures are tied. (Courtesy of Prof. Ahmed Shafik, MD.)

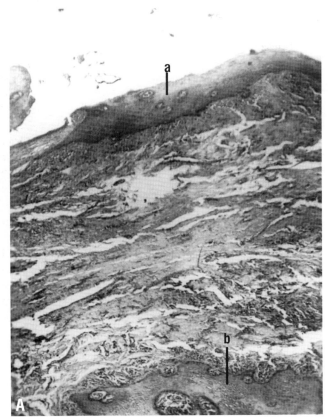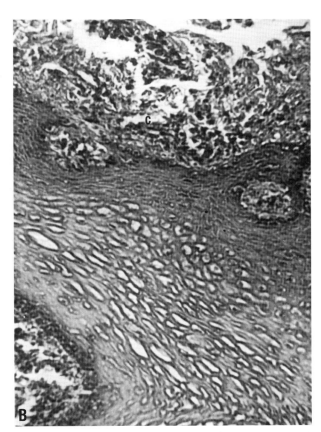

**FIG. 18-97.** Photomicrographs showing epithelial debris in the deep dermis of rectal neck of pruritus ani. The cells, arranged in sheets, are oval, swollen and vacuolated with the nucleus pushed aside. Lymphocytic aggregations are in the neighborhood of the epithelial debris. Haematoxylin and eosin. **A,** Magnification × 50. **B,** Magnification × 220. a, Epidermis. b, Epithelial cells. c, Lymphocytic aggregations. (Courtesy of Prof. Ahmed Shafik, MD.)

ation of the longitudinal rectal muscle coat, and the intermediate layer represents the downward prolongation of the levator plate, whereas the lateral muscle is the longitudinal extension of the top loop. The longitudinal muscle ends at the level of the lower border of the internal sphincter by a fibrous condensation called the central tendon (Figs. 18-76, 18-87). The tendon splits into multiple small fibrous septa which include a medial and a lateral septum as well as intermediate septa (see Fig. 18-81). The intermediate septa penetrate the base loop of the external anal sphincter, then they split and decussate to form the corrugator cutis ani which inserts into the perianal skin. The medial septum proceeds medially to attach to the anal lining between the internal sphincter and base loop of the external sphincter. The lateral septum passes laterally into the ischiorectal fossa.

## *Striated Musculature*

*Classically, the external anal sphincter has been de-*

*scribed as having deep, superficial, and subcutaneous parts. The deep part consists of circular fibers. The superficial part is elliptical, being attached to the tip of the coccyx posteriorly and to the perineal body anteriorly. The subcutaneous part is a circular ring of fibers.*

This description did not comply with the findings of Shafik's anatomic investigations,[163,282] which could demonstrate that the external anal sphincter is a triple loop system (Figs. 18-76, 18-92). The top loop consists of the deep portion of the external anal sphincter fused with the puborectalis muscle. It sends a downward prolongation which shares in the formation of the longitudinal muscle (Figs. 18-76, 18-92). The top loop forms a U-shaped ribbon around the upper rectal neck and is attached to the symphysis pubis. The intermediate loop is attached to the coccyx, and the base loop to the perianal skin anteriorly. Each of the 3 loops is enclosed in a separate fascial compartment (Fig. 18-76).

*The levator ani has been defined as consisting of ilio-*

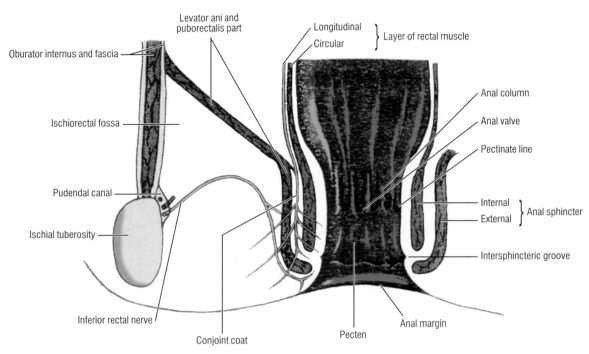

**FIG. 18-98.** The anorectal musculature. (Courtesy of Prof. Ahmed Shafik, MD.)

coccygeus, pubococcygeus, and puborectalis; their fibers are in continuity from the ischial spine to the body of the pubis, across the white line of the obturator fascia. The iliococcygeus portion arises from the posterior half of the white line and the ischial spine and inserts into the coccyx and the anococcygeal raphe. The pubococcygeus arises from the anterior half of the white line and the body of pubis and is inserted into the coccyx and anococcygeal raphe. The puborectalis is attached anteriorly to the pubic body, passes backwards around the anorectal junction and meets with fibers of the opposite side to form a U-shaped sling.

Shafik's studies[282] have confirmed that the levator ani consists of the pubococcygeus and iliococcygeus, but have revealed that the puborectalis belongs to the external anal sphincter, not to the levator ani:[282] the puborectalis fuses with the deep external anal sphincter to form the top loop of the external anal sphincter. The pubococcygeus is funnel-shaped (Fig. 18-76); it consists of a transverse and a vertical portion.[282] The transverse portion on both sides forms a platelike structure called the levator plate (Figs. 18-76, 18-77). At the anorectal junction, the levator plate bends sharply downwards to form the vertical portion called the anal suspensory sling.[282] The latter constitutes the middle layer of the longitudinal anal muscle. The levator plate is connected to the anorectal junction by a fibrous condensation called the hiatal ligament.

## Mechanism of Continence

A great deal of controversy has arisen as to the relative importance of the external and internal anal sphincters in the mechanism of anal continence. Thus, Goodsall[295] and Allingham[296] believed that the internal sphincter is a more important muscle than the external one, whereas Tuttle[297] and Lockhart-Mummery[298] claimed the reverse. This conflict was the result of inaccurate anatomic information gained at that time.[299] Milligan and Morgan's account[300] contributed somewhat to the clarity of the anatomy of the anal musculature.

Anal continence is a joint function of the external and internal anal sphincters; the former is responsible for voluntary continence, whereas the latter maintains involuntary continence.[142] Contrary to the views of investigators holding that the levator ani has a sphincteric action on the anorectal junction,[299,300] it acts as the rectal neck dilator.[301] Functioning mainly during defecation, the levator ani plays no role in anal continence. On contraction, the levator plate is elevated and retracted laterally, pulling the hiatal ligament which opens the rectal neck inlet[301] (Fig. 18-81). Furthermore, contraction of the anal suspensory sling of the levator muscle opens up and shortens the rectal neck.

The part played by the longitudinal muscle in anal

continence is minimal. The corrugations formed by the corrugator cutis, which result from the insertion of the longitudinal muscle into the perianal skin, help the base loop of the external anal sphincter induce an airtight anal occlusion.[105] The muscle's major role occurs during defecation. Its contraction results in shortening and opening of the rectal neck[105] (Fig. 18-81). Furthermore, it fixes the rectal neck during fecal descent to prevent anal prolapse.

The internal anal sphincter is responsible for involuntary continence. Being unstriated, it maintains continence for long periods. However, it cannot resist a call to stool or flatus; that is, it cannot maintain voluntary continence, because it is reflexively relaxed when the rectal detrusor contracts on entrance of stools or flatus. There is a reciprocal action between the detrusor and the internal sphincter: when one contracts, the other relaxes reflexively.[142,302] Accordingly, it is the reflex action that makes the internal sphincter relax and prevents it from opposing defecation. This is shown clinically by the fact that a patient with rectal inertia is continent, despite the rectum being full of stool and the external sphincter being relaxed. The explanation for this could well be that no reflex internal sphincter relaxation occurs, because the detrusor contraction is lost by inertia. Continence in such cases is maintained by the internal sphincter.

The external anal sphincter is responsible for voluntary continence. It contracts to resist a call to stool, or to interrupt or terminate the act of defecation.[163] It seems that the muscle induces continence by a double action:[163] (1) prevention of internal sphincter relaxation on detrusor contraction –an action effected by what Shafik refers to as the "voluntary inhibition reflex"– and (2) direct compression of the rectal neck, or the "mechanical action."

## *Voluntary Inhibition Reflex*

As stool enters the rectum, the detrusor contracts and the internal sphincter reflexively relaxes to unseal the rectal neck (Fig. 18-99). However, the neck does not open unless the external sphincter has voluntarily relaxed. If there is no desire to defecate, the external sphincter contracts, thereby mechanically preventing relaxation of the internal sphincter (Fig. 18-100). Failure of the internal sphincter to relax reflexively inhibits contraction of the detrusor which relaxes and dilates to accommodate the new contents.[163] Commonly the individual, while opposing defecation, senses the sudden detrusor relaxation which occurs due to failure of the internal sphincter to relax (a characteristic sensation, especially if the rectum contains gases); this is followed by loss of the desire to defecate.

Voluntary external sphincter contraction to prevent reflex internal sphincter relaxation, with subsequent inhibition of detrusor contraction, is what could be called "voluntary inhibition reflex."[163] The latter seems to be the main action responsible for voluntary continence; it leads to immediate detrusor relaxation and loss of the desire to defecate. For this reason, internal sphincter integrity is necessary not only for involuntary, but also for voluntary continence since the action of the voluntary inhibition reflex is mediated through it. Voluntary inhibition is further potentiated by the base loop contraction acting on the longitudinal muscle.[163] Thus, on external sphincter contraction, the base loop glides medially, stretching the longitudinal muscle tight by pulling on the fibrous prolongations penetrating the base loop substance. The tightened longitudinal muscle limits internal sphincter relaxation and thus augments the voluntary inhibition action.

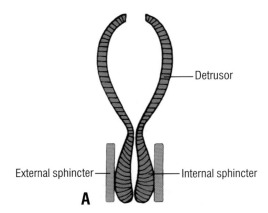 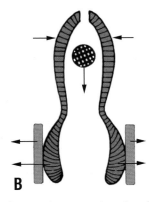

**Fig. 18-99.** External and internal sphincters at rest and during defecation. **A,** At rest: detrusor relaxed and internal sphincter involuntarily contracted. **B,** During defecation: detrusor contracted and external and internal sphincters relaxed. (Courtesy of Prof. Ahmed Shafik, MD.)

## Voluntary Mechanical Action

In addition to its voluntary inhibition reflex action, external sphincter contraction firmly seals the rectal neck by mechanical compression.[163] Being striated, the external sphincter cannot contract for a long period to maintain continence mechanically. The mechanical compression action is thus brief, and serves to occlude the rectal neck by the time the detrusor relaxes as a result of the action of the voluntary inhibition reflex. If the detrusor does not relax, the external sphincter tires out and relaxes, and defecation should occur. Once the detrusor relaxes and the desire for defecation wanes, the external sphincter relaxes and continence is then maintained by the internal sphincter. However, after some time, the loaded detrusor recontracts; if the desire to defecate is still opposed, the external sphincter contracts again. This process is repeated until either defecation is acceded to or a prolonged contraction of the unstriated detrusor tires out the striated — and briefly contracting — external sphincter which involuntarily relaxes, leading to internal sphincter relaxation and opening of the rectal neck.[163]

## Stress Defecation

In conditions of internal sphincter damage and resulting loss of the voluntary inhibition reflex, voluntary continence is induced only by the mechanical action of the external sphincter. Being striated, the external sphincter cannot contract long enough to withstand the uninhibited prolonged contraction of the loaded detrusor. Thus, detrusor contraction continues despite external sphincter contraction until the latter sphincter fatigues and relaxes

and the detrusor forces evacuation[163] (Fig. 18-101). Accordingly, in cases of internal sphincter damage, once the desire to defecate is initiated, evacuation should occur. This condition, which is referred to as "stress defecation," is observed in patients after internal sphincterotomy for anal fissure.[163] This not only underscores the importance of the internal sphincter in the mechanism of voluntary continence, but could also offer an explanation for the impaired control of flatus and liquid feces which occurs after internal sphincterotomy, as reported by Bennett and Goligher.[303]

## Single Loop Continence Theory

The external sphincter consists of three loops (Fig. 18-102): top, intermediate, and base. Each has its own attachments, direction of muscle bundles, and innervation, which are separate and different from the others.[164] Each loop also has its own fascial investment (Fig. 18-103). The top loop is directed forward, with an upward inclination to be attached to the symphysis pubis and the adjoining pubic bone; it is innervated by the inferior rectal branch of the pudendal nerve. The intermediate loop proceeds horizontally backward to gain attachment to the coccyx, and is supplied by the perineal branch of the fourth sacral nerve. The base loop is directed forward and slightly downward, and is attached anteriorly to the perianal skin in, and close to the midline; it is innervated by the inferior rectal nerve.

As a result of the arrangement of these parts of the external sphincter, and also because of the fact that each loop has its own innervation, any single loop can function as a sphincter separately.[163] Accordingly, the external sphincter action in continence can be achieved by the con-

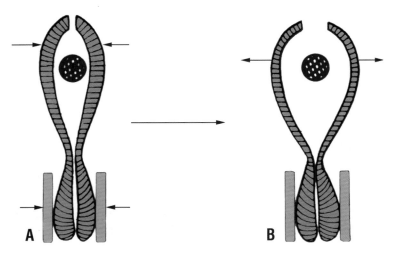

**FIG. 18-100.** Mechanism of voluntary inhibition reflex action to oppose a call to stool. **A,** Detrusor contraction with failure of internal sphincter relaxation due to voluntary external sphincter contraction. **B,** Reflex detrusor relaxation due to failure of internal sphincter relaxation (voluntary inhibition reflex action). (Courtesy of Prof. Ahmed Shafik, MD.)

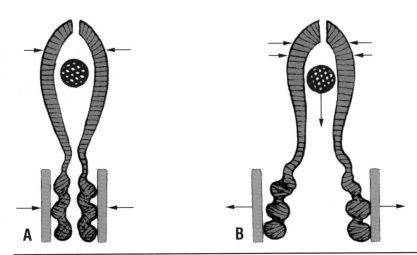

**FIG. 18-101.** Mechanism of stress defecation. **A,** Detrusor contraction with external sphincter contraction; internal sphincter is damaged. **B,** Detrusor continues contraction, uninhibited by the damaged internal sphincter; external sphincter fatigues, relaxes, and defecation occurs. (Courtesy of Prof. Ahmed Shafik, MD.)

traction of one singular element and not necessarily the three loops. This constitutes the basis of the "single loop continence" theory.[163] On contraction, a single loop induces continence by the action of the voluntary inhibition reflex and by mechanical occlusion. The latter action is significantly tight, as loop contraction is effected not only by direct compression but also by anal kinking.[164] The understanding of the "single loop continence" theory is of paramount surgical significance in planning for the treatment of anorectal abnormality, especially fistulas and incontinence. Thus, "unless all three of the loops are destroyed, continence can be maintained by any single loop."[163]

### Fallacy of the Anorectal Ring

The anorectal ring is the name given by Milligan and Morgan[300] to the muscular ring which encircles the anorectal junction, and is composed of the upper borders of the internal and external sphincters and puborectalis. It is claimed that this ring is responsible for anal continence and that its complete division results in incontinence.[299,300] In the light of recent studies, this ring represents only the upper border of the top loop of the external sphincter, and plays no specific role in the mechanism of anal continence in comparison to the intermediate and base loops.[164,301]

As has already been mentioned, anal continence is the result of the action of the voluntary inhibition reflex as well as of mechanical anal compression. These two actions could be achieved by any one of the three loops of the external sphincter, not necessarily the top, although the action of the top loop is most advantageous because of the natural kink at the rectal neck inlet which shares, although minimally, in the actual mechanism of anal continence.

The present view does not conflict with the opinion of other investigators[299,300] however, who hold that division of the anorectal ring in the treatment of high anal fistula leads to incontinence. The explanation could well be that in such

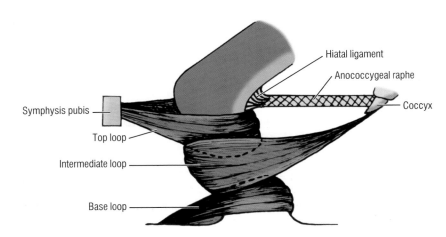

Symphysis pubis

Top loop

Intermediate loop

Base loop

Hiatal ligament

Anococcygeal raphe

Coccyx

**FIG. 18-102.** Triple loop system of external sphincter. (Modified from Shafik A. A new concept of the anatomy of the anal sphincter mechanism and the physiology of defecation. V. The rectal neck: Anatomy and function. Chir Gastroenterol 1977;11:319; with permission.)

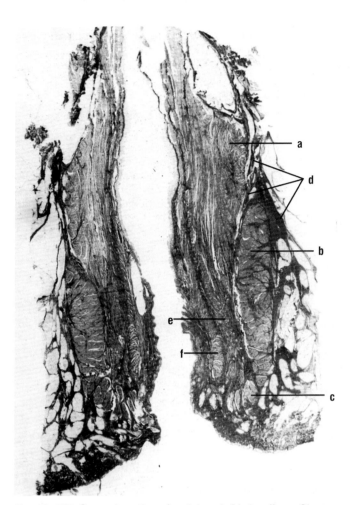

**FIG. 18-103.** Coronal section of rectal neck (Verhoeff-van Gieson; magnification × 6). Each of the three loops of the external sphincter has its own fascial covering. a, Top loop. b, Intermediate loop. c, Base loop. d, Fascial septa. e, Longitudinal muscle. f, Internal sphincter. (From Shafik A. A new concept of the anatomy of the anal sphincter mechanism and the physiology of defecation. I. The external anal sphincter. A triple-loop system. Invest Urol 1975;12:412-419; with permission.)

cases the intermediate and base loops have also been divided with the result that the integrity of all three of the loops has been destroyed, and incontinence is inevitable. Failure to realize this fact has led investigators to overestimate the role of the anorectal ring in anal continence. If one single loop, intermediate or base, could be spared in the treatment of high anal fistula, the patient will be continent in spite of division of the top loop.[163]

### Role of Internal Sphincter in Management of Anal Incontinence

The significant role of the internal sphincter in voluntary

continence should be considered in the repair of anal incontinence after traumatic damage of the external sphincter because frequently, in such cases, the internal sphincter is destroyed as well. A successful external sphincter repair should aim, however, at effecting not only mechanical occlusion but also voluntary inhibitory reflex action.[163] This necessitates repair of both the external and internal sphincters.

It seems that neglecting repair of the internal anal sphincter would explain the unsatisfactory operative results that are commonly obtained in such cases. In traumatic incontinence, the external and internal sphincters are commonly amalgamated at the injured site, in a mass of fibrous tissue. Internal sphincter injury would cause the rectal detrusor to lose its inhibitory component. Once the detrusor contracts, it immediately evacuates through the unguarded rectal neck. The operation practiced conventionally for repair of anal incontinence calls for suturing of the external sphincter;[304] whereas the internal sphincter is either ignored or included in the repair of the external sphincter. In both of these procedures the internal sphincter loses its voluntary inhibition reflex action as well as the ability to effect involuntary rectal neck closure.

A sound repair should free the internal sphincter from the external and suture each muscle separately. This allows the external sphincter to induce not only mechanical occlusion but also voluntary inhibition reflex action –mediated through the internal sphincter as described earlier.[163] Plastic operations for anal incontinence to supplement the external sphincter with muscle grafts or fascial slings[305] should also be planned to induce voluntary inhibition reflex action, rather than mechanical compression. Accordingly, the graft should be applied to surround the internal sphincter. Furthermore, in patients in whom tone of the anal sphincter is to be restored by electronic implants,[306] it is better to sew the electrodes to the internal sphincter than to the external. In the former, the voluntary inhibition reflex action is induced by direct stimulation and contraction of the internal sphincter.[163] This is more effective than applying the electrodes to the damaged external sphincter which lacks the efficient contraction to produce either mechanical compression or voluntary inhibition reflex action.

### Involuntary Action of the External Anal Sphincter

Studies of the histologic structure of the striated external anal sphincter following internal anal sphincter excision in dogs have revealed a distinct preponderance of smooth muscle fibers around the 10th postoperative month; this was confirmed by manometric and electromyographic experiments.[307,308] The increased nonstriated element in the external anal sphincter seems to be a structural-functional adaptation, meaning that the external anal sphincter, now a "compound muscle," takes on the otherwise lost involuntary function of the excised internal anal sphincter muscle.

## *Artificial Rectal Neck Pressure to Assist Anal Sphincteric Action*

In partial fecal incontinence when (for any of a variety of reasons) the rectal neck pressure has suffered a significant drop below normal, "filler"-injections into the anal submucosa produce an effect that can assist the diminished anal sphincteric activity by increasing, and eventually normalizing, the rectal neck pressure, thereby restoring fecal continence. There are two types of injections: perianal injection of polytetrafluoroethylene and perianal injection of autologous fat.

### Perianal Injection of Polytetrafluoroethylene

In the treatment of partial fecal incontinence,[309] the etiology of which may be idiopathic or following internal sphincterotomy, Teflon or polytef paste can be used. Five milliliters of polytef paste are injected, without anesthesia, into the rectal neck submucosa above the pectinate line, at both the 3 and 9 o'clock positions. Cure is usually achieved after the 1st injection or, in some cases, after repeat injections. Improvement is believed to be due to the increase in rectal neck pressure produced by the cushion effect of the polytef submucosal injection. The technique is simple, easy, and without complications. It is performed on an outpatient basis.[309]

### Perianal Injection of Autologous Fat

For the second type of injection, 50-60 ml of fat are harvested from the abdominal wall, thoroughly washed, and injected submucosally into the rectal neck at 3 and 9 o'clock positions.[310] The treatment is effective and achieves normalization of the pre-injection low rectal neck pressure. Occasional failures are due to insufficient washing of the fat or improper positioning of the needle; two to three repetitions of the injections achieves full fecal continence. The body fat is easily obtainable, biocompatible, and inexpensive. The technique is simple, easy, cost-effective, and performed on an outpatient basis.

## Mechanism of Defecation

The complexity of the mechanism of defecation seems to require a brief description before we look into the details of its anatomic, physiologic, and pathologic aspects. Then, having acquired a more profound understanding of the essential interrelations, we can probe the treatment modalities that have been developed.

The levator ani, which is the muscle of defecation,[282] is funnel-shaped, with a transverse part called the levator plate, and a vertical part called the suspensory sling[282] (see Fig. 18-76). The hiatal ligament connects the levator plate to the rectal neck.[301] The levator ani muscle is the rectal neck dilator. As a striated muscle, it contracts voluntarily at defecation to open the rectal neck to allow the stool to pass externally[311] (see Fig. 18-81). The puborectalis muscle is a U-shaped flat muscle that embraces the upper part of the rectal neck and acts as a constrictor muscle. It contracts to oppose, interrupt, or terminate the act of defecation.[282,301]

The concerted functions of the anorectal musculature at defecation are initiated and harmonized by voluntary impulses and reflex actions. When the rectal detrusor is distended with fecal mass and the stretch receptors are stimulated, the rectoanal-inhibitory reflex is initiated, and thus the rectal detrusor contracts and the internal sphincter relaxes. Detrusor contraction triggers two other reflexes: the rectopuborectalis reflex[312] and the rectolevator reflex.[313] Although acting simultaneously, these two reflexes have opposite functions: the rectolevator reflex effects a reflex levator contraction that opens the rectal neck, whereas at the same time, the puborectalis reflex actuates the reflex puborectalis contraction. Puborectalis contraction functions to seal the rectal neck, or keep it closed as impulses reach the conscious level to probe the circumstances for defecation. If time or circumstance is inopportune, the puborectalis continues voluntary contraction.

Voluntary puborectalis contraction evokes two reflex actions: the reflex levator relaxation through the levator-puborectalis reflex,[314] and the reflex detrusor relaxation by means of the voluntary inhibition reflex.[163] Furthermore, it aborts the rectoanal-inhibitory reflex which relaxes the internal sphincter. Hence, voluntary puborectalis contraction, through the voluntary inhibition reflex, prevents internal sphincter relaxation which results in reflex detrusor relaxation and waning of the urge to defecate (Fig. 18-100). However, as soon as the sensation of desire is felt, and circumstances are appropriate for defecation, the puborectalis muscle relaxes voluntarily and the detrusor evacuates its contents. This demonstrates that the act of defecation is under voluntary control despite the presence of reflex actions sharing the mechanism of defecation.

Thus, although the rectoanal-inhibitory and rectolevator reflexes function to open the rectal neck, the rectopuborectalis and the levator puborectalis reflexes keep the rectal neck closed until the decision for defecation has been taken. Straining at the start of defecation is a normal physiologic process and as such is part of the mechanism of defecation. By elevating the intraabdominal pressure, straining triggers the straining-levator reflex[315] which effects levator contraction and the opening of the rectal neck for spontaneous evacuation of the stools.

## Deflation Reflex: Role in Defecation

Contraction of the external anal sphincter on rectal "inflation" was reported in 1935 by Denny-Brown and Robertson[315] and was confirmed by other investigators.[316,317] Rectal inflation is accompanied by internal sphincter relaxation and momentary external sphincter contraction.[316,318,319] Shafik could demonstrate that the external sphincter contracts also upon rectal "deflation" through a reflex he calls "deflation reflex."[320]

The recto-anal inhibitory reflex comprises internal sphincter relaxation simultaneously with external sphincter contraction. It seems that the latter serves to close, momentarily, the rectal neck by the time the impulses reach the conscious decision whether to evacuate or not. If conditions are favorable, the external anal sphincter relaxes and defecation occurs. If the conditions are inopportune, external sphincter contraction continues preventing internal anal sphincter relaxation which leads to reflex rectal detrusor relaxation by means of the voluntary inhibition reflex.[163]

Reflex external anal sphincter contraction on rectal "deflation" is believed to play a role at defecation as well.[320] It functions to "interrupt" or "terminate" the act of defecation. Thus, at stool, the rectum contracts upon receiving fecal material from the sigmoid colon. The rectal neck opens and the rectal contents are delivered to the outside. Once the rectum is empty and becomes deflated, the external sphincter reflexively contracts.[320] To "interrupt" defecation, the base loop contraction of the external sphincter amputates the fecal column, expelling the lower portion. Following this, the rectal neck closes progressively upward by successive intermediate and top loop contractions, returning to the rectum any fecal material trapped in the rectal neck.[163] This process is repeated as long as the rectum receives fecal material from the sigmoid colon. At the end of defecation, reflex external sphincter contraction helps to "terminate" the act. The last fecal portion is pushed down the rectal neck to the outside by a process of "vermicular" contractions (Fig. 18-104) induced by the external sphincter triple loop system.[164]

### Voluntary Inhibition Reflex and the Deflation Reflex

The rectal detrusor and internal anal sphincter have a reciprocal action;[317,319] when one contracts, the other reflexively relaxes. Thus, at defecation, rectal detrusor contraction to evacuate its contents is associated with reflex internal sphincter relaxation and opening of the rectal neck. Detrusor contraction is involuntary and can be maintained for long periods without being exhausted. The internal sphincter is kept relaxed as long as the rectal detrusor remains contracted. However, at the end of detrusor contraction, the deflation reflex comes into action. Upon detrusor contraction and internal sphincter relaxation, and after the rectum is completely evacuated and deflated, the external anal sphincter reflexively contracts. External sphincter contraction impedes relaxation of the internal sphincter which leads to reflex detrusor relaxation.[163] Thus, the "deflation reflex" functions to terminate internal sphincter relaxation and detrusor contraction. Consequently, the detrusor relaxes to receive fresh fecal material or to terminate defecation.

### Role of the Deflation Reflex as a Diagnostic Tool

The deflation reflex may prove of diagnostic significance in defecation disorders. Detectable changes in latency and amplitude of the evoked response would indicate a defect in the reflex pathway such as a muscle or nerve damage from a disease of the spinal cord, spinal nerve roots, or peripheral nerves, or from a central lesion. The reflex may thus be incorporated as an investigative tool in the study of patients with anorectal disorders.

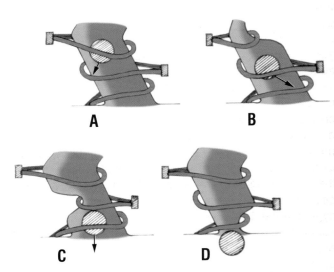

FIG. 18-104. Vermicular contractions of the external sphincter triple-loop. **A,** Fecal mass lies within the relaxed external sphincter. **B,** Top loop contraction and intermediate loop relaxation. **C,** Intermediate loop contraction and base loop relaxation. **D,** Base loop contraction. (Modified from Shafik A. A new concept of the anatomy of the anal sphincter mechanism and the physiology of defecation. 1. The external anal sphincter. A triple-loop system. Invest Urol 1975;12:412-419; with permission.)

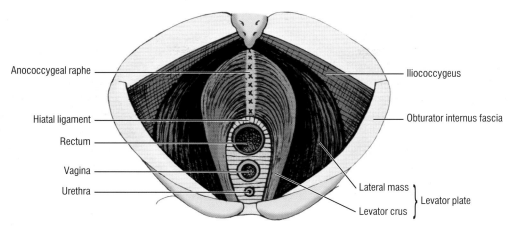

Fig. 18-105. Diagram illustrating the levator plate with its two lateral masses and two crura. (Courtesy of Prof. Ahmed Shafik, MD.)

## *Anatomic Components of the Mechanism of Defecation*

### Levator Plate

The levator plate muscle bundles are arranged into two main groups, each with its own attachments, direction, and function: a) the lateral bundles, which form the "lateral mass," and b) the medial bundles which form two "crura"[282] (Fig. 18-105).

The lateral mass is triangular in shape and arises with a wide base from the obturator internus fascia. The muscle bundles converge as they pass backward, with medial and downward inclination to be attached to the coccyx (Fig. 18-105). The lateral mass has a free lateral border separated from the iliococcygeus by a triangular gap.

The most medial fibers of the levator plate form two crura which bound the levator hiatus (Fig. 18-105). Each crus has its separate origin from the back of the lower part of the pubic body, about 2 cm above its lower border, and proceeds backward, with an upward inclination as a horizontal strip of fleshy bundles. In the midline posteriorly, the fleshy bundles of the two crura become tendinous and decussate in a crisscross pattern, forming the anococcygeal raphe. Laterally, each crus merges with the corresponding lateral mass. Medially, the inner borders of the two crura are connected to the intrahiatal structures along the hiatal ligament. The muscle bundles of the two crura are not directly attached to any of the pelvic viscera. Three patterns can be identified for the origin of the crura from the pubic body (Fig. 18-106): the classic pattern, crural overlap, and crural crossing.[282]

The classic pattern of origin of the levator crura (Fig. 18-106A) is the most common. The two crura arise from the body of the pubic bone almost side by side, without over-lap or crossing. The gap between the two crura at their origin is occupied by the puboprostatic or pubovesical ligaments.

In the crural overlap pattern (Figw. 18-106B, C), the proximal ends of the two crura overlap at their origin from the symphysis pubis. The crura may arise one above the other, or originate from a common tendinous origin at the back of the symphysis pubis and adjoining pubic bone, and then split into two slips.

In the crural "scissor" (crossing) (Fig. 18-106D), the right crus arises from the left pubic body and the left crus from the right one. They cross each other by overlapping one limb over the other or by interdigitation of the fibers from both limbs.

### Levator Tunnel

The intrahiatal structures, namely the rectal neck and the prostate in the male, and the rectal neck with vagina and urethra in the female, are ensheathed along their way down from the levator hiatus to the perineum in a muscular tube to which Shafik has applied the name "levator tunnel"[282] (Figs. 18-76, 18-77, 18-107, 18-108). The tunnel's posterior wall is longer than its anterior, due to the obliqueness of the levator plate. The length of the posterior wall in adults varies from 3 to 4 cm, and that of the anterior wall from 2.5 to 3 cm. The tunnel wall consists of two muscular coats of striated bundles (Figs. 18-76, 18-77, 18-109): an inner longitudinal coat formed by the suspensory sling, and an outer loop formed by the puborectalis.

The suspensory sling forms the inner coat of the levator tunnel. At the level of the levator hiatus, the levator plate bends sharply downward to form a vertical muscular cuff around the intrahiatal organs called the "suspensory sling"[301] (Figs. 18-76, 18-77, 18-107, 18-108). Detailed

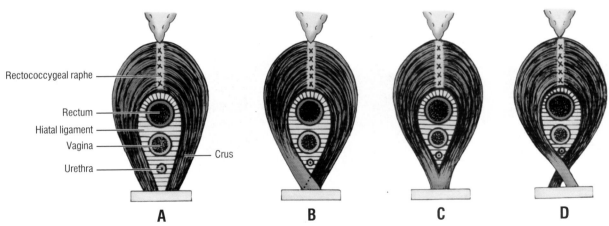

FIG. 18-106. Diagram illustrating crural patterns. **A,** Classic pattern. **B, C,** Crural overlap. **D,** Crural crossing. (Courtesy of Prof. Ahmed Shafik, MD.)

study of the latter sling has shown that it consists of longitudinally arranged striated muscle bundles impregnated with collagen. It is separated from the intrahiatal structures by a fascial septum which can be called the "tunnel septum."[282] From a descriptive viewpoint, the suspensory sling can be divided into two parts: anal and urethral.

The anal suspensory sling extends along the back and sides of the rectal neck. In the lower part, it fuses with the longitudinal muscle coat of the rectal neck, and then splits into multiple fibrous septa which penetrate the base loop of the external anal sphincter and insert into the perianal skin (see Fig. 18-76).

The urethral suspensory sling constitutes the anterior portion of the suspensory sling. It extends alongside the urethra and vagina in females, and the prostate in males. It ends by splitting into multiple septa which penetrate the substance of the external urethral sphincter. In females, it inserts in the skin around the external urethral meatus, whereas in males it merges with the intermuscular septa of the external urethral sphincter[282] (Fig. 18-107).

The outer loop of the tunnel wall consists of the puborectalis (Figs. 18-77, 18-109). As noted above, the muscle arises as a vertically oriented band by means of a tendinous attachment to the lower part of the symphysis pubis and adjoining pubic bone below the levator crural attachment. The aponeurotic origin gives rise to fleshy bundles, and the muscle proceeds backward with a downward inclination, underlying the inner border of the levator crura, and loops around the back of the rectal neck.[282] Behind the rectal neck, it becomes continuous with the corresponding muscle of the opposite side to form a U-shaped muscle, without intervention of the anococcygeal raphe.

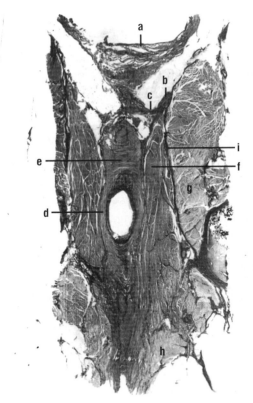

FIG. 18-107. Paracoronal section of vesical detrusor and neck in female cadaver (Verhoeff-Van Gieson stain, magnification × 5). a, Urinary bladder. b, Levator plate. c, Hiatal ligament. d, Longitudinal muscle. e, Internal sphincter. f, Suspensory sling. g, Puborectalis. h, External urethral sphincter. i, Tunnel septum. (From Shafik A. A new concept of the anatomy of the anal sphincter mechanism and the physiology of defecation. VIII. Levator hiatus and tunnel. Anatomy and function. Dis Colon Rectum 1979;22:539-549; with permission.)

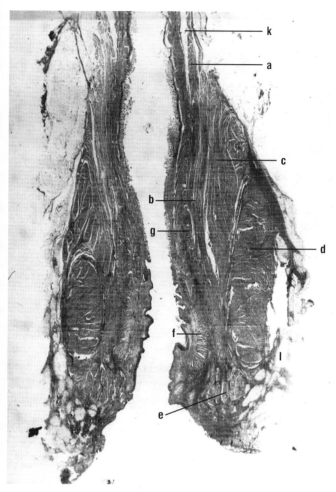

**FIG. 18-108.** Coronal section of the rectal neck shows the levator tunnel. a, Levator plate. b, Suspensory sling. c, Top loop (fused puborectalis and deep external anal sphincter). d, Intermediate loop of external anal sphincter. e, Base loop of external anal sphincter. f, Internal anal sphincter. g, Longitudinal anal muscle. k, Pelvirectal space. l, Ischiorectal (ischioanal) space (hematoxylin and eosin; magnification × 7). (From Shafik A. A new concept of the anatomy of the anal sphincter mechanism and the physiology of defecation. VIII. Levator hiatus and tunnel. Anatomy and function. Dis Colon Rectum 1979;22:539; with permission.)

In no part along its extent is the muscle attached to the levator plate.

As the puborectalis proceeds backward from its origin, it gives off muscle bundles to each intrahiatal organ forming the "individual" voluntary sphincters for these organs[282] (Fig. 18-109). In the male, the isolated puborectalis fibers surround the membranous urethra with a sheath of striated muscle bundles forming the external urethral sphincter (Figs. 18-110, 18-111). In the female, they give rise to the external urethral sphincter and, further back, provide the

vaginal tube with another muscular sheath, the vaginal sphincter. Posteriorly, the puborectalis, in both sexes, gives off loop fibers to embrace the rectal neck and to form the deep part of the external anal sphincter. However, the puborectalis and deep external anal sphincter were found fused together to such an extent that they could not be differentiated either morphologically or histologically; the conjoined muscle was termed "top loop."[169,301] The origin of the individual sphincters from the puborectalis muscle (PRM) could be demonstrated not only anatomically but also physiologically.

### Origin of External Anal, Urethral, Vaginal, and Prostatic Sphincters

An anatomic study[282] has demonstrated that the puborectalis muscle gives origin to the following sphincters: external anal (EAS), external urethral (EUS), prostatic (PS), and vaginal (VS). The response of EAS, EUS, PS, and VS to stimulation of the PRM was studied with the aim of physiologic validation of their anatomic origin from the PRM.[321] Twenty-eight healthy volunteers were examined (16 men, 12 women, mean age 40.6 ± 8.3 SD years).

The PRM was stimulated by a needle electrode. The response of the EAS and EUS was recorded by needle electrode, whereas the PS and VS were evaluated by manometric measuring of the urethral and vaginal pressures. Upon stimulation, the electromyogram (EMG) activity of the EAS and EUS increased, as did the prostatic urethral and vaginal pressures. There was no response to stimulation of the anesthetized PRM; this might indicate that the sphincters contract in response to PRM stimulation. The EMG recorded no latency, suggesting that the motor units of the EAS and EUS were simultaneously activated with those of the PRM and also that their muscle fibers seem to be directly derived from the PRM.

### Mass Contraction of the Pelvic Floor Muscles

The above-mentioned studies demonstrated both anatomically and physiologically that the EAS, EUS, PS, and VS and the bulbocavernosus muscle (BC) originate from the PRM. It is hypothesized that stimulation of any of these muscles would lead to contraction of all the others. Because the levator ani (pubococcygeus) muscle (LA) also has the same innervation as the previously discussed muscles, it is further suggested that it, too, contracts reflexively upon stimulation of any of these muscles. Shafik tested this hypothesis in 18 healthy volunteers.[322] EAS was stimulated and the response of the EUS, PRM, LA, and BC was determined. Each muscle was thereafter stimulated separately and the response of the other pelvic floor muscles was registered. Stimulation of any of the pelvic floor muscles effected an increased EMG activity of the rest of the mus-

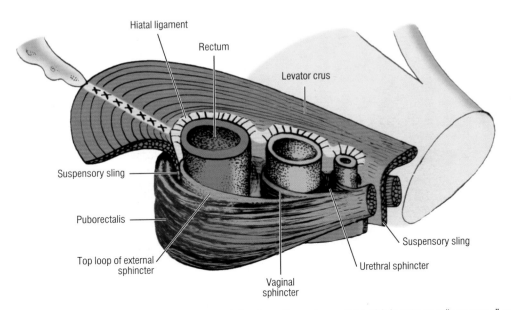

Hiatal ligament

Rectum

Levator crus

Suspensory sling

Puborectalis

Top loop of external
sphincter

Suspensory sling

Urethral sphincter

Vaginal
sphincter

**FIG. 18-109.** Diagram illustrating the "individual" sphincters arising from the puborectalis which acts as a "common" sphincter for the intrahiatal structures. (Courtesy of Prof. Ahmed Shafik, MD.)

cles.[322] The muscle contraction was instantaneous with no latency in any of the muscles except the LA EMG activity which showed a mean latency of 21.3 ± 6.6 ms. The response of the pelvic floor muscles seems to be attributable to muscle stimulation both directly and indirectly through activation of pudendal nerve fibers in the muscles. The study demonstrated that the pelvic floor muscles behave as one muscle; they contract or relax en masse. The "mass contraction" of the pelvic floor muscles might explain some of the physiologic phenomena that occur during pelvic organ evacuation. However, in addition to this mass contraction, a voluntary "selective" individual muscle activity exists by which each individual muscle would act independently of the others.[323]

### Hiatal Ligament

The levator tunnel is connected to the intrahiatal organs by a fascial condensation called the "hiatal ligament"[301] (Figs. 18-76, 18-77, 18-107). A detailed study[282] of the ligament has demonstrated that this structure arises circumferentially around the hiatal margin as a continuation of the fascia on the pelvic surface of the levator plate. The ligament has its origin slightly lateral to the inner edge of the levator plate over which it passes to fill the space between the levator plate and intrahiatal structures. In this space the pelvic fascia is condensed to form the hiatal ligament. The ligament splits fanwise into multiple septa which insert into the vesical neck and rectal neck inlet in both sexes as well as into the upper end of the vagina in females (Fig. 18-109). The inserting fibers penetrate the visceral fascia covering the intrahiatal organs, and

become continuous with the fibers of their intermuscular fascia; some fibers attach directly to the adventitia of these organs. This arrangement gives firmness to the ligamentous insertion.

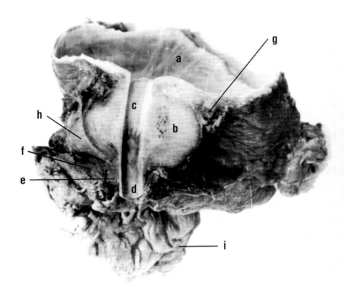

**FIG. 18-110.** Coronal section of the urinary bladder and prostate shows the levator tunnel. a, Urinary bladder. b, Prostate. c, Prostatic urethra. d, Membranous urethra. e, External urethral sphincter. f, Puborectalis. g, Levator plate. h, Suspensory sling inserted into external urethral sphincter. i, Rectal neck (opened). (Courtesy of Prof. Ahmed Shafik, MD.)

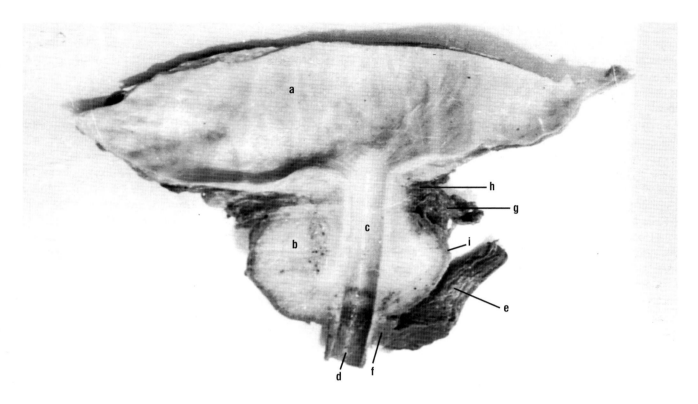

**FIG. 18-111.** Coronal section of the urinary bladder and prostate shows that the puborectalis gives rise to the external urethral sphincter. a, Urinary bladder. b, Prostate. c, Prostatic urethra. d, Membranous urethra. e, Puborectalis. f, External urethral sphincter. g, Levator plate. h, Hiatal ligament. i, Suspensory sling. (Courtesy of Prof. Ahmed Shafik, MD.)

Histologically, the hiatal ligament consists of elastic fibers intermingled with collagen. No muscle bundles were detected within the ligament. Anteriorly, the hiatal ligament fills the gap between the two levator crura at their origin, forming the puboprostatic or pubovesical ligament.[282] After giving rise to the hiatal ligament, the pelvic fascia over the levator plate continues downward as the "tunnel septum" (Figs. 18-76, 18-107) which lines the inner aspect of the levator tunnel.[282]

The pubovesical ligament represents only the anterior portion of the hiatal ligament.[282] It extends backward from the lower part of the symphysis pubis, between the two crural origins, to insert, in both sexes, into the vesical neck in a way similar to that of the hiatal ligament. Contrary to the view of investigators that the ligament in males is attached to the prostate, it was observed that the main insertion is into the vesical neck, with only a few fibers attaching to the prostate. Accordingly, the term "pubovesical" is more appropriate for the ligament in both sexes. In the classic crural pattern, the ligament is well formed as it stretches between the two separated crural origins. However, in crural overlap or scissors, the ligament was smaller and shorter. The pubovesical ligament, being a part of the hiatal ligament, shares with the latter its functional activity as will be mentioned later.

The tunnel septum (Figs. 18-76, 18-107) is the downward continuation of the fascia on the pelvic surface of the levator plate.[282] It lines the inner aspect of the levator tunnel and separates it from the fascia propria of the intrahiatal organs. It is loosely connected to these structures, being separated by a potential space filled with areolar tissue. It consists of collagen impregnated with a few elastic fibers. The septum not only separates the tunnel from its contents but demarcates the voluntary from the involuntary components of these contents. The understanding of this anatomic fact appears to be of major surgical importance because, with the line of cleavage along the tunnel septum, the intrahiatal structures could be mobilized from within the levator tunnel without injury to their voluntary sphincteric mechanism.[282,324]

### Physiologic Considerations of the Mechanism of Defecation

The levator plate (Fig. 18-105) consists of two zones

which seem to be functionally separate: a lateral "visceral support" zone represented by the two lateral masses, and a medial "dilator" zone represented by the two crura.[282] The two lateral masses are fixed muscular sheets which, on contraction, together with the iliococcygeus, become elevated and function to "support" the viscera. The two crura represent the functionally active components of the levator plate.

A previous study has shown a free passage, across the anococcygeal raphe, of the tendinous fibers of the two levators, denoting the existence of a "digastric pattern."[301] Such a pattern allows the two crura to contract simultaneously as a single sheet. On levator contraction, the two crura become elevated and laterally retracted, resulting in "dilatation" of the levator hiatus (Fig. 18-112). The dilator crural action seems to be an effect of the crisscross arrangement of the anococcygeal raphe, the presence of which prevents the crural constrictive action on the intrahiatal contents.[282] Thus, on crural contraction the anococcygeal raphe is shortened and broadened by the narrowing of the meshes between its fibers, with a resulting dilatation of the hiatus (Fig. 18-112).

If the crural muscle bundles were continuous on both sides without the intervention of the anococcygeal raphe, as is the case in the puborectalis, their contraction would constrict the intrahiatal structures. In the classical crural pattern, the separation of the two crura at their origin seems to provide them with the free mobility necessary for proper functioning. Deviation from the classical pattern occurred in 28%.[282] Crural overlap, or crossing, may interfere with the mechanism of hiatal action such that full hiatal dilatation required during the act of defecation or urination may not be achieved. Nevertheless, a good overlap seems to keep the intrahiatal structures in position more firmly, thus reducing the risk of prolapse.[282]

### Double Sphincteric Control

Each intrahiatal structure is provided with a double voluntary sphincteric apparatus: a) an "individual" organ sphincter derived from the puborectalis, which is specific for the organ, and b) a "common" tunnel sphincter, the bulk of the puborectalis, which acts on the intrahiatal organs collectively.[282,323] Thus, nature's way of providing separate sphincteric activity for the individual organs under the control of a common continent muscle secures not only an individual sphincteric function for the organ, but a harmonized action among the structures enclosed within the tunnel. Furthermore, the double sphincteric mechanism provided to each organ could be a guarantee of functional maintenance in case either of the two sphincters is damaged.[323] It is suggested that injury of either sphincter alone is not sufficient to induce incontinence of the concerned organ. Hence, unless both sphincters, the "individual" and "common," are destroyed, continence could be maintained by either.[282,323]

### Levator Complex

The levator tunnel seems to occupy an important role in the mechanisms of defecation and urination. It is provided with two striated muscle coats which differ in their morphologic structure and function: an inner longitudinal (the suspensory sling) which is a tunnel "dilator," and an outer loop (the puborectalis) which is a tunnel "constrictor."[282,301] The two coats

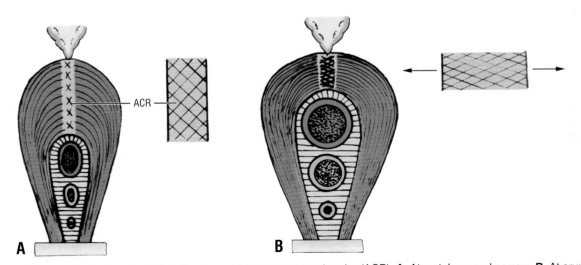

**Fig. 18-112.** Diagram illustrating the "dilator" action of the anococcygeal raphe (ACR). **A,** At rest: long and narrow. **B,** At crural contraction, anococcygeal raphe becomes short and broad (hiatal dilatation). (Courtesy of Prof. Ahmed Shafik, MD.)

act reciprocally: when one contracts, the other relaxes. During active contraction, the inner tunnel coat shares in opening the rectal or bladder necks, while the outer coat occludes them.

The levator crura (the functionally active components of the levator plate, as previously described) together with the levator tunnel and hiatal ligament form a "levator complex." This is structurally and functionally adapted to serve a dual function: a) to fix, and prevent herniation of, the intrahiatal organs, and b) to share in the mechanisms of defecation and urination.[282,301]

### ROLE OF THE LEVATOR COMPLEX IN INTRAHIATAL FIXATION.
The levator tunnel is connected to the intrahiatal structures through the hiatal ligament and along the attachment of its inner coat (the suspensory sling) to these structures. These two links not only bind the intrahiatal structures firmly to the levator tunnel, but also harmonize their action.[282,301] As the suspensory sling is a direct continuation of the levator plate, it slings the intrahiatal structures from the side wall of the pelvis. Thus, on levator contraction at stool or urination, the suspensory sling contracts, with a resultant shortening and widening of the levator tunnel. At the same time, it slings up and fixes the intrahiatal structures during evacuation of their contents: hence its name, the "suspensory sling."[301]

While the suspensory sling fixes the intrahiatal structures in a "vertical" plane, the hiatal ligament provides a "horizontal" suspension.[282,301] The rectal and vesical necks are continuously exposed to variations of intraabdominal tension due to respiratory movements and/or straining. The hiatal ligament constitutes a flexible connection between the levator tunnel and the intrahiatal structures. It allows for a certain degree of rectal and vesical neck mobility during respiration, defecation, and urination. Meanwhile, it seals the levator hiatus and prevents the intra-abdominal pressure from leaking through the hiatus to the intrahiatal organs, thus interfering with their functional activity. The hiatal ligament, thus, keeps the tunnel "pressure tight."[282] This mechanism is maintained as long as the intra-abdominal pressure is within physiologic limits. An increase beyond these limits, as in conditions of chronic straining, would tend to throw its load on the levator plate and tunnel, and eventually lead to prolapse of the intrahiatal structures.[282,301]

Thus, the anococcygeal raphe, being tendinous, becomes overstretched and subluxated under the effect of chronically increased tension. Consequently, the levator plate sags down, leading to pull and stretch of the hiatal ligament, as well as subluxation of the suspensory sling. The levator hiatus becomes widened and lowered such that the rectal and vesical necks lie above it and are di-

rectly exposed to the intraabdominal pressure action, which interferes with their stability and function. Sagging of the levator plate, and hiatal widening as well as hiatal ligament and suspensory sling subluxation result eventually in loss of support, slackening, and prolapse of the intrahiatal structures.[282,325]

### ROLE OF THE LEVATOR COMPLEX IN THE MECHANISM OF DEFECATION AND URINATION.
The defecation and urination mechanism has two components, intrinsic and extrinsic.[282] The intrinsic component involves the detrusor and its sphincter; it acts involuntarily, being composed of smooth muscle fibers. It is under the voluntary control of the extrinsic component which consists of the levator complex, the fibers of which are striated. The intrinsic component functions reflexively: as the detrusor, rectal, or vesical muscle contracts, the internal sphincter relaxes. However, continuation of the acts of defecation or urination depend essentially on the extrinsic component.

When defecation or urination is desired, the "common" tunnel sphincter (the puborectalis) and the "individual" sphincter specific for the organ to be evacuated are voluntarily relaxed. Straining is necessary to maintain the act of evacuation. The Valsalva maneuver elevates the intraabdominal pressure, thereby serving two purposes: a) it compresses and helps evacuation of the detrusor, and (b) it evokes the straining-levator[315] and straining-puborectalis reflexes.[326] The former tends to open the rectal or vesical neck while the latter closes it by the time signals reach the level of consciousness and the decision is made whether to evacuate or not. Although the intraabdominal pressure compresses the detrusor, it spares the rectal neck and urethra, inasmuch as they are located in the pressure-tight levator tunnel.

The levator plate is connected to the rectal and vesical necks along the hiatal ligament, and to the external sphincters (anal and urethral) through the suspensory sling.[282,301] On straining at stool or urination, the levator crura contract and are elevated and laterally retracted. In doing so, they pull the hiatal ligament, effecting traction to open the rectal neck inlet and bladder neck. Meanwhile the suspensory sling, a downward prolongation of the levator plate, contracts simultaneously with it. The contraction of the sling and plate has a twofold action: a) it shortens and widens the levator tunnel and, in turn, the rectal neck and urethra, and b) it pulls open the external sphincters (anal and urethral) by the action of the suspensory sling's terminal fibers which pass through the external urethral sphincter and base loop of the external anal sphincter.[282,301] The final result of levator contraction is that the rectal neck and/or vesical neck and urethra are opened for the rectum and/or bladder to evacuate their contents.

### Electromechanical Activity of the Rectum and Rectosigmoid Pacemaker

Rectal motility is complex, and is regulated and coordinated by motor and reflex actions.[273,312-315,326] Disturbances, of these mechanisms can lead to constipation. The "mass squeeze" contraction theory offers an explanation for rectal motility at defecation.[273] A single contraction wave, starting at the rectosigmoid junction, pushes the fecal matter from the rectum into the opened rectal neck; it is repeated until the rectum is completely evacuated. In dogs, the passage of an inflated balloon through the rectosigmoid junction caused a significant increase in rectal pressure; this response is absent in the anesthetized rectosigmoid junction, as well as in inertia-type constipation, whereas it is present in obstructive constipation.[266,271] A "pacemaker" has been suggested to exist in the rectosigmoid junction, organizing the motor activity of the rectum and defining its maximal contractile frequency.[269] This pacemaker may trigger rectal contraction when stimulated by stools traversing the rectosigmoid junction. In inertia constipation, the pacemaker seems to be disordered.[269,271]

Rectal myoelectrical activity is characterized by regular pacesetter potentials[266] (Fig. 18-113). Evidence supports the view that these potentials originate at the rectosigmoid junction and propagate distally.[266,271] Action potentials follow the pacesetter potentials, with rectal pressure increasing simultaneously, representing contractile activity. This provides additional evidence that the rectosigmoid junction could be the site of a pacemaker that evokes the pacesetter potentials. Animal studies have demonstrated that electrical stimulation applied to the rectosigmoid junction by an artificial pacemaker increases rectal pressure, but decreases rectal neck pressure.[266,271] An artificial pacemaker in the treatment of chronic constipation has been proven to be beneficial and effective.[269,271]

## ANATOMY-RELATED PATHOLOGIES AND TREATMENT

The importance of the anatomic and physiologic findings described above and the resulting conclusions became apparent when their impact on pelvic pathology — in particular, anorectal pathologic conditions — was probed. The newly acquired knowledge has replaced inadequate concepts of the etiologies of pathology with new ones applicable to many pelvic disorders. This knowledge has made essential contributions toward solving a variety of longstanding surgical problems.

### Intrahiatal Organ Mobilization from Within the Levator

With the understanding of the precise anatomy of the levator hiatus and tunnel, mobilization of intrahiatal organs can be performed safely, with preservation of voluntary sphincteric mechanism.[282,324] Thus, high rectal neck and lower rectal lesions can be approached per perineum by mobilizing the rectal neck and lower rectum from within the levator tunnel. Dissection extends between the longitudinal anal muscle and the suspensory sling and through the intersphincteric space, up to the pelvirectal space, the plane of cleavage being along the tunnel septum (see Fig. 18-78). The rectal neck and lower rectum can thus be cored out of the tunnel, pulled down, and brought outside the anal orifice so that any lesion within them can be managed easily, with sphincter preservation.[282,324]

Likewise, middle- or lower-third malignant rectal tumors can be excised radically by a combined abdominoperineal approach with sphincter preservation. The abdominal por-

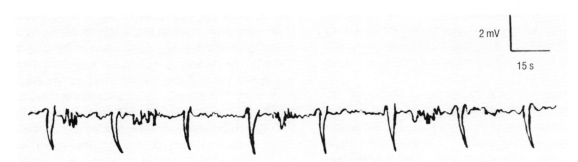

2 mV

15 s

**FIG. 18-113.** Electrorectogram from a normal subject showing pacesetter potentials followed randomly by action potentials. The frequency was calculated as cycles per minute. (Courtesy of Prof. Ahmed Shafik, MD.)

tion of the procedure is accomplished as usual, mobilizing the sigmoid and rectum down to the levator plate. The perineal part calls for coring out the rectal neck from within the levator tunnel in the way mentioned above.[324] The rectal neck, rectum, and sigmoid so mobilized are pulled outside the anal orifice and excised, and the colonic end is fixed to the perianal skin so as to be under the sphincteric control of the levator tunnel.[324]

It is suggested that by following the above-mentioned surgical principles, other intrahiatal organs (e.g., urethra, bladder, vagina, or uterus) can be mobilized and dealt with per perineum from within the levator tunnel, again with preservation of the sphincters.

## Reversion to Normal Defecation after End Colostomy

Comprehension of the interrelations described above has an important, and immediate, bearing on another aspect of sphincter "preservation." Electromyographic (EMG) studies of the perineal muscles after abdomino-perineal operation with end colostomy for rectal cancer have revealed in 50% of the cases that the levator ani and puborectalis muscles have been spared – as was also confirmed by gross anatomic and histologic examination of excised specimens.[327] Hence, advantage is taken of the presence of the muscles to reverse the otherwise permanent end colostomy by mobilizing and suturing the colonic stump to the perineal skin to lie under sphincteric control. Thus the fecal stream is diverted back to the perineal route to restore normal defecation and full fecal continence.

## Strainodynia

Excessive and exhaustive straining in defecation, even when the stools are soft and bulky, is a pathologic manifestation that Shafik refers to as "strainodynia."[328] Four types of strainodynia could be identified in his studies: "band," sphincter, levator, and detrusor.

### Band Strainodynia

'Band' strainodynia is more common in men. It presents with a stool of normal character, and is associated with elevated rectal neck pressure. Rectal neck biopsy reveals a fibrous band. Treatment by bandotomy results in adequate expansion of the rectal neck at defecation and thus relieves the problem.

### Sphincter Strainodynia

'Sphincter' strainodynia is a condition in which internal and external sphincters fail to relax (anismus), or their contraction (dyssynergia) on rectal contraction results in strainodynia. In constipation, the puborectalis and external anal sphincter muscles may contract, rather than relax, upon attempted defecation.[329-331] Contraction of the external anal sphincter with rectal distension is a condition Shafik has termed "detrusor-sphincter dyssynergia syndrome."[330] It has to be differentiated from the detrusor-rectal neck dyssynergia syndrome in which the internal anal sphincter contracts instead of relaxing on rectal distension.[332] Differentiation is made by recording EMG activity both of the external and internal sphincter on rectal distension. It is worth mentioning that the stools in both syndromes commonly are soft and bulky, although the main complaint is constipation. Fiber diet and laxatives do not improve either of the 2 syndromes. External sphincter myotomy in detrusor-sphincter dyssynergia syndrome and internal sphincter myectomy in detrusor-rectal neck dyssynergia syndrome relieve straining at defecation.[330,332]

### Levator Strainodynia

'Levator' strainodynia is due to levator ani muscle dysfunction which includes: levator dysfunction syndrome,[333] detrusor-levator dyssynergia syndrome,[334] and levator paradoxical syndrome.[335] Levator strainodynia occurs with repeatedly obstructing stools at defecation even though they have a normal character (i.e. soft and bulky). EMG of the levator ani muscle is diagnostic.

In the levator dysfunction syndrome, the levator ani muscle is subluxated and sags down; it shows no EMG activity at rest or on contraction.[333] Rectal prolapse may follow. Levatorplasty has satisfactory results.[333]

In the detrusor-levator dyssynergia syndrome, the levator muscle relaxes instead of exhibiting normal contraction on detrusor distension. EMG resting activity disappears, instead of increasing as occurs under normal physiologic conditions. There is no response to pharmacologic therapy, although biofeedback treatment may be beneficial.

With the levator 'paradoxical' syndrome,[335] the rectal neck pressure on straining is elevated instead of diminished. EMG here, too, is diagnostic. The levator muscle shows increased EMG activity on voluntary squeezing, and little or no activity on straining; whereas the normal levator EMG exhibits no change in resting activity on squeezing, and increased activity on straining. These results suggest that levator action is paradoxical. Normally, the levator muscle contracts to open the rectal neck at defecation; the paradoxical action results in failure of the rectal neck to open on straining at stool. Biofeedback treatment may also be useful for this condition.

### Detrusor Strainodynia

'Detrusor' strainodynia has a higher frequency of occurrence in women.[336] Pressure and EMG studies of anal sphincters and levator ani muscle are normal. Rectal detrusor retropulsion is evident. One hypothesis relates rectal retropulsion to an ectopic pacemaker in the rectal detrusor that generates abnormal impulses.[336] The pacemaker that regulates the rectal function seems to be located normally at the rectosigmoid junction.[269,271] Pharmacologic therapy fails to cure the condition while antegrade balloon expulsion training is successful.

## Oligofecorrhea

There are many known causes for oligofecorrhea, a term which can be applied to infrequent defecation, such as two or fewer weekly bowel movements.[337] "Idiopathic oligofecorrhea" is the category without a traceable cause. According to clinical and investigative data, oligofecorrhea presents in 3 different stages, which share major abnormal findings, such as high rectal neck resting pressure, reduced or absent rectoanal-inhibitory reflex, internal sphincter hypertrophy, and degenerated nerve plexus of the internal anal sphincter.[337] The abnormal innervation of the internal sphincter seems to interfere with the rectoanal-inhibitory reflex action, with a resulting failure of relaxation of the internal sphincter on rectal distension. The degenerative changes of the nerve plexus seem to affect mainly the parasympathetic supply, thereby producing predominantly sympathetic activity resulting in abnormal internal sphincter contraction, with an eventual result of muscle hypertrophy.

The 3 stages have criteria by which they are differentiated. In the deep intersphincteric groove category (stage 1), the lower end of the internal anal sphincter is thick and the intersphincteric groove is deeper than normal. Internal sphincterotomy has gratifying results.

In the everted intersphincteric groove category (stage 2), the intersphincteric groove lies outside the rectal neck orifice and is deeper than normal. The lower edge of the internal sphincter is thick and prominent and lies at the level of the external anal sphincter. It descends on straining to project as a cone outside the rectal neck outlet, producing the "cone sign."[337] Internal sphincterotomy results in improvement.

In cone anus (stage 3), the lower end of the internal sphincter protrudes as a cone without straining, outside the rectal neck orifice and below the lower edge of the external sphincter. On palpation, the sphincter is thicker and firmer than normal. The internal sphincter cone elongates on straining. Internal sphincter myotomy has resulted in improvement of all patients in this group.

## PHYSIOANATOMY OF THE HEMORRHOIDAL VENOUS PLEXUS AND RELATED PATHOLOGIC AND THERAPEUTIC POTENTIALS

The presence of a hemorrhoidal venous plexus at the level of both the submucosa and adventitia was demonstrated to extend over the entire length of the rectum and its neck.[338] This plexus constitutes the means of direct communication between the 3 rectal veins. The submucosal plexus (Fig. 18-114) consists of characteristic transverse venous rings, whereas the adventitial plexus (Fig. 18-115) is formed of intercommunicating oblique veins. Neither the fusiform, saccular, nor serpiginous dilatations of the anal submucosal plexus as described by Thomson[339] to be a regular feature of normal anatomy, nor the so-called corpus cavernosum recti by Stelzner[340] could be demonstrated. Contrary to views of some investigators[341,342] that the "collecting hemorrhoidal veins" (Fig. 18-116) lie in the columns of Morgagni, the study by Shafik and Mohi-El-Din[338] has revealed that they exist in the rectal adventitia. The columns are simply plicated mucosal folds that result from both the fusion of the wide hindgut with the narrow proctodeum and the tonic action of the rectal neck sphincters.

Two sites of portosystemic communication could be identified in the rectum: interhemorrhoidal and hemorrhoidogenital.[338] The first of these occurs between the three rectal veins, both submucosally and adventitially. The communication site was identified in the adventitia but not in the submucosa. The portal blood is shunted through this communication to the internal iliac vein. The second communication is through rectogenital collateral channels (Fig. 18-117) which connect the rectal venous plexus with the vesicoprostatic or vaginal plexuses. It seems that this portosystemic connection is extensive, because the urinary bladder, vagina, and uterus were opacified each time the inferior mesenteric vein was injected with barium sulfate.[338]

In contrast to investigators[341,342] who mention that the hemorrhoidal venous plexus is located in the lower rectum and anal canal, and is only submucosal in position, studies

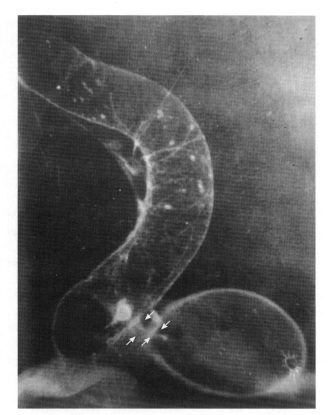

**FIG. 18-114.** Cadaveric specimen showing barium sulfate solution injected into inferior mesenteric vein. It demonstrates that the rectal submucosal plexus extends along the whole of the rectum including its neck and is arranged in transverse venous rings. Arrows indicate the hemorrhoidogenital veins connecting the hemorrhoidal with the vesicoprostatic venous plexus. (Courtesy of Prof. Ahmed Shafik, MD.)

by Shafik and Mohi-El-Din[338] have demonstrated that it not only extends along the whole rectum and its neck, but is both submucosal and adventitial. Being extensive, the plexus can absorb excess venous congestion along its entire length before it becomes varicose; likewise, the varicosity involves the entirety of the venous plexus and not only its lower submucous part. It simulates, in this respect, the diffuse congestion and varicosity of the pampiniform plexus in varicocele. This fact and the understanding that the portal hemorrhoidal blood can work its way to the systemic circulation through two portosystemic shunts (interrectal and rectogenital) tend to negate the theory of venous congestion in the lower part of the hemorrhoidal plexus as being the primary event in hemorrhoidogenesis.

Findings of Shafik and Mohi-El-Din[338] support the conclusion that hemorrhoids are a mucosal prolapse resulting primarily from the constricting effect of the anorectal band upon the rectal neck.[338] The observations explain the rarity

of hemorrhoids in portal hypertension, and are consistent with the incidence of hemorrhoids in bilharzial liver cirrhosis patients in Egypt, which does not differ from the incidence in subjects without bilharzial liver cirrhosis.[290,291] It also explains the rarity of rectal bleeding contrasted with esophageal bleeding in these patients.

## Porto-Systemic Circulation in the Rectum

Under normal physiologic conditions, the submucosal hemorrhoidal plexus drains into the adventitial plexus, which then drains into the 3 paired rectal veins: superior, middle, and inferior. Because of the submucosal and adventitial anastomoses of the three veins in the rectal neck, and due to the presence of the rectogenital veins, portal blood can drain into the systemic circulation – particularly when the rectum contracts at defecation. This was proved when contrast medium was injected into the rectal neck submucosa of nor-

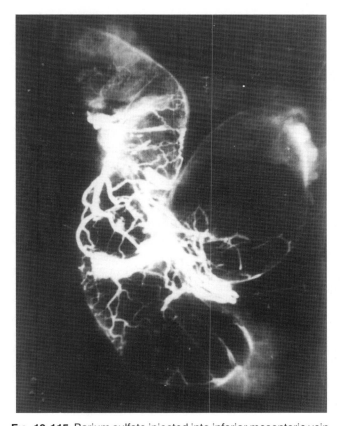

**FIG. 18-115.** Barium sulfate injected into inferior mesenteric vein. The oblique large veins are those of the adventitial plexus, whereas the upper small transverse veins belong to the submucosal plexus. The pectinate area shows the radiological blush. The bladder wall is opacified through the hemorrhoidogenital veins. (Courtesy of Prof. Ahmed Shafik, MD.)

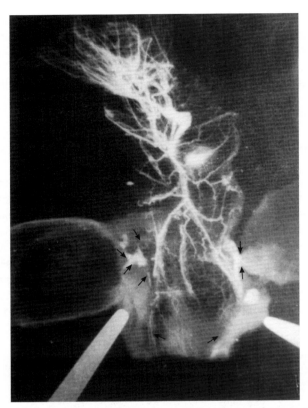

FIG. 18-116. Barium sulfate injected into inferior mesenteric vein. Rectum and urinary bladder were inflated, frozen, and bisected. Artery forceps points to urethra. Specimen shows "collecting veins." *Upper arrows* point to hemorrhoidogenital veins through which bladder wall is opacified. *Lower arrows* point to inferior hemorrhoidal plexus. (Courtesy of Prof. Ahmed Shafik, MD.)

mal living subjects: the dye appeared in the vesicoprostatic and vesicovaginal venous plexuses[343,344] (Fig. 18-118A & B).

Systemic blood cannot drain into the portal venous system, however. When either barium sulfate or blue plastic was injected into the deep dorsal vein of the penis, it could not be recovered in the hemorrhoidal plexus.[338] This is probably due to the presence of valves in the middle and inferior rectal veins which direct the blood to the systemic circulation, and not vice versa. Unlike elsewhere, portal blood shunted from the rectum and left colon to the systemic circulation seems to cause no toxicity problems from metabolic products, because this blood carries no nutrient materials.

## Rectourinary Syndrome

The venous channels that communicate between the rectum and genitourinary organs may provide explanation

for some of the previously unexplained pathologic lesions affecting these organs, such as idiopathic prostatitis, cystourethritis, vaginitis and cervicitis, recurrent bacteriuria, and others.[291,344-346] Portal blood is known to carry various organisms derived from the colon and rectum, notably *E. coli.* It appears that these organisms, under certain conditions, find their way through the communicating veins to the genitourinary organs and cause infection there. This is especially so if there is portal backflow, as occurs in portal hypertension, abdominal tumors, or pregnancy. Similarly, the anorectal congestion which is encountered with lesions like hemorrhoids, fissures, or abscesses is liable to result in congestion of genitourinary organs, which become readily infected from the organisms in the portal blood.

Rectal congestion from hemorrhoids also has been found to cause prostato-vesicular congestion, which in turn leads to idiopathic urethral discharge,[291] recurrent bacteriuria, and cervicitis.[345,346] Recurrent bacteriuria, cystourethritis, and recurrent cervicitis have *Escherichia coli* as their causative agent in the majority of cases. Bacteriologic examination of the organisms recovered

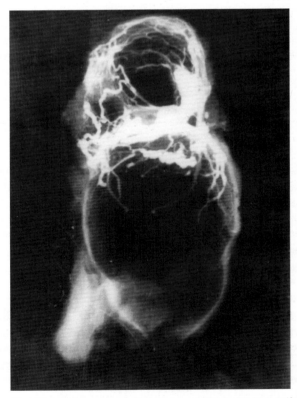

FIG. 18-117. Inferior mesenteric vein injected with barium sulfate. Rectum and urinary bladder inflated, frozen, and cut-sectioned. Specimen shows hemorrhoidogenital veins passing from rectal neck to vesical plexus. (Courtesy of Prof. Ahmed Shafik, MD.)

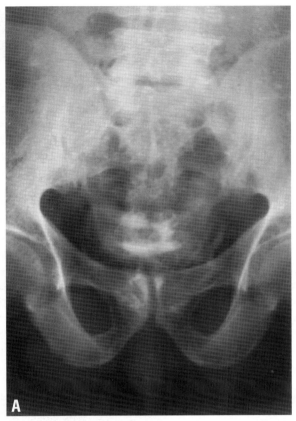
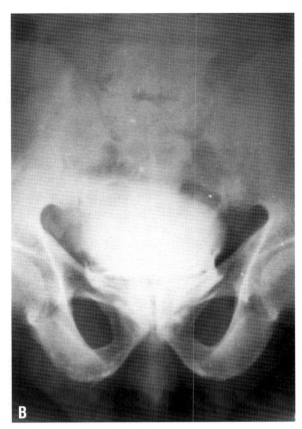

**FIG. 18-118.** Anal cystography in a living subject. **A,** Dye injected into lower rectal neck submucosa. X-ray, ten minutes after injection, showing dye outlining prostatic and lower vesical plexus. **B,** Whole urinary bladder opacified 30 minutes after injection. (From Shafik A. Anal cystography. New technique of cystography. Preliminary report. Urology 1984;23:313-316; with permission.)

from urine, cervix, and feces has demonstrated that they belong to the same serogroup.[345] Hemorrhoids, fissures, ulcers, and fistulas act as *E. coli* reservoirs, as well as leading to anorectal and genitourinary organ congestion. The *E. coli*-laden blood from the congested anal bacterial reservoirs passes through the communicating veins to the congested pelvic organs, causing their infection.[345,346] Treatment of the anal lesion, with or without obliteration of the rectogenital veins by sclerotherapy, is curative.[345]

Communicating veins also seem to play a vital role in genitourinary bilharziasis: schistosomal worms are either urinary (haematobium) or intestinal (mansoni). They mature in the intrahepatic portal venules. The male then carries the female worm in the gynecophoral canal and migrates down the portal vein and its mesenteric tributaries. *Schistosoma mansoni* worms, being bigger than the haematobium type, cannot proceed further and lay down their eggs in the colonic and rectal wall. The smaller schistosoma haematobium worms seem to continue their journey through the rectogenital veins to the vesico-prostatic or vaginal plexus

where the eggs are deposited in the pelvic genitourinary organs[338] – which would explain the mystery of the route adopted by this type of schistosoma to reach the genitourinary organs from the liver.

## Role of Pelvic Organ Venous Plexuses in Diagnostics

X-ray imaging can be used to demonstrate the configuration of the venous plexuses of the rectum and urogenital organs and the venous interconnections across the pelvic floor. Contrast medium injected into the anal submucosa diffuses from the site of injection through the vesico-prostatic plexus, outlining the prostate and the wall of the urinary bladder, but not its lumen. An anal cystography is obtained[343] (Fig. 18-118). By the same procedure, the dye reaches the vaginovesical plexus so that cystovaginohysterography can be performed[344] (Fig. 18-119).

## Role of the Rectogenital Veins for Chemotherapy in Pelvic Malignancies

Detection of the 2-6 small rectogenital veins described which communicate unidirectionally between the rectal veins and the vesicoprostatic or rectovaginal plexuses called for a method that would adequately exploit the prodigious potential of this anatomic route. The submucosal anal injection technique[338,347] was created for a direct anal or perineal approach.[348] It has developed into a landmark contribution from the point of view of nonsurgical and minimally invasive measures in the therapy of pelvic disorders, including advanced and metastatic stages of malignancies. The procedure is simple, easy, and of marked efficacy. For most of its applications it can be considered an office procedure.

Animal experiments had earlier shown that the anal route is adequate for administration of chemotherapy. The distribution of [14]C-labeled misonidazole, a radiation sensitizer, was studied in the serum and tissues of rats by comparison of the submucosal anal route with the oral route.[349] The drug concentration in the bladder tissue, relative to the serum, was highest by the anal route with a level of 8, and 5 times that of the serum 15 and 30 minutes, respectively, after administration. When the drug was administered orally, however, the drug concentration in the bladder tissue reached only one-fourth of, or a level equal to, the serum level in the same periods. In a similar experiment assessing the drug concentration in the uterus and vagina relative to serum, the submucosal anal route achieved a concentration of 10 and 8 times, respectively, of the serum level after 15 minutes. Oral administration in the same period of time produced a drug concentration of one-fifth and one-quarter the serum level.[350]

In view of these results, submucosal anal injection of chemotherapeutic agents was used with satisfactory results in the treatment of pelvic malignancies such as advanced vesical, prostatic, cervical, and rectal cancer.[347,351-353] No side effects were encountered. An essential advantage of this treatment modality is that there are no systemic effects of the therapeutic chemical agent, because a high drug concentration is achieved in the tumor while the serum drug concentration remains low. This was confirmed experimentally and by studies of methotrexate concentration in vesical and rectal tumor tissue and serum after anal injection compared to parenteral injection.[349,350,354] Chronic prostatitis is effectively treated via the submucosal anal route by injecting the appropriate antimicrobial agent as defined by sensitivity tests.[355]

## ARTERIAL PATTERN OF THE RECTUM AND ITS CLINICAL APPLICATION

The arterial supply of the rectum was studied in 32 cadavers by Shafik and Moustafa.[356] The superior rectal artery (SRA) (Fig. 18-120) and vein were found to be enclosed in a fibrous sheath which was connected to the posterior rectal surface by an anterior mesorectum containing the "transverse rectal branches," and to the sacrum by avascular posterior mesorectum. Small lymph nodes were scattered alongside the anterior mesorectum. The SRA gave rise to 4 branches: transverse rectal, descending rectal, rectosigmoid, and terminal. The transverse rectal arteries (Fig. 18-121) arose from the SRA in 24 specimens and from the descending rectal artery in 8. They were distributed to the upper half of the rectum. The rectosigmoid artery was distributed to the descending limb of the sigmoid colon and rectosigmoid junction. Examining terminal branches of the SRA in 32 cadavers, the authors

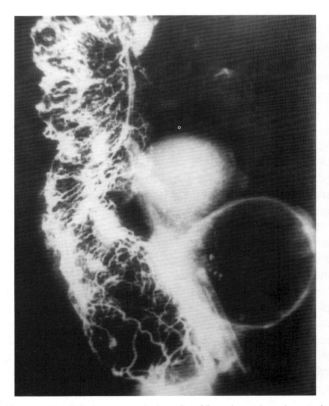

**FIG. 18-119.** Inferior mesenteric vein of female cadaveric specimen injected with barium sulfate. Vagina, uterus, and urinary bladder were opacified through hemorrhoidogenital veins. (Courtesy of Prof. Ahmed Shafik, MD.)

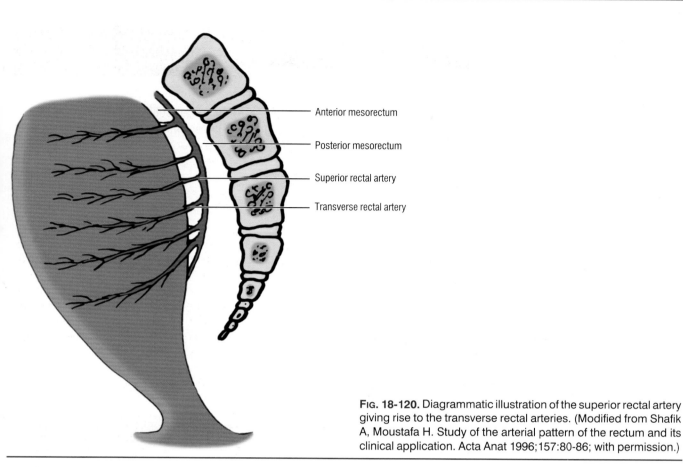

Anterior mesorectum

Posterior mesorectum

Superior rectal artery

Transverse rectal artery

**FIG. 18-120.** Diagrammatic illustration of the superior rectal artery giving rise to the transverse rectal arteries. (Modified from Shafik A, Moustafa H. Study of the arterial pattern of the rectum and its clinical application. Acta Anat 1996;157:80-86; with permission.)

found 2 branches in 21, and 3 branches in 11. The branches communicated in the lower half of the rectum. Inferior rectal arteries were present in all the dissected cadavers while middle rectal arteries could be identified in only 50% of the cadavers. Two arterial patterns were recognized: anular in the upper rectal half provided by the transverse rectal arteries, and plexiform in the lower half supplied by the SRA terminal branches.

The anterior mesorectum was vascular as it contained the transverse rectal arteries, whereas the posterior mesorectum was avascular.[356] These findings should be considered during rectal mobilization in operations for rectal prolapse or cancer to avoid excessive bleeding. In rectopexy for rectal prolapse,[357] the rectum is mobilized and this is preferably done through the posterior avascular mesorectum. Also mesorectum removal with rectal excision for rectal cancer reduces the recurrence rate.[358] To avoid bleeding, dissection is best performed in the posterior avascular plane. The pararectal lymph nodes existed alongside the anterior mesorectum. Their dissection necessitates excision of the superior rectal vessels and their mesenteries. This might explain the higher 5-year survival rate in rectal cancer when the mesorectum is included in the radical operation.[358] Removal of the mesorectum includes removal of the pararectal lymph nodes as well.

There were fewer branches of the SRA on the anterior rectal wall than on the posterior. The vascular branching diminished gradually from the posterior to the anterior aspect to the extent that a "bloodless line" is suggested to exist in the midline anteriorly (Figs. 18-120, 18-121). It is assumed that for this reason incisions in the posterior rectal wall heal faster than anterior wall incisions and, in addition, are less likely to leak. Incisions in the anterior rectal wall should have bleeding edges before being closed in order to avoid disruption and leak; they may be covered by a colostomy.

The rectosigmoid branch of the SRA constitutes a communication between the SRA and inferior mesenteric artery. The arterial pattern in the sigmoid colon and upper half of the rectum is segmental, and is provided by the transverse arterial rings which seem to constitute end arteries. The rectosigmoid artery might act to shunt the blood from the inferior mesenteric artery to the SRA in case of arterial interruption in the rectosigmoid area.

The middle rectal arteries seem to play a minor role in the arterial supply of the rectum as they are inconsistent.

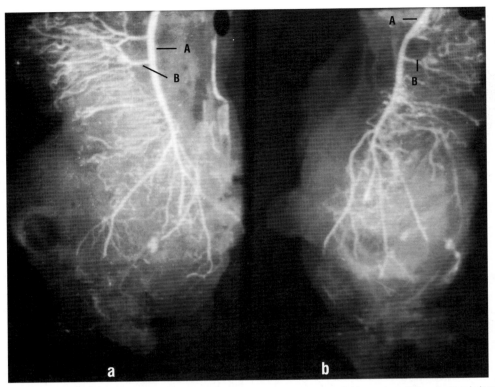

**Fig. 18-121.** Angiogram showing superior rectal artery (A) giving rise to transverse rectal branches (B). **a,** Lateral view. **b,** Anteroposterior view. Terminal branches of the transverse rectal arteries do not anastomose anteriorly and this results in the formation of a "bloodless line." The superior rectal artery terminates at the mid-rectum giving rise to 3 branches. (From Shafik A, Moustafa H. Study of the arterial pattern of the rectum and its clinical application. Acta Anat 1996;157: 80-86; with permission.)

Their low incidence has to be considered during rectal dissection in operations for rectal prolapse or cancer. This is in contrast to the inferior rectal arteries which were consistent in all the dissected specimens. They were distributed to the rectal neck. Anastomosis occurred between the 3 rectal arteries at the submucosal level.

## RECTUM: CONDUIT OR STORAGE ORGAN?

Most standard texts state that the rectum is usually empty.[359-362] However, the evidence upon which this statement is based is deficient. In a study by Shafik et al.,[363] stools were palpable in the lower rectum in 64.5% (31 of 48 subjects) and were demonstrated radiologically in 75% (12 of 16) (Fig. 18-122). In 3 of 16 subjects the stools were located in the rectum too high to be detected digitally, although they were demonstrated radiologically (Fig. 18-123). Stools situated more than 7.5 cm above the anal

verge are likely to be impalpable. The high location of the stools in the rectum seems to be peculiar. It is believed that the upper rectum can retain stools owing to the presence of the mucosal folds which may shelve the stools and keep them in the upper rectum. The higher stool frequency per week in subjects with an empty rectum as opposed to those with a full rectum is believed to be due to many factors including the type of diet and the response to the defecation reflex. Meanwhile the authors could not find a relation between the time elapsed since the last defecation and a full or an empty rectum.

The above study[363] demonstrated that the rectum may contain stools under normal physiologic conditions. This is in contrast to investigators who hold the view that the rectum is normally empty of feces and that, as the stools pass to the rectum from the sigmoid colon, the recto-anal inhibitory reflex is initiated and defecation occurs.[359-362] It is believed that the rectum receives the stools and stores them until they reach a certain volume which would stimulate the rectal stretch receptors and the defecation reflex. In such a case, digital rectal examination or radiography can detect stools in the rectum under normal physiologic conditions.

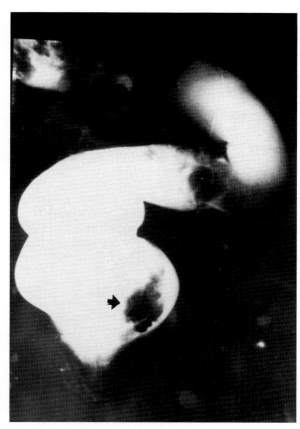

**FIG. 18-122.** Barium enema showing stools *(arrow)* in rectum. (From Shafik A, Ali YA, Afifi R. Is the rectum a conduit or storage organ? Int Surg 1997;82:194-197; with permission.)

Another explanation for the presence of stools in the rectum under normal physiologic conditions could be that the stools enter the rectum in a volume sufficient to initiate the defecation reflex. Should the circumstances be unfavourable for defecation, the external sphincter voluntarily contracts evoking the voluntary inhibition reflex which results in rectal relaxation and waning of the desire to defecate.[163] The defecation reflex might not return until an additional amount of feces enters the rectum; this can take several hours to occur, during which time the stools may be palpable in the rectum.

## PUDENDAL NERVE

The pudendal nerve is an important motor and sensory nerve to the pelvic organs and perineum. It provides supply for the anal and urethral sphincters, as well as cutaneous

and skeletal motor innervation of the penis and clitoris. Pudendal neuropathy or nerve injury leads to pathologic changes of these structures.[333,364-367] Pudendal nerve compression in the pudendal canal causes the pudendal canal syndrome (an entrapment syndrome) with a resulting incompetence of anal and urethral sphincters.[368-370] Electrode application to the pudendal nerve or to its roots or branches has been used for treatment of anal and urethral sphincter insufficiency.[371-376]

Sound knowledge of the precise anatomic location and pattern of the pudendal nerve and its roots and branches is essential to facilitate their detection. The localization of the nerve by its surgical anatomy has important diagnostic and therapeutic advantages in procedures such as confirmation of the diagnosis of pudendal canal syndrome or corroboration of indications for pudendal canal decompression operation.[368-370,377] Adequate anatomic knowledge and thorough screening studies of the pudendal nerve are imperative to:

- Expose the nerve in patients with pudendal canal syndrome wherein the roof of the canal is slit open to decompress the nerve[368-370,377-383]
- Decompress the nerve[368-370,377-383]
- Provide exposure for the positioning of electrodes for the performance of an accurate nerve stimulation
- Stimulate the nerve roots or branches for fecal and urinary incontinence or erectile dysfunction[371-377]
- Stimulate the nerve to assess its functional integrity and that of the pelvic floor musculature
- Determine pudendal nerve terminal motor latency[364]

The pudendal nerve arises from the anterior rami of S2-4, and is formed of three roots and two cords (Fig. 18-124).

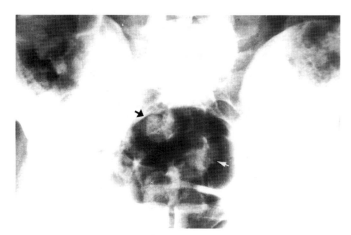

**FIG. 18-123.** Air insufflated into the rectum. Stools *(arrows)* are located above the upper rectal valve. (From Shafik A, Ali YA, Afifi R. Is the rectum a conduit or storage organ? Int Surg 1997;82:194-197; with permission.)

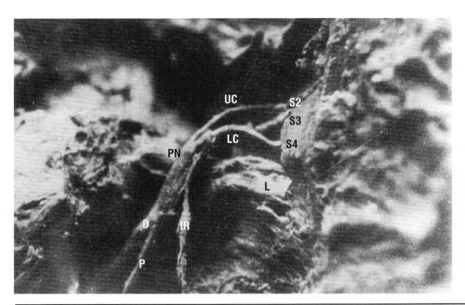

**FIG. 18-124.** Photograph of an adult cadaver showing the first root (S2) that passes downward and laterally to form the upper cord (UC). The second root (S3) passes downward to fuse with the third root (S4) forming the lower cord (LC). The two cords fuse together just above the sacrospinous ligament (L) to form the pudendal nerve (PN). IR, Inferior rectal nerve. P, Perineal nerve. D, Dorsal nerve of penis. (Courtesy of Prof. Ahmed Shafik, MD.)

It may take a contribution from S1 and S5 (Fig. 18-125). The first root continues as the upper cord while the 2nd and 3rd roots unite to form the lower cord. The 2 cords fuse to form the pudendal nerve.[384] In neurostimulation of the pudendal nerve, identification of the cords helps in applying the neuroprosthesis to the appropriate cords. The upper cord is longer and thinner than the lower; it was thick and shorter, however, when it received a contribution from S1. In all dissected cadavers, the pudendal nerve was formed by the merging of the two cords above the sacrospinous ligament before it crossed the pelvic surface of the ligament a short distance medial to the ischial spine.[384] In no specimen did the nerve cross the bony ischial spine. This is in contrast to the view of other investigators who state that the pudendal nerve passes behind the ischial spine.[385,386] For pudendal nerve block or stimulation, the needle or electrode has to be moved medially after locating the ischial spine, allowing for close apposition to the pudendal nerve.

The inferior rectal nerve originated from the pudendal nerve in the pudendal canal in 18 of 20 dissected cadavers (7 male, 13 female). In one, it arose from the pudendal nerve in the lesser sciatic foramen before entering the pudendal canal, and in another it arose directly from S3.[384] The inferior rectal nerve supplies the external anal sphincter and levator ani muscle. In pudendal canal syndrome, pudendal nerve compression in the pudendal canal leads to anal or scrotal pain, fecal or urinary incontinence and/or erectile dysfunction. Decompression of the pudendal canal relieves the symptoms.[368-370,377] It is highly probable that subjects in whom the inferior rectal nerve arises from the pudendal nerve proximal to the pudendal canal or from the pudendal

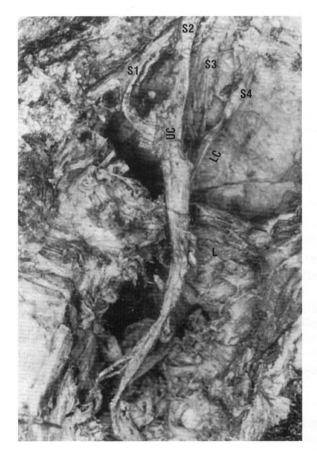

**FIG. 18-125.** Photograph of an adult cadaver showing the three roots (S2, S3, and S4) and the two cords (UC, upper cord, and LC, lower cord) of the pudendal nerve above the sacrospinous ligament (L). The upper cord receives a contribution from the first sacral root (S1). (Courtesy of Prof. Ahmed Shafik, MD.)

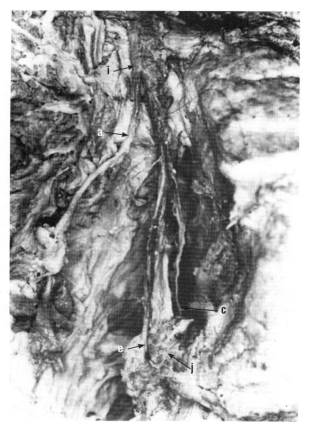

**FIG. 18-126.** Photograph of male cadaver showing the three branches of the right pudendal nerve (i) arising in the pudendal canal: inferior rectal nerve (e), perineal nerve (j), and dorsal nerve of penis (c). They show also the accessory rectal branch (a) which arises behind the sacrospinous ligament. (Courtesy of Prof. Ahmed Shafik, MD.)

nerve roots are spared the anorectal manifestations of the pudendal canal syndrome.[384]

In seven male cadavers the pudendal nerve gave off an "accessory rectal nerve" behind the sacrospinous ligament (Fig. 18-126), which innervated the levator ani muscle and perineal and perianal skin.[384] Juenemann et al.[385] dissected three male cadavers and reported a branch arising from the pudendal nerve, but described the nerve as innervating the transversus perinei and ischiocavernosus muscles. Shafik et al. failed to demonstrate the innervation of these muscles by the accessory rectal nerve, and it seems that the two branches are different. The finding of the accessory rectal nerve exclusively in male cadavers and not in the female is mysterious. The levator ani muscle in such cadavers was doubly innervated on its perineal surface by the inferior rectal nerve and the accessory rectal nerve. While the inferior rectal nerve arose in the pu-

dendal canal, the accessory rectal nerve arose above it and therefore might be spared the neuropathy of the other branches of the pudendal nerve in the pudendal canal syndrome.[384]

The pudendal nerve can be used to study the integrity of pelvic floor muscles, in biofeedback training, nerve blocks, stimulation trials to treat chronic incontinence, and in nerve conduction studies or evoked potential recordings.[384]

## Pudendal Canal

The anatomy of the pudendal canal (PC) (Fig. 18-127) was studied in 26 cadavers: 10 stillborn and 16 adult (mean age 48.2 years).[387] Two approaches were used to expose the PC: gluteal and perineal. The PC was an obliquely lying tube with a mean length of 0.8 cm in the stillborn and 1.6 cm in the adult cadavers. It started at a mean distance of 0.8 cm from the ischial spine in the stillborn and of 1.6 cm in the adult cadavers, and ended at a mean distance of 0.7 cm and 2.6 cm, respectively, from the lower border of the symphysis pubis. The PC wall was formed by splitting of the obturator fascia and not by the lunate fascia. The PC contained the pudendal nerve and vessels embedded in loose areolar tissue. The 3 branches of the neurovascular bundle arose inside the canal in all but 3 cadavers. The wall of the PC consisted of collagen and elastic fibers while that of the obturator fascia consisted of collagen only. The PC seems to be structurally adapted to serve certain functions.

### *Structural-Functional Adaptation of the Pudendal Canal*

The anatomic structure of the PC seems to provide it with maximum functional performance.[387] Thus, the loose areolar tissue in which the neurovascular bundle is embedded allows for changes in the vessel diameter in response to pelvic organ activities, especially during sexual arousal and erection, without blood supply embarrassment. The functional adaptation of the PC is further provided by its histologic structure. The crisscross plywood arrangement gives the PC wall a textile nature that allows the canal to change its shape in adaptation to pressure changes in the pudendal vessels. The PC can thus expand, giving the pudendal vessels a space to engorge during sexual arousal and intercourse. Meanwhile, the elastic fibers included in the wall effect spontaneous return of the PC to its original size by their elastic recoil. With such structure, the PC is suggested to be acting as a "pump" that assists venous return in the pudendal veins. Furthermore, the elastic fibers seem to prevent collagen

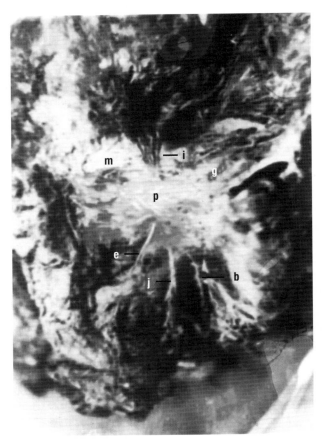

**FIG. 18-127.** Dissected cadaveric specimen showing the pudendal canal (p) with the pudendal nerve (i) entering it posteriorly and its branches leaving it anteriorly. m, Sacrospinous ligament. g, Obturator internus muscle. e, Inferior rectal nerve. b, Dorsal nerve of clitoris. j, Perineal nerve. (Courtesy of Prof. Ahmed Shafik, MD.)

overstretch and PC subluxation as a result of its continuous distension by vessel engorgement.

### Pulley Action of the Pudendal Canal

In the meantime, it appears that the PC acts as a "pulley" for the pudendal neurovascular bundle.[387] The latter, arising in the pelvis, passes through the PC on its journey to the ischiorectal fossa. It seems that the pulley action of the PC not only fixes the bundle during its travel to the pelvic floor muscles but also prevents it from being traumatized by the continuous movement of these muscles.

### *Pudendal Canal Syndrome*

The pulley action of the PC may be disrupted by dysfunctioning pelvic floor muscles or disordered defecation.

Thus in cases of levator dysfunction syndrome,[388] the levator muscle becomes subluxated and sags. This would lead to continuous pull on the neurovascular bundle with eventual occurrence of pudendal neuropathy and pudendal arteritis, a condition we call "pudendal canal syndrome."[368-370,377-383,389-391] This syndrome presents with the sensory and motor manifestations of the pudendal nerve such as fecal incontinence,[369,381,389] anal pain,[368] stress urinary incontinence,[390,391] erectile dysfunction,[377] and perineal hypoesthesia.[368-370,377-379,381-383,389-391] The PC syndrome is treated by PC decompression.[368-370,377-379,381-384, 390,391] The canal is slit open to release the pudendal vessels and nerve from their entrapment.

### *Pudendal Canal Decompression*

Surgeons exposing the PC must know its precise anatomy so they can avoid injury to the neurovascular bundle or its branches. The PC lies obliquely with its proximal end close to the ischial spine and its distal end lateral to, and level with, the inferior border of the symphysis pubis;[387] it is located a few centimeters above the ischial tuberosity. In view of these anatomic landmarks, the PC could be exposed through 2 routes: perineal,[368] and posterior.[378] In the perineal route (Fig. 18-128), the PC is exposed through a para-anal incision. The inferior rectal nerve is identified in the ischiorectal (ischioanal) fossa and taken as a guide to the pudendal nerve in the PC. The posterior approach to the PC (Fig. 18-129) is performed through a parasacral incision, dividing the underlying gluteus maximus muscle, exposing the pudendal nerve, and following it to the PC. However, the perineal approach was more satisfactory than the posterior because it is easier, simpler, and less time-consuming.

In conclusion, knowledge of the surgical anatomy of the PC is necessary not only for diagnostic purposes but also for designing a proper therapeutic approach.

## NEW METHODS OF INVESTIGATION

Although we have a great variety of diagnostic methods at our disposal, the need for qualitative improvement remains constant. This improvement need not necessarily be effected by more sophisticated instrumentation, however. With regard to the assessment of disorders of the anorectum, Shafik et al. have introduced approaches that are less sophisticated in that they simply put to use known

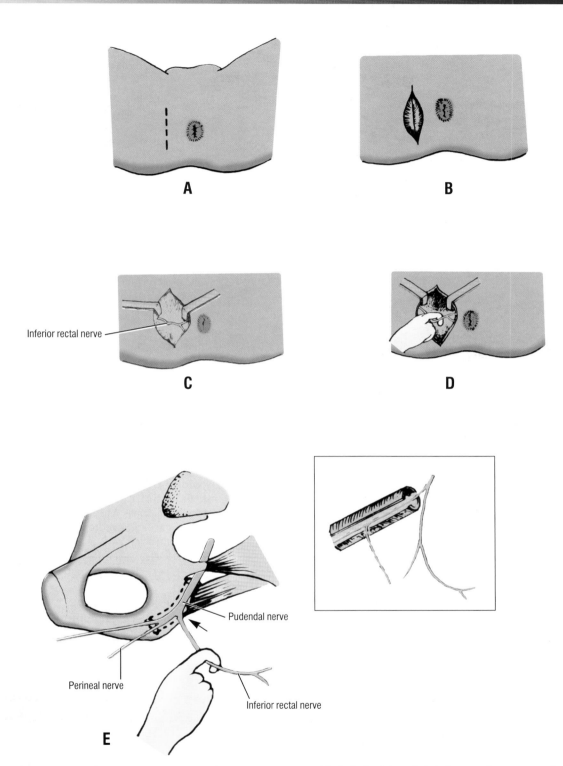

FIG. **18-128.** Pudendal canal decompression operation (anterior approach). **A, B,** Incision. **C,** Inferior rectal nerve crossing ischiorectal (ischioanal) fossa. **D,** Inferior rectal nerve hooked with index finger. **E,** Inferior rectal nerve followed to pudendal nerve. *Inset,* Pudendal nerve in and outside pudendal canal. (Courtesy of Prof. Ahmed Shafik, MD.)

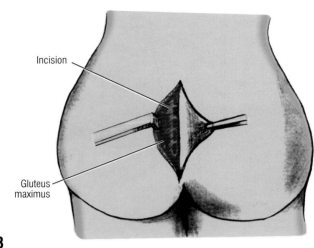

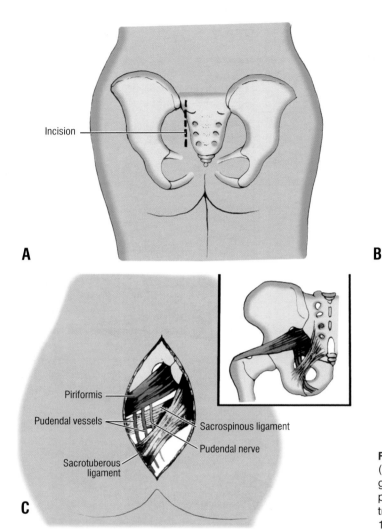

FIG. 18-129. Pudendal canal decompression operation (posterior approach). **A,** Parasacral incision. **B,** Division of gluteus maximus muscle. **C,** Pudendal nerve and vessels exposed. (Modified from Shafik A. The posterior approach in the treatment of pudendal canal syndrome. Coloproctology 1992; 14:310-315; with permission.)

anatomic or physiologic principles; yet they give excellent objective results in highly reliable and detailed ways.

## Fecoflowmetry

With respect to anorectal complaints, conventional examinations reveal little correlation between subjective symptoms and investigative results. This may be partly due to the fact that patients' assessment of their own defecation is frequently misleading. The main reason, however, is the inadequacy of these types of investigations to reveal exactly what occurs during defecation. Neither defecometry[392] nor the balloon expulsion test[393] are representative of the procedure of defecation in view of the minimal –if any– increase in voluntary abdominal pressure required with normal defecation as opposed to the significant rectal

expulsion pressure needed to expel the balloons.[393] In search of a method simulating natural rectal evacuation as closely as possible, Shafik and colleagues[394,395] introduced the fecoflowmeter, which produces an authentic and comprehensive record of the act of defecation in all its details.

The fecoflowmeter apparatus is based on weighing the defecated fluid; it consists of a weight transducer, amplifier, and oscillograph. The technique of fecoflowmetry is simple and noninvasive.[395] The patient is instructed to evacuate the bowel prior to examination by either defecation or enema. Then, with the patient in the left lateral position, a 1 L water enema is given slowly. The water is incubated at 37°C and instilled under gravity through a 14F catheter placed in the rectum 8-12 cm from the rectal neck orifice. The catheter is removed after enema administration. The subject is then asked to walk around, retain the enema as long as possi-

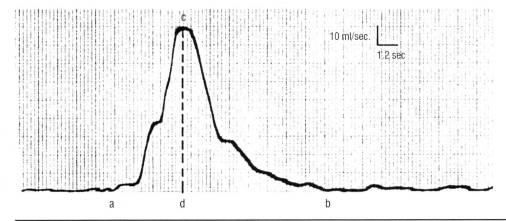

**FIG. 18-130.** Normal defecation flow curve. a-b, Defecation time (seconds). c-d, Maximum flow rate (ml/sec). a-d, Time to maximum flow (seconds). (Courtesy of Prof. Ahmed Shafik, MD.)

ble, and to sit on the commode of the fecoflowmeter when feeling the urge to defecate. The fecal flow rate is the product of rectal detrusor action against outlet resistance and measures the defecated volume passed per time unit.[395] Fecoflowmetry provides quantitative as well as qualitative data concerning the act of defecation. All objective parameters are assessed in one test. The defecated volume, the flow time, the time to maximum flow, as well as the mean and maximum flow rates are calculated from the defecation flow curve.[395] The shape of the normal curve reflects the dominance of an active detrusor and the modulation of a passive rectal neck. The ascending limb illustrates the rectal detrusor contraction, while the descending limb displays the function of the rectal neck.

The results of contrasting the fecoflowmetric parameters of chronically constipated patients to those of normal controls[394,395] have shown that the time to maximum flow is longer in the constipated group than in the normal group, while the mean and maximum flow rates are lower. The volume expelled is smaller in the constipated patients.

Furthermore, the time elapsing from the administration of the enema to the sensation of urgency is prolonged in the constipated group. The flow curve of the controls (Fig. 18-130) is characteristic:[395] It is obelisk-shaped. The ascending limb rises steeply and is commonly smooth. The descending limb has a tendency to be drawn out, but is also smooth. In contrast, the flow curve of constipated patients (Fig. 18-131) presents with a less steeply rising ascending limb and with fluctuation in flow intensity.[395] Also, pre-evacuation fluctuations are common. As the maximum flow is reached, a plateau may form. The descending limb commonly shows fluctuations.

## Reflex Reactions

The reflexes which are involved in the mechanisms of defecation and continence, namely recto-puborectalis reflex,[312] recto-levator reflex,[313] levator-puborectalis reflex,[314] straining-levator reflex,[315] straining-puborectalis reflex,[326] and levator-sphincter reflex[396] are additional investigative

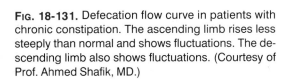

**FIG. 18-131.** Defecation flow curve in patients with chronic constipation. The ascending limb rises less steeply than normal and shows fluctuations. The descending limb also shows fluctuations. (Courtesy of Prof. Ahmed Shafik, MD.)

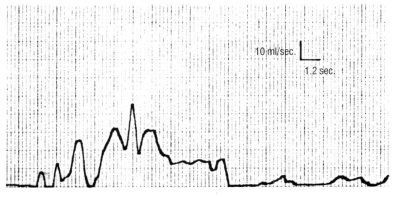

tools. They are reliable, objective, and substantial sources of information on the physiologic state of the pelvic floor muscles and of the nerves supplying them. Evaluation of the reflex actions of the pertinent musculature contributes to establishing a diagnosis in anorectal disorders with yet more accuracy, in a more comprehensive manner, and in less time because the approach is direct. The technique of evaluating the interrelationships between reflexes of the rectal area and the responses of the involved musculature follows an easily understood principle. A balloon-tipped catheter is introduced into the rectum and is attached to a pressure transducer. An electromyographic concentric needle electrode is inserted into the muscle that is to be investigated for its response to rectal balloon inflation. Detectable changes in the latency, duration, or motor unit action potentials of the evoked response may indicate a defect in the reflex pathway that could be an indication of muscular or nerve damage.

## Water Enema Test

Another simple office test, the so-called water enema test, was introduced for anorectal investigation.[397] At 37°C, 1.5 L of water is instilled under gravity into the rectum through a 16-gauge Nélaton catheter at a rate of 150 ml/min. The subject is asked to report the first rectal sensation as well as desire and urge to evacuate. The volume of water infused at the time of these occurrences is determined, and compared with standard values from controls. Defecation disorders can be identified with this easy and noninvasive office test.

## Inguinal Pelviscopy

Inguinal pelviscopy (Fig. 18-132) examines structures in the extra- and intraperitoneal pelvic cavity.[398] Through a 1 cm incision above the symphysis pubis, a Veress needle is inserted into the retropubic space, and gas is insufflated; the pelviscope is introduced through a second 1 cm incision in the area overlying the superficial inguinal ring and advanced in the inguinal canal to cross the deep inguinal ring into the extraperitoneal pelvic cavity. It is used to visualize and biopsy questionable masses in the pelvis. The approach is safe, because the entry is through a natural pathway, the inguinal canal; the examination is extraperitoneal.[398] It is direct, as the deep inguinal ring is near and represents a natural gateway to the pelvic cavity. Furthermore, extraperitoneal masses are difficult and hazardous to approach by the standard intraperitoneal laparoscopic technique. Inguinal pelviscopy can also deal with

intraperitoneal pelvic and abdominal lesions, when the instrument is made to pierce the peritoneum at the deep inguinal ring or close to the fallopian tube. It is most suitable for visualizing the ovaries, tubes, and uterus. These organs are close to the deep inguinal ring and can be approached either extra- or intraperitoneally or both. Inguinal pelviscopy is used not only for diagnostic purposes but also for some minor therapeutic procedures. Pelvic adhesions can be easily located and managed. Tubal sterilization is safely done. Small, simple cysts are aspirated and biopsied. With such a simple and safe technique, repeated inguinal pelviscopy allows pelvic lesions to be followed and surgery to be properly timed.

## Rectometry

Rectometry is a simple, noninvasive way of assessing rectal volume, pressure, and compliance at the first rectal and urge sensations in one test.[399] Carbon dioxide is infused into a balloon introduced into the rectum and connected to a pressure transducer. Simultaneous measurement of the rectal and intra-abdominal pressure is done, and a rectometrogram (Fig. 18-133) is obtained. It reads the volume of carbon dioxide infused and the intrarectal and detrusor pressure at both the first rectal and urge sensations. In addition to supplying information on the quantitative values, the curve configuration itself differentiates not only between normal and constipated subjects, but also between the obstructive and inertia types of constipation.[399] Apart from its diagnostic value, rectometry can be used to follow the effectiveness of drugs on detrusor function.

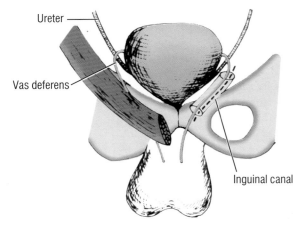

**Fig. 18-132.** Route to enter pelvic cavity *(dotted line)*. (Courtesy of Prof. Ahmed Shafik, MD.)

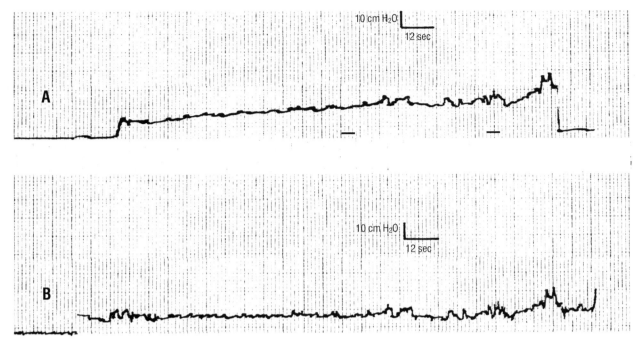

**FIG. 18-133. A,** Rectometrogram of normal evacuation. **B,** Intraabdominal pressure curve, showing slight increase of pressure at evacuation. First dash below tone limb denotes first rectal sensation, second dash denotes urge sensation. (From Shafik A, Moneim KA. Rectometry: A new method assessing rectal function. Coloproctology 1991;13:237-243; with permission.)

## Electrorectogram in Normal Subjects and in Rectal Pathologic Conditions

Electrorectography is a noninvasive and nonradiologic technique by which the electric activity of the rectum is recorded, using a silver/silver chloride electrode situated 1 cm from the tip of a 6F catheter which is applied to the rectal mucosa by suction.[266,267] The procedure could be included as a valuable method in assessing rectal detrusor efficiency and in diagnosing disorders and pathologic rectal conditions. In normal subjects, regular and reproducible pacesetter potentials are recorded with a mean frequency of 2.6 ± 0.4 cycle/min, amplitude of 1.9 ± 0.6 mV and velocity of 4.2 ± 0.9 cm/sec. They are followed randomly by action potentials[267] (see Fig. 18-113). In inertia constipation, pacesetter potentials are infrequent (bradyrectia) and action potentials are registered only occasionally. In obstructive constipation, regular and reproducible pacesetter potentials record a higher frequency and velocity than normal (tachyrectia).[400] In chronic proctitis, the pacesetter potentials frequency is higher, while amplitude and velocity are lower than normal. Action potentials have a higher frequency and amplitude.[401] In Hirschsprung's disease, pacesetter potentials or action

potentials are not recordable, and a "silent" reproducible electrorectogram is obtained.[402] Recently an electrorectogram has been recorded percutaneously;[268] likewise, percutaneous electrovesicography and electrovasography studies in normal and pathologic conditions have been carried out.[403,404]

## ANATOMIC COMPLICATIONS OF SURGERY OF ANORECTUM

### Chronic Anal Fissure and Hemorrhoids

Manual dilatation of the anus has been advocated for treatment of chronic anal fissure and hemorrhoids.[405,406] It is likely that it acts by disrupting the anorectal band described by Shafik[285] with a resulting release of the anal stenosis which seems to be responsible for the high rectal neck pressure that accompanies chronic anal fissure and hemorrhoids.[289,292]

The eight-finger dilatation may be accompanied by unpredictable sphincter damage.[342] Anorectal bandotomy[292] divides the band more accurately than manual dilatation and causes no sphincteric damage.

Internal anal sphincterotomy is widely used in the treatment of chronic anal fissure. Partial fecal incontinence, i.e. incontinence to fluid stools or flatus, occurs in approximately 25%. Fecal soiling may occur due to the "key-hole" deformity created by a posterior internal sphincterotomy, while lateral sphincterotomy might cause a less prominent groove and fewer control disorders than a posterior one. "Stress defecation"[163] or inability to hold stools for a long period might occur after internal sphincterotomy due to loss of the voluntary inhibition reflex as already mentioned.

Complications related to open or closed hemorrhoidectomy are few. Bleeding occurs in 4% of cases and is commonly of a secondary nature.[407]

Anal stenosis may be encountered due to excessive removal of anoderm. Fecal incontinence results from the destruction of sphincters during excision of the hemorrhoidal masses. It occurs in 0.4% of cases. Recurrence may occur from missed daughter or mother hemorrhoids.

## Fistula-in-Ano

The commonest complications of fistula operations are recurrence and functional disorders. Recurrence may be a true recurrence due to incomplete excision of the track or a "de novo" fistula due to infection of new areas of epithelial debris.[408] Functional disorders occur in the form of complete or partial fecal incontinence as a result of injury of the anal sphincters. Incontinence for solid stools was encountered in 3.4 % and for loose stools or flatus in 17% and 25%, respectively.[409] Fistulotomy may be associated with partial fecal incontinence since the internal anal sphincter is always divided in such operations. Fistulectomy injures the external anal sphincter more commonly than fistulotomy and thus has a higher incidence of incontinence. For this reason, fistulotomy is now more commonly practiced than fistulectomy.

## Rectal Prolapse

Both constipation with excessive straining (strainodynia) and fecal incontinence are frequently associated with rectal procidentia. Preceding studies have shown that procidentia is due to levator subluxation and sagging that might result from pregnancy trauma, strainodynia, or senility.[325] Levator sagging exposes the rectal neck to the direct action of the intraabdominal pressure. At stool, the increased intraabdominal pressure, acting on the rectal neck, obstructs the fecal stream with a resulting constipation.[333] In cases with advanced levator subluxation and sagging, the pudendal nerve is pulled down and stretched. This might lead to pudendal neuropathy and pudendal canal syndrome[368] which presents with fecal incontinence.[369]

Operations for cure of rectal prolapse are either perineal or abdominal. The anatomic complications of the abdominal rectopexy with or without sigmoidectomy are constipation which is attributable to the constricting action of the graft applied to the rectum. Furthermore, a preexisting constipation or fecal incontinence may not improve after rectopexy as the latter cures the rectal prolapse by mechanical fixation of the rectum without managing the disordered levator ani muscle.[410] Therefore, repair of the levator muscle should be an integral part in any operation for the cure of rectal prolapse.[410]

## Rectal Cancer

Today operations for rectal cancer are directed to sphincter-saving procedures. In tumors of the upper or middle third of the rectum, there is no problem with continence. Tumors of the lower third may compromise continence due to encroachment on the control mechanism, whether sphincteric or sensory. These patients complain commonly of fecal soiling.

Other complications that occur during abdominal dissection of the rectum are injury to the pelvic nerve leading to urinary and sexual disorders in the form of urinary retention, impotence, and ejaculatory failure. To avoid these complications, nerve-sparing operations are now adopted in many centers. Other anatomic complications include ureteric injuries and median sacral artery injury.

## Abdominoperineal Resection

The anatomic complications of abdominoperineal resection can be summarized as: (1) vascular injury, (2) organ injury, and (3) nerve injury.

Presacral veins, the left iliac vein, the middle rectal artery (if present), and the inferior hemorrhoidal vessels are subject to injury.

Trauma to the left ureter, duodenum, urinary bladder, and male urethra must be avoided. Other complications of abdominoperineal resection are: inadequate reconstruction of the peritoneal floor, small bowel obstruction, colostomy complications, rupture of the rectum, and contamination.

Injury to the sympathetic or parasympathetic nerves may result in bladder dysfunction, failure of ejaculation, impotence, and retention of urine.[41] The surgeon should remember that the pelvic splanchnics (nervi erigentes) penetrate the fascia of Waldeyer; therefore, the fascia of Waldeyer should be divided at the tip of the coccyx.

The ureter (and the lateral ligaments of the rectum) must be traced deep into the pelvis by careful dissection without elevation; after this, division of the colon and formation of the colostomy can be done. The pelvic peritoneum should be closed to avoid herniation and obstruction of the small bowel.

The perineal phase of the abdominoperineal dissection encounters the following structures: the pudendal vessels (which should be ligated), the levator plate (which should be excised widely), and the membranous urethra of the male (into which a Foley catheter is placed prior to surgery). Use sharp dissection to separate the prostate from the lower rectum. The perineum should be partially or completely closed; a suction drain is advisable.

# REFERENCES

1. Van Damme JPJ. Behavioral anatomy of the abdominal arteries. Surg Clin North Am 1993;73:699-725.

2. Ferguson JA, Parks AG. Cited in Rains AJH, Ritchie HD (eds). Bailey & Love's Short Practice of Surgery (18th ed). London: HK Lewis & Co, 1981, p. 1095.

3. Langman JM, Rowland R. The number and distribution of lymphoid follicles in the human large intestine. J Anat 1986;149: 189-194.

4. Okamota E, Ueda T. Embryogenesis of intramural ganglia of the gut and its relation to Hirschsprung's disease. J Pediatr Surg 1967;2: 437.

5. O'Rahilly R, Müller F. Human Embryology & Teratology (2nd ed). New York: Wiley-Liss, 1996, p. 234.

6. Rowe JS Jr, Skandalakis JE, Gray SW, Olafson RP, Steinmann RJ. The surgical anal canal. Contemp Surg 5:107-116, 1974.

7. Gross RE. The Surgery of Infancy and Childhood. Philadelphia: Saunders, 1958.

8. Davis DL, Poynter CWM. Congenital occlusions of the intestine. Surg Gynecol Obstet 1922;34:35.

9. Sturim HS, Ternberg JL. Congenital atresia of the colon. Surgery 1966;59:458.

10. Dalla Vecchia LK, Grosfeld JL, West KW, Rescorla FJ, Scherer LR, Engum SA. Intestinal atresia and stenosis: a 25-year experience with 277 cases. Arch Surg 1998;133:490-497.

11. Lambrecht W, Kluth D. Hereditary multiple atresias of the gastrointestinal tract: report of a case and review of the literature. J Pediatr Surg 1998;33:794-797.

12. Stone WD, Hendrix TR, Schuster MM. Aganglionosis of the entire colon in an adolescent. Gastroenterology 48:636-641, 1965.

13. Skandalakis JE, Gray SW. Embryology for Surgeons (2nd ed). Baltimore: Williams & Wilkins, 1994.

14. Lohlun J, Margolis M, Gorecki P, Schein M. Fecal impaction causing megarectum-producing colorectal catastrophes. A report of two cases. Dig Surg 2000;17:196-198.

15. Wulkan ML, Georgeson KE. Primary laparoscopic endorectal pull-through for Hirschsprung's disease in infants and children.

Semin Laparosc Surg 1998;5:9-13.

16. Balthazar EJ. Congenital positional anomalies of the colon: Radiographic diagnosis and clinical implications. Gastrointest Radiol 1977;2:41-47.

17. DePrima SJ, Hardy DC, Brant WE. Reversed intestinal rotation. Radiology 1985;157:603-604.

18. Prassopoulos P, Raissaki M, Daskalogiannaki M, Gourtsoyiannis N. Retropsoas positioned bowel: incidence and clinical relevance. J Comput Assisted Tomogr 1998;22:304-307.

19. Herman TE, Coplen D, Skinner M. Congenital short colon with imperforate anus. Pediatr Radiol 2000;30:243-246.

20. Wakhlu AK, Wakhlu A, Pandey A, Agarwal R, Tandon RK, Kureel SN. Congenital short colon. World J Surg 20:107-114, 1996.

21. Kim HL, Gow KW, Penner JG, Blair GK, Murphy JJ, Webber EM. Presentation of low anorectal malformations beyond the neonatal period. Pediatrics 2000;105:E68.

22. Connaughton JC, Poletti L, Broderick T, Sugerman HJ. Rectal duplication cyst with a large perineal hernia presenting as recurrent perineal abscesses. Surgery 124:926-928, 1998.

23. Susuki K, Baba M, Sasaki K. Two cases of non-rotation in adults: Its anatomical analysis. Clin Anat 1993;6:111-115.

24. Peveretos P, Krespis E, Polydorou A, Golematis B. Incontinence anale idiopathique: Cure chirurgicale [French]. J Chir (Paris) 1987; 124:399-402.

25. Gordon PH. Retrorectal tumors. In: Gordon PH, Nivatvongs S (eds.). Principles and Practice of Surgery for the Colon, Rectum, and Anus, St. Louis, MO: Quality Medical Publishing, Inc. 1992, pp. 383-400.

26. Williams PL, Warwick R, Dyson M, Bannister LH (eds). Gray's Anatomy (37th ed). Edinburgh: Churchill Livingstone, 1989, pp. 1774-1787, p. 194.

27. Goligher JC. Surgical anatomy of the colon, rectum and anal canal. In: Turell R (ed). Diseases of the Colon and Anorectum (2nd ed). Philadelphia: WB Saunders, 1969.

28. Saunders BP, Phillips RK, Williams CB. Intraoperative measurement of colonic anatomy and attachments with relevance to colonoscopy. Br J Surg 1995;82:1491-1493.

29. Sadahiro S, Ohmura T, Yamada Y, Saito T, Taki Y. Analysis of length and surface area of each segment of the large intestine according to age, sex, and physique. Surg Radiol Anat 1992;14: 251-257.

30. Steward J, Rankin FW. Blood supply of the large intestine: Its surgical considerations. Arch Surg 1933;26:843.

31. George R. Topography of the unpaired visceral branches of the abdominal aorta. J Anat 1935;69:196.

32. Michels NA, Siddharth P, Kornblith PL, Parke WW. The variant blood supply to the small and large intestine: its import in regional resections. J Int Coll Surg 1963;39:127.

33. Cheng B, Chen K, Gao S, Tu Z. Colon interposition. Recent Results Cancer Res 2000;155:151-160.

34. Furst H, Hartl WH, Lohe F, Schildberg FW. Colon interposition for esophageal replacement: an alternative technique based on the use of the right colon. Ann Surg 2000;231:173-178.

35. Griffiths JD. Surgical anatomy of the blood supply of the distal colon. Ann R Coll Surg 1956;19:241-256.

36. Van Damme JPJ, Bonte J. Vascular Anatomy in Abdominal Surgery. New York: Thieme Verlag, 1990.

37. Dworkin MJ, Allen-Mersh TG. Effect of inferior mesenteric

artery ligation on blood flow in the marginal artery - dependent sigmoid colon. J Am Coll Surg 1996;183:357-360.

38. Adachi Y, Kakisako K, Sato K, Shiraishi N, Miyahara M, Kitano S. Factors influencing bowel function after low anterior resection and sigmoid colectomy. Hepatogastroenterology 2000;47:155-158.

39. Haigh PI, Temple WJ. The gargantuan marginal artery sign: a case report of averting total necrosis of the small intestine. Surgery 123; 362-364, 1998.

40. Sudeck P. Ueber die Gefässversorgung des Mastdarmes in Hinsicht auf die operative Gangrän. Med Wschr (Muenchen) 1907;54:1314.

41. Goligher JC. Surgery of the Anus, Rectum and Colon (4th ed). London: Baillière Tindall, 1980.

42. Bertelli L, Lorenzini L, Bertelli E. The arterial vascularization of the large intestine: anatomical and radiological study. Surg Radiol Anat 1996;18(Suppl I):S1-S59.

43. Voiglio EJ, Boutillier du Retail C, Neidhardt JPH, Caillot JL, Barale F, Mertens P. Gastrocolic vein: Definition and report of two cases of avulsion. Surg Radiol Anat 1998;20:197-201.

44. Fishman SJ, Shamberger RC, Fox VL, Burrows PE. Endorectal pull-through abates gastrointestinal hemorrhage from colorectal venous malformations. J Pediatr Surg 2000;35:982-984.

45. Yada H, Sawai K, Taniguchi H, Hoshima M, Katoh M, Takahashi T. Analysis of vascular anatomy and lymph node metastases warrants radical segmental bowel resection for colon cancer. World J Surg 21:109-115, 1997.

46. Guyton AC, Hall JE. Textbook of Medical Physiology (9th ed). Philadelphia: WB Saunders Co, 1996.

47. Anson BJ, McVay CB. Surgical Anatomy (5th ed). Philadelphia: Saunders, 1971.

48. Pavlov S, Pétrov V. Sur l'anse sous-clavièr de l'artère sous-clavièr droite rétro-oesophagienne. Folia Med (Plovdiv) 1968;10:73-78.

49. Skandalakis JE. Volvulus of the cecum: clinical, anatomical and experimental work (thesis). Athens (Greece): University of Athens Medical School, 1949.

50. Treves F. The anatomy of the intestinal canal and peritoneum in man. Br Med J 1885;1:415.

51. Sappey PC. Traité d'Anatomie Descriptive (3rd ed). Paris: VA Delahaye et Cie., 1879. Cited in: DiDio LJA, Anderson MC. The "Sphincters" of the Digestive System: Anatomical, Functional and Surgical Considerations. Baltimore: Williams & Wilkins, 1968, p. 152.

52. DiDio LJA, Anderson MC. The "Sphincters" of the Digestive System: Anatomical, Functional and Surgical Considerations. Baltimore: Williams & Wilkins, 1968.

53. Kumar D, Phillips SF. The contribution of external ligamentous attachments to function of the ileocecal junction. Dis Colon Rectum 1987;30:410-416.

54. Bogers JJ, Van Marck E. The ileocecal junction. Histol Histopath 1993;8:561-566.

55. Gedgaudas-McClees, R Kristin. (Clinical Professor of Radiology, Saint Joseph's Hospital, Atlanta GA) Letter to: John E. Skandalakis. 1995 Dec 20.

56. Silverman PM, Kelvin FM, Baker ME, Cooper C. Computed tomography of the ileocecal region. Comput Med Imaging Graph 1988; 12:293-303.

57. Khope S, Rao PL. Cecal volvulus in a 2-month-old baby. J Pediatr Surg 1988;23:1038.

58. Shoop SA, Sackier JM. Laparoscopic cecopexy for cecal volvulus.

59. Frank AJ, Goffner LB, Fruauff AA, Losada RA. Cecal volvulus: The CT whirl sign. Abdom Imaging 1993;18:288-289.

60. Moore JH, Cintron Jr, Duarte B, Espinosa G, Abcarian H. Synchronous cecal and sigmoid volvulus: Report of a case (Review). Dis Colon Rectum 1992;35:803-805.

61. Theuer C, Cheadle WG. Volvulus of the colon. Am Surg 1991;57: 145-150.

62. VanderKolk W, Snyder CA, Figg DM. Cecal-colic adult intussusception as a cause of intestinal obstruction in Central Africa. World J Surg 20:341-344, 1996.

63. Lear TF, Gray SW, Milsap JH, Skandalakis JE. Benign lesions of the right colon. J Med Assoc Ga 60:271-275, 1971.

64. Astler VB, Miller EB, Snyder RS, McIntyre CH, Lillie RH. Benign surgical lesions of the cecum. Arch Surg 86:435, 1963.

65. Hatch KF, Blanchard DK, Hatch GF III, Wertheimer-Hatch L, Davis GB, Foster RS Jr, Skandalakis JE. Tumors of the appendix and colon. World J Surg 24:430-436, 2000.

66. Hatch KF, Blanchard DK, Hatch GF III, Wertheimer-Hatch L, Davis GB, Foster RS Jr, Skandalakis JE. Tumors of the rectum and anal canal. World J Surg 24:437-443, 2000.

67. Simon AM, Birnbaum BA, Jacobs JE. Isolated infarction of the cecum. Radiology 2000;214:513-516.

68. Nelson RL. Division of the colorectum into anatomic subsites: Why and where? J Surg Oncol 1998;69:1-3.

69. Poon RT-P, Chu K-W. Inflammatory cecal masses in patients presenting with appendicitis. World J Surg 1999;23:713-716.

70. Mann GN, Scoggins CR, Adkins B. Perforated cecal adenocarcinoma presenting as a thigh abscess. South Med J 90(9):949-951, 1997.

71. Skandalakis JE, Colborn GL, Skandalakis LJ. The embryology of the inguinofemoral area: an overview. Hernia 1:45-54, 1997.

72. Wolfer JA, Beaton LE, Anson BJ. Volvulus of the cecum: anatomical factors in its etiology. Report of a case. Surg Gynecol Obstet 1942;74:882.

73. Symington J. The relations of the peritoneum to the descending colon in the human subject. J Anat Physiol 1892;26:530.

74. Haskin PH, Teplick SK, Teplick JG, Haskin ME. Volvulus of the cecum and right colon. JAMA 1981;245:2433.

75. Rogers RL, Harford FJ. Mobile cecum syndrome. Dis Colon Rectum 1984;27:399-402.

76. Wright TP, Max MH. Cecal volvulus: review of 12 cases. South Med J 1988;81:1233-1235.

77. Ballantyne GH, Brandner MD, Beart RW Jr, Ilstrup DM. Volvulus of the colon: Incidence and mortality. Ann Surg 1985;202:83-92.

78. Rabinovici R, Simansky DA, Kaplan O, Mavor E, Manny J. Cecal volvulus [Review]. Dis Colon Rectum 1990;33:765-769.

79. Jones IT, Fazio VW. Colonic volvulus: Etiology and management [Review]. Dig Dis 1989;7:203-209.

80. Benacci JC, Wolff BG. Cecostomy. Therapeutic indications and results. Dis Colon Rectum 1995;38:530-534.

81. Marinella MA. Acute colonic pseudo-obstruction complicated by cecal perforation in a patient with Parkinson's disease. South Med J 1997;90(10):1023-1026.

82. Woodburne RT, Burkel WE. Essentials of Human Anatomy (9th ed). New York: Oxford University Press, 1994.

83. Charnsangavej C, DuBrow RA, Varma DGK, Herron DH, Robinson TJ, Whitley NO. CT of the mesocolon. Part 1. Anatomic

Case report and a review of the literature [Review]. Surg Endosc 1993;7:450-454.

considerations. Radiographics 1993;13:1035-1045.

84. Charnsangavej C, DuBrow RA, Varma DGK, Herron DH, Robinson TJ, Whitley NO. CT of the mesocolon. Part 2. Pathologic considerations. Radiographics 1993;13:1309-1322.

85. Robillard GL, Shapiro AL. Variational anatomy of the middle colic artery. J Int Coll Surg 1947;10:157.

86. Hollinshead WH. Anatomy for Surgeons (2nd ed). New York: Harper & Row, 1968, Volume 2, p. 497.

87. Horiuchi T, Shimomatsuya T, Uchinami M, Yoshida M, Amaya H, Aotake T, Chiba Y, Imamura Y. Retroperitoneoscopic excision of a mesenteric cyst. J Laparoendosc Adv Surg Tech (Part A) 2000;10;59-61.

88. Dixon AK, Henderson PJ, Oliver JL, Matthewson MH. Posteriorly situated retroperitoneal colon: A study using CT and MRI. Clin Anat 1993;6:269-274.

89. Hadar H, Gadoth N. Positional relations of colon and kidney determined by perirenal fat. Am J Roentgenol 1984;143:773-776.

90. Sherman JL, Hopper KD, Green AJ, Johns TT. The retrorenal colon on computed tomography: A normal variant. J Comput Assist Tomogr 1985;9:339-341.

91. Hopper KD, Maj MC, Sherman JL, Luethke JM. The retrorenal colon in the supine and prone patient. Radiology 1987;162:443-446.

92. Helms CA, Munk PL, Witt WS, Davis GW, Morris J, Onik G. Retrorenal colon: Implications for percutaneous diskectomy. Radiology 1989;171:864-865.

93. Prassopoulos PN, Gourtsoyiannis N, Cavouras D, Pantelidis N. A study of the variation of colonic positioning in the pararenal space as shown by computed tomography. Eur J Radiol 1990;10:44-47.

94. LeRoy AJ, Williams HJ, Bender CE, Segura JW, Patterson DE, Benson RC. Colon perforation following percutaneous nephrostomy and renal calculus removal. Radiology 1985;155:83-85.

95. Bonaldi G, Belloni G, Prosetti D, Moschini L. Percutaneous discectomy using Onik's method: 3 years' experience. Neuroradiology 1991;33:516-519.

96. Grant JCB, Basmajian JV. Grant's Method of Anatomy (7th ed). Baltimore: Williams & Wilkins, 1965, p. 258.

97. Manasse P. Die arterielle Gefässversorgung des S. Romanum in ihrer Bedetung für die operative Verlagerung desselben. Arch Klin Chir 1907;83:999.

98. Shafik A. Sigmoido-rectal junction reflex: role in the defecation mechanism. Clin Anat 9:391-394, 1996.

99. Anson BJ. An Atlas of Human Anatomy (2nd ed). Philadelphia: Saunders, 1963.

100. Vaez-Zadeh K, Dutz W. Ileosigmoid knotting. Ann Surg 1970; 172:1027.

101. Shafik A. A new concept of the anatomy of the anal sphincter mechanism and the physiology of defecation: IV. Anatomy of the perianal spaces. Invest Urol 13:424, 1976.

102. Milligan ETC, Morgan CN, Jones LE, Officer R. Surgical anatomy of the anal canal, and the operative treatment of haemorrhoids. Lancet 1937:2:1119.

103. Courtney H. Anatomy of the pelvic diaphragm and anorectal musculature as related to sphincter preservation in anorectal surgery. Am J Surg 1950;79:155.

104. Milligan ETC. The surgical anatomy and disorders of the perianal space. Proc R Soc Med 1943;36:365.

105. Shafik JA. A new concept of the anatomy of the anal sphincter mechanism and the physiology of defecation: III. The longitudinal anal muscle: Anatomy and role in anal sphincter mechanism. Invest Urol 1976;13:271.

106. Haagensen CD, Feind CR, Herter FP, Slanetz CA, Weinberg JA. The Lymphatics in Cancer. Philadelphia: Saunders, 1972.

107. Parks AG. Pathogenesis and treatment of fistula-in-ano. Br Med J 1961;1:463.

108. Jackman RJ, Clark PL III, Smith ND. Retrorectal tumors. JAMA 1951;145:956-962.

109. Heald RJ, Moran BJ. Embryology and anatomy of the rectum. Semin Surg Oncol 1998;15:66-71.

110. Heald RJ. The "Holy Plane" of rectal surgery. J R Soc Med 1988;81:503-508.

111. Konerding MA, Heintz A, Huhn P, Junginger T. [Rectal carcinoma. Optimizing therapy by knowledge of anatomy with special reference to the mesorectum]. [German] Zentralbl Chir 1999;124; 413-417.

112. Enker WE, Kafka NJ, Martz J. Planes of sharp pelvic dissection for primary, locally advanced, or recurrent rectal cancer. Semin Surg Oncol 2000;18:199-206.

113. Law WL, Chu KW, Ho JWC, Chan CW. Risk factors for anastomotic leakage after low anterior resection with total mesorectal excision. Am J Surg 2000;179:92-96.

114. Aeberhard P, Fasolini F, del Monte G. Anatomical basis and rationale of total mesorectal excision. Swiss Surg 1997;3:243-247.

115. Hohenberger W, Schick CH, Gohl J. Mesorectal lymph node dissection: is it beneficial? Langenbecks Arch Surg 1998;386:402-408.

116. Tiret E, Pocard M. [Total excision of the mesorectum and preservation of the genitourinary innervation in surgery of rectal cancer]. [French] Ann Chir 1999;53:507-514.

117. Leo E, Belli F, Andreola S, Gallino G, Bonfanti G, Ferro F, Zingaro E, Sirizotti G, Civelli E, Valvo F, Gios M, Brunelli C. Total rectal resection and complete mesorectum excision followed by coloendoanal anastomosis as the optimal treatment for low rectal cancer: the experience of the National Cancer Institute of Milano. Ann Surg Oncol 2000;7: 85-86 and 125-132.

118. Leong F. Selective total mesorectal excision for rectal cancer. Dis Colon Rectum 2000;43:1237-1240.

119. Tocchi A, Mazzoni G, Lepre L, Liotta G, Costa G, Agostini N, Miccini M, Scucchi L, Frati G, Tagliacozzo S. Total mesorectal excision and low rectal anastomosis for the treatment of rectal cancer and prevention of pelvic recurrences. Arch Surg 2001; 136:216-220.

120. Maurer CA, Renzulli P, Meyer JD, Buchler MW. [Rectal carcinoma. Optimizing therapy by partial or total mesorectum removal]. [German] Zentralbl Chir 1999;124:428-435.

121. Burke RM, Zavela D, Kaump DH. Significance of the anal gland. Am J Surg 1951;82:659.

122. Michels NA. Blood Supply and Anatomy of the Upper Abdominal Organs with a Descriptive Atlas. Philadelphia: Lippincott, 1955.

123. Boxall TA, Smart PJG, Griffiths JD. The blood supply of the distal segment of the rectum in anterior resection. Br J Surg 1962;50:399.

124. Last RJ. Anatomy: Regional and Applied (5th ed). Baltimore: Williams & Wilkins, 1972.

125. Vogel P, Klosterhalfen B. The surgical anatomy of the rectal and anal blood vessels [German]. Langenbecks Arch Chir 1988;373: 264-269.

126. Goligher JC. The blood supply to the sigmoid colon and rectum. Br J Surg 1949;37:157-162.

127. Batson OV. The function of the vertebral veins and their role in the spread of metastases. Ann Surg 1940;112:138.

128. Koch M, Weitz J, Kienle P, Benner A, Willeke F, Lehnert T, Herfarth C, von Knebel Doeberitz M. Comparative analysis of tumor cell dissemination in mesenteric, central, and peripheral venous blood in patients with colorectal cancer. Arch Surg 2001;136:85-89.

129. Ueno H, Mochizuki H, Fujimoto H, Hase K, Ichikura T. Autonomic nerve plexus involvement and prognosis in patients with rectal cancer. Br J Surg 2000;87:92-96.

130. Grinnell RS. Lymphatic metastases of carcinoma of the colon and rectum. Ann Surg 1950;131:494.

131. Morgan CN. Treatment of cancer of the rectum. Am J Surg 1968; 115:442.

132. Morgan CN. Carcinoma of the rectum. Ann R Coll Surg Engl 1965;36:73.

133. Williams ST, Beart RW Jr. Staging of colorectal cancer. Semin Surg Oncol 1992;8:89-93.

134. Granfield CA, Charnsangavej C, Dubrow RA, Varma DG, Curley SA, Whitley NO, Wallace S. Regional lymph node metastases in carcinoma of the left side of the colon and rectum: CT demonstration. AJR Am J Roentgenol 1992;159:757-761.

135. Madden JL, McVeigh GJ. The extension of operation in the treatment of carcinoma in the region of the splenic flexure. Surg Clin North Am 1954;34:523.

136. Block IR, Enquist IF. A more radical resection for carcinoma of the rectum in the female. Surg Gynecol Obstet 1964;119:1328.

137. Davies MRQ. Anatomy of the nerve supply of the rectum, bladder, and internal genitalia in anorectal dysgenesis in the male. J Pediatr Surg 32(4):536-541, 1997.

138. Duthie HL, Gairns FW. Sensory nerve endings and sensation in the axial region of man. Br J Surg 1960;47:38.

139. Stelzner F, Fritsch H, Fleischhauer K. The surgical anatomy of the genital nerves of the male and their preservation in excision of the rectum [German]. Chirurg 1989;60:228-234.

140. Williams JT, Slack WW. A prospective study of sexual function after major colorectal surgery. Br J Surg 1980;67:772-774.

141. Pearl RK, Monsen H, Abcarian H. Surgical anatomy of the pelvic autonomic nerves: A practical approach. Am Surg 1986;52(5): 236-237.

142. Gaston EA. The physiology of fecal continence. Surg Gynecol Obstet 1948;87:280.

143. Gunterberg B, Kewenter J, Petersen I, Stener B. Anorectal function after major resections of the sacrum with bilateral or unilateral sacrifice of sacral nerves. Br J Surg 1976;63:546-554.

144. Speakman CTM, Hoyle CHV, Kamm MA, Henry MM, Nicholls RJ, Burnstock G. Decreased sensitivity of muscarinic but not 5-hydroxytryptamine receptors of the internal anal sphincter in neurogenic faecal incontinence. Br J Surg 1992;79:829-832.

145. Sunderland S. Nerves and Nerve Injuries (2nd ed). Edinburgh: Churchill Livingstone, 1978, pp. 82-86.

146. Henry MM, Parks AG, Swash M. The pelvic floor musculature in the descending perineum syndrome. Br. J Surg 1982;69:470-472.

147. Fornell EKU, Berg G, Hallböök O, Matthiesen LS, Sjödahl R. Clinical consequences of anal sphincter rupture during vaginal delivery. J Am Coll Surg 1996;183:553-558.

148. Chifflet A. Surgery for cancer of the lower rectum: The perirectal fascia with reference to conservative surgery and technic. Dis Colon Rectum 1964;7:493.

149. Watson SJ, Loder PB, Halligan S, Bartram CI, Kamm MA, Phillips RKS. Transperineal repair of symptomatic rectocele with Marlex mesh: a clinical, physiological and radiologic assessment of treatment. J Am Coll Surg 183:257-261, 1996.

150. Merad F, Hay J-M, Fingerhut A, Yahchouchi E, Laborde Y, Pélissier E, Msika S, Flamant Y, The French Association for Surgical Research. Is prophylactic pelvic drainage useful after elective rectal or anal anastomosis? A multicenter controlled randomized trial. Surgery 1999;125:529-535.

151. Ross A, Rusnak C, Weinerman B, Kuechler P, Hayashi A, Mac Lachlan G, Frew E, Dunlop W. Recurrence and survival after surgical management of rectal cancer. Am J Surg 1999;177:392-395.

152. Siddharth P, Ravo B. Colorectal neurovasculature and anal sphincter. Surg Clin North Am 1988;68:1185-2000.

153. Healey JE Jr, Hodge J. Surgical Anatomy (2nd ed). Toronto: BC Decker, 1990, p. 262.

154. Azimuddin K, Stasik JJ, Rosen L, Riether RD, Khubchandani IT. Dieulafoy's lesion of the anal canal: a new clinical entity. Report of two cases. Dis Colon Rectum 2000;43:423-426.

155. Rao PM, Rhea JT, Wittenberg J, Warshaw AL. Misdiagnosis of primary epiploic appendagitis. Am J Surg 176:81-85, 1998.

156. Kuganeswaran E, Fisher JK. Giant sigmoid diverticulum: a rare manifestation of diverticular disease. South Med J 91(10):952-955, 1998.

157. Welton ML. Human colonic microvascular endothelial cells as a model of inflammatory bowel disease. Am J Surg 174:247-250, 1997.

158. Gordon PH, Nivatvongs S. Principles and Practice of Surgery for the Colon, Rectum, and Anus. St. Louis: Quality Medical Publishing, 1992, p. 7.

159. O'Kelly TJ, Brading A, Mortensen NJ. In vitro response of the human anal canal longitudinal muscle layer to cholinergic and adrenergic stimulation: evidence of sphincter specialization. Br J Surg 1993;80:1337-1341.

160. Delancey JO, Toglia MR, Perucchini D. Internal and external anal sphincter anatomy as it relates to midline obstetric lacerations. Obstet Gynecol 1997;90:924-927.

161. Haas PA, Fox TA Jr. The importance of the perianal connective tissue in the surgical anatomy and function of the anus. Dis Colon Rectum 1977;20:303-313.

162. Sangwan YP, Solla JA. Internal anal sphincter. Advances and insights. Dis Colon Rectum 1998;41:1297-1311.

163. Shafik A. A new concept of the anatomy of the anal sphincter mechanism and the physiology of defecation: IX. Single loop continence: A new theory of the mechanism of anal continence. Dis Colon Rectum 1980;23:37.

164. Shafik A. A new concept of the anatomy of the anal sphincter mechanism and the physiology of defecation. The external anal sphincter: A triple loop system. Invest Urol 1975;12:412

165. Oh C, Kark AE. Anatomy of the external anal sphincter. Br J Surg 1972;59:717.

166. Hollinshead WH. Anatomy for Surgeons. New York: Hoeber-Harper, 1956.

167. Kratzer GL, Dockerty MB. Histopathology of the anal ducts. Surg Gynecol Obstet 1947;84:333.

168. Klosterhalfen B. Offner F, Vogel P, Kirkpatrick CJ. Anatomic nature and surgical significance of anal sinus and anal intramuscular glands. Dis Colon Rectum 1991;34:156-160.

169. Heiken JP, Zuckerman GR, Balfe DM. The hypertrophied anal

papilla: recognition on air-contrast barium enema examinations. Radiology 1984;151:315-318.

170. Kusunoki M, Horai T, Sakanoue Y, Yanagi H, Yamamura T, Utsunomiya J. Giant hypertrophied anal papilla. Case report. Eur J Surg 1991;157:491-492.

171. Schutte AG, Tolentino MG. A second study of anal papillae. Dis Colon Rectum 1971;14:435.

172. Mollen RM, Kuijpers JH, van Hoek F. Effects of rectal mobilization and lateral ligament division on colonic and anorectal function. Dis Colon Rectum 2000;43:1283-1287.

173. Havenga K, DeRuiter MC, Enker WE, Welvaart K. Anatomical basic of autonomic nerve-preserving total mesorectal excision for rectal cancer. Br J Surg 1996;83:384-388.

174. Gorski T, Khubchandani IT, Stasik JJ, Riether R. Retrorectal carcinoid tumor. South Med J 1999;92:417-420.

175. Brasel KJ, Borgstrom DC, Weigelt JA. Management of penetrating colon trauma: A cost-utility analysis. Surgery 1999;125:471-479.

176. Curran TJ, Borzotta AP. Complications of primary repair of colon injury: literature review of 2,964 cases. Am J Surg 1999; 177:42-47.

177. McDaniel KP, Charnsangavej C, DuBrow RA, Varma DG, Granfield CA, Curley SA. Pathways of nodal metastasis in carcinomas of the cecum, ascending colon, and transverse colon: CT demonstration. AJR Am J Roentgenol 1993;161:61-64.

178. Lane JS, Sarkar R, Schmit PJ, Chandler CF, Thompson JE. Surgical approach to cecal diverticulitis. J Am Coll Surg 1999;188:629-634.

179. McDonald JM, Moonka R, Bell RH. Pathologic risk factors of occult malignancy in endoscopically unresectable colonic adenomas. Am J Surg 1999;177:384-387.

180. Lopez-Kostner F, Lavery IC, Hool GR, Rybicki LA, Fazio VW. Total mesorectal excision is not necessary for cancers of the upper rectum. Surgery 124:612-618, 1998.

181. Heald RJ, Smedh RK, Kald A, Sexton R, Moran BJ. Abdominoperineal excision of the rectum—an endangered operation. Dis Colon Rectum 1997;40:747-751.

182. Havenga K, Enker WE, Norstein J, Moriya Y, Heald RJ, van Houwelingen HC, van de Velde CJ. Improved survival and local control after total mesorectal excision or D3 lymphadenectomy in the treatment of primary rectal cancer: an international analysis of 1411 patients. Eur J Surg Oncol 1999;25:368-374.

183. Wimmer AP, Bouffard JP, Storms PR, Pilcher JA, Liang CY, DeGuide JJ. Primary colon cancer without gross mucosal tumor: unusual presentation of a common malignancy. South Med J 91(12):1173-1176, 1998.

184. Hayashi N, Egami H, Kai M, Kurusu Y, Takano S, Ogawa M. Notouch isolation technique reduces intraoperative shedding of tumor cells into the portal vein during resection of colorectal cancer. Surgery 1999;125:369-374.

185. Condon RV, Lamphier TA. Surgical considerations in mobilizing the hepatic flexure. Surg Gynecol Obstet 1950;90:623.

186. Phelan JT, Nadler SH. A technique of hemicolectomy for carcinoma of the right colon. Surg Gynecol Obstet 1968;126:355.

187. Koea JB, Conlon K, Paty PB, Guillem JG, Cohen AM. Pancreatic or duodenal resection or both for advanced carcinoma of the right colon: is it justified? Dis Colon Rectum 2000;43:460-465.

188. Dixon CF. Anterior resection for carcinoma low in the sigmoid and the rectosigmoid. Surgery 1944;15:367.

189. Barnes JP. A pull-through technique for rectal resection. Surg

Gynecol Obstet 1966;123:357.

190. Sharma P, Klaasen H. Duodenal seromyectomy in the management of adherent colonic carcinoma in elderly patients. Can J Surg 40(4):289-293, 1997.

191. Eisen LK, Cunningham JD, Aufses AH. Intussusception in adults: institutional review. J Am Coll Surg 1999;188:390-395.

192. Michelassi F, Hurst R. Restorative proctocolectomy with J-pouch ileoanal anastomosis. Arch Surg 2000;135:347-353.

193. ReMine SG, Dozois RR. Hartmann's procedure: Its use with complicated carcinomas of sigmoid colon and rectum. Arch Surg 1981; 116:630.

194. Bell GA. Closure of colostomy following sigmoid colon resection for perforated diverticulitis. Surg Gynecol Obstet 1980;150:85.

195. Bardoel JWJM, Stadelmann WK, Tobin GR, Werker PMN, Stremel RW, Kon M, Barker JH. Use of the rectus abdominis muscle for abdominal stoma sphincter construction: an anatomical feasibility study. Plast Reconstr Surg 2000;105:589-595.

196. Tschmelitsch J, Wykypiel H, Promegger R, Bodner E. Colostomy vs tube cecostomy for protection of a low anastomosis in rectal cancer. Arch Surg 1999;134:1385-1388.

197. Sakai Y, Nelson H, Larson D, Maidl L, Young-Fadok T, Ilstrup D. Temporary transverse colostomy vs loop ileostomy in diversion. Arch Surg 2001;136:338-342.

198. Hartmann H. Nouveau procede d'ablation des cancers de la partie terminale du colon pelvien. Strasbourg (France): Trentieme Congres de Chirurgie, 1921.

199. Belmonte C, Klas JV, Perez JJ, Wong WD, Rothenberger DA, Goldberg SM, Madoff RD. The Hartmann procedure: first choice or last resort in diverticular disease? Arch Surg 131:612-617, 1996.

200. Rosoff, L. Discussion. ReMine SG, Dozois RR. Hartmann's procedure: Its use with complicated carcinomas of sigmoid colon and rectum. Arch Surg 1981;116:630.

201. Liu CD, Rolandelli R, Ashley SW, Evans B, Shin M, McFadden DW. Laparoscopic surgery for inflammatory bowel disease. Am Surg 61(12):1054-1056, 1995.

202. Ichihara T, Nagahata Y, Nomura H, Fukumoto S, Urakawa T, Aoyama N, Kuroda Y. Laparoscopic lower anterior resection is equivalent to laparotomy for lower rectal cancer at the distal line of resection. Am J Surg 2000;179:97-98.

203. Reissman P, Cohen S, Weiss EG, Wexner SD. Laparoscopic colorectal surgery: ascending the learning curve. World J Surg 20: 277-282, 1996.

204. Leung KL, Kwok SPY, Lau WY, Meng WCS, Lam TY, Kwong KH, Chung CC, Li AKC. Laparoscopic-assisted resection of rectosigmoid carcinoma. Arch Surg 132:761-765, 1997.

205. Bouvet M, Mansfield PF, Skibber JM, Curley SA, Ellis LM, Giacco GG, Madary AR, Ota DM, Feig BW. Clinical, pathologic, and economic parameters of laparoscopic colon resection for cancer. Am J Surg 1998;176:554-558.

206. Targarona EM, Martínez J, Nadal A, Balagué C, Cardesa A, Pascual S, Trias M. Cancer dissemination during laparoscopic surgery: tubes, gas, and cells. World J Surg 22:55-61, 1998.

207. Tomita H, Marcello PW, Milsom JW. Laparoscopic surgery of the colon and rectum. World J Surg 1999;23:397-405.

208. Stocchi L, Nelson H. Laparoscopic colectomy for colon cancer: trial update. J Surg Oncol 1998;68:255-267.

209. Marubashi S, Hiroshi Y, Monden T, Hata T, Takahashi H, Fujita S, Kanoh T, Iwazawa T, Matsui S, Nakano Y, Tateishi H, Kinuta M, Takiguchi S, Okamura J. The usefulness, indications, and com-

plications of laparoscopy-assisted colectomy in comparison with those of open colectomy for colorectal carcinoma. Surg Today 2000;30:491-496.

210. Bussi M, Ferrero V, Riontino E, Gasparri G, Camandona M, Cortesina G. Problems in reconstructive surgery in the treatment of carcinoma of the hypopharyngoesophageal junction. J Surg Oncol 2000;74:130-133.

211. Soffer SZ, Rosen NG, Hong AR, Alexianu M, Pena A. Cloacal exstrophy: a unified management plan. J Pediatr Surg 2000;35:932-937.

212. Howell G, Caldamone A, Snyder H, Ziegler M, Ducket J. Optimal management of cloacal exstrophy. J Pediatr Surg 1983; 18:365-369.

213. Ricketts RR, Woodard JR, Zwiren GT, Andrews HG, Broecker BH. Modern treatment of cloacal exstrophy. J Pediatr Surg 1991;26:444-450.

214. Saunders BP, Masaki T, Sawada T, Halligan S, Phillips RK, Muto T, Williams CB. A peroperative comparison of Western and Oriental colonic anatomy and mesenteric attachments. Int J Colorectal Dis 1995;10:216-221.

215. Scoma JA. Salvati EP, Rubin RJ. Incidence of fistulas subsequent to anal abscesses. Dis Colon Rectum 1974;17:357.

216. Adams D, Kovalcik PJ. Fistula in ano. Surg Gynecol Obstet 1981; 153:731.

217. Nomikos IN. Anorectal abscesses: need for accurate anatomical localization of the disease. Clin Anat 10:239-244, 1997.

218. Argov S, Levandovsky O. Open lateral sphincterotomy is still the best treatment for chronic anal fissure. Am J Surg 2000;179:201-202.

219. Sharp FR. Patient selection and treatment modalities for chronic anal fissure. Am J Surg 171:512-515, 1996.

220. da Silva JH. Pilonidal cyst: cause and treatment. Dis Colon Rectum 2000;43:1146-1156.

221. Davis KA, Mock CN, Verasaci A, Lentrichia P. Malignant degeneration of pilonidal cysts. Am Surg 1994;60:200-204.

222. Herold A, Bruch HP. [Laparoscopic therapy of functional disorders of the rectum and pelvic floor]. [German] Langensbecks Arch Chir (Suppl Kongressband) 1997;114:905-908.

223. Schultz I, Mellgren A, Dolk A, Johansson C, Holmstrom B. Long-term results and functional outcome after Ripstein retropexy. Dis Colon Rectum 2000;43:35-43.

224. Blair S, Ellenhorn JD. Transanal excision for low rectal cancers is curative in early-stage disease with favorable histology. Am Surg 2000;66:817-820.

225. Agachan F, Reissman P, Pfeifer J, Weiss EG, Nogueras JJ, Wexner SD. Comparison of three perineal procedures for the treatment of rectal prolapse. South Med J 90(9):925-932, 1997.

226. Pikarsky AJ, Joo JS, Wexner SD, Weiss EG, Nogueras JJ, Agachan F, Iroatulam A. Recurrent rectal prolapse: what is the next good option? Dis Colon Rectum 2000;43:1273-1276.

227. Skandalakis LJ, Gadacz TR, Mansberger AR Jr, Mitchell WE Jr, Colborn GL, Skandalakis JE. Modern Hernia Repair. New York: Parthenon, 1996.

228. Dehni N, Cunningham C, Sarkis R, Parc R. Results of coloanal anastomosis for rectal cancer. Hepatogastroenterology 2000;47:323-326.

229. Read TE, Kodner IJ. Proctectomy and coloanal anastomosis for rectal cancer. Arch Surg 1999;134:670-677.

230. Di Matteo G, Mascagni D, Zeri KP, Torretta A, Di Matteo FM, Maturo A, Peparini N. Evaluation of anal function after surgery for rectal cancer. J Surg Oncol 2000;74:11-14.

231. Madoff RD, Baeten CG, Christiansen J, Rosen HR, Williams NS, Heine JA, Lehur PA, Lowry AC, Lubowski DZ, Matzel KE, Nicholls RJ, Seccia M, Thorson AG, Wexner SD, Wong WD. Standards for anal sphincter replacement. Dis Colon Rectum 2000;43:135-141.

232. Lamont JP, McCarty TM, Digan RD, Jacobson R, Tulanon P, Lichliter WE. Should locally excised $T_1$ rectal cancer receive adjuvant chemoradiation? Am J Surg 2000;180:402-406.

233. Gervaz P, Rotholtz N, Pisano M, Kaplan E, Secic M, Coucke P, Pikarsky A, Efron J, Weiss E, Wexner S. Quantitative short-term study of anal sphincter function after chemoradiation for rectal cancer. Arch Surg 2001;136:192-196.

234. Borgstein P, Meijer S. Historical perspective of lymphatic tumour spread and the emergence of the sentinel node concept. Eur J Surg Oncol 1998;24:85-89.

235. Saha S, Wiese D, Badin J, Beutler T, Nora D, Ganatra BK, Desai D, Kaushal S, Nagaraju M, Arora M, Singh T. Technical details of sentinel lymph node mapping in colorectal cancer and its impact on staging. Ann Surg Oncol 2000;7:82-84 and 120-124.

236. Schrock TR, DeVeney CW, Dunphy JE. Factors contributing to leakage of colonic anastomoses. Ann Surg 1973;177:513.

237. Welch CE, Ottinger LW, Welch JP: Manual of Lower Gastrointestinal Surgery. New York: Springer-Verlag, 1980.

238. Tocchi A, Mazzoni G, Lepre L, Costa G, Liotta G, Agostini N, Miccini M. Prospective evaluation of omentoplasty in preventing leakage of colorectal anastomosis. Dis Colon Rectum 2000;43:951-955.

239. Moran B, Heald R. Anastomotic leakage after colorectal anastomosis. Semin Surg Oncol 2000;18:244-248.

240. Patricio J, Bernades A, Nuno D, Falcao F, Silveira L. Surgical anatomy of the arterial blood supply of the human rectum. Surg Radiol Anat 1988;10:71-75.

241. Jansen A, Brummelkamp WH, Davies GAG, Klopper PJ, Keeman JN. Clinical application of magnetic rings in colorectal anastomosis. Surg Gynecol Obstet 1981;153:537.

242. Graham JW, Goligher JC. The management of accidental injuries and deliberate resections of the ureter during excision of the rectum. Br J Surg 1954;42:151.

243. Andersson A, Bergdahl L. Urologic complications following abdominoperineal resection of the rectum. Arch Surg 1976;111: 969.

244. Béland G. The abdominal surgeon and the ureter. Can J Surg 1979;22:540.

245. Kirkegaard P, Hjortrup A, Sanders S. Bladder dysfunction after low anterior resection for mid-rectal cancer. Am J Surg 1981;141:266.

246. Havenga K, Enker WE, McDermott K, Cohen AM, Minsky BD, Guillem J. Male and female sexual and urinary function after total mesorectal excision with autonomic nerve preservation for carcinoma of the rectum. J Am Coll Surg 182:495-502, 1996.

247. Mancini R, Cosimelli M, Filippini A, Tedesco M, Pugliese P, Marcellini M, Pietrangeli A, Lepiane P, Mascagni D, Cavaliere R, Di Matteo G. Nerve-sparing surgery in rectal cancer: feasibility and functional results. J Exper Clin Cancer Res 2000;19:35-40.

248. Goligher JC, Graham NG, DeDombal FT. Anastomotic dehiscence after anterior resection of rectum and sigmoid. Br J Surg 1970;57:109.

249. Chassin JL. Operative Strategy in General Surgery. New York:

Springer-Verlag 1980.

250. Hines JR, Harris GD. Colostomy and colostomy closure. Surg Clin North Am 1977;57:1379.

251. Varnell J, Pemberton LB. Risk factors in colostomy closure. Surgery 1981;89:683.

252. Stothert JC, Brubacher L, Simonowitz DA. Complications of emergency stoma formation. Arch Surg 1982;117:307.

253. Kasperk R, Klinge U, Schumpelick V. The repair of large parastomal hernias using a midline approach and a prosthetic mesh in the sublay position. Am J Surg 2000;179:186-188.

254. Nakai S, Yoshizawa H, Kobayashi S, Maeda K, Okumura Y. Anorectal and bladder function after sacrifice of the sacral nerves. Spine 2000;25:2234-2239.

255. Porter GA, O'Keefe GE, Yakimets WW. Inadvertent perforation of the rectum during abdominoperineal resection. Am J Surg 172:324-327, 1996.

256. Gedebou TM, Wong RA, Rappaport WD, Jaffe P, Kahsai D, Hunter GC. Clinical presentation and management of iatrogenic colon perforations. Am J Surg 172:454-458, 1996.

257. Church JM, Raudkivi PJ, Hill GL. The surgical anatomy of the rectum — a review with particular relevance to the hazards of rectal mobilisation. [Review]. Int J Colorectal Dis 1987;2:158-166.

258. Knoefel WT, Hosch SB, Hoyer B, Izbicki JR. The initial approach to anorectal abscesses: fistulotomy is safe and reduces the chance of recurrences. Dig Surg 2000;17:274-278.

259. Liberman H, Thorson AG. Anal stenosis. Am J Surg 2000;179:325-329.

260. Timaran CH, Sangwan YP, Solla JA. Adenocarcinoma in a hemorrhoidectomy specimen: case report and review of the literature. Am Surg 2000;66:789-792.

261. Bissett IP, Hill GL. Extrafascial excision of the rectum for cancer: a technique for the avoidance of the complications of rectal mobilization. Semin Surg Oncol 2000;18:207-215.

262. Ho YH, Tsang C, Tang CL, Nyam D, Eu KW, Seow-Choen F. Anal sphincter injuries from stapling instruments introduced transanally: randomized, controlled study with endoanal ultrasound and anorectal manometry. Dis Colon Rectum 2000;43:169-173.

263. Shafik A. Right colon flexure syndrome. Report of two cases. Coloproctology 1981;3:105-106.

264. Shafik A. Functional activity of the sigmoid colon and rectum: a study during fecal storage in the sigmoid. Coloproctology 1997;19:236-241.

265. Shafik A. The hypertonic rectosigmoid junction: description of a new clinicopathologic entity causing constipation. Surg Laparosc Endosc 1997;7:116-120.

266. Shafik A. Study of the electrical and mechanical activity of the rectum: an experimental study. Eur Surg Res 1994;26:87-93.

267. Shafik A. Study of the electromechanical activity of the rectum. II. Human study. Coloproctology 1993;15:215-221.

268. Shafik A, Nour A, Abdel-Fattah A. Transcutaneous electrorectography. Human electrorectogram from surface electrodes. Digestion 1995;56:479-482.

269. Shafik A. Rectosigmoid pacemaker: role in defecation mechanism and constipation. Dig Surg 1993;10:95-100.

270. Shafik A. Rectosigmoid pacemaker: role in defecation mechanism and constipation. (abstract) Dis Colon Rectum 1992;35:29-30.

271. Shafik A. Artificial pacemaker for rectal evacuation. Coloproctology 1992;14:96-98.

272. Shafik A, Moneim KA. Dynamic study of the rectal detrusor activity at defecation. Digestion 1991;49:167-174.

273. Shafik A, El-Sibai O, Moustafa R, Shafik I. Study of the mechanism of rectal motility. The "mass squeeze contraction." Arch Physiol Biochem 2002;109:418-423.

274. Shafik A. Artificial pacemaker for rectal evacuation. II. Role in patients with chronic idiopathic constipation. Proc 3rd Int Mtg Coloproct, Ivrea/Italy 1994, pp. 31-34.

275. Shafik A. Electrosigmoidogram, electrorectogram and their relation. Front Biosci 2 (1997), b12-16; PubMed No. 9294095.

276. Guyton AC, Hall JE. The gastrointestinal tract: nervous control, movement of food through the tract and blood flow. In: Guyton AC, Hall JE. (eds), Human Physiology and Mechanisms of Disease (6th ed). WB Saunders, Philadelphia 1997, pp. 511-523.

277. Shafik A. "Tube" and "marsupialization" colostomy: a simplified technique for colostomy. Am J Proct 1982;33:12-16.

278. Vesalius (1555). Quoted by Gabriel WB. The Principles and Practice of Rectal Surgery (5th ed). London: HK Lewis and Company, 1963, p. 15.

279. Last RJ: Anatomy, Regional and Applied. 5th Edition, reprint. Edinburgh & London: The English Language Book Society and Churchill Livingstone, 1973, p. 531.

280. Bill AH, Jr, Johnson RJ: Failure of migration of the rectal opening as a cause for most cases of imperforate anus. Surg Gynecol Obstet 1958;106:643.

281. Shafik A: A new concept of the anatomy of the anal sphincter mechanism and the physiology of defecation. V. The rectal neck: Anatomy and function. Chir Gastroenterol 1977;11:319-336.

282. Shafik A: A new concept of the anatomy of the anal sphincter mechanism and the physiology of defecation. VIII. Levator hiatus and tunnel. Anatomy and function. Dis Colon Rectum 1979;22:539-549.

283. Shafik A. A new concept of the anatomy of the anal sphincter mechanism and the physiology of defecation. XIX. The malformed rectum. A new theory of pathogenesis with simplified classification. Am J Proct Gastroent Col Rect Surg 1983;34:16-20.

284. Harding Rains AJ, David Ritchie H. In: Bailey and Love's Short Practice of Surgery. The esophagus (17th ed). The English Language Book Society & H.K. Lewis & Co. Ltd., 1979, p. 759.

285. Shafik A: A new concept of the anatomy of the anal sphincter mechanism and the physiology of defecation. X. Anorectal sinus and band: anatomical nature and surgical significance. Dis Colon Rectum 1980;23:170-179.

286. Shafik A: A new concept of the anatomy of the anal sphincter mechanism and the physiology of defecation. VII. Anal fistula: A simplified classification. Dis Colon Rectum 1979;22:408-414.

287. Shafik A: A new concept of the anatomy of the anal sphincter mechanism and the physiology of defecation. XXVI. Fistula-in-ano. A new theory of pathogenesis. Coloproctology 1988;10:148-156.

288. Shafik A, Abdel-Wahab E-S, El-Sibai O, Khalil A: Anorectal fistulae: Results of treatment with cauterization. Dig Surg 1994;11:16-19.

289. Shafik A: A new concept of the anatomy of the anal sphincter mechanism and the physiology of defecation. XV. Chronic anal fissure. A new theory of pathogenesis. Am J Surg 1982;144:262-268.

290. Shafik A: A new concept of the anatomy of the anal sphincter mechanism and the physiology of defecation. XXII. The pathogenesis of hemorrhoids and their treatment by anorectal bandotomy. J Clin Gastroent 1984;6:129-137.

291. Shafik A. Urethral discharge, constipation and hemorrhoids. New syndrome with report of 7 cases. Urology 1981;18:155-160.

292. Shafik A: A new concept of the anatomy of the anal sphincter mechanism and the physiology of defecation. XXVII. Treatment of hemorrhoids. Report of a technique. Am J Surg 1984;148:393-398.

293. Shafik A: A new concept of the anatomy of the anal sphincter mechanism and the physiology of defecation. XVI. Pruritus ani. A new theory of pathogenesis. Coloproctology 1981;3:239-243.

294. Shafik A: A new concept of the anatomy of the anal sphincter mechanism and the physiology of defecation. XXIII. An injection technique for the treatment of idiopathic pruritus ani. Int Surg 1990;75:43-46.

295. Goodsall DH, Miles WE: Diseases of the Anus and Rectum. London: Longmans, Green & Co. Part I, 1900-1905.

296. Allingham W, Allingham HW: The Diagnosis and Treatment of Diseases of the Rectum; Being a Practical Treatise on Fistula, Piles, Fissure and Painful Ulcer, Procidentia, Polypus, Stricture, Cancer, etc. London: Bailliere, Tindall and Cox, 1901.

297. Tuttle JP: A Treatise on Diseases of the Anus, Rectum and Pelvic Colon. New York: Appleton, 1902.

298. Lockhart-Mummery JP: Diseases of the Rectum and Colon and Their Surgical Treatment (2nd ed). Baltimore: William Wood, 1934.

299. Goligher JC: Surgery of the Anus, Rectum and Colon (3rd ed). London: Baillière Tindall, 1975, pp. 15, 17, 225.

300. Milligan ET, Morgan CN: Surgical anatomy of the anal canal with special reference to anorectal fistulae. Lancet 1934;2:1150, 1213.

301. Shafik A: A new concept of the anatomy of the anal sphincter mechanism and the physiology of defecation. II. Anatomy of the levator ani muscle with special reference to puborectalis. Invest Urol 1975;13:175-182.

302. Garry RC: The responses to stimulation of the caudal end of the large bowel in the cat. J Physiol 1933;78:208.

303. Bennett RC: Goligher JC. Results of internal sphincterotomy for anal fissure. Br Med J 1962;2:1500.

304. Parks AG, McPartlin JF: Late repair of injuries of the anal sphincter. Proc R Soc Med 1971;64:1187.

305. Mann A: Gracilis anoplasty: report of a successful case. Aust NZ J Surg 1970;39:405.

306. Caldwell KP: A new treatment of rectal prolapse. Proc R Soc Med 1965;58:792.

307. Shafik A, Gamal El-Din MA, El-Bagoury EM, Abdel Hamid Z, El-Said B, Metwalli S, Olfat E: A new concept of the anatomy of the anal sphincter mechanism and the physiology of defecation. The involuntary action of the external anal sphincter. Histologic study. Acta Anat 1990;138:359-363.

308. Shafik A, Gamal El-Din MA, El-Sibaei O, Abdel Hamid Z, El-Said B: Involuntary action of the external anal sphincter. Manometric and electromyographic studies. Eur Surg Res 1992;24: 188-196.

309. Shafik A: Polytetrafluoroethylene injection for the treatment of partial fecal incontinence. Int Surg 1993;78:159-161.

310. Shafik A: Perianal injection of autologous fat for treatment of sphincteric incontinence. Dis Colon Rectum 1995;38:583-587.

311. Shafik A: A new concept of the anatomy of the anal sphincter mechanism and the physiology of defecation. 17. Mechanism of defecation. Coloproctology 1982;4:49-54.

312. Shafik A: A new concept of the anatomy of the anal sphincter mechanism and the physiology of defecation. 42. Recto-pubo-rectalis reflex. Coloproctology 1990;12:170-172.

313. Shafik A. Recto-levator reflex. The description of a new reflex and its clinical application. Preliminary report. Clin Physiol Biochem 1993;10:13-17.

314. Shafik A: Levator-puborectalis reflex. The description of a new reflex and its clinical significance. Pract Gastroenterol 1991;15: 28-35.

315. Shafik A: Straining-levator reflex: the description of a new reflex and its clinical significance. Coloproctology 1991;13:314-319.

316. Denny-Brown D, Roberston EG. An investigation of the nervous control of defecation. Brain 1935;58: 256-310.

317. Schuster MM, Hookman P, Hendrix TR, Mendeloff AI. Simultaneous manometric recording of internal and external anal sphincter reflexes. Bull Johns Hopkins Hosp 1965;116:79-88.

318. Arhan P, Faverdin C, Persoz B, Devroede G, Dubois F, Dornic C, Pellerin D. Relationship between viscoelastic properties of the rectum and anal pressure in man. J Appl Physiol 1976;41:677-682.

319. Gowers WR. The autonomic action of the sphincter ani. Proc R Soc (London) 1877;26:77.

320. Shafik A. Deflation reflex. Description and clinical significance. Anat Rec 1997; 29: 405-408.

321. Shafik A. A study on the origin of the external anal, urethral, vaginal and prostatic sphincters. Int Urogynecol J 1997;8:126-129.

322. Shafik A. A new concept of the anatomy of the anal sphincter mechanism and the physiology of defecation: Mass contraction of the pelvic floor muscles. Int Urogynecol J 1998;9:28-32.

323. Shafik A. Pelvic double-sphincter control complex: Theory of pelvic organ continence with clinical application. Urology 1984; 23:611-618.

324. Shafik A: A new concept of the anatomy of the anal sphincter mechanism and the physiology of defecation. XII. Anorectal mobilization. A new surgical access to rectal lesions. Preliminary report. Am J Surg 1981;142:625-635.

325. Shafik A: A new concept of the anatomy of the anal sphincter mechanism and the physiology of defecation. XIII. Rectal prolapse. A concept of pathogenesis. Am J Proct Gastroent Col Rect Surg 1981;32:6.

326. Shafik A: Straining-puborectalis reflex: description and significance of a new reflex. Anat Rec 1991;229:281-284.

327. Shafik A: A new concept of the anatomy of the anal sphincter mechanism and the physiology of defecation. Reversion to normal defecation after combined operation and end colostomy for rectal cancer. Am J Surg 1986;15:278-284.

328. Shafik A: A new concept of the anatomy of the anal sphincter mechanism and the physiology of defecation. 31. Strainodynia: an etiopathologic study. J Clin Gastroenterol 1988;10:179-184.

329. Preston DM, Lennard-Jones JE: Anismus in chronic constipation. Dig Dis Sci 1985;30:413-418.

330. Shafik A: Detrusor-sphincter dyssynergia syndrome. A new syndrome and its treatment by external sphincter myotomy. Eur Surg Res 1990;22:243-248.

331. Turnbull GK, Lennard-Jones JE, Batram CL: Failure of rectal expulsion as a cause of constipation: why fiber and laxative sometimes fail. Lancet 1986;1:767-769.

332. Shafik A: Detrusor-rectal neck dyssynergia syndrome: a new syndrome with report of 9 cases. Int Surg 1991;76:241-244.

333. Shafik A: A new concept of the anatomy of the anal sphincter mechanism and the physiology of defecation. XVIII. The levator dysfunction syndrome: a new syndrome with report of 7 cases.

Coloproctology 1983;5:159-165.

334. Shafik A: Detrusor-levator dyssynergia syndrome: a new syndrome with report of 8 cases. Coloproctology 1990;12:369-373.

335. Shafik A: Levator paradoxical syndrome. A new syndrome. Proc 3rd Int Mtg Coloproctology (Ivrea, Italy) 1994, pp. 48-54.

336. Shafik A: Rectal detrusor retropulsion syndrome: report of 5 cases. Proc 2nd Int Mtg Coloproctology (Ivrea, Italy) 1992, pp. 69-77.

337. Shafik A: Idiopathic oligofecorrhea: a clinicopathologic entity. Pathogenesis and treatment. Digestion 1991;48:51-58.

338. Shafik A, Mohi-el-Din M. A new concept of the anatomy of the anal sphincter mechanism and the physiology of defaecation. XXIV. Haemorrhoidal venous plexuses: anatomy and role in haemorrhoids. Coloproctology 1985;7:291-296.

339. Thomson WAF: The nature of haemorrhoids. Br J Surg 1975; 62:542-552.

340. Stelzner F: Haemorrhoids and other diseases of the corpus cavernosum recti and the anal canal. Ger Med Mon 1963;8:177-182.

341. Goligher JC: Surgery of the Anus, Rectum and Colon. Baillière Tindall, London (5th ed). 1984, pp. 98-149.

342. Goldberg SM, Gordon PH, Nivatvongs S: Essentials of Anorectal Surgery. Philadelphia: Lippincott, 1980, pp. 69-85.

343. Shafik A: Anal cystography. New technique of cystography. Preliminary report. Urology 1984;23:313-316.

344. Shafik A, Mohi M: Pelvic organ venous communications. Anatomy and role in urogenital diseases. A new technique of cysto-vagino-hysterography. Am J Obstet Gynecol 1988;159:347-351.

345. Shafik A: Role of hemorrhoids in the pathogenesis of recurrent bacteriuria with a new approach for treatment. Eur Urol 1985;11: 392-396.

346. Shafik A, Saleh F, Twefik O, Abdel-Azim S, Saad R, Olfat E, Sharkawi A: The role of hemorrhoids in urinary tract infection: A clinicobacteriologic study. Pract Gastroenterol 1989;13:21-29.

347. Shafik A, Haddad S, Elwan F, El-Metnawi W, Olfat E: Anal submucosal injection: A new route for drug administration in pelvic malignancies. II. Methotrexate anal injection in the treatment of advanced bladder cancer (preliminary study). J Urol 1988;140:501.

348. Shafik A: Perineal versus anal submucosal injection of chemotherapeutic drugs. Eur Urol 1992;21:256. (Letter to the Editor).

349. Shafik A, El-Merzabani MM, El-Aaser AA, et al: Anal submucosal injection. A new route for drug administration in pelvic malignancies. I. Experimental study of misonidazole distribution in serum and tissues, with special reference to urinary bladder. Invest Radiol 1986;21:278-281.

350. Shafik A, El-Desouky G: Anal submucosal injection: A new route for drug administration in pelvic malignancies. III. Misonidazole distribution in serum, uterus and vagina: An experimental study. Gynecol Obstet Invest 1990;29:219-223.

351. Shafik A: Anal submucosal injection: A new route for drug administration in pelvic malignancies. V. Advanced prostatic cancer: results of methotrexate treatment using the anal route. Preliminary study. Eur Urol 1990;18:132-136.

352. Shafik A: Anal submucosal injection: A new route for drug administration in pelvic malignancies. IV. Submucosal anal injection in treatment of cancer of uterine cervix. Preliminary study. Am J Obstet Gynecol 1989;161: 69-72.

353. Shafik A, El-Metnawi W, El-sibai O. Treatment of advanced rectal cancer by anal submucosal injection. Eur J Surg Oncol 1999;25:76-81

354. Shafik A, El-Dawi M, El-Metnawy W. Anal submucosal injection:

methotrexate concentration in rectal tumor tissue and serum after anal compared with parenteral injection. Anti-Cancer Drugs 1994;5:650-654.

355. Shafik A: Anal submucosal injection: A new route for drug administration. VI. Chronic prostatitis: A new modality of treatment with report of eleven cases. Urology 1991;37:61.

356. Shafik A, Moustafa H. Study of the arterial pattern of the rectum and its clinical application. Acta Anat 1996;157:80-86.

357. Ripstein CB. Procidentia: definitive corrective surgery. Dis Colon Rectum 1972;15:334-336.

358. Heald RJ. Ryall RDH. Recurrence and survival after total mesorectal excision for rectal cancer. Lancet 1986;i:1479-1482.

359. Guyton AC. Movement of food through the alimentary tract. In: Guyton AC (ed). Human Physiology and Mechanics of Disease (4th ed). Philadelphia: WB Saunders, 1987, pp. 486-496.

360. Connell AM. The motility of the pelvic colon. I. Motility in normals and in patients with asymptomatic duodenal ulcer. Gut 1961;2:175-186.

361. Truelove SC. Movements of the large intestine. Physiol Rev 1966; 46:457-512.

362. Edwards DA, Beck ER. Movement of radiopacified feces during defecation. Am J Dig Dis 1971;16:709-711.

363. Shafik A, Ali YA, Afifi R. Is the rectum a conduit or storage organ? Int Surg 1997;82:194-197.

364. Kiff ES, Swash M: Slow conduction in pudendal nerves in idiopathic fecal (neurogenic) incontinence. Br J Surg 1984;71: 614-616.

365. Neil ME, Parks AG, Swash M: Physiological studies of the pelvic floor in idiopathic fecal incontinence and rectal prolapse. Br J Surg 1981;68:531-536.

366. Jones PN, Lubowski DZ, Swash M, Henry MM: Relationship between perineal descent and pudendal nerve incontinence. Int J Colorect Dis 1987;9:3-7.

367. Womack NR, Morrison JFB, Williams NS: The role of pelvic floor denervation in etiology of idiopathic fecal incontinence. Br J Surg 1986;73:404-408.

368. Shafik A: Pudendal canal syndrome. Description of a new syndrome and its treatment: Report of 7 cases. Coloproctology 1991; 13:102-110.

369. Shafik A: Pudendal canal decompression in the treatment of idiopathic fecal incontinence. Dig Surg 1992;9:265-271.

370. Shafik A: Chronic scrotalgia: Report of four cases with successful treatment. Pain Digest 1993;3:252-256.

371. Thuroff JW, Bazeed MA, Schmidt RA, Wiggin DM, Tanagho EA: Functional pattern of sacral root stimulation in dogs. I. Micturition. J Urol 1982;127:1031-1033.

372. Thuroff JW, Bazeed MA, Schmidt RA, Wiggin DM, Tanagho EA: Functional pattern of sacral root stimulation in dogs. II. Urethral closure. J Urol 1982;127:1034-1038.

373. Hohenfellner M, Paick JS, Trigo Rocha F, Schmidt RA, Kaula NF, Thuroff JW, Tanagho EA. Site of deafferentation and electrode placement for bladder stimulation: Clinical implication. J Urol 1992;147:1665-1669.

374. Shafik A: Pudendal nerve stimulation for anal and urethral sphincter control. Experimental study. Eur J Gastroenterol Hepatol 1994;6:345-349.

375. Shafik A: Perineal nerve stimulation for urinary sphincter control. Experimental study. Urol Res 1994;22:151-155.

376. Shafik A: Sacral root stimulation for controlled defecation. Eur

Surg Res 1995;27:63-68.

377. Shafik A: Pudendal canal decompression in the treatment of erectile dysfunction. Arch Androl 1994;32:141-149.

378. Shafik A. The posterior approach in the treatment of pudendal canal syndrome. Coloproctology 1992;14:310-315.

379. Shafik A. Role of pudendal canal syndrome in the etiology of fecal incontinence in rectal prolapse. Digestion 1997;58:489-493.

380. Shafik A. Pudendal artery syndrome presenting as ischemic proctitis. Report of 3 cases. Dig Surg 1996;13:53-58.

381. Shafik A. Pudendal canal decompression for the treatment of fecal incontinence in complete rectal prolapse. Am Surg 1996; 62:339-343.

382. Shafik A. Pudendal canal syndrome: a new etiological factor in prostatodynia and its treatment by pudendal canal decompression. Pain Dig 1998;8:32-36.

383. Shafik A. Pudendal canal syndrome as a cause of vulvodynia and its treatment by pudendal nerve decompression. Eur J Obstet Gynecol Reprod Biol 1998;80:215-220.

384. Shafik A, El-Sherif M, Youssef A, El-Sibai O: Surgical anatomy of the pudendal nerve and its clinical implications. Clin Anat 1995;8:110-115.

385. Juenemann KP, Lue TF, Schmidt RA, Tanagho EA: Clinical significance of sacral and pudendal nerve anatomy. J Urol 1988; 139:74-77.

386. Schmidt RA: Technique of pudendal nerve localization for block or stimulation. J Urol 1989;142:1528-1531.

387. Shafik A, Doss S. Pudendal canal: surgical anatomy and clinical implication. Am Surg 1999;65:176-180.

388. Shafik A. The levator dysfunction syndrome. A new syndrome with report of seven cases. Coloproctology 1983;5:159-165.

389. Shafik A. Pudendal canal decompression in the treatment of idiopathic fecal incontinence. Dis Colon Rectum 1993;36:17 (abstract).

390. Shafik A. Stress urinary incontinence: an alternative concept of pathogenesis. Int Urogynecol J 1994;5:3-11.

391. Shafik A. Pudendal canal decompression in the treatment of urinary stress incontinence. Int Urogynecol J 1994;5:215-220.

392. Lestar B, Penninckx FM, Kerremans RP: Defecometry: A new method for determining the parameters of rectal evacuation. Dis Colon Rectum 1989;32:197-201.

393. Barnes PR, Lennard-Jones JE: Patients with constipation of different types have difficulty in expelling a balloon from the rectum. Gut 1984;25:562-563.

394. Shafik A, Khalid A: Fecoflowmetry in defecation disorders. Pract Gastroenterol 1990;14:46-52.

395. Shafik A, Abdel-Moneim K: Fecoflowmetry: A new parameter assessing rectal function in normal and constipated subjects. Dis Colon Rectum 1993;36:35-42.

396. Shafik A: Levator-sphincter reflex. Description of a new reflex and its clinical significance. Coloproctology 1992;14:172-175.

397. Shafik A. Water enema test: a means of assessing rectal function. Pract Gastroenterol 1992;16:24J-24P.

398. Shafik A: Inguinal pelviscopy: A new approach for examining the pelvic organs. Gynecol Obstet Invest 1990;30:159-161.

399. Shafik A, Moneim KA. Rectometry: A new method assessing rectal function. Coloproctology 1991;13:237-243.

400. Shafik A: Electrorectography in chronic constipation. World J Surg 1995;19:772-775.

401. Shafik A: Electrorectogram in chronic proctitis. World J Surg 1993;17:675-679.

402. Shafik A: The electrorectogram in Hirschsprung's disease. A new diagnostic tool. Preliminary report. Pediatr Surg Int 1995;10: 478-480.

403. Shafik A, Abdel-Fattah A: Transcutaneous electrovesicography. Urologia 1995;62:371-374.

404. Shafik A: Electrovasography in normal and vasectomized men before and after vasectomy reversal. Int J Androl 1996;19:33-38.

405. Récamier M. Quoted by Maisonneure JG. Du traitement de la fissure a l'anus par la dilatation forcée. Gaz d'Hop (3rd series) 1849; 1:220.

406. Lord PH. Conservative management of hemorrhoids. Part II: Dilatation treatment. Clin Gastroenterol 1975;4:601-606.

407. Buls JG, Goldberg SM. Modern management of hemorrhoids. Surg Clin North Am 1978;58:469-479.

408. Shafik A. Recurrent anal fistula: is it a true recurrence or "de novo" fistula? Coloproctology 1995;17:249-253.

409. Marks CG, Ritchie JK. Anal fistulas at St Mark's Hospital. Br J Surg 1977;64:84-87.

410. Shafik A. Complete rectal prolapse: a technique for repair. Coloproctology 1987;9:345-352.

# Chapter *19*

# *Liver*

JOHN E. SKANDALAKIS, GENE D. BRANUM, GENE L. COLBORN,
PETROS MIRILAS, THOMAS A. WEIDMAN, LEE J. SKANDALAKIS,
ANDREW N. KINGSNORTH, PANAJIOTIS N. SKANDALAKIS,
ODYSSEAS ZORAS

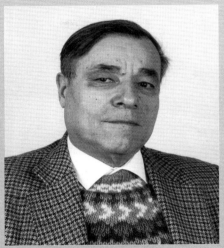

**Claude Couinaud (1922--)** formulated the surgical anatomy of the liver and hepatic segments.

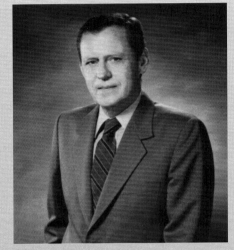

**Thomas Starzl (1926--)** performed the first successful transplantation of the liver.

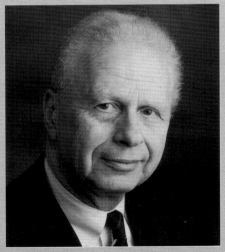

**Seymour I. Schwartz (1928--)** wrote of the beautiful book *Surgical Diseases of the Liver,* which was published in 1964.

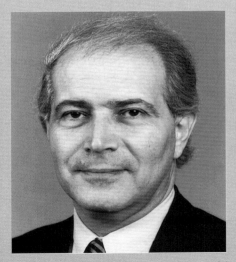

**Achilles A. Demetriou (1946--)** is Chairman of the Department of Surgery at Cedars-Sinai Medical Center, Los Angeles, and a pioneer of studies of hepatocyte implantation into the spleen.

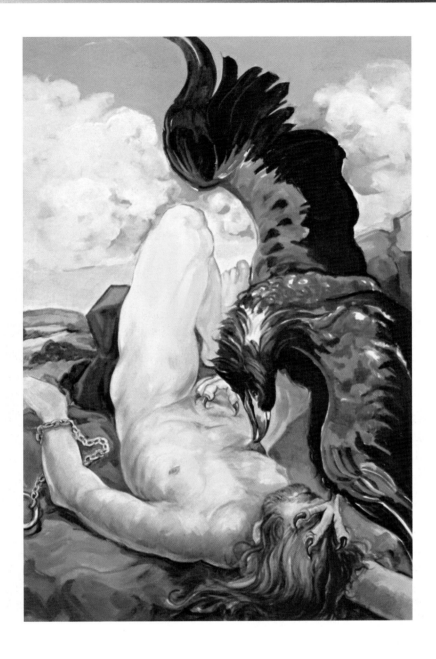

*John E. McClusky*

*And in ineluctable, painful bonds he fastened Prometheus*
*of the subtle mind, for he drove a stanchion through his middle. Also*
*he let loose on him the wing-spread eagle, and it was feeding*
*on his imperishable liver, which by night would grow back*
*to size from what the spread-winged bird had eaten in the daytime.*

**Hesiod, 750-700 B.C.***

*Hesiod, "Theogony," translated by Richard Lattimore, University of Michigan Press, Ann Arbor, 1959, p. 154, lines 522-526.

*...the liver is tender, full-blooded and solid and on account of these qualities is resistant to the movement of other organs. Thus wind, being obstructed by it, becomes more forceful and attacks the thing which obstructs it with great power. In the case of an organ such as the liver, which is both full-blooded and tender, it cannot but experience pain. For this reason, pain in the hepatic area is both exceedingly severe and frequently encountered.*

*Hippocrates*[1]

## HISTORY

The anatomic and surgical history of the liver is presented in Table 19-1.

## EMBRYOGENESIS

### Normal Development

The earliest appearance of the liver primordium occurs on Day 22 after conception. It appears at the superior intestinal portal, caudal and ventral to the heart. By Day 24, the hepatic diverticulum is growing into the transverse septum that, at this stage, contains the vitelline and umbilical veins. Differentiation of the components of the liver begins before the primordium becomes recognizable.

Using chick embryos, Croisille and LeDouarin[2] postulated three separate inductive processes acting on the endoderm (Fig. 19-1). First, lateral splanchnic mesoderm migrates anteriorly and fuses across the midline beneath the embryonic pharynx. This tissue, called hepatocardiac mesoderm, induces differentiation of the overlying endoderm cells at the anterior intestinal portal.

As the hepatic bud appears, the hepatic and cardiac mesenchyme become segregated. The second and third inductions occur when the hepatic mesenchyme stimulates the cells of the endodermal cords to differentiate into hepatocytes, and simultaneously the endodermal hepatocytes stimulate the mesenchyme to form the endothelial cells of the liver sinusoids.

The vitelline and umbilical veins divide into a plexus of vessels, and the invading endoderm cells move into the spaces around and between them.[3] This endodermal invasion in humans is not by cords of cells but by migration of individual endoderm cells. These endoderm cells do not maintain contact with each other, but mingle freely with mesenchyme cells of the transverse septum.

Elias[4,5] and Wilson and colleagues[6] suggested another source of liver parenchyma. They postulated that mesodermal celomic lining cells invading the transverse septum become indistinguishable from endodermal cells.

Bennett[7] presented three sets of events:
- Cell multiplication
- New and differentiated cells from the undifferentiated zygote
- New and differentiated cells with specific histology, function, and physiological destiny.

Bennett wrote that some gene activities, different proteins, and different functions of the cell are responsible for this embryonic differentiation. By differentiation, endodermal cells produce the liver diverticulum which produces liver cells.

Sherer[8] speculated that the development of the hepatic parenchyma depends on interaction of its epithelial and mesenchymal tissues.

By Day 32, most of the blood flow from the umbilical veins has been tapped by the parenchyma that surrounds the venous channels. These channels become the liver sinusoids. The right umbilical vein regresses in the sixth week. The left vein carries placental blood to the fetus until birth. Its remnant is the round ligament in the free edge of the falciform ligament. By Day 51, the intrahepatic veins have nearly attained the normal adult distribution and segmentation. The hepatic arteries and the bile duct do not advance as quickly toward their adult pattern. The investing cores of parenchyma, at first three to five cells thick, become reduced to a single cell layer near term.

## TABLE 19-1. Anatomic and Surgical History of the Liver

| | | |
|---|---|---|
| Mesopotamians | ca. 2000-3000 B.C. | Performed hepatic divination using clay models of sheep livers for instruction |
| Herophilus of Chalcedon (334-280 B.C.) | | First anatomic description of liver. Stated: "In some [animals] the liver does not have lobes at all but is round and undifferentiated. In some however it has two, in some more, and in many four and in some more lobes." Discovered mesenteric lacteals. |
| Erasistratus of Chios (310-250 B.C.) | | Described basic intrahepatic capillary bed while studying liver anatomy |
| Celsus | ca. 30 B.C. | Emphasized four-lobed liver in *De Re Medicina* |
| Rufus of Ephesus | 50 A.D. | Described five-lobed liver |
| Galen (130-210 A.D.) | | Documented Herophilus' and Erasistratus' anatomic findings. Claimed liver spreads like the five fingers of a hand. Defined liver as primary organ of sanguinification that converts chyle to blood. |
| Berengario da Carpi | 1522 | In *Isagogae Breves,* cautiously challenged Galen, claiming liver can have two, three, four, or five lobes |
| Andreas de Laguna | 1535 | Observed two, three, four, and five-lobed livers |
| Vesalius | 1538 1546 | Published *Tabulae Sex,* depicting a five-lobed liver Published *Fabrica,* showing a symmetric two-lobed liver |
| Fabricus Hildanus (1560-1634) | Early 17th century | Excised small piece of liver protruding from abdomen after knife wound |
| Gasparo Aselli | 1622 | Rediscovered mesenteric lacteals and claimed they drain into liver |
| Jan de Wale (Walaeus) | 1640 | Described capsule, later renamed Glisson's capsule |
| Johann Vesling | 1647 | First to report bifurcation of human portal vein |
| Jean Pecquet | 1647 | Described the thoracic duct while correctly claiming it terminates in subclavian vein. Conclusively proved that chyle is not transported to the liver, thus challenging notion that blood is made in liver. Published findings in 1651. |
| Olof Rudbeck | 1652 | Described course of lymphatics from liver to thoracic duct and venous systems during a royal gathering in Uppsala Castle of Sweden |
| Thomas Bartholin | 1652 | Further confirmed course of lymphatic drainage. Incorrectly noted that mesenteric lacteals carry lymph to the liver. Rudbeck corrected this error in 1653. |
| Francis Glisson | 1654 | Published *Anatomia Hepatis* describing capsule named for him. Provided detailed account of intrahepatic vasculature. |
| Marcello Malpighi | 1661 | Published *De Pulmonibus Epistolae,* describing hexagonal lobules in liver |
| Johan Jacob Wepfer | 1664 | Discovered that "acini," or lobules, exist in a pig's liver |
| Fredrick Ruysch | 1665 | Hypothesized that Malpighian lobules represent interconnections between portal and vascular system |
| Malpighi | 1666 | Published *De Viscerum Structura Exercitatio Anatomica* further describing hexagonal lobules. Confirmed belief that hepatic and portal veins are interconnected by capillary beds. |
| Gottfried Bidloo | 1685 | Published *Anatomia Humani Corporis,* writing of interconnected small units of liver |
| Albrecht von Haller | 1764 | Provided modern account of human liver. Divided it into right, left, anterior, and caudate lobes. |
| Francis Kiernan | 1833 | Established concept of "classic" liver lobule with a hepatic vein in the center and six hepatic triads at periphery |
| E. Brissuad & C. Sabourin | 1834 | Advocated concept of portal lobule with bile ducts in center |

## TABLE 19-1 (cont'd). Anatomic and Surgical History of the Liver

| | | |
|---|---|---|
| René-Joachin-Henri Dutrochet | 1838 | Described cytology of hepatocytes |
| J. McPherson | 1846 | Excised a small piece of liver from a spear wound |
| Joseph von Gerlach | 1849 | Postulated liver cord theory using terms "cords" and "trabeculae" to describe arrangement of hepatocytes in relation to bile capillaries (bile canaliculi) and vascular sinusoids |
| | 1854 | Noted presence of "bile caniculi" in liver |
| T.H. MacGillavry | 1865 | Reported finding space between surface of hepatocytes and sinusoidal endothelium; these later named spaces of Disse |
| Ewald Hering | 1866 | Considered liver parenchyma to be continuous mass of hepatocytes lined in a series of plates of one-celled thickness |
| Chrzonszczewsky | 1866 | Described relationship of hepatic arteries to central sinuses |
| Victor von Bruns | 1870 | Successfully excised a "nut-sized" section of liver from a fellow surgeon suffering from gunshot wounds |
| H. Tillmanns | 1879 | Removed wedge-shaped pieces of liver from 12 rabbits. Determined that degree of injury to liver depends on wound size and amount of hemorrhage. |
| Lawson Tait | 1880 | Reportedly first to use laparotomy for liver trauma |
| Themistokles Gluck | 1883 | Reported physiological data helping to establish concept that liver regenerates after surgery |
| P. Postemski | 1885 | Recommended suturing liver to control bleeding |
| A. Luis | 1886 | Removed an adenoma of liver the size of a "one-year-old child's head" |
| Carl von Langebuch | 1887 | Performed first successful subtotal left hepatectomy |
| Hugo Rex | 1888 | Described right and left lobes as being equal in size. Showed the plane of division is through bed of gallbladder and notch of inferior vena cava and not through falciform ligament. |
| L. McLane Tiffany | 1890 | Reported performing first American subtotal left hepatectomy |
| Emil Ponflick | 1890 | Using animal pathology experiments, found liver resections of up to 80% are non-fatal due to rapid and extensive regeneration |
| J. Disse | 1890 | Described perisinusoidal spaces bearing his name in an attempt to describe relations of lymph with liver |
| William Williams Keen | 1892 | Performed first successful liver resection in America (typical left hepatectomy). Reported his findings through the 1890s while documenting 76 cases of hepatectomies in world literature. Used his thumb to strip liver capsule. |
| M. Kousnetzoff & J. Pensky | 1896 | Devised suture method to stem liver hemorrhage using blunt needles, mattress sutures, and "guards" such as magnesium plates to overcome liver's friability |
| J. Cantlie | 1897 | Confirmed Rex's findings. Rex's lobular plane of division later named Cantlie's line. |
| W. Anschutz | 1903 | Advocated division of liver parenchyma with blunt objects to control bleeding |
| R. Kretz | 1905 | Reported work supporting Hering's one-cell thick parenchyma over Gerlach's two-cell thick model |
| Franklin Paine Mall | 1906 | Advocated Brissaud and Sabourin's "portal" lobule, and described the spaces surrounding the portal triads; these later named spaces of Mall |
| Hogarth Pringle | 1908 | Occluded portal triad with his finger and thumb ("Pringle Pinch") to temporarily control bleeding during liver surgery |
| W. Wendel | 1911 | Performed first subtotal right hepatectomy. Deliberately tied off right hepatic artery before resection. |
| Sir Archibald Hector McIndoe & V. Counsellor | 1927 | Studied intrahepatic ducts in 42 human livers. Confirmed bilateral symmetry established by Rex and Cantlie. |

**TABLE 19-1 *(cont'd)*. Anatomic and Surgical History of the Liver**

| | | |
|---|---|---|
| G. Caprio | 1931 | Performed first sub-total left hepatectomy under hilar ligation |
| L.B. Arey | 1932 | Further developed "portal" lobule concept by describing the coexistence of hepatic and portal lobules in seals |
| Ton That Tung | 1939 | Published paper describing primary parenchymatous transection during liver surgery |
| E.J. Donovan & T.V. Santulli | 1944 | Performed sub-total left hepatectomy for sarcoma while tying off left hepatic artery, left hepatic duct, and left portal vein of liver |
| C. Hjortsjö | 1948 | Using corrosion specimens and cholangiograms, originated concept that branching of the bilary ducts has a segmental pattern |
| Ronald William Raven | 1948 | Applied anatomic principles during a left segmentectomy by resecting through the falciform ligament |
| H. Elias | 1949 | Restated Hering's concept and further explained it in more than 30 papers during the ensuing 25 years |
| Owen Harding Wangensteen | 1949 | Performed first typical right hepatectomy to treat metastatic cancer |
| Julian Quattlebaum | 1952 | Performed typical right hepatectomy for primary adenoma. Used back of his scalpel as a parenchymal fracture technique. |
| A.M. Rappaport | 1952 | Proposed concept of "liver acinus" in which a cylindrical mass of hepatic tissue surrounds a portal triad. Indicated boundaries between sinuses are not visible. Doctoral thesis accepted in 1952, papers published in 1954 and 1958. |
| George T. Pack & Harvey W. Baker | 1952 | Performed total right hepatectomy; reported in 1953 |
| J.L. Lorat-Jacob & H.G. Robert | 1953 | Performed extended right hepatectomy (right trisegmentectomy) by thoracoabdominal approach using preliminary vascular control |
| John E. Healey & Paul C. Schroy | 1953 | Described segmental anatomy of liver based on patterns of bilary intrahepatic architecture. Reported liver is divided into five segments (medial, lateral, posterior, anterior, and caudate). |
| Claude Couinaud | 1954 | Affirmed segmental anatomy using internal vasculature and bilary architecture as a guide. Reported liver is divided into eight sections (I-VIII). |
| Charles Welch | 1955 | Performed first liver homotransplantation in dogs, confirming liver transplantation is possible |
| N.A. Goldsmith & R.T. Woodburne | 1957 | Described segmental anatomy after examining 33 human livers in vivo. Used "subsegment" nomenclature. |
| Tien-Yu Lin, Kuang-Yung Hsu, Chen-Min Hsieh, & Chi-Sen Chen | 1958 | Published paper describing modern "finger fracture" techniques used in resection |
| Thomas Starzl | 1963 | Attempted first orthotopic liver transplant in humans |
| R.N. McClelland & T. Shires | 1965 | Published paper describing the first "nonanatomical" resections |
| J.P. Heaney, W.R. Stanton, D.S. Halbert, J. Seidel, & T. Vice | 1966 | Advanced Pringle's occlusion principle by cross clamping aorta and inferior vena cava |
| Thomas Starzl | 1968 | Performed first successful human orthotopic liver transplant |
| T. Schrock, T. Baisdell, & C. Matthewson | 1968 | Isolated liver's vasculature with atriocaval shunting |
| Thomas Starzl | 1975 | Performed first reduced-size liver transplant |
| Henri Bismuth | 1980 | Performed first heterotopic liver transplant in humans |

**TABLE 19-1 (cont'd). Anatomic and Surgical History of the Liver**

| | | |
|---|---|---|
| Thomas Starzl | 1980 | Performed first extended left hepatectomy (left trisegmentectomy) |
| R. Pichlmayr & J. Broelsh | 1984 | Performed first split-liver transplant |
| S. Raia, J.R. Nery, & S. Mies | 1989 | Performed first living related-donor liver transplant |
| Richter et al. | 1990 | Introduced transjugular intrahepatic protosystemic stent-shunt (TIPS) into clinical practice; revolutionized management of difficult cases of esophagogastric variceal bleeding and other complications of portal hypertension |

*History table compiled by David A. McClusky III and John E. Skandalakis.*

**References**

McClusky DA III, Skandalakis LJ, Colborn GL, Skandalakis JE. Hepatic surgery and hepatic surgical anatomy: historical partners in progress. World J Surg 1997;21:330-342.

Popper H. Vienna and the liver. In Brunner H, Thaler H (eds). Hepatology: A Festschrift for Hans Popper. New York: Raven Press, 1985, pp. 1-14.

Richter GM, Noeldge G, Palmz JC. The transjugular intrahepatic protosystemic stent-shunt (TIPS): experience results of a pilot study. Cardiovasc Intervent Radiol 1990;13:200.

Growth of the liver makes it bulge out of the transverse septum so that the liver becomes a truly abdominal organ lying in the ventral mesentery. The bare area of the liver and diaphragm remains as an indication of the origin of the liver from the transverse septum. The asymmetry of the organ increases.

The intrahepatic bile ducts were long assumed to develop by extension of the extrahepatic ducts. It is now believed that the ducts differentiate from hepatic cells and join the extrahepatic duct system secondarily. The ducts appear first at the hilum and spread peripherally.[4,9] Bile may appear as early as the third month and is often in the intestine by the fifth month. By the ninth week, the liver embraces as much as 10% of body volume. Its relative size decreases to 5% by term.

The earliest source of blood in the embryo is the mesoderm of the yolk sac. Groups of stem cells, the blood islands, produce cells (primitive erythrocytes) that synthesize hemoglobin and retain their nuclei. Stem cells from the blood islands seed the liver and proliferate. Adult types of erythrocytes (RBCs), granulocytes, and platelets are produced in the liver between the ninth and 24th weeks of fetal life.

With the progress of ossification and the appearance of bone marrow, which will be seeded by stem cells from the liver, the liver structure shuts down its hemopoietic activity well before birth. The potential for blood production continues into adult life, expressing itself if the bone marrow fails to function. Galen was not entirely wrong in assigning a blood-forming function to the liver!

Initially the right lobe is smaller than the left lobe. Between birth and adulthood, the right lobe increases in size at the expense of the left lobe, which undergoes some peripheral degeneration[10] (Fig. 19-2).

The alterations in relative size of the left and right parts of the liver are accompanied by changes in the orientation and size of the upper abdominal arteries. In this regard, note that the hepatic artery is the largest branch of the celiac trunk in newborns. In adults the splenic artery is larger than the hepatic. In later development, the mass of the liver reduces and shifts to the right side. This results in decreased size of the hepatic artery and in the left-to-right orientation of the hepatic artery and the celiac trunk.[11]

REMEMBER:

• Around the middle of the 3rd week or at the beginning of the 4th week, the liver primordium (liver bud), gall-

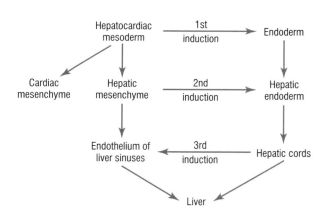

FIG. 19-1. Differentiation *(vertical arrows)* and induction *(horizontal arrows)* in the development of liver cords and sinuses in the embryo. (From Skandalakis JE, Gray SW (Eds). Embryology for Surgeons, 2nd Ed. Baltimore: Williams & Wilkins, 1994; with permission.)

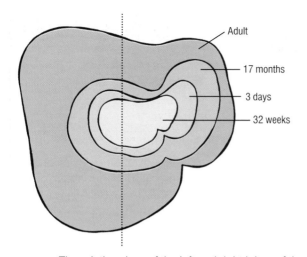

FIG. 19-2. The relative sizes of the left and right lobes of the liver in the fetus at 32 weeks; in the infant at 3 days and at 17 months; and in the adult. The dotted line represents the location of the main lobar fissure. (Modified from Healey JE Jr, Sterling JA. Segmental anatomy of the newborn liver. Ann NY Acad Sci 111:25-36, 1963; with permission.)

bladder, and biliary duct (gallbladder bud) arise as a ventral outgrowth from the distal end of the foregut.

- Early in the 5th week, the liver bud stalk is formed by proliferating cells. These cells start to infiltrate the transverse septum through the rays of its endodermal cells. This is an embryologic mesodermal (mesenchymal) entity between the pericardial cavity and the stalk of the yolk sac. The future hepatic stroma, the hemopoietic Kupffer cells, and the vessels are all of mesenchymal origin.
- At this same time, the connecting elements between the hepatic diverticulum and the already-formed duodenum form the bile duct. Later this produces the cystic duct and the gallbladder.
- Later the hepatic sinusoids (endothelium-lined spaces) are formed from the epithelial cells. These spaces now communicate by anastomosis with small vessels from the vitelline and umbilical veins.
- Around the 9th week, rapid hepatic growth causes the liver to account for 10% of the total fetal weight. The hemopoietic function and the multiple sinusoids are, most likely, responsible for this hepatomegaly. At birth, the liver weighs approximately 5% of the total body weight.
- Occlusion and canalization take place at the extrahepatic biliary system. These processes, however, are not responsible for extrahepatic biliary atresia.
- The ventral mesentery (mesogastrium) produces the:
  - Lesser omentum, formed by the gastrohepatic ligament and the hepatoduodenal ligament

- Falciform ligament from the ventral abdominal wall to the liver

    The hepatoduodenal ligament envelops the hepatic triad, and the falciform ligament hosts the left umbilical vein at its free border. The right umbilical vein disappears very early.
- According to Sergi et al.,[12] "the surface and the perimeter of the portal tracts, the longest axis of the migrating peripheral tubular structures, and the maturation of bile ducts follow a process continuous and active up to term, but they slow between the 20th and the 32nd week of gestation, when intraportal granulopoiesis of the liver is active."
- A higher proportion of umbilical blood is directed to the liver and less is shunted through the ductus venosus in the human fetus than in other animals.[13]

## Congenital Anomalies

Fig. 19-3 illustrates sites of the major congenital anomalies of the liver. Complete absence of the liver is rare and is not compatible with postnatal life. Absence of the left lobe of the liver has been detected in adults by radiography,[14] ultrasonogram, and CT scan;[15] this defect in itself produces no symptoms.

Kakitsubata et al.[16] reported segmental anomalies. They observed absence of the anterior segment of the right lobe in one patient and anomalies of the left lobe in three others. Ozgun and Warshauer[17] reported agenesis of the medial segment of the left lobe. Agenesis of the right lobe was reported by Morphett and Adam.[18] Klin et al.[19] reported a case of agenesis of the left lobe.

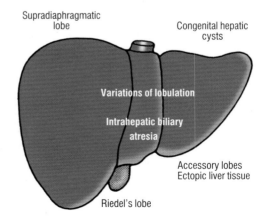

FIG. 19-3. Sites of the major anomalies of the liver. (Modified from Skandalakis JE, Gray SW (Eds). Embryology for Surgeons, 2nd Ed. Baltimore: Williams & Wilkins, 1994; with permission.)

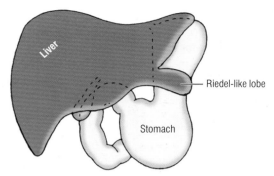

**FIG. 19-4.** An anomalous lobe on the left side of the liver resembling Riedel's lobe on the right side. (Modified from Dick J. Riedel's lobe and related partial hepatic enlargements. Guy Hosp Rep 100:270-277, 1951; with permission.)

## Transposition

Transposition of the liver is a manifestation of total or partial situs inversus viscerum. Diagnosis is suggested by a right-sided gastric air bubble on x-ray. Hepatic transposition is associated with transposition of the great vessels, tetralogy of Fallot, pulmonary stenosis, asplenia, duodenal stenosis or atresia, preduodenal portal vein, and biliary atresia. Mortality from associated malformations is as high as 50%.[20]

In three cases of situs inversus in adults without associated malformations, the arterial distribution was neither normal nor a true mirror image. Large intrahepatic anastomoses between right and left hepatic arteries were present.[21]

## Anomalous Lobes of the Liver

### Riedel's Lobe

An anomalous tongue of liver extending downward from the right lobe in ten female patients was described by Riedel[22] in 1888 (Figs. 19-3, 19-4, 19-5). Reitemeir and colleagues at the Mayo Clinic[23] reported 31 cases, all but one in women between 31 and 77 years of age. Using radionuclide imaging, Baum and colleagues[24] found Riedel's lobe in 19.4% of females and 6.1% of males. The hepatic tissue of the lobe was normal and often fixed to the colon at the hepatic flexure. In one patient, it produced partial colonic obstruction.[25] In a more recent case, El Haddad and colleagues[26] found total pyloric obstruction from a cystogastrocolic band that contained ectopic liver tissue. McGregor[27] considered such bands to represent persistent portions of the embryonic ventral mesentery. Similar tongues of hepatic tissue have been reported on the left.[28] The chief significance of Riedel's lobe is that it presents as an unexplained abdominal mass. If such a lobe is present, a liver scan or ultrasound will identify it.

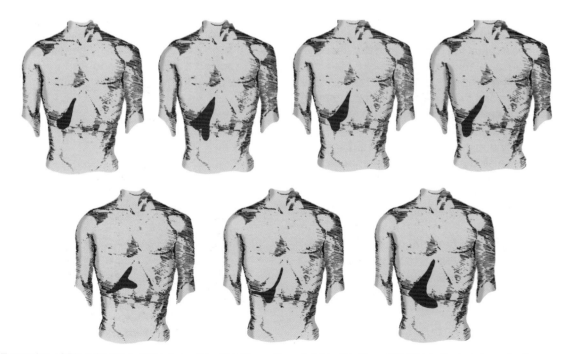

**FIG. 19-5.** Examples of Riedel's lobe of the liver. (Modified from Skandalakis JE, Gray SW (Eds). Embryology for Surgeons, 2nd Ed. Baltimore: Williams & Wilkins, 1994; with permission. Redrawn from Dick J. Riedel's lobe and related partial hepatic enlargements. Guy Hosp Rep 100:270-277, 1951.)

Gillard et al.[29] stated, "Although the identification of Riedel's lobe has been valuable on both clinical and anatomical grounds, the usefulness of the term is now perhaps limited because of its relative prevalence as shown by modern cross-sectional imaging."

### Supradiaphragmatic Liver

Four cases of liver tissue sequestered above the diaphragm in the right thorax have been reported in living patients. In each case, the ectopic mass was attached to the liver by a pedicle passing through a small aperture in the diaphragm without a hernial sac (Fig. 19-6). The pedicle contained branches of the hepatic artery, portal vein, and bile duct, and, in one patient, the gallbladder. All cases were asymptomatic except one.[30]

Because the liver forms within the transverse septum, it is surprising that portions of the liver above the diaphragm are not more common. Mendoza et al.[31] reported hepatic tissue in the lung.

### Accessory and Ectopic Lobes of the Liver

Heterotopic nodules of liver tissue have been described on the surface of the gallbladder,[32] in the gallbladder wall,[33] associated with the pancreas,[34] and in an adrenal gland,[25] splenic capsule,[35] and omphalocele.[36]

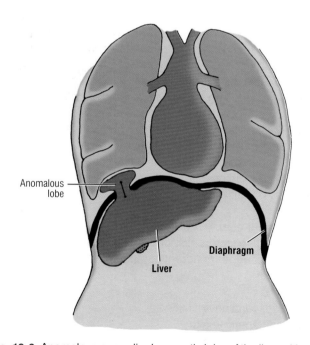

Anomalous lobe

Diaphragm

Liver

**FIG. 19-6.** Anomalous supradiaphragmatic lobe of the liver with a pedicle passing through the diaphragm, carrying an artery, a vein and a bile duct. (Modified from Skandalakis JE, Gray SW (Eds). Embryology for Surgeons, 2nd Ed. Baltimore: Williams & Wilkins, 1994; with permission.)

### *Mesenchymal Hamartoma*

First described in 1903 by Maresch,[37] mesenchymal hamartoma is a rare, usually asymptomatic tumor of the liver. It appears shortly after birth or later in adult life[38-40] as a rapidly enlarging mass in the right upper quadrant. Such a tumor can weigh as much as 3 kg and can cause respiratory embarrassment by its sheer size. Shuto and colleagues[41] mentioned the appearance of 30 cases of such tumors in the Japanese literature and about 100 cases in English-language reports. These authors reported a case of bilateral lobectomy excluding the caudate lobe for giant mesenchymal hepatic hamartoma.

The tumor consists of loose fibrous connective tissue with multiple cysts ranging in size from microscopic to several centimeters in diameter. Some tumors are largely cystic; others are predominantly fibrous. If the tumor is pedicled, a simple resection will be effective. A broader attachment may require lobectomy. We have found no reports of recurrence after operation.

### *Intrahepatic Biliary Atresia*

In this defect, there is absence of interlobular bile ducts, with or without patent extrahepatic bile ducts. Bile canaliculi are present. Whether the defect is congenital and an extension of extrahepatic biliary atresia, or acquired following hepatitis is unresolved. At the present time the most acceptable etiology is progressive fibrosis and destruction of the epithelial elements by viral, toxic, or immunologic mechanism.

Intrahepatic biliary atresia was first described in 1951[42] and is less common than extrahepatic biliary atresia. Most affected individuals die before the age of four years; however, some have lived as long as 13 years.[43] Longmire[44] believed that there may be varying degrees of hypoplasia. It is difficult to explain the long survival time if atresia is complete. At present, liver transplantation offers the greatest hope for effective treatment of intrahepatic biliary atresia.

### *Cysts*

Congenital solitary nonparasitic cysts of the liver were reported by Quillin and McAlister[45] and Karia et al.[46] These are very rare cysts presenting as abdominal masses.

Koperna et al.[47] concluded that laparoscopic fenestration of nonparasitic hepatic cysts should replace the conventional surgical technique.

### *Congenital Hepatic Fibrosis*

Congenital hepatic fibrosis is an anomaly that has not

been well established. Desmet[48] postulates that congenital fibrosis is secondary to faulty development of interlobular bile ducts due to destructive cholangiopathy. Sung et al.[49] and Lipschitz et al.[50] each reported a case.

Bands of fibrous tissue with linear and circular degeneration, lined with bile duct epithelium as a simple entity but usually associated with pancreatic or renal anomalies, were reported by Murray-Lyon et al.[51] as congenital hepatic fibrosis. Annand et al.[52] presented this anomaly associated with polycystic renal disease.

### Vascular Malformations

Congenital vascular malformation of the liver ranging from solitary hemangiomas to multiple hemangioendotheliomas are now being discovered with increased frequency. The increase is due to the widespread use of prenatal and neonatal ultrasound.

Gedaly et al.[53] stated that cavernous hemangiomas of the liver can be removed safely by either hepatic resection or enucleation. Enucleation is associated with fewer intraabdominal complications and should be the technique of choice when tumor location and technical factors favor enucleation.

## SURGICAL ANATOMY

## Physical Characteristics and Topography

### Weight

The human liver is the largest solid organ of the body, weighing about 150 g at birth. The weight of the liver of the adult male ranges from 1.4 kg to 1.8 kg, and the adult female from 1.2 kg to 1.4 kg.[54] The actual weight varies with the individual's age, sex, somatotype, and state of health.

Because of the role of the liver in blood formation during fetal life, the organ at birth contributes 4% to 5% to body weight. In the newborn infant, the liver bulges both the left and right hypochondrium. The effect of the weight of the liver on the location of the infant's center of gravity may be an important factor in the development of the ability to attain upright posture and locomotion.

### Shape

The liver is wedge-shaped. Its average transverse dia-

meter is 20 cm to 23 cm and its anteroposterior diameter is 10 cm to 12.5 cm at the area of the upper pole of the right kidney.[55] The craniocaudal span at the right midclavicular line has been measured by scintigram,[56] percussion,[57] extremely soft percussion, and ultrasound.[58] The ultrasound technique provides consistently higher values than do other methods of measurement. The effect of the liver on the percussion note evoked extends above the actual upper limit of the organ. Thus the upper border lies slightly below the line along which the percussion note changes.[59]

Extension of the inferior border of the liver below the costal margin can occur incidental to disorders other than liver enlargement. If a liver possesses a long, thin anterior inferior edge or a so-called "Riedel's lobe," the organ may be considered enlarged. The liver may also descend after weight loss.

### Location and Extent

In the adult, the liver fills the right hypochondrium and the epigastric regions. It extends inferiorly into the right lumbar region and occupies part of the left hypochondrium, reaching to the left lateral line. The liver is covered by ribs and costal cartilages, except in the epigastric region where it reaches the anterior abdominal wall just below the infrasternal notch.

The right side of the liver is closely applied to the costal muscle fibers and the central tendon of the right leaf of the diaphragm. The left lobe (the apex of the "wedge") reaches for a variable distance into the left upper part of the abdominal cavity, abutting the left leaf of the diaphragm.

The right lobe of the liver apposes the bony thoracic wall. Convenient sites for transthoracic puncture for liver biopsy are present in the anterior axillary line at the seventh to ninth interspaces, always one interspace below the upper limit of liver dullness. Ultrasound guidance is increasingly used to obtain an appropriate window for percutaneous biopsy.

Flament et al.[60] reported the following anatomic and nonanatomic factors responsible for the fixation of the liver at the right upper quadrant of the abdomen.

*Anatomic*
- Inferior vena cava
- Suprahepatic veins
- Several ligaments such as the round ligament and coronary ligament
- Peritoneal folds

*Nonanatomic*
- Positive intraabdominal pressure

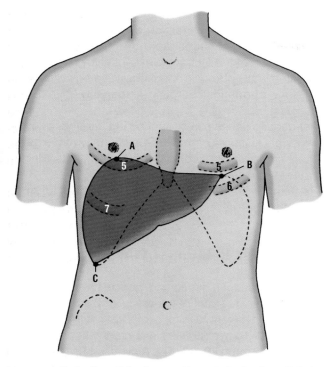

FIG. **19-7.** Projection of the liver on the anterior body wall. Points A-C are the usual landmarks by which the position can be established. (Modified from Skandalakis JE, Gray SW, Rowe JS Jr. Anatomical Complications in General Surgery. New York: McGraw-Hill, 1983; with permission.)

## *Outlines of the Liver on the Anterior Body Wall*

See Figure 19-7 to trace the outline of the liver on the anterior body wall:

- **Point A** is 1 cm (about one-half fingerwidth) below the right nipple at the level of the fifth rib
- **Point B** is located approximately 2 cm (about one-finger-width) inferior to and medial to the left nipple, at the level of the left fifth intercostal space
- **Point C** is in the right costal margin at the anterior axillary line

Lockhart et al.[61] charted the approximate rib levels of the liver, lungs, and pleurae (Fig. 19-8).

The gallbladder attaches to the visceral surface of the liver and moves with it. The fundus usually projects below the liver margin and lies in contact with the anterior abdominal wall near the intersection of the ninth costal cartilage and the lateral border of the rectus sheath.

## *Individual Location*

In broad-chested individuals, the left side of the liver is more prominent than in slender individuals. In the latter, the organ is disposed principally to the right of the mid-sagittal plane and can extend considerably below the right costal margin.

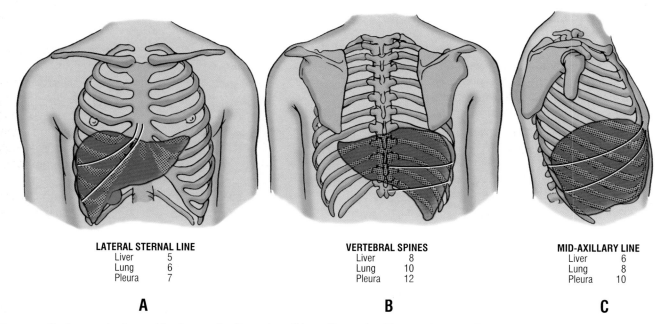

| LATERAL STERNAL LINE | | VERTEBRAL SPINES | | MID-AXILLARY LINE | |
|---|---|---|---|---|---|
| Liver | 5 | Liver | 8 | Liver | 6 |
| Lung | 6 | Lung | 10 | Lung | 8 |
| Pleura | 7 | Pleura | 12 | Pleura | 10 |
| **A** | | **B** | | **C** | |

FIG. **19-8.** Surface projections of the liver on the thoracic wall from **A**) anterior, **B**) posterior, and **C**) lateral views. The inferior limits of the lung parenchyma and the parietal pleura are noted beneath each figure and illustrated for comparison with the liver projections. (Modified from Skandalakis LJ, Gray SW, Colborn GL, Skandalakis JE. Surgical anatomy of the liver and associated extrahepatic structures: Part 2. Contemp Surg 30:26-38, 1987; with permission.)

## Motion and Activity

The position of the liver in the body is not static.[59] The liver moves up and down with the diaphragm and rotates during respiration. It rotates backward when an individual lies down in the supine position. The upper surface of the liver can move upward from 1 cm to 10 cm when full expiration follows deep inspiration. The most cranial level attained by the upper border of the liver during quiet respiration shows great individual variation and reflects the type of diaphragm — high, intermediate, or low. These facts should be kept in mind when interpreting radiographic images. Fig. 19-8 summarizes the typical bony relationships of the superior extent of the liver and the inferior extent of the lungs and parietal pleura.

REMEMBER:
- The healthy adult liver weighs between 1.0 kg and 2.0 kg.
- Dimensions of the liver are as follows:
- Anteroposteriorly, the distance extends 10.0 cm to 12.5 cm from the area related to the anterior abdominal wall to its rounded posterior surface
  - The transverse diameter is 20.0 cm to 25.5 cm from the right paracolic gutter to the midpoint of the left diaphragmatic leaflet
  - The anteroinferior edge stretches vertically 15.0 cm to 17.5 cm to the top of the dome of the right hepatic lobe
- According to Gelfand,[62] the obscurity of the hepatic borders on x-ray is due to the specific gravity of the liver (1.05). This is almost the same as all other "water density" tissues such as the diaphragm and gastrointestinal wall. The presence of fat helps prevent the blending of the liver margins with other organs. The same author stated that the anatomic relations between hepatic substance and fat are extremely important for radiographic determination of the hepatic borders.
- The shadow of the inferior border expressed on x-rays is due to the combined effects of the amount of retroperitoneal fat, habitus of the patient, and "hepatic angle" (junction between lateral and inferior hepatic borders).

## Surgical Considerations

- The procedure to be performed and body habitus of the patient dictate the selection of the incision. Most surgeons use a long bilateral subcostal incision with perixiphoid extension for major hepatic resections. Combined with newer retraction systems, this incision provides wide and deep exposure. Recent reports show renewed interest in right thoracoabdominal ap-

proaches to large right lobe lesions. However, the surgeon should use the incision with which he or she is most familiar and comfortable.
- Preparation of the GI tract is essential for surgery with hepatomegaly of known or unknown etiology or in cases of prior abdominal surgery (especially in cirrhotic patients).
- Perihepatic adhesions should be cut carefully to avoid injury of Glisson's capsule. Occasionally these adhesions are vascular or contain minute bile ducts. Electric cautery is advised.
- Remember the relation of the liver to the diaphragm above and the several anatomic entities below.

## Topographic Relations of the Liver

Although wedge-shaped and, hence, having three surfaces, the liver is "a cast of the cavity in which it grows."[63] Thus, it is convenient to think of this cast of the upper abdomen as having two surfaces, diaphragmatic and visceral (Figs. 19-9 through 19-12). The radiologist uses this concept.[59] The diaphragmatic surface is molded by the diaphragm. The visceral surface bears impressions from the stomach, duodenum, transverse colon, and, a beautiful radiologic landmark, the right kidney.

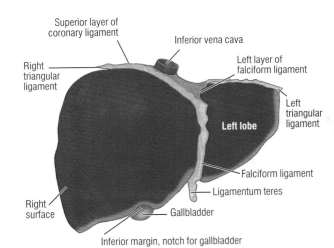

**FIG. 19-9.** Diaphragmatic aspect of the liver illustrating features of the anterior and superior surfaces. This specimen from a broadchested, muscular (mesomorphic habitus) individual is seen also in Figures 19-11 and 19-12. The liver measured 21 cm transversely, 20.3 cm vertically, and 14.6 cm in thickness. (Modified from Skandalakis LJ, Gray SW, Colborn GL, Skandalakis JE. Surgical anatomy of the liver and associated extrahepatic structures: Part 2. Contemp Surg 30:26-38, 1987; with permission.)

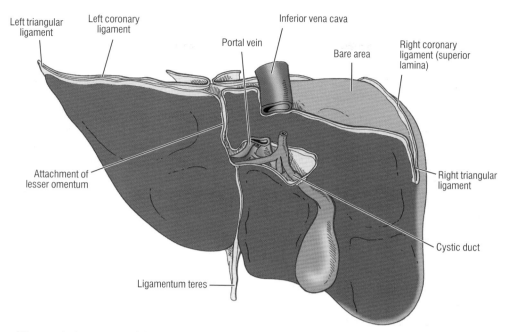

**FIG. 19-10.** Diagram of the posterior aspect of the liver to show the arrangement of the peritoneal attachments. Note the horizontal course of the left branch of the portal vein and the comparatively short course of the right branch.

## Diaphragmatic Surface

The diaphragmatic surface may be divided into superior, posterior, anterior, and right portions.

- **Superior:** The superior portion is related to the diaphragm and the following organs from right to left: right pleura and lung, pericardium and heart (cardiac impression), left pleura and lung. The superior surface is covered with peritoneum except where, more dorsally, the superior reflection of the coronary ligament bounds the bare area of the liver.
- **Posterior:** The posterior portion is related to the dia-

phragm and lower ribs. It contains the greater part of the bare area and the sulcus of the inferior vena cava (IVC).
- **Anterior:** The anterior part is related to the diaphragm and costal margin, xiphoid process, the abdominal wall, and the sixth to tenth ribs on the right.
- **Right:** The right portion is related to the diaphragm and the seventh to eleventh ribs. It is a lateral continuation of the posterior portion.

The diaphragmatic surface separates from the visceral surface at the inferior border. This surface is blunt, rounded, and unmarked posteriorly but sharp anteriorly. The clinician palpates this sharp anterior portion. However, the

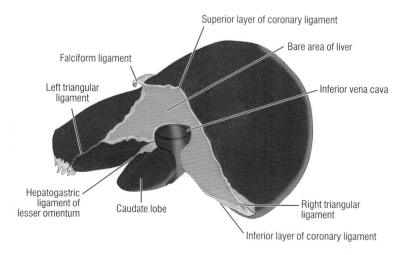

**FIG. 19-11.** Posterior aspect of the liver. The distinction between the left and right layers of the falciform ligament is slightly exaggerated to emphasize the contributions of these to the left triangular ligament and coronary ligament, respectively. (Modified from Skandalakis LJ, Gray SW, Colborn GL, Skandalakis JE. Surgical anatomy of the liver and associated extrahepatic structures: Part 2. Contemp Surg 30:26-38, 1987; with permission.)

liver "edge" seen in a plain x-ray is the rounded posterior border. This is not a true border but represents the interface of the posterior aspect of the right lobe of the liver with retroperitoneal fat.

Anteriorly, the inferior border of the liver is marked by two notches to the right of the median plane. These are:

- Deep notch accommodating the ligamentum teres (Fig. 19-9, Fig. 19-10)
- Shallow notch allowing space for the gallbladder (Fig. 19-9)

More details of the radiology of the liver can be found in the excellent works of Whalen,[59] Gamsu and associates,[64] and Meyers.[65]

### Falciform Ligament

The anterior surface of the liver is covered entirely by peritoneum except at the sagittal line of attachment of the falciform ligament (Fig. 19-11). The falciform ligament extends from the anterior surface of the liver to the diaphragm and the anterior abdominal wall and is disposed at a variable distance to the right of the midline. It contains the ligamentum teres (Figs. 19-9 and 19-10), the obliterated left umbilical vein. The ligamentum is typically accompanied by one or more paraumbilical veins in the adult. Remember that the right umbilical vein is "lost in space" very early. But in a study of 340 liver cirrhosis patients, Ibukuro et al.[64] reported the hepatic falciform ligament artery (HFLA) as follows:

> The HFLA was demonstrated in 26 (7.6%) of the 340 patients on angiography. Two HFLAs were observed in one patient. The origin was the middle hepatic artery (A4) in 16 cases, the superior branch of the middle hepatic artery in three, the inferior branch of the middle hepatic artery in two, the inferior branch of the left hepatic artery (A3) in three, and the confluence of A3 and A4 in three cases.

Baba et al.[67] stated that the pathway of the hepatic falciform artery should be recognized before chemoembolization of the middle or left hepatic artery.

The left leaf of the falciform ligament continues laterally where, superiorly, it becomes the left triangular ligament (Figs. 19-9, 19-10). This ligament consists of the two fused layers of peritoneum from the anterior and posterior surfaces of the left lobe. It suspends the left lateral segment from the diaphragm. If the left triangular ligament is divided, the lateral segment of the left lobe becomes freely mobile. The medial inferior aspect of the left triangular ligament is continuous with the anterior layer of the lesser omentum (Fig. 19-10).

The presence of blood vessels, aberrant bile ducts, cords of hepatocytes, and nerves in the free edge of the left triangular ligament has long been known.[68] More recently, Gao and Roberts[69] showed that biliary ducts may be found in 80% to 90% of individuals examined, liver cords in 60%, nerve bundles in 80%, and blood vessels are always present. When sectioning the ligament, the surgeon must watch for bleeding and bile leakage.[70]

The right leaf of the falciform ligament diverges at the superior aspect of the liver, successively forming the superior layer of the coronary ligament (Fig. 19-9, Fig. 19-11), right triangular ligament (Fig. 19-10), and inferior layer of the coronary ligament. To the left of the midline, it forms the posterior layer of the lesser omentum.

### *Visceral Surface*

In contrast to the smooth, rounded, generally convex shape of its parietal surface, the visceral surface of the liver (Fig. 19-12) is distinctly concave in form with variably distinct impressions from adjacent organs, intervening fat, and connective tissues, both posteriorly and inferiorly.

In addition to the contours attributable to other organs, the visceral surface is characterized by indentations that outline the porta hepatis, gateway to the liver (Fig. 19-13). These landmarks form a capital "H" (Hepar) configuration in many individuals, although they can also resemble a capital "K."

The right limb of the "H" bordering the porta is formed anteriorly by the fossa for the gallbladder and posteriorly by the fossa for the inferior vena cava. The left limb is formed anteriorly by the fissure for the round ligament and posteriorly by the fissure for the ligamentum venosum. The porta hepatis forms the crossbar of the "H." Posterior to the crossbar is the caudate lobe; anterior to the crossbar is the quadrate lobe.

The visceral surface relates to several organs; we will describe them from right to left. The hepatic flexure of the colon and part of the transverse colon are related to the anterior one-third of the visceral surface of the right lobe, passing behind the sharp, anterior inferior margin of the liver. The colic impression (Fig. 19-12) begins at the right lobe and ends at the quadrate lobe.

Behind the colic impression is the renal impression (Fig. 19-12, Fig. 19-13), produced by the right kidney and right adrenal gland. Fat, connective tissue, and peritoneum intervene between these organs and the liver. The right adrenal gland is in contact with the bare area of the liver.

The gallbladder lies in a fossa (Fig. 19-13) just beneath the anterior inferior border of the liver. To the left of the gallbladder is a depression for the first and second portions of the duodenum. Posterior to the gallbladder fossa is the fossa for the inferior vena cava.

Posteriorly and to the left of the ligamentum venosum

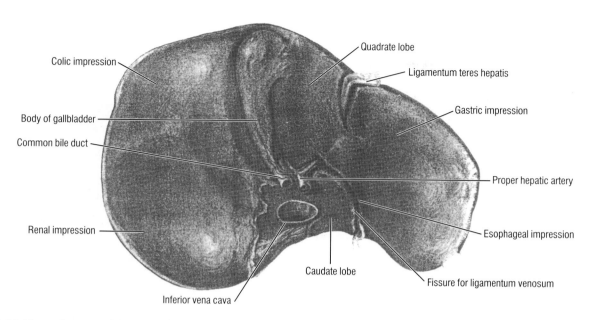

Colic impression
Quadrate lobe
Ligamentum teres hepatis
Body of gallbladder
Gastric impression
Common bile duct
Proper hepatic artery
Renal impression
Esophageal impression
Caudate lobe
Fissure for ligamentum venosum
Inferior vena cava

**FIG. 19-12.** Visceral aspect of the liver. The inferior margin of the anterior surface is uppermost in the figure. The major impressions on the liver made by the stomach, colon, and right kidney are seen clearly. A bridge of hepatic parenchyma bridges the groove for the ligamentum venosum in this specimen. (Modified from Skandalakis LJ, Gray SW, Colborn GL, Skandalakis JE. Surgical anatomy of the liver and associated extrahepatic structures: Part 2. Contemp Surg 30:26-38, 1987; with permission.)

(the posterior limb of the "H"), one can see a small impression for the abdominal esophagus. Almost the entire visceral surface of the left lobe is in contact with the stomach, forming the gastric impression (Fig. 19-12, Fig. 19-13).

## Surgical Considerations

- The right lobe of the liver has a convex surface and right lateral surface. The convex surface is subdivided into superior and anterior. The superior convex surface relates to the right hemidiaphragm covered by peritoneum below and pleura above, the right pleural cavity, and the lower lobe of the right lung. The anterior convex surface relates to the right costal margin and right upper abdominal wall. The right lateral surface relates to the right costodiaphragmatic recess and to the right thoracic wall from the 7th to 11th ribs.
- The left lobe of the liver relates to the diaphragm. Under normal conditions and for all practical purposes, the left lobe is not related to the left upper abdominal wall.
- We have seen a few patients with echinococcal cysts of the right lobe of the liver penetrate through the right hemidiaphragm and into the lower lobe of the right lung. These cysts evacuated into the bronchial tree and the patient coughed out the material. The pathway for evacuation of the cyst created by adhesions of the anatomic

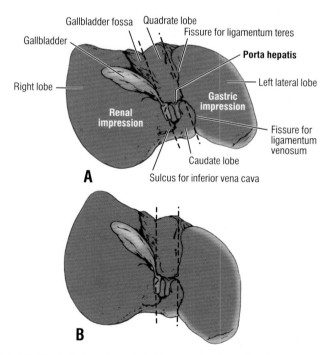

Gallbladder fossa    Quadrate lobe
Fissure for ligamentum teres
Gallbladder
**Porta hepatis**
Right lobe
Left lateral lobe
**Gastric impression**
**Renal impression**
Fissure for ligamentum venosum
Caudate lobe
**A**    Sulcus for inferior vena cava

**B**

**FIG. 19-13.** Porta hepatis and features of the visceral surface of the liver. **A.** Typical orientation of the "H" configuration of the portal structures. **B.** Common but incorrect depiction of relationship of "H"-parallel with the mid-sagittal plane of the body. (Modified from Skandalakis LJ, Gray SW, Colborn GL, Skandalakis JE. Surgical anatomy of the liver and associated extrahepatic structures: Part 2. Contemp Surg 30:26-38, 1987; with permission.)

entities involved is a magnificent phenomenon of nature.

- Percutaneous needle biopsy of a solid or cystic mass at the superior convex of the right lobe will penetrate pleura, diaphragm, and peritoneum. For further details, see the section that follows considering supra- and infra-hepatic collection.
- Pathology of the anterior convex surface may be reached by a needle penetrating only the peritoneum.

## *Peritoneal Relations*

An imaginary cross-sectional plane passing through the transverse mesocolon defines a supracolic and an infracolic compartment of the peritoneal cavity. Within the supracolic compartment lie the liver and its attachments. These define the right and left suprahepatic (subdiaphragmatic or subphrenic) and right and left subhepatic spaces.

### Ventral Mesogastrium

The supracolic compartment is the most difficult area of the abdomen to conceptualize. Our description is based on the work of Livingstone,[71] Ochsner and Graves,[72] Mitchell,[73] Autio,[74] Boyd,[75] Meyers,[76] and Whalen.[59]

Early in embryonic development, both a dorsal and a ventral mesentery are present. All the ventral mesentery except the foregut disappears. The persisting ventral mesentery extends from the abdominal esophagus to the umbilicus. It contains liver, stomach, and the first 2 cm of the duodenum. The liver divides this mesentery in two, forming the falciform ligament anteriorly and the lesser omentum posteriorly.

As noted earlier, the falciform ligament passes obliquely from the umbilicus to the superior surface of the left lobe of the liver. Here it marks the fissure between the medial and lateral segments of the left lobe (Fig. 19-14). In its free edge, the falciform ligament contains the remnant of the proximal part of the left umbilical vein, the round ligament of the liver or ligamentum teres. The right umbilical vein disappears early in development. The left vein returns placental blood to the fetus and closes soon after birth. In adults, the left umbilical vein may remain patent for much of its length.[77] The terminal portion of this vein is retained as the ligamentum venosum, a structure connecting the left branch of the portal vein with the left hepatic vein.

We have seen two cases in which the falciform ligament was only partially attached to the anterior abdominal wall. This created a hiatus through which a loop of intestine might have passed, causing a partial or complete small bowel incarceration.

The leaves of the falciform ligament separate as they reach the liver to form the superior layer of the coronary ligament (Fig. 19-15). Laterally, the layers reflect back medi-

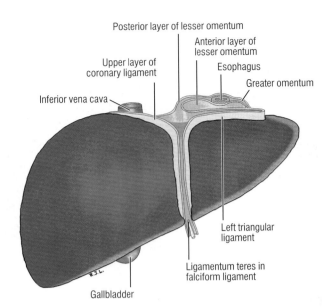

**FIG. 19-14.** Anterior view of the liver. The esophagus is pulled upwards from its normal position behind the left lobe to show the peritoneal attachments. All peritoneal edges seen here are attached to the diaphragm. (Modified from Last RJ. Anatomy: Regional and Applied, 5th Ed. Baltimore: Williams & Wilkins, 1972; with permission.)

ally to form the right and left triangular ligaments. They are not symmetrical. The right is more posterior and lateral. The left is more superior and medial. On the left, the anterior and posterior layers are almost in apposition until they reach the abdominal esophagus. On the right, the layers diverge as they approach the inferior vena cava. This wide separation is often surgically termed the "right coronary ligament" (Fig. 19-16). There are not distinctly separate right and left coronary ligaments, but the terms are convenient for the surgeon who is exploring the gastroesophageal junction.

In spite of the convenience of the terminology, however, the concept of a "right" and a "left" coronary ligament has to be corrected. Only a left triangular ligament and the complex of coronary and right triangular ligaments exist. To be accurate we should name the layers of the coronary ligament "superior" rather than "anterior" and "inferior" rather than "posterior." Furthermore the liberal use of the term "ligament" to describe mesothelium-covered conduits to and from the respective organs has to be revised; actually these are peritoneal attachments or reflections. We suggest use of "left triangular peritoneal attachment" of the liver instead of "left triangular ligament" and "coronary peritoneal attachment" of the liver instead of "coronary ligament."

Nevertheless, the old terminology is so ingrained in our thinking and writing that we continue to use it and it will be found within this text. We do hope, though, that our recom-

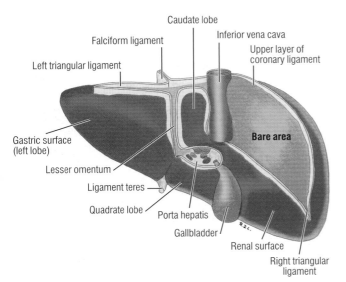

Caudate lobe
Falciform ligament
Inferior vena cava
Upper layer of
coronary ligament
Left triangular ligament
**Bare area**
Gastric surface
(left lobe)
Lesser omentum
Ligament teres
Quadrate lobe
Porta hepatis
Gallbladder
Renal surface
Right triangular
ligament

**FIG. 19-15.** Posterior view of the liver. The under surface of the organ, sloping down to the anterior border, is visible from this aspect. The peritoneal attachments are shown. The cut edges around the porta hepatis and in the lower part of the lesser omentum are attached to the lesser curvature of the stomach; all other peritoneal edges seen here are attached to the diaphragm. (Modified from Last RJ. Anatomy: Regional and Applied, 5th Ed. Baltimore: Williams & Wilkins, 1972; with permission.)

ments. The hepatogastric ligament extends from the porta hepatis to the lesser curvature of the stomach and the abdominal esophagus. The ligament encloses the gastroesophageal junction on the right and the two leaves rejoin on the left as the gastrosplenic ligament, a portion of the embryonic dorsal mesentery. The posterior leaf does not reach the gastroesophageal junction. Therefore, the small bare area on the posterior wall of the stomach lies on the left crus of the diaphragm and is related to the left adrenal gland and the left gastric artery and vein.[78] The abdominal esophagus is covered partially by peritoneum in front and on its left lateral wall.

The hepatogastric ligament contains the left gastric artery and vein and the hepatic division of the left vagal trunk. Occasionally, it may contain the right gastric artery and vein and both vagal trunks. In about one-fourth of subjects, it contains an aberrant left hepatic artery that arises from the left gastric artery.[79]

The hepatoduodenal ligament extends between the liver and the first portion of the duodenum and is continuous with the right border of the hepatogastric ligament. It contains the common bile duct, hepatic artery, and portal vein as well as the hepatic plexus and lymph nodes. Consider this ligament as the mesentery of the portal triad. It also forms the anterior boundary of the epiploic foramen of Winslow.

mended terminology will be adopted and will come into everyday usage.

The posterior component of the ventral mesentery forms the lesser omentum (Fig. 19-16). This may be divided into the proximal hepatogastric and distal hepatoduodenal liga-

### Dorsal Mesogastrium

Unlike the ventral mesentery, the primitive dorsal mesentery persists in the adult. In the supracolic compartment, it forms the greater omentum (Fig. 19-16). Initially, the fetal dorsal mesentery extended from the dorsal border of the

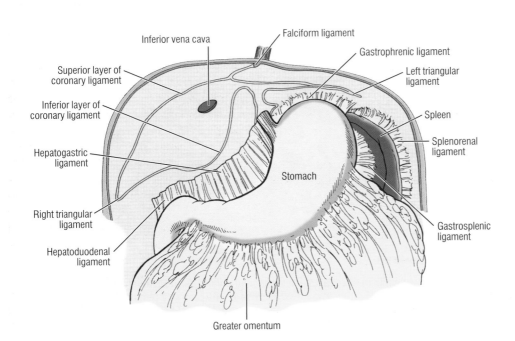

Inferior vena cava
Falciform ligament
Gastrophrenic ligament
Superior layer of
coronary ligament
Left triangular
ligament
Inferior layer of
coronary ligament
Spleen
Hepatogastric
ligament
Splenorenal
ligament
Stomach
Right triangular
ligament
Hepatoduodenal
ligament
Gastrosplenic
ligament
Greater omentum

**FIG. 19-16.** Peritoneal reflections of the stomach, gastroesophageal junction, and bare area of the diaphragm.

stomach to the midline of the posterior abdominal wall. This simple relationship changes as a result of the 90° counterclockwise rotation of the stomach and the development of the spleen.

The embryonic dorsal mesentery of the supracolic compartment may be divided into the following three parts.

- Upper, the gastrophrenic ligament
- Middle, the gastrosplenic ligament
- Lower, the gastrocolic ligament

In addition, the middle portion is interrupted by the spleen to form posteriorly the splenorenal ligament (Fig. 19-16).

### Surgical Considerations

- The falciform ligament may be cut with impunity if necessary. The cut should be made between proximal and distal ligations to avoid bleeding from a patent round ligament (left umbilical vein).
- The left coronary ligament, including its lateral end or triangular ligament, may be also sacrificed without negative consequences using electrocautery. However, the surgeon should remember not to be overenthusiastic when cutting this ligament medially, as one may encounter the left hepatic vein in this area.
- The right triangular, superior, and inferior coronary ligaments may be cut successfully using electrocautery. The superior right coronary ligament is cut with ease. Then, by anterior and caudal elevation of the right lobe, the inferior right coronary ligament is incised carefully to the

foramen of Winslow. At that point the right lobe is mobilized.

- The hepatogastric ligament is routinely divided during mobilization of the liver or stomach. The surgeon must take care to preserve a dominant left hepatic artery that travels through the ligament if a right hepatic lobectomy is planned, if the patient has cirrhosis, or if the patient has had prior interruption of the right hepatic artery. Division of the artery in these circumstances may lead to ischemia and insufficiency of the left lobe.

## Perihepatic Spaces

Among the several spaces that the peritoneum forms in the supracolic compartment are those above and below the liver. These are extremely important to the radiologist and the surgeon. We follow the nomenclature of Whalen[59] and of Ochsner and DeBakey[80] in part, realizing that it is arbitrary.

### Suprahepatic Spaces

A portion of the superior surface of the liver and a corresponding portion of the inferior surface of the diaphragm are in direct contact with one another without being covered by peritoneum. This area of contact is the "bare area." Its margins are the falciform, coronary, and left and right triangular ligaments of the liver (Fig. 19-15, Fig. 19-16, Fig. 19-17).

Except over its bare area, the serous surfaces of the

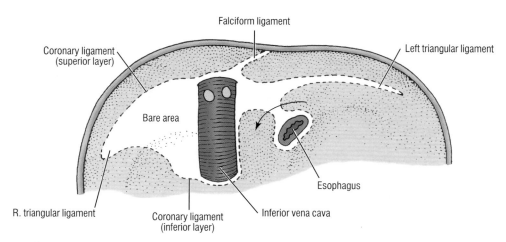

Coronary ligament (superior layer) · Falciform ligament · Left triangular ligament · Bare area · Esophagus · R. triangular ligament · Coronary ligament (inferior layer) · Inferior vena cava

**FIG. 19-17.** The inferior surface of the diaphragm showing the peritoneal attachments of the liver *(dashed lines)*. Within the boundaries of these attachments is the "bare area" of the liver and the diaphragm. The arrow represents the pathway behind the abdominal esophagus where surgeons may pass a finger through the inferior layer of the coronary ligament. (Modified from Gray SW, Rowe JS Jr, Skandalakis JE. Surgical anatomy of the gastroesophageal junction. Am Surg 45(9):575-587, 1979; with permission.)

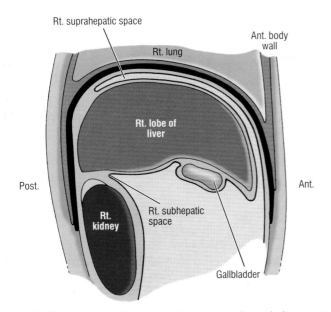

**FIG. 19-18.** Diagrammatic parasagittal section through the upper abdomen showing the potential right suprahepatic and subhepatic spaces. The thick black line represents the diaphragm. (Modified from Skandalakis JE, Gray SW, Rowe JS Jr. Anatomical Complications in General Surgery. New York: McGraw-Hill, 1983; with permission.)

liver and diaphragm are side by side and separated by a potential space. This potential space may become the site of intraperitoneal fluid collection and of suprahepatic (subphrenic) abscess.

The suprahepatic potential space is divided into right and left spaces by the falciform ligament. The right suprahepatic space (Fig. 19-18) lies between the diaphragm and the anterosuperior surface of the right lobe and the medial segment of the left lobe of the liver. The boundaries are:
- Left — falciform ligament
- Posterior — right superior coronary and right triangular ligaments
- Inferior — right lobe and medial segment of the left lobe of the liver

The space opens into the general peritoneal cavity anteriorly and inferiorly.

The corresponding suprahepatic space on the left (Fig. 19-19) is between the diaphragm and the superior surface of the lateral segment of the left lobe of the liver and the fundus of the stomach. To the right, the left suprahepatic space is bounded by the falciform ligament and, posteriorly, by the left coronary and triangular ligaments. Anteriorly and laterally, the space communicates with the infrahepatic space and the general peritoneal cavity. On the left, the anterior and posterior leaves of the coro-

nary ligament are side by side. The left triangular ligament separates the anterior and superior suprahepatic spaces.

Min et al.[81] report that the posterior left suprahepatic space is located anterior and superior to the lesser sac, with inferior continuation to the gastrohepatic space. These authors emphasize that the left posterior suprahepatic space and the lesser sac are separated by the lesser omentum and the stomach.

Each suprahepatic space may be divided into anterior and posterior portions. The distinction is unimportant in the absence of disease. On the right, fluid may collect or an abscess may form between the liver and diaphragm anteriorly just beneath the sternum (right anterior suprahepatic abscess) (Fig. 19-20). Or an abscess may form at the reflection of the superior leaf of the coronary ligament (right posterior suprahepatic abscess) (Fig. 19-21). The single space of the anatomist may be divided by pseudomembranes into two spaces.

The left suprahepatic space may be similarly compartmentalized by pseudomembranes between the liver and diaphragm or the abdominal wall (Fig. 19-22, Fig. 19-23). The left suprahepatic and left anterior infrahepatic spaces are not separated anatomically, but they may become separate pathologically by pseudomembranes. Large accumulations of fluid may extend into the sub-

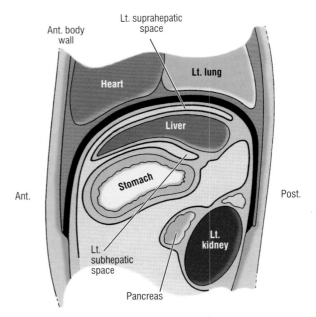

**FIG. 19-19.** Diagrammatic parasagittal section through the trunk showing the potential left suprahepatic and subhepatic spaces. (Modified from Skandalakis JE, Gray SW, Rowe JS Jr. Anatomical Complications in General Surgery. New York: McGraw-Hill, 1983; with permission.)

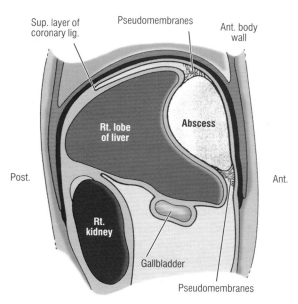

**FIG. 19-20.** Relations of an abscess in the anterior portion of the right suprahepatic space. (Modified from Skandalakis JE, Gray SW, Rowe JS Jr. Anatomical Complications in General Surgery. New York: McGraw-Hill, 1983; with permission.)

hepatic space where the stomach, spleen, and liver participate in walling off the infection. The diaphragm is usually elevated over the abscess or fluid collection.

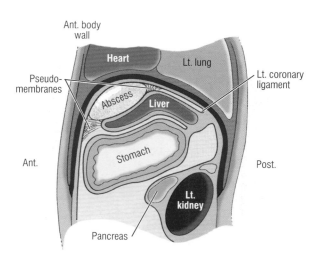

**FIG. 19-22.** Relations of an abscess in the anterior portion of the left suprahepatic space. (Modified from Skandalakis JE, Gray SW, Rowe JS Jr. Anatomical Complications in General Surgery. New York: McGraw-Hill, 1983; with permission.)

Anteriorly, a surgical approach from beneath the costal margin presents no anatomic complications. Posteriorly, the approach must be by an incision at the level of the spinous process of the first lumbar vertebra. This method avoids the pleura. The pleura and the twelfth rib are related at the vertebral spine. Thus the surgeon must avoid traversing the bed of the twelfth rib.

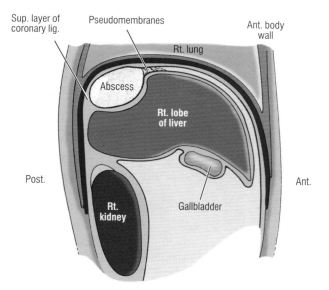

**FIG. 19-21.** Relations of an abscess in the posterior portion of the right suprahepatic space. (Modified from Skandalakis JE, Gray SW, Rowe JS Jr. Anatomical Complications in General Surgery. New York: McGraw-Hill, 1983; with permission.)

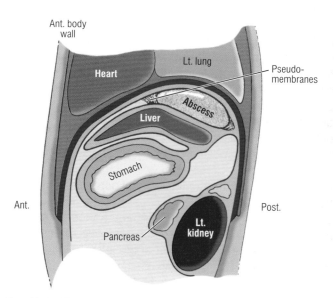

**FIG. 19-23.** Relations of an abscess in the posterior portion of the left suprahepatic space. (Modified from Skandalakis JE, Gray SW, Rowe JS Jr. Anatomical Complications in General Surgery. New York: McGraw-Hill, 1983; with permission.)

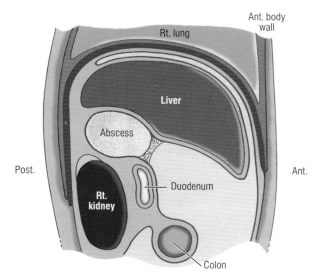

**FIG. 19-24.** Relations of an abscess in the right infrahepatic space. (Modified from Skandalakis JE, Gray SW, Rowe JS Jr. Anatomical Complications in General Surgery. New York: McGraw-Hill, 1983; with permission.)

## *Infrahepatic Spaces*

The right infrahepatic space (Fig. 19-24) (subhepatic space, hepatorenal space, pouch of Morison) is bounded superiorly and anteriorly by the right lobe and medial segment of the left lobe of the liver and the gallbladder. It is limited superiorly and posteriorly by the inferior layer of the coronary ligament and the posterior layer of the right triangular ligament. Inferiorly, the space opens into the general peritoneal cavity and is partly bounded by the hepatic flexure of the colon and the transverse mesocolon and, medially, by the hepatoduodenal ligament. The right suprahepatic space communicates with the right infrahepatic space in three places: the margin of the right lobe of the liver; the right triangular ligament; and a small space, the quadrangular space of Mitchell. The quadrangular space is bounded above by the quadrate lobe of the liver, below by the transverse colon, on the left by the falciform ligament, and on the right by the gallbladder. The coronary ligament suspends the liver not from above but from the dorsum. The left triangular ligament suspends the left lobe not from the apex of the diaphragm but from the dorsal aspect of the diaphragm.[75]

The left infrahepatic space (Fig. 19-25) may be divided into the smaller antegastric space and the larger lesser sac of the peritoneum.

### Antegastric Space

The anterior space lies between the left lobe of the liver above and the stomach below and behind (Fig. 19-25).

The boundaries are:

- Superior and anterior, the left lobe of the liver and the anterior abdominal wall
- Posterior, the stomach and lesser omentum
- Inferiorly, the middle third of the transverse colon.

This space has been termed "perigastric," but this is misleading; "paragastric" might be better. This space is entirely anterior to the stomach. Hollinshead[82] believes it is merely part of the left suprahepatic (subphrenic) space in general.

### Lesser Sac

The lesser sac of the peritoneum becomes, by the terminology used here, the left posterior infrahepatic space. This is a valid concept. For practical purposes, our two preferred terms are the "lesser sac" or the "omental bursa."

## *Extraperitoneal Spaces*

There are two potential extraperitoneal spaces in which abscesses can occur. On the right, abscesses may form over the bare area of the liver that is outlined by the falciform, coronary, and triangular ligaments (Fig. 19-17). On the left, they may occur in a poorly defined space that is bounded by the distal pancreas, the descending (left) colon, the upper pole of the left kidney, the left adrenal gland, Gerota's perirenal fascia, and fat. Altemeier and

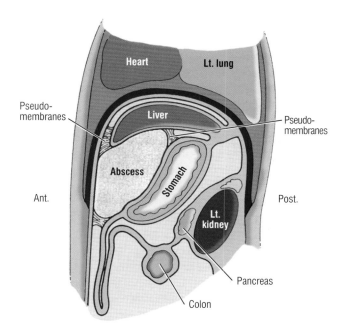

**FIG. 19-25.** Relations of an abscess in the left infrahepatic space. (Modified from Skandalakis JE, Gray SW, Rowe JS Jr. Anatomical Complications in General Surgery. New York: McGraw-Hill, 1983; with permission.)

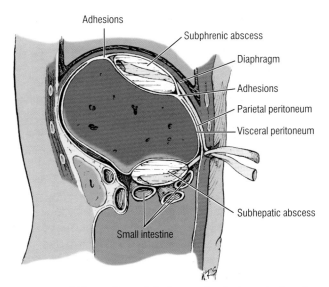

FIG. 19-26. Extraperitoneal drainage of anterior subphrenic and subhepatic abscesses. Schematic position of drains. Note the position of the drain for subphrenic abscesses between parietal peritoenum and diaphragm. The drain tract to the subhepatic abscess is walled off from the rest of the peritoneal cavity by adhesions between the loops of small intestine. (Modified from Hau T. Drainage of hepatic, subphrenic, and subhepatic abscesses. In: Nyhus LM, Baker RJ, eds. Mastery of Surgery, 2nd Ed. Boston: Little, Brown, 1992; with permission.)

Alexander[83] discuss these and other sites of retroperitoneal abscesses.

### Surgical Considerations

- Ultrasonography, CT scan, or MRI will help the surgeon decide whether to use the closed or open method in the treatment of a perihepatic abscess.
- Percutaneous needle-guided drainage (closed method) may be achieved by guiding the needle into the abscess cavity, advancing a wire into the cavity, dilating the tract around the wire with successively larger dilators, and placing a self-retaining catheter into the cavity or cavities.
- Open method
  - Drain a right anterior subphrenic (suprahepatic) abscess using a small right subcostal incision to establish an extraperitoneal route (Fig. 19-26).
  - Reach a right posterior subphrenic abscess (suprahepatic or infrahepatic) using a posterior route through the bed of the already excised 12th rib. Push the right kidney and the right adrenal gland downward (Fig. 19-27).
  - Approach a left anterior suprahepatic or infrahepatic abscess (Fig. 19-28) anteriorly using a small LUQ incision and proceeding intra- or extraperitoneally.
  - A left posterior suprahepatic or infrahepatic abscess

can be approached as on the right posterior, pushing the peritoneum down over the spleen and the gastric fundus. This forms a space between these two organs and the diaphragm.

## Lobes and Segments of the Liver

### Bases of Hepatic Segmentation

On first inspection, the liver appears to be divided into a large right portion and a much smaller left portion. The apparent plane of division (left fissure) passes through the falciform ligament, the round ligament, and the ligamentum venosum. Unfortunately, this apparent division does not correspond to the internal distribution of bile ducts and blood vessels (Figs. 19-29, 19-30, 19-31, 19-32).

**Actual Structure**

Injection and corrosion preparations, first made by Hjortsjo in 1951[84] and independently by Healey and Schroy in 1953,[68] clearly show that the true right and left lobes of the liver are about the same size. Further, the lobes are separated by a plane called the median fissure that passes through the bed of the gallbladder below and the fossa of the inferior vena cava above (Fig. 19-29).

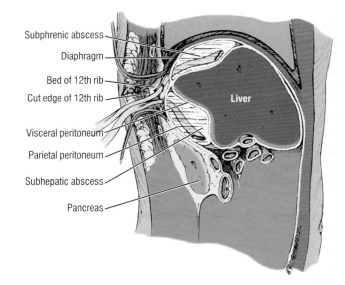

FIG. 19-27. Extraperitoneal drainage of posterior subphrenic and subhepatic abscesses. Schematic position of the drains passing through the bed of the twelfth rib. Neither drain violates the peritoneal cavity. (Modified from Hau T. Drainage of hepatic, subphrenic, and subhepatic abscesses. In: Nyhus LM, Baker RJ, eds. Mastery of Surgery, 2nd Ed. Boston: Little, Brown, 1992; with permission.)

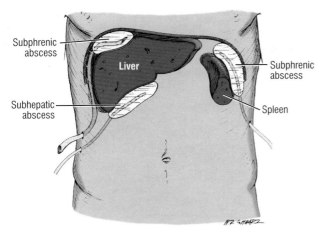

FIG. 19-28. Transperitoneal drainage of subphrenic and subhepatic abscesses. Schematic position of drains. (Modified from Hau T. Drainage of hepatic, subphrenic, and subhepatic abscesses. In: Nyhus LM, Baker RJ, eds. Mastery of Surgery, 2nd Ed. Boston: Little, Brown, 1992; with permission.)

## True Left Lobe and True Right Lobe

The true left lobe consists of a left medial segment and a left lateral segment (Fig. 19-29). The latter is the "left lobe" of older anatomic descriptions. Each of these two segments can be further divided into superior and inferior subsegments on the basis of the distribution of the bile ducts, hepatic arteries, and portal veins.

The true right lobe is divided by the right fissure into anterior and posterior segments. The plane of this fissure corresponds to the line of the eighth intercostal space. Each segment of the right lobe can be subdivided into superior and inferior subsegments.

**QUADRATE LOBE.** The quadrate "lobe" is a portion of the inferior half or so of the medial segment of the left lobe (Figs. 19-12, 19-13, 19-15, 19-33A & B). According to Sales et al.,[85] it lies to the right of the falciform ligament, anterior to the hilum, and to the left of the gallbladder. It is related to the pylorus and the first portion of the duodenum.

**CAUDATE LOBE.** The caudate lobe is a separate region divided by the interlobar plane into right and left subsegments. Its bile ducts, arteries, and portal veins arise from both right and left main branches. Hence, the plane between the true right and left lobes passes through the middle of the caudate lobe. The right portion of the caudate lobe is continuous with the true right lobe by the caudate process, or tuber. This process forms the superior boundary of the epiploic foramen. The caudate lobe is drained by two small, fairly constant hepatic veins that enter the left side of the vena cava. Names such as cau-

date and quadrate "lobes" are mentioned for convenience. They are not true lobes.

Padbury and Azoulay[86] report the segmental anatomy of the liver as two hemilivers and a dorsal or caudate lobe (or Couinaud's segment I). Segments II-IV form the left hemiliver. Segments V-VIII form the right hemiliver. (If we were to follow our own terminology, we would refer to them as "subsegments" II-IV and V-VIII rather than "segments," but we follow Couinaud's usage.)

Dodds et al.[87] studied the caudate lobe from an embryologic, anatomic and pathologic standpoint. They report the following.

- The caudate lobe may be hypertrophic (enlarged) secondary to liver cirrhosis, occlusion of the hepatic veins due to greater blood flow, and other focal lesions.
- The caudal margin of the caudate lobe often attaches by a narrow connection to a papillary process. On CT, this may be identified as a large lymph node.

NOTE: The caudate (spigelian) lobe is the "third liver" of Bismuth.[88] This terminology is used because the lobe has independent vascularization that receives branches from the right and left sides of the portal vein and hepatic artery, and its veins drain directly into the IVC.

Brown et al.[89] emphasized the anatomic distinction of the caudate lobe from the left and right hepatic lobes. It is located between the IVC posteriorly, the left and right hepatic lobes anteriorly and superiorly, and the main portal vein inferiorly (Fig. 19-34, Fig. 19-35).

To be more specific, we quote Heloury et al.[90] They define the caudate lobe as "...bounded ...by the IVC on the right, by the fissure of the ligamentum venosum on the left, and by the hilum of the liver below and in front." These authors report that the lobe is characterized by great morphologic variation. We strongly advise the study of their article.

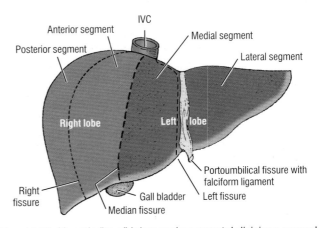

FIG. 19-29. Hepatic "true" lobar and segmental divisions according to Ger. (Modified from Skandalakis JE. Liver anatomy [letter to the editor]. South Med J 73:1096, 1980.)

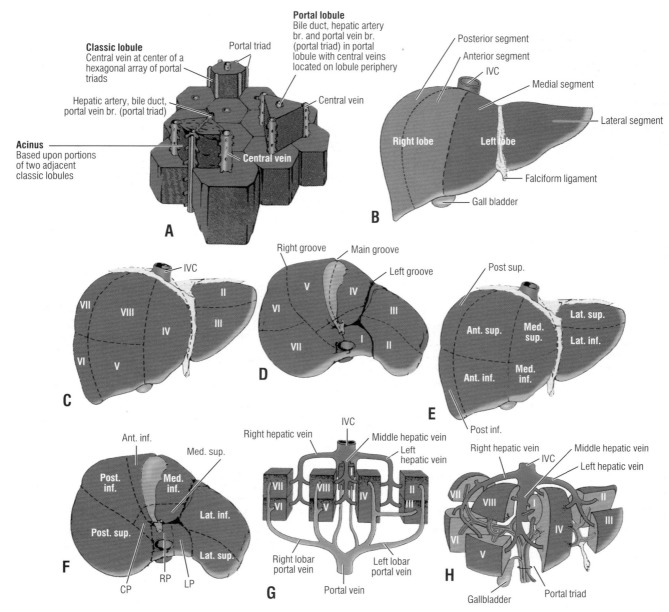

**FIG. 19-30. A.** Three concepts of the liver lobule. The "classic" lobule, with central veins and peripheral hepatic triads; the "portal" lobule, centered on the hepatic triads; and the hepatic acinus. Both the central vein and the hepatic traids are peripheral. It is the concept of the acinus that has proved to be the most useful for understanding liver functions. **B.** Modern concept of the lobes and segments of the human liver. **C** to **F.** Projection of liver lobes and segments based on the distribution of intrahepatic ducts and blood vessels. **C** and **D.** Terminology of Couinaud (1954). **E** and **F.** Terminology of Healey and Schroy (1953). (CP, caudate process; RP and LP, right and left portions of the caudate lobe). **G.** Highly diagrammatic presentation of the segmental functional anatomy of the liver emphasizing portal distribution and hepatic veins. **H.** Exploded segmental view of the liver emphasizing the intrahepatic anatomy and hepatic veins. (**A,** Modified from Gray SW, Skandalakis JE, Colborn GL, Skandalakis LJ. Surgical anatomy of the liver and associated extrahepatic structures. Part 1. Contemp Surg 1987;30(4):37-47. **B,** Modified from Skandalakis JE. Liver anatomy [letter to the editor]. South Med J 1980;73:1096. **C-F,** Modified from Skandalakis JE, Gray SW, Skandalakis LJ, Colborn GL. Surgical anatomy of the liver and associated extrahepatic structures. Part 2. Contemp Surg 1987;30(5):26-38. **G, H,** Modified from Skandalakis JE, Gray SW (eds). Embryology for Surgeons, 2nd Ed. Baltimore: Williams & Wilkins, 1994. With permission.)

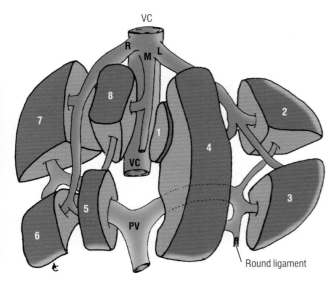

**FIG. 19-31.** Exploded diagrammatic sketch of the liver. The umbilical fissure separates the anatomic left lobe (segments 2 and 3) from the right lobe (segments 4-8). The middle hepatic vein runs within the main portal fissure (Cantlie's line), which separates the left liver (segments 2 to 4) from the right liver (segments 5 to 8). The hepatic veins are distributed on an intersegmental basis. VC, vena cava; R, right; M, middle; L, left hepatic veins, and 1, caudate lobe. (From Czerniak A, Lotan G, Hiss Y, Shemesh E, Avigad I, Wolfstein I. The feasibility of in vivo resection of the left lobe of the liver and its use for transplantation. Transplantation 1989;48:26; with permission.)

Schwartz[91] made the following points about the anatomy of the caudate lobe.

- The caudate lobe is not a true lobe.
- The caudate lobe is generally regarded as that portion of the liver between the line of Cantlie and the line corresponding to the falciform ligament.
- It is posterior to an imaginary horizontal line in the porta hepatis.
- It is divided arbitrarily and without good landmarks into the caudate lobe proper and a caudate process extending to the right lobe of the liver.
- Its biliary drainage is usually into both right and left duct systems.
- In most instances its arterial supply is from both right and left hepatic arterial branches. It originates totally from the right hepatic artery in 35% of cases and from the left hepatic artery in 12%.
- In the Couinaud[92] nomenclature, the caudate lobe makes up segment I.
- According to Couinaud,[92] its position varies with respect to the portal bifurcation and therefore may belong to only the left or right lobe, or it may belong to both.

We quote from Kogure et al.[93] on their dissection studies of the human liver:

> The caudate lobe exhibited distinct portal segmentation with a portal fissure that was indicated internally by the proper hepatic vein and externally by the notch at the caudal edge of the caudate lobe.

Hepatic segmental anatomy was also described in detail by Healey and Schroy,[68] Healey,[94] and Couinaud[92] (Fig. 19-30B-E).

Using computed tomography scans to evaluate patients for resection of focal lesions, Rieker et al.[95] found that the segmental anatomy of the liver using the planes of hepatic veins and portal trunks according to Couinaud was not an accurate tool for the presurgical localization of all liver lesions.

In 1957, Goldsmith and Woodburne[96] presented another segmental terminology and nomenclature. For all practical purposes and "anatomically" at least, the paper of Goldsmith and Woodburne agreed with those of Healey and Schroy,[68] Healey[94] and Couinaud[92] regarding hepatic segmentation. Therefore, all are correct, but because of different nomenclature, the surgical descriptions of liver resections are confusing.

Onishi et al.[97] studied the surgical anatomy of the medial segment (segment 4) of the liver. They categorized two main types and several subtypes of bile duct branches, and the morphology of the portal vein, middle hepatic vein, and middle hepatic artery. They stated that knowledge of the topographic anatomy of the ducts and vessels will facilitate resection of the medial segment.

We quote from Cho et al.[98] on the surgical anatomy of the right anterosuperior area (segment 8) of the liver:

> In most of the patients, the dorsal branches of segment 8 supplied the dorsocranial area of the right lobe posterior to the right hepatic vein. The paracaval portion of the caudate lobe was limited to below the interval between the middle and right hepatic veins in the majority of patients who showed medial branches of segment 8 arising near the porta hepatis. Recognition of this vascular anatomy is clinically important for preoperative evaluation of hepatic tumors in segment 8 because it may contribute to a safer surgical approach.

### Bismuth System and the Fissures

Soyer[99] urged that the Bismuth system be accepted worldwide to put an end to ongoing confusion. Soyer's table (Table 19-2) is self-explanatory.

What is the Bismuth system (Figs. 19-36, 19-37, 19-38)? In 1982, Bismuth[88] combined Couinaud's[92] cadaveric and Goldsmith and Woodburne's[96] in vivo systems. Bismuth used the three vertical fissures (the homes of the three hepatic veins) and a single transverse fissure to di-

## Anatomic Nomenclature

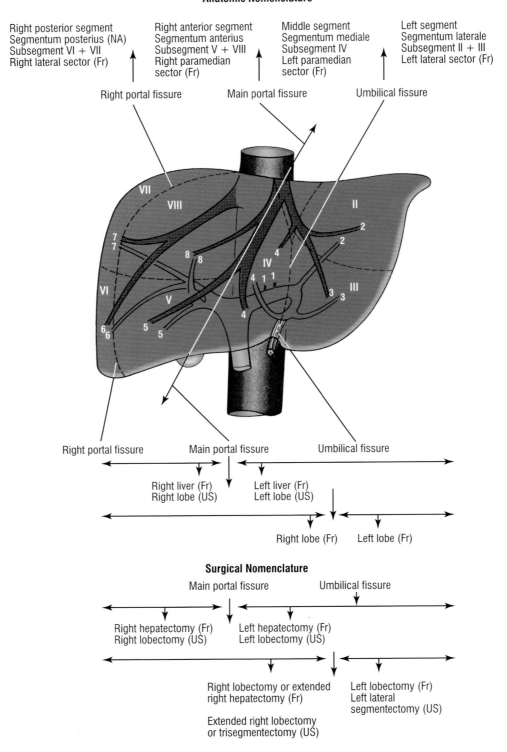

Right posterior segment
Segmentum posterius (NA)
Subsegment VI + VII
Right lateral sector (Fr)

Right anterior segment
Segmentum anterius
Subsegment V + VIII
Right paramedian
sector (Fr)

Middle segment
Segmentum mediale
Subsegment IV
Left paramedian
sector (Fr)

Left segment
Segmentum laterale
Subsegment II + III
Left lateral sector (Fr)

Right portal fissure

Main portal fissure

Umbilical fissure

Right portal fissure

Main portal fissure

Umbilical fissure

Right liver (Fr)
Right lobe (US)

Left liver (Fr)
Left lobe (US)

Right lobe (Fr)

Left lobe (Fr)

### Surgical Nomenclature

Main portal fissure

Umbilical fissure

Right hepatectomy (Fr)
Right lobectomy (US)

Left hepatectomy (Fr)
Left lobectomy (US)

Right lobectomy or extended
right hepatectomy (Fr)

Extended right lobectomy
or trisegmentectomy (US)

Left lobectomy (Fr)
Left lateral
segmentectomy (US)

**Fig. 19-32.** Differences in anatomic and surgical nomenclature of the liver. The division into lobes is based on external features. The division into segments is based on the intrahepatic ramifications of the hepatic veins and the portal elements. (Fr = French, US = American, NA = Nomina Anatomica). *Editor's note: The main portal fissure is also called the median fissure or the line of Rex. The umbilical fissure is also called the left fissure.* (Modified from Van Damme JPJ. Behavioral anatomy of the abdominal arteries. Surg Clin North Am 73(4):699-725, 1993; with permission.)

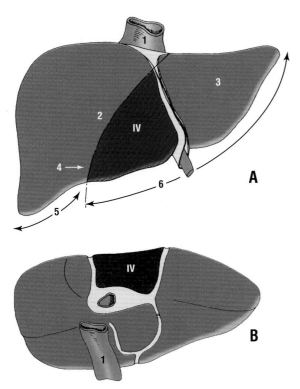

**FIG. 19-33.** Morphology of the liver. **A.** Anterior view: 1. inferior vena cava, 2. right lobe, 3. left lobe, 4. fissura portalis sagittalis, 5. right liver, 6. left liver; **B.** Inferior view: 1. inferior vena cava. *Editor's note: The "left lobe" is, in modern terminology, the lateral segment of the left lobe. Segment IV is the medial segment of the left lobe.* (Modified from Sales JP, Hannoun L, Sichez JP, Honiger J, Levy E. Surgical anatomy of liver segment IV. Anat Clin 1984;6:295; with permission.)

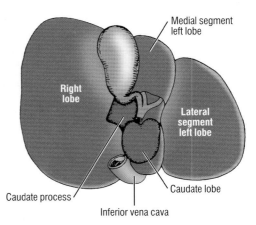

**FIG. 19-34.** Diagrammatic illustration of the undersurface of the liver. The caudate lobe is distinct from the left and right hepatic lobes and is interposed between the inferior vena cava posteriorly and the left hepatic lobe anteriorly and superiorly. (Modified from Brown BM, Filly RA, Callen PW. Ultrasonographic anatomy of the caudate lobe. J Ultrasound Med 1982; 1:189; with permission.)

- Left
  - Left lateral superior subsegment (segment II)
  - Left lateral inferior subsegment (segment III)
  - Left medial subsegment (segment IV)
- Right
  - Right anterior inferior subsegment (segment V)
  - Right anterior superior subsegment (segment VIII)

vide the liver into seven subsegments. He counted the caudate lobe separately. Adding the caudate lobe to the seven sub-segments produces eight hepatic subsegments in toto – two functional lobes (right and left) separated by the middle hepatic vein. The right has an anterior and a posterior segment separated by the right hepatic vein. The left has a medial and a lateral segment separated by the left hepatic vein.

The transverse fissure is an imaginary line through the right and left portal branches. *Note:* Although readers will see horizontal lines dividing the right lobe and lateral segment of the left lobe into superior and inferior subsegments (Fig. 19-30C), illustrations in this book and other books tend not to label the "transverse fissure." This is because there are no definite landmarks by which to place it, and because it is a morphologic rather than functional division.

The transverse fissure subdivides the segments into the following seven subsegments (Fig. 19-31):

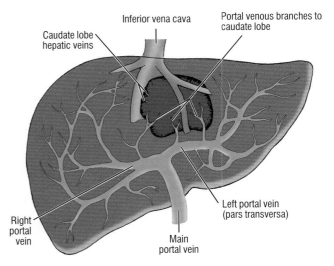

**FIG. 19-35.** Diagrammatic illustration demonstrating the caudate lobe and its portal venous blood supply and hepatic venous drainage. (Modified from Brown BM, Filly RA, Callen PW. Ultrasonographic anatomy of the caudate lobe. J Ultrasound Med 1982;1:189; with permission.)

**TABLE 19-2. Anatomic Segments of the Liver and Corresponding Nomenclature**

| Anatomic Subsegment | Nomenclature | | |
| --- | --- | --- | --- |
| | Couinaud | Bismuth | Goldsmith and Woodburne |
| Caudate lobe | I | I | Caudate lobe |
| Left lateral superior subsegment | II | II | Left lateral segment |
| Left lateral inferior subsegment | III | III | |
| Left medial subsegment | IV | IVa, IVb | Left medial segment |
| Right anterior inferior subsegment | V | V | Right anterior segment |
| Right anterior superior subsegment | VIII | VIII | |
| Right posterior inferior subsegment | VI | VI | Right posterior segment |
| Right posterior superior subsegment | VII | VII | |

*Source:* Soyer P. Segmental anatomy of the liver: utility of a nomenclature accepted worldwide. AJR 1993;161:572; with permission.

– Right posterior inferior subsegment (segment VI)
– Right posterior superior subsegment (segment VII)

Adding the caudate lobe (segment 1), to the seven subsegments embraces all eight subsegments.

The lobes and segments are hepatic masses supplied by specific branches of bile ducts, hepatic arteries, and portal veins. In the fissures or intervals between adjacent lobes and segments lie tributaries of the hepatic veins (Fig. 19-39). These are intersegmental, and each drains portions of two adjacent segments. The hepatic veins do not follow branches of the biliary tree.

The intrahepatic arrangement of hepatic veins with respect to biliary, portal venous, and arterial branches is reminiscent of the intrapulmonic distribution of vessels. In the lungs, the pulmonary veins run between lobes; whereas the bronchi, bronchial arteries, and pulmonary arterial branches run within distinct bronchopulmonary segments.

By definition, the vertical fissures are planes that divide the liver along the pathways of the three hepatic veins. We use the term "fissure," although Bismuth used the word "scissura."

**RIGHT FISSURE.** The right fissure (Fig. 19-38) is an oblique 40° imaginary line at the anterior surface of the right functional lobe of the liver. According to Couinaud,[92] it starts in

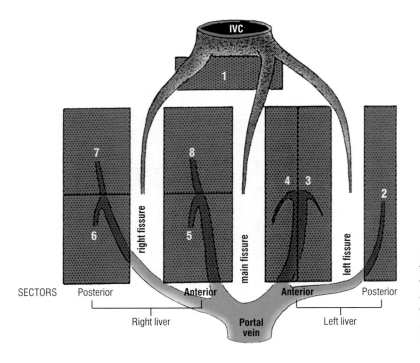

**FIG. 19-36.** Bismuth's schematic representation of the functional anatomy of the liver: 3 main hepatic veins divide the liver into 4 sectors, each receiving a portal pedicle. Hepatic veins and portal pedicles are intertwined as the fingers of the 2 hands. (Modified from Bismuth H. Surgical anatomy of the liver. Recent Results Cancer Res 100:179-184, 1986; with permission.)

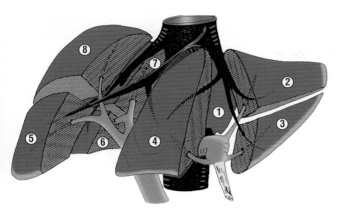

**FIG. 19-37.** The functional division of the liver and the hepatic segmentation (in vivo position of the liver). (Modified from Bismuth H. Surgical anatomy of the liver. Recent Results Cancer Res 100:179-184, 1986; with permission.)

the middle of the anterior border between the right angle and the right side of the gallbladder and extends to the confluence between the right hepatic vein and the inferior vena cava posteriorly.

Ton That Tung[100] stated that anatomically this fissure corresponds to a line parallel to the right lateral edge of the liver, but located three finger breadths more anteriorly.

The right hepatic vein is located within the vicinity of this imaginary fissure. We have frequently observed a variably distinct notch in the inferior margin of the right lobe, a notch that coincided with the inferior extent of the right fissure.

**MIDDLE FISSURE.** The middle fissure (Fig. 19-38) is an oblique, 75° imaginary line at the anterior surface of the

liver which connects the left side of the fossa for the gallbladder and the IVC. The middle hepatic vein is located in the vicinity of this line and, therefore, between the right and left functional hepatic lobes.

Oran and Memis[101] demonstrated that in 11.1% (2 of 18) of patients, part of hepatic segment IV had a blood supply from the right hepatic artery. They concluded that there is no coincidence between the arterial watershed line between the right and left hepatic artery areas and the middle fissure of Couinaud's segmental anatomy.

**LEFT FISSURE.** The left fissure is located within the left functional lobe of the liver, in the superior aspect of the umbilical fissure, just to the left of the line of attachment of the falciform ligament (Fig. 19-29). It separates the lobe into lateral and medial segments. The left hepatic vein is located along this line. In most cases, the middle hepatic vein drains into the left hepatic vein. Occasionally it is very close to the upper part of the vein near the inferior vena cava (IVC).

### Ger's Description of the Fissures

Ger[102] includes a fourth fissure in his description of the lobes and segments of the liver. Even though Ger's concept is similar to Bismuth's, it is so useful to the surgeon that we include it here in its entirety (Fig. 19-29).

*RIGHT FISSURE. This fissure commences at the right margin of the inferior vena cava and follows the attachment of the right superior coronary ligament to about 3 to 4 cm from the junction of the latter with the right infe-*

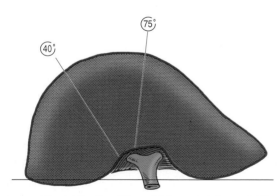

**FIG. 19-38.** The obliquity of the middle and right portal fissures. Relationship to the horizontal plane (in degrees) shown in circles. (Modified from Blumgart LH, Baer HU, Czerniak A, Zimmermann A, Dennison AR. Extended left hepatectomy: technical aspects of an evolving procedure. Br J Surg 1993;80: 903; with permission.)

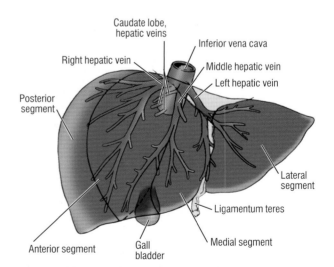

**FIG. 19-39.** Diagram of the intrahepatic distribution of the hepatic veins. These veins lie between lobes and segments rather than within them. (Modified from Skandalakis LJ, Gray SW, Colborn GL, Skandalakis JE. Surgical anatomy of the liver and associated extrahepatic structures: Part 2. Contemp Surg 30:26-38, 1987; with permission.)

**TABLE 19-3. Relations of Resections to Vascular and Ductal Structures**

| Resection | Line of Incision | Vascular and Ductal Structures Divided | Vascular and Ductal Structures Preserved |
|---|---|---|---|
| Right hepatic lobectomy (segments V, VI, VII, VIII) | Gallbladder fossa to IVC | Right hepatic vein; right branch of hepatic pedicle<br>Branches entering middle hepatic vein from right; accessory veins from segments VI and VII | Middle and left hepatic veins; left branch hepatic pedicle |
| Extended right hepatic lobectomy (segments IV, V, VI, VII, VIII) | 1 cm to right of portoumbilical fissure | Right and middle hepatic veins; right branch of hepatic pedicle and branches of left hepatic pedicle to segment IV | Left hepatic vein; left branch hepatic pedicle, including branches to segments II and III |
| Right lateral lobectomy (segments VI and VII) | Right fissure | Right hepatic vein, posterior division; right hepatic pedicle | Middle and left hepatic veins, anterior division; right hepatic pedicle |
| Left hepatic lobectomy (segments II, III, IV) | 1 cm to left of median fissure | Left hepatic vein and tributaries entering middle hepatic vein from left; left branch hepatic pedicle | Middle hepatic vein |
| Left lateral lobectomy (segments II and III) | 1 cm to left of portoumbilical fissure | Left hepatic vein before junction with the middle hepatic vein; branches of hepatic pedicle to segments II and III | Middle hepatic vein; left branch of hepatic pedicle, including branches to segment IV |
| Mesohepatectomy/ median hepatectomy (segments IV, V, VIII) | 1 cm to right of portoumbilical fissure, 1 cm to left of right fissure; inferiorly obliquely to hilum, leftward to 1 cm from portoumbilical fissure, to anterior margin of liver | Middle hepatic vein, branches joining left side of right hepatic vein, anterior division; right branch hepatic pedicle, left branch hepatic pedicle to segment IV, cystic duct, and artery | Right and left hepatic veins, posterior division; right branch hepatic pedicle, left branch hepatic pedicle |

*Source:* Ger R. Surgical anatomy of the liver. Surg Clin North Am 1989;69:179; with permission.

*rior layer. The fissure then curves anteriorly to a point on the inferior margin about midway between the gallbladder fossa and the right margin of the liver. Passing posteriorly, the fissure follows a line that runs parallel to the gallbladder fossa and crosses the caudate process to reach the right side of the inferior vena cava. Lying almost in the coronal plane, the fissure contains the right hepatic vein, with branches passing anteriorly to segments V and VIII and posteriorly to segments VI and VII.*

*MEDIAN FISSURE. This fissure passes from the gallbladder fossa to the left margin of the inferior vena cava.*

*Posteroinferiorly, the fissure is represented by a line from the gallbladder fossa to the main bifurcation of the hepatic pedicle (portal triad) and, thence, to the retrohepatic inferior vena cava.*

*LEFT FISSURE. This fissure runs from the left side of the inferior vena cava to a point between the dorsal one third and ventral two thirds of the left margin of the liver. Inferiorly, the fissure passes to the commencement of the ligamentum venosum.*

*PORTOUMBILICAL FISSURE. This fissure is marked superficially by the attachment of the falciform ligament, which contains the ligamentum teres hepatis in its inferior border. Angled less generously than the right fissure, it meets the inferior margin of the liver at an angle of about 50°.*

In a small number of instances, the relationship between the left fissure and the portoumbilical fissure may vary. In most cases the left fissure is to the right of the portoumbilical fissure. However, occasionally the left fissure is just inside the ligamentum teres and falciform ligament or just to the left of the duo.

Ger[102] presented a table (Table 19-3) of resections related to the vascular and ductal structures of the liver. Blumgart et al.[103] also presented a table (Table 19-4) showing anatomic classification of the five types of major resection.

Of the planes dividing these lobes and segments, only the one between the medial and lateral segments of the left lobe commonly marks the surface of the liver.

In retrospect, the fact that the portal vein and the hep-

**TABLE 19-4. Anatomical Classification of Major Hepatic Resections**

| Couinaud[1] | Goldsmith and Woodburn[2] |
| --- | --- |
| Right hepatectomy (segments V, VI, VII and VIII) | Right hepatic lobectomy |
| Left hepatectomy (segments II, III and IV) | Left hepatic lobectomy |
| Right lobectomy (segments IV, V, VI, VII and VIII; sometimes also segment I) | Extended right hepatic lobectomy |
| Left lobectomy (segments II and III) | Left lateral segmentectomy |
| Extended left hepatectomy (segments II, III, IV, V and VIII; sometimes also segment I) | Extended left lobectomy |

Right lobectomy (extended right hepatic lobectomy) has also been referred to as right trisegmentectomy and this term in commonly found in the literature. Similarly, extended left hepatectomy is referred to as left hepatic trisegmentectomy.[3]

**References**
1. Couinaud C. Le Foie. Etudes Anatomiques et Chirurgicales. Paris: Masson, 1957.
2. Goldsmith NA, Woodburn RT. The surgical anatomy pertaining to liver resection. Surg Gynecol Obstet 105:310-318, 1957.
3. Starzl TE, Iwatsuki S, Shaw BW, et al. Left hepatic trisegmentectomy. Surg Gynecol Obstet 55:21-27, 1982.

*Source:* Blumgart LH, Baer HU, Czerniak A, Zimmermann A, Dennison AR. Extended left hepatectomy: technical aspects of an evolving procedure. Br J Surg 1993;80:903; with permission.

atic ducts and arteries bifurcate and send branches of nearly equal size to the right and left might have provided a clue to the lobar structure. By overlooking the clue, we are reminded that appearances can be deceiving, and that careful analysis is always important.

**Rise and Demise of Segment IX**

For several years Couinaud and his colleagues, as well as several other investigators, referred to an area of the dorsal sector of the liver close to the inferior vena cava as "segment IX." But the existence of this segment was short-lived when, in 2002, Couinaud and his associates[104] published the following conclusion:

> *Because no separate veins, arteries, or ducts can be defined for the right paracaval portion of the posterior liver and because pedicles cross the proposed division between the right and left caudate, the concept of segment IX is abandoned.*

We advise the interested reader to study the "genesis" and "death" of segment IX in articles published by none other than the "father of hepatic segmentation" – Couinaud – and several other investigators.[105-108]

**Interlobar Anastomoses**

With the true lobar anatomy of the liver established, the question of interlobar anastomoses presents itself. The accepted view was that except in the caudate lobe,[109] connections between bile ducts or blood vessels of the right and left lobes are few, inconstant, and insignificant.[68,96,110-112]

In 1977, Mays[113] challenged these views, using radiographic techniques in living human subjects. Mays was able to show that an occluded left hepatic artery fills with blood from the right side and vice versa. He also noted that, "...when the common hepatic artery was interrupted, inferior phrenic and pancreaticoduodenal collaterals reconstituted intrahepatic arterial blood flow. These anastomoses could not be observed in the cadaver."

## *Orientation of Hepatic Lobes in Sectional Imaging*

The visceral surface of the liver faces inferiorly, posteriorly, and to the left. This orientation is a composite of the two oblique planes impressed upon the liver by the midline position of the vertebral column and the deep paravertebral gutters disposed on either side of the column.

As expressed by Schneck,[114] the vertebral column forms a longitudinal ridge-line within the abdominal cavity. The column's forward portion of the lordotic lumbar curve of the column causes this ridge-line to arch anteriorly behind the liver. The posterior portions of the lower ribs cause the right and left paravertebral gutters to deepen considerably.

The right paravertebral gutter principally houses the large, rounded dextral aspect of the liver. The right kidney and right adrenal gland lie behind the right lobe on the sloping lateral aspect of the lumbar vertebrae. The left paravertebral gutter is relatively crowded with various organs, including the esophagus, body of the stomach, tail of the pancreas, spleen, left kidney, and left adrenal gland. This anteriorly displaces the left side of the liver. The pylorus, duodenum, and head and body of the pancreas are displaced forward as they approach or cross in front of the vertebral column.

The importance of the in situ obliquity of the liver's visceral surface is best appreciated when viewing tomographic sections of the liver and attempting to identify hepatic lobes and segments in the sections. The majority of textbook and atlas illustrations of the liver's external features and their relationships to internal hepatic segmentation are often misleading or inaccurate. The liver is not shown in its true anatomic orientation.

The falciform ligament is often shown as a midline structure passing in the midsagittal plane from the abdominal wall to the anterior surface of the liver. Likewise, the long axis of the H-shaped features of the porta hepatis is shown as parallel with the midsagittal plane of the body (Fig. 19-13). In fact, the left side of the liver is displaced both anteriorly and to the right by the vertebral column and viscera. This causes the falciform ligament, ligamentum teres, and portal indentation to shift markedly toward the right in most individuals. In cross-sectional imaging, the fissure for the ligamentum teres lies at the right midclavicular line in many cases. The fissure for the ligamentum venosum and the lesser omentum lies roughly parallel with a coronal plane of the abdomen.

In cadaveric sections or computer-generated images, intrahepatic fissures can be used to approximate the margins of the intrahepatic lobes and their primary segments.[115] This process can be facilitated by observing other features, such as the hepatic veins (disposed roughly intersegmentally), ligaments, inferior vena cava, and gallbladder (Figs. 19-40, 19-41).

In upper abdominal transverse sections, the fissure for the ligamentum venosum departs obliquely from the left intersegmental fissure (left fissure) toward a coronal plane with the lesser omentum in front of the caudate lobe (Fig. 19-40A-C). The caudate lobe separates the left lobe anteriorly and the left lobe from the right lobe posteriorly and to the right.

To approximate the interlobar (median) fissure between the right and left lobes draw a line between the left margin of the bed of the gallbladder and the sulcus for the IVC. The superior recess of the bed of the gallbladder can often be seen above the gallbladder as a space containing fat, the portal vein, and small vessels (Fig. 19-40C). The right lobe is situated posterior to and to the right of the line. The medial lobe lies anteriorly and to the left. In the intermediate level sections, the porta hepatis and caudate process separate the left and right lobes.

The intersegmental fissure (right fissure) between the right anterior and right posterior segments can be roughly defined by one of two methods. Either place a line over the right hepatic vein running between the two segments or construct a line midway between the anterior and posterior branches of the right portal vein (Fig. 19-40D, E). The surface marking of this plane may correspond to the line of the 7th or 8th rib.

The left intersegmental fissure (left fissure) between the medial and lateral segments of the left lobe is usually readily visible in lower transverse sections through the liver (Fig. 19-40D). This fissure contains the ligamentum teres and some fat. It may vary in orientation from parallel with the midsagittal abdominal plane to 45° or greater to the right of that plane.

In sagittal sections through the middle of the liver, such as images computer-reconstructed from transverse sections, observe the lateral segment of the left lobe anterior and to the left of the quadrate lobe (Fig. 19-41). The lateral segment is also anterior to the caudate lobe in such sections. From a study of sagittal images, one readily understands how intermediate level transverse sections can pass through the quadrate and caudate lobes at the same level. Sagittal sections through the bed of the gallbladder often reveal the quadrate lobe's location anterior to the right lobe. See the transverse section shown in Fig. 19-40C.

Sagittal sections through the right side of the liver reveal the roughly coronal plane assumed by the right hepatic vein as it passes inferiorly between the anterior and posterior segments of the right lobe (Fig. 19-41D).

Bismuth and Garden[116] state that Anglo-Saxon terminology such as lobectomy, segmentectomy, etc., is anatomically wrong. Perhaps so, but we have used this terminology anyway, because of its general acceptance and usage in the medical literature.

## Intrahepatic Architecture

The hepatic arteries branch repeatedly to form interlobular arteries in the hepatic triads, with branches to the structures of the triad and to the sinusoids at varying distances between the periphery and the central vein. The portal vein similarly branches to form interlobular veins that open into the sinusoids.

The sinusoids receive both venous (75 percent) and arterial (25 percent) blood. In the center of the lobule, the radially arranged sinusoids open into a central vein. The central vein emerges at the end of the lobule to become a sublobular tributary of a hepatic vein. The hepatic veins empty into the inferior vena cava.

### Hepatocytes

Hepatocytes (Fig. 19-42) range in diameter from 20 to 30 micrometers and have a life span of about five months. Liver cells are seen to lie in plates such that between adjacent cells are the bile canaliculi into which project some microvilli. Paralleling the plates of liver cells are the hepatic sinusoids, the walls of which are composed of endothelial cells and stellate sinusoidal macrophages (Kupfer cells). The endothelial cells are generously fenestrated, and there are numerous, large gaps between adjacent cells of the sinusoidal walls. Between the sinusoids and the basal sides of the plates of hepatic cells is the perisinusoidal space (of Disse). Microvilli of the hepatocytes project into this space.

Due to the large gaps between adjacent sinusoidal

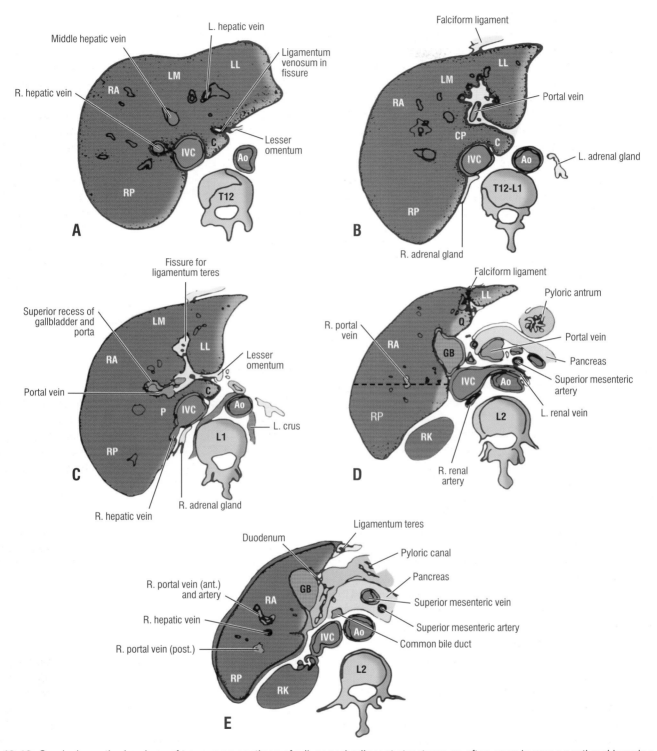

**FIG. 19-40.** Semischematic drawings of transverse sections of a liver and adjacent structures as often seen in cross-sectional imaging showing in situ relations of liver segments. Sections **A-B** proceed from superior to inferior, as indicated by vertebral levels. The dotted line in **D** approximates the line of separation between the anterior and posterior segments of the right lobe. Ao, aorta; C, caudate lobe; CP, caudate process; GB, gallbladder; IVC, inferior vena cava; LL, left lateral segment; LM, left medial segment; Q, quadrate lobe; RA, right anterior segment; RK, right kidney; RP, right posterior segment. (From Skandalakis LJ, Gray SW, Colborn GL, Skandalakis JE. Surgical anatomy of the liver and associated extrahepatic structures: Part 2. Contemp Surg 30:26-38, 1987; with permission.)

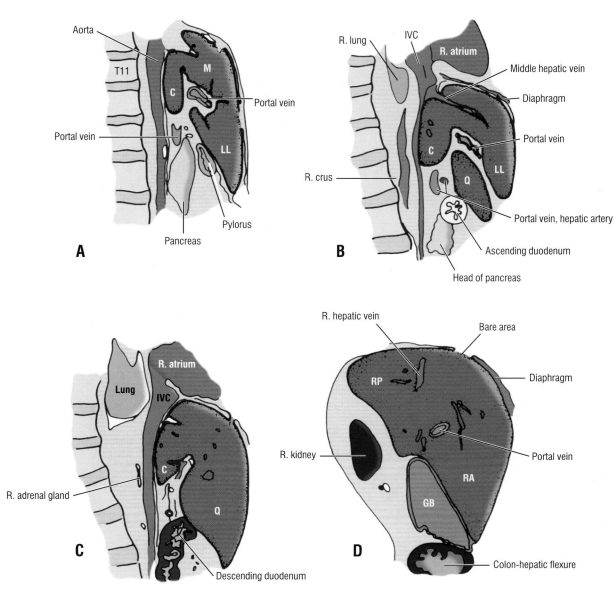

**FIG. 19-41.** Semischematic drawings of sagittal sections of a liver depicting relations of liver segments. **A,** Midsagittal section passing through liver and aorta. **B, C,** Sagittal sections through inferior vena cava. **D,** Sagittal section through the right side of the liver and the gallbladder. Abbreviations as in Fig. 19-40; M, medial. (Modified from Skandalakis LJ, Gray SW, Colborn GL, Skandalakis JE. Surgical anatomy of the liver and associated extrahepatic structures: Part 2. Contemp Surg 30:26-38, 1987; with permission.)

cells and the absence of a continuous basal lamina, no significant barrier exists between the blood plasma in the sinusoids and the hepatocyte membrane. Proteins and lipoproteins synthesized by the hepatocytes are transferred into the blood in the perisinusoidal space. This is the pathway for the endocrine secretions of the liver. In the perisinusoidal space is a cell type called the lipocyte or adipose cell (also known as Ito cell) which serves as a storage site for vitamin A. When depleted of lipid, these cells resemble fibroblasts and secrete collagen type III (reticular fibers) which forms a stroma. An increase in the latter fibers may be an early sign of hepatic response to toxins and can lead to fibrosis. Two to four other surfaces of the hepatocytes are in contact with adjacent liver cells of the plates.

### Bile Secretion

Between the adjacent hepatocytes is a tubular space, the bile canaliculus or bile capillary (Fig. 19-42). The

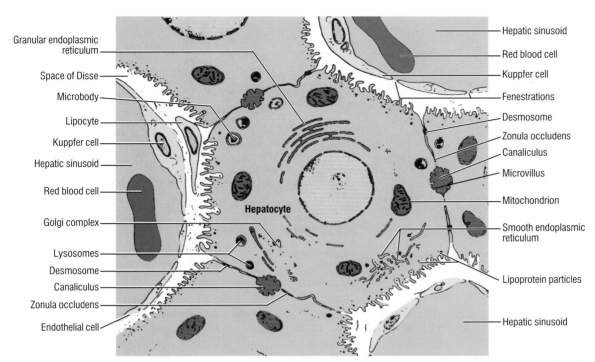

Granular endoplasmic reticulum
Space of Disse
Microbody
Lipocyte
Kuppfer cell
Hepatic sinusoid
Red blood cell
Golgi complex
Lysosomes
Desmosome
Canaliculus
Zonula occludens
Endothelial cell

Hepatocyte

Hepatic sinusoid
Red blood cell
Kuppfer cell
Fenestrations
Desmosome
Zonula occludens
Canaliculus
Microvillus
Mitochondrion
Smooth endoplasmic reticulum
Lipoprotein particles
Hepatic sinusoid

FIG. 19-42. Diagram of a liver cell (hepatocyte) and its relation to an adjacent cell (right) and to liver sinusoids. (Modified from Skandalakis LJ, Gray SW, Colborn GL, Skandalakis JE. Surgical anatomy of the liver and associated extrahepatic structures: Part 3. Contemp Surg 30:15-23, 1987; with permission.)

space contains a few short microvilli from the bordering hepatocytes. On either side of the canaliculus, the hepatocytes are held together by gap junctions and desmosomes.

Bile is secreted into the canaliculi and carried from the center of the lobule to the periphery; thus it flows in a direction counter to that of the incoming blood of the liver. At the periphery of the lobule, the canaliculi continue as the ductules of Hering, small channels bordered in part proximally by hepatocytes and much smaller cuboidal cells. From there on, the hepatocytes of the ductules are replaced entirely by cuboidal cells in the terminal biliary vessels. These slender channels drain into the bile ducts of the portal triad, which form the tributaries of the intrahepatic biliary tract.

## *Vascular Distribution*

Two blood vessels, the hepatic artery and the portal vein, supply the liver. About one-fourth of the blood and one-half the oxygen come by way of the hepatic artery. The remainder is carried by the portal vein.[117] Blood from these two sources mingles in the blood sinusoids of the liver parenchyma and is drained by tributaries of the hepatic veins. These veins open into the inferior vena cava.

The hepatic artery, portal vein, and intrahepatic bile ducts are arranged in a lobar pattern with dichotomous branching into segment vessels that, in turn, divide into area vessels. Because of their similar distribution, the terminology of the three systems is much the same. The general pattern applicable to all three is shown in Fig. 19-43. The branching of the left portal vein differs somewhat from this pattern. The hepatic veins, which drain the liver, in contrast, follow an interlobar pattern of distribution (Fig. 19-39).

Ohkubo[118] described dissection findings of an absent right gastric vein with an aberrant left gastric vein which directly drained into the liver. He considered the aberrant left gastric vein an important portal collateral pathway, corresponding to the phylogenetic and ontogenetic "left portal vein."

## Hepatic Vasculature (Fig. 19-44)

The fundamental studies of the intrahepatic pattern of the hepatic artery are those of Healey and colleagues,[110] Couinaud,[92] Michels,[111] and Suzuki and colleagues.[119]

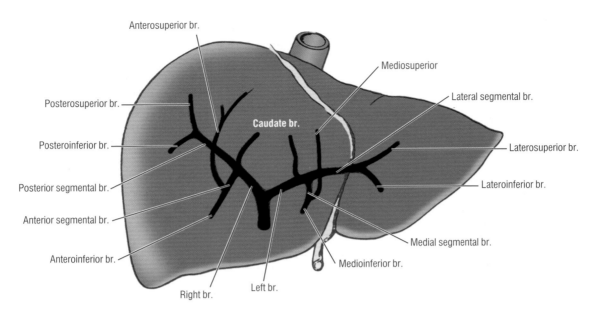

**FIG. 19-43.** Terminology of the branches of the hepatic artery, portal vein, and tributaries of the bile ducts, which all branch similarly (in most cases). (Modified from Skandalakis LJ, Gray SW, Colborn GL, Skandalakis JE. Surgical anatomy of the liver and associated extrahepatic structures: Part 3. Contemp Surg 30:15-23, 1987; with permission.)

## Proper Hepatic Artery

In the usual pattern, the common hepatic artery arises from the celiac trunk. After giving origin to the gastroduodenal artery, the hepatic artery continues as the proper hepatic artery in the hepatoduodenal ligament. In this ligament, the proper hepatic artery lies to the left of the common bile and hepatic ducts and anterior to the portal vein. It divides into right and left hepatic (lobar) arteries before it enters the porta.

## Right Hepatic Artery

The right hepatic (lobar) artery passes to the right, usually posterior to the hepatic duct but occasionally anterior to it. The cystic artery generally arises from the right hepatic in the hepatocystic triangle located between the cystic duct and the common hepatic duct.

The right hepatic artery bifurcates to form the anterior and posterior segment arteries. This division may take place within the liver or extrahepatically in the porta. The segment arteries divide, in turn, into superior and inferior area arteries that run with and are, generally, inferior to the bile ducts serving the same area.[120]

The anterior segmental branch of the right hepatic artery is more tortuous than the posterior segmental branch. After passing downward toward the neck of the gallbladder, it turns abruptly upward to accompany the bile duct of the anterior segment. In the downward part of its course near the gallbladder fossa, the anterior segment branch can be vulnerable to injury during operative procedures on the gallbladder.[120]

## Left Hepatic Artery

The left hepatic artery is shorter than the right because

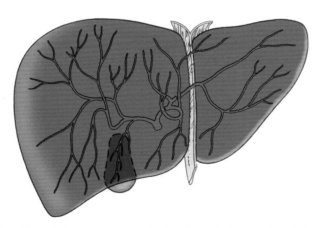

**FIG. 19-44.** Diagram to show the intrahepatic distribution of the hepatic artery. Note the "returning loop" of the left branch at the junction of medial and lateral segments. It is liable to injury here during left lateral segmentectomy. (Modified from Dawson JL. Anatomy. In: Wright R, Alberti AGMM, Karran S, Millward-Sadler GH (eds). Liver and Biliary Diseases. Philadelphia: Saunders, 1979; with permission.)

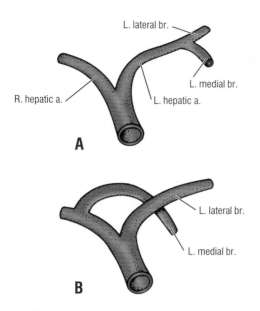

**FIG. 19-45.** Hepatic arteries. **A.** Usual pattern of segmental hepatic arteries. **B.** Anomalous origin of the left medial segmental artery from the right hepatic artery, crossing the midline to reach the medial segment of the left lobe. This may be encountered in 25 percent of individuals. (Modified from Skandalakis JE, Gray SW, Rowe JS Jr. Anatomical Complications in General Surgery. New York: McGraw-Hill, 1983; with permission.)

the right and left hepatic arteries arise to the left of the interlobar (median) fissure. In about 40 percent of Healey's subjects,[121] the left hepatic artery ended at its bifurcation into medial and lateral segmental arteries (Fig. 19-45, Fig. 19-46A). In 35 percent, however, the lateral segmental artery divided into laterosuperior and lateroinferior branches to the right of the intersegmental fissure (right fissure). In these the medial segmental artery arose from the lateroinferior branch (Fig. 19-46B). In addition, in 25 per-

cent of subjects, the medial and lateral segmental arteries arose separately from the proper hepatic artery so that there was no true left hepatic artery. In such cases, the left medial segmental artery arose from the right hepatic artery, crossing the midline to reach the left medial lobe (Fig. 19-46C). A similar configuration on the right was less common.

The medial segmental artery passes into the substance of the quadrate lobe. In 70 percent of specimens, it divided into two superior and two inferior area arteries. In 30 percent, various combinations occurred in which two or more area arteries arose from a common trunk. The other area arteries arose separately from the medial segmental artery.

### *Lateral Segmental Artery*

The lateral segmental artery usually divides into its superior and inferior branches along the line of the left intersegmental fissure or, variably, to the right of the fissure. The arterial branches run with the bile ducts serving these areas and may course either just above or below them.

### *Caudate Lobe Arteries*

The configuration of arteries to the caudate lobe of the liver varies. Typically, one artery arises from the right hepatic artery and supplies the caudate process and right side of the caudate lobe. A similar vessel from the left hepatic artery supplies the left side of the lobe. The arteries may number one (23 percent), two (45 percent), three (30 percent), or four (two percent), as reported by Healey et al.[110] The caudate lobe is supplied entirely by the right hepatic artery in 35 percent of cases and by the left hepatic artery in 12 percent.[120]

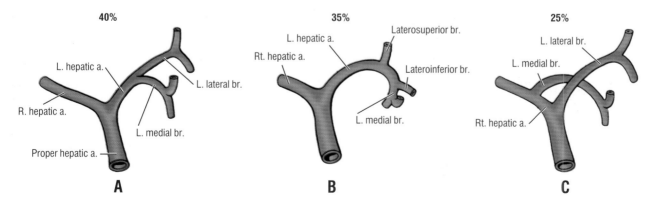

**FIG. 19-46. A, B, C.** Variations in the branching of the left hepatic artery. In **C,** the left medial branch arises from the right hepatic artery, crossing the interlobar (median) fissure to do so. (Modified from Skandalakis LJ, Gray SW, Colborn GL, Skandalakis JE. Surgical anatomy of the liver and associated extrahepatic structures: Part 3. Contemp Surg 30:15-23, 1987; with permission.)

## Arterial Supply

Branches of the hepatic arteries have long been considered to be end arteries. Small and inconstant anastomoses between arterial branches outside the liver parenchyma have been reported.[110] The most important anastomoses are in the connective tissue of the capsule and its intrahepatic reflections.

More than ninety years ago, von Haberer[122] showed that ligation of the common hepatic artery proximal to the gastroduodenal artery produced no liver changes. Ligation distal to the gastroduodenal artery usually, but not always, resulted in liver necrosis.[123]

Distal ligation of a lobar artery beyond the branches to the subcapsular plexus always results in lobar ischemia and necrosis. Graham and Cannell[124] concluded that the more distal the ligation of the artery, the greater the probability of liver necrosis. Bengmark and Rosengren[125] and Mays and colleagues[113,126,127] disputed the concept that hepatic arteries are end arteries in humans. They agreed that anastomoses cannot be seen in arteriograms of normal living individuals or in injection preparations of cadavers, but that such anastomoses arise *de novo* in the presence of hepatic artery ligation. Such collaterals between segmental arteries within the liver may appear 10 hours to 15 hours after ligation.

Survival of a liver segment following arterial ligation is the result of all the following:

- Increased extraction of oxygen from portal venous blood[128]
- Extrahepatic collateral circulation
- Intrahepatic collateral circulation formed in response to the ligation

Mays[113] reported that the hepatic necrosis seen in experimental animals after arterial ligation is due to species differences and that animal models do not behave in the same manner as human beings.

## Intrahepatic Portal Venous Network

The portal vein divides into left and right lobar branches at the porta before entering the liver. The portal lobar veins lie posterior to the hepatic arteries and the bile ducts. This relationship to the arteries and ducts is preserved in the intrahepatic distribution of the vessels.

### Right Portal Vein

The branches of the right portal vein (Fig. 19-47) follow the pattern of distribution of the right hepatic duct and right hepatic artery. The right portal vein is short and typically divides into anterior and posterior segmental vessels. Each of these subdivides into superior and inferior subsegmental branches. The right portal vein sends a small branch to the caudate process and the right side of the caudate lobe. The right portal system is more variable than the left.

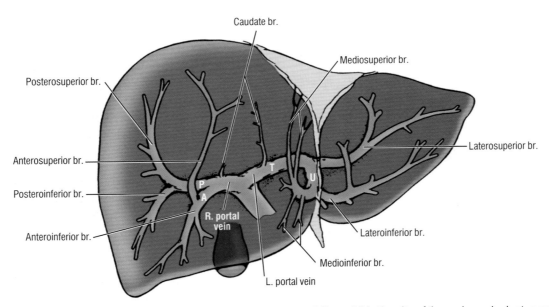

**FIG. 19-47.** Intrahepatic distribution of the hepatic portal vein. The pars umbilicus (U) is the site of the embryonic ductus venosus. T, pars transversus; P, posterior segment; A, anterior segment. (Modified from Skandalakis LJ, Gray SW, Colborn GL, Skandalakis JE. Surgical anatomy of the liver and associated extrahepatic structures: Part 3. Contemp Surg 30:15-23, 1987; with permission.)

## Left Portal Vein

The left portal vein (Fig. 19-47) is longer than the right. It begins in the hepatic portal as the pars transversa and courses to the left. It turns inferiorly in the liver's left lateral fissure at the umbilical fossa and is the markedly dilated pars umbilicus. As the vein enters the left lobe it is joined by the paraumbilical veins (of Sappey) and the ligamentum teres hepati, the nearly obliterated and functionless remnants of the left umbilical vein. The left hepatic vein goes on to be connected to the inferior vena cava by the ligamentum venosum, a vestige of the ductus venosus. The small extrahepatic section of the left branch, from which veins to the quadrate and left lobes arise, is a persistent part of the left umbilical vein.

The distribution of the left portal vein differs from the typical branching pattern of the left hepatic artery and bile duct in the following ways.[68]

- The superior and inferior subsegmental veins of the lateral segment arise from the left side of the pars umbilicus of the left portal vein.
- The medial segmental veins arise from the right side of the pars umbilicus of the left portal vein. Usually, one common mediosuperior and medioinferior trunk arises from the umbilical portion.

In the majority of cases, the left portal vein provides one branch to the left side of the caudate (segment I) lobe. This branch arises from the pars transversus.

REMEMBER

- The right portal vein divides into two parts: anterior and posterior. The anterior branch of the right portal vein further subdivides into ascending (for segment VIII) and descending (for segment V). The posterior branch also divides into ascending (for segment VII) and descending (for segment VI).
- The left portal vein also displays a unique subdivision. Two branches from its lateral side supply segments II and III. The vein, however, continues to supply segment IV.

## *Hepatic Veins*

The hepatic veins lie in the planes that divide the lobes and segments of the liver. Thus, they are intersegmental (Fig. 19-39) and drain parts of adjacent segments. This is in contrast to the hepatic arteries, portal veins, and tributaries of the bile ducts (Fig. 19-43) which define these areas of the liver.

Surgical implications of this arrangement are that in a right lobectomy the line of resection should be placed just to the right of the interlobar plane; in a left lobectomy, it should be just to the left.

The hepatic veins arise as central veins of the liver lobules. They coalesce to form interlobular veins, several orders of collecting veins, and right, middle, and left hepatic veins that emerge from the liver to enter the inferior vena cava.

### Right Hepatic Vein

The right hepatic vein lies in the right fissure and drains the:

- Superior and inferior areas of the right posterior segment
- Superior area of the anterior segment

### Middle Hepatic Vein

The middle hepatic vein lies in the median fissure and drains the:

- Anteroinferior area of the right lobe
- Medial inferior area of the left lobe

### Left Hepatic Vein

The left hepatic vein lies in the upper part of the left fissure and drains the:

- Left lateral segment
- Superior area of the medial segment

A variable number of small veins entering the vena cava directly drain the:

- Caudate lobe
- Posterior segment of the right lobe (inconstant)

REMEMBER

- The right hepatic vein drains segments V, VI, VII, and partially drains segment VIII.
- The middle hepatic vein drains segments IV, V, and VIII.
- The left hepatic vein drains segments II and III and partially drains segment IV.
- The multiple accessory hepatic veins drain mostly into the right hepatic vein. These are short and variable, and must be carefully ligated.

Nakamura and Tsuzuki[129] reported the anatomy of the common trunk of the middle and left hepatic veins. Figure 19-48 represents their findings.

In more than half of subjects, the left and middle hepatic veins join and enter the vena cava as a single vein less than 1 cm below the diaphragm. Nakamura and Tsuzuki[129] found, in addition to the three major veins, up to 50 small dorsal hepatic veins entering the vena cava. Only about 14 of the veins were of significant size. For evaluation, these authors assumed that 1 cm of vein, free from tributaries, would be adequate for successful ligation. By their standard, the right hepatic vein could be ligated in 51 of 83 cadavers examined (61.4 percent). The left vein could be ligated in only nine specimens (10.8 percent). The hepatic veins could be exposed by dividing

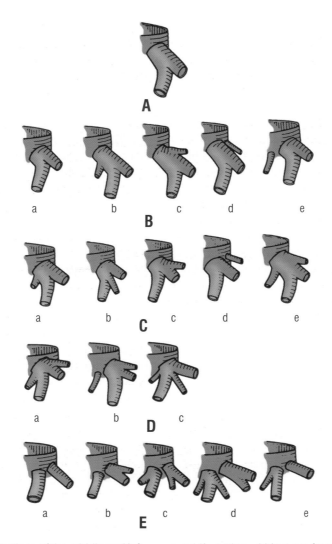

**FIG. 19-48.** Various patterns of ramifications of the middle and left hepatic vein. **A,** Type I, 9 (10.8 percent), has no ramification within less than 1 cm from the inferior vena cava. **B,** Type II, 35 (42.2 percent), has two ramifications within 1 cm from the inferior vena cava. a, Type IIa, 22 (26.5 percent), has the middle and left hepatic vein. b, Type IIb, 6 (7.2 percent), has a right anterosuperior vein. c, Type IIc, 5 (6 percent), has a left superior vein. d, Type IId, 1 (1.2 percent), has an independent left superior vein and the common trunk. e, Type IIe, 1 (1.2 percent), has an independent right anterosuperior vein and the common trunk. **C,** Type III, 22 (26.5 percent), has a trifurcation within 1 cm from the inferior vena cava. a, Type IIIa, 5 (6 percent), has a trifurcation consisting of the right anterosuperior, middle, and left hepatic veins. b, Type IIIb, 8 (9.6 percent), has a trifurcation consisting of the middle, left, and left superior veins. c, Type IIIc, 4 (4.8 percent), has a trifurcation consisting of the middle, left medial, and left hepatic veins. d, Type IIId, 3 (3.6 percent), has an independent left superior vein and the common trunk of the middle and left hepatic veins. e, Type IIIe, 2 (2.4 percent), has a trifurcation consisting of the right anterosuperior, common trunk of the middle and left hepatic veins, and the left superior vein. **D,** Type IV, 4 (4.8 percent), has a quadrifurcation within 1 cm from the inferior vena cava. a, Type IVa, 2 (2.4 percent), has a quadrifurcation consisting of the right anterosuperior, middle, left medial, and left hepatic veins. b, Type IVb, 1 (1.2 percent), has an independent right anterosuperior vein and a trifurcation consisting of the middle, left, and left superior veins. c, Type IVc, 1 (1.2 percent), has a quadrifurcation consisting of the right anterosuperior, middle, and left superior veins. **E,** Type V, 13 (15.7 percent), has the independent middle and left hepatic veins. a, Type Va, 6 (7.2 percent), has the independent middle and left hepatic vein without ramification. b, Type Vb, 3 (3.6 percent), has the middle and left hepatic veins with left superior vein. c, Type Vc, 2 (2.4 percent), has the middle hepatic vein with right anterosuperior vein and the left hepatic vein with left medial vein. d, Type Vd, 1 (1.2 percent), has the middle hepatic vein with right anterosuperior and left medial veins and the left hepatic vein. e, Type Ve, 1 (1.2 percent), has the middle hepatic vein with right anterosuperior and the left hepatic veins. (Modified from Nakamura S, Tsuzuki T. Surgical anatomy of the hepatic veins and the inferior vena cava. Surg Gynecol Obstet 152:43-50, 1981; with permission.)

the triangular and coronary ligaments and retracting the right lobe downward and to the left and the left lobe downward and to the right.

The intrahepatic venous network, formed by the incoming portal blood and outgoing hepatic blood, is intimately related to the liver cell. Ger[102] stated that a perivascular fibrous sheath envelops the portal network within the liver, a network consisting of branches of the portal vein, hepatic artery, and bile duct. No such fibrous sheath surrounds the hepatic veins and their tributaries; indeed, one can differentiate the hepatic vein tributaries from the other vessels in the liver by magnetic resonance imaging, due to the difference in contrast attributable to the presence or absence of the fibrous sheath. The hepatic veins receive blood directly from the liver sinusoids by way of central veins of the liver lobules, carrying both portal venous blood and hepatic arterial flow. The sinusoids lie immediately adjacent to the hepatic cells. The absence of a protective fibrous investment leaves the hepatic veins unprotected and prone to bleeding in hepatic trauma.

## Intrahepatic Biliary System

The bile canaliculi join to form ductules (canals of Hering) which are lined with cuboidal epithelial cells. These are not hepatocytes and have a complete basal lamina. The ductules open into interlobular bile ducts which form part of the portal triads. The interlobular ducts join to form right and left lobar ducts which join at the hilum to form the extrahepatic common hepatic duct (Fig. 19-49).

### Right Biliary Tree

The right biliary tree (Fig. 19-50) originates in the four areas of the right lobe. The branches take their names from their locations: anterosuperior, anteroinferior, posterosuperior, and posteroinferior. These area ducts join to form anterior and posterior segment ducts that, in turn, form the right hepatic duct. Some variations occur in the biliary vessels of the right lobe.

### Left Biliary Tree (Fig. 19-51)

The left hepatic duct usually forms by the confluence of the ducts of the medial and lateral segments. Healey and Schroy[68] describe 14 possible arrangements of the left medial segment ducts of which nine were actually present among their 100 specimens.

The laterosuperior biliary duct may extend upward into the left triangular ligament, as Healey and Schroy[68] noted. The frequency of occurrence of aberrant biliary and blood vessels in the proximal one-third of the ligament may exceed 80 percent in human livers, according to data of Gao and Roberts.[69] They further observed that 60 percent of the specimens they studied contained rudimentary liver cords, perhaps retained after developmental regression of the left lobe. Biliary leakage and bleeding may occur subsequent to surgical division of the left triangular ligament if adequate preventive precautions are not taken.

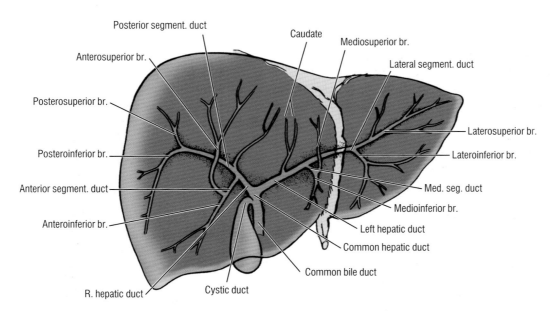

**FIG. 19-49.** Intrahepatic distribution of the bile ducts. (From Skandalakis LJ, Gray SW, Colborn GL, Skandalakis JE. Surgical anatomy of the liver and associated extrahepatic structures: Part 3. Contemp Surg 30:15-23, 1987; with permission.)

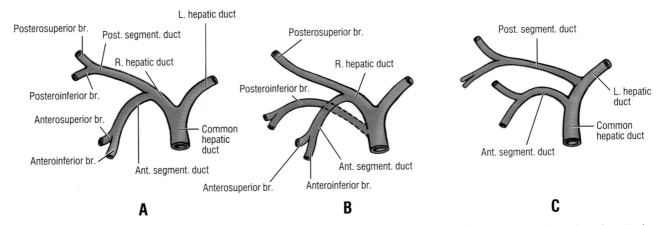

FIG. 19-50. Variations of the tributaries of the right hepatic duct. **A,** Usual pattern in which the right hepatic duct receives the anterior and posterior segment ducts. **B,** Alternate pattern in which the posteroinferior area duct enters the common hepatic duct. **C,** Anterior and posterior segment ducts enter the left hepatic duct; the right hepatic duct is absent. (Modified from Skandalakis LJ, Gray SW, Colborn GL, Skandalakis JE. Surgical anatomy of the liver and associated extrahepatic structures: Part 3. Contemp Surg 30:15-23, 1987; with permission.)

### Caudate Lobe

The tributaries of the right and left hepatic ducts drain the caudate lobe. A separate duct serves the caudate process, draining into the right hepatic duct.

Variations of hepatic duct confluence and of the intrahepatic ductal system are shown in Figs. 19-52, 19-53.

REMEMBER
- The right hepatic duct drains segments V, VI, VII and VIII.
- The left hepatic duct drains segments II, III, IV.
- The caudate lobe (segment I) drains to both right and left hepatic ducts.

Meyers et al.[130] reported that low insertion of hepatic segmental duct VII-VIII is an important cause of major biliary injury or misdiagnosis. They emphasized that knowledge of the topographic anatomy is paramount in avoiding such injury or misdiagnosis.

### IVC and Liver

The anatomic entities related to the IVC, from cranial to caudal, are:
1. Epiploic foramen: IVC forms its posterior boundary
2. Groove between right and caudate lobes: This occasionally becomes intrahepatic tunnel
3. Right diaphragmatic crus posterior to the IVC
4. Right adrenal gland and right adrenal vein posterior to the IVC
5. Central tendon
6. Right atrium of the heart

The IVC may be exposed after mobilizing the right lobe of the liver, careful suture ligation of the right adrenal vein, and several other small named and unnamed veins.

According to Sing and colleagues,[131] measurement of vena caval diameter and anatomy may be performed bedside in critically ill patients using carbon dioxide as a contrast agent.

Ger[102] enriched the surgical profession with a classic presentation of the relations of resections to vascular and ductal structures (see Table 19-3). This table illustrates our surgical considerations.

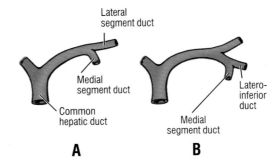

FIG. 19-51. Variations of the left hepatic duct. **A,** Usual pattern in which the left hepatic duct is formed by the confluence of the medial and lateral segment ducts. **B,** The medial segment duct may enter the lateroinferior duct. The medial segment duct is usually doubled. (Modified from Skandalakis LJ, Gray SW, Colborn GL, Skandalakis JE. Surgical anatomy of the liver and associated extrahepatic structures: Part 3. Contemp Surg 30:15-23, 1987; with permission.)

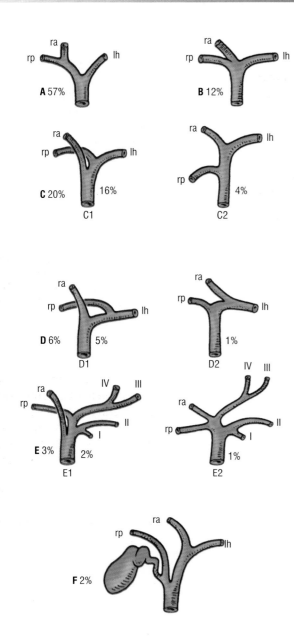

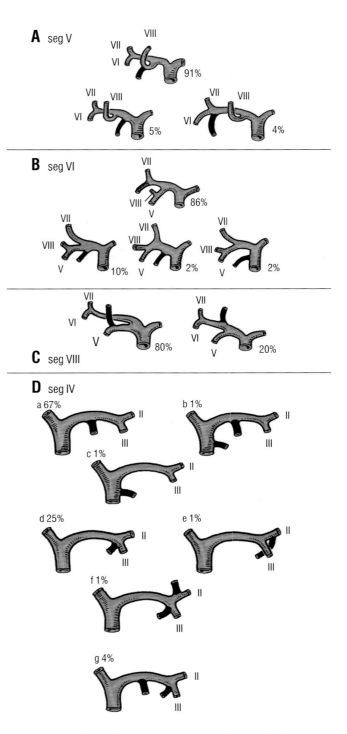

**FIG. 19-52.** Main variations of the hepatic duct confluence (Couinaud 1957[185]). **A,** Typical anatomy of the confluence. **B,** Triple confluence. **C,** Ectopic drainage of a right sectoral duct into the common hepatic duct: C1, right anterior duct draining into the common hepatic duct; C2, right posterior ducts draining into the common hepatic duct. **D,** Ectopic drainage of a right sectoral duct into the left hepatic ductal system: D1, right posterior sectoral duct draining into the left hepatic ductal system; D2, right anterior sectoral duct draining into the left hepatic ductal system. **E,** Absence of the hepatic duct confluence. **F,** Absence of right hepatic duct and ectropic drainage of the right posterior duct into the cystic duct. ra, right anterior; rp, right posterior; lh, left hepatic. (Modified from Smadja C, Blumgart LH. The biliary tract and the anatomy of biliary exposure. In: Blumgart LH (ed). Surgery of the Liver and Biliary Tract. New York, Churchill Livingstone, 1988, pp. 11-22; with permission.)

**FIG. 19-53.** A sketch to show the main variations of the intrahepatic ductal system (Healey and Schroy 1953[68]): **A.** variations of segment V, **B.** variations of segment VI, **C.** variations of segment VIII, **D.** variations of segment IV. Note that there is no variation of drainage of segments II, III and VII. (Modified from Smadja C, Blumgart LH. The biliary tract and the anatomy of biliary exposure. In: Blumgart LH (ed). Surgery of the Liver and Biliary Tract. New York, Churchill Livingstone, 1988, pp. 11-22; with permission.)

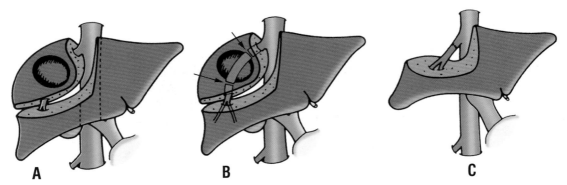

FIG. 19-54. Diagrams showing the procedure from isolation of the hepatic veins to completion of direct anastomosis. **A,** Skeletonization of the right hepatic vein. **B,** Sites for cutting the right hepatic vein are shown by arrows. **C,** Completion of direct anastomosis. (Modified from Nakamura S, Suzuki S, Hachiya T, Ochiai H, Konno H, Baba S. Direct hepatic vein anastomosis during hepatectomy for colorectal liver metastases. Am J Surg 174(3):331-333, 1997; with permission.)

## *Surgical Considerations*

- Hepatic arteries are not end arteries. In humans, intra-hepatic, translobar, and subcapsular collateral circulation develops within 24 hours after ligation of the right or left hepatic artery.

- The subcostal, right inferior phrenic, and pancreatico-duodenal arteries provide collateral intrahepatic circulation after ligation of the common hepatic artery in humans. In rare cases, ligation of the right or left artery may be necessary for control of arterial hemorrhage. More often, the Pringle maneuver or total vascular isolation of the porta hepatis and suprahepatic and infrahepatic vena cavae allows for direct repair of vascular injuries or resection, if necessary.

- The portal vein may be ligated in human beings, but repair is preferred because the mortality rate with ligation is much higher.

- When it is necessary for the portal vein to be excised in extended liver surgery, Lorf et al.[132] have used the excised hepatic vein to reconstruct the portal vein.

- Temporary occlusion of the total afferent blood supply (hepatic artery and portal vein) may be tolerated in humans for 30 to 45 minutes routinely and for periods up to 60 minutes if the body is cooled and no concurrent liver disease is present. Wang et al.[133] reported that the safest method of hepatic vascular clamping is 60 minutes of intermittent ischemia consisting of 6 cycles of 10 minutes interrupted by 5 minutes of reperfusion. Vascular occlusion in a cirrhotic liver is fraught with danger. Man et al.[134] concluded that the safe and effective upper limit of tolerance of the liver to intermittent Pringle maneuver is 120 minutes.

- Nakamura et al.[135] removed the right and middle hepatic veins during total resection of segments VII and VIII, and

partial resection of segments V and VI including the caudate lobe, and reported successful direct hepatic vein anastomosis (Fig. 19-54).

- Grazi et al.[136] reported that total vascular exclusion to control blood inflow to the liver during hepatic surgery must have a limited role, but it can be useful in cases of liver trauma.

- Malassagne et al.[137] recommended selective vascular clamping for major hepatectomies in selected patients with peripheral hepatic tumors.

- Evans et al.[138] stated that total vascular exclusion is a safe hemodynamic procedure for liver resection, even in patients older than 70 years, as long as clamp times do not exceed 45 minutes.

- Segmental hepatic vein ligation may be done without hepatic resection.

- Ligation of both branches of the hepatic artery and portal vein may be performed in liver trauma in extremely rare cases. Ligate the artery first. If good results are not obtained, then ligate the branch of the portal vein to that lobe. A significant percentage of hepatic necrosis will ensue, but the patient is likely to survive.

- Ligation of an extrahepatic duct produces atrophy of the corresponding lobe and will likely be complicated by cholangitis until the atrophy is complete. Repair is preferred.

- Remember that approximately 10 percent of human beings have some type of anomaly of the biliary tract.

- Due to unknown factors, the liver regenerates within four to six months.

- Ten to twenty percent of normal liver tissue is sufficient to maintain life.

- To prevent stricture formation, do not devascularize the anterior surface of the CBD.

# Lymphatics of the Liver

The liver sinusoids (Fig. 19-42) have an endothelial lining composed of flattened squamous cells and stellate macrophages (Kupffer cells). This endothelial layer is separated from the surrounding hepatocytes by a narrow perivascular space (of Disse) partially filled by microvilli of the hepatocytes.

The openings in this endothelial lining of sinusoids in humans allow the passage of blood plasma and chylomicrons. Cellular elements cannot pass. These openings are usually considered discontinuities of the endothelium. Others[139] believe they are fenestrae in the endothelial cells. There are no closing membranes in the fenestrae and no basal lamina in human sinusoids.

The perivascular space of Disse (Fig. 19-42) is the source of lymph produced by the liver. The flow is toward the portal triads at the periphery of the lobule. Here the lymph is collected in the slightly larger space of Mall around the vessels of the triad.

The spaces of Disse and Mall are tissue spaces, not lymphatic vessels. The true endothelium-lined lymphatic vessels originate in the connective tissue around the portal triad. They presumably end blindly in the space of Mall because retrograde injections of lymphatic vessels do not pass from the lymphatics to the spaces.

The lymphatics of the liver are usually divided into superficial or subcapsular and deep or portal systems. Hardy and associates[140] wrote that the hepatic lymphatics form a single functional unit.

## *Superficial Lymphatics*

The superficial lymphatics (Fig. 19-55) lie near the surface of the liver beneath the serosa and within Glisson's capsule. Five pathways were described by Rouviere,[141] with later modifications.

These five pathways extend from the:
- Anterior and right superior surfaces of the liver through the sternocostal foramen (of Morgagni) to anterior phrenic nodes
- Posterior and superior surfaces through the caval hiatus to middle (lateral) phrenic nodes
- Posterior surface of the left lateral segment to the paracardial group of left gastric nodes
- Posterior surface of the right lobe to celiac nodes by way of nodes of the inferior phrenic artery
- Entire anterior margin of the liver and the entire visceral surface to hepatic nodes

A summary of connections of the phrenic nodes is provided in Table 19-5.

## *Deep Lymphatics*

The deep lymphatics (Fig. 19-56) carry the greater part of the lymphatic outflow and drain to:
- Middle (lateral) phrenic nodes of the diaphragm, following tributaries of the hepatic veins to the vena cava and ascending through the caval hiatus
- Nodes of the porta hepatis following portal vein branches.

There is free communication between the superficial and deep lymphatic systems.

Fahim and associates[142] state that the lymphatic drainage of the right lobe, gallbladder, and extrahepatic biliary system pass through pericholedochal nodes. These include the hiatal (epiploic) and superior pancreatoduodenal nodes. The lymph from the left lobe flows to nodes along the hepatic artery.

Therefore, the transdiaphragmatic hepatic drainage reaches the internal mammary and diaphragmatic lymph nodes. Lymph reaches the right lymphatic duct, partly via the tracheobronchial lymph nodes.[54]

# Nerve Supply to the Liver

The liver and biliary ducts receive sympathetic and parasympathetic fibers from the anterior hepatic plexus around the hepatic artery and the posterior hepatic plexus around the portal vein (Fig. 19-57).

The sympathetic fibers arise from thoracic spinal cord segments 7 to 10. The parasympathetic efferent fibers arise from the hepatic division of the anterior and posterior vagal trunks. Some fibers appear to arise from the right phrenic nerve[143] and others may enter the liver by following the hepatic veins.[144] The phrenic nerve supply via its C3, 4, 5 roots is probably the basis of shoulder pain in biliary colic.[145]

The most obvious of the hepatic nerves is the hepatic division of the anterior vagal trunk (Fig. 19-58). The nerve structure may be single or multiple as it passes through the lesser omentum.[146] After passing through the hepatogastric ligament near the fissure for the ligamentum venosum, this division branches extensively with the biliary vessels.

Galen saw the hepatic division of the anterior vagal trunk and speculated about the need for a nerve to the liver, an organ that has neither movement nor sensation.[147] We are only a little better informed today. Section of this nerve produces ill-defined and often contradictory effects.

The hepatic branch of the posterior vagal trunk passes, in part, through the celiac plexus. Its branches then accompany the hepatic artery to the liver. Hess and Tamm[145]

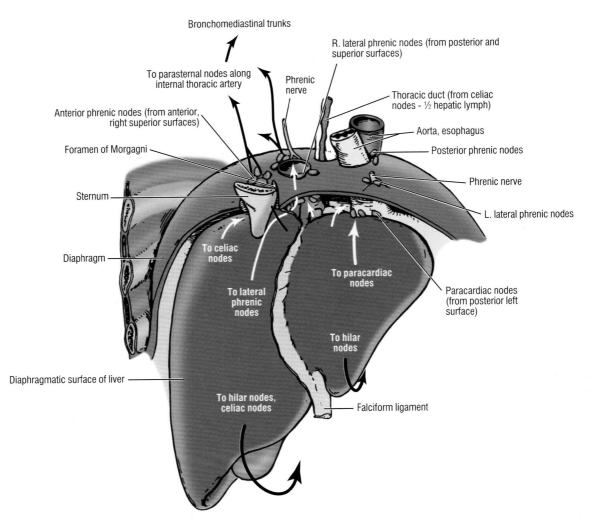

**Fig. 19-55.** Superficial lymphatic drainage of the liver. About one-half of the drainage is to the thoracic duct. (Modified from Skandalakis LJ, Gray SW, Colborn GL, Skandalakis JE. Surgical anatomy of the liver and associated extrahepatic structures: Part 3. Contemp Surg 30:15-23, 1987; with permission.)

| TABLE 19-5. The Phrenic Lymph Nodes | | | |
|---|---|---|---|
| | **Anterior Group** | **Middle Group** | **Posterior Group** |
| Number | 2-3 | 2-3 | 2-3 |
| Location | Behind, on either side of the xiphoid | With the right phrenic nerve | Crura of the diaphragm |
| Drainage from (afferent) | Convex surface of liver, diaphragm and anterior abdominal wall | Middle of diaphragm, right portion of convex surface of liver, deep lymphatics of the region of the hepatic vein | Posterior part of diaphragm, lymphatic from middle phrenic group |
| Drainage to (efferent) | Sternal nodes | Posterior phrenic nodes | Lumbar nodes, posterior mediastinal nodes, celiac nodes |

*Source:* Colborn GL, Skandalakis LJ, Gray SW, Skandalakis JE. Surgical anatomy of the liver and associated extrahepatic structures: Part 3. Contemp Surg 30:15-23, 1987; with permission.

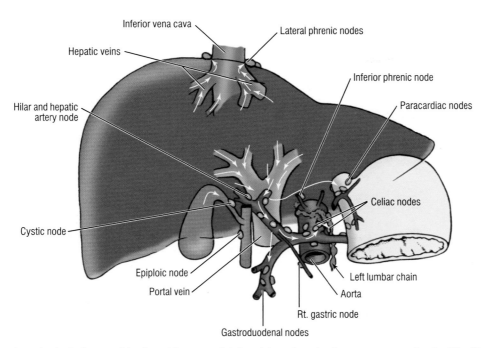

Fig. **19-56.** Deep lymphatic drainage of the liver. The superficial and deep lymphatics anastomose freely. (Modified from Skandalakis LJ, Gray SW, Colborn GL, Skandalakis JE. Surgical anatomy of the liver and associated extrahepatic structures: Part 3. Contemp Surg 30:15-23, 1987; with permission.)

report that the right vagus nerve (posterior trunk) provides the principal source of parasympathetic fibers to the biliary passages, including the sphincter of Oddi.

According to Jungermann[148] and Friedman,[149] the intrahepatic autonomic nerves regulate blood flow and liver metabolism. Afferent nerves connect chemoreceptors, osmoreceptors, and baroreceptors. These nerves have vasomotor regulation and play a role in controlling metabolic hepatic function.[150,151]

Sutherland[152] studied the intrinsic innervation of the liver. He reported that peritoneal folds associated with the liver are the pathways that myelinated and non-myelinated fibers use to reach the liver.

Meguid et al.[153] state that a liver that had not been denervated might inhibit the release of dopamine in the lateral hypothalamus, and this might play an inhibitory role in the regulation of food intake.

Within the liver, perivascular nerve fibers terminate on smooth muscle fibers in the media of arterioles and venules. There is little doubt that adrenergic fibers produce vasomotor responses, but there is some question whether hepatic parenchymal cells receive nerve fibers. Nobin, Moghimzedeh, and their colleagues[154,155] found innervated hepatic cells in humans and other primates but not in mice or rats. Kyosola and associates[156] could not confirm the presence of nerve fibers distributed to hepatocytes in human livers.

Sawchenko and Friedman[157] reviewed the evidence for the direct innervation of intralobular hepatic cells. They

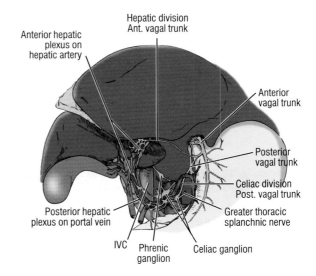

Fig. **19-57.** The distribution of vagus nerve fibers in the thorax and upper abdomen. The hepatic division of the anterior vagus trunk contains parasympathetic and sensory fibers to the liver. The intrahepatic course of these is not well known. (Modified from Skandalakis LJ, Colborn GL, Gray SW, Skandalakis JE. Surgical anatomy of the liver and extrahepatic biliary tract. In: Nyhus LM, Baker RJ, eds. Mastery of Surgery, 2nd Ed. Boston: Little, Brown, 1992; with permission.)

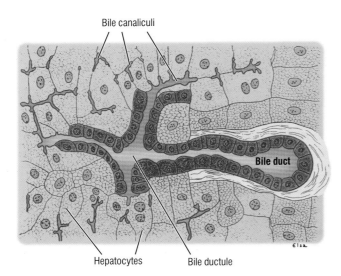

Bile canaliculi

Bile duct

Hepatocytes    Bile ductule

**FIG. 19-58.** Transition from bile canaliculi of the liver cords to bile ducts of the hepatic triads. (Modified from Junqueira LC, Carneiro J, Kelley RO. Basic Histology, 9th Ed. Stamford, Conn: Appleton & Lange, 1998; with permission.)

concluded that "...modern light microscopic studies do provide ample evidence of fibers circumscribing, and probably terminating upon, hepatocytes."

Amenta et al.[158] found cholinergic fibers associated with extrahepatic and intrahepatic hepatic arteries, portal veins, and hepatic veins. They found a few cholinergic fibers innervating the parenchyma and sinusoids of the liver in humans. Fibers have been reported travelling through the perivascular spaces of Disse, ending on hepatocytes and even on Kupffer cells,[159] and fat storage cells.[160] The existence of an intrinsic nerve plexus corresponding to that of the gastrointestinal wall was suggested by Burnett and colleagues;[143] however, ganglion cells have not been found.

Contrary to Galen's view that the liver has no sensation,[147] it now appears that 75 to 90 percent of vagal fibers in the abdomen are afferent and almost all of them unmyelinated. Specific receptors have not been recognized, but osmoreceptors, ionic receptors, baroreceptors, and metabolic receptors are considered to exist in the liver.[157]

## Glissonian Sheaths

While lecturing in Egypt, the senior author of this chapter, Dr. John Skandalakis, had the opportunity to hear a very interesting paper, *Surgical Anatomy of the Glissonian Sheaths: A Prerequisite for Hepatic Resection and Liver Transplantation.* He proposed that the authors, Ramadan M. El-Gharbawy, Moustafa M. El-Hennawi, Farouk A.

Mekky, Ossama A. El-Deeb, and Mohamed K. El-Saiedy of the Departments of Anatomy and General Surgery of the Faculty of Medicine, Alexandria University, publish their work in this book, and we are grateful that they agreed.

***ABSTRACT.*** *A complete knowledge of the anatomic variations in arterial supply, bile duct, portal, and hepatic venous anatomy, as well as the segmental anatomy of the liver, is an essential prerequisite for hepatic resection and liver transplantation. Twenty normal fresh human livers were injected with colored latex and dissected to study the glissonian sheaths of the eight hepatic segments. Segment I had three sheaths that entered the anterior surface of the lower end of the segment. The glissonian sheaths of segments II, III, and the lower part of segment IV arose constantly in the fissure for ligamentum teres from the left main sheath. The upper part of segment IV had its sheath in the porta hepatis in ten specimens from the left main sheath and from the right anterior sector sheath in the other ten specimens. The right main sheath bifurcated into the right anterior and the right posterior sector sheaths. The right anterior sector sheath gave the sheaths of segments V and VIII. The right posterior sector sheath gave the sheaths of segments VI and VII exhibiting two patterns of distribution.*

***INTRODUCTION.*** *Hepatic resection for primary tumors and metastases has gained increasing support as it represents the only chance to improve long-term survival of selected patients.[161-164] In the last three decades, extensive hepatic resection has become a safe operative procedure.[165] In patients with impaired hepatic function, preservation of hepatic parenchyma is an important consideration during resection.[166] These resections, whether extensive or segmental, could be performed on the anatomic basis of the liver.[165]*

*Liver transplantation has developed into a major effort to support patients with advanced liver disease. Although the techniques have been standardized, it remains a difficult and complex procedure. A complete knowledge of the anatomic variations in arterial supply, bile duct, portal and hepatic venous anatomy, as well as the segmental anatomy of the liver, is an essential prerequisite to developing the surgical skills for this form of surgery.[54]*

*The capsule of the liver (Glisson's capsule) condenses around the hepatic trinity structures and surrounds them as they enter the liver substance. Thus each bile duct, hepatic artery, and portal vein unit is surrounded by a fibrous sheath which is called the "glissonian sheath." When approached from within the liver substance, the sheaths simplify ligation of the hepatic trinity and if the sheath to a particular segment is ligated it will contain contain structures passing to or from that segment only. Ligation of the individual sheaths is therefore not only simpler but safer.[167]*

The present study aimed at studying the glissonian sheaths of the eight hepatic segments.

**MATERIAL AND METHODS.** *Twenty normal fresh human livers were used in the present study. Ten of them were harvested from adult cadavers brought to the Anatomy Department, Alexandria Faculty of Medicine prior to injection with the fixative. The other ten were livers of stillborns obtained from the Department of Obstetrics, Alexandria Faculty of Medicine. The portal vein and the common bile duct were ligated and divided behind the neck of the pancreas. The hepatic artery was ligated and divided at its origin from the celiac trunk, and also the accessory or replacing hepatic arteries were ligated and divided at suitable lengths from the liver if they were present. The inferior vena cava was ligated and divided above the renal veins and at the level of the right atrium, and the segment in between was removed with the liver. The liver was then taken out of the cadaver.*

*The portal vein, the bile duct, the hepatic artery(ies), and the inferior vena cava were cannulated and perfused with normal saline to wash out their contents. The liver was then perfused with 500 mL of three percent formol saline and left for four hours taking care not to squeeze it. After that the bile duct, the hepatic artery(ies), the portal vein, and the inferior vena cava were injected with colored latex in that order.*

*After the injection was completed, the liver was wrapped with a towel soaked with a wetting fluid[168] and refrigerated for 24-48 hours. The livers were dissected starting at the porta hepatis. The right and left main glissonian sheaths were*

identified. Their segmental branches were followed, then the sheaths were opened and their contents were studied, photographed, and documented.

**RESULTS. Glissonian sheaths of the right and left lobes.** *The glissonian sheaths of the right lobe (right main sheath) and of the left lobe (left main sheath) arose from the structures of portal trinity in the right end of the porta hepatis (Figs. 19-59, 19-60).*

The RIGHT MAIN SHEATH. *The right main sheath contained the right branches of the portal vein, the hepatic artery proper and the right hepatic duct. It arose from the structures of portal trinity in the right end of the porta hepatis and passed to the right into the parenchyma of the right lobe to bifurcate into the right anterior and right posterior sector sheaths (Figs. 19-60, 19-61).*

THE LEFT MAIN SHEATH. *This fascial sheath contained the branches of the portal vein, the hepatic artery, and the bile ducts of the left lobe of the liver. The sheath passed to the left end of the porta hepatis then anteroinferiorly in the fissure for ligamentum teres. In all specimens, the whole course of the left main sheath was extrahepatic (Figs. 19-60, 19-61).*

**Glissonian sheaths of segment I.** *Segment I had three sheaths in all specimens (Figs. 19-61, 19-62). One, to the left, entered the anteroinferior aspect of the papillary pro-*

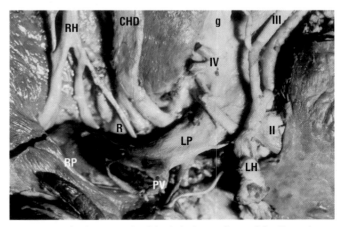

FIG. 19-60. A photograph of the inferior surface of the liver showing the contents of the right main and left main sheaths. The right main sheath passes immediately into the parenchyma. The course of the left main sheath is wholly extrahepatic. PV, portal vein; LP, left branch of portal vein; LH, left branch of hepatic artery; R, right hepatic duct; III, contents of segment III's sheath; IV, contents of lower part of segment IV's sheath; RH, right branch of hepatic artery; RP, right branch of portal vein; CHD, common hepatic duct; II, contents of segment II's sheath; g, ligamentum teres. (Courtesy of El-Gharbawy, El-Hennawi, Mekky, El-Deeb, El-Saiedy.)

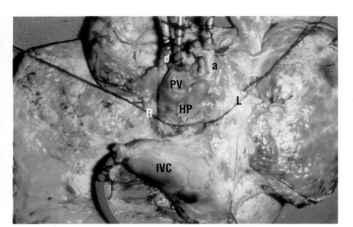

FIG. 19-59. A photograph showing the posterior surface of the hilar plate (HP) after encircling the right main (R) and left main (L) sheaths with silk threads. PV, portal vein; d, bile duct; a, hepatic artery proper; IVC, inferior vena cava. (Courtesy of El-Gharbawy, El-Hennawi, Mekky, El-Deeb, El-Saiedy.)

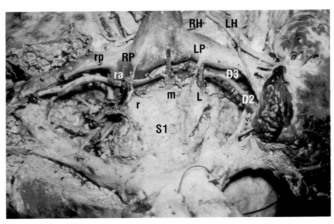

**FIG. 19-61.** A photograph showing the contents of the right main and left main sheaths. The contents of the right main sheath divide into the contents of the right anterior and right posterior sector sheaths. RH, right branch of hepatic artery proper; RP, right branch of portal vein; D2 & D3, bile ducts in the left main sheath; rp, contents of the right posterior sector sheath; r, m, L, contents of the right, middle and the left sheaths of segment I (S1); LH, left branch of the hepatic artery proper; LP, left branch of the portal vein; ra, contents of the right anterior sector sheath. (Courtesy of El-Gharbawy, El-Hennawi, Mekky, El-Deeb, El-Saiedy.)

cess. Its vein arose from the adjacent side of the left branch of the portal vein. Its artery arose from the branch of the left branch of the hepatic artery going to the lower part of segment IV in 16 specimens (80%) and from a replacing hepatic artery arising from the left gastric artery in the remaining four (20%). The artery crossed posterior to the left portal branch. Its duct joined the posterosuperior aspect of the duct to segment II.

The middle sheath entered the middle of the antero-inferior aspect of the lower end of the segment. Its vein arose from the posterior surface of the bifurcation of the portal vein. Its artery arose from the branch of the right branch of the hepatic artery running medial to the portal branch of the sheath of the right anterior sector. Its duct joined the posterosuperior aspect of the duct to segment II.

One, to the right, entered the anteroinferior aspect of the caudate process. Its vein arose from the adjacent side of the right branch of the portal vein. Its artery arose from the artery going to segment VII. Its duct joined the beginning of the stem of the duct to both segment VI and VII.

**Glissonian sheath of segment II.** Segment II had one sheath in all specimens (Figs. 19-63, 19-64, 19-65, 19-66). The sheath arose from the left main sheath at the left end of the porta hepatis, where the inferior end of the fissure for ligamentum venosum met the posterosuperior end of the fissure for ligamentum teres. On reaching the left end of the porta hepatis, the left branch of the portal vein gave several branches (avg. 3 ± 0.75) where it changed its direction to

run in the bottom of the fissure for ligamentum teres. These formed the portal component of segment II sheath.

The duct draining segment II received the ducts of the left and middle sheaths of segment I and joined the right hepatic duct in 16 specimens. In the remaining 4 specimens it received, in addition to the ducts of the left and middle sheaths of segment I, a duct from segment III. The artery of segment II sheath arose from the left branch of the hepatic artery proper in 16 specimens (80%) and from a replacing hepatic artery in 4 specimens (20%). This replacing hepatic artery, when present, arose from the left gastric artery near the cardia and ran in the lesser omentum to reach the fissure for ligamentum venosum skirting its left bank. In these four specimens the replacing hepatic artery provided the artery of the left sheath of segment I.

**Glissonian sheath of segment III.** Segment III had one sheath in all specimens (Figs. 19-63, 19-64, 19-65, 19-66). The sheath was found in the bottom of the fissure for ligamentum teres on the left side of the attachment of the round ligament with the left branch of the portal vein. The number of the portal branches in the sheath was 3 ± 0.17. The artery of the sheath arose from the left branch of the hepatic artery proper in 16 specimens (80%) and from a replacing hepatic artery in 4 specimens (20%). The latter arose from the left gastric artery and passed in the gastrohepatic ligament (lesser omentum) to the fissure for ligamentum venosum. It skirted the left banks of the fissures for ligament venosum and teres passing posterior to the portal branches to segment II providing the artery to that segment and continued to reach the sheath of segment III and became its artery.

The duct of segment III was present posterosuperior to the portal branches of the segment. In eight specimens it

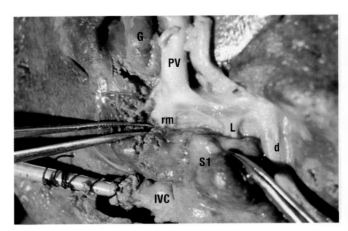

**FIG. 19-62.** A photograph of the inferior surface of a stillborn's liver showing the three glissonian sheaths (right [r]. middle [m] and left [L] of segment I [S1]). PV, portal vein; d, ductus venosus; IVC, inferior vena cava; G, gallbladder. (Courtesy of El-Gharbawy, El-Hennawi, Mekky, El-Deeb, El-Saiedy.)

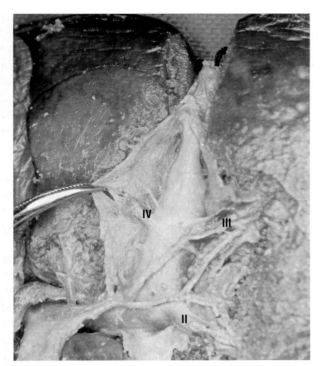

FIG. 19-63. A photograph of a stillborn's liver showing the contents of the glissonian sheaths of segments II, III, and lower part of IV. (Courtesy of El-Gharbawy, El-Hennawi, Mekky, El-Deeb, El-Saiedy.)

followed the left side of the portal branch superiorly to pass anterior to the portal branches of segment II, then it curved to the right traversing the porta hepatis postero-superior to the left portal branch. This configuration was called by the author "curved duct pattern." In another

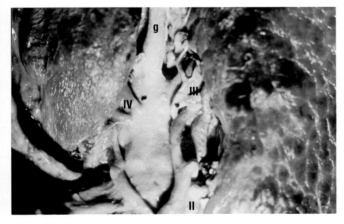

FIG. 19-64. A photograph of the inferior surface of the liver showing the course and contents of the left main sheath, the contents of the sheaths of segments II, III and lower part of IV and round ligament (g). (Courtesy of El-Gharbawy, El-Hennawi, Mekky, El-Deeb, El-Saiedy.)

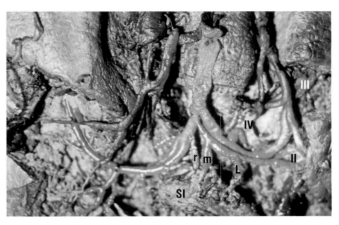

FIG. 19-65. A photograph showing the arteries and ducts of the sheaths of segments II, III, and lower part of IV. The ducts of the right (r), the middle (m), and the left (L) sheaths of segment I (SI) are also shown. (Courtesy of El-Gharbawy, El-Hennawi, Mekky, El-Deeb, El-Saiedy.)

eight specimens (40%) the duct passed directly to the right anterior to the left portal branch to reach the porta hepatis. This configuration was called by the author "straight duct pattern." In the remaining four specimens (20%), the segment was drained by two ducts that passed to the porta hepatis anterior to the left portal branch and one superior to the other. This configuration was called by the author "double duct pattern."

**Glissonian sheaths of segment IV.** The lower part of segment IV received its sheath in the fissure for ligamentum teres, nearly opposite to the sheath of segment III in all specimens. This sheath contained 3 to 7 portal branches (mean 5 ± 0.92) that arose from the left portal branch just before it became continuous with the round ligament. The

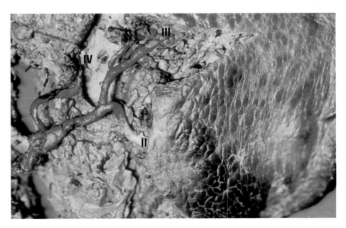

FIG. 19-66. A photograph showing the arteries of the sheaths of segments II, III, and lower part of IV. (Courtesy of El-Gharbawy, El-Hennawi, Mekky, El-Deeb, El-Saiedy.)

*artery in the sheath arose from the left branch of the hepatic artery proper in all specimens. Its duct joined the duct of segment III in 16 specimens (80%). In four specimens (20%), where segment III was drained by two ducts, the duct of the lower part of segment IV joined the inferior one (Figs. 19-63, 19-64, 19-65, 19-66).*

*The sheath of the upper part of segment IV in ten specimens (50%) originated in the porta hepatis. The portal branches arose from the left portal branch. The artery arose from the left branch of the hepatic artery. The duct joined that draining segment III. In the other ten specimens the sheath originated from the sheath of the right anterior sector "segments V and VIII." In these ten specimens (50%), the branches of the right branch of the portal vein and the right branch of the hepatic artery to the right anterior sector were the source of the blood supply to the upper part of segment IV. The duct joined that of the anterior sector (Figs. 19-67 and 19-68).*

**Glissonian sheath of the right anterior sector.** *The sheath passed from the end of the right main sheath anteriorly (Figs. 19-61 and 19-69) to provide 1 to 3 sheaths (2.05 ± 0.99) to segment V and one sheath for segment VIII in all specimens. In addition it provided 1 to 2 sheaths (1.3 ± 0.23) to the upper part of segment IV in ten specimens (50%) (Figs. 19-67 and 19-68).*

**Glissonian sheaths of segments V and VIII.** *The right anterior sector sheath was the origin of the sheaths of segment V. In all specimens (Figs. 19-67, 19-68, 19-69) the segment had 1 to 3 sheaths (2.05 ± 0.99). In all livers, segment VIII received single sheath (Figs. 19-67, 19-68, and 19-69).*

**Glissonian sheath of the right posterior sector.** *The right posterior sector sheath passed to the right and posteriorly from the point of bifurcation of the right·main sheath (Fig. 19-61).*

**Glissonian sheaths of segments VI & VII.** *The right posterior sector sheath was the origin of the sheaths of segments VI and VII in all specimens. In the present study, the manner in which the right posterior sector was distributed to both segments could be classified into two patterns.*

*In the first, the right posterior sector sheath bifurcated into the sheaths of segments VI and VII. This pattern was encountered in three adult livers and in all the stillborns' livers (65%) (Figs. 19-69, 19-70, and 19-71).*

*The second pattern was encountered in seven adults' livers (35%). The right posterior sector sheath ran first towards the inferior border, then to the right, and, lastly, superiorly; i.e., it ran a curved course in segments VI and VII respectively. It gave several branches to either segment from its convex border. Segment VI received 3 to 5 branches (4 ± 0.66) and segment VII received 4 to 7 (5.28 ± 1.24) (Fig. 19-72).*

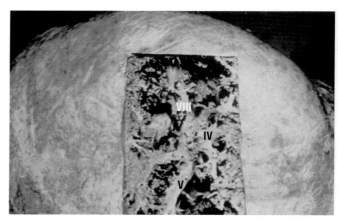

**FIG. 19-67.** A photograph showing the anterior surface of an adult's liver. The parenchyma was removed to show the glissonian sheaths of segments V, VIII, and the upper part of IV. (Courtesy of El-Gharbawy, El-Hennawi, Mekky, El-Deeb, El-Saiedy.)

**DISCUSSION.** *The sheaths of segment I arose from the posterior aspects of the right main and left main sheaths and entered the anteroinferior aspect of the lower end of the segment. This critical anatomical location of the sheaths, in addition to the presence of the segment on the posterior surface of the liver behind the upper part of segment IV and its direct venous drainage into the inferior vena cava, made Launois and Jamieson[167] regard segment I difficult to excise. Ton That Tung[169] and Bismuth and Houssin[170] had proposed excising segments II and III to gain access to segment I. Launois and Jamieson[167] had proposed excision of segments I and IV together.*

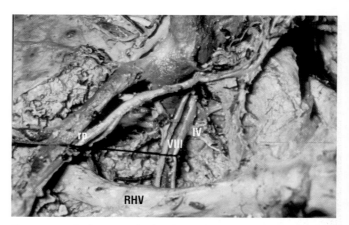

**FIG. 19-68.** A photograph showing the components of the glissonian sheaths of segment VIII and the upper part of segment IV. RHV, right hepatic vein; rp, components of right posterior sector. (Courtesy of El-Gharbawy, El-Hennawi, Mekky, El-Deeb, El-Saiedy.)

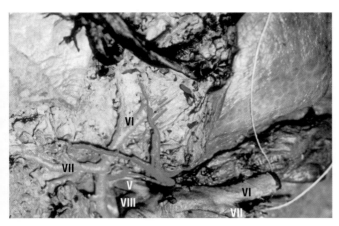

**FIG. 19-69.** A photograph showing the portal branches of segments V and VIII arising from the portal branch of the right anterior sector. The portal branch of the right posterior sector has been retracted to the left and its branches to segments VI and VII are shown. The ducts and arteries of segments VI & VII are also shown. (Courtesy of El-Gharbawy, El-Hennawi, Mekky, El-Deeb, El-Saiedy.)

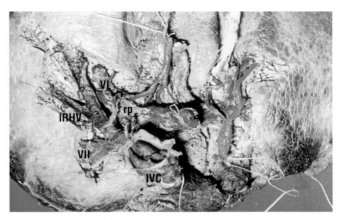

**FIG. 19-71.** A photograph of an adult's liver showing the first pattern of the right posterior (rp) sector sheath. It bifurcated into the sheaths of segments VI and VII. The inferior right hepatic vein (IRHV) was severed from the inferior vena cava (IVC) and retracted to expose the point of bifurcation. (Courtesy of El-Gharbawy, El-Hennawi, Mekky, El-Deeb, El-Saiedy.)

*Segment II had single sheath in all specimens. It arose from the left main sheath when the latter left the left end of the porta hepatis to run in the fissure for ligamentum teres. The banks of the fissure can be easily and safely forced apart to expose the origin of segment II sheath.[171] Segment II can be excised alone. On doing segmentectomy II, the operator has to dissect the sheath of segment II in the liver substance 1 cm to the left of its origin. In this way the duct and the artery of segment III are safeguarded if they are coursing along the left side of the left portal branch.*

*In the present study segment III received single sheath that arose from the left side of the left main sheath where it became continuous with the round ligament in the fissure for ligamentum teres. The origin of the sheath was extrahepatic and constant in all specimens, and the round ligament served as a guide to its site. Launois and Jamieson[167] mentioned that there might be one, two, or even three glissonian sheaths to segment III.*

*The extrahepatic origin and the constant location of the sheaths of segments II and III, the peripheral position of the segments, and their easily identifiable borders on the*

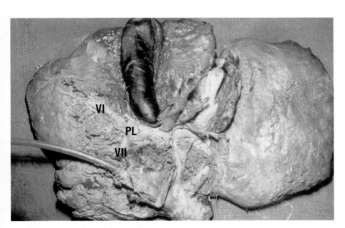

**FIG. 19-70.** A photograph of a stillborn's liver showing the first pattern of the right posterior (PL) sector sheath. It bifurcated into the sheaths of segments VI and VII. (Courtesy of El-Gharbawy, El-Hennawi, Mekky, El-Deeb, El-Saiedy.)

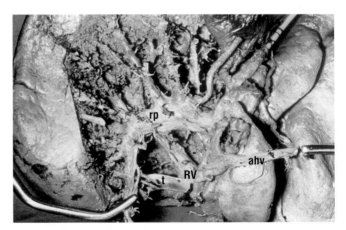

**FIG. 19-72.** A photograph of an adult's liver showing the second pattern of the right posterior (rp) sector sheath. An accessory hepatic vein (ahv) is cut and retracted. Two tributaries (t) of the right hepatic vein (RV) are shown. (Courtesy of El-Gharbawy, El-Hennawi, Mekky, El-Deeb, El-Saiedy.)

*anterosuperior surface (falciform ligament) and postero-inferior surface (fissures venosum and teres) could explain why segmentectomy II and III is a straightforward operation.*[167]

*Segment IV is formed of two parts. Its lower part, i.e., the quadrate lobe, is well circumscribed. The sheath of this lower part arose constantly in the fissure for ligamentum teres from the right side of the left main sheath just proximal to the attachment of the latter with the round ligament so resection of the quadrate lobe is a straightforward segmentectomy. The sheaths of the upper part arose from the left main sheath in the porta hepatis in ten specimens and from the right anterior sector sheath in the other ten. This upper part is bounded above by two major structures, i.e., the middle and left hepatic veins, and lies in front of segment I separated from it by the dorsal fissure whose plane has to be guessed during resection of this upper part. This might explain why the resection of this part is difficult.*[167]

*The right main sheath bifurcated into the sheaths of the right anterior and the right posterior sectors inside the liver substance. The right main sheath could be dissected in the porta hepatis and controlled with a tape in right hepatectomy.*[167]

*The right main sheath branched into the sheaths of the right anterior and the right posterior sectors inside the liver parenchyma. This fact is the basis of the "posterior approach" adopted by the French surgeons in segmentectomies of the right lobe of the liver. They dissect the right anterior sector sheath through the inferior surface of the liver prior to parenchymatous transection and clamp it with the hepatic pedicle unclamped. The right anterior sector became cyanosed and its right and left borders delineate the right and main hepatic fissures respectively.*[167,172]

*The sheath of the right anterior sector ran antero-posterior. It gave 1 to 3 sheaths to segment V that ran anteroinferiorly and single sheath to segment VIII. Launois and Jamieson[167] stated that the glissonian sheaths of segment V are usually 1 to 3 in number, anteroposterior in direction, straight, and never recurrent. They also reported two sheaths for segment VIII. To the best of the investigators' knowledge, the branches of the right anterior sector sheath to the upper part of segment IV were not mentioned before and need further confirmation.*

*The right posterior sector sheath had two patterns of distribution. In the first pattern (65%) it bifurcated into the sheaths of segments VI and VII. This means that either segment can be resected alone safely. In the second pattern (35%) the sector's sheath ran a curved course first through segment VI, then through segment VII. It had several segmental branches that arose from its convex border. In this case resection of segment VI jeopardizes the blood supply of segment VII.*

*In the present study, segment VI had single sheath in 65% of specimens and received 3 to 5 sheaths in 35% of specimens. According to Launois and Jamieson,[167] the number of cases in which a single glissonian sheath supplies segment VII is probably less than half and there are often two or even three sheaths, with the first arising from the right main sheath. On excising segment VII, they expressed the importance of leaving all the sheaths that are recurrent or posterior, as they supply segment VI. This could be clearly explained by the second pattern of distribution described in the present study.*

*Segment VII received single sheath in 65% of specimens and had 4 to 7 sheaths in the remaining 35%. Launois and Jamieson[167] stated that segment VII is usually supplied by a single sheath.*

## HISTOLOGY AND PHYSIOLOGY

The liver is the main metabolic organ of the body. It is composed of parenchyma (hepatocytes) and its supporting connective tissue stroma. The exocrine secretion of the hepatocytes is bile. The bile passes into intercellular bile canaliculi; these open into bile ducts. Endocrine secretions into the bloodstream include glucose, plasma proteins, and lipoproteins. Important metabolic activities of the hepatocytes are:

- converting glucose to glycogen and vice versa
- degrading steroid hormones
- detoxifying toxic substances and drugs
- utilizing lipids in lipoprotein synthesis

Each hepatocyte borders on a bile canaliculus and on one or more blood sinusoids. Overall, the liver is composed of parenchymal units arranged in six-sided prisms about 0.7 mm × 2.0 mm in size (Fig. 19-30A). These units are the "classic" liver lobules but not the functional lobules. In the center of the prisms are the tributaries of the hepatic veins. On the edges of the prisms are the three elements of the hepatic triad. They are the:

- Branches of the bile ducts
- Hepatic arteries
- Hepatic portal vein

The hepatic portal vein is surrounded by connective tissue that continues at the porta with the connective tissue of the fibrous (Glisson's) capsule of the liver. Three to six triads are associated with each unit.

The liver cells (hepatocytes) of the unit are arranged in fenestrated plates disposed radially from the central vein to the periphery. The spaces between the plates are occupied by the liver sinusoids, the walls of which are formed by a discontinuous endothelium. This endothelium lies on the microvilli of the hepatocyte forming a perivascular space (of Disse) (Fig. 19-42). Because the discontinuities of the endothelium are smaller than erythrocytes, the space of Disse contains macromolecules but not blood cells. Fixed macrophages (Kupffer cells) are associated with the endothelial cells of the sinusoid. Stellate "fat storing" cells are also present in the perivascular spaces.

According to Sasse et al.,[173] each hepatocyte has a vascular pole responsible for an ingestive sense and a biliary pole responsible for secretory function.

The biliary tract begins with the bile canaliculi (Fig. 19-42). These canaliculi are bounded by two or three hepatocytes and range from about 0.5 μm to 1.0 μm in diameter. They form a polyhedral network between hepatocytes. The network is continuous from lobule to lobule and is without blind ends. With the light microscope, the canaliculi appear to be lined by a membrane. This appearance is due to adenosine triphosphate activity in the hepatocyte at the surface of the canaliculus.

The canaliculus is bounded by the plasma membrane of two or more hepatocytes from which short, stubby microvilli project into the lumen. On either side of the canaliculus, adjacent hepatocytes are attached to one another by a zonula occludens. Thus, the bile is confined to the bile canaliculus and can move only toward the periphery of the lobule.

As the canaliculi approach the periphery, small ducts lined with cuboidal epithelium appear; these are the bile ductules (Hering's canals) (Fig. 19-58). As these enter the connective tissue of the portal triad, they become true bile ducts of the triads. The lining of the duct is a regular cuboidal or columnar epithelium and the duct is covered by a sheath of connective tissue.

The classic liver lobule (Fig. 19-30A) exhibits a hexagonal shape. The portal tract area (or radicle) at each "corner" contains portal vein branches, the hepatic artery, bile ducts, lymphatics, and connective tissue. The central vein lies within the center of the lobule. Within the lobule are portal vein and hepatic artery branches entering and anastomosing with thin-walled sinusoids. These extend from the radicle to the central vein of the lobule. This vein opens into the sublobular veins that drain into hepatic veins, and these open into the inferior vena cava. Trabeculae are plates of hepatocytes radiating from central vein to edge of the lobule.

"True" ducts of Luschka are in the hepatic surface. These are ductlike structures which may connect with bile ducts but never open into gallbladder lumen.

The surgical physiology of the liver may be summarized in Merrell's[174] beautiful table (Table 19-6).

The capacity of the liver to regenerate is well-known. This enigmatic act has been appreciated for many centuries. Even after a 75 to 90 percent hepatectomy, a liver possessing a normal remnant may fully regenerate within weeks or months.[175] The mechanism of regeneration is highly hypothetical; however, it is known that hepatocytes proliferate first, and nonparenchymal cells appear later. Insulin, glucagon, epidermal growth factor, and other elements may possibly be involved.

Holley[176] reported that growth factors and hormones may act by invoking the same intracellular growth-control mechanisms affected by nutrients. Barker and colleagues[177] and Lambotte and Tagliaferri,[178] all of the University of Louvain in Belgium, are engaged in ongoing studies of in vivo "priming" and "progression" factors as well as the synthesis of DNA in liver regeneration following partial hepatectomy.

After experimenting in rats, Hashimoto and Sanjo[179] stated that functional liver capacity was minimal during parenchymal cell mitosis in the regenerating liver. The same authors observed that functional restoration after two-thirds hepatectomy was delayed in comparison with morphologic restoration in rats.

## TABLE 19-6. Hepatic Functions

**Filtration (i.e. reticuloendothelial system)**
    Process incoming substrate & vitamins

**Metabolic homeostasis**
    *Fundamental mechanisms*
        Capture
        Maintenance of intracellular metabolism
        Storage
        Release

    *Metabolic substrates*
        Carbohydrates — modulate glucose
        Lipids — modulate free fatty acids
        Amino acids — modulate amino acid pools

**Specific protein synthesis**

| Coagulation | { | Fibrinogen<br>Prothrombin<br>VII, IX, X |
|---|---|---|
| Carrier proteins | { | Albumin<br>Transferrin<br>Lipoprotein |

**Lipid phase metabolism**
    Drug metabolism
    Bile formation
    Lysosomal and nonlysosomal transport

*Source:* Clark JH III, Wood RP. Hepatic physiology. *In:* Miller TA (ed). Physiologic Basis of Modern Surgical Care (2nd ed). St. Louis: CV Mosby, 1998, pp. 491-511; with permission.

## SURGERY

*The liver, because of its unforgiving and extraordinarily difficult surgical anatomy and complex physiology, will remain the Mount Everest of organs for surgeons. It is no place for the fainthearted, perhaps, but it will continue to challenge the bright and the bold.*

*James H. Foster[180]*

## Exploration of the Abdomen

Upon entering the abdomen, if a pathologic diagnosis is needed prior to proceeding, perform a needle biopsy or wedge biopsy of the liver as soon as possible. This avoids any changes in the liver due to injury by instruments or the effects of the anesthetic drugs. As a rule, the biopsy should be taken far away from the area of the gallbladder, especially if there are pathologic processes involving the gallbladder that might affect the adjacent liver tissue. Ultrasonographic examination may be performed to identify the area of pathology if necessary.

Exploration should begin with the omentum, transverse colon, and mesocolon, which should be withdrawn from the abdomen and positioned between a warm pack outside and the upper part of the incision. The hand should pass down to the pelvis to palpate the left colon, male or female pelvic organs, urinary bladder, great vessels, and the anatomic entities within the retroperitoneal space.

The surgeon may choose to palpate the right colon at this time or after examining the small intestine and its mesentery from the ligament of Treitz to the ileocecal valve. We do not object to retrograde examination from the valve to the ligament. Examine part of the second, third, and fourth parts of the duodenum. Observe the relation of the superior mesenteric artery to the third part of the duodenum. Harvest any abnormal lymph nodes and send them for examination while mobilization of the liver begins.

The pancreas must now be palpated. The inspection of the infracolic compartment concludes with examination of the abdominal wall for hernias, omphalomesenteric anomalies, and urachal cysts.

Replace the omentum and transverse colon and its mesentery in the abdomen. Inspect the supracolic compartment from the right, starting by palpating the right kidney, duodenum, head of the pancreas, and pylorus. The stomach, up to and including the gastroesophageal junction, should be felt. Palpate the spleen with great care; the peritoneal attachments are short and the splenic capsule is easily torn.

## Exploration of the Liver

The entire liver and biliary tract must be methodically evaluated. Examine the inferior surface of the diaphragm prior to the actual hepatic exploration. The area of suspected pathology should be the last to be examined. Intraoperative ultrasonography is the most accurate method for examination of the liver and should be performed routinely.

Palpate the lateral segment of the liver by passing the hand to the left of the falciform ligament and move backward until the fingertips reach the coronary and left triangular ligaments. Similarly, the hand may be passed to the right of the falciform ligament, moving backward to palpate the coronary and right triangular ligaments. Palpate the falciform and splenorenal ligaments. Occasionally the base of the falciform ligament is not fused with the abdominal wall, leaving a hiatus through which a loop of intestine may herniate.

We quote from Takao and Kawarada[181] on the hepatic hilar area:

*It is important to understand the main variations of the biliary and vascular elements inside the plate system for hilar bile duct carcinoma because all variations of these elements occur in this plate system. The plate system consists of the hilar plate, cystic plate, and umbilical plate which cover the extrahepatic vascular system and are fused with the hepatoduodenal ligament. The bile duct and vascular system that penetrate the plate system form Glisson's capsule in the liver, but the caudate branch and the medial segmental branch are exceptions. The bile duct and hepatic artery accompanying the plate system can be exfoliated from the portal vein with numerous lymph ducts and nerves. The bile ducts in the right hepatic lobe are classified into 4 types, and the standard type is present in 53-72% of cases. In the left bile duct, the medial segmental bile duct is connected in the vicinity of the hilar area in 35.5% of cases, and these cases should be treated the same as the caudate lobe in hilar bile duct carcinoma. Generally, there is little main variation of the portal vein (16-26%), but more variation in the hepatic artery (31-33%). During surgery for hilar bile duct carcinoma, it is important to observe the plate system and the many variations of the bile duct vascular system.*

## The Surgeon and the Liver in the Operating Room

It is not within the scope of this chapter to discuss details of liver pathology. We will, however, describe the gross appearance of some hepatic pathology collectively, but not specifically. We hope this will help the surgeon make the right decision in the operating room.

The dilemma of the surgeon is whether to perform a partial hepatectomy and thus cure the patient if the lesion is benign, to palliate the patient for a longer or shorter period if the lesion is malignant, or whether to leave the patient alone. The patient's history and laboratory reports will help the surgeon decide.

Another dilemma is the choice of an open or needle biopsy. Nearly all common pathologic entities can currently be distinguished by their appearance on imaging studies (CT, spiral CT, MRI, arteriograms, etc.). Biopsies may be done for confirmation but are not always necessary. Remember that a small hemangioma will bleed copiously, and the aspiration of an *Echinococcus* cyst of the liver may produce a fatal anaphylactic reaction.

Tables 19-7 and 19-8 list anatomic differential diagnosis of the liver and gallbladder and ducts in the operating room. We present these tables with mixed feelings, since the gross appearance of a hepatocellular carcinoma, for example, overlaps the gross appearance of a cholangiocarcinoma. Liver cell adenoma, focal nodular hyperplasia, and hemangioma may have the same or different appearance. If the anatomist, with the aid of the pathologist, can help the surgeon differentiate between benign and malignant lesions, the patient is the beneficiary.

The surgeon goes to the operating room with a definite strategy. His or her armamentarium includes a variety of diagnostic procedures, which, along with their complications, are described below.

The surgery of the liver consists of biopsies; suture of lacerations; right hepatectomy (lobectomy), typical or extended; left hepatectomy (lobectomy), typical or extended; segmentectomy; removal or drainage of cysts; and total or partial transplantation.

Czerniak et al.[182] reported the following. [*Authors' note:* For clarity, we would replace all occurrences of the term "left lobe" with "segments II and III."]

> The anatomical possibility of resecting the left lobe of the liver (segments II and III) in living subjects and using it for transplantation was evaluated. A group of 60 cadaveric livers were dissected at autopsy. The vascular and biliary elements of the left lobe were isolated and the lobe was resected and evaluated for possible grafting.
>
> The left lobe was 12% to 28% (mean 19.4%) of the liver mass. An extrahepatic segment of the left hepatic vein was isolated in 95% of specimens. Arterial blood supply to the left lobe consisted of a single artery (92%) or two arteries (8%).
>
> A single portal vein segment to the left lobe (type I)

was found in 35% livers. Portal vein branches originated from a common orifice (type II, 35%) or separately (type III, 30%) from the left portal vein, and in these instances, preparation of a portal segment necessitated partial section of the left portal vein wall.

> Biliary drainage was extrahepatic in 56 livers and consisted of a single duct (type I, 78%), or two ducts (type II, 15%).
>
> The resected left lobe was evaluated as satisfactory (single hepatic vein and artery, types I or II portal vein, type I bile duct) in 48% of cases, while a less-satisfactory lobe (type III portal vein or type II bile duct) was obtained in 33%.
>
> It was found anatomically difficult or impossible to resect the left lobe for possible transplantation in 11 (19%) liver specimens.

However, Kazemier et al.[183] disagreed "strikingly" with Czerniak and colleagues. Table 19-9 is Kazemier's summary of the differences between the results of his team's study of 39 corrosion casts and Czerniak's dissection of 60 human cadaveric livers along the umbilical fissure.

The reply of Czerniak et al.[184] to Kazemier et al. follows verbatim.

> ...We suggest that the difference in the technique used (dissection vs. the cast method) may explain the discrepancy between the results of our study and the study of Kazemier et al. Michels[78] in his detailed dissection study of 200 livers, has found a single artery to the left lobe in 88.5% of cases. Couinaud[185] reports the portal blood supply to segments II and III to consist of a single portal vein branch in 96% and 31%, respectively. A type I portal vein (though not named as such) is also described (Couinaud). In the same study, and based on dissection of 100 livers, a single bile duct draining the left lobe was found in 77% of livers.[185] These results are comparable with ours.
>
> There are often ducts and vessels coming from the liver substance underlying the umbilical fissure and the fossa for the ligamentum venosum,[78] and it may be difficult to ascertain the relationship between these structures and the various structures of the left lobe by the cast method.
>
> Moreover, using the cast method, judgement about the various planes of resection of the liver parenchyma as being within or adjacent to the umbilical fissure, is only approximate.[186] Kazemier et al.[183] have found a single artery to the left lobe in 59% and a type I bile duct in 56% of the 39 livers examined. However, when they examined a plane that is presumed to be to the right of the umbilical fissure, a single artery supplying the graft was obtained in 77%, and a single biliary

## TABLE 19-7. Anatomic Differential Diagnosis of the Liver in the Operating Room

**PATHOLOGY**

I. Abscesses
   A. Pyogenic
      Abscesses usually small and multiple; may be solitary and multilocular. According to Schwartz (1984) a solitary abscess is usually in the right lobe.
   B. Amebic
      Single large abscesses usually in the right lobe on either hepatic surface. Aspiration will give the characteristic chocolate-like or "anchovy paste" fluid. Variable; may be multiple.

II. Cirrhosis
   A. Cirrhosis (micronodular)
      Hepatomegaly with minute nodules and panhepatic fibrosis. The liver is a dark brown color if hemosiderosis is present; tan or yellow if fatty metamorphosis has occurred.
   B. Cirrhosis (macronodular)
      Liver, large or small, with large nodules

III. Cysts
   A. Nonparasitic
      Solitary, usually at the anterior inferior surface of the right lobe, containing crystal clear fluid or brown-yellow semiliquid material. Traumatic cysts are single without epithelium and filled with bile (Schwartz, 1964). Polycystic cysts are usually throughout the liver but they may be limited to the right lobe. They have a honeycomb appearance. About one half of patients will have polycystic kidneys also.
   B. Parasitic Hydatid (Echinococcus)
      1. E. granulosus
         85% are superficial in the right lobe. The cystic wall consists of an outer (adventitia) and an inner (germinative) membrane. The cysts contain clear fluid at high pressure.
      2. E. multilocularis (alveolar)
         There is no capsule or cystic wall. Multiple minute cysts with gelatinous rather than fluid contents. They infiltrate the surrounding tissue.

IV. Tumors
   A. Benign
      May or may not be encapsulated. May be large or small, discrete or nodular, well defined or ill defined, single or multiple, often subscapular.
   B. Malignant
      1. Primary
         Single or multiple masses or nodules in one or both lobes of the liver. Hepatomegaly may be present. Cirrhotic appearance is usual. The tumor may be nodular, massive or diffuse. If firm and whitish and in the periphery of the liver, consider cholangiocarcioma. Portal vein thrombosis in malignant hepatoma has been reported (Albacete et al. 1967).
      2. Metastatic – superficial
         Discrete yellow or grayish nodules, or centrally necrosed, under the hepatic capsule, but very visible. Hepatomegaly. Lesions mimic fibrous scars, tubercular nodules, nodular hyperplasia, bile duct adenoma, syphylitic nodules, etc.
      3. Metastatic – deep
         Lesions deep in the liver parenchyma without visible nodules. The absence of visible nodules on the surface does not rule out metastatic disease (Goligher, 1941).

**References**
Schwartz SI. Liver. In: Schwartz SI, Shires GT, Spencer FC, Storer EH (eds). Principles of Surgery. New York: McGraw-Hill, 1984.
Schwartz SI. Surgical Diseases of the Liver. New York: McGraw-Hill, 1964.
Albacete RA, Matthews MJ, Saini N. Portal vein thromboses in malignant hepatoma. Ann Intern Med 67:337, 1967.
Goligher JC. Surgery of the Anus, Rectum and Colon, 5th Ed. London: Balliere Tindall, 1984, p. 450.

branch in 95% of cases. When one considers the possible discrepancies in the planes of resection between the two studies, these results approximate ours (92% and 78%, respectively).

Based on our dissection studies, we suggest that the plane of resection of the liver should be within the umbilical fissure. Using this plane, both an accurate extrahepatic dissection and preparation of the portal structures to the left lobe, and an avoidance of damage to segment IV structures can be achieved.

## TABLE 19-8. Anatomic Differential Diagnosis of the Gallbladder and Ducts in the Operating Room

**PATHOLOGY**

I. Cholecystitis

A. Acute calculus

The gallbladder is red and edematous and is distended due to cystic duct obstruction secondary to an impacted stone. The color is black if gangrene is present. Perforation may have occurred with evidence of local bile peritonitis. After aspiration the gallstones are palpable under the thick, hypertrophic, edematous wall. Large lymph nodes are present. Pus is present with pyogenic membranes. The ducts, particularly the common bile duct, are covered by the edematous gastrohepatic omentum and the duct may be inflamed sympathetically. If the epiploic foramen is obliterated secondary to edema, stones may be palpated in the common bile duct. Remember: gallstone ileus. Jaundice may be present. A large solitary calculus in Hartmann's pouch may distend the gallbladder with mucocele, hydrops or empyema.

B. Acute acalculus — 10%

As above but without stones. Perforation is frequent.

C. Chronic calculus

The wall may be thickened, but stones are palpable. Jaundice, adhesions and enlarged lymph nodes may be present. The common bile duct may be dilated due to distal obstruction. The gallbladder may be normal or shrunken.

D. Chronic acalculus

As above but without stones.

E. Choledocholithiasis

Impaction at the lower end. Jaundice may be present; the common bile duct may be dilated. Remember two synchronous impactions: cystic duct and ampulla of Vater. The results are jaundice and mucocele or empyema. The presence of stones does not proclude malignancy. Check the head of the pancreas and the porta hepatis. Remember: a stone may produce acute pancreatitis.

F. Cancer of gallbladder

Metastases to choledochal lymph nodes. Rarely a cause of obstruction by compression.

G. Other pathology of the common bile duct

With cancer of the head of the pancreas the common duct is dilated, thin walled and bluish. With distal cancer the gallbladder is usually distended, the common duct is not affected with chronic pancreatitis; jaundice may be present. The common bile duct and the gallbladder are distended, edematous and pale.

However, the scientific battle for the anatomy of the noble organ continues.

Kazemier et al.,[187] analyzing 60 corrosion casts of human cadaveric livers for dissection planes for transplantation, reported the following (Table 19-10).

*...Our anatomical study suggests that cutting plane A (in the umbilical fissure, just left of Rex' sinus) necessitates the highest average total number of arterial, portal, and biliary anastomoses (6.4) for a viable (left) graft in liver transplantation using SG [split grafting] or*

## TABLE 19-9. Anatomy of Supplying and Draining Structures of Couinaud Segments II and III (Resection at Plane in Umbilical Fissure)

|  | Czerniak et al.[178] (n = 60) | Kazemier et al.[179] (n = 39) |
|---|---|---|
| Arterial blood supply to segments II and III: |  |  |
| 1 Artery | 92% | 59% |
| >1 Artery | 8% | 41% |
| Portal blood supply to segments II and III: |  |  |
| Type I (single portal vein to segments II and III) | 35% | 0% |
| Type II (common orifice of portal vein branches to segments II and III) | 35% | 0% |
| Type III (separate orifices of portal vein branches to segments II and III) | 30% | 100% |
| Biliary drainage of segments II and III: |  |  |
| Type I (single duct) | 78% | 56% |
| Type II (two ducts) | 15% | 44% |

*Source:* Kazemier G, Hesselink EJ, Terpstra OT. Hepatic anatomy. Transplantation 1990;49:1029; with permission.

LRG [living related grafting] techniques. Cutting plane B [in the umbilical fissure, through Rex' sinus, by a longitudinal section of the left portal vein wall] reduces this number significantly (4.2). Both planes have the advantage of creating a small wound surface in the liver at the place of resection. Both cutting planes leave segment IV attached to the right liver half (SG) or to the donor (LRG), including a volume reduction of only two small segments (segments II and III), but transection of arterial and/or biliary branches to segment IV in 17% and 20%, respectively, limited the number of viable segments IV. Plane B requires the additional reconstruction of the left portal vein (Rex' sinus) to ensure sufficient portal blood flow to segment IV. Cutting plane C (in the liver hilum, just left of the arterial, portal, and biliary bifurcations) has the clear advantage of the lowest average total number of arterial, portal, and biliary anastomoses for a viable (left) graft (3.1), but it also creates the largest wound surface in the liver and in the case of LRG it will reduce the amount of liver tissue left with the donor by three segments (II, III, and IV). However, using plane C, vasculobiliary branches to segment II and III can be denuded, by dissecting and removing the parenchyma of segment IV.[188] Thereby one achieves sufficient length of these branches, thus facilitating the anastomosing procedure of the (left) graft in the recipient. In this way only one arterial, one portal, and one biliary anastomosis of branches with acceptable length and diameter remain. In conclusion, cutting plane C, in the liver hilum seems to be the best option to split a liver into two parts for transplantation purposes using SG or LRG techniques. When using this plane, a relatively large wound surface is created

and the functional liver mass in the living donor is reduced by segments II, III, and IV. In the clinical setting this plane has proven to be a usable one, regarding several reports.[188-190]

Blumgart et al.[103] (whose colleagues included Czerniak) presented the anatomic entities involved in left extended hepatectomy. It is not within the scope of this book to describe the technique. The interested reader should refer to the book of Blumgart, *Surgery of the Liver and Biliary Tract.*[191]

Czerniak et al.[192] proposed a direct approach to the hepatic veins in left hepatectomy. Their work is based upon Elias and Petty,[193] Goldsmith and Woodburne,[96] Banner and Brasfield,[194] Baird and Britton,[195] Depinto et al.,[196] Nakamura and Tsuzuki,[129] Castaing et al.,[197] and Ou and Herman.[198]

Czerniak and colleagues advised that the anatomy of the veins in most instances is extrahepatic, but fixed to the left lobe of the liver and IVC by an avascular fibroareolar tissue. The authors advised, "once a plane is made between them and the liver, their true extrahepatic nature is disclosed."[192]

The authors have seen this avascular tissue in the laboratory covered occasionally by a very thin stroma of hepatic tissue. This is confusing for the surgeon. Of course, Czerniak et al.[182] emphasized this dissection in vivo.

Nery et al.[199] studied the surgical anatomy and blood supply of the left biliary tree and the use of the lateral segment of the left lobe for transplantation, which is quite adequate for living donation. Their study demonstrated the following.

• The hepatic arteries had the usual origin (Table 19-11).
• The left bile duct and its tributaries did not receive any

**TABLE 19-10. Average Number of Arterial, Portal, Biliary, and Total (= A + P + B) Anastomoses (±SD; range) to be Made at Three Different Cutting Planes in the Left Liver to Create a Viable (Left) Graft for SG and LRG Purposes**

| Cutting Plane | Average Number of Anastomoses (±SD; Range) | | | |
| | Arterial | Portal | Biliary | Total |
|---|---|---|---|---|
| A | 2.0 (±0.66; 1-4) | 2.3 (±0.51; 2-4) | 2.1 (±0.58; 1-3) | 6.4 (±1.32; 4-12) |
| B | 1.6 (±0.62; 1-4) | 1.0 (±0.0) | 1.6 (±0.52; 1-3) | 4.2 (±0.90; 3-7)* |
| C | 1.1 (±0.34; 1-2) | 1.0 (±0.0) | 1.0 (±0.0) | 3.1 (±0.34; 3-4)[†,‡] |

Note. (A) In the umbilical fissure, just left of Rex' sinus; (B) in the umbilical fissure, through Rex' sinus; (C) in the liver hilum, just left of the arterial, portal, and biliary bifurcations.
*vs A: $P < .001$.
[†]vs A: $P < .001$.
[‡]vs B: $P < .001$.
SG, Split graft; LRG, Living related graft.

*Source:* Kazemier G, Hesselink EJ, Lange JF, Terpstra OT. Dividing the liver for the purpose of split grafting or living related grafting: a search for the best cutting plane. Transplant Proc 1991;23:1545; with permission.

| n | Origin | Segmental Branches |
|---|--------|-------------------|
| 36 | LHA | II, III, IV |
| 16 | LHA | II, III |
|    | RHA | IV |
| 07 | LHA | II, III, IV, IV |
| 06 | LHA | II, III, III, IV |
| 05 | LHA | II, III, III |
|    | RHA | IV |
| 01 | LHA | II, II, III, IV |
| 01 | LHA | II, II, II, III, IV |
| 01 | LHA | II, II, II, III, III, IV |
| 01 | LHA | II, III, III, IV, IV |
| 01 | LHA | II, III, IV |
|    | RHA | IV |
| 01 | LHA | II, III |
|    | RHA | IV, IV |
| 01 | LHA | III |
|    | RHA | II, IV |
| 01 | LHA | II, II, III, III |
|    | RHA | IV |

**TABLE 19-11. Extra-hepatic Segmental Arteries to the Left Hepatic Lobe According to Origin. Multiple Branches to a Single Segment are Underlined**

Total: 78

LHA, Left hepatic artery; RHA, Right hepatic artery.

*Source:* Nery JR, Frasson E, Rilo HLR, Purceli E, Barros MFA, Neto JB, Mies S, Raia S, Belzer FO. Surgical anatomy and blood supply of the left biliary tree pertaining to partial liver grafts from living donors. Transplantation Proc 1990;22: 1492; with permission.

contributions from the portal system.

- The left biliary tree had 13 variations. In 85.9%, the left hepatic duct was long; in 14.1%, it was very short (Fig. 19-73).
- The left hepatic artery was the main and only artery of the lateral segment of the left lobe.
- The surgeon must avoid entering the hilar plate too close to the bile duct wall.
- Angiographic studies are essential to verify the arterial anatomy.

Couinaud and Houssin[200] reported that blind partition of the right and left lobes to obtain two transplants is problematic because of left arterial and right ductal variations. These authors advised the following procedures.

- Arteriography and cholangiography prior to surgery for mapping and protecting arterial and biliary networks
- The following three surgical maneuvers
  - Resection of segment IV when arterio-biliary duplications are present
  - Attribution of the common hepatic artery at its duplication
  - Partial attribution of the common hepatic duct at the side of the biliary duplication

Couinaud,[201] in a calculation spreading to six digits, showed the "vanity" of attempting to classify the multiple variations of the right ductal system, and advised cholangiography. In a discussion appended to that article, Hureau reminds the hepatic surgeon to search beyond the "ideal" and "average" subject of the textbook to best operate on a given patient's own "personal anatomy." Houssin and colleagues (including Couinaud)[202] reported similar findings.

Portography or ultrasonography to detect absence of portal vein bifurcation has been used by Couinaud.[199] He reported five occurrences of this anomaly (1.9 percent frequency). Three figures (Figs. 19-74, 19-75, 19-76) demonstrate this rare anomaly.

Characteristically, portal vein bifurcation absence manifests with a "huge portal ring."[203] The large vein turns toward the right. After reaching the umbilical fissure, it sends the usual branches, ending at the caudate lobe. Thus, there is no left portal vein. The author advises total vascular bypass, skeletonization of the portal vein, and resection. Another technique consists of deep interruption of the portal stem in the hilum, division of the main portal fissure at the right margin of the middle hepatic vein, and transection of the transverse portion of the portal ring.

In a further publication, Couinaud[204] stated that partition of the right and left lobes maintains segment IV's association with the right lobe. However, this interrupts its portal vessels springing from the left portal pedicle. In a large series, he reported a 12.15 percent rate of preservation of the bile ducts. The segment had a good blood supply from the segmental artery (originating from the right hepatic stem) in 10.75 percent. The author also stated that disruption of both arterial and portal branches produces a potentially fatal necrosis of segment IV (a "sword of Damocles"). According to Couinaud, the segment should be resected, since its survival is rarely possible. He terms maltreatment of segment IV in liver transplantation "un scandale"[204] in the ancient Hebrew sense of "stumbling block." Couinaud's philosophy of transplantation is illustrated in Figures 19-77 through 19-80.

Couinaud's paper "Surgical approach to the dorsal section of the liver,"[205] painstakingly explains why the triangular ligaments, the coronary ligament, and the inferior vena cava present "formidable but illusory barriers," and is a classic. We advise all hepatobiliary surgeons to familiarize themselves with its contents.

Couinaud,[206] the patriarch of intrahepatic anatomy, reported variations in liver morphology and vasculobiliary elements (Figs. 19-81 through 19-85). We quote Couinaud's summary in toto.

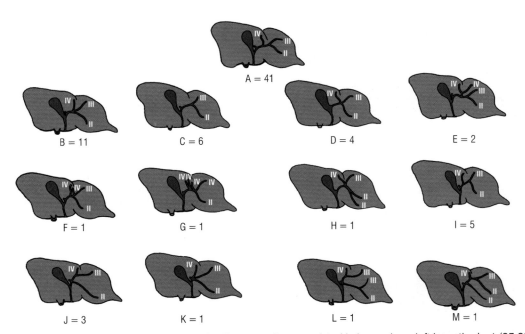

FIG. 19-73. Morphologic patterns of the extra-hepatic left biliary tree. Patterns A to H show a long left hepatic duct (85.9%), while I to M have a very short or absent left hepatic duct (14.1%). Morphologic identification previous to dissection will help to avoid injury to segmental ducts during graft resection. Numbers represent the number of specimens that contained the depicted pattern in a study of 78 livers. (Modified from Nery JR, Frasson E, Rilo HLR, Purceli E, Barros MFA, Neto JB, Mies S, Raia S, Belzer FO. Surgical anatomy and blood supply of the left biliary tree pertaining to partial liver grafts from living donors. Transplantation Proc 1990;22:1492; with permission.)

*In transplantation of the whole liver, the variable shape of the organ can exceptionally be the source of difficulties, as in the rare cases of situs inversus. Arterial variants may be the source of great difficulties. Among the biliary variants, the low junction of the right and left hepatic ducts in the main portal pedicle, and especially the cysto-hepatic ducts (entrance of a right duct into the gallbladder or the cystic duct) are particularly important, with a frequency ranging from 2% to 15% of the cases. Right liver-left liver, or right liver-left lobe bipartition is now a well controlled technique. Right lobe, left lobe bipartition should never be performed. The left hepatic vein is attributed to the left transplant (left liver or left lobe). In case of duplication of the left vein, the terminal portion of the middle vein is attributed to the left transplant, and the continuity of the middle vein with the inferior vena cava must be reconstructed. The middle vein is always attributed to the right transplant. When the portal bifurcation is missing, usually bipartition is impossible. When the right portal vein is duplicated, the portal stem is attributed to the right liver. Duplications of right and left arteries and ducts make difficulties. A thorough preoperative investigation is necessary in case of a living donor. Cholangiography and arteriography on the back table are essential to achieve an ex vivo bi-*

*partition. The surgeon then disposes of three manoeuvres: resection of segment IV, attribution of a short segment of the main duct on the side of a biliary duplication, attribution of the main hepatic artery (or the celiac axis) on the side of an arterial duplication. In*

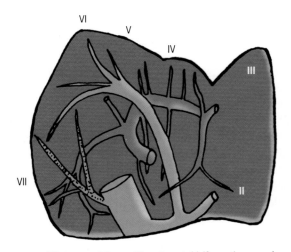

FIG. 19-74. Diagram of liver without portal bifurcation as observed by Couinaud. (Modified from Couinaud C. Absence de la bifurcation porte. J Chir (Paris) 130(3):111-115, 1993; with permission.)

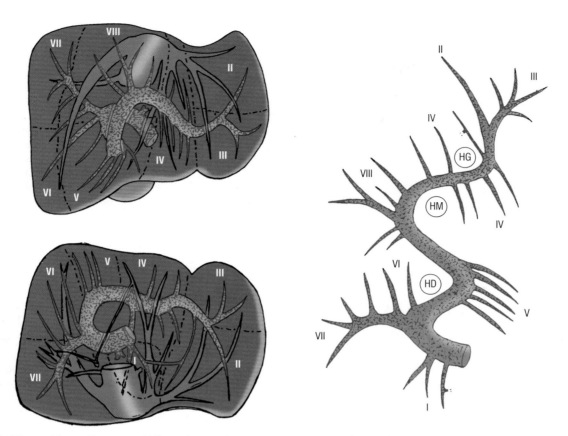

**FIG. 19-75.** Views of liver without portal bifurcation as observed by Agossou-Voyème. HG, left hepatic segment; HM, middle hepatic segment; HD, right hepatic segment. (Modified from Couinaud C. Absence de la bifurcation porte. J Chir (Paris) 130(3):111-115, 1993; with permission.)

*vivo harvesting of a left transplant (left liver or left lobe) is possible in 86% of cases, ex vivo is possible in 95.70% of cases. Tripartition of the liver is not yet a controlled technique.*

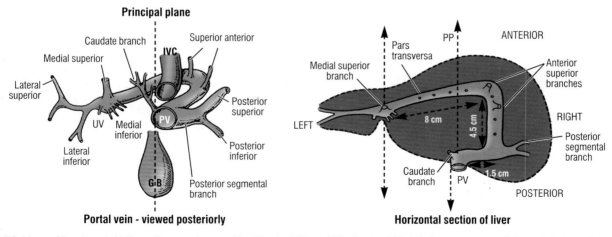

**FIG. 19-76.** Liver without portal bifurcation as observed by Hardy. UV, umbilical vein; IVC, inferior vena cava; GB, gallbladder; PV, portal vein; PP, principal plane. (Modified from Couinaud C. Absence de la bifurcation porte. J Chir (Paris) 130(3):111-115, 1993; with permission.)

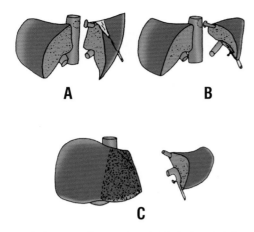

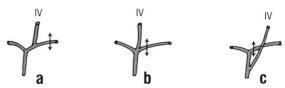

FIG. **19-79.** Biliary canals of segment IV. **a,** The canal enters near the upper biliary confluent. **b,** The canal terminates in the upper confluent. **c,** The canal becomes the primary pathway. Sectioning the left hepatic canal to the left of the segment IV canal preserves the biliary tree of the right lobe. (Modified from Couinaud C. (A "scandal": segment IV and liver transplantation). (French) J Chir (Paris) 1993;130:443; with permission.)

FIG. **19-77.** Modalities of bipartition. **A,** Right liver-left liver bipartition. The inferior vena cava is conserved on the right transplant; the left hepatic vein (with a cuff of inferior vena cava, if necessary, occluding the orifice with a venous patch graft) drains the left transplant. The caudate lobe is usually sacrificed. The division is performed along the main portal fissure. **B,** Right liver-left lobe bipartition. Segment IV is amputated. The division is performed along the umbilical fissure. **C,** Right lobe-left lobe bipartition is prohibited. The portal elements of segment IV (shown with dotted shading) are derived from the left paramedian pedicle situated in the inferior part of the umbilical fissure and are interrupted when segment IV remained attached to the right liver, resulting in necrosis of this segment. (From Couinaud C. (A "scandal": segment IV and liver transplantation). (French) J Chir (Paris) 1993;130:443; with permission.)

## *Hepatic Resections*

For our discussion of hepatic resections, Figures 19-86, 19-87, and 19-88 will serve as orientation. The triumph of hepatic surgery and anatomic resection of hepatic lobes and segments prompts us to quote Meyers,[207] who employs a logical approach to remembering the segmental sections (Figure 19-88):

> *The following logic can be employed to remember the segmental sections: The caudate lobe is its own segment (segment I) and is located posteriorly. In a clockwise order beginning from the top, segments II and III determine the tissue left of the falciform ligament (i.e., the left lateral segment in the American system). Segment IV corresponds to the tissue between the falciform ligament and Cantlie's line or the middle hepatic vein (and corresponds to the left medial segment). Segment IV is sometimes divided into part A, a superior part, and part B, an inferior part.*

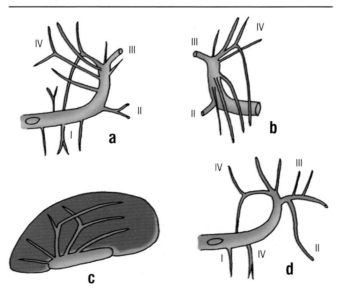

FIG. **19-78.** Portal veins of segment IV. **a,** Inferior view, anterior margin of the liver upward. **b,** Superior view. **c,** Sagittal section, anterior margin of the liver to the left. **d,** Inferior view. A deep posterior vein arises from the left portal vein. The separation of segment IV from the left portal pedicle interrupts all portal branches. (Modified from Couinaud C. (A "scandal": segment IV and liver transplantation). (French) J Chir (Paris) 1993;130:443; with permission.)

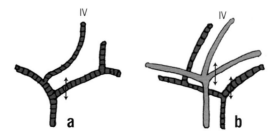

FIG. **19-80.** The segment IV artery arises from the right hepatic artery. **a,** The main artery vascularizes the right lobe after right-left partition (10.75 percent incidence). **b,** Preservation of both arterial and biliary duct function after right-left partition occurs in only 2.15 percent of livers. (Modified from Couinaud C. (A "scandal": segment IV and liver transplantation). (French) J Chir (Paris) 1993;130:443; with permission.)

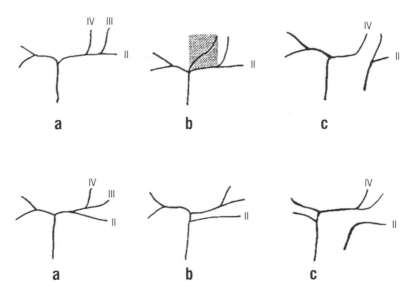

**FIG. 19-81.** *Upper:* Type (II+III) and IV left arterial or biliary distribution is shown in **a** through **c. a,** The elements of segments II and III have a common trunk into which drain the elements of segment IV. When the latter are close to the bifurcation, the bile duct or left hepatic artery is short. Such a left-sided distribution was observed in 36 out of 93 cases for the artery and in 69 out of 93 cases for the bile duct. **b,** The element of segment IV drains into the right-left bifurcation or lower down, in the main duct, resulting in duplication of the left elements. This distribution was observed in 44 out of 93 cases for the artery and 8 out of 93 cases for the bile duct. In 5 out of 93 cases, the artery of segment IV was derived from the right artery and/or bile duct for a left transplant which, in this case, is the left lobe. **c,** A left hepatic artery, arising from the left gastric artery and supplying the left lobe, constitutes this type of duplication: a left liver transplant is obtained by collecting the celiac trunk (which is excluded in vivo), or a left lobe transplant is obtained by amputating segment IV: 16 out of 93 cases. *Lower:* Type (III+IV) and II left arterial or biliary distribution is shown in **a** through **c. a,** The elements of segments III and IV have a common trunk into which drain the elements of segment II. When left cut is short: this distribution was observed in 5 out of 93 cases for the artery and in 14 out of 93 cases for the bile duct. **b,** The element of segment II drains into the bifurcation or lower down, in the main duct, resulting in duplication of the left elements: observed in 2 out of 93 cases for the bile duct. Amputation of segment IV does not allow a single artery or bile duct to be obtained for a left lobe transplant and this type of distribution excludes in vivo transplant collection. **c,** A left hepatic artery, arising from the left gastric artery and only supplying segment II, constitutes this type of duplication: 5 out of 93 cases. (From Couinaud C. Anatomie intra-hépatique: application à la transplantation du foie. Ann Radiol 37(5):323-333, 1994; with permission.)

*Segments V, VI, VII, and VIII continue according to this clockwise labeling. The gallbladder fossa lies between segments IV and V. The figure depicts the internal vascular skeleton, which is confirmed with intraoperative ultrasonography.*

Except for the sulcus, which divides the lateral segments (II, III) and medial segment (IV) of the left lobe, the diaphragmatic surface of the liver gives little indication of its internal lobulation.

In resection, the following segments are removed:
• Right hepatic lobectomy: V, VI, VII, and VIII (Fig. 19-89)
• Left hepatic lobectomy: II, III, and IV (Fig. 19-90).
• Left lateral segmentectomy: II and III (Fig. 19-91)
• Right trisegmentectomy: IV, V, VI, VII, VIII and I (Fig. 19-92)
• Several other combinations

The basic plan of blood vessels within the liver is subject to many variations. Thus, preoperative aortic, celiac, or selective hepatic arteriography must be performed and the films studied carefully before attempting any surgical procedure. The main arterial trunk to the medial segment arises from the right hepatic artery and passes to the left across the midline in about 25 percent of individuals. Precede ligation of any arterial branch with manual occlusion and observation of the limits of color change in the tissue.

Because interlobar and intersegmental spaces are occupied by the hepatic veins (Fig. 19-93), it is necessary to transect the liver in a paralobular or parasegmental plane. Liver transection patterns are as follows.
• Right of the middle vein for a right lobectomy
• Right of the left vein for trisegmentectomy
• Left of the right vein for a left lobectomy
• Left of the middle vein for a lateral segmentectomy

This is especially important in the true interlobar (umbilical) fissure, where vessels and bile ducts may lie in the fissure and return to the medial lobe more distally.

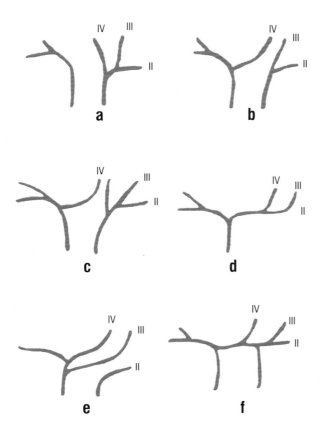

FIG. 19-82. Left hepatic artery derived from the left gastric artery. **a**, Supplying the whole left liver = solitary artery (5 out of 93 cases). **b**, Supplying the left lobe = type (II+III) and IV duplication (16 out of 93 cases). **c**, Supplying the left lobe and part of segment IV (1 out of 93 cases). **d, e**, Only supplying segment II = type (III+IV) and II duplication (7 out of 93 cases). **f**, Anastomosed with the normal middle hepatic artery (2 out of 93 cases). (From Couinaud C. Anatomie intra-hépatique: application â la transplantation du foie. Ann Radiol 37(5): 323-333, 1994; with permission.)

## Right Lobectomy

For a right lobectomy or for a trisegmental lobectomy[208,209] ("extended" right lobectomy[210,211]), use a right subcostal incision. It may be continued upward into the thorax or paraxiphoid or to the left, if necessary.

Incise the right triangular and coronary ligaments so that the right lobe may be retracted. Divide all ligamentous attachments of the liver to allow complete mobilization and visualization of all hepatic structures. In a "true" right or left lobectomy, the gallbladder must be sacrificed.

Dissection begins at the hilum. Ligate branches of the hepatic artery, portal vein, and bile duct of the lobe to be removed, and preserve the interlobar hepatic veins. Use blunt dissection throughout.

The line of the interlobar fissure (line of Rex, median fissure) extends from the gallbladder fossa below to the infe-

rior vena cava above. The dissection must pass to the right of the middle hepatic vein to preserve drainage of segment IV (Fig. 19-89). Ligate the right hepatic vein extrahepatically before transection of the liver.[129]

## Left Lobectomy

If the left lobe is to be resected, ligate the left hepatic artery, portal vein, and bile duct. Sectioning of the triangular ligament permits mobilization of the left lobe. Transection should follow a line from the left side of the fossa of the gallbladder to the left side of the fossa of the inferior vena cava (Fig. 19-94). Expose and ligate the left and middle hepatic veins within the liver or extrahepatically at the vena cava after ultrasonic confirmation of the precise anatomy.

In most cases, the left and middle hepatic veins form a common trunk before emerging from the liver.[194,212] It may be best to ligate the hepatic veins at the end of the dissection to be sure of ligating only the veins from the resected segments.[213] A left resection may be lobar, segmental, or even wedge-shaped for a superficially located

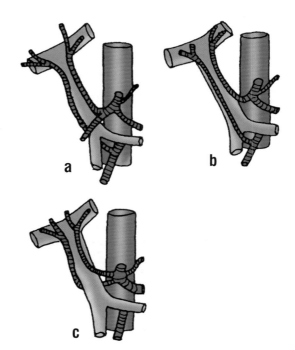

FIG. 19-83. Right hepatic artery arising from the superior mesenteric artery or celiac trunk. **a**, Right hepatic artery according to the classical definition. **b**, A right hepatic artery arising from the superior mesenteric artery may ascend anterior to the portal trunk. **c**, A right hepatic artery arising from the celiac trunk may cross over behind the portal trunk (according to Michels, this is always the case when the celiac trunk gives two branches to the liver). (Modified from Couinaud C. Anatomie intra-hépatique application â la transplantation du foie. Ann Radiol 37(5):323-333, 1994; with permission.)

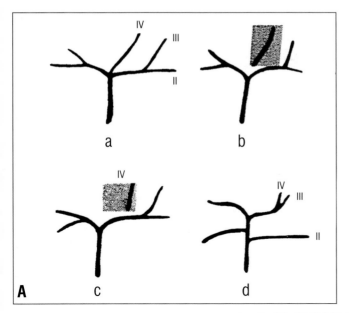

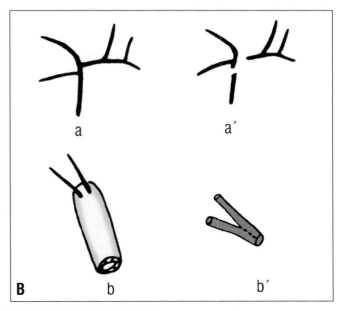

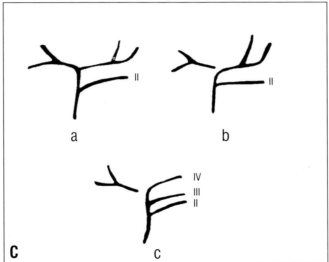

FIG. 19-84. The surgeon's 3 assets. **A)** The surgeon's first asset: resection of segment IV. In the case of a type (II+III) and IV duplication of a left element (a), resection of segment IV results in a left lobe with a single pedicle (b). This resection may also be performed exclusively to reduce the volume of an excessively large left liver for a child (c). In a type (III+IV) and II duplication, resection of segment IV does not allow a single pedicle to be obtained for the left lobe, but IV is possible (d). **B)** The second asset: the common hepatic duct. (a and a´) A segment of common hepatic duct is retained on the side of the duplication. On the right side, a double anastomosis onto a jejunal loop or, when possible, a side-to-side biliary anastomosis may be preferred (b and b´). **C)** The third asset: common hepatic artery. The common hepatic artery is retained on the side of an arterial duplication (b) or triplication (c). (Modified from Couinaud C. Anatomie intra-hépatique: application â la transplantation du foie. Ann Radiol 37(5):323-333, 1994; with permission.)

tumor. Povoski et al.[214] found extended left hepatectomy "a viable resectional technique for large, strategically placed left-sided and central hepatic lesions that extend rightward to involve the right anterior sectorial portal pedicular structures."

### Left Lateral Segmentectomy

A left lateral segmentectomy (Fig. 19-91) consists of the removal of segments II and III. These segments are lateral to the falciform ligament. Segment IV remains in situ.

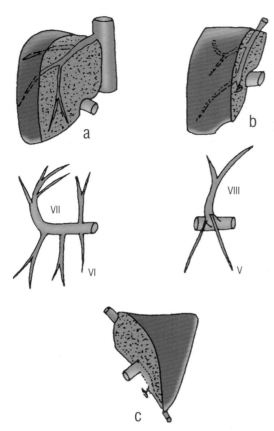

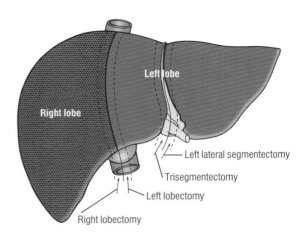

**FIG. 19-86.** Planes of transection of the liver for lobectomy and segmentectomy. Trisegmentectomy includes anterior and posterior segments of the right lobe and the medial segment of the left lobe. (Modified from Skandalakis JE, Gray SW, Rowe JS Jr. Anatomical Complications in General Surgery. New York: McGraw-Hill, 1983; with permission.)

**FIG. 19-85.** Tripartition of the liver. **a,** Right lateral sector with lateral pedicle in its sheath and the inferior vena cava. The right hepatic vein is in the right portal fissure. *Below diagram "a":* right lateral pedicle. **b,** Right paramedian sector with the right portal pedicle in its sheath and the middle hepatic vein. The middle hepatic vein is in the principal portal fissure. *Below diagram "b":* diagram showing procurement of the right portal pedicle. **c,** Left lobe with left portal pedicle and left hepatic vein. (Modified from Couinaud C. Anatomie intra-hépatique: application à la transplantation du foie. Ann Radiol 37(5):323-333, 1994; with permission.)

## Liver Resection and Trauma

The treatment of traumatic liver injury has seen rapid evolution since the early 1980s. In 1989 the American Association for the Surgery of Trauma (AAST) developed the liver injuries scale now in use[216] (Table 19-12). Seventy to ninety percent of liver injuries are grade I or II and may be managed nonoperatively. The utility of CT scanning in liver trauma cannot be overstated. Patients with subcapsular or intrahepatic hematomas who previously might have undergone exploration can now be safely managed with close observation and serial CT scans.

## Trisegmentectomy

A right "extended" lobectomy (trisegmentectomy) (Fig. 19-92) is similar, but the liver is transected just to the right of the falciform ligament. The middle hepatic vein must be ligated, since the medial segment is to be removed. Take extreme care to preserve the left hepatic vein, as the middle vein typically joins it prior to its junction with the vena cava.

## Mesohepatectomy

Wu et al.[215] reported that even though mesohepatectomy (removal of segments IV, V, and VIII) is time-consuming, its advantages justify its use for selected patients with centrally located large hepatocellular carcinoma.

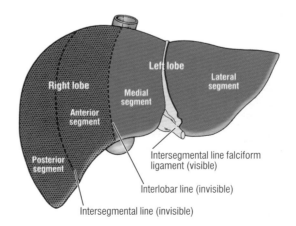

**FIG. 19-87.** The true lobulation and segmentation of the liver: diaphragmatic surface. (Modified from Skandalakis JE, Gray SW, Rowe JS Jr. Anatomical Complications in General Surgery. New York: McGraw-Hill, 1983; with permission.)

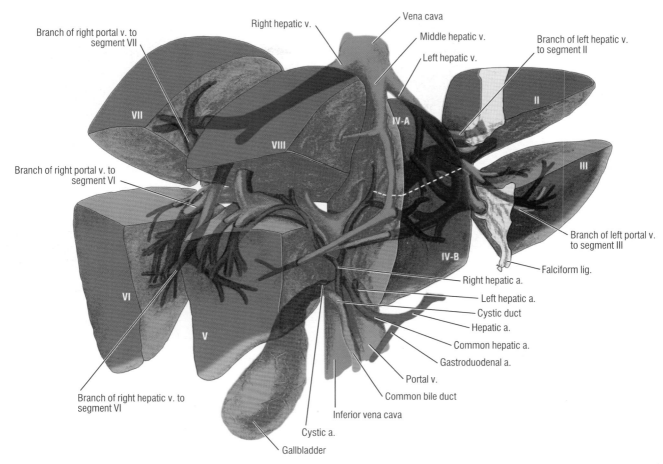

**Fig. 19-88.** Subsegmentation of the liver. Segment I is not shown. (Modified from Meyers WC. Segmental hepatic resection. In: Sabiston DC Jr. Atlas of General Surgery. Philadelphia: WB Saunders, 1994, p. 535; with permission.)

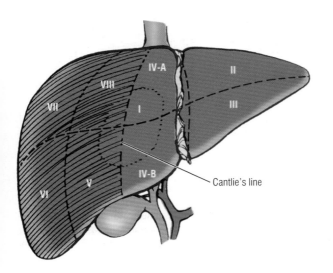

**Fig. 19-89.** Right hepatic lobectomy: shaded segments are removed. (Modified from Meyers WC. Segmental hepatic resection. In: Sabiston DC Jr. Atlas of General Surgery. Philadelphia: WB Saunders, 1994, p. 536; with permission.)

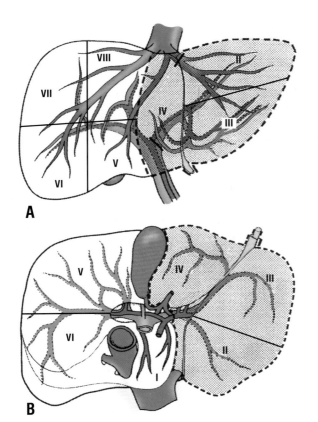

**A**

**B**

**FIG. 19-90.** Left hepatectomy (left lobectomy): shaded segments are removed. **A.** Anterior view. **B.** Inferior view. (Modified from Bismuth H, Garden OJ. Regular and extended right and left hepatectomy for cancer. In: Nyhus LM, Baker RJ, eds. Mastery of Surgery, 2nd Ed. Boston: Little, Brown, 1992; with permission.)

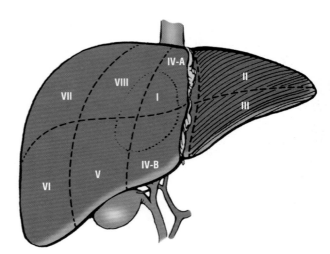

**FIG. 19-91.** Left lateral segmentectomy: shaded segments are removed. (Modified from Meyers WC. Segmental hepatic resection. In: Sabiston DC Jr. Atlas of General Surgery. Philadelphia: WB Saunders, 1994, p. 536; with permission.)

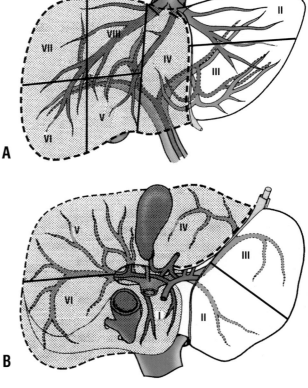

**A**

**B**

**FIG. 19-92.** Extended right hepatectomy: shaded segments are removed. **A.** Anterior view. **B.** Inferior view. (Modified from Bismuth H, Garden OJ. Regular and extended right and left hepatectomy for cancer. In: Nyhus LM, Baker RJ, eds. Mastery of Surgery, 2nd Ed. Boston: Little, Brown, 1992; with permission.)

Fang et al.[217] reported that the presence of pooling contrast material within the hepatic parenchyma on computed tomography indicates active bleeding. Angiography should help in the decision whether to perform emergency exploratory laparotomy.

Pursuant to progress in prehospital care, patients often arrive *in extremis* but alive with enormous hepatic injuries. This has led to a resurgence in the use of perihepatic packing for the early management of complex liver injuries.[218-220] Packing and reexploration work best when:

- Used early in an operation
- The patient is cold, coagulopathic, and needs further resuscitation prior to undertaking a complex hepatic repair, or
- A specific injury has been identified that will require complex repair but the patient is coagulopathic

Hepatic resection is safe when performed electively. Formal hepatic resection for trauma, however, carries a high mortality rate. Cogbill and associates reported a rate

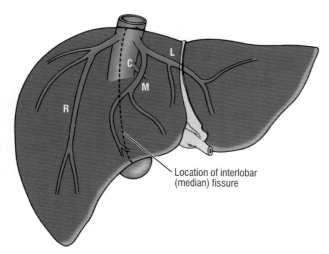

**FIG. 19-93.** Diagram of the intrahepatic distribution of the hepatic veins. Note that they are interlobular rather than lobular. C = caudate, L = left, M = medial, R = right. (Modified from Skandalakis JE, Gray SW, Rowe JS Jr. Anatomical Complications in General Surgery. New York: McGraw-Hill, 1983; with permission.)

of formal hepatic resection of 0.89 percent with a mortality rate of 58 percent,[221] though other authors have reported lower mortality rates.[222,223] In the Hollins and Littell series of 281 patients, 42 (14 percent) underwent hepatic resection and 83 percent of those underwent resectional debridement.[224] The mortality for the entire group was 21 percent.

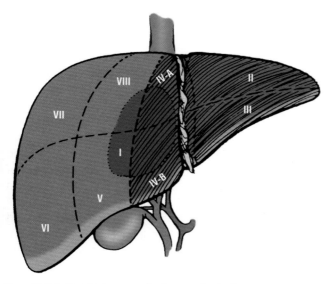

**FIG. 19-94.** Right trisegmentectomy: shaded segments are removed. (From Meyers WC. Segmental hepatic resection. In: Sabiston DC Jr. Atlas of General Surgery. Philadelphia: WB Saunders, 1994, p. 536; with permission.)

Extensive experience by American trauma surgeons indicates that formal hepatic resection for trauma is rare. Resectional debridement is more common and is often required to approach the site of a specific injury. The finger fracture technique is useful in this approach. Portal occlusion is safe in otherwise healthy trauma patients for up to an hour. Madding and Kennedy[112] proposed only the following two reasons for formal lobectomy in trauma. The reasons are:

- Blunt or penetrating injuries resulting in extensive devitalization of a major portion of the right lobe
- Damage to the hepatic veins or vena cava requiring right lobectomy for visualization and repair

Pachter et al.[225] would modify these to the following cases:

- Total destruction of normal hepatic parenchyma
- Injury extensive enough to preclude perihepatic packing
- Resection was performed by the injury itself and can be quickly completed using several additional clamps
- Hepatic resection is the only method of controlling exsanguinating hemorrhage.

**TABLE 19-12. Liver Injury Scale (1994 Revision)**

| Grade[a] | | Injury Description |
|---|---|---|
| I | Hematoma | Subcapsular, <10% surface area |
| | Laceration | Capsular tear, <1 cm parenchymal depth |
| II | Hematoma | Subcapsular, 10-50% surface area; intraparenchymal, <10 cm in diameter |
| | Laceration | 1-3 cm parenchymal depth, <10 cm in length |
| III | Hematoma | Subcapsular, >50% surface area or expanding; ruptured subcapsular of parenchymal hematoma |
| | | Intraparenchymal hematoma >10 cm or expanding |
| | Laceration | >3 cm parenchymal depth |
| IV | Laceration | Parenchymal disruption involving 25-75% of hepatic lobe or 1-3 Couinaud's segments within a single lobe |
| V | Laceration | Parenchymal disruption involving >75% of hepatic lobe or >3 Couinaud's segments within a single lobe |
| | Vascular | Juxtahepatic venous injuries; i.e., retrohepatic vena cava/central major hepatic veins |
| VI | Vascular | Hepatic avulsion |

[a]Advance one grade for multiple injuries, up to grade III.

*Source:* Moore EE, Cogbill TH, Jurkovich GJ, Shackford SR, Malangoni MA, Champion HR. Organ injury scaling: spleen and liver (1994 revision). J Trauma 1995;38:323-324; with permission.

During the past decade numerous specialized techniques in the management of hepatic trauma have been developed. These are beautifully reviewed by Pachter and colleagues.[225]

### Liver Resection for Cancer

Liver resection is the best therapy available for primary or metastatic lesions in the liver, and the only therapy with a chance for cure. The five-year survival rates for resection of liver-colorectal metastases are 25 to 39 percent with a current mortality rate from the operation of less than 5 percent.[226-228] Five-year survival rates in resection for hepatoma range from 12 percent to 39 percent. The operative mortality rate is slightly higher because of the incidence of cirrhosis in patients with hepatoma.[229] Mortality risk rises when factors such as progressive cholangitis, elevated serum creatine, elevated serum bilirubin, high operative blood loss and vena cava resection are found in combination.[230] Palliative resection offers no benefit if curative resection cannot be performed.

The size ratio of future liver remnant to preoperative liver volume may relate to biochemical and clinical outcome parameters. In an excellent paper, Vauthey and colleagues[231] found the correlation to be a useful method to evaluate response to portal vein embolization and a predictor of outcomes prior to extended liver resection.

Newer techniques, most significantly intraoperative ultrasonography, are critical for the safe performance of hepatic resection. Moreover, nonresectional techniques such as cryoablative therapy and microwave coagulation are under study and may offer significant advances in tumor ablation.

Bakalakos et al.[232] reported that patients with unilobar metastatic disease and certain patients with bilobar hepatic metastasis can achieve longterm survival after undergoing surgical resection with tumor-free margins.

Another study by Bakalakos et al.[233] found that patients with liver metastasis from colorectal cancer whose preoperative carcino-embryonic antigen level was 30 ng/mL are more likely to be resectable and have the longest survival. Wigmore et al.[234] found no evidence to support a differential pattern of hepatic metastasis related to the location of the primary colorectal cancer.

D'Angelica et al.[235] stated that patients with metastatic colorectal cancer who are disease-free 5 years after hepatic resection are likely to have been cured. These authors encouraged aggressive followup, including further surgery if recurrence takes place, because chances for longterm survival are good. The perspective of Bismuth and Majno[236] must be added: "Today the limitation to survival in primary and metastatic liver cancer lies not in the surgical technique but in the difficulty of dealing with microscopic and extrahepatic disease."

Weimann et al.[237] reported that nuclear medicine helps differentiate hepatic hemangioma and focal nodular hyperplasia from adenoma, which assists the surgeon in determining the appropriateness of surgery.

Based on studies of adult rats, Smail et al.[238] concluded that the organs responsible for increasing the levels of nitric oxide after trauma and hemorrhagic shock might be the liver and small intestine. They advised use of specific inhibitors for reduction of nitric acid.

To avoid the occurrence of postoperative liver failure, Miyazaki et al.[239] advised limited resection of segments I and IV for hepatic hilar cholangiocarcinoma.

Roayaie et al.[240] advised aggressive surgical approach with tumorfree margins in patients with intrahepatic cholangiocarcinoma.

Iwatsuki et al.[241] stated that both hepatic resection and liver transplantation offer satisfactory longterm survival for hilar cholangiocarcinoma.

Scientific techniques are helping us in the operating room. Delbeke et al.[242] reported the possibility of differentiation and evaluation of benign and malignant tumors of the liver by doing positron emission tomography using [$^{18}$F] fluorodeoxyglucose. However, limitations of this evaluation include false-positive results in a minority of hepatic abscesses and false-negative results in a minority of hepatocellular carcinoma.

Hepatocellular carcinoma (HCC) is the most common solid organ tumor worldwide, responsible for more than 1 million deaths annually.[243]

We quote Bilimoria et al.[244]:

> *Death caused by HCC is rare beyond 5 years after resection of HCC in the absence of fibrosis or cirrhosis. The data suggest that chronic liver disease acts as a field of cancerization contributing to new HCC. These patients may benefit from therapies directed at the underlying liver disease.*

However, Nakajima et al.[245] state that repeat resection for recurrent HCC has a low disease-free survival rate.

Billingsley et al.[246] recommended segmental hepatic resection for patients with metastatic neoplasms and hepatocellular carcinoma. A commentary by Meyers and Chari[247] in the same issue about this description of the progress in hepatic resection by Billingsley et al. stated that they make it sound so clear and simple that it may encourage inexperienced surgeons to attempt it. Meyers and Chari remind surgeons that hepatic resection must be done by experienced hands.

Yamamoto et al.[248] isolate and remove the caudate lobe of the liver by an anterior transhepatic approach by separating the hepatic parenchyma along the interlobar plane and anatomic identification of the right margin of the caudate lobe.

We quote from Azoulay et al.[249]:

*The anterior approach is useful for massive liver resection. It minimizes the risk of tumor rupture with spillage into the peritoneal cavity and hemorrhage from freeing vascularized adhesions or damaging the right hepatic vein or the retrohepatic vena cava. It also avoids the need for rotation of the huge right liver toward the remnant liver, preventing warm ischemia of the latter use of congestion or pedicle torsion.*

Yamamoto et al.[250] treated a huge liver tumor involving all of the hepatic venous confluence and the inferior vena cava by in situ pedicle resection in a left trisegmentectomy of the liver with right hepatic vein reconstruction.

Midorikawa et al.[251] stated that hepatectomy for the impaired liver is now as safe a procedure as for the normal liver, provided their overall guidelines are followed.

Twelfth rib resection as a posterior direct approach was used by Bosscha et al.[252] to treat subphrenic abscesses in cases of failure of percutaneous drainage, abandonment of percutaneous drainage in view of a too high risk of perforation of adjacent organs, or contamination of the pleural space, or an inaccessible abdomen.

Guidelines for minimally invasive hepatic surgery for malignant processes were proposed by Katkhouda and Mavor[253]:

*Open surgery is the treatment of choice when primary tumors are malignant, located posteriorly, or in proximity to major hepatic vasculature. Laparoscopic resection of liver metastases with a safety margin of 1 cm, when the total number is less than four, is not unreasonable and can be offered to patients without evidence of extrahepatic disease.*

Minimally invasive adjuvant therapies for the treatment of primary and secondary malignant hepatic tumors may have clinical results which exceed conventional chemotherapy or radiation therapy. Radio-frequency ablation, microwave ablation, laser ablation, cryoablation, ethanol ablation, and chemoembolization are acceptable for nonsurgical patients and may one day challenge surgical resection as the treatment of choice for patients with limited hepatic tumors.[254]

## *Operative Management of Portal Hypertension*

Numerous options are available for managing acute or refractory bleeding from esophageal varices. Factors including underlying liver disease, comorbid conditions, and the experience and expertise of the local physicians and surgeons determine the most appropriate therapies. Medical therapies include β-blockers for prophylaxis and vasopressin or somatostatin infusion for acute bleeding. Endoscopic sclerotherapy or variceal banding can be used for either acute bleeding or to prevent rebleeding. Liver transplantation is the most radical and definitive therapy in appropriate candidates.

### Distal Splenorenal Shunt

Surgical treatment of patients with bleeding varices or varices at risk to rebleed has changed in the past three decades. The side-to-side or end-to-side portacaval shunt was the primary option for portal decompression until the 1970s. Dean Warren and his colleagues[255-257] then developed the distal splenorenal shunt (DSRS). This procedure selectively decompresses the esophageal and gastric varices while maintaining antegrade portal perfusion. This procedure has undergone numerous refinements and long term evaluation. The re-bleeding rate at three years to five years following DSRS is approximately six percent. The operative mortality in series from the past five years ranges from zero percent to 15 percent. Encephalopathy, extremely common after portacaval shunt, occurs in only 15 percent of patients and is typically easily controlled with restriction of protein intake and lactulose administration.

### Small-Bore Portacaval H-Graft

The small-bore portacaval H-graft is formed using a reinforced 8-mm polytetrafluoroethylene (PTFE) graft between the portal vein and vena cava.[258] It decompresses the portal vein less completely, but it decreases portal pressure and maintains antegrade flow to the liver. This procedure is technically easier than DSRS, although the rate of flow reversal in the portal vein is higher and perioperative complications are similar.

### Transjugular Intrahepatic Portasystemic Shunt

Transjugular intrahepatic portasystemic shunt (TIPS)[259] is the newest method of treating portal hypertension by shunting portal blood to the systemic circulation. Using the jugular vein, a wire passes from the hepatic vein into a portal vein branch that is then dilated and stented with an expandable metal stent. This procedure forms a functional side-to-side portacaval shunt that decompresses the portal vein and, therefore, the esophageal and gastric varices. TIPS shows a success rate of at least 90 percent in reducing the portal vein-to-hepatic vein gradient to less than 12 mm Hg. The early re-bleeding rate is roughly equivalent to that of DSRS and significantly lower than sclerotherapy. Follow-up periods of 18 months to 24 months, however, show high rates (40 percent to 70 percent) of shunt stenosis or thrombosis.[260]

A randomized clinical trial is needed to determine the exact role of TIPS in the armamentarium of portal decompression techniques. At present the procedure is not recommended for definitive portal decompression in patients with Child A cirrhosis and good hepatic function[256] (Table 19-13). The technique is currently best suited for patients with Child C cirrhosis who are waiting for liver transplantation or who bleed from the varices but are at high risk for a surgical procedure. Patients with Child B cirrhosis occupy an intermediate category and the best longterm treatment for these patients remains unknown.

### Hepatic Injuries

Demetriades et al.[261] stated that selected patients with isolated grades I and II gunshot injuries to the liver can be managed nonoperatively.

Moore[262] wrote that the previously cited study by Demetriades et al. adds useful data to support selective nonoperative management of gunshot wounds to the liver. He contends, however, that candidates for observation are infrequent and that surgeons using this approach must be aware of the risks and have the resources to address potential complications.

## ANATOMIC COMPLICATIONS

## Complications of Some Diagnostic Procedures

### Open (Wedge) Biopsy

A wedge biopsy can be obtained through a mini-laparotomy or during another surgical procedure. Bleeding is the only complication, and it is easily controlled.

### Percutaneous (Needle) Biopsy

The colon is the organ most frequently perforated during percutaneous biopsy. In such a procedure, pancreatic and renal tissue occasionally appear. Pneumothorax is said to occur once in about 800 biopsies.[263] A summary of the possible complications is presented in Table 19-14.

Hemorrhage and peritonitis are the most frequent complications of needle biopsy, with intrahepatic hematoma and perforation of organs in addition to the colon also possible.

Millward-Sadler and Whorwell[264] have reported mortality rates in several large series beginning in the 1950s. In 1992, they estimated rates to be approximately 0.01 percent (one death per 10,000 biopsies), whereas some years earlier they had found the rate to be 0.1 percent (one death per 1,000 biopsies). In 1994, Schwartz[265] concluded that the overall mortality rate was 0.8 percent, with pain, pneumothorax, hemorrhage, and bile peritonitis the most common complications. Among uncommon complications is needle fracture during biopsy.[266,267]

## Anatomic Complications of Liver Surgery

### Vascular Injury

#### Hepatic Vein

When a hepatic vein occludes, it might be anticipated that the tissue drained by it would demand resection. Mays[113] stated that this is unnecessary in humans because of the anastomoses between the left and right hepatic veins. He cited two reports of hepatic vein ligation when most of the affected liver survived. In one patient, the left hepatic vein was ligated;[268] in the other, the middle and left hepatic veins were ligated.[196] Segmental hepatic vein ligation without hepatic resection avoids the tedious construction of a vena caval shunt, a procedure usually requir-

| TABLE 19-13. Child's Classification of Hepatic Reserve | | | |
|---|---|---|---|
| Criteria | Good A | Moderate B | Poor C |
| Serum bilirubin (mg%) | <2.0 | 2.0-3.0 | >3.0 |
| Serum albumin (g%) | >3.5 | 3.0-3.5 | <3.0 |
| Ascites | None | Easily controlled | Poorly controlled |
| Encephalopathy | None | Minimal | Advanced, "coma" |
| Nutrition | Excellent | Good | Poor, muscle wasting |

*Source:* Richardson JD, Gardner B. Gastrointestinal bleeding. In: Polk HC Jr, Gardner B, Stone HH. Basic Surgery, 4th Ed. St. Louis: Quality Medical Publishing, 1993; with permission.

## TABLE 19-14. Complications of Percutaneous (Needle) Biopsy

| Organ Injury | Result |
| --- | --- |
| Colon | Peritonitis[1] |
| Right kindey | Peritonitis[1] |
| Pancreas | Pancreatitis |
| Diaphragm | Pain |
| Lung or pleura | Pneumothorax[6], hemothorax |
| Gallbladder or bile ducts | Bile peritonitis[3], hemobilia |
| Hematoma between chest wall and liver | Hemorrhage |
| Intercostal artery or veins | Hemorrhage[4] |
| **Intrahepatic Injury** | |
| Hepatic artery, vein or portal vein | Hemorrhage, hematoma[2] |
| Bile ducts | Bile peritonitis |
| **General Complications** | |
| | Infections of needle track |
| | Needle fracture |
| | Pain[5] |
| | Shock |

1. Injury to abdominal viscera is rare (Terry, 1952).
2. Three cases of intrahepatic hematoma have been described by Rainer (1974).
3. Six cases have been reported by Madden (1961).
4. Hemorrhage is the most frequent complication and the major cause of death following needle biopsy.
5. Pain is more frequently associated with the use of the Vim-Silverman needle (20 percent) than with the Menghini needle (3.2 percent), though the specimen is smaller with the latter instrument (Schwartz, 1964).
6. One case in 2000 biopsies (Brown, 1961).

### References

Brown CH. Needle biopsy of the liver. Am J Diag Dis 6:269, 1961.
Madden RE. Complications of needle biopsy of the liver. Arch Surg 83:778, 1961.
Rainer DR, van Heertum RL, Johnson LF. Intrahepatic hematoma: A complication of percutaneous liver biopsy. Gastroenterology 67:284, 1974.
Schwartz SI. Surgical Diseases of the Liver. New York: McGraw-Hill, 1964.
Terry RB. Risks of needle biopsy of the liver. Br Med J 1:1102, 1952.

ing the facilities of a large medical center and a skilled surgeon. In experienced hands, intraoperative ultrasonography and detailed anatomic knowledge can prevent the vast majority of hepatic venous occlusions.

## Portal Vein

The umbilical portion of the portal vein lies within the umbilical fissure. In a left lateral segmental resection, incise the liver 1 cm to the left of the fissure.

Ligation of the left or right portal vein following injury to the liver has been successful in some patients,[269-272] but the mortality rate from portal vein injuries is still about 50 per-

cent.[273] Stone[274] reported 15 survivors among 20 patients undergoing emergency portal vein ligations.

Pachter and associates[275] feel that portal vein ligation, even with its risk of portal hypertension and intestinal infarction, may be safer than immediate shunting procedures, which risk encephalopathy. "Severe hepatic trauma limited to one lobe of the liver is the main indication for ligating both the portal vein and hepatic artery supplying the injured lobe. The artery should be ligated first. If this fails to stop hemorrhage, then the branch of the portal vein to that lobe should be ligated."[113] Resectional debridement may then be necessary to remove devitalized tissue.

## Hepatic Artery

If possible, repair inadvertent ligation of a lobar hepatic artery. With good supportive care, the patient usually survives even if blood flow cannot be restored. Kim and colleagues[276] found 50 deaths among 322 hepatic artery occlusions. Twenty-seven deaths were from accidental ligation during major operations. Ligation was the direct cause of death in only 12 cases. Using these figures, the mortality could be said to be less than 4 percent.

The degree of hepatic ischemia depends on the location of the hepatic artery ligation. Ligation proximal to the gastroduodenal artery or even proximal to the origin of the right gastric artery will probably not result in liver ischemia. In some individuals, if the ligation is distal to the right gastric artery, an aberrant hepatic artery may provide the sole supply of oxygenated blood to the liver. Ligation of the left hepatic artery seems to carry a higher mortality rate than does ligation of the right artery. No valid reason is known.

The surgeon performing a formal lobectomy must remember that in as many as 25 percent of individuals, the left medial segmental artery (segment IV) arises from the right hepatic artery.[110] Sectioning of the right hepatic artery for a right lobectomy could result in arterial ischemia of the left medial segment.

## Summary of Ligation of Hepatic Vessels

### HEPATIC VEINS

- Lobar or segmental hepatic vein ligation is feasible.
- Hepatic resection following ligation of a hepatic vein is not always necessary.

### PORTAL VEIN

- Portal veins may be ligated without fatality. The hepatic sinusoids of the adjacent lobules provide intersegmental communication. There are few true anastomoses between venous branches.
- Reduction in portal blood flow increases hepatic artery

blood flow. The reverse is not true.
- Atrophy follows portal vein ligation.
- Ligation of both lobar hepatic artery and portal vein results in atrophy without necrosis.
- Following a radical pancreaticoduodenal resection, the portal vein should not be ligated. Portal blood flow must be restored by a shunt or a replacement graft.

### HEPATIC ARTERY

- Hepatic arteries are not end arteries in vivo. Ligation of a right or left hepatic artery results in translobar and subcapsular collateral circulation within 24 hours.
- After proximal ligation of the common hepatic artery, the right gastric and gastroduodenal arteries will maintain hepatic blood flow.
- Hepatic artery ligation is well-tolerated. Death following such ligation is not usually the result of the artery ligation.
- Cholecystectomy must always accompany hepatic artery ligation.

## Organ Injury

### Bile Ducts

Accidental section of a segmental bile duct requires immediate repair, proximal and distal ligation of the severed duct, or resection of the segment. Ligation of a segmental bile duct produces jaundice, hypocholic stools and urine, and enlargement of the lobe of the liver on the side of the obstruction.[277] Braasch and colleagues[278] reported atrophy of the obstructed segment. Possibly initial hypertrophy is followed later by atrophy. It is curious that unilateral lobar obstruction produces jaundice, while unilateral lobectomy does not. One would expect the unaffected lobe to prevent the occurrence of jaundice.

Lo et al.[279] recommended the following for avoiding biliary complications after hepatic resection: 1) Preresection cholangiography for left-sided hepatectomy, and 2) early surgical intervention for leakage of the common bile duct. Tables 19-15 and 19-16 demonstrate the incidence and sites of complications.

### Other Organs

Most of the organs of the upper abdomen are close enough to the liver that resection of that organ provides many opportunities for inadvertent injury.

## Complications of DSRS, Portacaval H-graft, and TIPS

### Vascular Injury

- The splenic vein has many branches draining the pan-

creas. Failure to carefully ligate these leads to significant bleeding. The splenic vein may be torn during this dissection, preventing its use.
- Angulation, distortion, and tension are the chief dangers in forming the splenorenal or H-graft anastomoses.
- Multiple vascular complications may occur during or following TIPS procedures. These include perforation or tearing of the portal vein or vena cava, formation of a portobiliary fistula with resultant hemobilia, or stent migration into the superior mesenteric vein with eventual thrombosis.
- During exposure of the portal vein for portacaval H-graft, anomalous or variant hepatic arteries or collateral veins may be ligated. This can lead to segmental ischemia that might be well-tolerated in noncirrhotic patients, but dangerous or fatal in a patient with marginal hepatic reserve.
- During DSRS, failure to adequately ligate retroperitoneal lymphatics when exposing the renal vein may cause chylous ascites. This may require drainage and may become infected.

### Organ Injury

Segmental liver ischemia may follow accidental injury to an aberrant hepatic artery.

---

**TABLE 19-15. Types of Hepatic Resection and Incidence of Biliary Complications**

| Operation | No. of Patients (No. of Concomitant Caudate Resections) | | Biliary Complication, No. of Patients (%) | |
|---|---|---|---|---|
| Major* | | | | |
| Right hemihepatectomy | 118 | (9) | 11 | (9.3) |
| Right extended hepatectomy | 32 | (2) | 1 | (3.1) |
| Right trisegmentectomy | 30 | (7) | 2 | (6.7) |
| Left hemihepatectomy | 32 | (4) | 6 | (18.8) |
| Left extended hepatectomy | 14 | (2) | 3 | (21.4) |
| Left trisegmentectomy | 3 | (0) | 2 | (66.7) |
| Minor† | | | | |
| Left lateral segmentectomy | 61 | (0) | 2 | (3) |
| Segmentectomy | 25 | (0) | 0 | (0) |
| Subsegmentectomy | 32 | (0) | 1 | (3.1) |

*Includes 229 patients.
†Includes 118 patients

*Source:* Lo C-M, Fan S-T, Liu C-L, Lai ECS, Wong J. Biliary complications after hepatic resection: risk factors, management, and outcome. Arch Surg 133:156-161, 1998; with permission.

**TABLE 19-16. Site of Biliary Leakage According to Different Types of Hepatic Resection**

| Site | Type of Resection, No. of Patients | | |
|------|-------------|------------|-------|
| | Right-sided* | Left-sided* | Minor |
| Hepatic duct stump | 4 | 2 | 0 |
| Bilioenteric anastomosis | 1 | 3 | 0 |
| Common hepatic duct | 1 | 2 | 0 |
| Raw surface of liver | 1 | 1 | 0 |
| T-tube insertion | 1 | 0 | 0 |
| Unknown | 6 | 3 | 3 |
| **Total** | **14** | **11** | **3** |

*Includes hemihepatectomy, extended hepatectomy, and trisegment-ectomy.

*Source:* Lo C-M, Fan S-T, Liu C-L, Lai ECS, Wong J. Biliary complications after hepatic resection: risk factors, management, and outcome. Arch Surg 133:156-161, 1998; with permission.

# SURGICAL ANATOMY OF LIVER TRANSPLANTATION

The following description of preparation of the donor liver is anatomic rather than technical, and does not include the physiologic basis of the procedure. The description of donor total hepatectomy is based on the papers of Starzl and colleagues,[280] Shaw and colleagues,[281] Gordon and colleagues,[282] Quinones-Baldrich and colleagues,[283] and Ekberg and associates.[284]

## *Freeing and Preparing the Donor Liver*

The following steps free the donor liver and prepare it for placement in the recipient (Fig. 19-95).

1. Make a long midline incision from the suprasternal notch to the symphysis pubis to provide maximum exposure.
2. Inspect the liver for good color and texture.
3. Look for anomalies of the extrahepatic blood vessels. Specifically, look for aberrant accessory or replacing hepatic arteries arising from the left gastric or the superior mesenteric artery. (See below for procedure in the presence of an aberrant right hepatic artery).
4. Dissect the celiac axis very close to the aorta if possible, with ligation and division of the left gastric and splenic arteries.
5. Ligate and divide the gastroduodenal and right gastric arteries.
6. Open the gallbladder and wash out the extrahepatic biliary tree. Remove the gallbladder, then mobilize and transect the common bile duct.
7. Locate the portal vein under the gastroduodenal artery. Isolate and clean the vein as far as the junction of the splenic and superior mesenteric veins.
8. Cannulate and ligate the splenic vein close to the spleen.
9. Locate and encircle the superior mesenteric vein. Divide the neck of the pancreas if necessary.
10. Ligate the inferior mesenteric artery.
11. Divide, cannulate, and ligate the aorta above the bifurcation.
12. Divide, cannulate, and ligate the inferior vena cava above the junction of the iliac veins.
13. Wash out the organs with cold preservation solution.
14. Ligate the lumbar vessels.
15. Ligate the superior mesenteric artery and vein.
16. Clamp the aorta as for a graft nephrectomy.
17. Detach the celiac axis from the aorta with an aortic patch or full aortic circumference (Fig. 19-96).
18. Dissect the suprahepatic vena cava free with a cuff of the caval hiatus of the diaphragm.
19. Cut the posterior attachments of the liver.
20. Ligate the right adrenal veins.
21. Remove the liver and ligate tributaries of the inferior vena cava.

The operator must remember that the arterial supply is "abnormal" in almost half of patients encountered. The dictum must be accepted, whether right or wrong, that all hepatic arteries are end arteries and that accessory as well as replacing arteries must be preserved.

We can do no better than to use the words of Gordon and associates[282] who describe their method for forming a common channel when the hepatic arterial supply arises from the celiac axis and the superior mesenteric artery:

*If a left gastric branch to the left lobe can be seen and palpated in the gastrohepatic ligament lying beneath the left lobe of the liver, it can be preserved by dissecting the vessel back to its origin from the main left gastric artery which in turn is preserved to its origin from the celiac axis.*

*If a right hepatic artery arises from the superior mesenteric artery, it can be located by its pulsation posterior to the portal vein and common duct. Its origin from the superior mesenteric artery is usually found just beneath the splenic vein near its junction with the portal vein. Division of the splenic vein for insertion of a portal perfusion cannula also facilitates exposure for*

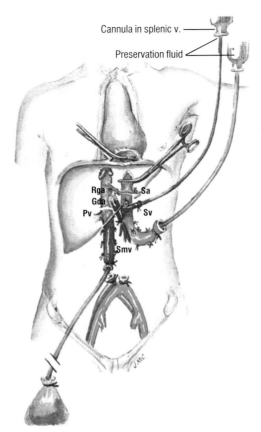

Cannula in splenic v.

Preservation fluid

Rga
Gda
Pv
Sa
Sv
Smv

FIG. 19-95. Transplantation of the liver. *In situ* perfusion method of Starzl and associates. This is suitable for removal of liver and kidneys from the same donor. Rga = right gastric artery; Gda = gastroduodenal artery; Sa, Sv = splenic artery and vein; PV = portal vein; Smv = superior mesenteric vein. (Modified from Starzl TE, Hakala TR, Shaw BW Jr, Hardesty RL, Rosenthal TJ, Griffith BP, Iwatsuki S, Bahnson HT. A flexible procedure for multiple cadaveric organ procurement. Surg Gynecol Obstet 158:223, 1984; with permission.)

*the superior mesenteric artery and the origin of a right hepatic branch. The superior mesenteric artery is dissected from its beginning at the aorta to at least one cm beyond the origin of the anomalous right hepatic artery. The origin of the celiac axis also is dissected clean at the aorta.*

*The technique of cold perfusion and preservation has been described. A patch of anterior aortic wall containing the origin of both the celiac axis and the superior mesenteric artery is removed. This preserves the entire hepatic arterial supply and is first in reconstruction of a common channel. As the patch is cut, the aortic origins of the renal arteries are noted and avoided. These are in close proximity to the origin of the superior mesenteric artery.*

## Components of Hepatic Transplantation

From a surgicoanatomic standpoint, Dodson[285] divides the surgical components of hepatic transplantation into the following three areas.
- Donor hepatectomy
- Recipient hepatectomy
- Implantation of donor liver

We advise very strongly that the student of hepatic transplantation study carefully the above-referenced excellent paper of Dodson.

Bismuth et al.[189] reported that the liver can be divided into two hemilivers for transplantation. The line of division is the main fissure. The hemilivers are the right with segments V, VI, VII, and VIII, and the left with segments II, III, and IV. Bismuth and coworkers also advised resection of the caudate lobe (segment I).

Srinivasan et al.[286] transplanted only segment III of the liver (monosegment liver transplantation) to six babies with liver failure, with an 83.3% success rate.

## Couinaud's Approach

Couinaud[287] presented a simplified method for controlled left hepatectomy. In 1994,[206] he discussed the intrahepatic anatomy in relation to transplantation. He emphasized variations in shape, arterial, and biliary variants, and the cystohepatic ducts. Couinard stated that right lobe/left lobe bipartition should never be performed. A left transplant (left liver or left lobe) should include the left hepatic vein. A right transplant should include the middle hepatic vein. Preoperative investigation should cover absence of portal bifurcation, duplication of the right portal vein, and duplication of both right and left hepatic arteries and ducts. The authors of this chapter strongly advise the study of these articles written by the father of segmental hepatic anatomy.

In 1995, Thompson et al.[288] criticized the Couinaud technique of hepatic resection as presented in his 1985 article on controlled left hepatectomy.[287] They considered this technique unsafe unless biliary anatomic variants are stringently excluded prior to right or left hepatic lobectomy.

Our comment is that embryology and anatomy must always be fellow travelers. Evaluation prior to surgery and in the operating room of every case must proceed without ANY acceptance of ANY assumption. This is essential! We owe as much to our patients and to Couinaud.

Hardy and Jones[289] found hepatic artery anomalies in 38.5 percent of prospective donor livers in their sample. However, arterial anastomosis may be carried out successfully in transplantations from these livers.

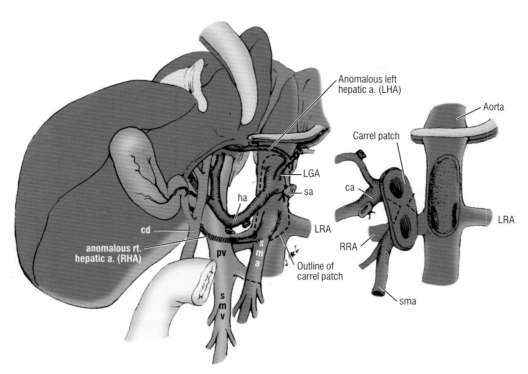

**FIG. 19-96.** Liver transplantation in the presence of an aberrant blood supply to the donor liver. Shown is a right "accessory" artery arising from the superior mesenteric artery, a left "accessory" artery arising from the left gastric artery, and a "normal" common hepatic artery arising from the celiac trunk. A patch of donor aorta containing the origin of the celiac trunk and the superior mesenteric artery is placed in the wall of the recipient aorta. The donor superior mesenteric artery distal to the aberrant hepatic artery is anastomosed to the recipient hepatic artery. LHA, RHA = left and right "accessory" hepatic arteries; cd = common bile duct; ha = common hepatic artery; LGA = left gastric artery; sma, smv = superior mesenteric artery and vein; pv = portal vein; LRA, RRA = left and right renal arteries; ca = celiac axis; sa = splenic artery. (Modified from Gordon RD, Shaw BW, Iwatsuki S, Todo S, Starzl TE. A simplified technique for revascularization of homographs of the liver with a variant right hepatic artery from the superior mesenteric artery. Surg Gynecol Obstet 160:474, 1985; with permission.)

## *Living-Related Donor Procedure*

When reconstructing the hepatic vein on living-related donor liver transplantation patients, Egawa et al.[290] advised wide end-to-side anastomosis between the donor hepatic vein and cuffs consisting of the recipient middle and left hepatic veins and an incision to the inferior vena cava.

Marcos et al.[291] studied the anatomic variations of the right lobe in living donor transplantation:

> *Anatomical variations of the right lobe can be accommodated without donor complications or complex reconstruction. Previous transplantation and transjugular intrahepatic portosystemic shunt do not significantly complicate right lobe transplantation. Microvascular arterial anastomosis is not necessary, and vascular complications should be infrequent. Biliary complications can be minimized with stenting.*

Pomfret et al.[292] stress the need for careful evaluation of potential living donors, since significant donor morbidity is encountered even with careful selection.

## *Treatment of Postoperative Ascites*

We quote from Cirera et al.[293]:

> *[M]assive ascites after liver transplantation is relatively uncommon but associated with increased morbidity and mortality and is primarily related to difficulties of hepatic venous drainage. Measurement of hepatic vein and atrial pressures to detect a significant gradient and correct possible alterations in hepatic vein outflow should be the first approach in the management of these patients.*

Neuberger[294] summed up the current status of liver transplantation:

> *One of the major challenges facing the transplant community is the shortage of donor organs: imagi-*

*native approaches to overcome this problem include more effective use of marginal donor livers, splitting livers and development of living related transplants. While advances have been made in the field of xenotransplantation, there remain many hurdles to be overcome before this approach can be introduced into human transplantation.*

### Treatment of Postoperative Stenosis

Azoulay et al.[295] reported that postoperative stenosis of the portal vein after hepatic transplantation may be treated by balloon dilatation through an iliac vein.

## Editorial Comment

*The past several decades have led to major advances in the field of liver surgery. Improvements in imaging techniques, better management of the critically ill, and improvements in the treatment of organ transplant rejection have all played a role, but a major contribution has come from a better understanding of the surgical anatomy of the liver and improved techniques in liver surgery. The advances have led to some major success in the surgical treatment of hepatic malignancies, hepatic trauma, hepatic failure, and portal hypertension.*

*In many major medical centers hepatic malignancies, both primary hepatocellular carcinomas and secondary metastatic lesions at up to 4 or 5 sites from colorectal carcinoma, are currently being resected with operative mortality rates of less than 5% and five-year survival rates of 25% to 35%. There needs to be thorough evaluation to determine the extent of the intrahepatic tumor, to exclude the presence of extrahepatic metastases, and to determine functional hepatic reserve. Potential candidates for resection of liver malignancies are patients with good hepatic function, no limiting co-morbid disease, no evidence of extrahepatic tumor, and tumors that do not encroach on both the right and left portal trunks. The tumor may yield itself to resection either according to the segmental anatomy well described in this chapter or even through non-anatomic resections that cross the defined anatomic boundaries. A critical component of success in the resection of hepatic malignancies has been the ability to obtain a 1 to 2 cm margin of normal tissue around the tumor.*

*The liver is commonly injured in blunt and penetrating abdominal trauma. Injuries may vary from simple capsular tears and lacerations that quickly stop bleeding to extensive parenchymal fractures that may include bile duct disruption, hepatic artery injury, venous injuries, and/or*

*tearing of the hepatic veins from the vena cava. Most liver injuries stop bleeding spontaneously and require no specific therapy, and drainage is unnecessary unless there is a laceration deep into the parenchyma. More major injuries require control of the bleeding, removal of devitalized tissue, and the establishment of adequate drainage because of the high probability of bile duct injury and postoperative biliary leakage. In severe liver injury the first priority is resuscitation of the patient. Bleeding may need to be controlled initially by either a Pringle maneuver or packing the liver tightly. If a bleeding laceration will not respond to local control measures it may need to be explored in order to ligate specific vessels and biliary radicals. If bleeding continues despite attempted ligation of parenchymal vessels the porta hepatis may be occluded by the Pringle maneuver. If the bleeding stops with the Pringle maneuver it is presumed to be parenchymal bleeding coming from the portal vein and/or the hepatic artery. If the rate of bleeding is unchanged by the Pringle maneuver, that may mean that it not parenchymal bleeding but bleeding that is coming from the hepatic veins and/or the vena cava. As indicated in this chapter accessory right and left hepatic arteries do not travel through the porta hepatis, and if they are present may need to be occluded separately.*

*Alternatives for the control of major parenchymal lacerations with persistent bleeding are resectional debridement (sometimes aided by an intermittent Pringle maneuver) or ligation of the hepatic artery. Retrohepatic bleeding from the vena cava or hepatic veins is a difficult and high risk problem. Alternative approaches are the placement of an intracaval shunt for partial vascular isolation while permitting venous return to the heart, or total venous isolation with perhaps better visualization but with reduced venous return to the heart. If parenchymal*

## Editorial Comment *(cont'd)*

*liver bleeding or hepatic vein bleeding cannot be readily controlled and/or if the patient is difficult to resuscitate, is hypothermic or coagulopathic, better success rates have been obtained with packing of the right upper quadrant and taking the patient to an intensive care unit for further resuscitation than with persistent attempts to obtain surgical control. The patient is returned to the operating room after 24 to 72 hours for removal of the packs and appropriate surgery in a stabilized patient.*

*Hepatic transplantation has progressed remarkably over the past decade. Generally accepted survival rates are 75% at one year and 65% at five years. Recent advances in partial liver transplantation have permitted living donor transplants. The most common causes of hepatic failure leading to transplantation are postnecrotic cirrhosis, primary biliary cirrhosis, alcoholic cirrhosis, primary sclerosing cholangitis, and biliary atresia. For non-neoplastic diseases the cause of the liver failure is less important to success than the patient's condition at transplantation. Success rates are lower for patients who require support in an intensive care unit just prior to their transplantation. Success rates are higher for patients who have less neurologic impairment, less malnutrition, less prolongation of the serum prothrombin time, and lower levels of bilirubin at the time of transplantation. The results of transplantation for hepatic neoplasms are relatively poor overall but are quite acceptable for a few well defined subgroups such as: small hepatomas of favorable histology without vascular invasion or nodal metastases, hepatoblastomas, he-*

*mangioendotheliomas, and a few neuroendocrine tumors. The results following hepatic transplantation for cholangiocarcinomas and metastatic tumors such as colon and breast have been uniformly poor.*

*This chapter describes the anatomy of the advances in the surgical treatment of portal hypertension over the past several decades. The venous phase of mesenteric angiography can aid in the selection of the appropriate surgical procedure for shunting the portal blood. However, in most centers surgery for portal hypertension has become much less common. Vasopressin and sclerotherapy have proved to be effective for the treatment of acute bleeding. Serial sclerotherapy or banding of the varices in the esophagus have permitted the avoidance of major surgery in many patients, particularly in children. In patients with poor hepatic function transplantation is a potential option, however the availability of cadaver organs for transplantation is limited. Despite the improvements in the management of portal hypertension and the great success in a few, most patients with portal hypertension eventually die from the complications of progressive liver failure. The goal should be the prevention of the liver diseases that lead to portal hypertension. The hepatitis B vaccine is a partial solution for one cause of viral hepatitis, but other antiviral vaccines and treatments need to be developed, as well as a wide variety of public health measures to control the many causes of liver damage that lead to portal hypertension. (RSF Jr)*

# REFERENCES

1. Hippocrates. Tradition in Medicine. In: Lloyd GER (ed). Chadwick J, Mann WN (trans). Hippocratic Writings. New York: Viking Penguin, 1983, pp. 85-6.
2. Croisille Y, Le Douarin NM. Development and regeneration of the liver. In: De Haan RL, Urspung H, eds. Organogenesis. New York: Holt, Rinehart & Winston, 1965.
3. Lipp W. Die Entwicklung der Parenchymarchitektur der Leber. Verh Anat Ges 50:241-249, 1952.
4. Elias H. Origin and early development of the liver in various vertebrates. Acta Hepat 3:1-56, 1955.
5. Elias H. Appositional growth of the embryonic liver. Rev Int Hepat 14:317-322, 1964.
6. Wilson JW, Groat CS, Leduc EH. Histogenesis of the liver. Ann NY Acad Sci 111:8-24, 1963.
7. Bennett D. Modern views of embryonic development and differentiation. In: Javitt NB, ed. Neonatal Hepatitis and Biliary Atresia: an International Workshop. Bethesda: National Institutes of Health, March 21-23, 1977.
8. Sherer GK. Vasculogenic mechanisms and epithelio-mesenchymal specificity in endodermal organs. In: Feinberg RN, Sherer GK, Auerbach R. eds. The Development of the Vascular System. Basel: Karger, 1991.
9. Horstmann E. Entwicklung und entwicklungsbedingungen des in-

trahepatischen Gallengangsystems. Arch Entwicklungsmech Organ 139:363-392, 1939.

10. Healey JE Jr, Sterling JA. Segmental anatomy of the newborn liver. Ann NY Acad Sci 111:25-36, 1963.

11. Van Damme JPJ, Bonte J. The branches of the celiac trunk. Acta Anat 122:110, 1985.

12. Sergi C, Adam S, Kahl P, Otto HF. The remodeling of the primitive human biliary system. Early Hum Dev 2000;58:167-178.

13. Kiserud T, Rasmussen S, Skulstad S. Blood flow and the degree of shunting through the ductus venosus in the human fetus. Am J Obstet Gynecol 2000;182:147-153.

14. Merrill GG. Complete absence of left lobe of liver. Arch Pathol 42:232, 1946.

15. Belton RL, VanZandt TF. Congenital absence of the left lobe of the liver: a radiologic diagnosis. Radiology 147:184, 1983.

16. Kakitsubata Y, Kakitsubata S, Asada K, Ochiai R, Watanabe K. MR imaging of anomalous lobes of the liver. Acta Radiol 34(4):417-419, 1993.

17. Ozgun B, Warshauer DM. Absent medial segment of the left hepatic lobe: CT appearance. J Comput Assist Tomogr 16(4):666-668, 1992.

18. Morphett A, Adam A. Agenesis of the right lobe of the liver: diagnosis by computed tomography. Australas Radiol 36(1):68-69, 1992.

19. Klin B, Efrati Y, Vinograd I. Case report: selective occipital lobe hydrocephalus and agenesis of the left lobe of the liver in congenital myotonic dystrophy. Clin Radiol 46(4):284-285, 1992.

20. Fonkalsrud EW, Tompkins R, Clatworthy HW. Abdominal manifestations of situs inversus in infants and children. Arch Surg 92:791, 1966.

21. Ion A, Tiberiu CG. Anatomical features of the liver in situs inversus. Acta Anat 112:353, 1982.

22. Riedel BMKL. Uber den zungenformigen Fortsatz des rechten Leberlappens und seine pathognostische Bedeutung fur die Erkrankung der Gallenblase nebst Bemerkungen uber Gallensteinoperationen. Berlin Klin Wschr 25:577, 1888.

23. Reitemeier RJ, Butt HR, Bagenstoss AH. Riedel's lobe of the liver. Gastroenterology 34:1090, 1958.

24. Baum S, Locko RC, d'Avignon MB. Functional anatomy and radionuclide imaging: Riedel's lobe of the liver. Anat Clin 4:121, 1982.

25. Cullen TS. Accessory lobes of the liver. Arch Surg 11:718, 1925.

26. El Haddad MJY, Currie ABM, Honeyman M. Pyloric obstruction by ectopic liver tissue. Br J Surg 72:917, 1985.

27. McGregor AL, Du Plessis DJ. A Synopsis of Surgical Anatomy, 10th Ed. Baltimore: Williams and Wilkins, 1969.

28. van der Reis L, Clark AG, McPhee VG. Congenital hepatomegaly. Calif Med 85:41, 1956.

29. Gillard JH, Patel MC, Abrahams PH, Dixon AK. Riedel's lobe of the liver: fact or fiction? Clin Anat 11:47-49, 1998.

30. Organ CH, Hayes DF. Supradiaphragmatic right liver lobe and gallbladder. Arch Surg 115:989, 1980.

31. Mendoza A, Voland J, Wolf P, Benirschke K. Supradiaphragmatic liver in the lung. Arch Pathol Lab Med 110(11):1085-1086, 1986.

32. Bassis ML, Izenstark JL. Ectopic liver: its occurrence in the gallbladder. Arch Surg 73:204, 1956.

33. Horanyi J, Fusy F. Nebenpankreas in der Gallenblasenwand. Zbl Chir 88:1414, 1963.

34. Davies JNP. Accessory liver in Africans. Br Med J 2:736, 1946.

35. Heid GJ, von Haam E. Hepatic heterology in the splenic capsule. Arch Pathol 46:377, 1948.

36. Fock G. Ectopic liver in omphalocele. Acta Paediat 52:288, 1963.

37. Maresch R. A lymphangioma of the liver. Z Heilk 24:39, 1903.

38. Drachenberg CB, Papadimitriou JC, Rivero MA, Wood C. Distinctive case. Adult mesenchymal hamartoma of the liver: report of a case with light microscopic, FNA cytology, immunohistochemistry, and ultrastructural studies and review of the literature. [Review]. Mod Pathol 4(3):392-395, 1991.

39. Chau KY, Ho JW, Wu PC, Yuen WK. Mesenchymal hamartoma of liver in a man: comparison with cases in infants. J Clin Pathol 47(9):864-866, 1994.

40. Wada M, Ohashi E, Jin H, Nishikawa M, Shintani S, Yamashita M, Kano M, Yamanaka N, Nishigami T, Shimoyama T. Mesenchymal hamartoma of the liver: report of an adult case and review of the literature. [Review]. Intern Med 31(12):1370-1375, 1992.

41. Shuto T, Kinoshita H. Yamada C, Hirohashi K, Shiokawa C, Kubo S, Fujio N, Kobayashi Y. Bilateral lobectomy excluding the caudate lobe for giant mesenchymal hamartoma of the liver. Surgery 113(2):215-222, 1993.

42. Ahrens EH Jr, Harris RC, MacMahon HE. Atresia of the intrahepatic bile ducts. Pediatrics 8:628, 1951.

43. Krovetz LJ. Intrahepatic biliary atresia. J Lancet 79:228, 1959.

44. Longmire WP. Congenital biliary hypoplasia. Ann Surg 159:335, 1964.

45. Quillin SP, McAlister WH. Congenital solitary nonparasitic cyst of the liver in a newborn. Pediatr Radiol 22(7):543-544, 1992.

46. Karia M, Dasgupta TK, Sharma V, Chaudhuri MM, Mazumder DN. Symptomatic solitary giant congenital cysts of liver. Indian J Gastroenterol 11(3):136-138, 1992.

47. Koperna T, Vogl S, Satzinger U, Schulz F. Nonparasitic cysts of the liver: results and options of surgical treatment. World J Surg 21:850-855, 1997.

48. Desmet VJ. What is congenital hepatic fibrosis? [Review]. Histopathology 20(6):465-477, 1992.

49. Sung JM, Huang JJ, Lin XZ, Ruaan MK, Lin CY, Chang TT, Shu HF, Chow NH. Caroli's disease and congenital hepatic fibrosis associated with polycystic kidney disease. A case presenting with acute focal bacterial nephritis. Clin Nephrol 38(6):324-328, 1992.

50. Lipschitz B, Berdon WE, Defelice AR, Levy J. Association of congenital hepatic fibrosis with autosomal dominant polycystic kidney disease. Report of a family with review of literature. [Review]. Pediatr Radiol 23(2):131-133, 1993.

51. Murray-Lyon IM, Ochendan BG, Williams R. Congenital hepatic fibrosis: is it a single clinical entity? Gastroenterology 64:653-656, 1973.

52. Annand SK, Chan JG, Liberman E. Polycystic disease and hepatic fibrosis in children. Am J Dis Child 129:810-825, 1975.

53. Gedaly R, Pomposelli JJ, Pomfret EA, Lewis WD, Jenkins RL. Cavernous hemangioma of the liver. Arch Surg 134:407-411, 1999.

54. Williams PL. Gray's Anatomy, 38th ed. New York: Churchill Livingstone, 1995.

55. Kennedy PA, Madding GF. Surgical anatomy of the liver. Surg Clin North Am 1977;57:233.

56. Naftalis J, Leevy CM. Clinical estimation of liver size. Am J Dig Dis 1963;8:236.

57. Castell DO, O'Brien KD, Muench H, Chalmers TC. Estimation of liver size by percussion in normal individuals. Ann Intern Med 1969;70:1183.

58. Sapira JD, Williamson DL. How big is the normal liver? Arch Intern Med 1979;139:971.

59. Whalen JP. Radiology of the Abdomen: Anatomic Basis. Philadelphia: Lea and Febiger, 1976.

60. Flament JB, Delattre JF, Hidden G. The mechanisms responsible for stabilising the liver. Anat Clin 4:125-135, 1982.

61. Lockhart RD, Hamilton GF, Fyfe FW. Anatomy of the Human Body. Philadelphia: JB Lippincott, 1959.

62. Gelfand DW. Anatomy of the liver. Radiol Clin North Am 1980; 18:187.

63. Last RJ. Anatomy: Regional and Applied. 7th ed. Edinburgh: Churchill Livingstone, 1984.

64. Gamsu G, Webb WR, Sheldon P, Kaufman L, Crooks LE. Nuclear magnetic resonance imaging of the thorax. Radiology 147:473, 1983.

65. Meyers MA. Dynamic Radiology of the Abdomen. 4th ed. New York: Springer-Verlag, 1994.

66. Ibukuro K, Tsukiyama T, Mori K, Inoue Y. Hepatic falciform ligament artery: angiographic anatomy and clinical importance. Surg Radiol Anat 20:367-371, 1998.

67. Baba Y, Miyazono N, Ueno K, Kanetsuki I, Nishi H, Inoue H, Nakajo M. Hepatic falciform artery. Angiographic findings in 25 patients. Acta Radiol 2000;41:329-333.

68. Healey JE Jr, Schroy PC. Anatomy of the biliary ducts within the human liver: analysis of the prevailing pattern of branchings and the major variations of the biliary ducts. Arch Surg 1953;66:599.

69. Gao XH, Roberts A. The left triangular ligament of the liver and the structures in its free edge (appendix fibrosa hepatis) in Chinese and Canadian cadavers. Am Surg 1986;52:246.

70. Rapant V, Hromada JA. A contribution to the surgical significance of aberrant hepatic ducts. Ann Surg 1950;132:253.

71. Livingstone EM. A Clinical Study of the Abdominal Cavity and Peritoneum. New York: Hoeber, 1933.

72. Ochsner A, Graves AM. Subphrenic abscesses: analysis of 3372 collected and personal cases. Ann Surg 1933;98:961.

73. Mitchell GAG. Spread of acute intraperitoneal effusions. Br J Surg 1940;28:291.

74. Autio G. The spread of intraperitoneal infections: studies with roentgen contrast medium. Acta Chir Scand (suppl) 1964;321:1.

75. Boyd DP. The subphrenic spaces and the emperor's new robes, New Engl J Med 1966;275:913.

76. Meyers MA. The spread and localization of acute intraperitoneal effusions. Radiology 1970;95:547.

77. Silva YJ. In vivo use of human umbilical vessels and the ductus venosus arantii. Surg Gynecol Obstet 1979;148:595.

78. Michels NA. Blood Supply and Anatomy of the Upper Abdominal Organs, Philadelphia: Lippincott, 1955.

79. Gray SW, Rowe JS Jr, Skandalakis JE. Surgical anatomy of the gastroesophageal junction. Am Surg 1979;45:575.

80. Ochsner A, DeBakey M. Subphrenic abscesses: collective review and an analysis of 3608 collected and personal cases. Surg Gynecol Obstet (Int Abstr Surg Suppl) 1938;66:426.

81. Min PQ, Yang ZG, Lei QF, Gao XH, Long WS, Jiang SM, Zhou DM. Peritoneal reflections of left perihepatic region: radiologic-anatomic study. Radiology 1992;182:553.

82. Hollinshead WH. Anatomy for Surgeons. New York: Paul B. Hoeber, 1956

83. Altemeier WA, Alexander JW. Retroperitoneal abscess. Arch Surg 1961;83:512.

84. Hjortsjo CH. The topography of the intrahepatic duct system. Acta Anat 1951;11:599.

85. Sales JP, Hannoun L, Sichez JP, Honiger J, Levy E. Surgical anatomy of liver segment IV. Anat Clin 1984;6:295.

86. Padbury R, Azoulay D. Anatomy. In: Toouli J (ed) Surgery of the Biliary Tract. New York: Churchill Livingstone, 1993, pp. 3-19.

87. Dodds WJ, Erickson SJ, Taylor AJ, Lawson TL, Stewart ET. Caudate lobe of the liver: anatomy, embryology, and pathology. AJR 1990;154:87.

88. Bismuth H. Surgical anatomy and anatomical surgery of the liver. World J Surg 1982;6:3.

89. Brown BM, Filly RA, Callen PW. Ultrasonographic anatomy of the caudate lobe. J Ultrasound Med 1982;1:189.

90. Heloury Y, Leborgne J, Rogez JM, Robert R, Barbin JY, Hureau J. The caudate lobe of the liver. Surg Radiol Anat 1988;10:83.

91. Schwartz SI. Resection of the caudate lobe of the liver. (Editorial). J Am Coll Surg 184:75-76, 1997.

92. Couinaud C. Lobes et segments hepatiques: note sur l'architecture anatomique et chirurgicale du foie. Presse Med 1953;62:709.

93. Kogure K, Kuwano H, Fujimaki N, Makuuchi M. Relation among portal segmentation, proper hepatic vein, and external notch of the caudate lobe in the human liver. Ann Surg 2000;231:223-228.

94. Healey JE. Clinical anatomic aspects of radical hepatic surgery. J Int Coll Surg 1954;22:542.

95. Rieker O, Mildenberger P, Hintze C, Schunk K, Otto G, Thelen M. [Segmental anatomy of the liver in computed tomography: do we localize the lesion accurately?]. ROFO 2000;172:147-152.

96. Goldsmith NA, Woodburne RT. Surgical anatomy pertaining to liver resection. Surg Gynecol Obstet 1957;105:310.

97. Onishi H, Kawarada Y, Das BC, Nakano, Gadzijev EM, Ravnik D, Isaji S. Surgical anatomy of the medial segment (S4) of the liver with special reference to bile ducts and vessels. Hepatogastroenterology 2000;47:143-150.

98. Cho A, Okazumi S, Takayama W, Takeda A, Iwasaki K, Sasagawa S, Natsume T, Kono T, Kondo S, Ochiai T, Ryu M. Anatomy of the right anterosuperior area (segment 8) of the liver: evaluation with helical CT during arterial portography. Radiology 2000;214:491-495.

99. Soyer P. Segmental anatomy of the liver: utility of a nomenclature accepted worldwide. AJR 1993;161:572.

100. Ton That Tung. La vascularisation veineuse du foie et ses applications aux résections hépatiques. (Thesis). Hanoi, 1939.

101. Oran I, Memis A. The watershed between right and left hepatic artery territories: findings on CT scans after transcatheter oily chemoembolization of hepatic tumors. A preliminary report. Surg Radiol Anat 20:355-360, 1998.

102. Ger R. Surgical anatomy of the liver. Surg Clin North Am 1989; 69:179.

103. Blumgart LH, Baer HU, Czerniak A, Zimmermann A, Dennison AR. Extended left hepatectomy: technical aspects of an evolving procedure. Br J Surg 1993;80:903.

104. Abdalla EK, Vauthey JN, Couinaud C. The caudate lobe of the liver: implications of embryology and anatomy for surgery. Surg Oncol Clin North Am 2002 Oct; 11(4):835-848.

105. Couinaud C. (Surgical approach to the dorsal section of the liver). (French) Chirurgie 1993-1994;119(9):485-488.

106. Couinaud C. (Dorsal sector of the liver). (French) Chirurgie 1998 Feb; 123(1):8-15.

107. Filipponi F, Romagnoli P, Mosca F, Couinaud C. The dorsal sec-

tor of human liver: embryological, anatomical and clinical relevance. Hepatogastroenterology 2000 Nov-Dec; 47(36):1726-1731.

108. Gadžijev EM, Ravnik D, Stanisavljevič D, Trotovšek B. Venous drainage of the dorsal sector of the liver: differences between segments I and IX. Surg Radiol Anat 1997; 19:79-83.

109. Michels NA. The hepatic, cystic and retroduodenal arteries and their relations to the biliary ducts. Ann Surg 1951;133:503.

110. Healey JE Jr, Schroy PC, Sorensen RJ. The intrahepatic distribution of the hepatic artery in man. J Int Coll Surg 1953;20:133.

111. Michels NA. Newer anatomy of the liver and variant blood supply and collateral circulation. Am J Surg 1966;112:337.

112. Madding GF, Kennedy PA. Trauma to the Liver. Philadelphia: WB Saunders, 1965.

113. Mays ET. Vascular occlusion. Surg Clin North Am 1977;57:291.

114. Schneck CD. The anatomical basis of abdominopelvic sectional imaging. In: Ultrasound in Inflammatory Disease (Clinics in Diagnostic Ultrasound, Vol II). New York: Churchill Livingstone, 1983.

115. Baron RL, Freeny PC, Moss AA. The liver. In: Moss AA, Gamsu G, Gerant K. Computed Tomography of the Body. Philadelphia: WB Saunders, 1983.

116. Bismuth H, Garden OJ. Regular and extended right and left hepatectomy for cancer. In: Nyhus LM, Baker RJ. Mastery of Surgery. 2nd ed. Boston: Little, Brown; 1992, pp. 864-72.

117. Dawson JL. Anatomy. In: Wright R, Alberti AGMM, Karran S, Millward-Sadler GH (eds). Liver and Biliary Diseases. Philadelphia: Saunders, 1979.

118. Ohkubo M. Aberrant left gastric vein directly draining into the liver. Clin Anat 2000;13:134-137.

119. Suzuki T, Nakayasu A, Kauabe K, Takeda H, Honjo I. Surgical significance of anatomic variations of the hepatic artery. Am J Surg 1971;122:505.

120. Healey JE Jr, Schwartz SI. Surgical anatomy. In: Schwartz SI. Surgical Diseases of the Liver. New York: McGraw-Hill, 1964.

121. Healey JE Jr. Vascular anatomy of the liver. Ann NY Acad Sci 1970;170:8.

122. von Haberer H. Experimentelle Unterbindung der Leberarterie. Arch Klin Chir 1905;78:557.

123. Edgecombe P, Garner C. Accidental ligation of the hepatic artery and its treatment. Can Med Assoc J 1951;64:518.

124. Graham RR, Cannell D. Accidental ligation of hepatic artery. Br J Surg 1933;20:566.

125. Bengmark S, Rosengren K. Angiographic study of the collateral circulation to the liver after ligation of the hepatic arteries in man. Am J Surg 1970;119:620.

126. Mays ET, Wheeler CS. Demonstration of collateral arterial flow after interruption of hepatic arteries in man. New Engl J Med 1974;290:993.

127. Mays ET, Conti S, Fallahzadeh H, Rosenblatt M. Hepatic artery ligation. Surgery 1979;86:536.

128. Tygstrup N, Winkler K, Meelemgaard K. Determination of the hepatic arterial blood flow and oxygen supply in man by clamping the hepatic artery during surgery. J Clin Invest 1962;41:447.

129. Nakamura S, Tsuzuki T. Surgical anatomy of the hepatic veins and the inferior vena cava. Surg Gynecol Obstet 152:43-50, 1981.

130. Meyers WC, Peterseim DS, Pappas TN, Schauer PR, Eubanks S, Murray E, Suhocki P. Low insertion of hepatic segmental duct VII-VIII is an important cause of major biliary injury or misdiagnosis. Am J Surg 171:187-191, 1996.

131. Sing RF, Stackhouse DJ, Jacobs DG, Heniford BT. Safety and accuracy of bedside carbon dioxide cavography for insertion of inferior vena cava filters in the intensive care unit. J Am Coll Surg 2001;192:168-171.

132. Lorf T, Hanack U, Ringe B. Portal vein replacement by hepatic vein transposition. Am J Surg 174:353-354, 1997.

133. Wang M, Sakon M, Umeshita K, Miyoshi H, Taniguchi K, Kishimoto S, Imajoh-Ohmi S, Monden M. Determination of a safe vascular clamping method for liver surgery. Arch Surg 133: 983-987, 1998.

134. Man K, Fan ST, Ng IOL, Lo CM, Liu CL, Yu WC, Wong J. Tolerance of the liver to intermittent Pringle Maneuver in hepatectomy for liver tumors. Arch Surg 134:533-539, 1999.

135. Nakamura S, Suzuki S, Hachiya T, Ochiai H, Konno H, Baba S. Direct hepatic vein anastomosis during hepatectomy for colorectal liver metastases. Am J Surg 174(3):331-333, 1997.

136. Grazi GL, Mazziotti A, Jovine E, Pierangeli F, Ercolani G, Gallucci A, Cavallari A. Total vascular exclusion of the liver during hepatic surgery. Arch Surg 132:1104-1109, 1997.

137. Malassagne B, Cherqui D, Alon R, Brunetti F, Humeres R, Fagniez PL. Safety of selective vascular clamping for major hepatectomies. J Am Coll Surg 187:482-486, 1998.

138. Evans PM, Vogt DP, Mayes JT III, Henderson JM, Walsh RM. Liver resection using total vascular exclusion. Surgery 124:807-815, 1998.

139. Wisse E. An electron microscope study of the fenestrated endothelial lining of rat liver sinusoids. J Ultrastruct Res 1970:31:125.

140. Hardy KJ, Wheatley IC, Anderson AIE, Bond RJ. The lymph nodes of the porta hepatis. Surg Gynecol Obstet 1976;143:225.

141. Rouviere H. Anatomy of the Human Lymphatic System. Tobias MJ (trans). Ann Arbor MI: Edwards Brothers, 1938.

142. Fahim RB, McDonald JR, Richards JC, Ferns DO. Carcinoma of the gallbladder: a study of its modes of spread. Ann Surg 1962; 156:114.

143. Burnett W, Cairns FW, Bacsich P. Innervation of the extrahepatic biliary system. Ann Surg 1964;159:8.

144. Honjo I, Hasebe S. Studies on the intrahepatic nerves in the cirrhotic liver. Rev Int Hepat 1965;15:595.

145. Hess W, Tamm H. Surgery of the Biliary Passages and the Pancreas. Princeton NJ: D. Van Nostrand, 1965.

146. Skandalakis LJ, Gray SW, Skandalakis JE. The history of surgical anatomy of the vagus nerve. Surg Gynecol Obstet 1986;162:75.

147. Galen C. On the Usefulness of the Parts of the Body. May MT (trans) New York: Cornell University Press, 1968.

148. Jungermann K. Regulation von Stoffwechsel und Hämodynamik der Leber durch die hepatischen Nerven. Z Gastroenterol 1987; 25(suppl 1):44.

149. Friedman MI. Hepatic nerve function. In: Hue L, Schachter D, Shafritz DA (eds). The Liver: Biology and Pathobiology. New York: Raven Press, 1988, pp.949-59.

150. De Wulf H, Carton H. Neural control of glycogen metabolism. In: Hue L, van de Werve G (eds). Short Term Regulation of Liver Metabolism. Amsterdam: Elsevier North Holland, 1981.

151. Shimazu T. Central nervous system regulation of liver and adipose tissue metabolism. Diabetologia 1981;20:343.

152. Sutherland SD. The intrinsic innervation of the liver. Rev Int Hepat 1965;15:569.

153. Meguid MM, Yang ZJ, Bellinger LL, Gleason JR, Koseki M,

Laviano A, Oler A. Innervated liver plays an inhibitory role in re-gulation of food intake. Surgery 1996;119:202.

154. Nobin A, Baumgarten HG, Falck B, Ingemansson S, Moghimzadeh E, Rosengren E. Organization of the sympathetic innervation in liver tissue from monkey and man. Cell Tissue Res 1978; 195:371.

155. Moghimzadeh E, Nobin A, Rosengren E. Fluorescence micros-copical and chemical characterization of the adrenergic innerva-tion in mammalian liver tissue. Cell Tissue Res 1983;230:605.

156. Kyosola K, Penttila O, Ihamaki T, Varis K, Salaspuro M. Adren-ergic innervation of the human liver: a fluorescence histochemical analysis of clinical liver biopsy specimens. Scand J Gastroenterol 1985;20:254.

157. Sawchenko PE, Friedman MI: Sensory functions of the liver: a re-view. Am J Physiol 1979;236:R5.

158. Amenta F, Cavallotti C, Ferrante F, Tonelli F. Cholinergic nerves in the human liver. Histochem J 1981;13:419.

159. Forssman WG, Ito S. Hepatocyte innervation in primates. J Cell Biol 1977;73:299.

160. Ito T, Shibasaki S. Electron microscopy study on the hepatic sin-usoidal wall and the fat-storing cells in the normal human liver. Arch Histol Jpn Niigata Jpn 1968;29:137.

161. Tan KC, Rela M, Ryder SD, Rizzi PM, Karani J, Portmann B, Heaton ND, Howard ER, Williams R. Experience of orthotopic liver transplantation and hepatic resection for hepatocellular car-cinoma of less than 8 cm in patients with cirrhosis. Br J Surg 1995; 82:253-6.

162. Cherqui D, Alon R, Piedbois P, Duvoux C, Dhumeaux D, Julien M, Fagniez PL. Combined liver transplantation and pancreato-duodenectomy for irresectable hilar bile duct carcinoma. Br J Surg 1995, 82: 397-8.

163. Karajia ND, Rees M, Schache D, Heald RJ. Hepatic resection for colorectal secondaries. Br J Surg 1990; 77:27-9.

164. Doci R, Gennari L, Bignami P, Montalto F, Morabito A, Bozzetti F, Bonalumi MG. Morbidity and mortality after hepatic resection of metastases from colorectal cancer. Br J Surg 1995; 82:377-81.

165. Makuuchi M, Hasegawa H, Yamazaki S. Ultrasonically guided subsegmentectomy. Surg Gynecol Obstet 1985; 161:346-50.

166. Makuuchi M, Hasegawa H, Yamazaki S, Takayasu K. Four new hepatectomy procedures for resection of the right hepatic vein and preservation of the inferior right hepatic vein. Surg Gynecol Obstet 1987; 164:69-72.

167. Launois B, Jamieson GG. Modern operative techniques in liver surgery. Churchill Livingstone: Edinburgh; 1993; 9-89.

168. Tompsett DH. Anatomical Techniques, 2nd ed. Edinburgh: E & S Livingstone 1970; 180-1.

169. Ton That Tung. Les resections et mineures du foie. Masson: Paris 1979. Quoted from Launois B, Jamieson GG. Modern operative techniques in liver surgery. Churchill Livingstone: Edinburgh; 1993; 9-110.

170. Bismuth H, Houssin D. Major and minor segmentectomies "Réglées" in liver surgery. World J Surg. 1982; 6:10.

171. Blumgart LH. Hilar and intrahepatic biliary enteric anastomosis. Surg Clin North Am 1994;74(4):845-63.

172. Schwartz SI. Hepatic resection. In: Maingot's Abdominal Operations, 9th ed. USA: Prentice-Hall International Inc. Vol. 111, 1990; 1273-4.

173. Sasse D, Spornitz UM, Maly IP. Liver architecture. Enzyme 1992;46:8.

174. Merrell RC. Hepatic physiology. In: Miller TA (ed). Physiologic

175. Meyers WC. Anatomy and physiology. In: Sabiston DC Jr. Textbook of Surgery 15th ed. Philadelphia: WB Saunders, 1996, pp. 1046-1061.

176. Holley RW. Control of growth mammalian cells in cell culture. Nature 1975;258:487.

177. Barker A, Baranski A, Lambotte L. Study of the control of liver re-generation: partial hepatectomy followed by auxilliary liver trans-plantation. Hepatology 1993;18(Pt.2):163A.

178. Lambotte L, Tagliaferri E. Liver regeneration after temporary partial hepatectomy. Gastroenterology 1993;104(Pt. 2):A934.

179. Hashimoto M, Sanjo K. Functional capacity of the liver after two-thirds partial hepatectomy in the rat. Surgery 121:690-697, 1997.

180. Foster JH. History of liver surgery. Arch Surg 126:381-387, 1991.

181. Takao H, Kawarada Y. [Surgical anatomy of the hepatic hilar area]. J Jpn Surg Soc 2000;101:386-392.

182. Czerniak A, Lotan G, Hiss Y, Shemesh E, Avigad I, Wolfstein I. The feasibility of in vivo resection of the left lobe of the liver and its use for transplantation. Transplantation 1989;48:26.

183. Kazemier G, Hesselink EJ, Terpstra OT. Hepatic anatomy. Trans-plantation 1990;49:1029.

184. Czerniak A, Lotan G, Hiss Y, Shemesh E, Avigad I, Wolfstein I. Reply to Kazemier et al. Transplantation 1990;49:1030.

185. Couinaud C. Le Foie: Etudes Anatomiques et Chirurgicales. Paris: Masson, 1957.

186. Hobsley M. Intrahepatic anatomy: a surgical evaluation. Br J Surg 1958;45:635.

187. Kazemier G, Hesselink EJ, Lange JF, Terpstra OT. Dividing the liver for the purpose of split grafting or living related grafting: a search for the best cutting plane. Transplant Proc 1991;23:1545.

188. Strong RW, Lynch SV, Ong TH, Matsunami H, Koido Y, Bal-derson GA. Successful liver transplantation from a living donor to her son. New Engl J Med 1990;322:1505.

189. Bismuth H, Morino M, Castaing D, Gillon MC, Descorps Declere A, Saliba F, Samuel D. Emergency orthotopic liver transplantation in two patients using one donor liver. Br J Surg 76(7): 722-724, 1989.

190. Merz B. Two new approaches to liver transplantation: one organ, two patients ...two organs, one patient (news). JAMA 1989;262: 14, Jul 7.

191. Blumgart LH (ed). Surgery of the Liver and Biliary Tract. New York, Churchill Livingstone, 1988.

192. Czerniak A, Shabtai M, Avigad I, Ayalon A. A direct approach to the left and middle hepatic veins during left-sided hepatectomy. Surg Gynecol Obstet 1993;177:303.

193. Elias H, Petty D. Gross anatomy of the blood vessels and ducts within the human liver. Am J Anat 1952;90:59.

194. Banner RL, Brasfield RD. Surgical anatomy of the hepatic veins. Cancer 1958;11:22.

195. Baird RA, Britton RC. The surgical anatomy of the hepatic veins. J Surg Res 1973;15:345.

196. Depinto DJ, Nucha SJ, Powers PC. Major hepatic vein ligation ne-cessitated by blunt abdominal trauma. Ann Surg 1976;183:243.

197. Castaing D, Kunstlinger F, Habib N, Bismuth H. Intraoperative sonography study of the liver. Am J Surg 1985;149:576.

198. Ou QJ, Herman RE. Hepatic vein ligation and preservation of liver segments in major resections. Arch Surg 1987;122:1198.

199. Nery JR, Frasson E, Rilo HLR, Purceli E, Barros MFA, Neto JB, Mies S, Raia S, Belzer FO. Surgical anatomy and blood supply of

the left biliary tree pertaining to partial liver grafts from living donors. Transplantation Proc 1990;22:1492.

200. Couinaud C, Houssin D. (Bisection of the liver for transplantation. Simplification of the method). (French) Chirurgie 1992; 118:217.

201. Couinaud C. (Variations of the right bile ducts. The futility of complete anatomical classifications). (French) Chirurgie 1993-1994;119:354.

202. Houssin D, Boillot O, Soubrane O, Couinaud C, Pitre J, Ozier Y, Devictor D, Bernard O, Chapuis Y. Controlled liver splitting for transplantation in two recipients: technique, results and perspectives. Br J Surg 1993;80:75.

203. Couinaud C. (Absence of portal bifurcation). (French) J Chir (Paris) 1993;130:111.

204. Couinaud C. (A "scandal": segment IV and liver transplantation). (French) J Chir (Paris) 1993;130:443.

205. Couinaud C. (Surgical approach to the dorsal section of the liver). (French) Chirurgie 1993-1994;119:485.

206. Couinaud C. (Intrahepatic anatomy: application to liver transplantation). (French) Ann Radiol (Paris) 1994;37:323.

207. Meyers WC. Segmental hepatic resection. In: Sabiston DC Jr. Atlas of General Surgery. Philadelphia: WB Saunders, 1994, p. 535.

208. Starzl TE, Bell RH, Beart RW, Putnam CW. Hepatic trisegmentectomy and other liver resections. Surg Gynecol Obstet 1975;141:429-437.

209. Starzl TE, Koep LJ, Weil R III, Lilly JR, Putnam CW, Aldrete JA. Right trisegmentectomy for hepatic neoplasms. Surg Gynecol Obstet 1980;150:208-214.

210. Pack GT, Miller TR, Brasfield RD. Total right hepatic lobectomy for cancer of the gallbladder. Ann Surg 142:6, 1955.

211. Erath HG Jr, Sawyers JL, O'Neill JA Jr, Adkins RB Jr. Major hepatic resection. South Med J 74:653, 1981.

212. Mays ET. Bursting injuries to the liver. Arch Surg 93:92, 1966.

213. Raffucci FL, Ramirez-Schon G. Management of tumors of the liver. Surg Gynecol Obstet 130:371, 1970.

214. Povoski SP, Fong Y, Blumgart LH. Extended left hepatectomy. World J Surg 1999;23:1289-1293.

215. Wu CC, Ho WL, Chen JT, Tang CS, Yeh DC, Liu TJ, P'eng FK. Mesohepatectomy for centrally located hepatocellular carcinoma: an appraisal of a rare procedure. J Am Coll Surg 188:508-515, 1999.

216. Moore EE, Shackford SR, Pachter HL, et al. Organ injury scaling: spleen, liver and kidney. J Trauma 29:1664, 1989.

217. Fang JF, Chen RJ, Wong YC, Lin BC, Hsu YB, Kao JL, Kao YC. Pooling of contrast material on computed tomography mandates aggressive management of blunt hepatic injury. Am J Surg 176: 315-319, 1998.

218. Feliciano DV, Mattox KL, Birch JM. Packing for control of hepatic hemorrhage: 58 consecutive patients. J Trauma 26:738, 1986.

219. Svoboda JA, Peter ET, Dan CU, et al. Severe liver trauma in the face of coagulopathy —a case for temporary packing and early re-exploration. Am J Surg 144:717, 1982.

220. Beal SL. Fatal hepatic hemorrhage: an unresolved problem in the management of complex liver injuries. J Trauma 30:163, 1990.

221. Cogbill TH, Moore EE, Jurkovich GJ, et al. Severe hepatic trauma: a multi-center experience with 1,335 liver injuries. J Trauma 28: 1433, 1988.

222. Balasegaram M, Joishy SK. Hepatic resection: the logical approach to surgical management of major trauma to the liver. Am J Surg 142:580, 1981.

223. Blumgart LH, Drury JK, Wood CB. Hepatic resection for trauma, tumour, and biliary obstruction. Br J Surg 66:762, 1979.

224. Hollands MJ, Little JM. The role of hepatic resection in the management of blunt liver trauma. World J Surg 14:478, 1990.

225. Pachter HL, Spencer FC, Hofstetter SR, et al. Significant trends in the treatment of hepatic trauma: experience with 411 injuries. Ann Surg 215:492, 1992.

226. Gayowski TJ, Iwatsuki S, Madariaga JR, et al. Experience in hepatic resection for metastatic colorectal cancer: analysis of clinical and pathologic risk factors. Surgery 116:703-711, 1994.

227. Rosen CB, Nagorney DM, Taswell HF. Perioperative blood transfusion and determinants of survival after liver resection for metastatic colorectal carcinoma. Ann Surg 216:493-505, 1992.

228. Scheele J, Stangl R, Altendorf-Hofmann A, et al. Indicators of prognosis after hepatic resection for colorectal secondaries. Surgery 110:13-29, 1991.

229. Farmer DG, Rososve MH, Shaked A. Current treatment for hepatocellular carcinoma. Ann Surg 219:236-247, 1994.

230. Melendez J, Ferri E, Zwillman M, Fischer M, DeMatteo R, Leung D, Jarnagin W, Fong Y, Blumgart LH. Extended hepatic resection: a 6-year retrospective study of risk factors for perioperative mortality. J Am Coll Surg 2001;192:47-53.

231. Vauthey JN, Chaoui A, Do KA, Bilimoria MM, Fenstermacher MJ, Charnsangavej C, Hicks M, Alsfasser G, Lauwers G, Hawkins IF, Caridi J. Standardized measurement of future liver remnant prior to extended liver resection: methodology and clinical associations. Surgery 2000;127:512-519.

232. Bakalakos EA, Kim JA, Young DC, Martin EW Jr. Determinants of survival following hepatic resection for metastatic colorectal cancer. World J Surg 22:399-405, 1998.

233. Bakalakos EA, Burak WE, Young DC, Martin EW Jr. Is carcinoembryonic antigen useful in the follow-up management of patients with colorectal liver metastases? Am J Surg 177:2-6, 1999.

234. Wigmore SJ, Madhavan K, Redhead DN, Currie EJ, Garden OJ. Distribution of colorectal liver metastases in patients referred for hepatic resection. Cancer 2000;89:285-287.

235. D'Angelica M, Brennan MF, Fortner JG, Cohen AM, Blumgart LH, Fong Y. Ninety-six five-year survivors after liver resection for metastatic colorectal cancer. J Am Coll Surg 185:554-559, 1997.

236. Bismuth H, Majno PE. Hepatobiliary surgery. J Hepatol 2000; 32:208-224.

237. Weimann A, Ringe B, Klempnauer J, Lamesch P, Gratz KF, Prokop M, Maschek H, Tusch G, Pichlmayr R. Benign liver tumors: differential diagnosis and indications for surgery. World J Surg 21:983-991, 1997.

238. Smail N, Catania RA, Wang P, Cioffi WG, Bland KI, Chaudry IH. Gut and liver: the organs responsible for increased nitric oxide production after trauma-hemorrhage and resuscitation. Arch Surg 133:399-405, 1998.

239. Miyazaki M, Ito H, Nakagawa K, Ambiru S, Shimizu H, Shimizu Y, Okuno A, Nozawa S, Nukui Y, Yoshitomi H, Nakajima N. Segments I and IV resection as a new approach for hepatic hilar cholangiocarcinoma. Am J Surg 175:229-231, 1998.

240. Roayaie S, Guarrera JV, Ye MQ, Thung SN, Emre S, Fishbein TM, Guy SR, Sheiner PA, Miller CM, Schwartz ME. Aggressive surgical treatment of intrahepatic cholangiocarcinoma: predictors of outcomes. J Am Coll Surg 187:365-372, 1998.

241. Iwatsuki S, Todo S, Marsh JW, Madariaga JR, Lee RG, Dvorchik

I, Fung JJ, Starzl TE. Treatment of hilar cholangiocarcinoma (Klatskin tumors) with hepatic resection or transplantation. J Am Coll Surg 187:358-364, 1998.

242. Delbeke D, Martin WH, Sandler MP, Chapman WC, Wright JK Jr, Pinson CW. Evaluation of benign vs malignant hepatic lesions with positron emission tomography. Arch Surg 133:510-516, 1998.

243. Fong Y, Kemeny N, Lawrence TS. Cancer of the liver and biliary tree. In: DeVita VT Jr, Hellman S, Rosenberg SA (eds). Cancer: Principles & Practice of Oncology (6th ed). Philadelphia: Lippincott Williams & Wilkins, 2001, pp. 1162-1203.

244. Bilimoria MM, Lauwers GY, Doherty DA, Nagorney DM, Belghiti J, Do KA, Regimbeau JM, Ellis LM, Curley SA, Ikai I, Yamaoka Y, Vauthey JN. Underlying liver disease, not tumor factors, predicts long-term survival after resection of hepatocellular carcinoma. Arch Surg 2001;136:528-535.

245. Nakajima Y, Ko S, Kanamura T, Nagao M, Kanehiro H, Hisanaga M, Aomatsu Y, Ikeda N, Nakano H. Repeat liver resection for hepatocellular carcinoma. J Am Coll Surg 2001;192: 339-344.

246. Billingsley KG, Jarnagin WR, Fong Y, Blumgart LH. Segment-oriented hepatic resection in the management of malignant neoplasms of the liver. J Am Coll Surg 187:471-481, 1998.

247. Meyers WC, Chari RS. We've come a long way, baby! [Editorial] J Am Coll Surg 187:534-535, 1998.

248. Yamamoto J, Kosuge T, Shimada K, Yamasaki S, Takayama T, Makuuchi M. Anterior transhepatic approach for isolated resection of the caudate lobe of the liver. World J Surg 23:97-101, 1999.

249. Azoulay D, Marin-Hargreaves G, Castaing D, Adam R, Savier E, Bismuth H. The anterior approach: the right way for right massive hepatectomy. J Am Coll Surg 2001;192:412-417.

250. Yamamoto Y, Terajima H, Ishikawa Y, Uchinami H, Taura K, Nakajima A, Yonezawa K, Yamamoto N, Ikai I, Yamaoka Y. In situ pedicle resection in left trisegmentectomy of the liver combined with reconstruction of the right hepatic vein to an inferior vena caval segment transpositioned from the infrahepatic portion. J Am Coll Surg 2001;192:137-141.

251. Midorikawa Y, Kubota K, Takayama T, Toyoda H, Ijichi M, Torzilli G, Mori M, Makuuchi M. A comparative study of postoperative complications after hepatectomy in patients with and without chronic liver disease. Surg 1999;126:484-91.

252. Bosscha K, Roukema AJ, van Vroonhoven TJ, van der Werken C. Twelfth rib resection: a direct posterior surgical approach for subphrenic abscesses. Eur J Surg 2000;166:119-122.

253. Katkhouda N, Mavor E. Laparoscopic management of benign liver disease. Surg Clin North Am 2000;80:1203-1211.

254. Dodd GD III, Soulen MC, Kane RA, Livraghi T, Lees WR, Yamashita Y, Gillams AR, Karahan OI, Rhim H. Minimally invasive treatment of malignant hepatic tumors: at the threshold of a major breakthrough. Radiogr 2000;20:9-27.

255. Warren WD, Zeppa R, Fomon JJ: Selective transplenic decompression of gastroesophageal varices by distal splenorenal shunt. Ann Surg 166:437, 1967.

256. Warren WD, Salam AA, Hutson D, et al.: Selective distal splenorenal shunt: Technique and results of operation. Arch Surg 108: 307, 1974.

257. Warren WD, Millikan WJ Jr, Henderson JM, et al.: Ten years' portal hypertensive surgery at Emory: Results and new perspective. Ann Surg 195:530, 1982.

258. Sarfeh IJ, Rypins EB, Mason GR.: A systemic appraisal of portcaval H-graft diameters. Ann Surg 204:356, 1986.

259. LaBerge JM, Ring EJ, Gordon RL, et al.: Creation of transjugular intrahepatic portosystemic shunts with the wallstent endoprosthesis: results in 100 patients. Radiology 187:413, 1993.

260. Shiffman ML, Jeffers L, Hoofnagle JH, et al.: The role of transjugular intrahepatic portosystemic shunt for treatment of portal hypertension and its complications: a conference sponsored by the National Digestive Diseases Advisory Board. Hepatology 22:1591, 1995.

261. Demetriades D, Gomez H, Chahwan S, Charalambides K, Velmahos G, Murray J, Asensio J, Berne TV. Gunshot injuries to the liver: the role of selective nonoperative management. J Am Coll Surg 1999;188:343.

262. Moore EE. When is nonoperative management of a gunshot wound to the liver appropriate? J Am Coll Surg 188:427-428, 1999.

263. Brown CH. Needle biopsy of the liver. Am J Dig Dis 6:269, 1961.

264. Millward-Sadler GH, Whorwell PJ. Liver biopsy: methods, diagnostic value and interpretation. In: Wright's Liver and Biliary Disease. 3rd ed. Millward-Sadler GH, Wright R, Arthur MJP (eds). Philadelphia: WB Saunders, 1992, pp. 476-97.

265. Schwartz SI. The liver. In: Principles of Surgery. 6th ed. Schwartz SI (ed). New York: McGraw-Hill, 1994, pp. 1319-66.

266. Purow E, Grosberg SJ, Wapnick S. Menghini needle fracture after attempted liver biopsy. Gastroenterology 1977;73:1404.

267. Piccinino F, Sagnelli E, Pasquale G. Complications following percutaneous liver biopsy. J Hepatol 1986;2:165.

268. Feldman EA. Injury to the hepatic vein. Am J Surg 111:244, 1966.

269. Brewer GE. Hydatid cyst of the liver with ligature of the portal vein. Ann Surg 47:619, 1908.

270. Colp R. The treatment of pylephlebitis of appendicular origin. Surg Gynecol Obstet 43:627, 1926.

271. Child C, Holswade G, McClure R, Gore A, O'Neil EA. Pancreaticoduodenectomy with resection of the portal vein in the macaca mulatta monkey and in man. Surg Gynecol Obstet 94:31, 1952.

272. Honjo I, Suzuki T, Ozawa K, Takasan H, Kitamura O, Ishikawa T. Ligation of a branch of the portal vein for carcinoma of the liver. Am J Surg 130:296, 1975.

273. Busuttil RW, Kitahama A, Cerise E, McFadden M, Lo R, Longmire WP. Management of blunt and penetrating injuries to the porta hepatis. Ann Surg 191:641, 1980.

274. Stone HH. Discussion, in Busuttil RW et al. Management of blunt and penetrating injuries to the porta hepatis. Ann Surg 191:641, 1980.

275. Pachter HL, Drager S, Godfrey N, LeFleur R. Traumatic injuries of the portal vein: the role of acute ligation. Ann Surg 189:383, 1979.

276. Kim DK, Kinne DW, and Fortner JG. Occlusion of the hepatic artery in man. Surg Gynecol Obstet 136:966, 1973.

277. Braasch JW, Preble HE. Unilateral hepatic duct obstruction. Ann Surg 158:17, 1963.

278. Braasch JW, Whitcomb FF Jr, Watkins E Jr, Maguire RR, Khazei AM. Segmental obstruction of the bile duct. Surg Gynecol Obstet 134:915, 1972.

279. Lo C-M, Fan S-T, Liu C-L, Lai ECS, Wong J. Biliary complications after hepatic resection: risk factors, management, and outcome. Arch Surg 133:156-161, 1998.

280. Starzl TE, Hakala TR, Shaw BW Jr, Hardesty RL, Rosenthal TJ, Griffith BP, Iwatsuki S, Bahnson HT. A flexible procedure for multiple cadaveric organ procurement. Surg Gynecol Obstet

1984;158:223-230.

281. Shaw BW, Iwatsuki S, Starzl TE. Alternative methods of arterialization of the hepatic graft. Surg Gynecol Obest 1984;159: 491.

282. Gordon RD, Shaw BW, Iwatsuki S, Todo S, Starzl TE. A simplified technique for revascularization of homographs of the liver with a variant right hepatic artery from the superior mesenteric artery. Surg Gynecol Obest 1985;160:475.

283. Quinones-Baldrich WJ, Memsic L, Ramming K, Hiatt J, Busuttil R. Branch patch arterialization of hepatic grafts. Surg Gynecol Obstet 1986;162: 489.

284. Ekberg H, Tranberg KG, Anderson R, Jeppsson B, Bengmark S. Major liver resection: perioperative course and management. Surgery 1986;100:1.

285. Dodson TF. Surgical anatomy of hepatic transplantation. Surg Clin North Am 1993;73:645.

286. Srinivasan P, Vilca-Melendez H, Muiesan P, Prachalias A, Heaton ND, Rela M. Liver transplantation with monosegments. Surg 1999;126:10-12.

287. Couinaud C. A simplified method for controlled left hepatectomy. Surgery 1985;97:358.

288. Thompson EC, Grier JF, Gholson CF, McDonald JC. A critical review of the Couinaud technique of hepatic resection. Arch Surg 1995;130:553.

289. Hardy KJ, Jones RM. Hepatic artery anatomy in relation to reconstruction in liver transplantation: some unusual variations. Aust NZ J Surg 1994;64:437.

290. Egawa H, Inomata Y, Uemoto S, Asonuma K, Kiuchi T, Okajima H, Yamaoka Y, Tanaka K. Hepatic vein reconstruction in 152 living-related donor liver transplantation patients. Surgery 121: 250-257, 1997.

291. Marcos A, Ham JM, Fisher RA, Olzinski AT, Posner MP. Surgical management of anatomical variations of the right lobe in living donor liver transplantation. Ann Surg 2000;231:824-831.

292. Pomfret EA, Pompselli JJ, Lewis D, Gordon FD, Burns DL, Lally A, Raptopoulos V, Jenkins RL. Live donor adult liver transplantation using right lobe grafts. Arch Surg 2001;136:425-433.

293. Cirera I, Navasa M, Rimola A, Garcia-Pagan JC, Grande L, Garcia-Valdecasas JC, Fuster J, Bosch J, Rodes J. Ascites after liver transplantation. Liver Transplant 2000;6:157-162.

294. Neuberger J. Liver transplantation. J Hepatol 2000;32:198-207.

295. Azoulay D, Castaing D, Ahchong K, Adam R, Bismuth H. A minimally invasive approach to the treatment of stenosis of the portal vein after hepatic transplantation. Surg Gynecol Obstet 1993; 176: 599.

# Chapter 20

# Extrahepatic Biliary Tract and Gallbladder

JOHN E. SKANDALAKIS, GENE D. BRANUM, GENE L. COLBORN,
THOMAS A. WEIDMAN, PANAJIOTIS N. SKANDALAKIS,
LEE J. SKANDALAKIS, ODYSSEAS ZORAS

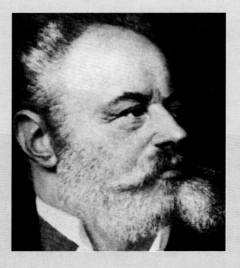

**Carl Johan August Langenbuch (1846-1901)**
performed the first cholecystectomy.

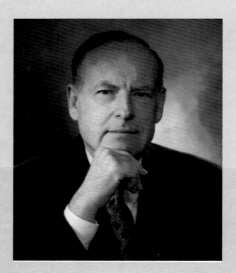

**James A. O'Neill Jr. (1933--)** wrote an excellent
paper about choledochal cysts.

*The discovery of the means to visualize the human gallbladder was a case of the old dictum that chance favors the prepared mind. After nearly five months of disappointing results, Cole finally saw a gallbladder shadow on the x-ray... "As soon as I [Cole] saw the film I called Dr. Graham, who was working late as usual. We stood there admiring the dripping film with a white blob in the center, as if we had found a treasure chest full of gold. After a few moments of silence he slapped me on the back and announced enthusiastically, 'Well Warren, we have a muskie on the line, and if the line doesn't break or the boat capsize, we should land him.'"*

*Warren Cole and Evarts Graham*[1]

*Young surgeons who are not yet familiar with the handling of an anatomically abnormal cystic blood supply need to be more aware of the precise anatomy of the extrahepatic biliary tree.*

*Suzuki et al.*[2]

## HISTORY

The anatomic and surgical history of the extrahepatic biliary tract and gallbladder is shown in Table 20-1.

## EMBRYOGENESIS

### Normal Development

The genesis of the extrahepatic biliary duct system and gallbladder may, perhaps, be the responsibility of the distal portion of the hepatic diverticulum. By the end of the 4th week, it has produced the cystic duct and gallbladder primordium. The common bile duct and the hepatic ducts may be seen at the beginning of the 5th week. The solid stage of the ducts takes place during the 5th week. The ducts elongate to reach the liver, progressively forming at this time. Slow ductal recanalization occurs approximately from the 6th through 12th weeks. Human fetal gallbladder contractility in the second half of pregnancy has been reported, although its physiological role is unknown.[3]

Gallstones are among fetal gallbladder anomalies that have been reported.[4]

## Variations and Congenital Anomalies of the Gallbladder

In an ultrasonographic study of 1823 patients, Senecail et al.[5] found morphologic variations and abnormalities in more than 33% of gallbladders, topographic variations in approximately 3.5%, and 3 cases of duplication.

Sites of potential malformations of the extrahepatic biliary tract and common bile duct are shown in Fig. 20-1. Anomalies are shown in Tables 20-2 and 20-3.

### Absence of the Gallbladder

Occasionally the gallbladder (and usually the cystic duct as well) is absent or vestigial (Fig. 20-2). The absence must be confirmed by ruling out an intrahepatic gallbladder or a left-sided gallbladder. A history of gallbladder disease with previous cholecystectomy is not in itself sufficient to establish absence of the organ. In at least three cases, a gallbladder was removed and the incision closed without discovery of the presence of a second gallbladder.[2]

**TABLE 20-1. Anatomic and Surgical History of the Extrahepatic Biliary Tract and Gallbladder**

| | | |
|---|---|---|
| Aristotle (384-322 B.C.) | | Mentioned absence of gallbladder in animals |
| Galen (ca. A.D. 130-200) | | Stated that humans have a single bile duct, or perhaps paired bile ducts |
| Berengario da Carpi | 1522 | Agreed with Galen. Wrote, "Sometimes a man lacks a gallbladder; he is then of infirm health and a shorter life." |
| De Laguna | 1535 | Agreed with Galen |
| Vesalius | 1543 | Did not accept concept of Galen |
| Fallopius | 1606 | Denied concept of Galen |
| Bergman | 1701 | First definite case of absence of human gallbladder |
| Vater | 1723 | First report of dilatation of common bile duct |
| Morgagni | 1769 | Reported deformations of the gallbladder; may have been first to see torsion of the gallbladder |
| Home | 1813 | Described biliary atresia |
| Bobbs | 1867 | Described hydrops of gallbladder and performed first successful removal of gallstones |
| Von Wyss | 1870 | Studied variations of the common bile duct |
| Nitze | 1877 | Introduction of cystoscope |
| Calot | 1891 | Original description of cholecystohepatic triangle (Triangle of Calot) |
| Swain | 1894 | Performed first successful operation for cystic dilatation of the bile duct, a cholecystojejunostomy |
| Eppinger | 1902 | Studied cholestasis |
| Dévé | 1903 | First description of gallbladder completely submerged in the liver substance (intrahepatic gallbladder) |
| Yllpö | 1913 | Reported extrahepatic biliary atresia due to embryonic developmental arrest |
| Reich | 1918 | Produced first roentgenography of biliary tree by injecting bismuth paste and petrolatum into an external fistula |
| Beall and Jagoda | 1921 | Obtained incidental opacification of the biliary tract during upper GI series performed with barium and buttermilk |
| Bakes | 1923 | First report of intraoperative endoscopic visualization of the bile ducts; used ampullary dilators which are now known as Bakes' dilators |
| Neugebauer | 1924 | First preoperative diagnosis of cystic dilatation of the common bile duct |
| Boyden | 1926 | Studied duplication of the gallbladder |
| Ladd | 1928 | First successful repair of biliary atresia |
| Ginzburg and Benjamin; Gabriel | 1930 | Simultaneous studies of biliary tract with Lipiodol injections |
| Mirizzi | 1931 | First operative cholangiography |
| Boyden | 1932 | Reviewed reports from 1800-1932 of bile ducts entering the stomach |
| Hicken, Best, and Hunt | 1936 | Performed operative cholangiography through the cystic duct stump |
| Babcock | 1937 | Used cystoscope to visualize interior of gallbladder |
| McIver | 1941 | Visualization of bile duct, showing stone |
| Porcher and Caroli | 1948 | Designed device for operative cholangiography |
| Mirizzi | 1948 | Reported syndrome of a long cystic duct with impacted stone (Mirizzi's syndrome) |
| Ahrens | 1951 | First description of intrahepatic biliary atresia |
| Mallet-Guy | 1952 | Attempted to establish operative cholangiography as a routine procedure |
| Wildegans | 1953 | Instrumental in development of observation choledochoscope and operating-observation choledochoscope |
| Healey and Schroy | 1953 | Studied intrahepatic anatomy of bile ducts |

## TABLE 20-1 *(cont'd)*. Anatomic and Surgical History of the Extrahepatic Biliary Tract and Gallbladder

| | | |
|---|---|---|
| Boyden | 1957 | Described relationship of sphincter of Oddi to common bile duct |
| Kasai | 1957 | Described treatment of "noncorrectable" cases of biliary atresia by hepatic portoenterostomy. Report published in Japanese in 1957, in English in 1968. |
| Alonso-Lej et al. | 1959 | Presented first classification system for choledochal cysts (described 3 types) |
| Myers et al. | 1962 | Cinefluorographic observation of the common bile duct |
| Kune | 1964 | Described surgical anatomy of common bile duct |
| Klatskin | 1965 | Described adenocarcinoma at hepatic duct bifurcation (Klatskin tumors) [Altemeier had described same structures in 1957] |
| Hering | 1972 | Described the connecting link between bile canaliculi and ductules |
| Todani et al. | 1977 | Developed current standard classification of cystic dilatation of the common bile duct |
| Harlaftis et al. | 1977 | Reviewed the literature of gallbladder duplication |
| Northover and Terblanche | 1978 | First description of retroportal artery |
| Frimdberg | 1978 | Performed laparoscopic cholecystotomy in pigs |
| Toouli et al. | 1982 to 1986 | Studied normal and abnormal function of sphincter of Oddi |
| Filipi, Mall, and Reosma | 1985 | Performed first animal laparoscopic cholecystectomy |
| Mühe | 1985 | Successfully treated patients by laparoscopic cholecystectomy |
| Mouret | 1987 | Generally credited with first human laparoscopic cholecystectomy |
| Petelim | 1991 | Performed laparoscopic choledochocholithotomy |
| Cotton et al. | 1991 1994 1995 | Studied risks and benefits of endoscopic sphincterotomy for bile stones in elderly high-risk patients and healthy young patients with normal-sized ducts |
| O'Neill | 1992 | Wrote classic monograph on choledochal cysts |
| Hintze et al. | 1997 | Successfully treated post-gastrojejunostomy patients endoscopically for biliary disease |

*History table compiled by David A. McClusky III and John E. Skandalakis.*

### References

Cotton PB, Geenen JE, Sherman S, Cunningham JT, Howell D, Carr-Locke DL, Nickl NJ, Hawes RH, Lehman GA, Ferrari A, Slivka A, Lichtenstein DR, Baillie J, Jowell PS, Lail LM, Evangelou H, Bosco JJ, Hanson BL, Hoffman BJ, Rahaman SM, Male R. Endoscopic sphincterotomy for stones by experts is safe, even in younger patients with normal ducts. Ann Surg 1998;227:201-204.

Davis CJ. A history of endoscopic surgery. Surg Laparosc Endosc 1992;2(1):16-23.

Diekhoff EJ. Altemeier tumors? [letter] Am J Surg 1993;166:570-571.

Hintze RE, Adler A, Veltzke W, Abou-Rebyeh H. Endoscopic access to the papilla of Vater for endoscopic retrograde cholangiopancreatography in patients with Billroth II or Roux-en-Y gastrojejunostomy. Endoscopy 1997;29:68-73.

Hintze RE, Veltzke W, Adler A, Abou-Rebyeh H. Endoscopic sphincterotomy using an S-shaped sphincterotome in patients with Billroth II or Roux-en-Y gastrojejunostomy. Endoscopy 1997;29:74-78.

LaRusso NF (ed). Gallbladder and Bile Ducts. Philadelphia: Current Medicine, 1997.

Nagy AG, Poulin EC, Girotti MJ, Litwin DEM, Mamazza J. History of laparoscopic surgery. Can J Surg 1992;35:271-274.

Popper H. Vienna and the liver. In: Brunner H, Thaler H (eds). Hepatology: A Festschrift for Hans Popper. New York: Raven Press, 1985, pp. 1-14.

Schein CJ, Stern WZ, Jacobson HG. The Common Bile Duct. Springfield IL: Charles C Thomas, 1966.

Skandalakis JE, Gray SW. Embryology for Surgeons (2nd ed). Baltimore: Williams & Wilkins, 1994.

Toouli J (ed). Surgery of the Biliary Tract. New York: Churchill Livingstone, 1993.

Di Vita et al.[7] reported agenesis of the gallbladder associated with lithiasis of the common bile duct. This rare congenital malformation is frequently associated with other anomalies.

It was suggested by Wilson and Deitrich[8] that absence of the gallbladder may be a familial trait. Ultrasonography now makes it possible to detect the absence of the organ in individuals without gallbladder disease. Sarli et al.[9] recommend preoperative cholangiography and laparoscopic exploration completed by laparoscopic sonography as adequate

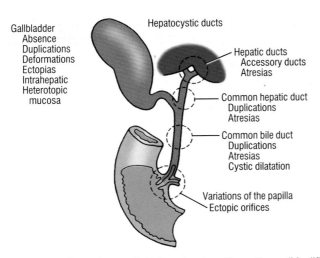

Gallbladder
  Absence
  Duplications
  Deformations
  Ectopias
  Intrahepatic
  Heterotopic
    mucosa

Hepatocystic ducts

Hepatic ducts
  Accessory ducts
  Atresias

Common hepatic duct
  Duplications
  Atresias

Common bile duct
  Duplications
  Atresias
  Cystic dilatation

Variations of the papilla
  Ectopic orifices

FIG. 20-1. Sites of potential biliary tract malformations. (Modified from Skandalakis JE, Gray SW. Embryology for Surgeons (2nd ed). Baltimore: Williams & Wilkins, 1994; with permission.)

modalities to diagnose gallbladder agenesis. Gotohda et al.[10] stated that if the gallbladder is not visualized by imaging techniques, laparoscopy should be performed before laparotomy.

## Multiple Gallbladders

A double gallbladder in a human was found at autopsy by Blasius in 1674[11]; the first such anomaly to be recorded from observation of a living patient was in 1911.[12] Harlaftis et al. reviewed 297 reports of double gallbladder and eight reports of triple gallbladder.[6] Of these anomalies, 142 were described adequately. Triple gallbladders can each have an individual cystic duct or all share the same duct. Variably, two of the gallbladders can share a duct, and the third have a separate duct.

Multiple gallbladders form a continuous spectrum of malformations, from an externally normal organ with an in-

## TABLE 20-2. Anomalies of the Extrahepatic Biliary Ducts and the Gallbladder

| Anomaly | Prenatal Age at Onset | First Appearance | Sex Chiefly Affected | Relative Frequency | Remarks |
|---|---|---|---|---|---|
| Extrahepatic biliary atresia | Acquired | Soon after birth | Equal | Rare | Most likely infectious or environmental; not genetic or congenital |
| Variation of the hepatic ducts | 5th week | None | Equal | Very common | |
| Accessory hepatic duct | 4th week? | None | Equal | Common | |
| Duplication of common hepatic duct | 4th week? | None | ? | ? | |
| Subvesicular and hepatocystic ducts | 6th week | None | ? | Rare | Anomaly not well established |
| Variations of the common bile duct | 4th week | None | ? | Common | |
| Cystic dilatations of common bile duct | Unknown | Any age | Female | Rare (most common in Japanese) | |
| Duplication of common bile duct | 4th-5th week | None | ? | Very rare | |
| Absence of gallbladder | 4th week | Adulthood, if ever | Female | Rare | |
| Duplication of gallbladder | 4th week | None | Equal | Rare | |
| Deformation of gallbladder | 6th week | None | Equal | Uncommon | |
| Left-sided gallbladder | 4th week? | None | ? | Very rare | |
| Intrahepatic gallbladder | 2nd month | None | ? | Rare | |
| Mobile gallbladder | 2nd month | Late adulthood, if ever | Female | Rare | Symptoms result from torsion |
| Heterotopic mucosa in gallbladder | 4th week? | None | ? | Very rare | |
| Adenomyoma of gallbladder | 6th week? | Late adulthood, if ever | Female | Rare | |
| Anomalies of cystic duct | 5th week | None | ? | Common | |

*Source:* Skandalakis JE, Gray SW (Eds). Embryology for Surgeons, 2nd Ed. Baltimore: Williams & Wilkins, 1994; with permission.

## TABLE 20-3. Symptoms, Diagnosis, and Treatment of Anomalies of the Biliary Tract

| Anomaly | Pathology | Symptoms | Diagnosis | Treatment | Remarks |
|---|---|---|---|---|---|
| Extrahepatic biliary atresia | | Early: Persistent progressive jaundice  Late: Enlarging abdomen; white stools | Elevated serum billirubin; biopsy to confirm presence of intrahepatic ducts; operative cholangiogram | Anastomosis where possible: Hepatocholedochostomy; Choledochoduodenostomy; Cholecystoduodenostomy or Kasai portoenterostomy (various modifications) | 80% will ultimately require liver transplant |
| Variations of hepatic ducts | | Asymptomatic | Incidental radiographic or surgical finding | None required | |
| Accessory hepatic duct | | Asymptomatic | Incidental radiographic or surgical finding | None required | |
| Duplication of common hepatic duct | | Asymptomatic | Incidental radiographic or surgical finding | | |
| Subvesicular and hepatocystic ducts | | Abdominal distension | Identified only at autopsy | | Possible source of hepatic cysts |
| Variations of common bile duct | | Asymptomatic | Incidental radiographic or surgical finding | | |
| Cystic dilatation of hepatic and common bile ducts | | Early: jaundice | IV cholangiogram, abdominal ultrasound; ERCP | Cystectomy with Roux-en-Y; common hepaticojejunostomy | Source of malignancy if not totally resected |
| Duplication of common bile duct | | Asymptomatic | Incidental radiographic or surgical finding | | |

ERCP, endoscopic retrograde cholangiopancreatography

*Table continues on the next page*

**Table 20-3** *(cont'd)*. **Symptoms, Diagnosis, and Treatment of Anomalies of the Biliary Tract**

| Anomaly | Pathology | Symptoms | Diagnosis | Treatment | Remarks |
|---|---|---|---|---|---|
| Ectopic orifice of common bile duct | | Asymptomatic | Usually at surgery or autopsy | | |
| Absence of gallbladder | | Asymptomatic | Absence on x-ray film not diagnostic; preoperative diagnosis not possible | | |
| Duplication of gallbladder | | Asymptomatic | Recognizable on radiography | | |
| Deformations of gallbladder | | Asymptomatic | May be recognized on radiography | | May be result of cholecystitis and not of congenital origin |
| Abnormal positions of gallbladder | | | | | |
|     Left sided | | Asymptomatic | May be outside the radiographic field, hence not visualized | | |
|     Intrahepatic | | Asymptomatic | Visualized radiographically; apparently absent at operation | | |
|     Mobile | | Symptoms of torsion or strangulation | At surgery | | |
| Absence of cystic duct (sessile gallbladder) | | Asymptomatic | Incidental radiographic or surgical finding | | |
| Anomalies of junction of cystic and common bile ducts | | Asymptomatic | Incidental finding at surgery | | May predispose to lithiasis |

*Source:* Skandalakis JE, Gray SW (Eds). Embryology for Surgeons, 2nd Ed. Baltimore: Williams & Wilkins, 1994; with permission.

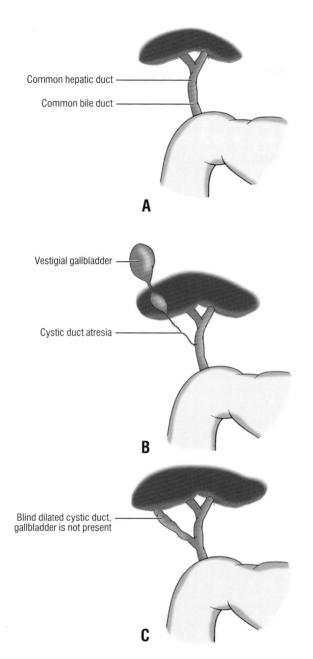

A

B

C

**FIG. 20-2.** Anomalies of gallbladder. **A,** Complete absence of gallbladder and cystic duct. **B,** Vestigial gallbladder and cystic duct atresia. **C,** Blind, dilated cystic duct without gallbladder.

Labels (Fig. 20-2):
- Common hepatic duct
- Common bile duct
- Vestigial gallbladder
- Cystic duct atresia
- Blind dilated cystic duct, gallbladder is not present

ternal longitudinal septum to the most widely separated accessory gallbladders. For practical purposes, the anomalies can be categorized into six basic types.[6,13,14] Three types belong to the split primordium group and three belong to the accessory gallbladder group. All are described below.

### Split Primordium Group

In a split primordium, multiple gallbladder elements drain to the common bile duct by means of a single cystic duct. The three types follow.

- **Septate gallbladder.** A longitudinal septum divides the gallbladder into two chambers. There may be no external trace of the septum or there may be a fundic cleft extending toward the neck (11.3%) (Figs. 20-3A, 20-3B).
- **Bilobate "V" gallbladder.** Two gallbladders, separated at the fundus, are joined at the neck by a single, normal cystic duct (8.5%) (Fig. 20-3C).
- **"Y" duplication.** Two separate gallbladders are present. Their respective cystic ducts join to form a common cystic duct before entering the common bile duct (25.3%) (Figs. 20-3D, 20-3E).

### Accessory Gallbladder Group

- **Ductular "H" duplication.** The cystic duct and accessory cystic duct enter the common bile duct separately. This is the most frequent type (47.2%) (Figs. 20-4A - 20-4C).
- **Trabecular duplication.** The accessory cystic duct enters a branch of the right hepatic duct within the liver (2.1%) (Fig. 20-4D). Rarely, the cystic duct is duplicated without duplication of the gallbladder (Fig. 20-4E).
- **Triple gallbladder.** Various combinations may be present (5.6%).

Gallbladder duplication is reported more often in women than in men (1.7:1), but the incidence of duplication is

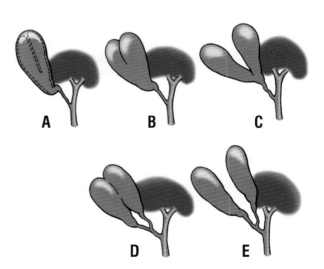

A     B     C

D     E

**FIG. 20-3.** Types of double gallbladder arising from a split primordium. See text for explanation. (Modified from Colborn GL, Skandalakis LJ, Gray SW, Skandalakis JE. Surgical anatomy of the liver and associated extrahepatic structures. Part 5: Variations and anomalies. Contemp Surg 1987;31(2):27-39; with permission.)

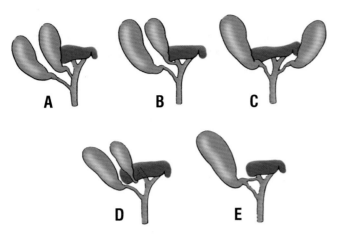

**FIG. 20-4.** Types of "accessory" gallbladder. See text for explanation. (Modified from Colborn GL, Skandalakis LJ, Gray SW, Skandalakis JE. Surgical anatomy of the liver and associated extrahepatic structures. Part 5: Variations and anomalies. Contemp Surg 1987;31(2): 27-39; with permission.)

probably more nearly equal. The disparity might be attributed to the greater incidence of gallbladder disease in women. When disease is present, both gallbladders are usually affected if they are intimately connected, less frequently if separation is complete.

Ultrasound is the best diagnostic test for double gallbladder and is useful in both healthy and diseased states.[15] Previously, oral or intravenous cholecystogram failed to detect duplication preoperatively in 60% of cases.[6] Nuclear medicine scan may identify double gallbladder, but if cystic duct obstruction is present it will fail to demonstrate one or both organs. Symptoms of gallbladder disease in a patient who has previously undergone cholecystectomy can suggest the presence of a second organ or of cystic duct remnant syndrome.[16]

### Left-Sided Gallbladder

Rarely, a gallbladder is found on the inferior surface of the left lobe of the liver. In such cases, the cystic duct enters the common bile duct from the left. There is no associated functional disorder. Ultrasonography should detect this anomaly, but the radiologist must be alert.

### Intrahepatic Gallbladder

An intrahepatic gallbladder is submerged in the liver and gives the appearance of absence of the gallbladder. CT scan or ultrasonography may provide its only evidence. A high percentage of occurrence of lithiasis is associated with this anomaly.

### Mobile Gallbladder

At the opposite extreme from intrahepatic gallbladder is the occasional mobile gallbladder, attached to the liver by a mesentery. Such a gallbladder is susceptible to torsion and strangulation. Otherwise, it causes no symptoms.

## Vascular Anomalies

### Congenital Portocaval Shunt

A portal vein entering the inferior vena cava was first publicly described in 1793.[17] This "natural" portocaval shunt is, perhaps, the result of persisting supracardinal veins[18] and is an anomaly of the formation of the vena cava rather than of portal vein development. The condition is compatible with life.

### Preduodenal Portal Vein

In 1921, Knight[19] described a patient in whom the portal vein crossed the duodenum anteriorly instead of posteriorly. In the next 40 years, 13 more cases were recorded. In Knight's case, there was no history of symptoms; however, duodenal compression has resulted from such an anomalous vein.[20]

The portal vein develops from the primitive paired vitelline veins (Fig. 20-5A) that arise on the yolk sac and pass up the body stalk to enter the developing heart. They reach their greatest development in the fourth week. Two extrahepatic cross-connections develop between the paired vessels. The cranial anastomosis lies behind the duodenum and the caudal anastomosis passes in front of the duodenum. Normally the cranial, retroduodenal anastomosis persists as the portal vein (Fig. 20-5B). Abnormally the caudal, preduodenal anastomosis can become the portal vein (Fig. 20-5C).

### Failure of Portal Vein to Bifurcate

Hardy and Jones[21] reported failure of the portal vein to bifurcate and emphasized the surgical significance of this anomaly.

### Congenital Absence of Portal Vein

Congenital absence of the portal vein is a very rare anomaly in which the intestinal and splenic venous drainage bypasses the liver, draining into the inferior vena cava. The absence of portal flow may cause nodular regenerative hyperplasia of the liver.[22]

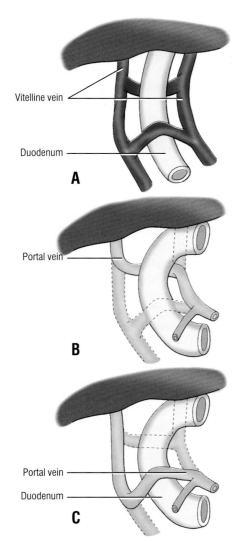

FIG. **20-5.** Embryonic origin of preduodenal portal vein. **A,** Two extrahepatic communications between vitelline veins early in sixth week of gestation. **B,** Normal development. Cranial, post-duodenal communicating vein persists as part of portal vein. **C,** Anomalous development. Caudal, preduodenal communicating vein persists while cranial vein disappears.

### Anomalous Pulmonary Veins

Anomalous pulmonary veins that pierce the diaphragm and enter the portal system are found occasionally. At least 37 cases were reported by Leal del Rosal and colleagues.[23] Such veins compose about 15% of all anomalous pulmonary vein drainage. This anomaly results in a left-to-right shunt that is usually compensated for by a patent foramen ovale providing a right-to-left shunt. This malformation is caused by failure of the pulmonary vein to tap the pulmonary plexus, combined with persistence of a connec-

tion with the splanchnic plexus in the fifth week.[24] Successful correction of this anomaly by anastomosing the pulmonary channel to the left atrium was reported by Woodwark and colleagues.[25]

## Variations and Anomalies of the Biliary Ducts

### Extrahepatic Biliary Atresia

Congenital biliary atresia is the most serious malformation of the biliary tract. A short segment, an entire duct, or the whole system may be atretic. All possible combinations may be encountered. Most of these have been described by Thompson[26] and Holmes[27] (Fig. 20-6). The atretic duct may be hypoplastic,[28] stenosed, or reduced to a fibrous band that is easily overlooked by the surgeon.

From a purely embryologic viewpoint, if a liver has formed from the hepatic primordium, agenesis of structures other than those of the cystic diverticulum (the gallbladder and cystic ducts) is hard to imagine. In other words, the hepatic ducts and the common hepatic ducts have formed, even if in a greatly reduced state. Even when no remnant of the hepatic ducts can be identified, no true "agenesis" of these ducts has occurred.

Hepatic biliary ductular atresias may be divided into three groups:

- The first type includes patent proximal hepatic ducts and occluded distal ducts. Patency may occur in any portion of the right or left hepatic duct as it emerges from the liver. This atresia is called "correctable" (Figs. 20-6A-C).
- The second type includes occluded proximal ducts. No portion of the emerging hepatic duct is patent. This atresia is called "noncorrectable" (Figs. 20-6D-F).
- The third type includes the presence of intrahepatic atresia. In this form of atresia, the extrahepatic ducts may be present or absent. The mechanism of intrahepatic atresia remains obscure[29] and the condition is as yet noncorrectable. It requires early liver transplantation (Fig. 20-6G).

Three explanations may be offered to explain biliary atresia.

- Recanalization of the solid cords of epithelium may fail. This developmental arrest of the duct system occurs in the sixth prenatal week.[30]
- The epithelium may fail to proliferate fast enough to keep up with the elongation of the ducts during the fifth week. The ducts become attenuated and finally break, resulting in a complete loss of ductal continuity.[24]
- Late prenatal or early postnatal inflammatory liver disease

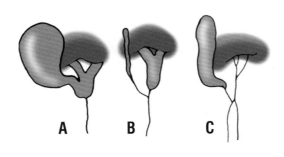

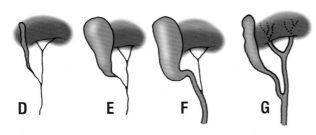

**FIG. 20-6.** Atresias of biliary tract. **A-F,** Extrahepatic biliary atresias. **G,** Intrahepatic atresia with normal extrahepatic ducts. Defects **A-C** are "correctable"; at least one patent duct emerges from the liver. **D-G** are termed "noncorrectable." (Modified from Skandalakis JE, Gray SW. Embryology for Surgeons. 2nd ed. Baltimore: Williams & Wilkins, 1994; with permission.)

can result in fibrosis of part or all of the duct system.[31]

Surgery is the only treatment for unfortunate children with extrahepatic biliary atresia. The surgical procedure is decided upon in the operating room.

Hashimoto et al.[32] reported their modification of hepatic portoenterostomy (Kasai operation) for biliary atresia, using the Cavitron ultrasonic suction aspirator. Persistent biliary drainage resulted in 77% of their cases.

### *Congenital Dilatation of the Common Bile Duct (Choledochal Cysts)*

A local balloon-shaped or cylindrical enlargement of the common bile duct is probably congenital. Symptoms of obstruction are the result of the dilatation rather than its cause. Several explanations for these dilatations have been offered. None seems adequate.[24]

The first classification of these dilatations is that of Alonso-Lej et al.[33] in 1959, who described three types of choledochal cysts. In 1984, Todani[26] described a modification of this system that included five types (Fig. 20-7). A classic monograph on the topic was written by O'Neill[35] in 1992; we urge the interested student to study O'Neill's excellent work.

Todani's classification of five types of choledochal cysts is summarized as follows.

- *I*, Solitary fusiform extrahepatic cyst. Single cystic dilatation of the common bile duct (80-90% of cases)
- *II*, Extrahepatic supraduodenal diverticulum. Double gallbladder, with one element sessile without cystic duct. Epithelial lining is that of normal gallbladder, according to Vohman and Brown [personal communication from Vohman and Brown to J.E. Skandalakis, 1987] (3%)
- *III*, Intraduodenal diverticulum/choledochocele. Cystic biliary dilatation within the duodenal wall (5%)
- *IV*, Any combination of multiple cysts, i.e., types I, II, III (10%)
  - *IVA*, Fusiform extra- and intrahepatic cysts. Combination of types I and II
  - *IVB*, Multiple extrahepatic cysts. Combination of type I with multiple intrahepatic cysts
- *V*, Caroli's disease/multiple intrahepatic cysts (very rare)

Among 58 patients with choledochal cysts reported by Todani and colleagues,[34] 46 had cystic dilatations (type I). The enlargements were cylindrical in 12 patients. The pancreaticocholedochal junction was abnormal in most of these patients.

Type I is the most common (90-95%), according to O'Neill.[36] These cysts are either saccular or fusiform dilatations of the extrahepatic biliary ductal system. O'Neill wrote that choledochoceles, which are type III, have two forms, as shown in Figure 20-8. They are more commonly found in the duodenum, but occasionally occur in the head of the pancreas.

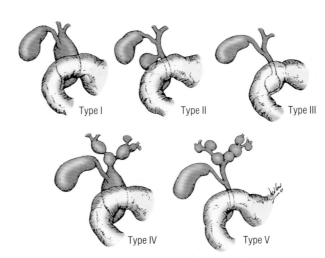

**FIG. 20-7.** Five general forms of choledochal cyst found by cholangiography as originally described by Todani.[34] (Modified from Taylor LA, Ross AJ III. Abdominal masses. *In* Walker WA, Durie PR, Hamilton JR, Walker-Smith JA, Walkins JB (eds). Pediatric Gastrointestinal Disease (2nd ed). St. Louis: Mosby, 1996;227-240; with permission.)

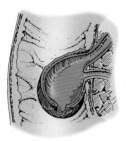 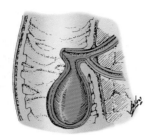

Type 1                    Type 2

FIG. 20-8. Two generally encountered forms of choledochocele (type I more common). (Modified from O'Neill JA Jr. Choledochal cyst. Curr Probl Surg 1992;29:361-410; with permission.)

Histopathologically, choledochal cysts have the following characteristics according to O'Neill[36]:

- Thick-walled structure of dense connective tissue with some strands of smooth muscle
- Chronic inflammatory process in older patients, but minimal in patients younger than 8-10 years
- The biliary mucosa is acellular and in rare cases sparse islands of columnar epithelium and microscopic bile ducts are present
- Malignancy is rare in childhood but common in adults as a form of adenosquamous carcinoma or occasionally small cell cancer

It is probable that the two most common causes of choledochal cyst formation are, according to O'Neill,[36]

- Congenital abnormal insertion of the pancreatic duct into the common bile duct resulting in reflux of trypsin and other pancreatic enzymes into the common bile duct (CBD)
- Obstruction of the distal CBD, perhaps with primary weakening

For adult patients with anomalous junction of pancreaticobiliary ductal system (AJPBDS) without bile duct dilatation, Tanaka et al.[37] recommended prophylactic cholecystectomy even if no malignant lesion is found in the gallbladder. They make this recommendation because patients with AJPBDS have a high incidence of gallbladder cancer as well as poor prognosis. Tuech et al.[38] reported a case of gallbladder carcinoma in a patient with pancreatobiliary maljunction without dilatation of the biliary tract. They urged resection of the extrahepatic biliary tract rather than cholecystectomy alone to prevent bile duct carcinoma in these patients.

Caudle and Dimler[39] pointed out that the classic symptoms of pain, jaundice, and palpable mass are often absent in ductular dilatation. Diagnosis may be attained easily by sonography, endoscopic retrograde cholangio-

pancreatography (ERCP), and iminodiacetic acid scans. These authors also remarked on the occurrence of anomalies of the junction of the bile duct and the pancreatic ducts. They are not convinced that these are of etiologic significance.

Sugiyama et al.[40] cautioned that associated pancreatic disease and an abnormal pancreatogram may be associated with anomalous pancreaticobiliary junction (APBJ). While cholecystectomy alone may be adequate for APBJ without choledochal cyst, APBJ with cyst requires cyst excision.

REMEMBER:

Choledochal cysts are most common in adult females, who complain about biliary tract symptomatology or perhaps pancreatitis. A right upper quadrant mass with pain and jaundice in infants suggests a choledochal cyst. Diagnosis is established by ultrasonography, CT scan, and cholangiography.[41]

The following questions about choledochal cysts remain unanswered.

- Why are there so many cases in Asia?
- Do Asians living in the West have a higher incidence than the general population?
- Why do some cases of abnormal junction show no dilatation of the common bile duct?
- Since the sphincteric apparatus of Boyden does not exist in an abnormal junction, why is there no clinical picture of pancreatitis and histologic changes in the pancreas in the first month of life?
- Is type II a congenital dilatation or a double gallbladder with minimal cystic duct or without cystic duct?

Yoshida et al.[42] stated that the congenital anomaly of APBJ outside the sphincter of Oddi without dilatation of the extrahepatic biliary system appears to be an important risk factor responsible for the genesis of carcinoma of the gallbladder. There have been some favorable outcomes for patients with gallbladder carcinoma associated with APBJ. However, Vitetta et al.[43] raised the possibility that carcinoma of the gallbladder is an age-dependent malignancy, present mostly in females, intimately associated with long term benign gallstone disease.

## Miscellaneous Asymptomatic Anomalies

Some of the many variations encountered in the biliary tract are shown in Figures 20-9 to 20-15. Some of these variations may be more prone to lithiasis than the normal configuration. Their chief interest is to the surgeon, who must be aware of the possible occurrence of these and other variations rather than trying to make the findings at operation fit a "normal" pattern. An anomaly or variation

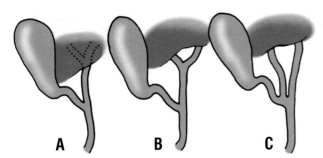

FIG. 20-9. Variations of hepatic ducts. **A,** Intrahepatic union of right and left hepatic ducts. **B,** Extrahepatic (normal) union of hepatic ducts. **C,** Distal union of hepatic ducts resulting in absence of common hepatic duct. (Modified from Skandalakis JE, Gray SW. Embryology for Surgeons. 2nd ed. Baltimore: Williams & Wilkins, 1994; with permission.)

must be recognized as such; the surgeon should never attempt to explain abnormal findings as "normal." This is especially critical in laparoscopic surgery and reinforces the importance of cholangiography.

REMEMBER:
- In most cases, the portal vein, hepatic artery, and biliary duct are fellow travelers within the hepatic parenchyma.
- The hepatic veins do not follow the triad within the liver parenchyma: they pass between segments or subsegments.
- The triad is enveloped extrahepatically and intrahepatically by a thin fibrous sheath. This structure is a continuation of the endoabdominal fascia. Characteristically, the hepatic veins are not protected by this special envelope. This explains their tendency to tear easily. The connective tissue envelope also allows one to differentiate the former structures from hepatic veins by ultrasound and MRI (magnetic resonance imaging).
- The right hepatic vein can be exposed by division of the retrocaval ligament which connects segments I and VII.
- Lumbar veins do not enter the retrohepatic part of the IVC.
- The line of Rex (gallbladder to IVC) divides the liver into two equal functional lobes.
- There are no external landmarks for the division created by the line of Rex.
- There is confusion in the literature about the true anatomy of the quadrate and caudate lobes. All the various opinions may be correct from a surgical standpoint. However, in a right functional lobectomy, large parts of both the caudate and the quadrate lobes are transected. For all practical purposes, the caudate lobe (segment I) belongs to both the right and left functional lobes. The

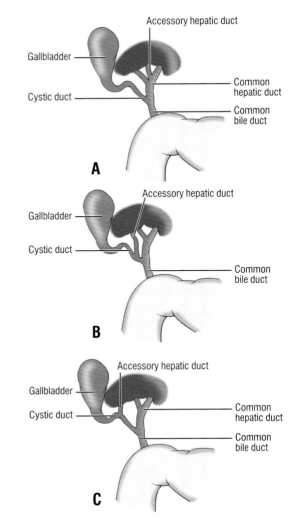

FIG. 20-10. Accessory hepatic ducts.

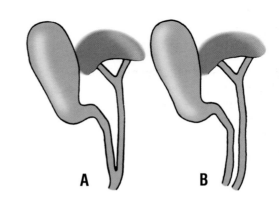

FIG. 20-11. Variations of common bile duct. **A,** Low junction of cystic and common hepatic ducts results in shortened common bile duct. **B,** Absence of a common bile duct. (Modified from Skandalakis JE, Gray SW. Embryology for Surgeons (2nd ed). Baltimore: Williams & Wilkins, 1994; with permission.)

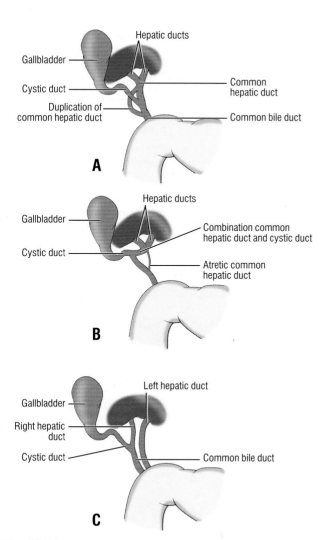

FIG. 20-12. **A,** Duplication of common hepatic duct; case of Michels.[44] **B,** Duplication of common hepatic duct; case of Nygren and Barnes.[229] Duplication is patent. Normally located duct is atretic. **C,** May be called "absence" of common hepatic duct or "duplication" of common bile duct.

quadrate lobe belongs to the medial segment of the left lobe (segment IV).

• The right and left coronary ligaments are quite different. The right is composed of two leaflets, anterior and posterior. The left is composed only of a seemingly singular leaflet. The left anterior and posterior leaflets are either fused or separated by a small layer of fibrofatty tissue containing small vessels and bile ducts. Therefore, always ligate the left triangular and coronary ligaments. Also, remember that the left hepatic vein can be injured during the division of the left ligament, resulting in massive hemorrhage and a fatal outcome.

## SURGICAL ANATOMY

## Extrahepatic Triad and Extrahepatic Hepatic Veins

The extrahepatic triad consists of the hepatic artery,

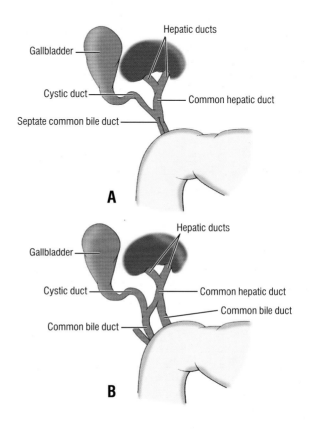

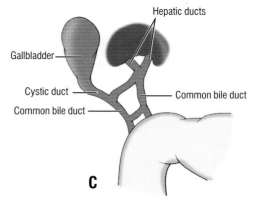

FIG. 20-13. Duplications of common bile duct. **A,** Double and parallel lumina of common bile duct. **B,** "X" type of anastomosis between duplicated bile ducts. **C,** "X" and "H" types of anastomosis between duplicated bile ducts.

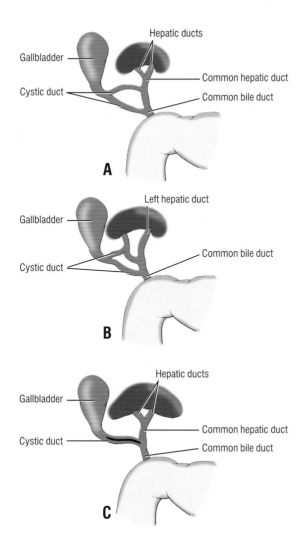

**FIG. 20-14.** Duplications of cystic duct without duplication of gallbladder. **A,** Both cystic ducts enter common hepatic duct. **B,** Accessory cystic duct opening into right hepatic duct. **C,** Double-barreled duplication of cystic duct.

hepatic portal vein, and hepatic duct (Fig. 20-16). The course of the cystic artery and variations of the cystic artery are considered in the section "Vessels of the Gallbladder and Biliary Tract."

## Blood Vessels

### Hepatic Artery, Common Hepatic Artery, and Proper Hepatic Artery

The hepatic artery (Fig. 20-16) provides 25% of the afferent blood supply to the liver, as well as about 50% of the oxygen. The hepatic arterial supply is derived from the celiac trunk in 55% of subjects.[44] In 45%, the common hep-

atic artery, the right hepatic, or the left hepatic may arise from vessels other than the celiac trunk (aberrant hepatic arteries).

The common hepatic artery takes origin from the celiac trunk in the majority of individuals: 83.2% according to Daseler and colleagues;[45] 86% according to Van Damme and Bonte (Figs. 20-17 and 20-18).[46] In other cases, it may arise from the superior mesenteric artery (2.9%), from the aorta (1.1%), from the left gastric artery (0.54%), or even from rarer sources, according to Van Damme and Bonte.

In 75% of the 200 specimens of Michels,[44] the gastroduodenal artery arose from the distal horizontal portion of the common hepatic artery. The right gastric artery arose from the common or proper hepatic in about 40% of these cases and from the left hepatic artery with similar frequency. In other specimens, the right gastric artery took origin from another hepatic branch (11%) or from the gastroduodenal artery (8%).

Concerning the overall behavior of the normal hepatic arteries, Van Damme wrote the following;[47] we concur with his rules.

*By definition, the normal common hepatic artery becomes the proper hepatic artery at the point where the gastroduodenal artery begins. According to most textbooks, the proper hepatic artery divides into a right and a left hepatic branch but variations are legion. We find no reason to consider a middle hepatic branch as*

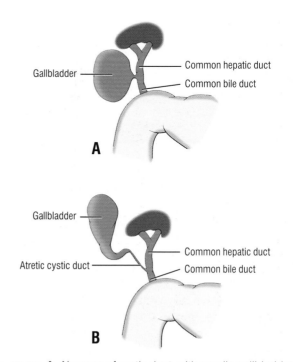

**FIG. 20-15. A,** Absence of cystic duct, with sessile gallbladder. **B,** Atretic cystic duct with normal gallbladder.

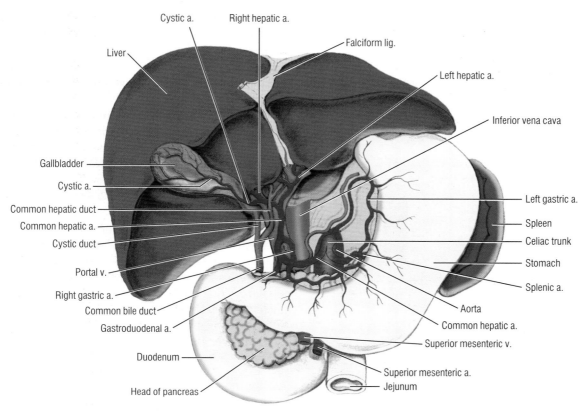

**FIG. 20-16.** Origin and branches of the celiac trunk. (Modified from Gray SW, Skandalakis JE. Atlas of Surgical Anatomy for General Surgeons. Baltimore: Williams & Wilkins, 1983; with permission.)

Michels[44] did, because this only increases the confusion. We have summarized the behavior of the hepatic artery in three rules. First, the hepatic artery may divide into its right and left hepatic branches at any point between the liver hilum and the origin of the hepatic artery itself [Fig. 20-18]. If it divides exactly at the site of origin of the gastroduodenal artery, there is no proper hepatic artery. If it splits at the origin of the hepatic artery itself, there is not even a common hepatic artery.

Second, the gastroduodenal artery always arises at a fixed point at the transition of the mobile and fixed segments of the first part of the duodenum. Consequently, the origin of the gastroduodenal artery is determined by the hepatic vessel that passes at this site, whatever the divisional pattern of the hepatic artery may be. Third, if a normal common hepatic artery bifurcates very early, medial to the portal vein [Fig. 20-18], the right branch will pass behind the portal vein; the pulsations can be palpated through the hiatus of Winslow.

When arising from the common source, the typical common hepatic artery (Fig. 20-19A) runs horizontally along the upper border of the head of the pancreas and then turns upward to ascend between the layers of the lesser omentum. The peritoneum of the posterior wall of the omental bursa covers the horizontal portion of the artery. The hepatoduodenal ligament envelops the ascending portion, which lies in front of the epiploic foramen (of Winslow) to the left of the common bile duct and anterior to the portal vein.

**Aberrant Hepatic Arteries**

There is confusion in the literature regarding the terms aberrant, replacing, and accessory arteries. Aberrant hepatic arteries occur frequently (46% according to Van Damme;[47] 45% according to Suzuki et al;[48] 43% according to Healey et al;[49] 41.5% according to Michels[44]) as shown in Figs. 20-19B-D. Aberrant or atypical hepatic arteries are often described as "replacing" arteries if the artery arises entirely from some source other than the celiac arterial distribution. In such cases, the replacing artery can supply the entire liver or an entire lobe of the liver. Atypical hepatic arteries are often, if erroneously, referred to as "accessory" hepatic arteries if they arise from some aberrant source

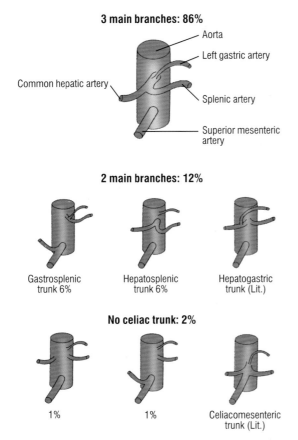

**3 main branches: 86%**

Aorta

Left gastric artery

Common hepatic artery

Splenic artery

Superior mesenteric artery

**2 main branches: 12%**

Gastrosplenic trunk 6%

Hepatosplenic trunk 6%

Hepatogastric trunk (Lit.)

**No celiac trunk: 2%**

1%

1%

Celiacomesenteric trunk (Lit.)

**Fig. 20-17.** Division of celiac trunk. *(Lit.),* reported in medical literature. (Modified from Van Damme JP, Bonte J. Atresia splenica and the blood supply of the spleen (splen). Probl Gen Surg 1990;7:18-27, with permission.)

As one might reasonably predict, various combinations of "replacing" or "accessory" hepatic arteries can occur in the same individual. For instance, in 2% of cases a replaced right hepatic may exist together with an accessory left hepatic in the same person, or the configuration may be reversed.[50]

Feigl and colleagues[54] distinguished the following types of anastomoses between the celiac artery and the superior mesenteric artery: 1) direct connection; 2) anastomoses with the hepatic artery; 3) anastomoses following pre- or postnatal stenosis; and 4) the pancreatic arcades. Two of the authors of this chapter (JES and GLC) have independently observed instances of an accessory right hepatic artery that arose from the superior mesenteric artery and terminated in a normal right hepatic artery of celiac origin. It must be emphasized, however, that such collateral vessels are seen only infrequently. Almost all "accessory" hepatic arteries exposed surgically should be considered functionally essential to the survival of liver tissue.

In a study of the anatomic variations in the vascular supply to the liver in 1000 donor liver arteries used for trans-

and are additive to lobar branches derived from the celiac hepatic arteries (Fig. 20-19B). Except in unusual cases, truly "accessory" arteries do not exist, because they are providing the primary arterial supply to a specific part of the liver, whether it be a lobe, segment, or subsegment of parenchyma.

The common hepatic artery may arise from the superior mesenteric, the aorta, the left gastric, or other sources, as noted above. The left hepatic artery arises in 25-30% of cases from the left gastric artery.[46,50] These include a totally "replacing" left hepatic artery in 10% and an "accessory" left hepatic artery in about 15% of cases.

The right hepatic artery originates from the superior mesenteric in about 17%[50,51] of cases. Of these, 11% represent total replacement (Fig. 20-19D), and about 7% are "accessory" in nature. The middle hepatic artery arises with nearly equal frequency from the left or right hepatic artery, although it is more often depicted as arising from the left hepatic artery.[52,53]

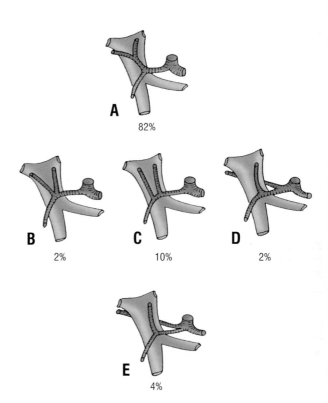

**A**

82%

**B**

2%

**C**

10%

**D**

2%

**E**

4%

**Fig. 20-18.** Variations of hepatic artery. **A,** Normal pattern, 82%. **B-D,** Absence of proper hepatic artery, 14%. **E,** Absence of common hepatic artery and proper hepatic artery, 4%. (Modified from Van Damme JP, Bonte J. Vascular Anatomy in Abdominal Surgery. New York: Thieme, 1990; with permission.)

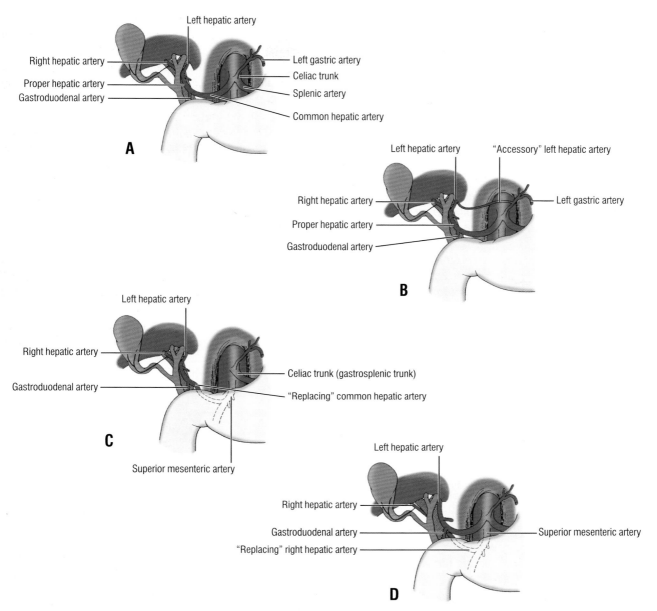

FIG. 20-19. Aberrant hepatic arteries. **A,** "Normal" hepatic artery arises from celiac trunk. **B,** "Accessory" left hepatic artery arises from left gastric artery. **C,** "Replacing" common hepatic artery arises from superior mesenteric artery. **D,** "Replacing" right hepatic artery arises from superior mesenteric artery.

plantation, Hiatt et al.[55] reported the arterial patterns in order of frequency as follows:

- Normal type (common hepatic artery arising from the celiac axis to form the gastroduodenal and proper hepatic arteries, and the proper hepatic dividing distally into right and left branches): 757 cases
- Replaced or accessory right hepatic from SMA: 106 cases
- Replaced or accessory left hepatic from left gastric: 97 cases

- Both right hepatic (from SMA) and left hepatic (from left gastric) arising abnormally: 23 cases
- Entire common hepatic artery from SMA: 15 cases
- Common hepatic artery from aorta: 2 cases

Weimann et al.[56] stated that an aberrant left hepatic artery arising from the left gastric artery may be protected if the left gastric artery is ligated distal to the origin of the hepatic branch.

If one traces aberrant arteries backward, that is, from within the liver, the path will reveal the "replacing" arteries to be lobar arteries with aberrant origin but with normal distribution.

Van Damme's[47] findings and thoughts about aberrant hepatic arteries follow:

> Aberrant hepatic branches are found in 46% of the preparations [dissection, postmortem arteriography, and corrosion]: a right one in 24% and a left one in 30%; in 8% there is both a right and a left aberrant hepatic branch. We do not follow Michels[44] in distinguishing between accessory and replaced aberrant hepatic branches, because this distinction is very difficult to make during surgery and because even the "accessory" branches are usually the only supply for a specific segment. An aberrant right hepatic branch from the superior mesenteric artery (20%) always runs behind the pancreas and behind the portal vein and always supplies a cystic artery. Its ligation should always be followed by cholecystectomy. From behind the portal vein it runs through the intercholedochohepatic triangle and usually crosses under the bile ducts before it enters the liver posterolateral to the hepatic duct [Fig. 20-20A]. Exceptionally, it may turn in the intercholedochohepatic triangle toward the anterior side of the portal vein and continue like a normal hepatic artery [Fig. 20-20B]. During surgery, this aberrant branch is to be found in the intercholedochohepatic triangle and in the triangle between the cystic and hepatic ducts. Through the hiatus of Winslow it can be palpated behind the portal vein. After a Kocher maneuver its pulsations can be felt behind the head.

> The aberrant left hepatic branch (30%) always arises from the left gastric artery. It runs in the cranial part of the lesser omentum where it is endangered during gastrectomy and hiatal hernia repair. It enters the liver through the fissure of the venous ligament. It often gives off branches to the stomach and to the esophagus.

We quote from Rygaard et al.[57]:

> From a surgical point of view it is important to know the gross anatomy of the hepatic arteries before an intervention on the liver and pancreas. Thus, when the right hepatic artery arises from the superior mesenteric artery, it may pass through the pancreatic head. Particulars about this variant are of great value prior to pancreatectomy and hemihepatectomy. Information to the effect that the left hepatic artery originates from the left gastric artery may allow rapid dissection of the porta hepatis in hemihepatectomy. Ligation or embolization of hepatic arteries in the treatment of liver trauma, hepatic tumor or lesions of the hepatic vessels such as aneurysm, arteriovenous fistula or hemobilia require detailed angiographic analysis.

### Hepatic Portal Vein

The hepatic portal vein provides 75% of the blood and about 50% of the oxygen reaching the liver. The portal vein (Fig. 20-21) is formed by the confluence of the superior mesenteric vein and the splenic vein behind the neck of the pancreas. However, the inferior mesenteric vein may enter the splenic vein, superior mesenteric vein, or their junction. In these cases the portal vein is thought of as being formed by the junction of all three. Table 20-4 indicates some studies of these variations.

Toward the liver, the portal vein lies in front of the inferior vena cava. The common bile duct is on the right, and the proper hepatic artery is on the left. In the absence of disease, the portal vein and the superior mesenteric vein can be easily separated from the posterior surface of the pancreas.

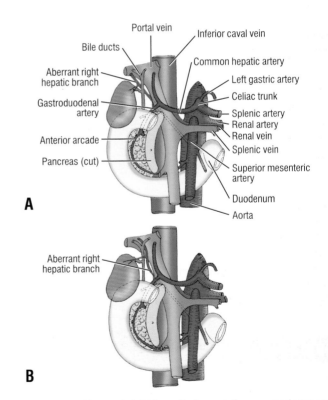

FIG. 20-20. Aberrant right hepatic branch from superior mesenteric artery runs behind pancreas and behind portal vein. **A,** Branch appears in intercholedochohepatic area and continues behind choledochus. **B,** Same branch turns upward to run upon portal vein, behaving like normal right hepatic branch. (Modified from Van Damme JP, Bonte J. Vascular Anatomy in Abdominal Surgery. New York: Thieme, 1990; with permission.)

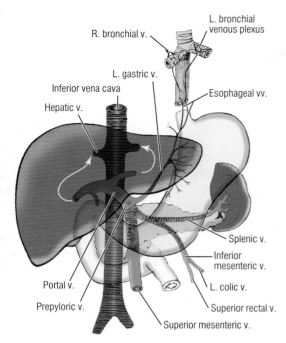

**FIG. 20-21.** Portal vein and major tributaries. (Modified from O'Rahilly RO. Gardner-Gray-O'Rahilly Anatomy (5th ed). Philadelphia: WB Saunders, 1986; with permission.)

The portal vein is 7-10 cm long and 0.8-1.4 cm in diameter and is without valves. At the porta hepatis, it bifurcates into right and left portal veins. Its further course in the liver is discussed in the chapter on the liver in the section on hepatic portal veins.

The inferior mesenteric vein ends with approximately equal frequency in the splenic vein, the superior mesenteric vein, or the portal vein. Either the splenic vein or the portal vein receives the coronary (left gastric) vein as well. The portal vein receives an accessory pancreatic vein on the left and the superior pancreaticoduodenal and the pyloric veins on the right.

In 17 of 23 subjects the senior author of this chapter (JES) dissected, the left gastric vein entered the portal vein;

in six, it entered the splenic vein. Healey and Schwartz[51] observed a portal termination of the left gastric vein in 83% of their specimens. Where drainage was into the portal vein, the left gastric vein lay in the hepatogastric ligament.

### Hepatic Veins (Upper Portas)

The liver is drained by a series of dorsal hepatic veins. They are located in the area aptly called "the upper hilum"[58] by Rodney Smith. There are 3 major veins — the right, middle, and left hepatic— and from 10 to 50 smaller veins opening into the inferior vena cava.[59]

The extrahepatic length of the three major veins varies from 0.5 cm to 1.5 cm. The right hepatic vein (Fig. 20-22) is the largest. It lies in the right segmental fissure, draining the entire posterior segment and the superior area of the anterior segment of the right lobe.

The middle hepatic vein lies in the main lobar fissure. It drains the inferior area of the anterior segment of the right lobe and the inferior area of the medial segment of the left lobe.

The left hepatic vein lies in the upper part of the left segmental fissure. It drains the superior area of the medial segment and all of the lateral segment. In about 60% of individuals, the left and middle veins unite to enter the inferior vena cava as a single vein.[51] The length of the common trunk is 1-2 cm. Nakamura and Tsuzuki[59] found a common trunk in 70 of 83 autopsies. They state that 1 cm of vein without tributaries was sufficient for successful ligation. By their standards, the right vein could have been ligated in 60% of the cadavers examined. The middle and left veins could have been ligated in only 11%. Any surgeon contemplating procedures in this area should study Nakamura and Tsuzuki's findings.

The right hepatic vein enters the inferior vena cava. In some individuals a significant segment of the right vein may course in a retrohepatic position, where it is especially vulnerable to posterior incisions at the level of the 12th rib or other surgical approaches designed to treat upper posterior abdominal injuries or pathology. The left hepatic vein may also enter the inferior vena cava directly. This vein

| Investigator, # of Cases | Inferior Mesenteric Vein Enters: | | | |
|---|---|---|---|---|
| | Splenic v. | SMV | Junction of Splenic/SMV | Other |
| Treves (100) | 18% | 36% | 44% | 2% |
| Douglass et al. (92) | 38% | 29.3% | 32.7% | — |
| Purcell et al. (100) | 28% | 53% | 3% | 16% |

**TABLE 20-4. Participation of the Inferior Mesenteric Vein in the Formation of the Hepatic Portal Vein**

SMV, Superior mesenteric vein.

Data from Hollinshead WH. Anatomy for Surgeons, Vol. 2. New York: Hoeber-Harper, 1961, pp. 454-455.

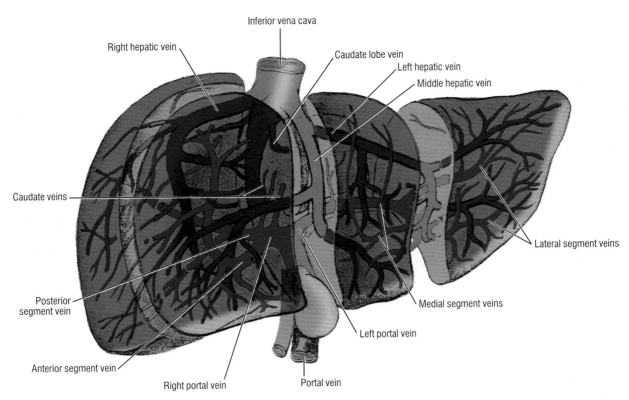

**FIG. 20-22.** Portal venous supply. (Modified from Healy JE Jr, Hodge J. Surgical Anatomy (2nd ed). Philadelphia: Decker, 1990; with permission.)

may be torn during operations at the gastroesophageal junction when the left triangular ligament is incised. The middle hepatic vein enters into the left hepatic vein.

Of the smaller veins, one or two constant vessels drain the caudate lobe and enter the inferior vena cava on the left side. Several inconstant veins draining the posterior segment of the right lobe enter the right posterolateral aspect of the inferior vena cava.[60]

As noted previously, the number of these small veins may vary from 10 to as many as 50. Between 5 and 10 of these will require ligation during hepatic resections.[59]

Cavalcanti et al.[61] reported a large number of muscular and collagenous fibers present on the walls of the hepatic veins at the level of the junction with the inferior vena cava. They consider this a sphincterlike formation that may play some physiological role in controlling hepatic circulation.

## Extrahepatic Biliary Tract

The right and left lobes of the liver are drained by ducts originating as bile canaliculi in the lobules. The canaliculi empty into the canals of Hering in the interlobular triads. The canals of Hering are collected into ducts draining the hepatic areas, the four hepatic segment ducts, and finally, outside the liver, the right and left hepatic ducts.

### Right Hepatic Duct

The right hepatic duct is formed by the union of the anterior and posterior segment ducts at the porta hepatis. This pattern was present in 72% of specimens examined by Healey and Schroy[62] as shown in Fig. 20-23A. In the remainder, the posterior segment duct (or, rarely, the anterior segment duct) (Figs. 20-23B, 20-23C) crossed the segmental fissure to empty into the left hepatic duct or one of its tributaries. In these cases, the right hepatic duct is absent. The average length of the right hepatic duct, when present, is 0.9 cm.

### Left Hepatic Duct

The left hepatic duct is usually (67% of Healey and Schroy's[62] specimens) formed by the union of the medial and lateral segment ducts (Fig. 20-24A), although the medial segment duct sometimes enters the inferolateral duct (Fig. 20-24B). The union of the two area ducts is in line with the left segmental fissure (50%), to the right of the fissure (42%), or to the left of the fissure (8%).

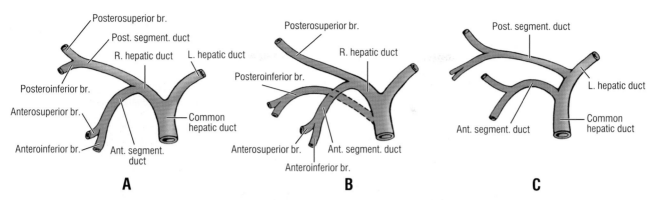

FIG. 20-23. Variations in tributaries to right hepatic duct. **A,** Usual pattern. Right hepatic duct receives anterior and posterior segment ducts. **B,** Alternate pattern. Posteroinferior area duct enters common hepatic duct. **C,** Anterior and posterior segment ducts enter left hepatic duct. Right hepatic duct absent. (Modified from Colborn GL, Skandalakis LJ, Gray SW, Skandalakis JE. Surgical anatomy of the liver and associated extrahepatic structures. Part 3: Surgical anatomy of the liver. Contemp Surg 1987;30(6):15-23; with permission.)

The average length of the left hepatic duct is 1.7 cm.[62] Usually the right and left hepatic ducts are of equal size. In patients with chronic obstructive biliary disease, the left duct, for unknown reasons, is larger than the right duct.[63] Drainage of the medial segment duct is shown in Fig. 20-25.

### Common Hepatic Duct

The common hepatic duct (Fig. 20-26) is formed by the union of the right and left hepatic ducts in the porta at the transverse fissure of the liver. Its lower end is defined as its junction with the cystic duct. The distance between these points varies from 1.0 cm to 7.5 cm. The diameter of the

duct is about 0.4 cm.

Several arteries are found in relation to the extrahepatic biliary tract. Many of these may lie anterior or posterior to

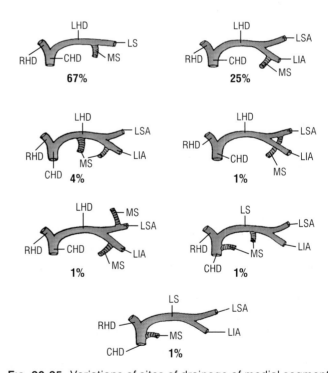

FIG. 20-25. Variations of sites of drainage of medial segment duct. CHD, Common hepatic duct; RHD, Right hepatic duct; LHD, Left hepatic duct; LS, Lateral segment duct; MS, Medial segment duct; LSA, Lateral superior area duct; LIA, Lateral inferior area duct. (Modified from Healey JE Jr, Schroy PC. Anatomy of the biliary ducts within the human liver: analysis of the prevailing pattern of branchings and the major variations of the biliary ducts. Arch Surg 1953;66:599; with permission.)

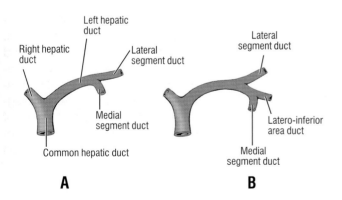

FIG. 20-24. Variations of left hepatic duct. **A,** Usual pattern. Left hepatic duct forms by confluence of medial and lateral segment ducts. **B,** Medial segment duct may enter inferolateral duct. Medial segment duct is usually double. (Modified from Colborn GL, Skandalakis LJ, Gray SW, Skandalakis JE. Surgical anatomy of the liver and associated extrahepatic structures. Part 3: Surgical anatomy of the liver. Contemp Surg 1987;30 (6):15-23; with permission.)

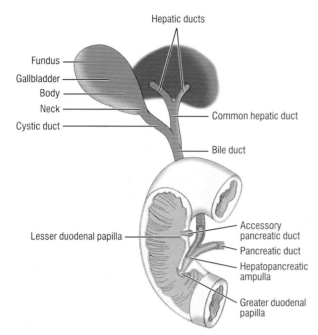

Fundus
Gallbladder
Body
Neck
Cystic duct

Hepatic ducts

Common hepatic duct

Bile duct

Lesser duodenal papilla

Accessory pancreatic duct
Pancreatic duct
Hepatopancreatic ampulla
Greater duodenal papilla

**FIG. 20-26.** Location of common hepatic duct. (After O'Rahilly RO. Gardner-Gray-O'Rahilly Anatomy (5th ed). Philadelphia: WB Saunders, 1986; with permission.)

**TABLE 20-5. Segments of the Biliary Tract and the Frequency of Arteries Lying Anterior to Them**

| Segment | Artery Anterior | Percent Frequency |
|---|---|---|
| Right and left hepatic ducts | Right hepatic artery | 12-15 |
| | Cystic artery | <5 |
| Common hepatic duct | Cystic artery | 15-24 |
| | Right hepatic artery | 11-19 |
| | Common hepatic artery | <5 |
| Supraduodenal common bile duct | Anterior artery to CBD | 50 |
| | Posterosuperior pancreaticoduodenal artery | 12.5 |
| | Gastroduodenal artery | 5.7-20* |
| | Right gastric artery | <5 |
| | Common hepatic artery | <5 |
| | Cystic artery | <5 |
| | Right hepatic artery | <5 |
| Retroduodenal common bile duct | Posterosuperior pancreaticoduodenal artery | 76-87.5 |
| | Supraduodenal artery | 11.4 |

*In another 36 percent, the gastroduodenal artery lay on the left border of the common bile duct (Maingot, 1974).
CBD, Common bile duct.

*Source:* Skandalakis JE, Gray SW, Rowe JS Jr. Anatomical Complications in General Surgery. New York: McGraw-Hill, 1983. Data from Johnston and Anson. Surg Gynecol Obstet 94:669, 1952, and others; with permission.

the ducts. The frequency with which they lie anterior to the ducts is summarized in Table 20-5.

## Cystic Duct

The cystic duct contains a series of 5 to 12 crescent-shaped folds of mucosa similar to those seen in the neck of the gallbladder. These form the so-called spiral valve of Heister. The length of the cystic duct and the manner in which it joins the common hepatic duct vary.

The pressure of secretion from the mucous glands in the cystic duct is higher than the secretion pressure of bile. The intracholecystic result of prolonged obstruction of the extrahepatic biliary tree proximal to the cystic duct is white "bile," composed only of mucus.

The cystic duct joins the hepatic duct at an angle of about 40° in 64-75% of individuals (Fig. 20-27A). In 17-23%, the cystic duct parallels the hepatic duct for a longer or shorter distance and may even enter the duodenum separately. This is called "absence" of the common bile duct, and is shown in Fig. 20-27F. In 8-13%, the cystic duct may pass inferior to or superior to the common hepatic duct to enter the latter on the left side[64-66] as shown in Figs. 20-27B, C. In the parallel type of junction, the common duct is at risk from the surgeon attempting to ligate the cystic duct. If the long parallel portion of the cystic duct is left in place, cystic duct remnant syndrome with various sequelae may result. Less frequently, the gallbladder is sessile

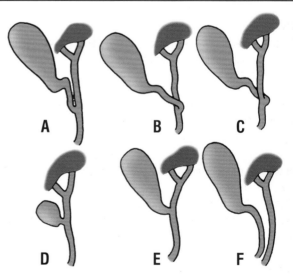

**A** **B** **C**

**D** **E** **F**

**FIG. 20-27.** Variations of cystic duct. **A,** Cystic duct parallels common bile duct before entering it. **B-C,** Cystic duct crosses common bile duct and enters it on left. **D-E,** Short cystic duct. **F,** Long cystic duct enters duodenum. This can also be called absence of common bile duct (separate entrance of common hepatic duct and cystic duct into duodenum). (Modified from Skandalakis JE, Gray SW. Embryology for Surgeons (2nd ed). Baltimore: Williams & Wilkins, 1994; with permission.)

with little or no cystic duct (Figs. 20-27D, E).

The cystic duct should be prepared well. The duct should be ligated such that it avoids a long cystic duct remnant, but at the same time avoiding ligation so close that the common bile duct is injured.

In his doctoral thesis about the cystic duct remnant and the postcholecystectomy syndrome, Droulias[16] concluded:

1. *A relatively long cystic duct remnant can be the cause of postcholecystectomy symptoms, sometimes quite severe, by being the site of chronic inflammation, lithiasis or neuroma formation. Rarely, it can cause kinking of the common bile duct or reflex spasm of Oddi.*

2. *Re-exploration and excision of the remnant is indicated after thorough study of the patient, provided the symptoms are severe enough to interfere with normal life and work.*

3. *Should the remnant be found quite long or diseased during re-operations on the biliary tree or pancreas it must be excised.*

4. *Prevention can be achieved by meticulous dissection of the cystic duct at cholecystectomy and ligation 2-3 mm from the junction with the common bile duct.*

5. *It seems probable that regeneration of the gallbladder after complete cholecystectomy in humans, dogs and monkeys does not take place.*

## Gallbladder

The gallbladder is 7-10 cm long and has a capacity of 30-50 ml. It is located on the visceral surface of the liver in a shallow fossa at the plane dividing the right lobe from the medial segment of the left lobe (the GB-IVC line). In other words, the gallbladder fossa is found at the junction of the quadrate lobe (segment IV) and the right lobe of the liver along the line of Rex. The gallbladder is separated from the liver by the connective tissue of Glisson's capsule. Anteriorly, the peritoneum of the gallbladder is continuous with that of the liver.

The gallbladder can be divided into fundus, body, infundibulum, neck, and cystic duct (Fig. 20-28). However, these divisions are arbitrary and imprecise; some classifications omit the infundibulum. From a surgical standpoint (when performing cholecystectomy, cholangiogram, etc.), it makes no difference which classification you choose. The following paragraphs describe the fundus, body, infundibulum, and neck; the cystic duct was described above.

**Fundus.** The fundus is usually located at the angle of the ninth costal cartilage with the right border of the rectus

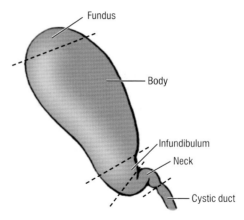

**Fig. 20-28.** Arbitrary divisions of gallbladder. (Modified from Skandalakis LJ, Gray SW, Colborn GL, Skandalakis JE. Surgical anatomy of the liver and associated extrahepatic structures. Part 4: Surgical anatomy of the hepatic vessels and the extrahepatic biliary tract. Contemp Surg 1987;31(1):25-36; with permission.)

sheath and to the left of the hepatic flexure of the colon. It is completely covered by peritoneum, because it projects beyond the lower border of the liver.

A partial folding of the fundus may result in the "Phrygian cap" deformity (Fig. 20-29A), named by Bartel[67] after the Greek term for the liberty cap, the widely used symbol of the French Revolution. Two to six percent of gallbladders have this shape. The deformation may or may not be visible from the outside. When seen radiographically, many cases appear to be caused by defective musculature of the fundus.[66] It was suggested that such gallbladders may be at higher risk for lithiasis,[68] but this has not been confirmed.

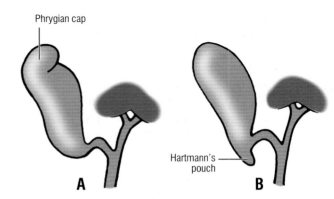

**Fig. 20-29.** Deformations of gallbladder. **A,** "Phrygian cap" deformity, showing partial folding of tip of fundus. **B,** Hartmann's pouch of infundibulum. (Modified from Skandalakis JE, Gray SW. Embryology for Surgeons (2nd ed). Baltimore: Williams & Wilkins, 1994; with permission.)

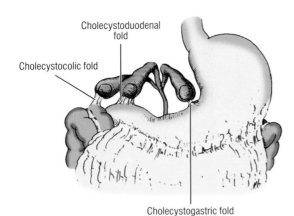

Cholecystoduodenal fold

Cholecystocolic fold

Cholecystogastric fold

FIG. 20-30. Inconstant or rare peritoneal folds of gallbladder to duodenum, colon, or stomach. Their presence is often associated with biliary fistulas. (Modified from Skandalakis JE, Gray SW, Skandalakis LJ. Surgical anatomy of intestinal obstruction. In: Fielding LP, Welch J (eds). Intestinal Obstruction. New York, Churchill Livingstone, 1987, pp. 14-32; with permission.)

BODY. The body of the gallbladder is in contact with the first and second portions of the duodenum and occupies the gallbladder fossa of the liver. The body is also related to the transverse colon. Only in the rare presence of a mesentery (wandering gallbladder), a prerequisite for acute torsion, is the body completely covered by peritoneum.

Occasionally in the operating room and in the laboratory, we have seen several inconstant or anomalous peritoneal (lesser omental) folds from the gallbladder to the duodenum, colon, or stomach (Fig. 20-30) in that order of frequency.

The peritoneal folds may be associated with the pathway of a large gallstone ulcerating from the gallbladder into the intestinal tract. The duodenal path is the most common; the gastric path is the rarest. We do not know if there is a relationship between these folds and the corresponding fistulous tracts of gallstone ileus. However, it is possible that the folds predispose to fistulas.[69]

INFUNDIBULUM. The infundibulum is the angulated posterior portion of the body between the neck and the point of entrance of the cystic artery. When this portion is dilated, with eccentric bulging of its medial aspect, it is called a Hartmann's pouch (Fig. 20-29B) (though it was originally described by Broca). Many have regarded it as a constant feature; Kaiser[70] considered it to be a normal constitutional characteristic of a short stocky habitus. Davies and Harding[71] have determined that it is consistently a sequela of pathological states, especially dilatation. It may be im-

portant to note that when this pouch achieves considerable size, the cystic duct arises from its upper left aspect rather than from what appears to be the apex of the gallbladder. The pouch is often associated with chronic or acute inflammation due to lithiasis and often accompanies a stone impacted in the infundibulum.

NECK. The narrow neck (cervix) curves up and forward and then sharply back and downward forming an S to become the cystic duct. The junction of the neck and the cystic duct is said to be indicated by a constriction.[72] The cystic artery is found in this region coursing in the loose connective tissue that attaches the neck of the gallbladder to the liver.

The mucosa lining the neck is a spiral ridge said to be a spiral valve, but not to be confused with the spiral valve of the cystic duct (the valve of Heister). When the neck becomes distended, this spiral gives its surface a spiral groove. The neck lies in the free border of the hepatoduodenal ligament. The ridges of the valve of Heister, in addition to the previously mentioned constriction, interfere with the passage of an instrument and may stop the passage of gallstones.

Following removal of the gallbladder, there is sometimes leakage of bile from small bile ducts in the gallbladder bed. (There has been disagreement as to whether these ducts [hepatocystic ducts] enter the gallbladder. Michels[44] was unable to find such ducts in his 500 carefully dissected specimens. He found branches from the right hepatic duct in the gallbladder bed but the branches did not communicate with the gallbladder.) The small bile ducts may cause postoperative bile leakage if they are injured.

Lindner and Green[73] and Wayson and Foster[74] expressed opposing views on the existence of hepatocystic ducts, citing personal experience and hepatic embryology to prove their cases. Because the presence of a cystic vein is an extremely rare phenomenon, Lindner and Green state that there are multiple small veins that drain into the liver parenchyma. They indicate that minute bile canaliculi may drain directly from the hepatic parenchyma into the gallbladder. Wayson and Foster considered these vessels to be postinflammatory artifacts.

### Common Bile Duct (Ductus Choledochus)

The common bile duct begins at the union of the cystic and common hepatic ducts and ends at the papilla of Vater in the second part of the duodenum. It varies in length from 5 cm to 15 cm, depending on the actual position of the ductal union. In 22%, the common hepatic and cystic ducts, on average, run parallel for 17 mm before the ducts actually unite.[66] The average diameter is about 6 mm.

The common bile duct can be divided into four portions

or segments (Fig. 20-31): supraduodenal, retroduodenal, pancreatic, and intramural.

The *supraduodenal portion* of the common bile duct lies between the layers of the hepatoduodenal ligament in front of the epiploic foramen of Winslow, to the right or left of the hepatic artery, and anterior to the portal vein. Its length is 2-5 cm.[73]

The distal part of the supraduodenal portion is related to the posterior superior pancreaticoduodenal (PSPD) artery, which has a retroduodenal location and which crosses the duct first anteriorly and then posteriorly. This artery is not to be confused with the supraduodenal artery, which also may pass anterior to the common bile duct. In the majority of cases the retroportal artery joins the PSPD artery, but it may join the right hepatic artery directly and send branches to the common duct en route. The PSPD artery is easily injured while exploring the common duct.[44]

If the junction of the cystic and common hepatic ducts is low, the supraduodenal segment is short or even absent. Large lymph nodes may be fixed to the right side of the supraduodenal segment.

The *retroduodenal portion* of the common bile duct is between the superior margin of the first portion of the duodenum and the superior margin of the head of the pancreas. It is 1-3.5 cm long. The duct may be free or partially fixed to the duodenum.

The gastroduodenal artery lies to the left. The PSPD artery lies anterior to the common bile duct. The middle colic artery lies anterior to the common bile duct and other arteries.

Prudhomme et al.[75] reported the following relationships of the bile duct and retroduodenal arteries after studying 35 bloc specimens of normal cadavers.

*The distances between the gastroduodenal artery (GDA), the pylorus, and the bile duct were measured in the sagittal plane. The origin and course of the posterior superior pancreaticoduodenal artery (PSPD) in relation to the bile duct were studied. The relation of the GDA and the bile duct were divisible into four types: in Type 1 (n=22) the two structures separated progressively, the artery being on the left of the bile ducts; in Type 2: (n=7) the structures approached each other without crossing; Type 3: (n=5) the GDA crossed in front of the bile duct at the level of the first part of the duodenum (D1); Type 4: (n=1) the GDA crossed the bile duct below D1 and ran along its right border. The PSPD originated at the posterior face of D1 in 20% of cases (n=7) and crossed the anterior surface of the bile duct at the posterior surface of D1. In four cases there was no pancreatic tissue between the PSPD and the bile duct. It follows that the risk of injury to the bile duct when securing hemostasis by transfixing a bleed-*

*ing duodenal ulcer in the D1 segment is great when the arterial structures (GDA and PSPD) cross the bile duct. This risk is increased when there is no pancreatic tissue between them.*

Dorrance et al.[76] reported that acquired absence of the cystic duct secondary to inflammatory process of an impacted gallstone in Hartmann's pouch may occur with some frequency. Therefore, the surgeon should be extremely careful to avoid injuring the common bile duct. However, a problem remains if the cystic duct is congenitally absent or has become obliterated secondary to inflammatory processes.

The *pancreatic portion* of the common bile duct extends from the upper margin of the head of the pancreas to the point of entrance into the duodenum. It passes downward to the right, posterior to the pancreas or within the pancreatic parenchyma.

From a series of 200 specimens, Smanio[77] described five patterns of the relation of the common bile duct and the pancreas (Fig. 20-32). Other variations include a prepancreatic common bile duct; seven cases were found among 550 bodies examined.[44] The senior author of this chapter (JES) has seen a case in which the bile duct was

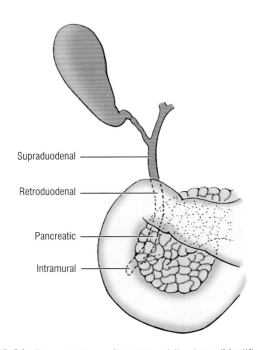

**FIG. 20-31.** Four portions of common bile duct. (Modified from Skandalakis LJ, Gray SW, Colborn GL, Skandalakis JE. Surgical anatomy of the liver and associated extrahepatic structures. Part 4: Surgical anatomy of the hepatic vessels and the extrahepatic biliary tract. Contemp Surg 1987;31(1):25-36; with permission.)

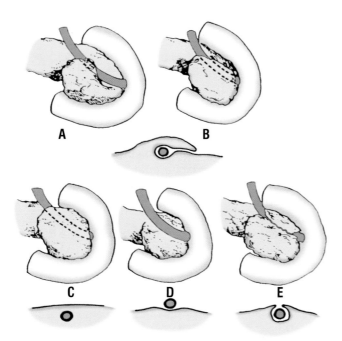

FIG. 20-32. Five variations of third portion of common bile duct to pancreas. **A-B,** Bile duct partially covered by tongue of pancreatic tissue (44%). **C,** Bile duct completely covered by pancreas (30%). **D,** Bile duct completely uncovered. It lies on posterior surface of pancreas (16.5%). **E,** Bile duct covered by two tongues of pancreatic tissue (9%). (After Smanio T. Varying relations of the common bile duct with the posterior face of the pancreas in negroes and white persons. J Int Coll Surg 1954;22:150-173. Modified from Skandalakis JE, Gray SW. Embryology for Surgeons, 2nd ed. Baltimore: Williams & Wilkins, 1994; with permission.)

The common bile duct and the pancreatic duct end at the papilla of Vater on the posteromedial wall of the second part of the duodenum, just to the right of the second or third lumbar vertebra. Rarely, the bile duct enters at another location (Fig. 20-34).

Variations in the distance between the pancreaticobiliary junction and the tip of the papilla are the result of developmental processes.[81] In the embryo, the main pancreatic duct arises as a branch of the common bile duct that, in turn, arises from the duodenum. As the duodenum increases in size, it absorbs the proximal bile duct up to its junction with the pancreatic duct. When the resorption is minimal, there is a long ampulla and the junction is high or even extramural. Increased resorption shortens the ampulla; maximum resorption results in separate orifices for the common bile and pancreatic ducts. Michels[44] classified the types of junctions, as shown in Figure 20-35.

Opie[82] suggested that a gallstone impacted in the papilla might, in the presence of a long ampulla, permit bile to reflux into the pancreatic duct and produce pancreatitis. This "common channel" theory was supported by Dragstedt and colleagues[83] and revived by Doubilet and Mulholland.[84] Silen[85] questioned the frequency of this cause of pancreatitis. He observed that the pancreatic secretory pressure is usually higher than that of the liver. Although reflux pancreatitis is real, the frequency of its origin from

completely extrapancreatic and near the renal vein.

The PSPD artery crosses the pancreatic portion of the common bile duct. It first passes ventral to the duct at the point of origin of the artery from the gastroduodenal artery, and then passes dorsal to the duct just before the latter reaches the pancreas.

The duct may be in intimate contact with the duodenum for 0.8-2.2 cm before entering the wall.[78] Lytle[79] reported that the pancreatic groove or tunnel occupied by the duct may be palpated using the Kocher maneuver. The groove is located in front of the right renal vein.

The *intramural portion* of the common bile duct takes an oblique path averaging 1.5 cm through the duodenal wall[80] (Fig. 20-33). Here it receives the main pancreatic duct inferiorly. The two ducts usually lie side-by-side with a common adventitia for several millimeters. The diameter of both ducts decreases within the duodenal wall.[80] The septum between the ducts is reduced to a thin mucosal membrane before the ducts become confluent.

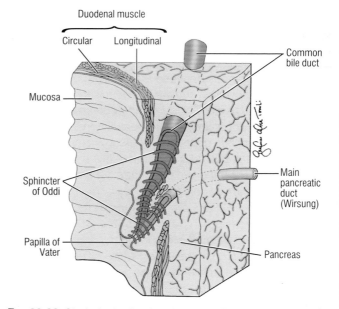

FIG. 20-33. Choledochoduodenal junction. The sphincteric muscle is predominately circular in orientation. It extends beyond the wall of the duodenum and for a short distance along the pancreatic duct. (After Toouli J. Sphincter of Oddi motility. Br J Surg 1984;71:251-256; with permission.)

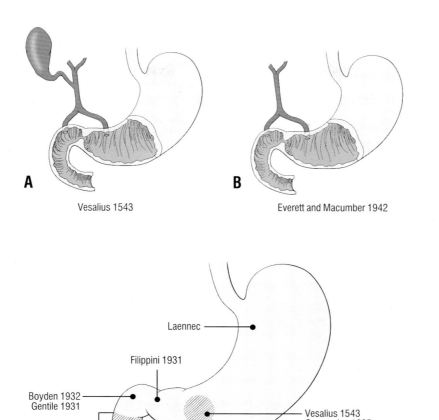

**FIG. 20-34.** Duplication of common bile duct. One duct enters stomach. **A,** Case of Vesalius.[230] **B,** Case of Everett and Macumber.[231] Gallbladder and cystic duct absent. **C,** Sites of ectopic openings of common bile duct.[232]

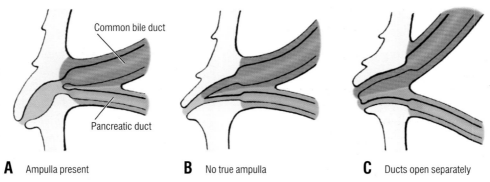

**FIG. 20-35.** Variations of opening of common bile duct and pancreatic duct into duodenum. **A,** Junction of ducts is high. Common channel may or may not be dilated to form ampulla (85%). **B,** Common channel is short. No ampulla present (5%). **C,** Common bile and pancreatic ducts enter duodenum separately. No ampulla present (9%). (Modified from Skandalakis LJ, Gray SW, Colborn GL, Skandalakis JE. Surgical anatomy of the liver and associated extrahepatic structures. Part 4: Surgical anatomy of the hepatic vessels and the extrahepatic biliary tract. Contemp Surg 1987;31(1):25-36; with permission.)

ampullary obstruction is still controversial and largely unsupported by animal models.

Fuzhou et al.[86] reported that anomalous junction of pancreaticobiliary ducts (AJPB) is related to pancreatitis. They conclude that AJPB is an anatomic factor inducing pancreatitis. Another study by Fuzhou et al.[87] found that endoscopic nasobiliary drainage (ENBD) can prevent the development of severe acute pancreatitis in patients with mild acute pancreatitis. A thin tube is inserted into the bile duct with the help of a duodenoscope (Fig. 20-36A). According to the researchers, the gallstones leave the common pancreaticobiliary channels (Fig. 20-36B), and the bile drains directly into the duodenum (Fig. 20-36C). They speculate that because the tube curves in a U-shaped course around the ampulla of Vater (Fig. 20-36D), the tube pulls the ampulla to relieve its obstruction resulting from edema, inflammation, or stricture.

Richer et al.[88] advised that a long common channel in excess of 15 mm is associated with a higher incidence of carcinoma of the gallbladder or the bile duct.

## Vessels of the Gallbladder and Biliary Tract

### Arteries

The cystic artery usually arises from the right hepatic artery as it traverses the hepatocystic triangle to the right of the common hepatic duct (Fig. 20-37A). The lymph node of Calot usually lies just superficial to the position of the cystic artery in the cystic triangle, and can be a good guide to finding and ligating it. Reaching the gallbladder behind the common hepatic duct, the cystic artery usually branches into an anterior superficial branch and a posterior deep branch. These branches anastomose and send arterial twigs to the adjacent liver. Remember in this context that in approximately one third of cases the right hepatic artery arises from the superior mesenteric artery. The cystic artery may arise from the left hepatic artery (Fig. 20-37B) or the gastroduodenal artery (Fig. 20-37C).

In approximately 25% of subjects, the superficial and deep branches arise separately (Fig. 20-37D). The deep branch usually comes from the right hepatic artery, but two of the authors of this chapter (GLC and JES) have observed a number of cases in which it arose directly from the superior mesenteric artery. The superficial branch may spring from the right hepatic, left hepatic, gastroduodenal, or retroduodenal artery.[89] Each possible origin and its frequency are shown in Table 20-6.

In an exhaustive study of the cystic artery, Michels[44] described 12 types of double cystic arteries; consult his book for details. Less common than duplications is a recurrence of the superficial branch. The artery first supplies the fundus, then turns downward to branch over the body of the gallbladder[90] as shown in Figs. 20-37D, E.

Again we wish to quote Van Damme.[47] This time we present his beautiful description of the behavior of the cystic artery.

*The behavior of the cystic artery can be summarized using the following three general rules.*

- *A cystic artery arising to the right of the bile ducts from the right hepatic branch is found in the triangle between the hepatic and cystic ducts.*
- *A second cystic artery that arises to the left of the bile ducts usually runs anterior to the bile ducts.*
- *If the posterior pancreaticoduodenal arcade arises from a normal gastroduodenal artery, it lies in front of the ductus choledochus. If it arises from a vessel behind the pancreatic head, it also passes behind the ductus choledochus. This is important to remember during choledochotomy and pancreaticoduodenectomy.*

Balija et al.[91] presented a laparoscopic visualization and classification of the cystic artery (Figs. 20-38 to 20-42).

Chen et al.[92] reported autopsy findings on the origin and course of the cystic artery:

*The cystic artery arises from many possible origins; the right hepatic artery is the most common origin (76.6%). The Calot triangle (hepatocystic triangle), which is an important imaginary referent area for biliary surgery, is bounded by the common hepatic duct (CHD), the cystic duct, and the cystic artery. Of all the cystic arteries, 86.1% coursed through the Calot triangle, and 100% of the cystic arteries originating from the right hepatic artery coursed through the Calot triangle. However, only 54% of the cystic arteries that originated from the left, bifurcation, proper, and common hepatic arteries ran through the triangle. None of the cystic arteries that originated from the gastroduodenal, celiac, superior mesentery, or superior pancreaticoduodenal arteries passed through the triangle. Furthermore, 72.7% of the cystic arteries that originated from the right hepatic artery ran beneath the CHD as they entered the Calot triangle; the others ran anterior to the CHD. Of the cystic arteries that arose from locations other than the right hepatic artery, 29.4% ran posterior to the CHD, and 11.8% ran anterior to the CHD.*

The extrahepatic bile ducts in most individuals are supplied from the cystic artery above and from the posterior superior pancreaticoduodenal artery below. Shapiro and

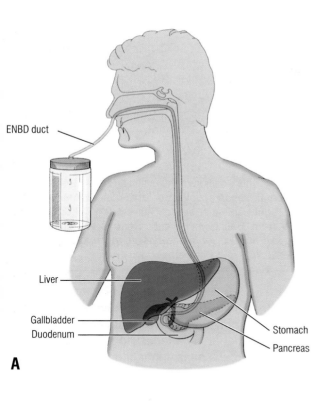

ENBD duct

Liver

Gallbladder
Duodenum

Stomach
Pancreas

**A**

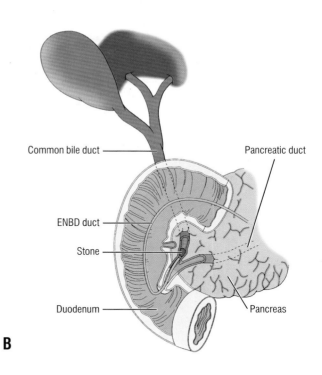

Common bile duct

Pancreatic duct

ENBD duct

Stone

Duodenum

Pancreas

**B**

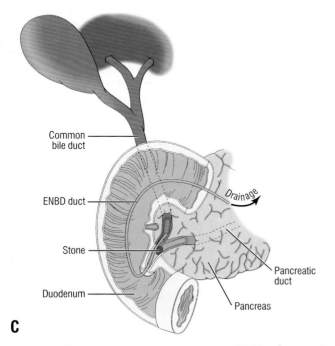

Common
bile duct

ENBD duct

Stone

Duodenum

Drainage

Pancreatic
duct

Pancreas

**C**

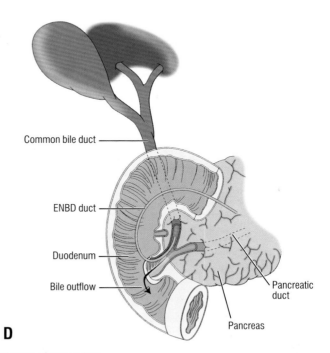

Common bile duct

ENBD duct

Duodenum

Bile outflow

Pancreatic
duct

Pancreas

**D**

FIG. 20-36. Endoscopic nasobiliary drainage (ENBD). See text for description of procedure.

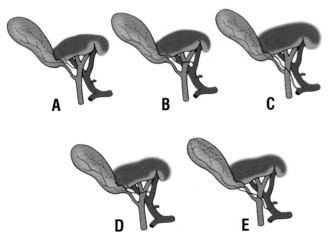

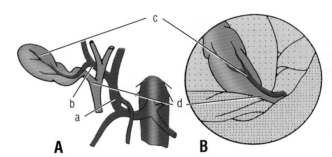

**FIG. 20-37.** Variations of origin and course of cystic artery. **A,** Cystic artery arises from right hepatic artery (74.7%). **B,** Cystic artery arises from left hepatic artery and passes anterior to common hepatic duct (20.5%). **C,** Cystic artery arises from gastroduodenal artery (2.5%). **D-E,** Recurrent cystic arteries reach fundus of gallbladder and descend toward neck (rare). In the remainder (approximately 2.3%, not shown), cystic artery arises from a variety of other arteries. (Modified from Skandalakis LJ, Gray SW, Colborn GL, Skandalakis JE. Surgical anatomy of the liver and associated extrahepatic structures. Part 4: Surgical anatomy of the hepatic vessels and the extrahepatic biliary tract. Contemp Surg 1987;31(1):25-36; with permission.)

**FIG. 20-38.** Normal position of the cystic artery. **A,** Conventional visualization. **B,** Laparoscopic visualization. a, Common hepatic artery; b, Right hepatic artery; c, Cystic artery; d, Cystic duct. (Modified from Balija M, Huis M, Nikolię V, Stulhofer M. Laparoscopic visualization of the cystic artery anatomy. World J Surg 1999;23:703-707; with permission.)

Robillard[93] described several variations in this pattern. The upper supply from the cystic artery is relatively constant. The lower supply may be from the hepatic, gastroduodenal, or supraduodenal arteries.

The epicholedochal arterial plexus of the common bile duct is derived from the retroduodenal or posterior superior pancreaticoduodenal arteries[94] (Figs. 20-43, 20-44). The collateral circulation is enhanced by two intramural plexuses (Fig. 20-45). These may be compressed between the edematous mucosa and the external tough fibrous coat in pathologic conditions such as cholangitis or common bile duct obstruction secondary to choledocholithiasis. Appleby[95] emphasized that the surface of the common bile duct should be protected to prevent iatrogenic ischemia as well as to avoid venous bleeding.

### Veins

The hepatic surface of the gallbladder is drained by numerous small veins passing through the gallbladder bed that break up into capillaries within the liver. They do not

**TABLE 20-6. Origin of the Cystic Artery**

| Origin | Anson (676) | Michels (200) | Moosman (482) |
|---|---|---|---|
| | | Percent | |
| Right hepatic artery | | | |
|   Normal | 61.4 | 76 | 72 |
|   Aberrant (accessory) | 10.2 | 13.5 | 15 |
|   Aberrant (replacing) | 3.1 | — | — |
| Left hepatic artery | 5.9 | 4 | 3 |
| Common hepatic artery | 14.9* | 3 | 5 |
| Gastroduodenal artery | 2.5 | 4 | 2 |
| Other | 1.0 | rare | 3 |
| | 100.5 | 99 | 100 |

*Includes "bifurcation" of artery.

*Source:* Skandalakis LJ, Gray SW, Colborn GL, Skandalakis JE. Surgical anatomy of the liver and associated extrahepatic structures. Contemp Surg 31(4):25-36, 1987; with permission.

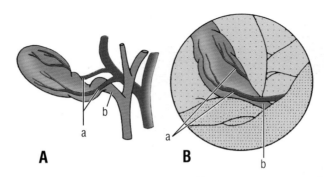

**FIG. 20-39.** Double cystic artery. **A,** Conventional visualization. **B,** Laparoscopic visualization. a, Double cystic arteries; b, Cystic duct. (Modified from Balija M, Huis M, Nikolię V, Stulhofer M. Laparoscopic visualization of the cystic artery anatomy. World J Surg 1999;23:703-707; with permission.)

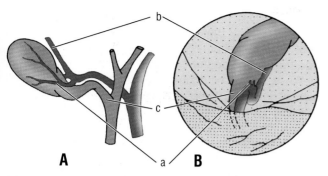

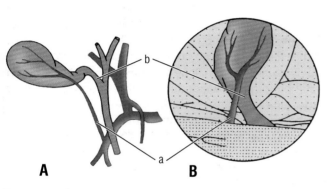

**FIG. 20-40.** "Large cystic artery." **A,** Conventional visualization. **B,** Laparoscopic visualization. a, Cystic artery (or cystic arteries); b, Aberrant right hepatic artery; c, Cystic duct. (Modified from Balija M, Huis M, Nikolić V, Štulhofer M. Laparoscopic visualization of the cystic artery anatomy. World J Surg 1999;23:703-707; with permission.)

**FIG. 20-41.** Cystic artery originating from the gastroduodenal artery. **A,** Conventional visualization. **B,** Laparoscopic visualization. a, Cystic artery; b, Cystic duct. (Modified from Balija M, Huis M, Nikolić V, Štulhofer M. Laparoscopic visualization of the cystic artery anatomy. World J Surg 1999; 23:703-707; with permission.)

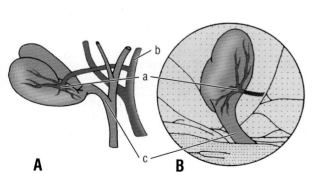

**FIG. 20-42.** Cystic artery originating from the left hepatic artery. **A,** Conventional visualization. **B,** Laparoscopic visualization. a, Cystic artery originating from the left hepatic artery; b, Left hepatic artery; c, Cystic duct. (Modified from Balija M, Huis M, Nikolić V, Štulhofer M. Laparoscopic visualization of the cystic artery anatomy. World J Surg 1999;23:703-707; with permission.)

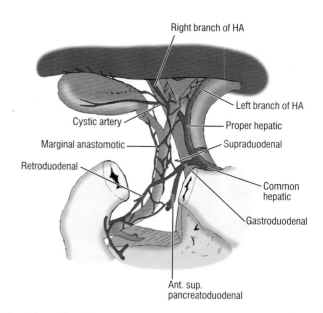

**FIG. 20-43.** Arterial blood supply of extrahepatic biliary tract showing epicholedochal arterial plexus. HA, Hepatic artery. (Modified from Toouli J (ed). Surgery of the Biliary Tract. New York: Churchill Livingstone, 1993; with permission.)

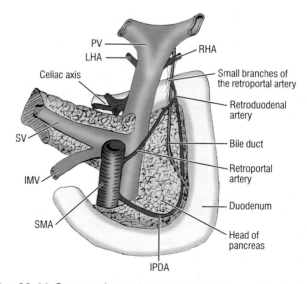

**FIG. 20-44.** Course of retroduodenal and retroportal arteries (posterior view). PV, Portal vein. LHA, Left hepatic artery. RHA, Right hepatic artery. SV, Splenic vein. IMV, Inferior mesenteric vein. SMA, Superior mesenteric artery. IPDA, Inferior pancreaticoduodenal artery. (Modified from Toouli J (ed). Surgery of the Biliary Tract. New York: Churchill Livingstone, 1993; with permission.)

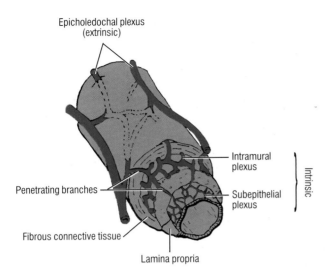

FIG. 20-45. Arterial blood supply of extrahepatic biliary tract showing epicholedochal arterial plexus. (Modified from Toouli J (ed). Surgery of the Biliary Tract. New York: Churchill Livingstone, 1993; with permission.)

form a single "cystic vein." Veins from the hepatic surface drain directly into the liver. Veins on the free surface open directly or follow the hepatic ducts into the liver.

From the peritoneal surface, one vein usually drains the fundus and body and other veins drain the neck and upper portions of the cystic duct as well as the hepatic ducts. These small veins enter the liver together with ascending veins from the common bile duct[96] as shown in Fig. 20-46. These veins rarely open into extrahepatic portal veins.[97] This is not an important portosystemic shunt.

Sugita et al.[98] recommended the use of computed tomography during angiography to detect cystic vein inflow portions of the intrahepatic vessels, identifying possible areas of micrometastasis of gallbladder cancer.

## Lymphatics of the Biliary Tract

The lymphatic drainage of the gallbladder has been well documented from the studies by Clermont,[99] Rouviere,[100] Fahim and colleagues,[101] and Ito et al.[102]

Long collecting trunks drain the lymphatic plexus of the fundus and body of the gallbladder (Figs. 20-47 and 20-48). The trunks are on the right and left borders (lateral and medial borders of the gallbladder wall) and are connected by an oblique trunk to form a large "N" on the surface. The trunks on the left drain into the cystic node, which lies in the angle formed by the cystic and common hepatic ducts. The trunks on the right follow the cystic duct, passing without entering the cystic node. These vessels and the ef-

ferent vessels of the cystic node drain to the node of the anterior border of the epiploic foramen, called the "hiatal node" by Fahim et al.,[101] and to the superior pancreaticoduodenal nodes on the common bile duct. As shown in Fig. 20-48, there is no drainage upward to the liver.[99] For all practical purposes, lymphatics of the gallbladder and hepatic ducts have the same lymphatic drainage.

Ito et al.[102] divided the lymphatic drainage of the gallbladder into the following three pathways.

• The cholecystoretropancreatic pathway is the main pathway. It terminates in a large node at the retroportal segment, designated as the principal retroportal lymph node.

• The cholecystoceliac pathway at the left of the hepatoduodenal ligament ends at the celiac nodes.

• The cholecystomesenteric pathway passes to the left and front of the portal vein and terminates at the superior mesenteric lymph nodes.

Near the left renal vein all pathways converge with the abdomino-aortic lymph nodes.

The hiatal node also drains the wall of the extrahepatic bile ducts and the right lobe of the liver. It, in turn, drains to the superior pancreaticoduodenal node. From the latter node, efferents pass to preaortic and celiac nodes or, by way of several small posterior pancreaticoduodenal nodes, to reach nodes at the origin of the superior mesenteric artery from the aorta.

Enlarged metastatic lymph nodes may cause jaundice by obstructing the common bile duct.[45] However, the likelihood of this is minimized by some writers.[103]

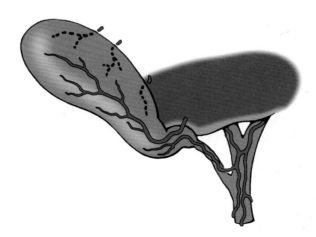

FIG. 20-46. Venous drainage of gallbladder and cystic duct. (Modified from Skandalakis LJ, Gray SW, Colborn GL, Skandalakis JE. Surgical anatomy of the liver and associated extrahepatic structures. Part 4: Surgical anatomy of the hepatic vessels and the extrahepatic biliary tract. Contemp Surg 1987;31(1):25-36; with permission.)

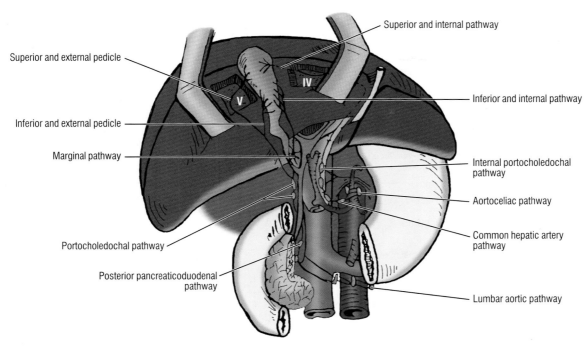

**FIG. 20-47.** Intra- and extrahepatic lymphatic drainage of gallbladder. (Modified from Toouli J (ed). Surgery of the Biliary Tract. New York: Churchill Livingstone, 1993; with permission.)

Kurosaki et al.[104] reported the following results about the mode of lymphatic spread in carcinoma of the bile duct.

*The frequency of lymphatic spread of carcinomas in the proximal, middle, and distal bile ducts, excluding seven T1 tumors, was 48%, 67%, and 56%, respectively. With regard to the mode of lymphatic spread: (1) a metastatic pathway along the common hepatic artery predominated over that to the retropancreatic area in the proximal duct carcinoma group; (2) in the middle duct carcinoma group, metastatic lymph nodes were distributed widely, involving nodes around the superior mesenteric artery or at the para-aortic area; and (3) in the distal duct carcinoma group, metastatic nodes generally were localized around the head of the pancreas (Figs. 20-49, 20-50).*

Malignancy of the hepatic duct confluence was studied by Jarnagin et al.[105] Since complete excision of tumors in this area is not always possible, various palliative measures must be considered. Doglietto et al.[106] found palliative endoscopic stenting a safe and efficient procedure for inoperable extrahepatic bile duct cancer. Kobayashi et al.[107] found that residual bile duct carcinoma occurred in patients with pancreaticobiliary maljunction who had undergone excision of extrahepatic bile ducts, and recommended careful long-term follow-up.

# Innervation of the Gallbladder and Biliary Tract

Parasympathetic (vagal) and general visceral sensory fibers from the hepatic division of the anterior vagal trunk

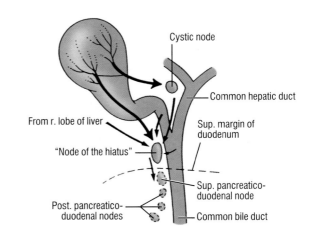

**FIG. 20-48.** Lymphatic drainage of gallbladder and biliary tract. Left lateral wall of gallbladder drains to cystic node and then to "node of the hiatus." Right lateral wall drains directly to hiatal node. (Modified from Skandalakis JE, Gray SW, Rowe JS Jr. Anatomical Complications in General Surgery. New York: McGraw-Hill, 1983; with permission.)

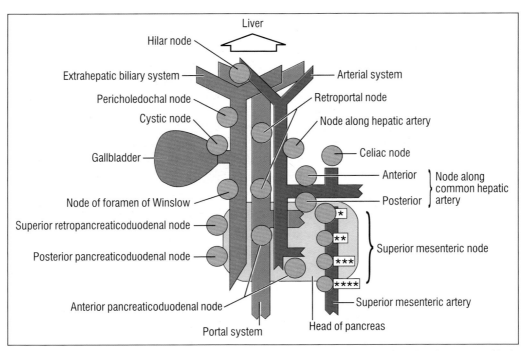

**FIG. 20-49.** Anatomic configuration of lymph nodes around head of pancreas and in hepatoduodenal ligament. Nodes along superior mesenteric artery are subdivided into four groups: * Node near origin of superior mesenteric artery; ** Node around origin of inferior pancreaticoduodenal artery; *** Node around origin of middle colic artery; **** Node around origin of first jejunal artery. (Modified from Kurosaki I, Tsukada K, Hatakeyama K, Muto T. The mode of lymphatic spread in carcinoma of the bile duct. Am J Surg 1996;172:239-243; with permission.)

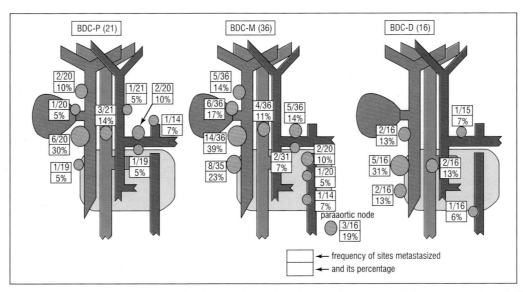

**FIG. 20-50.** Comparison of modes of lymphatic spread according to location of primary tumor (T1 tumors excluded). BDC-P, Proximal bile duct carcinoma. BDC-M, Middle bile duct carcinoma. BDC-D, Distal bile duct carcinoma. (Modified from Kurosaki I, Tsukada K, Hatakeyama K, Muto T. The mode of lymphatic spread in carcinoma of the bile duct. Am J Surg 1996;172:239-243; with permission.)

and the celiac division of the posterior vagal trunk follow the hepatic artery and its branches to the extrahepatic bile ducts and the gallbladder.

Preganglionic sympathetics and visceral afferent fibers for pain reach the celiac plexus by way of the greater thoracic splanchnic nerves. The autonomic fibers synapse in the celiac ganglia, and postganglionic and sensory fibers pass into the hepatic plexuses to reach the liver.

Fibers from the right phrenic nerve travel by way of the phrenic, celiac, and hepatic plexuses to reach the gallbladder. Many of these fibers are afferent and may account for the pain referred to the right hypochondrium and radiating to the back between the shoulder blades in some patients with gallbladder diseases.

Burnett and associates[108] demonstrated three nerve plexuses: subserous, muscular, and mucosal. The ganglion cells in each nerve plexus decrease in number from subserous to mucosal levels. In comparison with the myenteric plexus of the gut, the subserous plexus ganglia are larger and spaced farther apart. In spite of this well developed nerve supply, there are relatively few smooth muscle cells in the ducts.[109] Petkov[110] reported a distinct nerve to the sphincter of the common bile duct in 92% of the cases he studied.

## Hepatocystic Triangle, Triangle of Calot, and Area of Moosman

The hepatocystic triangle is formed by the proximal part of the gallbladder and cystic duct to the right, the common hepatic duct to the left, and the margin of the right lobe of the liver superiorly. The triangle originally described by Calot[111] defined the upper boundary as the cystic artery. The area included in the triangle has enlarged over the years[112] as shown in Fig. 20-51. The area of Moosman[113] is a circular area 30 mm in diameter; it fits into the hepatocystic duct angle.[114]

Within the boundaries of the triangle as it is now defined and of Moosman's area are several structures that must be identified before they are ligated and sectioned: the right hepatic artery, common bile duct, aberrant hepatic artery (if present), and cystic artery.

After its origin from the proper hepatic, the right hepatic artery enters the hepatocystic triangle by crossing posterior to the common hepatic duct in 85% of cases. The right hepatic artery or one of its branches passes anterior to the duct in 15%.[44,51] It lies parallel with the cystic duct for a short distance, then turns upward to enter the liver. Saint[115] emphasized the presence of an epicholodochal venous plexus that helps the surgeon to

identify the common bile duct. There is no such venous plexus on the surface of the cystic duct. The right hepatic artery lay within 1 cm of the duct in 20% of cadavers examined by Moosman[116] and might have been mistaken for the cystic artery. As a general rule, no artery more than 0.3 cm in diameter in the triangle will be a cystic artery.

An aberrant right hepatic artery was present in 18% of Moosman's[116] specimens. In 83% of these, the aberrant artery gave rise to the cystic artery within the triangle.

In most individuals (96%), the cystic artery is found in the hepatocystic triangle.[116] In 80%, the origin of the artery from a normal or aberrant right hepatic artery is within the triangle.[44] In a few cases, the origin of the right hepatic artery is to the left of the common hepatic duct. Hence, it enters the triangle by passing in front of the duct. A similar course is followed in the rare cases in which the cystic artery originates in the left hepatic artery. Where the artery arises from the common hepatic artery or gastroduodenal artery, it enters the triangle from below.

Among 220 cadavers examined by Michels,[44] the cystic artery was double in 50 and triple in one. Michels described 20 possible patterns of the origin of double cystic arteries. Three of the possible arrangements have never been reported.

Bergamaschi and Ignjatovic[117] reported on the surgical ramifications of the occurrence of multiple anatomic structures within Calot's triangle. Inadvertent ligation of variant

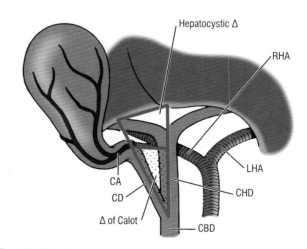

FIG. 20-51. Hepatocystic triangle and triangle of Calot. Upper boundary of hepatocystic triangle is inferior border of liver. CA, Cystic artery. CD, Cystic duct. CHD, Common hepatic duct. CBD, Common bile duct. LHA/RHA, Left and right hepatic arteries. (Modified from Skandalakis JE, Gray SW, Rowe JS Jr. Anatomical Complications in General Surgery. New York: McGraw-Hill, 1983; with permission.)

veins or bile ducts may complicate laparoscopic cholecystectomy.

Stremple[114] estimated that 85% of all variations in the hepatic pedicle are found in Moosman's area, and 50% of these variations are a potential hazard during cholecystectomy.

## HISTOLOGY

The bile ducts are composed of an external fibrous layer of connective tissue, a few thin smooth muscle layers (longitudinal, oblique, and circular), and an internal layer of mucosa of columnar epithelium.

Opening into the cystic duct are the true ducts of Luschka. These are found in the connective tissue between the neck of the gallbladder and liver, but they open into the lumen of the cystic duct, not that of the gallbladder. These are histologically the same as intrahepatic bile ducts and may be the remnants of aberrant embryonic ducts.

The gallbladder wall is formed, from external to internal, by the following layers:
- Serosa
- Adventitia
- Fibromuscular layers
- Mucosa

Serosa is the typical visceral peritoneum formed by mesothelium on the surface with loose connective tissue directly beneath.

Adventitia is a layer of dense connective tissue that is found external to the muscularis externa where the gallbladder is attached to the surface of the liver. The adventitia contains large blood vessels, autonomic fibers for innervation of muscularis externa and blood vessels, a rich lymphatic network, and a plethora of elastic fibers and adipose tissue.

Fibromuscular layers comprise many elastic and collagen fibers among bundles of smooth muscle cells. No muscularis mucosa or submucosa is found in the gallbladder.

Mucosa is distinguished by having very tall, slender columnar epithelial cells. While no glands are found in the mucosa, this layer is thrown into elaborate folds which on first inspection give the impression of glands. These folds form deep diverticula of the mucosa and have been identified as "Rokitansky-Aschoff sinuses"; in some cases, these extend through the muscularis externa. Bacteria have been known to accumulate in these folds, and chronic inflammation may develop.

## PHYSIOLOGY

Bile, produced by hepatocytes, drains into the hepatic canaliculi. It travels from the terminal bile ducts to the right and left hepatic ducts. Then it moves to the common hepatic duct. The majority of the bile goes from the common hepatic duct through the cystic duct to the gallbladder, drains to the common bile duct, and then to the duodenum. The remainder of the bile goes to the common bile duct, then to the duodenum, bypassing the gallbladder.

Bile production is such that 250 ml to 1,500 ml of bile enters the duodenum each day. The gallbladder has a capacity ranging from 15 to 60 ml (average approximately 35 ml). The gallbladder concentrates bile by absorbing sodium, chloride, and bicarbonate ions and water such that bile salts can be concentrated 5 to 250 times. Potassium ions are concentrated as the water is absorbed; further concentration results from simple diffusion. Bile contains significant amounts of carbonate and calcium ions. The epithelium secretes hydrogen ions, and the carbonate ions are converted to bicarbonate. Calcium and bicarbonate ions are absorbed by the epithelial cells and, thus, calcium carbonate precipitation in the gallbladder is avoided.

The hormone cholecystokinin causes contraction of the gallbladder muscle, forcing bile out. Stimulation from the vagus nerve also causes the gallbladder to contract. The sphincteric apparatus of Oddi becomes inhibited in the presence of cholecystokinin and relaxes as a reaction to gallbladder contraction.[118] All of these actions force bile into the common bile duct and the duodenum.

## SURGERY OF THE EXTRAHEPATIC BILIARY TRACT AND GALLBLADDER

Prior to surgery, if possible, the gallbladder should be studied and diagnosis of the disease should be made using some of the following tools:
- Abdominal x-rays
- Oral cholecystogram
- Abdominal ultrasonography
- Hepatobiliary scintigraph

While transabdominal ultrasonography will demonstrate polypoid lesions of the gallbladder, Azuma and colleagues[119] recommend endoscopic ultrasonography for differential diagnosis of gallbladder polyps.

## Exploration of the Gallbladder and Ducts

To explore the gallbladder and ducts first inspect and palpate the liver. Then place the patient in a reversed Trendelenburg position to permit the viscera to descend. Gallstones in the gallbladder can be felt because they will be in the most dependent position.

When the hepatic triad and lesser omentum are palpated, enlarged lymph nodes may be found. Large stones in the common bile duct can occasionally be felt. Tumors of the porta hepatis or of the head of the pancreas can be discovered with careful palpation. The pulsation of the hepatic artery and a normal or dilated common bile duct can be seen. Remember that obstruction can be present without dilatation of the duct.[120]

To palpate the distal common bile duct, kocherization of the duodenum is necessary. This is accomplished by mobilizing the hepatic flexure of the colon and incising the peritoneum lateral to the second part of the duodenum. The left index and middle fingers are inserted posteriorly while the left thumb is positioned anteriorly. In this way, the common duct and a possible stone or tumor can be palpated, and the duodenum and the head of the pancreas can be evaluated (Table 20-7).

## Surgical Procedures

### *Open Cholecystectomy*

Routinely, the anterior leaf of the hepatoduodenal ligament is incised over the hepatocystic triangle and the underlying structures are revealed. In more difficult cases, where adhesions from inflammation or previous surgery have obscured normal relationships, greater efforts are required. Three techniques follow.

- The hepatic flexure of the colon and the duodenum may be mobilized to the left.
- The liver may be retracted to the right. This puts slight tension on the biliary ducts and opens the epiploic foramen of Winslow, providing better orientation of the field.
- When dissecting the gallbladder away from the liver bed, one may expose the cystic artery by rotating the gallbladder to the left. This also exposes the common hepatic duct, the right and left hepatic ducts, and the cystic duct. Performing this maneuver provides one of the advantages of removing the gallbladder from the fundus downward.

Occasionally the gallbladder bed bleeds profusely. The

**TABLE 20-7. The Anatomy of Differential Diagnosis in the Operating Room**

| Pathology | Pancreas | Gallbladder/Common Bile Duct |
|---|---|---|
| Carcinoma of the pancreas | Discrete mass in head (67%); less often in body or tail (33%). Body and tail distal to tumor are pale, indurated, rounder; tail is retracted from splenic hilum. Distal pancreatic duct is dilated and palpable along ventral surface of gland. With more ductal dilation, duct of Wirsung becomes centrally located. | With CA of head, common duct is dilated, thin-walled and bluish. Gallbladder is usually distended with distal CA, common duct is not involved. |
| Carcinoma of ampulla of Vater | Marble-like structure projecting from medial wall of duodenum. If duct of Wirsung is obstructed (20-25%) then pancreas is as above. | Same as above |
| Chronic pancreatitis | If the duct of Wirsung is obstructed, then the duct is palpable and the pancreas is rounded, pale and indurated as in cancer | If jaundice is present, then the gallbladder and common bile duct are distended, thick-walled, edematous and pale. Hepatogastric ligament is inflamed. |
| Penetrating duodenal ulcer | Localized induration in the head of the pancreas, without obstruction of the pancreatic duct. No pancreatic changes. | No jaundice. No dilation of gallbladder or common bile duct. |
| Impacted stone | Stone in the head of the pancreas without projecting into the lumen of the duodenal induration around the stone. No pancreatic changes. | Gallstones in 93% cases. Gallbladder and common bile duct rarely distended. |

*Source:* Skandalakis JE, Gray SW, Rowe JS, Skandalakis LJ. Anatomical complications of pancreatic surgery, Part 2. Contemp Surg 15(6):21-50, 1979; with permission.

use of suction and diathermy is advisable. The gallbladder bed may be filled with omentum and a drain placed over the omentum (not between the bed and the omentum).

Subserous excision of the gallbladder, first advocated by Bickham,[121] is still a useful procedure.[122] In this procedure, the lamina propria of loose connective tissue is used as the plane of dissection. This at once removes the entire mucosa and leaves the surface of the liver uninjured.

Many surgeons, when removing the gallbladder, prefer to begin in the hepatocystic triangle. After incision of the anterior leaf of the hepatoduodenal ligament, the cystic artery and duct are identified, ligated, and transected. The gallbladder can then be dissected from its bed from below upward. This procedure has the following advantages:

- Early identification and ligation of the cystic duct prevents cystic or gallbladder stones from being milked into the common bile duct
- Early ligation of the cystic artery reduces blood loss to a minimum

An alternative procedure is to begin at the fundus of the gallbladder and dissect downward toward the neck. Blood loss may be reduced if branches of the cystic artery and veins are clamped or cauterized. When freeing up the cystic artery, one must be aware of a small branch from it to the cystic duct that can occasion bleeding if avulsed. Similarly, stones may be kept from descending by early ligation of the cystic duct. When there is doubt about the anatomy, an operating room cholangiogram is indicated.

Herman[123] advocated the following procedure for cholecystectomy.

1. Dissection of the gallbladder
2. Exposure of the cystic duct and its union with the common bile duct
3. An operating room cholangiogram
4. Dissection and ligation of the cystic duct and removal of the gallbladder

Regardless of the direction of the procedure, the junction of the cystic and common hepatic ducts should be identified. A short cystic duct may cause inadvertent injury to the common bile duct, but a long cystic duct remnant may produce the cystic duct remnant syndrome, which is similar to gallbladder disease secondary to lithiasis.

Seale and Ledet[124] reported good results with primary closure of the common bile duct following minicholecystectomy.

Davis et al.[125] advised percutaneous cholecystostomy for the treatment of patients with suspected acute cholecystitis. Kim et al.[126] found percutaneous gallbladder drainage a safe and effective emergency procedure for acute cholecystitis, allowing delayed laparoscopic cholecystectomy.

Bouvert's syndrome, which is obstruction of the gastric outlet or the first and (partially) second part of the duodenum including the duodenal bulb by a giant gallstone, occurs in 1-3% of all cholecystoenteric fistulas.[127]

Routine drainage of the subhepatic space after cholecystectomy has been debated in the past. Some authors have supported the practice as preventative against postoperative bile collection. Recent studies show that routine drainage results in increased hospital stay, higher postoperative fever, slower progression to a regular diet, and a higher rate of postoperative complications. Ronaghan and colleagues[128] showed that drainage should be used only where contamination, hemorrhage, bile leakage, or inflammation are present. Henry and Carey[129] emphasized that the proper timing of drainage is important. Attempting drainage too early fails to solve the problem and waiting too long exposes the patient to excess risk of systemic infection.

When carcinoma of the gallbladder is present, Ogura et al.[130] have recommended extensive hepatic resection if the malignancy invades the liver at the gallbladder fossa. Chijiwa et al.[131] urged radical surgery to treat T2 carcinoma of the gallbladder, with the presence of lymph node metastasis and/or perineural invasion suggesting a need for further post-surgical treatment. Azuma et al.[132] stated that intraoperative ultrasonography and frozen section examination are useful in the diagnosis of the depth of invasion of carcinoma of the gallbladder. Furukawa et al.[133] stated that differentiation between benign and malignant polypoid lesions in the gallbladder may be reliably identified, therefore cholecystectomy is not necessary. This may be so, but the authors of this chapter advise cholecystectomy.

According to Pati o and Quintero,[134] patients with asymptomatic cholelithiasis may have elective cholecystectomy, a safe procedure with low morbidity and mortality. Some patients, however, are at high risk for developing complications of their asymptomatic disease, and surgery in these patients may be technically difficult and involve high morbidity and mortality. The authors present the following criteria for identifying those high-risk patients:

- Life expectancy >20 years
- Calculi >2 cm in diameter
- Calculi <3 mm and patent cystic duct
- Radiopaque calculi
- Polyps in the gallbladder
- Nonfunctioning gallbladder
- Calcified gallbladder
- Concomitant diabetes
- Women <60 years
- Individuals in geographic regions with a high prevalence of gallbladder cancer

We quote from Merriam et al.:[135] "Older male patients

## Editorial Comment

*Open cholecystectomy has a long history and had become a relatively safe procedure in the United States by the 1990s. A geographically based study found an overall mortality rate of 0.17%, morbidity rate of 15%, and an estimated incidence of bile duct injuries of 0.2%. The mortality rate for elective cholecystectomy was 0.2%.[136] Another study from the 1980s found a mortality rate of 0.5%.[137] These mortality figures can be compared to the published data from earlier decades that showed open cholecystectomy mortality rates of 1.8 percent.[138] For elective open cholecystectomy the usual period of hospitalization post-operatively is 2 to 4 days. The more recent open cholecystectomy data are the standard against which newer operative procedures, such as laparoscopic cholecystectomy, need to be compared. (RSF Jr)*

(age older than 50 years) with history of cardiovascular disease, leukocytosis greater than 17,000 white blood cells/mL, and acute cholecystitis have increased risk of gallbladder gangrene and conversion of laparoscopic cholecystectomy to open cholecystectomy."

## *Laparoscopic Cholecystectomy*

*It should always be remembered that a well performed operation outside a trial setting is always more beneficial than a poorly conducted operation within a trial setting.*

**Alastair R. Brown[139]**

Regarding the earliest history of laparoscopic cholecystectomy, McKernan[140] has written:

*The first laparoscopic cholecystectomy was done by a German shortly after Semm performed laparoscopic appendectomy in 1982. On September 12, 1985, Erich Muhe, in Boblingen, Germany, performed a laparoscopic cholecystectomy by looking through the scope (without video optics). A piece of bicycle tubing was used as a large cannula through which the gallbladder was removed. His license was revoked shortly thereafter.*

Laparoscopic cholecystectomy was reintroduced to the surgical profession by DuBois, Mouret, and Périssat in 1988.[141] Since then, the laparoscopic technique has become the treatment of choice for symptomatic gallstones. Lujan et al.[142] stated that laparoscopic cholecystectomy for the treatment of acute cholecystitis is a safe and valid procedure with a low rate of complications.

Perissat[143] stated:

*The end of this century has witnessed a profound and definitive change in our surgical profession, a true revolution indeed. This change is comparable to that experienced by our elders by the end of the nineteenth century when surgery started to obey the laws of asepsis. Laparoscopic cholecystectomy, born during the years 1987-1988, will be remembered as the discovery that triggered this revolution.[144]*

The role of laparoscopic cholecystectomy in the treatment of gallbladder cancer is still evolving. Whalen et al.[145] reported the following about patients whose cancer was accidentally resected between 1985 and 1988 (immediate prelaparoscopic era) and from 1992 to 1995 (when laparoscopic cholecystectomy was well established):

*The widespread adoption of laparoscopic cholecystectomy did not worsen the survival of patients with gallbladder cancer, and patients with serendipitously treated gallbladder cancers did not have a worse survival after laparoscopic manipulation than after a standard open cholecystectomy. The laparoscopic aspects of operative manipulation of a gallbladder with cancer in it do not appear to be a proximate cause of the poor prognosis of this disease.*

Schwesinger et al.[146] presented the algorithm shown in Fig. 20-52 which includes laparoscopic management of acute cholecystitis.

In reference to laparoscopic common bile duct exploration, Crawford and Phillips[147] stated:

*Although still controversial, laparoscopic common bile duct exploration has been shown to be safe, applicable, and cost-effective in the treatment of choledocholithiasis.*

Jawad et al.[148] advised laparoscopic cholecystectomy for infants and children as the procedure of choice for gallstones.

Cholecystostomy is performed rarely today, but occasionally it is a necessity. As was emphasized several years ago by Skandalakis and Jones:[149] "Cholecystostomy should not be considered a mark of inferior surgical skill, but rather a sign of mature surgical judgment."

Sugiyama et al.[150] reported that cholecystostomy may be a definitive procedure for acalculus cholecystitis in elderly patients.

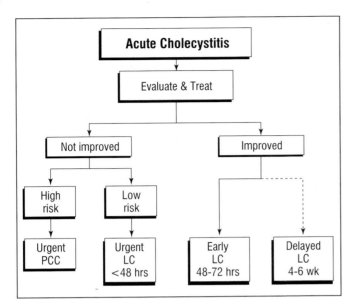

**FIG. 20-52.** Simplified algorithmic approach to the management of patients with acute cholecystitis. The dotted line represents an acceptable alternative strategy. PCC, percutaneous cholecystostomy. LC, laparoscopic cholecystectomy. (From Schwesinger WH, Sirinek KR, Strodel III WE. Laparoscopic cholecystectomy for biliary tract emergencies: State of the art. World J Surg 1999;23:334-342; with permission.)

A study by Misawa et al.[151] found that patients "with large branches of the middle hepatic vein close to the gallbladder bed are at risk of hemorrhage during laparoscopic cholecystectomy and should be identified preoperatively with ultrasound."

## Common Bile Duct Surgery

Although the diameter of the common bile duct increases in the presence of obstruction, there is no sharp dividing line between normal and obstructed ducts that can be applied in all cases.

Madden[152] provided good indicators for cholangiography or exploration of the duct in stone disease. The following list is based on his indicators:
- Recent or present jaundice (cholangiography)
- Dilatation of the common bile duct (7 mm ultrasonographically or 10 mm at direct visualization) (cholangiography)
- Multiple stones in the gallbladder together with a large cystic duct (cholangiography)
- Aspiration of murky bile from the duct (cholangiography)
- Presence of a palpable stone (exploration)
- Roentgenographic visualization of a stone (exploration)
- When in doubt, explore!

The ability to mobilize the common bile duct depends on the pathology and the scarring from previous operations. Lahey and Pyrtek[153] were able to obtain 2-5 cm in length by mobilizing the distal common bile duct from the undersurface of the pancreas. Since the duct may be intrapancreatic (see Fig. 20-32), the pancreas and duodenum should be mobilized. In about 70 percent of patients, the duct is free on the surface of the pancreas or is covered by a tongue of pancreatic tissue that leaves a cleavage plane between pancreas and duct (Figs. 20-32B-E). In the remaining cases, the pancreas may have to be mobilized because the duct is entirely covered by pancreatic tissue.

Cole and associates[154] were skeptical of mobilization of the distal common bile duct as a means of repairing strictures. They avoided all end-to-end anastomosis in favor of a Roux-en-Y procedure when more than 1 cm of the duct needed replacement. Avoidance of end-to-end anastomosis has become current standard practice, using instead a Roux-en-Y hepato- or choledochojejunostomy in virtually all bile duct reconstructions.

As to common bile duct malignant processes, Gerhards et al.[155] reported that absence of multifocality, diploid-type tumors and negative proximal bile duct margin histopathologies are significant factors prognostic of long-term survival for patients with carcinoma of the proximal bile duct (Klatskin tumors).

We quote from Blom and Schwartz[156] on the surgical treatment of Klatskin tumors:

*Curative resection could be achieved in approximately one third of patients who had cholangiocarcinoma, and should be the goal of treatment. Survival is significantly improved in those patients who are considered to have resectable tumors and who undergo removal of all gross disease. Palliative surgical treatments also revealed a survival advantage over nonoperative therapies.*

Sutherland et al.[157] stated that the Hepp-Couinaud hepaticojejunostomy without stenting is a reliable procedure for repair of postcholecystectomy stricture of bile ducts.

Nakayama et al.[158] advised that because it is usually not possible to determine whether strictures of the proximal bile duct are malignant or benign, they should be presumed malignant and treated accordingly.

## Common Bile Duct Stones

Thistle[159] presents the pathophysiology of bile duct stones as follows:
- Primary stones (less common, frequent recurrence, no pharmacologic response, difficult surgery)

- Intrahepatic
  "Pure" cholesterol
  Black mixed cholesterol
  Brown
- Extrahepatic
  Brown
- Secondary stones (common, easy to treat surgically)
  Black bilirubin polymer
  "Pure" cholesterol
  Mixed cholesterol
  Brown and other rare

Liu et al.[160] reported that the treatment of primary biliary stones was satisfactorily achieved by a systematic, aggressive approach consisting of hepatic resection, frequent construction of a hepaticocutaneous jejunostomy, and postoperative choledochoscopy.

González-Koch and Nervi[161] reported that although there is no primary indication to use solvents (chenodeoxycholic acid, ursodeoxycholic acid, monooctanoin, methyl tert-butyl ether) on common bile duct stones, due to their adverse reaction and their limited success in comparison with lithotripsy, the use of solvents may be indicated in a small group of patients in whom invasive or surgical treatment is risky or may fail.

Raraty et al.[162] advised that the treatment of acute cholangitis and pancreatitis secondary to common bile duct stones consists of systemic antibiotics and early removal of the obstructing stones by endoscopic retrograde cholangiopancreatography and endoscopic sphincterotomy. Cholecystectomy may be used prophylactically to prevent recurring episodes of gallstone pancreatitis.

We quote from Poon et al.[163]:

> Endoscopic sphincterotomy for biliary drainage and stone removal, followed by interval laparoscopic cholecystectomy, is a safe and effective approach for managing gallstone cholangitis. Patients with gallbladder left in situ after endoscopic sphincterotomy have an increased risk of biliary symptoms. Laparoscopic cholecystectomy should be recommended after endoscopic management of cholangitis except in patients with prohibitive surgical risks.

De Aretxabala and Bahamondes[164] advised that side-to-side choledochoduodenostomy with wide stoma is a safe procedure in selected patients with common bile duct stones and with minimal complications (5%). One complication is sump syndrome, which consists of bile duct contamination, cholangitis, and even secondary biliary cirrhosis.

Stuart et al.[165] stated that laparoscopic cholangiogram is safe, quick, and detects common bile duct stones.

Csendes et al.[166] stated that open choledochostomy has a definite place for the surgical treatment of bile duct stones, together with endoscopic retrograde cholangiopancreatography, papillotomy, and laparoscopic common bile duct exploration.

Navarrete et al.[167] reported their experience with 373 patients in whom residual choledocholithiasis was effectively treated by the percutaneous approach in the presence of a T-tube, with low morbidity and mortality.

Seitz et al.[168] reported that therapeutic endoscopic papillary balloon dilatation is an alternative procedure to endoscopic papillotomy for extraction of small common bile duct stones, but that further study is required before its routine use can be recommended.

Both Giurgiu et al.[169] and Shuchlieb et al.[170] reported that laparoscopic common bile duct exploration is an effective method for treatment of choledocholithiasis, the latter stressing the necessity of a laparoscopist who is skillful and who has good equipment. In his commentary on Shuchlieb, Fielding[171] stated, "Laparoscopic common bile duct exploration is the logical extension of the great revolution of laparoscopic cholecystectomy. It provides an all-in-one treatment for most patients with common bile duct (CBD) stones and avoids the need for preoperative endoscopic retrograde cholangiopancreatography (ERCP) in most patients."

## *Choledochal Cyst Surgery*

For treatment of choledochal cysts type I, the preferred procedure is excision of the cyst and Roux-en-Y hepaticojejunostomy (Figs. 20-53, 20-54).

Excision of the diverticulum only is the the accepted procedure of choice today for the treatment of type II choledochal cysts.

Duodenal choledochoceles (type III) are treated by duodenotomy with unroofing of the cyst, reapproximation of the mucosa with interrupted absorbable sutures, and sphincteroplasty. Pancreatic choledochoceles may require pancreaticoduodenectomy.

For type IV cysts, the treatment of choice is complete excision or hepatic lobectomy.

Caroli's disease (type V cyst) is treated by partial hepatic lobectomy when localized. Unroofing and drainage into a Roux loop should be performed as needed. Conservative treatment is advised when diffuse cystic disease is present.

When intrahepatic bile duct stenosis is present in patients with choledochal cysts, Ando et al.[172] advised resection of the stenotic ducts and performing a Roux-en-Y end-to-side anastomosis.

Type I

Type II

Type III

EXCISION, ROUX-EN-Y
  HEPATICOJEJUNOSTOMY
EXCISION, HEPATICODUODENOSTOMY
Roux-en-Y choledochocysto-
  jejunostomy
Choledochocystoduodenostomy

EXCISION

TRANSDUODENAL EXCISION
Transduodenal sphincteroplasty
Endoscopic sphincterotomy

Type IVA

Type IVB

Type V
(Caroli's disease)

Extrahepatic component
  EXCISION, ROUX-EN-Y HEPATICO-
    JEJUNOSTOMY
  EXCISION, HEPATICODUODENOSTOMY
Intrahepatic component
  Hepatic resection ±
    Roux-en-Y hepaticojejunostomy
Transhepatic intubation

EXCISION, ROUX-EN-Y
  HEPATICOJEJUNOSTOMY OR
  HEPATICODUODENOSTOMY
± transduodenal sphincteroplasty

HEPATIC RESECTION
Roux-en-Y intrahepatic
  cholangiojejunostomy
Transhepatic intubation

**FIG. 20-53.** Surgical options for treatment of choledochal cysts. (Preferred treatment in capital letters.) (Modified from Nagorney DM. Choledochal cysts in adult life. In: Blumgart LH (ed). Surgery of the Liver and Biliary Tract, vol 2. New York: Churchill Livingstone, 1988; with permission.)

Ishibashi et al.[173] reported that malignant change was not observed after total or subtotal excision in their series studying 48 patients over a 21-year period.

Hamada et al.[174] reported a case of choledochal cyst diagnosed at the 29th week of gestation with rapid cystic enlargement and gastric outlet obstruction after delivery. Temporary external drainage was performed and, at the age of 81 days, cystic excision and hepaticoduodenostomy.

Weyant et al.[175] review the literature on choledochal cysts in adults and describe two cases. They emphasize that, if possible, complete excision of the cyst should be performed to prevent malignancy.

Tanaka et al.[37] recommended prophylactic cholecystectomy in patients with anomalous junction of the pancreatobiliary ductal system but without dilatation. This recommendation is made to avoid future malignancy in a population that has a relatively high risk of developing biliary tract cancer.

Multiple carcinomas of the biliary tract in a patient with pancreaticobiliary maljunction and congenital choledochal

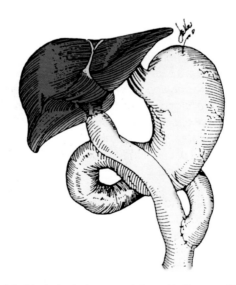

**FIG. 20-54.** Choledochal cyst excision with Roux-en-Y hepaticojejunostomy, the preferred method of operative management. (Modified from O'Neill JA Jr. Choledochal cyst. Curr Prob Surg 1992;19:361-410; with permission.)

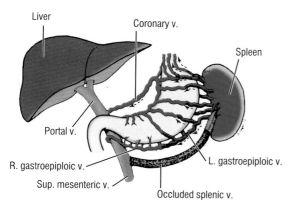

**FIG. 20-55.** Diagrammatic representation of collateral circulation characteristic of isolated occlusion of the splenic vein. (Modified from Salam AA, Warren WD. Anatomic basis of the surgical treatment of portal hypertension. Surg Clin North Am 1974;54:1247-1257; with permission.)

dilatation have been reported.[176]

Although we have recommended the writings of O'Neill[35,36] previously, they cannot be praised highly enough. They are a storehouse of information, and should be consulted by the surgeon of the extrahepatic biliary tract.

### *Portal Hypertension*

By definition, portal hypertension is produced by an increase in resistance of the portal blood flow secondary to cirrhosis of the liver in most cases, or secondary to splenic vein thrombosis (Fig. 20-55), with formation of collateral circulation between the portal and systemic venous networks.

Anatomically, submucosal varices are developed in the proximal stomach and distal esophagus. Hematemesis, ascites, hypersplenism, and encephalopathy may be the sequelae of this clinical entity. Among the choice of treatments are selective distal splenorenal shunt (Fig. 20-56), mesorenal interposition shunt (Fig. 20-57), and several other procedures.

Wind et al.[177] reported that with portal hypertension there are splenorenal and gastrorenal anastomoses, some of which are situated posteriorly in the left subphrenic compartment. The incidence of spontaneous splenorenal shunts is approximately 17%, and their anatomic pathway is as follows: the gastric collateral vein is connected to the left renal vein via the inferior vein of the left crus of the diaphragm and the middle capsular vein.

## ANATOMIC COMPLICATIONS

### Diagnostic Procedures

For complications of open (wedge) biopsy and percutaneous (needle) biopsy, please consult the chapter on the liver.

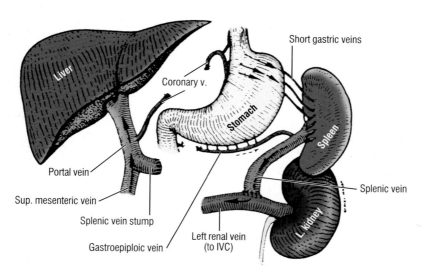

**FIG. 20-56.** Diagrammatic illustration of the selective distal splenorenal shunt. (Modified from Salam AA, Warren WD. Anatomic basis of the surgical treatment of portal hypertension. Surg Clin North Am 1974;54:1247-1257; with permission.)

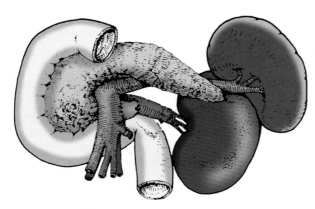

FIG. 20-57. Diagrammatic illustration of the mesorenal interposition shunt. (Modified from Salam AA, Warren WD. Anatomic basis of the surgical treatment of portal hypertension. Surg Clin North Am 1974;54:1247-1257; with permission.)

## Percutaneous Transhepatic Cholangiography (PTC)

Most of the organs that may be injured by needle biopsy are also at risk from percutaneous transhepatic cholangiography (PTC). Hemorrhage, bile peritonitis, and septicemia are the chief dangers.

## Endoscopic Retrograde Cholangiopancreatography (ERCP)

Cholangitis,[178] duodenal perforation, pancreatitis, pancreatic sepsis, and pseudocyst formation are among possible complications of endoscopic retrograde cholangiopancreatography (ERCP). The instrument may injure the common bile duct, the main pancreatic duct, or the duodenal papilla.

## Angiography

Although duplex Doppler sonography and MRI have lessened the need for invasive investigation, angiography still provides critical diagnostic information for carefully selected patients. Angiography may increase ongoing gastrointestinal bleeding and may increase existing renal or hepatic insufficiency. Contrast medium should not exceed 1 g of iodine per kilogram of body weight.[179]

## Choledochoscopy (Cholangioscopy)

Injury to bile ducts, duodenum, pancreas, or liver is always possible, though uncommon, during choledochoscopy. The incidence of wound infection is not increased by endoscopy. Schebesta and colleagues[180] reported a case of operative choledochoscopy resulting in aspiration of gastric contents into the tracheobronchial apparatus.

## Peritoneoscopy

Reynolds and Cowan[181] list the following complications from peritoneoscopy:
- Air embolism by accidental injection of air into liver or large abdominal veins
- Internal bleeding from vessels at puncture site or from vessels in adhesions
- Bleeding from associated liver biopsy
- Perforation of intestines adherent to the anterior body wall
- Injury to abdominal viscera
- Tearing of an adhesion containing a large blood vessel
- Puncture of an unsuspected ovarian cyst

Reynolds and Cowan reported only twelve major complications among 2400 peritoneoscopies over 30 years (0.5 percent). Other large series[182] had complication rates as high as 2.5 percent.

# Surgical Procedures

## Cholecystectomy, Common Bile Duct Surgery, and Sphincteroplasty

### General Considerations

Matolo[183] estimated that about 500,000 operations for biliary tract disease are performed in the United States each year, and he wrote that "nearly 10,000 deaths result from complications or treatment of diseases of the biliary system." A great many of these deaths result from anatomic complications following surgery in elderly patients with comorbid conditions.

Procedures of biliary tract surgery are many and complicated. The hazards in each procedure are similar, however. Here we consider the anatomic complications that are common to the following three procedures: cholecystectomy, surgery of the common bile duct, and sphincteroplasty.

REMEMBER:
- Isolate and study the structure you intend to cut or ligate.
- Identify the common hepatic duct, the cystic duct, and the common bile duct.
- Do a cholangiogram if in doubt.

Injuries associated with laparoscopic cholecystectomy will be presented later in this chapter.

## Vascular Injury

The most obvious danger is that of hemorrhage from the many large blood vessels lying anterior to the biliary tree. Such vessels are inconstant in number and location. The posterior superior pancreaticoduodenal artery, anterior to the retroduodenal portion of the common bile duct, is the vessel most frequently encountered.

All the vessels listed in Table 20-5 are subject to possible injury.

The following list of variations in the cystic artery may help one avoid common pitfalls.

- The cystic artery may be single or double, short or long.
- It may pass anterior or posterior to the right and left hepatic ducts, the common hepatic duct, or the common bile duct.
- It may be large, mimicking a small right hepatic artery.
- It may bifurcate at the neck of the gallbladder, or the two arteries may have separate origins.

Injury to the portal vein[184] or the inferior vena cava[185] is a serious complication. These vessels must, of course, be repaired at once.

Bleeding from veins of the gallbladder bed or from veins of the common bile duct is a minor complication.

A second vascular complication of biliary surgery is ischemia to the liver from unintended ligation of the right hepatic artery or an accessory or replacing aberrant right hepatic artery. Interference with the blood supply of the common bile duct may result in ischemia and stricture.[93,94] Other surgeons feel that the blood supply is good and that collateral circulation will prevent local ischemia.[186]

Parke and associates,[94] working on fetal and neonatal specimens, concluded that in spite of an apparently abundant blood supply, the common bile duct should not be skeletonized for more than 2 cm. The combination of ischemia and bile leakage is a danger recognized decades ago by Dragstedt.[187]

## Injury to the Biliary Tract

Jaundice, biliary fistula, and bile peritonitis with pain and fever will follow iatrogenic injury to the biliary ductal system (Fig. 20-58). Glenn[188] reviewed 100 cases of such iatrogenic injury.

Injury to any part of the extrahepatic biliary tree may result in bile leakage, which leads to bile peritonitis. A small, insidious bile leak is probably a greater danger than leakage from an inadvertently cut major duct, because the small leak may go undetected. Small bile ducts in the bed of the gallbladder and small accessory hepatic ducts are easily overlooked and cut. Loosening of the ligation of the cystic duct stump is a possible source of postoperative bile peritonitis.[189]

The common bile duct itself may be injured if one attempts to pass a probe through it without a preoperative cholangiogram. Fixation of the duct from disease or adhesion from prior surgery may result in unexpected sharp angulation.[190]

An anatomic classification of bile duct strictures was presented by Bismuth:[191]

*Since the length of the superior biliary stump is a determinant factor in biliary repair, a classification of postoperative biliary strictures according to the level where healthy biliary mucosa can be found may be proposed. Cholangiography is indispensable to precise knowledge of the level of the stricture. We have classified postoperative strictures of the common bile duct into five types (Fig. 20-59).*

- *Type 1. Low common hepatic duct stricture: the hepatic stump is longer than 2 cm.*
- *Type 2. Middle common hepatic duct stricture: the hepatic stump is less than 2 cm.*
- *Type 3. High stricture or hilar stricture preserving the biliary confluence: the hepatic duct does not exist any more. The stricture reaches the confluence of the right and left hepatic ducts but communication between the two branches is preserved across the confluence.*
- *Type 4. Hilar structure interrupts the confluence: communication between the left and right branches*

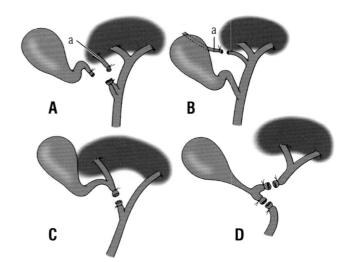

**FIG. 20-58.** Possible iatrogenic injuries to biliary tract. **A,** Ligation of an accessory hepatic duct (a) together with cystic duct. **B,** Ligation of an accessory hepatic duct (a) instead of cystic duct. **C,** Ligation of right hepatic duct below anomalous entry of cystic duct. **D,** Short cystic duct under tension may angulate common bile duct. One or both limbs may be inadvertently ligated. (Modified from Skandalakis JE, Gray SW, Rowe JS Jr. Anatomical Complications in General Surgery. New York: McGraw-Hill, 1983; with permission.)

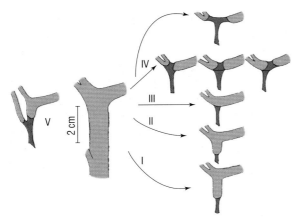

FIG. 20-59. The different types of postoperative strictures classified according to the length of the superior end. Three landmarks are used: 2 cm under the biliary confluence, the inferior level of the confluence, and roof of the confluence. Type 1: Low stricture. Type 2: Middle stricture. Type 3: High stricture (hilar stricture) preserving the biliary confluence. Type 4: High stricture (hilar stricture) interrupting the biliary confluence. Type 5: Apart, stricture on an anomalous union of the sectorial right branches. (Modified from Bismuth H. Postoperative strictures of the bile duct. In: Blumgart LH (ed). The Biliary Tract. Edinburgh: Churchill Livingstone, 1982, pp. 209-218; with permission.)

*no longer exists. If the fibrotic scar joining the two branches is thin, then they may remain in continuity, but if the process has destroyed an important part of the ductal tissue, the right and left hepatic ducts may be separated by 1-2 cm.*

- *Type 5. When the trauma has involved an anomalous distribution of the segmental right branches ('convergence étagée,' i.e., separate junction of posterior right sectorial duct below the major confluence), one of these two ducts can be separated from the biliary tract by the stricture.*

Lillimoe et al.[192] summarized the treatment of postoperative biliary strictures:

> *Major bile duct injuries and postoperative bile duct strictures remain a considerable surgical challenge. Management with preoperative cholangiography to delineate the anatomy and placement of percutaneous biliary catheters, followed by surgical reconstruction with a Roux-en-Y hepaticojejunostomy, is associated with a successful outcome in up to 98% of patients.*

### Injury to Other Organs

Efforts to dissect the distal common bile duct from the pancreas or to mobilize it may result in injury to the pancreas. Retraction of the liver to obtain a better approach to the right and left hepatic duct may tear the liver. Other structures to be protected are the stomach, duodenum, and hepatic flexure of the colon.

### Inadequate Procedures

The following inadequate procedures may result in iatrogenic injury.

- Leaving a long cystic duct stump may lead to cystic duct remnant syndrome.
- Failing to securely ligate the stump of the cystic duct may produce bile leakage.[193]
- Failure to recognize a dilated common bile duct that contains stones may lead to cholangitis or pancreatitis.

### *Laparoscopic Cholecystectomy*

The anatomic complications of laparoscopic cholecystectomy are similar to those of the open removal of the gallbladder. According to Morgenstern et al.,[194] injury to the common bile duct was less than 0.2% with the open method. The same authors reported bile duct injuries with laparoscopic cholecystectomy of 0.58% in 1284 operations performed between 1989 and 1991, and 0.50% in 1143 operations performed between 1992 and 1994. Moore and Bennett of the Southern Surgeons Club[195] stated that an individual surgeon had a 1.7% bile duct injury rate in his or her first 15-20 laparoscopic cholecystectomies, decreasing to 0.17% after 50 operations.

We agree with Morgenstern and colleagues[194] that laparoscopic cholecystectomy will continue to pose a problem in biliary tract surgery. Certainly the "learning curve," both institutional and individual, may explain some of the difference in outcome. The fact remains that the chance of injury to the bile duct is greater in laparoscopic cholecystectomy than in open gallbladder surgery.

The literature indicates differing views concerning operating room cholangiogram for recognition of bile duct injury. Morgenstern et al.[194] stated, "The early recognition and repair of ductal injuries in our cases, with successful outcomes in all cases, lends emphasis to the importance of the operative cholangiogram." Lorimer et al.[196] reported that intraoperative cholangiography is not essential. We agree with Morgenstern's analysis, while at the same time applauding Lorimer's plea for "meticulous demonstration of anatomic detail at operation."

We advocate routine fluoroscopic cholangiography in any surgeon's first fifty laparoscopic cholecystectomies and subsequently in any case where inflammation, questionable anatomy, leak of golden "hepatic" bile, or "aberrant" structures are encountered. Woods et al.[197] demonstrated that cholangiography can prevent a minor biliary injury from becoming a disastrous resection of the

extrahepatic biliary tree —the "classic" laparoscopic cholecystectomy injury.

We quote from Organ and Porter:[198]

*The role of laparoscopic surgery continues to be
defined as data from outcomes research becomes
available. Through a medical record review, Wherry
and colleagues[199] analysed the outcomes of laparoscopic cholecystectomies performed at 94 US military
hospitals between January 1993 and May 1994. Of
10458 cholecystectomies, 9130 (87%) were performed laparoscopically. This is an increase from the
65.9% rate of cholecystectomies performed laparoscopically between July 1990 and May 1992 when the
procedure was being introduced into the military
health services system.[200] Complete medical records
were obtained for 9054 patients who underwent laparoscopic cholecystectomy. The conversion rate to
an open procedure was slightly less than 10%. The 30-
day postoperative morbidity rate, including bile duct,
bowel, and vascular injuries, was 6.09%; the 30-day
postoperative mortality rate was 0.13%*

For all practical purposes the complications of laparoscopic cholecystectomy are the same as those of open
cholecystectomy. However, the incidence of complications is higher in laparoscopic cholecystectomy and the
severity of the bile duct injuries is greater.

There is no question, as Hunter[201] wrote, that cholecystectomy is a triumph of laparoscopic surgery. Nonetheless the procedure can be associated with tragic and
catastrophic ductal injuries. These injuries take place because of the surgeon's inexperience and because of congenital ductal anomalies and variations which are
extremely difficult to recognize during the procedure. The
extrahepatic biliary system is a topographicoanatomic
area notorious for anomalies.

Sarli et al.[202] reported 131 cases of gallbladder perforation during laparoscopic cholecystectomy out of 1127
cases (11.6%).

Aoki et al.[203] advised that repair of the injured peritoneum at trocar sites during laparoscopic cholecystectomy may reduce the frequency of wound metastasis in
cases of unexpected carcinoma of the gallbladder.

## Editorial Comment

*In the United States laparoscopic cholecystectomy has
become the procedure of choice for elective cholecystectomy. It is clearly preferred by patients over open cholecystectomy as postoperative pain is less, incisions are
smaller, hospitalization is shorter, and there is earlier
return to full activity. Early experience showed a high incidence of bile duct injuries and there is clearly a learning
curve relative to safe performance of the procedure.
Within a few years after the widespread performance of
laparoscopic cholecystectomy reports of large series from
the United States, Canada, and Europe showed that laparoscopic cholecystectomy can be performed with morbidity rates ranging from 3% to 10% and mortality rates
of 0.1% and less.[208-212] However, bile duct injury rates
were 0.2% to 0.6%, and it is possible that some injuries go
unreported. It would appear that the risk of biliary duct injury in laparoscopic cholecystectomy is about twice that
of open cholecystectomy. However, mortality rates and
overall morbidity rates appear to be lower for laparoscopic
cholecystectomy than for open cholecystectomy.*

*The challenge is to further reduce the risk of bile duct*

*injury. This risk can be reduced by knowledge of the surgi-
cal anatomy and its variations as described in this text, by
good visualization, by defining the anatomy before structures are divided, by the use of intraoperative cholangiography where there is any question about the anatomy
and/or anatomic structures are not clearly visible, and by
conversion to open cholecystectomy when it appears to be
the safer technique. In performing open cholecystectomy
the technique that I always used for both "difficult" and
"easy" cholecystectomies was to start at the fundus and
dissect the gallbladder from the liver bed prior to dissecting
the cystic duct. It is then possible to have a 360-degree view
of all of the structures in Calot's triangle before ligation or
transection. This approach minimizes the possibility of
misidentification of biliary ductal structures. Until recently
the instrumentation to make such an approach the procedure of choice in laparoscopic cholecystectomy was not
available. Use of the Harmonic Scalpel® makes a fundus
down approach very feasible in laparoscopic cholecystectomy and is currently undergoing clinical evaluation. (RSF
Jr)*

## Editorial Comment

*I believe that there are three alternatives for the management of choledocholithiasis, rather than two. At least this is true in some centers. In addition to laparoscopic and open procedures there are endoscopic procedures, endoscopic retrograde cholangiopancreatography (ERCP) with endoscopic sphincteroplasty. Some endoscopists (but certainly not all) have very high success rates and low morbidity rates for endoscopic management of choledocholithiasis. If those skills are available at a medical center and the laparoscopic surgeon is not skilled at laparoscopic common bile duct exploration, then it may be prudent to discontinue the procedure after the cholecystectomy and have the choledocholithiasis managed endoscopically a few days later. (RSF Jr.)*

Z'graggen et al.[204] stated that laparoscopic cholecystectomy on an undiagnosed adenocarcinoma of the gallbladder has a high incidence of recurrences at the port site, followed by death.

Aru et al.[205] reported that endoscopic retrograde cholangiopancreatography (ERCP) resolves isolated bile leaks, but iatrogenic strictures after laparoscopic cholecystectomy often require surgical treatment after ERCP.

Hannan et al.[206] recommended that "efforts be undertaken to carefully examine the choice of procedure for patients requiring cholecystectomies and to be sure that patients entering each hospital in which the procedure is performed have access to a sufficient number of surgeons trained to perform the procedure laparoscopically."

Machi et al.[207] recommended both laparoscopic ultrasonography and operative cholangiography during laparoscopic cholecystectomy.

Rosenthal et al.[213] reported that the choice of technique (open or laparoscopic) used in management of choledocholithiasis depends on the patient's condition, associated diseases, secondary complications of gallstones, and, above all, the good training and skill of the surgeon.

Habib et al.[214] concluded that gangrenous cholecystitis encountered in patients with acute cholecystitis was not a predictive factor in a laparoscopic approach being converted to open surgery.

NOTE: In the following material, repetition of information is intended to emphasize its importance.

## Bile Duct Injuries

Extrahepatic bile duct injuries are iatrogenic and virtually all are preventable (Table 20-8). They may involve any part of the extrahepatic biliary tract. Local or generalized bile peritonitis is the result of these injuries.

Careful dissection of the presumed cystic duct is essential. The surgeon should be familiar with this anatomic entity and able to identify both junctions of the cystic duct: the one to the gallbladder and, especially, the one to the common hepatic duct. The junction is exposed after dissecting approximately 1 cm above and 1 cm below the junction.

Nahrwold[215] stated that the junction of the three ducts (common hepatic duct, cystic duct, common bile duct) should serve as the primary anatomic landmark for all biliary tract operations. Nahrwold also supports the use of intraoperative cholangiography.

Ductal injuries can be recognized during surgery, in the operating room after surgery by observing bile leak or cholangiogram, or after surgery by the formation of ascites secondary to bile peritonitis. If injury is recognized at the time of surgery, an incomplete transection may undergo primary repair over a stent or T tube.

After studying 12,397 patients who had undergone laparoscopic cholecystectomy, Scott et al.[216] reported the following:

• Major bile duct injury: 0.3%

### TABLE 20-8. Techniques to Avoid Injury During Laparoscopic Cholecystectomy

Clear, unobstructed view of the infundibulum/triangle of Calot

Firm cephalad retraction of the fundus, inferior and lateral retraction of the infundibulum

Dissect fat/areolar tissue from infundibulum toward common duct, never vice versa

Visualize absolutely the cystic duct-gallbladder junction with no other intervening tissue

Cholangiography to confirm anatomy and rule out other pathology

Accessory/anomalous ducts are rare; do not over-call

A ductal structure wider than a standard clip is the common duct until proven otherwise

Never cauterize or clip blindly to control bleeding

Irrigate as often as necessary to clear the operative field and optimize visualization

Six to eight clips are the routine maximum; the need for more should lead to conversion

Asking oneself if one should convert to open surgery probably means one should

*Source:* Branum GD, Pappas TN. Complications of laparoscopic cholecystectomy. In Pappas TN, Schwartz LB, Eubanks S, eds. Atlas of Laparoscopic Surgery. Philadelphia: Current Medicine, 1996, pp. 2-11; with permission.

- Minor bile duct injury: 0.1%
- Bile leak: 0.4%
- Overall morbidity: 4%
- Mortality: 0.08%

These rates compare favorably with published reports for open cholecystectomy and indicate that laparoscopic cholecystectomy offers a viable alternative to conventional cholecystectomy.

A classification of laparoscopic bile duct injuries provided by Strasberg et al.[217] also includes 5 types, as follows (Figs. 20-60, 20-61).

- *Type A:* Bile leak from a minor duct still in continuity with the common bile duct.
- *Type B:* Occlusion of part of biliary tree.
- *Type C:* Bile leak from duct not in communication with common bile duct.
- *Type D:* Lateral injury to extrahepatic bile ducts.
- *Type E:* Circumferential injury of major bile ducts (Bismuth class 1 to 5).

Causes of laparoscopic biliary injuries as classified by Strasberg et al. are shown in Table 20-9.

Deziel et al.[211] reported the following for treatment of laparoscopic cholecystectomy complications: Laparotomy for the treatment of complications was required by 1.2% of patients. The mean rate of bile duct injury (excluding the cystic duct) was 0.6%. The most lethal complications included bowel injuries in 0.14% and vascular injuries in 0.25%. The most common origin of postoperative bile leak (0.3%) was from the cystic duct.

Beyer et al.[218] discussed the mode of treatment of biliary tract disease by minimally invasive procedures, emphasizing the nonoperative treatment of bile duct injuries, namely:

- Cholangiography for diagnosis of the biliary tract injury
- Balloon dilatation for treatment of the biliary stricture
- Biliary drainage to allow decompression of the biliary system, which is essential for uncomplicated healing
- Percutaneous drainage of fluid collections associated with bile duct injury

REMEMBER:
- The gallbladder bed is the most common site of bile leakage.
- Other potential sites of leakage are:
  - Posterolateral surface of the common hepatic duct, near its junction with the cystic duct
  - Posterior surface of the intrahepatic portion of the common bile duct

    Both of these injuries are difficult to recognize at the time of surgery, according to Nahrwold.[215]
- Liquidation or partial excision of the common hepatic duct or common bile duct are also iatrogenic injuries.

They are caused by:
- Too much traction of the cystic duct
- Poor anatomic dissection
- Incorrect use of clamps to stop bleeding
- If in doubt, perform an operating room cholangiogram and act as appropriate. You can:
  - Remove the ligation and insert a T tube
  - Perform primary repair (end to end anastomosis), or
  - Perform Roux-en-Y choledochojejunostomy

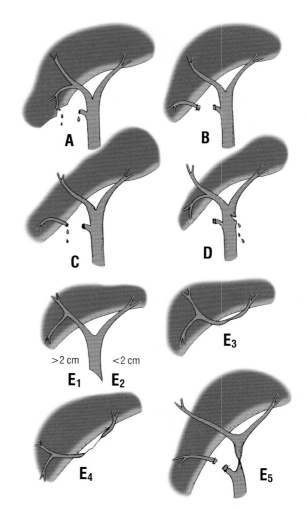

FIG. 20-60. Proposed classification of laparoscopic injuries to the biliary tract. The injuries Type **A** to **E** are illustrated. Type **E** injuries are subdivided according to the Bismuth classification. Type **A** injuries originate from small bile ducts that are entered in the liver bed or from the cystic duct. Type **B** and **C** injuries almost always involve aberrant right hepatic ducts. Type **A, C, D,** and some **E** injuries may cause bilomas or fistulas. Type **B** and other Type **E** injuries occlude the biliary tree and bilomas do not occur. (Modified from Strasberg SM, Hertl M, Soper NJ. An analysis of the problem of biliary injury during laparoscopic cholecystectomy. J Am Coll Surg 1995;180:101-125; with permission.)

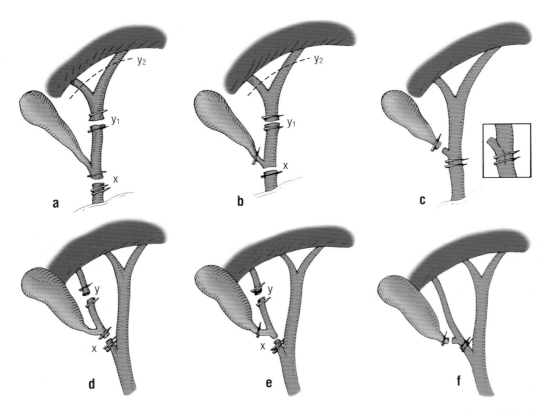

FIG. 20-61. Patterns of biliary injury. [Note: Type E injuries are illustrated also in Fig. 20-60.] **a,** "classical" Type E injury in which the common duct is divided between clips (point X). The ductal system is divided again later to remove the gallbladder (point Y1). **b** and **c** are variants of the injury. **d, e,** and **f** represent variants of injury to aberrant right hepatic duct, producing Type B and C injuries. (Modified from Strasberg SM, Hertl M, Soper NJ. An analysis of the problem of biliary injury during laparoscopic cholecystectomy. J Am Coll Surg 1995;180:101-125; with permission.

## Vascular Injuries

Ligate the cystic artery or its two branches (anterior and posterior) close to the gallbladder wall. Although there have been reports of ligation with good results, the hepatic artery and portal vein should be repaired immediately.[215]

---

### TABLE 20-9. Classification of Causes of Laparoscopic Biliary Injuries

Misidentification of bile ducts as the cystic duct
  Misidentification of common bile duct as cystic duct*
  Misidentification of aberrant right duct as cystic duct*
Technical causes
  Failure to securely occlude cystic duct*
  Too deep plane of dissection on liver bed*
  Injudicious use of thermal energy* to dissect, control bleeding, or divide tissue
  Tenting injury of cystic duct
  Injudicious use of clips to control bleeding
  Injuries due to improper techniques of ductal exploration

---

*Common causes of injury in laparoscopic cholecystectomy.

*Source:* Strasbert SM, Hertl M, Soper NJ. An analysis of the problem of biliary injury during laparoscopic cholecystectomy. J Am Coll Surg 180:101-125, 1995; with permission.

## Gallstone Spillage

Horton and Florence[219] report abscess formation secondary to dropped gallstones complicating laparoscopic cholecystectomy. Eisenstat[220] reported abdominal wall abscess secondary to gallstone spillage during laparoscopic cholecystectomy. According to Kakani and Bhullar,[141] gallstone spillage can be avoided by removing the gallbladder intact. This avoids future intraabdominal abscess and such rare complications as cholelithoptosis or cholelithorrhea. Of course, small bowel adhesions are present. Gerlinzani et al.[221] remind us that the loss of gallstones and their retention in the abdominal cavity should be noted in the description of the surgical procedure.

## Rare Complications

SUBCUTANEOUS EMPHYSEMA. According to Kent,[222] subcutaneous emphysema may be secondary to $CO_2$ pneu-

## Editorial Comment

*As indicated in the text, some endoscopists are highly skilled at laparoscopic management of retained stones. (RSF Jr.)*

moperitoneum. Hypercarbia and acidosis may also be present. Hyperventilation and elimination of the $CO_2$ pneumoperitoneum is the treatment of choice. Rarely patients may require conversion to $N_2$ insufflation. A chest film may reveal the presence of pneumothorax that, if present, should be treated by tube thoracostomy.

**HYDROCELE.** Kauer et al.[223] reported the formation of a hydrocele following laparoscopic cholecystectomy. The hydrocele was probably produced by high intraabdominal pressure. This resulted when extended pneumoperitoneum opened the obliterated processus vaginalis.

**SUBTOTAL CHOLECYSTECTOMY.** Inadvertent subtotal laparoscopic cholecystectomy with bilious ascites was reported by Blackard and Baron.[224] Exploratory laparoscopy with removal of a gallbladder remnant containing stones and drainage of the biliary ascites was performed with good results. Cottier et al.[225] and Bickel and Shtamler[226] cited specific presurgical indications for the performance of subtotal laparoscopic cholecystectomy in selected high risk patients.

**RETAINED STONES.** Retained stones should be avoided if at all possible. An operating room cholangiogram will detect virtually all common bile duct stones. When stones are detected, common bile duct exploration and removal of the stones is the procedure of choice and may be accomplished by laparoscopic or open surgery.

### Trocar Insertion

Thompson et al.[227] reported two instances of IVC injuries during insertion of trocar for laparoscopic cholecystectomy.

Suzuki et al.[228] studied port site recurrence of carcinoma of the gallbladder after laparoscopic cholecystectomy.

## REFERENCES

1. Connaughton D. Warren Cole, MD, and the Ascent of Scientific Surgery. Chicago: The Warren and Clara Cole Foundation, 1991.
2. Suzuki M, Akaishi S, Rikiyama T, Naitoh T, Rahman MM, Matsuno S. Laparoscopic cholecystectomy, Calot's triangle, and variations in cystic arterial supply. Surg Endosc 2000;14:141-144.
3. Tanaka Y, Senoh D, Hata T. Is there a human fetal gallbladder contractility during pregnancy? Hum Reprod 2000;15:1400-1402.
4. Muller R, Dohmann S, Kordts U. [Fetal gallbladder and gallstones]. Ultraschall Med 2000;21:142-144.
5. Senecail B, Texier F, Kergastel I, Patin-Philippe L. [Anatomic variability and congenital anomalies of the gallbladder: ultrasonographic study of 1823 patients]. Morphologie 2000;84:35-39.
6. Harlaftis N, Gray SW, Skandalakis JE. Multiple gallbladders. Surgery 1977;145:928-934.
7. Di Vita G, Sciume C, Lauria Lauria G, Patti R. [Agenesis of the gallbladder]. G Chir 2000;21:33-36.
8. Wilson JW, Deitrich JE. Agenesis of the gallbladder: case report and familial investigation. Surgery 1986;99:106.
9. Sarli L, Violi V, Gobbi S. Laparoscopic diagnosis of gallbladder agenesis. Surg Endosc (Online) 2000;14:373.
10. Gotohda N, Itano S, Horiki S, Endo A, Nakao A. Terada N, Tanaka N. Gallbladder agenesis with no other biliary tract abnormality: report of a case and review of the literature. J Hepato Biliary Pancreatic Surg 2000;7:327-330.
11. Blasius G. Observata anatomica in homine, simia, equo. Amsterdam: Gaasbeeck, 1674.
12. Sherren J. A double gallbladder removed by operation. Ann Surg 1911;54:204.
13. Harlaftis N, Gray SW, Olafson RP, Skandalakis JE. Three cases of unsuspected double gallbladder. Am Surg 42(3):178-180, 1976.
14. Gray SW, Olafson RP, Skandalakis JE, Harlaftis N. Developmental origin of the double gallbladder. Contemp Surg 4(5):71-76, 1974.
15. Diaz MJ, Fowler W, Hnatow BJ. Congenital gallbladder duplication: preoperative diagnosis by ultrasonography. Gastrointest Radiol 16:198-200, 1991.
16. Droulias KA. The cystic duct remnant as cause of the postcholecystectomy syndrome. [In Greek; summary in English]. Doctoral thesis at University of Athens, Athens, Greece, 1979.
17. Abernethy J. Account of two instances of uncommon formation in the viscera of the human body. Philosoph Trans 1809;17:296 (paper presented in 1793).
18. Edwards EA. Clinical anatomy of the lesser varieties of the inferior vena cava. Angiology 1951;2:85.
19. Knight HO. An anomalous portal vein with its surgical dangers. Ann Surg 1921;74:697.
20. Boles ET Jr, Smith B. Preduodenal portal vein. Pediatrics 1961;28:805.
21. Hardy KJ, Jones RMcL. Failure of the portal vein to bifurcate. Surgery 121:226-228, 1997.
22. Grazioli L, Alberti D, Olivetti L, Rigamonti W, Codazzi F, Matricardi L, Fugazzola C, Chiesa A. Congenital absence of portal vein with nodular regenerative hyperplasia of the liver. Eur Radiol 2000;10:820-825.
23. Leal del Rosal P, Marquez Monter H, Avila L, Arce Gomez F. Anomalous entry of the pulmonary veins into the umbilical vein and the vena portae: presentation of a case and the autopsy findings. Rev Med Hosp Gen (Mex) 1962;25:535.
24. Skandalakis JE, Gray SW. Embryology for Surgeons. 2nd ed. Baltimore: Williams & Wilkins, 1994.
25. Woodwark GM, Vince DJ, Ashmore PG. Total anomalous pul-

monary venous return to the portal vein. J Thorac Cardiovasc Surg 1963;445:662.

26. Thompson J. On congenital obliteration of the bile ducts. Edinb Med J 1891;37:523.

27. Holmes JB. Congenital obliteration of the bile ducts: diagnosis and suggestions for treatment. Am J Dis Child 1916;11:405.

28. Longmire WP. Congenital biliary hypoplasia. Ann Surg 1964;159:335.

29. Witzleben CL. Bile duct paucity ("intrahepatic atresia"). Perspect Pediatr Pathol 1982;7:185.

30. Bremer JL. Congenital Anomalies of the Viscera. Cambridge: Harvard University Press, 1944.

31. Holder TM, Ashcraft KW. The effects of bile duct ligation and inflammation in the fetus. J Pediatr Surg 1967;2:35.

32. Hashimoto T, Otobe Y, Shimizu Y, Suzuki T, Nakamura T, Hayashi S, Matsuo Y, Sato M, Manabe T. A modification of hepatic portoenterostomy (Kasai operation) for biliary atresia. J Am Coll Surg 185:548-553, 1997.

33. Alonso-Lej F, Rever WB Jr, Pessagno DJ. Congenital choledochal cyst, with a report of 2, and an analysis of 94 cases. Int Abst Surg 1959;108:1.

34. Todani T, Watanabe Y, Fujii T, Toki A, Uemura S, Koike Y. Congenital choledochal cyst with intrahepatic involvement. Arch Surg 1984;119:1038.

35. O'Neill JA Jr. Choledochal cyst. Curr Probl Surg 1992;29:361-410.

36. O'Neill JA Jr. Choledochal cyst. In: O'Neill JA Jr, Rowe MI, Grosfeld JL, Fonkalsrud EW, Coran AG. Pediatric Surgery (5th ed). St. Louis: Mosby, 1998, pp. 1483-1493.

37. Tanaka K, Ikoma A, Hamada N, Nishida S, Kadono J, Taira A. Biliary tract cancer accompanied by anomalous junction of pancreaticobiliary ductal system in adults. Am J Surg 175:218-220, 1998.

38. Tuech JJ, Pessaux P, Aube C, Regenet N, Cervi C, Bergamaschi R, Arnaud JP. Cancer of the gallbladder associated with pancreatobiliary maljunction without bile duct dilatation in a European patient. J Hepato Biliary Panc Surg 2000;7:336-338.

39. Caudle SO, Dimler M. The current management of choledochal cyst. Am Surg 1986;52:76.

40. Sugiyama M, Atomi Y, Kuroda A. Pancreatic disorders associated with anomalous pancreaticobiliary junction. Surgery 1999;126:492-497.

41. Lipsett PA, Segev DL, Colombani PM. Biliary atresia and biliary cysts. Ballières Clin Gastroenterol 1997;11:619-641.

42. Yoshida T, Shibata K, Matsumoto T, Sasaki A, Hirose R, Kitano S. Carcinoma of the gallbladder associated with anomalous junction of the pancreaticobiliary duct in adults. J Am Coll Surg 1999;189:57-62.

43. Vitetta L, Sali A, Little P, Mrazek L. Gallstones and gall bladder carcinoma. Aust NZ J Surg 200;70:667-673.

44. Michels NA. Blood Supply and Anatomy of the Upper Abdominal Organs. Philadelphia: Lippincott, 1955.

45. Daseler E, Anson B, Hambley W, Reiman A. Cystic artery and constituents of the hepatic pedicle. Surg Gynecol Obstet 1947;85:47.

46. Van Damme JP, Bonte J. The branches of the celiac trunk. Acta Anat 1985;122:110.

47. Van Damme JP. Behavioral anatomy of the abdominal arteries. Surg Clin North Am 73(4):699-725, 1993.

48. Suzuki T, Nakayasu A, Kauabe K, Takeda H, Honjo I. Surgical significance of anatomic variations of the hepatic artery. Am J Surg 1971;122:505.

49. Healey JE Jr, Schroy PC, Sorensen RJ. The intrahepatic distribution of the hepatic artery in man. J Int Coll Surg 1953;20:133.

50. Michels NA. Newer anatomy of the liver and variant blood supply and collateral circulation. Am J Surg 1966;112:337.

51. Healey JE Jr, Schwartz SI. Surgical anatomy. In: Schwartz SI (ed) Surgical Diseases of the Liver. New York McGraw-Hill, 1964.

52. von Haller A. Icones Anatomicae. Gottingen: Vandenhoeck, 1756.

53. Tiedemann F. Tabulae Arteriarum Corporis Humani. Karlsruhe: Müller, 1822.

54. Feigl W, Firbas W, Sinzinger H, Wicke L. Various forms of the celiac trunk and its anastomoses with the superior mesenteric artery [German]. Acta Anat 1975;92(2):272-284.

55. Hiatt JR, Gabbay J, Busuttil RW. Surgical anatomy of the hepatic artery in 1000 cases. Ann Surg 1994;220:50.

56. Weimann A, Meyer HJ, Mauz S, Ringe B, Jahne J, Pichlmayr R. Anatomische Verlaufsvariationen de Arteria hepatica sinistra. Chirurg 1991;62:552.

57. Rygaard H, Forrest M, Mygind T, Baden H. Anatomic variants of the hepatic arteries. Acta Radiol Diag 1986;27:425-427.

58. McGregor AL, Du Plessis DJ. A Synopsis of Surgical Anatomy. 10th ed. Baltimore: Williams & Wilkins, 1969, p. 529.

59. Nakamura S, Tsuzuki T. Surgical anatomy of the hepatic veins and the inferior vena cava. Surg Gynecol Obstet 1981;152:43.

60. Kennedy PA, Madding GF. Surgical anatomy of the liver. Surg Clin North Am 1977;57:233.

61. Cavalcanti JS, Andrade LP, Moreira IE, Rietra PH, Oliveira ML. A morphological and functional study of the cavo-hepatic junction in the human. Surg Radiol Anat 17:311-314, 1995.

62. Healey JE Jr, Schroy PC. Anatomy of the biliary ducts within the human liver: analysis of the prevailing pattern of branchings and the major variations of the biliary ducts. Arch Surg 1953;66:599.

63. Hermann RE. Manual of Surgery of the Gallbladder, Bile Duct and Endocrine Pancreas. New York: Springer-Verlag, 1979.

64. Braasch JW. Congenital anomalies of the gallbladder and bile ducts. Surg Clin North Am 1958;38:627.

65. Johnston EV, Anson BJ. Variations in the formation and vascular relationships of the bile ducts. Surg Gynecol Obstet 1952;94:669.

66. Newman HF, Northrup JD. Extrahepatic biliary tract anatomy. West J Surg Obstet Gynecol 1963;71:59.

67. Bartel J. Cholelithiasis und Korperkonstitution cholelithotripsie. Frankfurt Z Pathol 1916;19:206.

68. Flannery MG, Caster MP. Congenital abnormalities of the gallbladder: 101 cases. Int Abstr Surg 1956:103:439.

69. Skandalakis JE, Gray SW, Skandalakis LJ. Surgical anatomy of intestinal obstruction. In: Fielding LP, Welch J (eds). Intestinal Obstruction. New York, Churchill Livingstone, 1987, pp. 14-32.

70. Kaiser E. Congenital and acquired changes in gallbladder form. Am J Dig Dis 1961;6:938.

71. Davies F, Harding HE. Pouch of Hartmann. Lancet 1:193-195, 1942.

72. Williams PL. Gray's Anatomy (38th ed). New York: Churchill Livingstone, 1995, p. 1811.

73. Lindner HH, Green RB. Embryology and surgical anatomy of the extrahepatic biliary tract. Surg Clin North Am 1964;44:1273.

74. Wayson EE, Foster JH. Surgical anatomy of the liver. Surg Clin North Am 1964;44:1263.

75. Prudhomme M, Canovas F, Godlewski G, Bonnel F. The relationship of the bile duct and the retroduodenal arteries and their importance in the surgical treatment of hemorrhagic duodenal ulcer. Surg Radiol Anat 19:227-230, 1997.

76. Dorrance HR, Lingam MK, Hair A, Oien K, O'Dwyer PJ. Acquired abnormalities of the biliary tract from chronic gallstone disease. J Am Coll Surg 1999;189:269-273.

77. Smanio T. Varying relations of the common bile duct with the posterior face of the pancreas in Negroes and white persons. J Int Coll Surg 1954;22:150.

78. Kune GA. Surgical anatomy of the common bile duct. Arch Surg 1964;89:995.

79. Lytle WJ. The common bile duct groove in the pancreas. Br J Surg 1959;47:209.

80. Dowdy GS Jr. The Biliary Tract. Philadelphia: Lea and Febiger, 1969.

81. Schwegler RA Jr, Boyden EA. The development of the pars intestinalis of the common bile duct in the human fetus, with special reference to the origin of the ampulla of Vater and the sphincter of Oddi. Anat Rec 1937;67:441.

82. Opie EL. Etiology of acute hemorrhage pancreatitis. Bull Johns Hopkins Hosp 1901;12:182.

83. Dragstedt LR, Haymond HE, Ellis JC. Pathogenesis of acute pancreatitis (acute pancreatic necrosis). Arch Surg 1934;28:232.

84. Doubilet H, Mulholland JH. Eight years study of pancreatitis and sphincteroplasty. JAMA 1956;160:521.

85. Silen W. Pancreas. In: Schwartz SI (ed). Principles of Surgery. New York: McGraw-Hill, 1974.

86. Fuzhou T, Maoxu W, Jianzhong W. Is anomalous junction of pancreaticobiliary duct related to pancreatitis. J Chin Surg 33:345-347, 1995.

87. Fuzhou T, Darong H, Maoxu W. Prevention from exacerbation with endoscopic nasobiliary drainage in patients with acute pancreatitis – a prospective randomized trial. J Clin Surg 1995;33:345-347.

88. Richer JP, Faure JP, Morichau-Beauchant M, Dugue T, Maillot N, Kamina P, Carretier M. Anomalous pancreatico-biliary ductal union with cystic dilatation of the bile duct. Surg Radiol Anat 20:139-142, 1998.

89. Dowdy GS Jr, Waldron GW, Brown WG. Surgical anatomy of the pancreatobiliary ductal system. Arch Surg 1962; 84:93.

90. Nikolić V. Artere cystique recurrente. Bull Assoc Anat 1967;136:739.

91. Balija M, Huis M, Nikolić V, Štulhofer M. Laparoscopic visualization of the cystic artery anatomy. World J Surg 1999;23: 703-707.

92. Chen TH, Shyu JF, Chen CH, Ma KH, Wu CW, Lui WY, Liu JC. Variations of the cystic artery in Chinese adults. Surg Laparosc Endosc Percutaneous Tech 2000;10:154-157.

93. Shapiro AL, Robillard GL. The arterial blood supply of the common and hepatic bile ducts with reference to the problems of common duct injury and repair: based on a series of twenty-three dissections. Surgery 1948;23:1.

94. Parke WW, Michels NA, Ghosh GM. Blood supply of the common bile duct. Surg Gynecol Obstet 1963:117:47.

95. Appleby LH. Indwelling common duct tubes. J Int Coll Surg 1959; 31:631.

96. Petren T. Die extrahepatischen Gallenwegsvenen und ihre pathologisch-anatomische Bedeutung. Verh Dtsch Anat Ges 1932;41:139.

97. Douglass BE, Baggenstoss AH, Hollinshead WH. The anatomy of the portal vein and its tributaries. Surg Gynecol Obstet 1950;91:562.

98. Sugita M, Ryu M, Satake M, Kinoshita T, Konishi M, Inoue K, Shimada H. Intrahepatic inflow areas of the drainage vein of the gallbladder: analysis by angio-CT. Surgery 2000;128:417-421.

99. Clermont D. Lymphatiques des voies biliares. Toulouse Med 1909; 814:114.

100. Rouviere H. Anatomy of the Human Lymphatic System. Tobias MJ (transl). Ann Arbor MI: Edwards Brothers, 1938.

101. Fahim RB, McDonald JR, Richards JC, Ferns DO. Carcinoma of the gallbladder: a study of its modes of spread. Ann Surg 1962;156:114.

102. Ito M, Mishima Y, Sato T. An anatomical study of the lymphatic drainage of the gallbladder. Surg Radiol Anat 1991;13:89.

103. Dawson JL, Normal K. Anatomy. In: Liver and Biliary Disease. Wright R, Alberti AGMM, Karran S, Millward-Sadler GH (eds). Philadelphia: Saunders, 1979.

104. Kurosaki I, Tsukada K, Hatakeyama K, Muto T. The mode of lymphatic spread in carcinoma of the bile duct. Am J Surg 172:239-243, 1996.

105. Jarnagin WR, Burke E, Powers C, Fong Y, Blumgart LH. Intrahepatic biliary enteric bypass provides effective palliation in selected patients with malignant obstruction at the hepatic duct confluence. Am J Surg 1998;175:453-460.

106. Doglietto GB, Alfieri S, Pacelli F, Mutignani M, Costamagna G, Carriero C, Di Giorgio A, Papa V. Extrahepatic bile duct carcinoma: a western experience with 118 consecutive patients. Hepatogastroenterology 2000;47:349-354.

107. Kobayashi S, Asano T, Yamasaki M, Kenmochi T, Nakagohri T, Ochiai T. Risk of bile duct carcinogenesis after excision of extrahepatic bile ducts in pancreaticobiliary maljunction. Surgery 1999;126:939-944.

108. Burnett W, Cairns FW, Bacsich P. Innervation of the extrahepatic biliary system. Ann Surg 1964;159:8.

109. Mahour GH, Wakim KG, Soule FH, Ferris DO. Structure of the common bile duct in man: presence or absence of smooth muscle. Ann Surg 1967;166:91.

110. Petkov P. Anatomotopographic investigations on the anterior hepatic nerve plexus. Scripta Scient Med (Varna) 1968;7:95.

111. Calot JF. De la cholécystomie. (Thesis) Paris, 1890, No. 25, p. 50.

112. Rocko JM, Swan KG, DiGioia JM. Calot's triangle revisited. Surg Gynecol Obstet 1981;153:410.

113. Moosman DA, Coller FA. Prevention of traumatic injury to the bile ducts: a study of the structures of the cystohepatic angle encountered in cholecystectomy and supraduodenal choledochostomy. Am J Surg 1951;32:132.

114. Stremple JF. The need for careful operative dissection in Moosman's area during cholecystectomy. Surg Gynecol Obstet 1986; 163:169.

115. Saint JH. The epicholedochal venous plexus and its importance as a means of identifying the common duct during operations on the extrahepatic biliary tract. Br J Surg 1961;48:489.

116. Moosman DA. Where and how to find the cystic artery during cholecystectomy. Surg Gynecol Obstet 1975;141:769.

117. Bergamaschi R, Ignjatovic D. More than two structures in Calot's triangle: a postmortem study. Surg Endosc 2000;14:354-357.

118. Guyton AC. Textbook of Medical Physiology (7th ed). Phila-

delphia: WB Saunders, 1986.

119. Azuma T, Yoshikawa T, Araida T, Takasaki K. Differential diagnosis of polypoid lesions of the gallbladder by endoscopic ultrasonography. Am J Surg 2001;181:65-70.

120. Beinart C, Efremidis S, Cohen B, Mitty HA. Obstruction without dilation. JAMA 1981;245:353.

121. Bickham WS. Operative Surgery IV. Philadelphia: Saunders, 1924.

122. Schein CJ, Hurwitt ES. A safe technique for the difficult cholecystectomy utilizing intravesical manipulation. Surg Gynecol Obstet 102:112, 1956.

123. Hermann RE. A plea for a safer technique of cholecystectomies. Surgery 79:609, 1976.

124. Seale AK, Ledet WP. Primary common bile duct closure. Arch Surg 1999;134:22-24.

125. Davis CA, Landercasper J, Gundersen LH, Lambert PJ. Effective use of percutaneous cholecystostomy in high-risk surgical patients. Arch Surg 1999;134:727-732.

126. Kim KH, Sung CK, Park BK, Kim WK, Oh CW, Kim KS. Percutaneous gallbladder drainage for delayed laparoscopic cholecystectomy in patients with acute cholecystitis. Am J Surg 2000;179:111-113.

127. Bottari M, Pallio S, Scribano E. Pyloroduodenal obstruction by a gallstone: Bouvert's syndrome. Gastrointest Endosc 1988;34:440-441.

128. Ronaghan JE, Miller SF, Finley RK Jr, Jones LM, Elliott DW. A statistical analysis of drainage versus nondrainage for elective cholecystectomy. Surg Gynecol Obstet 1986;162:253.

129. Henry ML, Carey LC. Complications of cholecystectomy. Surg Clin North Am 1983;63:1191.

130. Ogura Y, Tabata M, Kawarada Y, Mizumoto R. Effect of hepatic invasion on the choice of hepatic resection for advanced carcinoma of the gallbladder: histologic analysis of 32 surgical cases. World J Surg 22:262-267, 1998.

131. Chijiwa K, Nakano K, Ueda J, Noshiro H, Nagai E, Yamaguchi K, Tanaka M. Surgical treatment of patients with T2 gallbladder carcinoma invading the subserosal layer. J Am Coll Surg 2001;192:600-607.

132. Azuma T, Yoshikawa T, Araida T, Takasaki K. Intraoperative evaluation of the depth of invasion of gallbladder cancer. Am J Surg 178:381-384, 1999.

133. Furukawa H, Kosuge T, Shimada K, Yamamoto J, Kanai Y, Mukai K, Iwata R, Ushio K. Small polypoid lesions of the gallbladder: Differential diagnosis and surgical indications by helical computed tomography. Arch Surg 1998;133:735-739.

134. Patiño JF, Quintero GA. Asymptomatic cholelithiasis revisited. World J Surg 1998;22:1119-1124.

135. Merriam LT, Kanaan SA, Dawes LG, Angelos P, Prystowsky JB, Rege RV, Joehl RJ. Gangrenous cholecystitis: analysis of risk factors and experience with laparoscopic cholecystectomy. Surgery 1999;126:680-686.

136. Roslyn JJ, Binns GS, Hughes EF, Saunders-Kirkwood K, Zinner MJ, Cates JA. Open cholecystectomy: a contemporary analysis of 42,474 patients. Ann Surg 218:129-137, 1993.

137. Ganey JB, Johnson PA Jr, Prillamen PE, McSwain GR. Cholecystectomy: clinical experience with a large series. Am J Surg 151:352-357, 1986.

138. Glenn F. Trends in surgical treatment of calculous disease of the biliary tract. Surg Gynecol Obstet 140:877-884, 1975.

139. Brown AR. Invited commentary. Sarli L, Pietra N, Sansebastiano G, Cattaneo G, Costi R, Grattarola M, Peracchia A. Reduced postoperative morbidity after elective laparoscopic cholecystectomy: stratified matched case-control study. World J Surg 1997;21:872-879.

140. McKernan B. Origin of laparoscopic cholecystectomy in the USA: Personal experience. World J Surg 1999;23:332-333.

141. Kakani PR, Bhullar IS. Complications of spilled gallstones during laparoscopic cholecystectomy. Contemp Surg 1993;43:357.

142. Lujan JA, Parrilla P, Robles R, Marin P, Torralba JA, Garcia-Ayllon J. Laparoscopic cholecystectomy vs open cholecystectomy in the treatment of acute cholecystitis. Arch Surg 133:173-175, 1998.

143. Perissat J. Laparoscopic cholecystectomy, a treatment for gallstones: From idea to reality. World J Surg 1999;23:328-331.

144. Tompkins RK. Laparoscopic cholecystectomy: Threat or opportunity? Arch Surg 1990;125:1245.

145. Whalen GF, Bird I, Tanski W, Russell JC, Clive J. Laparoscopic cholecystectomy does not demonstrably decrease survival of patients with serendipitously treated gallbladder cancer. J Am Coll Surg 2001;192:189-195.

146. Schwesinger WH, Sirinek KR, Strodel WE. Laparoscopic cholecystectomy for biliary tract emergencies: state of the art. World J Surg 1999;23:334-42.

147. Crawford DL, Phillips EH. Laparoscopic common bile duct exploration. World J Surg1999;23;1999.

148. Jawad AJ, Kurban K, El-Bakry A, Al-Rabeeah A, Seraj M, Ammar A. Laparoscopic cholecystectomy for cholelithiasis during infancy and childhood: cost analysis and review of current indications. World J Surg 22:69-74, 1998.

149. Skandalakis JE, Jones CS. Management of acute cholecystitis. J Med Assoc Ga 47(2):79-82, 1958.

150. Sugiyama M, Tokuhara M, Atomi Y. Is percutaneous cholecystostomy the optimal treatment for acute cholecystitis in the very elderly? World J Surg 22:459-463, 1998.

151. Misawa T, Koike M, Suzuki K, Unemura Y, Murai R, Yoshida K, Kobayashi S, Yamazaki Y. Ultrasonographic assessment of the risk of injury to branches of the middle hepatic vein during laparoscopic cholecystectomy. Am J Surg 178:418-421, 1999.

152. Madden J. Atlas of Technics in Surgery, vol 1. New York: Appleton-Century-Crofts, 1964.

153. Lahey FH, Pyrtek LJ. Experience with the operative management of 280 strictures of the bile ducts with a description of a new method and a complete follow-up study of the end results in 229 of the cases. Surg Gynecol Obstet 91:25, 1950.

154. Cole WH, Irenus C Jr, Reynolds JT. Strictures of the common bile duct: Studies in 122 cases. Ann Surg 142:537, 1955.

155. Gerhards MF, van Gulik TM, Bosma A, ten Hooper-Neumann H, Verbeek PCM, Gonzalez DG, de Wit LT, Gouma DJ. Long-term survival after resection of proximal bile duct carcinoma (Klatskin tumors). World J Surg 1999;23:91-96.

156. Blom D, Schwartz SI. Surgical treatment and outcomes in carcinoma of the extrahepatic bile ducts. Arch Surg 2001;136:209-214.

157. Sutherland F, Launois B, Stanescu H, Campion JP, Spiliopoulos Y, Stasik C. A refined approach to the repair of postcholecystectomy bile duct strictures. Arch Surg 1999:134:299-302.

158. Nakayama A, Imamura H, Shimada R, Miyagawa S, Makuuchi M, Kawasaki S. Proximal bile duct stricture disguised as malignant neoplasm. Surgery 1999;125:514-521.

159. Thistle JL. Pathophysiology of bile duct stones. World J Surg 1998; 22:1114-1118.

160. Liu C-L, Fan S-T, Wong J. Primary biliary stones: diagnosis and management. World J Surg 1998;22:1162-1166.

161. González-Koch A, Nervi F. Medical management of common bile duct stones. World J Surg 1998;22:1145-1150.

162. Raraty MGT, Finch M, Neoptolemos JP. Acute cholangitis and pancreatitis secondary to common duct stones: management update. World J Surg 1998;22:1155-1161.

163. Poon RTP, Liu CL, Lo CM, Lam CM, Yuen WK, Yeung C, Fan ST, Wong J. Management of gallstone cholangitis in the era of laparoscopic cholecystectomy. Arch Surg 2001;136:11-16.

164. de Aretxabala X, Bahamondes JC. Choledochoduodenostomy for common bile duct stones. World J Surg 1998;22:1171-1174.

165. Stuart SA, Simpson TIG, Alvord LA, Williams MD. Routine intraoperative laparoscopic cholangiography. Am J Surg 1998;176: 632-637.

166. Csendes A, Burdiles P, Diaz JC. Present role of classic open choledochostomy in the surgical treatment of patients with common bile duct stones. World J Surg 1998;22:1167-1170.

167. Navarrete CG, Castillo CT, Castillo PY. Choledocholithiasis: percutaneous treatment. World J Surg 1998;22:1151-1154.

168. Seitz U, Bapaye A, Bohnacker S, Navarrete C, Maydeo A, Soehendra N. Advances in therapeutic endoscopic treatment of common bile duct stones. World J Surg 1998;22:1133-1144.

169. Giurgiu DI, Margulies DR, Carroll BJ, Gabbay J, Iida A, Takagi S, Fallas MJ, Phillips EH. Laparoscopic common bile duct exploration. Arch Surg 1999;134:839-844.

170. Shuchleib S, Chousleb A, Mondragon A, Torices E, Licona A, Cervantes J. Laparoscopic common bile duct exploration. World J Surg 1999;23:698-702.

171. Fielding GA. Invited commentary. Shuchleib S, Chousleb A, Mondragon A, Torices E, Licona A, Cervantes J. Laparoscopic common bile duct exploration. World J Surg 1999;23:698-702, p. 701-702.

172. Ando H, Kaneko K, Ito F, Seo T, Ito T. Operative treatment of congenital stenoses of the intrahepatic bile ducts in patients with choledochal cysts. Am J Surg 173:491-494, 1997.

173. Ishibashi T, Kasahara K, Yasuda Y, Nagai H, Makino S, Kanazawa K. Malignant change in the biliary tract after excision of choledochal cyst. Br J Surg 84(12):1687-1691, 1997.

174. Hamada Y, Tanano A, Sato M, Kato Y, Hioki K. Rapid enlargement of a choledochal cyst: antenatal diagnosis and delayed primary excision. Pediatr Surg Int 13(5-6):419-421, 1998.

175. Weyant MJ, Maluccio MA, Bertagnolli MM, Daly JM. Choledochal cysts in adults: a report of two cases and review of the literature. Am J Gastroenterol 93(12):2580-2583, 1998.

176. Okamura K, Hayakawa H, Kuze M, Takahashi K, Kosaka A, Mizumoto R, Katsuta R. Triple carcinomas of the biliary tract associated with congenital choledochal dilatation and pancreaticobiliary maljunction. J Gastroenterol 2000;35:465-471.

177. Wind P, Alves A. Chevallier JM, Gillot C, Sales JP, Sauvanet A, Cuénod CA, Vilgrain V, Cugnenc PH, Delmas V. Anatomy of spontaneous splenorenal and gastrorenal venous anastomoses: review of the literature. Surg Radiol Anat 20:129-134, 1998.

178. Bilbao MK, Dotler CT, Lee TG, Katon RM. Complications of endoscopic retrograde cholangiopancreatography: a study of 10000 cases. Gastroenterology 1976;70:314.

179. Dick R. Angiography. In: Wright's Liver and Biliary Disease. 3rd ed. Millward-Sadler GH, Wright R, Arthur MJP (eds). Philadelphia: WB Saunders, 1992, pp. 582-94.

180. Schebesta AG, Sporr D, O'Leary J, Moulton J. Gastric aspiration associated with operative choledochoscopy. Anaesth Intensive Care 1983;11:257.

181. Reynolds TB, Cowan RE. Peritoneoscopy. In: Wright's Liver and Biliary Disease. 3rd ed. Millward-Sadler GH, Wright R, Arthur MJP (eds). Philadelphia: WB Saunders, 1992, pp. 636-647.

182. Bruehl W. Zwischenfalle und Komplikationen bei der Laraskopie und gezielten Leber punktion. Dtsch Med Woch 1966; 91:2297.

183. Matolo NM. Symposium on biliary tract disease (foreword). Surg Clin North Am 61:763, 1981.

184. Tchirkow G, Silver SC. Injury to the portal vein: A hazard during common bile duct exploration. Arch Surg 113:745, 1978.

185. Wyndham NR. Gross damage to the portal vein and hepatic artery during cholecystectomy. Aust N Z J Surg 25:292, 1956.

186. Douglass TC, Lounsbury BF, Cutter WW, Wetzel N. An experimental study of healing in the common bile duct. Surg Gynecol Obstet 91:301, 1950.

187. Dragstedt LR, Woodward ER. Transduodenal reconstruction of the bile ducts. Surg Gynecol Obstet 94:53, 1952.

188. Glenn F. Iatrogenic injuries to the biliary ductal system. Surg Gynecol Obstet 146:430-434, 1978.

189. Kune GA. Bile duct injury during cholecystectomy: Causes, prevention and surgical repair in 1979. Aust N Z J Surg 49:35, 1979.

190. Hicken NF, Coray QB, Franz B. Anatomic variations of the extrahepatic biliary system as seen by cholangiographic studies. Surg Gynecol Obstet 88:577, 1949.

191. Bismuth H. Postoperative strictures of the bile duct. In: Blumgart LH (ed). The Biliary Tract. Edinburgh: Churchill Livingstone, 1982, pp. 209-218.

192. Lillimoe KD, Melton GB, Cameron JL, Pitt HA, Campbell KA, Talamini MA, Sauter PA, Coleman J, Yeo CJ. Postoperative bile duct strictures: management and outcome in the 1990s. Ann Surg 2000;232:430-441.

193. Chandar VP, Hookman P. Choledochocolonic fistula through a cystic duct remnant: A case report. Am J Gastroenterol 74:179, 1980.

194. Morgenstern L, McGrath MF, Carroll BJ, Paz-Partlow M, Berci G. Continuing hazards of the learning curve in laparoscopic cholecystectomy. Am Surg 1995;61:914.

195. Moore MJ, Bennett CL. The learning curve for laparoscopic cholecystectomy: The Southern Surgeons Club. Am J Surg 1995; 170:55.

196. Lorimer JW, Fairfull-Smith RJ. Intraoperative cholangiography is not essential to avoid duct injuries during laparoscopic cholecystectomy. Am J Surg 1995;169:344.

197. Woods MS, Traverso LW, Kozerek RA, Donohue JH, Fletcher DR, Hunter JG, Oddsdottir M, Rossi RL, Tsao J, Windsor J. Biliary tract complications of laparoscopic cholecystectomy are detected more frequently with routine intraoperative cholangiography. Surg Endosc 9:1076-1080, 1995.

198. Organ CH Jr, Porter JM. General surgery. JAMA 1998;280:495-496.

199. Wherry DC, Marohn MR, Malanoski MP, Hetz SP, Rich NM. An external audit of laparoscopic cholecystectomy in the steady state performed in medical treatment facilities of the Department of Defense. Ann Surg 1996;224:145-154.

200. Wherry DC, Rob CG, Marohn MR, Rich NM. An external audit of laparoscopic cholecystectomy performed in medical treatment facilities of the Department of Defense. Ann Surg 1994;220:626-634.

201. Hunter JG. Advanced laparoscopic surgery. Am J Surg 173:14-18, 1997.

202. Sarli L, Pietra N, Costi R, Grattarola M. Gallbladder perforation during laparoscopic cholecystectomy. World J Surg 1999;23: 1186-1190.

203. Aoki Y, Shimura H, Li H, Mizumoto K, Date K, Tanaka M. A model of port-site metastases of gallbladder cancer: The influence of peritoneal injury and its repair on abdominal wall metastases. Surgery 1999;125:553-559.

204. Z'graggen K, Birrer S, Maurer CA, Wehrli H, Klaiber C, Baer HU. Incidence of port site recurrence after laparoscoic cholecystectomy for preoperatively unsuspected gallbladder carcinoma. Surgery 1998;124:831-838.

205. Aru GM, Davis CR Jr, Elliott NL, Morris SJ. Endoscopic retrograde cholangiopancreatography in the treatment of bile leaks and bile duct strictures after laparoscopic cholecystectomy. South Med J 90(7):705-708, 1997.

206. Hannan EL, Imperato PJ, Nenner RP, Starr H. Laparoscopic and open cholecystectomy in New York State: mortality, complications, and choice of procedure. Surgery 125:223-231, 1999.

207. Machi J, Tateishi T, Oishi AJ, Furumoto NL, Oishi RH, Uchida S, Sigel B. Laparoscopic ultrasonography versus operative cholangiography during laparoscopic cholecystectomy: review of the literature and a comparison with open intraoperative ultrasonography. J Am Coll Surg 1999;188:361-367.

208. Barkun JS, Barkun AN, Meakins JL. Laparoscopic versus open cholecystectomy: The Canadian experience. Am J Surg 1993;165: 455-458.

209. Perissat J. Laparoscopic cholecystectomy: The European experience. Am J Surg 1993;165:444-449.

210. Gadacz TR. U.S. experience with laparoscopic cholecystectomy. Am J Surg 1993: 165:450-454.

211. Deziel DJ, Millikan KW, Economou SG, Doolas A, Ko S-T, Airan MC. Complications of laparoscopic cholecystectomy: a national survey of 4292 hospitals and an analysis of 77,604 cases. Am J Surg 1992;165:9-14.

212. Jatzko GR, Lisborg PH, Pertl AM, Stettner HM. Multivariate comparison of complications after laparoscopic cholecystectomy and open cholecystectomy. Ann Surg 221:381-386, 1995.

213. Rosenthal RJ, Rossi RL, Martin RF. Options and strategies for the management of choledocholithiasis. World J Surg 1998;22: 1125-1132.

214. Habib FA, Kolachalam RB, Khilnani R, Preventza O, Mittal VK. Role of laparoscopic cholecystectomy in the management of gangrenous cholecystitis. Am J Surg 2001;181:71-75.

215. Nahrwold DL. Complications of biliary tract surgery and trauma. In: Greenfield LJ. Complications in Surgery and Trauma. 2nd ed. Philadelphia: JB Lippincott, 1990, pp. 547-58.

216. Scott TR, Zucker KA, Bailey RW. Laparoscopic cholecystectomy: a review of 12,397 patients. Surg Laparosc Endosc 2(3):191-198, 1992.

217. Strasberg SM, Hertl M, Soper NJ. An analysis of the problem of biliary injury during laparoscopic cholecystectomy. J Am Coll Surg 1995;180:101-125.

218. Beyer AJ III, Delcore R, Cheung LY. Nonoperative treatment of biliary tract disease. Arch Surg 1998;133:1172-1176.

219. Horton M, Florence MG. Unusual abscess patterns following dropped gallstones during laparoscopic cholecystectomy. Am J Surg 1998;175:375-379.

220. Eisenstat S. Abdominal wall abscess due to spilled gallstones. Surg Laparosc Endosc 1993;3:485-486.

221. Gerlinzani S, Tos M, Gornati R, Molteni B, Poliziani D, Taschieri AM. Is the loss of gallstones during laparoscopic cholecystectomy an underestimated complication? Surg Endosc (Online) 2000;14: 373-374.

222. Kent RB III. Subcutaneous emphysema and hypercarbia following laparoscopic cholecystectomy. Arch Surg 1991;126:1154.

223. Kauer W, Brune I, Feussner H, Hartung R, Siewert JR. Hydrocele following laparoscopic cholecystectomy. Endoscopy 1993; 25:372.

224. Blackard WG Jr, Baron TH. Leaking gallbladder remnant with cholelithiasis complicating laparoscopic cholecystectomy. South Med J 1995;88:1166.

225. Cottier DJ, McKay C, Anderson JR. Subtotal cholecystectomy. Br J Surg 1991;78:1326.

226. Bickel A, Shtamler B. Laparoscopic subtotal cholecystectomy. J Laparoendosc Surg 1993;3:365.

227. Thompson JE, Bock R, Lowe DK, Moody WE III. Vena cava injuries during laparoscopic cholecystectomy. Surg Laparosc Endosc 6(3):221-223, 1996.

228. Suzuki K, Kimura T, Hashimoto H, Nishihira T, Ogawa H. Port site recurrence of gallbladder cancer after laparoscopic surgery: two case reports of long-term survival. Surg Laparosc Endosc Percutaneous Tech 2000;10:86-88.

229. Nygren EJ, Barnes WA. Atresia of the common hepatic duct with shunt via an accessory duct. Arch Surg 68:337, 1954.

230. Vesalius A. De Humani Corporis Fabrica Libri Septum. Basileae, 1543.

231. Everett C, Macumber HE. Anomalous distribution of the extrahepatic biliary ducts. Ann Surg 115:472, 1942.

232. Boyden EA. The problem of the double ductus choledochus: an interpretation of an accessory bile duct found attached to the pars superior of the duodenum. Anat Rec 55:71, 1932.

# Chapter *21*

# *Pancreas*

JOHN E. SKANDALAKIS, LEE J. SKANDALAKIS,
ANDREW N. KINGSNORTH, GENE L. COLBORN,
THOMAS A. WEIDMAN, PANAJIOTIS N. SKANDALAKIS

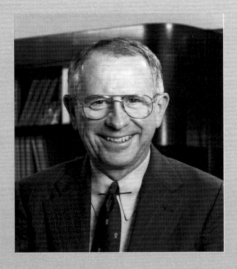

**John L. Cameron (1936-)** is Professor of Surgery at Johns Hopkins University School of Medicine, Director of Surgery at Johns Hopkins Hospital, and author of the excellent book *Current Surgical Therapy.*

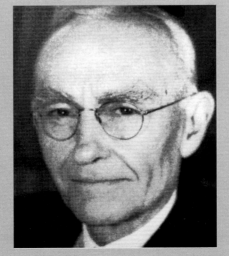

**Allen O. Whipple (1885-1963),** together with Parsons and Mullins, performed the first successful pancreaticoduodenectomy.

*The pancreas, more than any other abdominal organ, continues to provide fascinating surgical frontiers, in both the basic sciences as well as in clinical medicine as the structure and functions of ductal, acinar and islet cell components undergo further amazing detailed analysis.*

*W. P. Longmire Jr.*[1]

## HISTORY

The anatomic and surgical history of the pancreas is summarized in Table 21-1.

## EMBRYOGENESIS

### Normal Development

Two pancreatic primordia (anlagen), the dorsal and ventral (Fig. 21-1), are responsible for the genesis of the pancreas. At the end of the fourth week, on the 26th day, the dorsal pancreatic primordium arises from the dorsal side of the duodenum. The ventral primordium arises somewhat later, on the 32nd day, from the base of the hepatic diverticulum, near the bile duct. Contact between the two pancreatic primordia takes place at about 37 days. Their fusion occurs at the end of the sixth week, the ventral primordium locating below and behind the dorsal. The ventral primordium differentiates into part of the head and uncinate process of the pancreas.

After the fusion of the two primordia, their principal ducts anastomose. This allows the proximal part of the duct of Wirsung from the ventral pancreas to join the common bile duct (CBD), perhaps on the 32nd day, also contributing to the formation of the ampulla of Vater. The terminal portion of the duct of Wirsung is therefore formed by the duct of the ventral pancreas. The distal portion of the duct of the dorsal pancreas is retained as most of the main duct (Fig. 21-1). The duct of Santorini represents the proximal part of the duct of the dorsal pancreas. Remember, the ventral pancreas forms the duct of Wirsung and part of the uncinate process and head.

The dorsal pancreas forms the remainder of the uncinate process and head, plus the body and tail. The secretory acini appear during the third month, and the islands of Langerhans arise from the acini approximately at the end of the third month. Secretion of insulin is taking place around the 5th month. Parenchymal cells are also responsible for glucagon-secreting cells and somatostatin-secreting cells.

Two populations of endodermal cells develop: those that form ducts and acini, and those that form islet cells. Ducts and acini form first, but islet primordia bud off ducts as soon as they are formed. The approximate time of functional awakening of both endocrine and exocrine components is perhaps 10 to 12 weeks.

Polak et al.[2] stated that the patterns of endocrine differentiation and epithelial proliferation observed within the human pancreas early in development suggest that the mesenchyme plays a role in these phenomena.

Debas[3] hypothesizes that the endocrine pancreatic cells derive from the endodermal lining of the primitive gut (mesenchyme of the foregut), not from the endodermal neural crest. The presence of mesenchyme regulates the development of a pancreas with exocrine structures, ducts, and mature islet cells.

The only critical morphologic events are rotation and fusion of the pancreatic primordia. Malrotation of the ventral primordium in the fifth week results in an anular pancreas. Fusion in the seventh week produces several possible variations of ductal patterns. Around the sixth week, the pancreas lies within the dorsal mesentery.

The classic concept of ansa pancreatica (that is, that a loop is formed between an inferior branch of the dorsal pancreatic duct and an inferior branch of the ventral duct) is challenged by Suda et al.[4] There was, from the observations of Suda and colleagues, fusion between an inferior branch of the dorsal pancreatic duct and the ventral pancreatic duct.

## TABLE 21-1. Anatomic and Surgical History of the Pancreas

| | | |
|---|---|---|
| Egypt | ca. 1500 B.C. | The Ebers Papyrus described diabetes |
| Herophilus of Chalcedon (334-280 B.C.) | | Noted the existence of the pancreas |
| Erasistratus of Chios (319-250 B.C.) | | Also mentioned the pancreas but was unsure of its function |
| Aretaeus (A.D. 81-138) | | First to use the term diabetes |
| Rufus of Ephesus | ca. A.D. 100 | Thought the pancreas was part of the omentum. First to use the term "pankreas" (all flesh). |
| Galen (131-200 A.D.) | | Described the pancreas as glandular and identified its arterial and venous supplies |
| Da Carpi | 1522 | Wrote of a glandular pancreas that in the pig was edible ("Brisaro" or sweetbreads) |
| Edwardes | 1532 | Thought that lymphatic vessels were physically supported by the pancreas |
| Massa | 1536 | Wrote that the pancreas served as a pad "upon which the mouth of the stomach rests lest it touch the hard surface of the vertebrae without a buffer between." |
| Vesalius | 1541 | Provided illustrations of the pancreas offering pictures of its vasculature. Agreed with Galen on its glandular nature and disagreed with Rufus on its relationship with the omentum. |
| Wirsung | 1642 | Discovered the main pancreatic duct (Wirsung's duct) |
| Wharton | 1656 | Noted that the pancreas was similar to salivary glands |
| DeGraaf | 1664 | Collected pancreatic juices through a cannulated duct of a dog in order to study pancreatic function |
| Willis | 1674 | Noted that patients suffering from what he called "diabetes mellitus" produced sweet urine |
| Brunner | 1683 | Partially pancreatectomized dogs in vivisection experiments |
| Bidloo | 1685 | Provided a description of the duodenal papillae, the junction of the pancreatic and common bile ducts, and the hepatopancreatic ampulla |
| Vater | 1720 | Redescribed the duodenal papilla originally described by Bidloo; it is now commonly called the papilla of Vater |
| Santorini | 1724 | Observed the main and accessory duodenal papillae along with their associated pancreatic ducts. The accessory duct now bears his eponym (Santorini's duct). |
| Winslow | 1732 | Described the epiploic (omental) foramen (foramen of Winslow) |
| Morgagni | 1769 | First described pancreatoadenocarcinoma |
| Soemmering | 1791 | Described the glandular nature of the pancreas. Labeled it "Bauchspeicheldrüse" (abdominal salivary gland). |
| Bernard | 1849 to 1856 | Performed several experiments establishing the role of the pancreas during digestion. Showed that pancreatic juice emulsifies fatty foods into fatty acids and glycerin, converts starches into sugars, and breaks down proteins that pass undissolved through the stomach. |
| Treitz | 1853 | Located the retropancreatic fascia and Treitz's band |
| Langerhans | 1869 | Noted the presence of small polygonal, non-granulated cells with round nuclei scattered (like islands) throughout the parenchyma. These were named the islets of Langerhans by Laguesse in 1893. |
| Danilevsky | 1872 | Discovered trypsin |
| Kühne | 1874 | Isolated trypsin |
| MacBurney | 1878 | Used a duodenotomy and papillotomy to remove calculi in the papilla |
| Thiersch | 1881 | Drained a fluctuating tumor of the abdomen resulting in a spontaneously closing pancreatic fistula |
| Kühne and Lea | 1882 | Described the capillary network surrounding pancreatic islet cells |

## TABLE 21-1 *(cont'd)*. Anatomic and Surgical History of the Pancreas

| | | |
|---|---|---|
| Bozeman | 1882 | Removed a 20 pound pancreatic cyst |
| Trendelenburg | 1882 | In the process of excising a sarcoma he removed the tail of the pancreas and the spleen |
| von Winiwarter | 1882 | First operation for pancreatic adenocarcinoma |
| Capparelli | 1883 | Drained a pancreatic cyst using an external fistula |
| Gussenbauer | 1883 | Marsupialized a pancreatic pseudocyst |
| Oddi | 1887 | Observed and described the sphincter of the hepatopancreatic ampulla (sphincter of Oddi) |
| Toldt | 1889 | Described the Toldt fascia |
| Fitz | 1889 | Provided the first complete description of acute pancreatitis |
| von Mering and Minkowski | 1889 | Discerned that pancreatectomized dogs developed fatal diabetes |
| Ruggi | 1889 | Removed an adenosarcoma in the tail of the pancreas |
| Minkowski | 1892 | Implanted autogenous pancreatic grafts in pancreatectomized dogs. They did not develop glycosuria until the grafts were removed. |
| Laguesse | 1893 | Suggested that hormones were secreted from the "islots de langerhans" in discussing their capillary networks |
| Kocher | 1895 | Advocated using a choledochoduodenostomy after removing periampullary and choledochal calculi |
| Halsted | 1898 | Removed part of the duodenum along with the pancreas to treat an ampullary carcinoma. Implantation of the pancreatic and common bile duct into a portion of the duodenum followed. |
| Codivilla | 1898 | Treated pancreatic cancer with a pancreatoduodenectomy (resected the duodenum, head of the pancreas, and pylorus, then closed the duodenal stump) followed by a cholecysto-jejunostomy and a gastroenterostomy-en-Y |
| Mayo-Robson | 1900 | Removed a cylindrical portion of the duodenum along with a carcinoma of the ampulla |
| Opie | 1901 | Established the common-channel theory of pancreatitis stating that Wirsung's duct entered the common bile duct proximal to their duodenal entrance. Hypothesized that any stone wedged against the sphincter of this channel could cause bile to flow into the pancreas and pancreatic juice to flow into the biliary tract producing pancreatitis or cholecystitis. In the same report he noted that the islets of Langerhans were associated with diabetes because patients with hyalinized islet cells developed the disease. |
| Ssoboleff | 1902 | Observed that acinar tissue atrophied after ligation of the pancreatic duct while islet tissue remained unchanged |
| Bayliss and Starling | 1902 | Discovered secretin |
| Nicholls | 1902 | Reported a simple pancreatic adenoma involving islet tissue |
| Kocher | 1903 | Developed a method of duodenal mobilization (Kocher's maneuver) later used to enhance access to the duodenal papilla of Vater |
| Fabozzi | 1903 | First to describe islet cell carcinoma |
| Desjardins | 1907 | Performed a cadaveric two-stage procedure to excise the head of the pancreas and the duodenum |
| Svelzer | 1908 | Induced hypoglycemia using an isolated pancreatic extract |
| Lane | 1908 | Differentiated alpha and beta islet cells |
| Sauvé | 1908 | Advocated a one-stage procedure similar to Desjardins' |
| Navarro | 1908 | Performed a papillectomy |
| De Meyer | 1909 | Named Laguesse's hypothetical islet hormone "insuline" |
| Coffey | 1909 | Advocated the implantation of the pancreatic stump (the tail in this case) into the distal end of the resected duodenum after pancreatoduodenectomy |
| Kausch | 1909 | Performed the first successful pancreatoduodenectomy |
| Ombredanne | 1911 | Anastomosed a pancreatic cyst to the duodenum |

**TABLE 21-1 *(cont'd)*. Anatomic and Surgical History of the Pancreas**

| | | |
|---|---|---|
| Kausch | 1912 | First successful two-stage pancreatoduodenectomy |
| Hirschel | 1914 | Connected the common bile duct to the duodenum using a rubber tube after a one-stage partial pancreatoduodenectomy. The patient died one year later. |
| Dragstedt | 1918 | Proved that experimental animals could survive total duodenectomy |
| Banting and Best | 1922 | Isolated "insuline" from islet secretions of dog pancreas |
| Tetani | 1922 | Performed a successful two-stage pancreatoduodenectomy involving a posterior gastrojejunostomy and division of the common duct with a choledochoduodenostomy in the lower end of the duodenum in the first stage. After jaundice subsided, the second stage brought about the resection of duodenum and pancreas 2 cm beyond the ampullary growth with the head of the pancreas implanted into the lower end of the duodenum. |
| S. Harris | 1923 | Suggested that spontaneous hyperinsulinism was possible after noticing it in non-diabetic patients given an overdosage of insulin |
| Wilder | 1927 | Noticed a case of hyperinsulism in a patient with an islet cell tumor |
| Elman | 1927 | Invented the serum amylase test |
| Mayo | 1927 | First operated on a nonresectable metastatic malignant insulinoma |
| R. Graham | 1929 | Removed a benign pancreatic adenoma to successfully treat hyperinsulism |
| Whipple | 1930 | Offered his triad in insulinoma: 1) symptoms of hypoglycemia during fasting; 2) serum glucose less than 50 mg/dL; 3) with administration of exogenous glucose the hypoglycemic symptoms disappear |
| Whipple/ Parsons/ Mullins | 1935 | Published the results of their two-stage procedure for ampullary carcinoma. A cholecysto-gastrostomy was done in the first stage while a duodenectomy was done in the second. They were among the first to use silk suture instead of catgut (which was dissolved by pancreatic enzymes). |
| Whipple | 1935 | Performed a two-stage operation involving a cholecystojejunostomy in the first stage and a total duodenectomy and excision of much of the head of the pancreas in the second |
| Brunschwig | 1937 | Successfully performed a radical pancreatoduodenectomy for carcinoma of the head of the pancreas |
| Whipple | 1940 | Performed a one-stage excision of the entire head of the pancreas with total duodenectomy with 10-year survival |
| Waugh and Clagett | 1943 | Implanted the tail of the pancreas into the posterior wall of the stomach augmenting Whipple's procedure |
| Rockey | 1943 | Performed the first total pancreatectomy |
| Fallis and Szilagyi | 1944 | Performed the first successful total pancreatectomy for pancreatic cancer |
| Clagett | 1944 | Unsuccessfully treated pancreatitis with a total pancreatectomy |
| Zollinger and Ellison | 1955 | Reported four cases in which patients possessed an exaggerated gastric acidity as well as tumors of the alpha islet cells (producing gastrin) |
| Barrett and Bowers | 1957 | Described the 95% pancreatectomy |
| Watts | 1963 | Successfully treated acute fulminant pancreatitis with a total pancreatectomy |
| Doubilet and Mulholland | 1965 | Advocated sphincterectomy to treat acute pancreatitis |
| Kelly and Lillehei | 1966 | First clinical pancreas transplant |
| Fortner | 1973 | Introduced the regional pancreatectomy (total pancreatectomy, resection of the pancreatic segment of the portal vein, subtotal gastrectomy and regional lymph node dissection for type I, and extending to resect the hepatic and superior mesenteric arteries in type II) |
| Kelly, Acosta | 1974 | Reported gallstone migration through the ampulla of Vater initiating pancreatitis |
| Traverso and Longmire | 1978 | Introduced the pylorus-preserving pancreatoduodenectomy |

**TABLE 21-1 (cont'd). Anatomic and Surgical History of the Pancreas**

| | | |
|---|---|---|
| Safrany | 1980 | Performed early endoscopic papillotomy to remove calculi in the papilla |
| Ishida et al. | 1981 | Early report of laparoscopic pancreatic biopsy |
| Jordan | 1987 | Advocated anastomosis of the first and third portions of the duodenum after resection of the head of the pancreas |
| Beger et al. | 1988 | Described necrosectomy in management of necrotizing pancreatitis |
| Neoptolemos et al. | 1988 | Randomized trial of endoscopic retrograde cholangiopancreatography (ERCP) and endoscopic sphincterotomy |
| Warshaw et al. | 1990 | Study showed that laparoscopy for assessment of pancreatic cancer compared favorably with other methods |
| Sarr et al. | 1991 | Described necrosectomy in management of necrotizing pancreatitis |

Source: McClusky DA III, Skandalakis LJ, Colborn GL, Skandalakis JE. Harbinger or hermit? Pancreatic anatomy and surgery through the ages. Part III. World J Surg 2002; 26:1512-1524; with permission.

**References**

Beger HG, Büchler M, Bittner R, Block S, Nevalainen T, Roscher R. Necrosectomy and postoperative local lavage in necrotizing pancreatitis. Br J Surg 1988;75:207-212.

Cameron JL. Current Surgical Therapy (5th ed). St. Louis: Mosby, 1995, pp. 414, 465.

Ishida H, Furukawa Y, Kuroda H, Kobayashi M, Tsuneoka K. Laparoscopic observation and biopsy of the pancreas. Endoscopy 1981;13:68-73.

Lo CY, van Heerden JA, Thompson GB, Grant CS, Söreide JA, Harmsen WS. Islet cell carcinoma of the pancreas. World J Surg 1996;20:878-884.

Neoptolemos JP, Carr-Locke DL, London NJ, Bailey IA, James D, Fossard DP. Controlled trial of urgent endoscopic retrograde cholangiopancreatography and endoscopic sphincterotomy versus conservative treatment for acute pancreatitis due to gallstones. Lancet 1988;2:979-983.

Praderi RC. History of pancreatic surgery. In: Trede M, Carter DC (eds). Surgery of the Pancreas. New York: Churchill Livingtone, 1993, pp. 3-15.

Rhoads JE, Folin LS. The history of surgery of the pancreas. In: Howard JM, Jordan GL, Reber HA (eds.) Surgical Diseases of the Pancreas. Philadelphia: Lea and Febiger, 1987, pp. 3-10.

Sarr MG, Nagorney DM, Mucha P Jr., Farnell MB, Johnson CD. Acute necrotizing pancreatitis: management by planned, staged pancreatic necrosectomy/debridement and delayed primary wound closure over drains. Br J Surg 1991;78:576-581.

Tan HP, Smith J, Garberoglio CA. Pancreatic adenocarcinoma: An update. J Am Coll Surg 1996;183:164-184.

Warshaw AL, Gu ZY, Wittenberg J, Waltman AC. Preoperative staging and assessment of resectability of pancreatic cancer. Arch Surg 1990;125:230-233.

Whipple AO. A historical sketch of the pancreas. In: Howard JM, Jordan GL (eds.) Surgical Diseases of the Pancreas. Philadelphia: JB Lippincott, 1960, pp. 1-8.

We include here Table 21-2 from *Embryology for Surgeons*[5] and the quotation that accompanies it:

> It is not within the scope of this book to give details on fetal physiology nor to discuss ontogeny and phylogeny; however, we wish to include in the form of a table the ontogeny of the gastrointestinal peptides from the excellent chapter of Leung and Lebenthal.[6] This shows the approximate time of appearance of the peptides in various tissues of the human fetus.

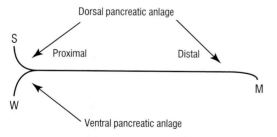

FIG 21-1. Embryogenesis of proximal and distal pancreatic duct (highly diagrammatic). S, Duct of Santorini; W, Duct of Wirsung; M, Main pancreatic duct. (From Skandalakis LJ, Rowe JS Jr., Gray SW, Skandalakis JE. Surgical embryology and anatomy of the pancreas. Surg Clin North Am 1993;73:661-697; with permission.)

## Congenital Anomalies

There are many congenital anomalies of the pancreas (Table 21-3). This chapter cannot present all of them but will briefly discuss the following: pancreas divisum, anular pancreas, pancreatic gallbladder, ectopic and accessory pancreas, intraperitoneal pancreas, gastrinomas, and insulinomas. The interested student is advised to study *Embryology for Surgeons*.[5]

### Pancreas Divisum

Failure of the dorsal and ventral pancreatic primordia (anlagen) to fuse may result in separate draining of the

### TABLE 21-2. Ontogeny of the Gastrointestinal Peptides

| Peptide | Age of Earliest Appearance (Weeks) | |
|---|---|---|
| Glucagon | 6 | (pancreas) |
| Insulin | 10 | (pancreas) |
| Somatostatin | 8 | (pancreas) |
| Somatostatin | 9-11 | (intestine) |
| Pancreatic polypeptide | 8-9 | (pancreas) |
| Gastrin | 10-11 | (duodenum) |
| Cholecystokinin | 10 | (duodenum) |
| Secretin | 8 | (duodenum) |
| GIP* | 8-10 | (duodenum and jejunum) |
| VIP† | 8-9 | (fundus and duodenum) |
| VIP | 10 | (VIP-nerve fibers) |
| Neurotensin | 12 | (jejunum, ileum, colon) |
| Motilin | 8-11 | (duodenum, jejunum) |
| Substance P | 18-25 | (brainstem) |
| Bombesin | 12 | (bronchus) |

*Gastric inhibitory polypeptide.
†Vasoactive intestinal peptide.

*Source:* Leung YK, Lebenthal E. Gastrointestinal peptides: physiology, ontogeny, and clinical significance. In: Lebenthal E (ed). Human Gastrointestinal Development. New York: Raven, 1989, pp. 41-98; with permission.

ducts of Wirsung and Santorini. This condition is called "pancreas divisum" or "isolated ventral pancreas." About 12 percent of patients with pancreatitis have pancreas divisum demonstrated on ERCP (endoscopic retrograde cholangiopancreatography), but only 3 percent of patients who have pancreatography for other reasons have the anomaly. This suggests that pancreas divisum predisposes to attacks of acute pancreatitis.[7-10] Pancreatitis may occur secondary to stenosis or obstruction of one or both ducts. Stenting may relieve the symptoms of patients with chronic pancreatitis.[11,12] To avoid the formation of stones, sphincteroplasty of both ducts and cholecystectomy is the current procedure of choice. Neblett and O'Neill[13] advised that patients with more distal ductal obstruction or ductal ectasia may benefit from pancreaticojejunostomy. Kamisawa et al.[14] presented what may be the first report of carcinoma associated with anular pancreas coexistent with pancreas divisum.

### Anular Pancreas

An anular pancreas (Fig. 21-2) is a thin, flat band of normal pancreatic tissue surrounding the second part of the duodenum and continuing into the head of the pancreas on either side. The band may be partially or wholly free from the duodenum, or the pancreatic tissue may penetrate the duodenal muscularis. The ring of pancreatic tissue contains a large duct that usually enters the main pancreatic duct. This, however, occasionally enters the duodenum independently.

The anular pancreas' developmental course is not known. Is the ventral anlage totally responsible because of its early division into two parts? Perhaps the left part follows an opposite direction and produces the constricting ring. Or is early fusion of the ventral pancreatic tip with the dorsal pancreas responsible for this anomaly? Nobukawa et al.[15] described an anular pancreas originating from paired ventral pancreata, with a ring formation originating from the left lobe.

Duodenal stenosis at the level of the pancreatic ring is typical. If obstruction at the site of the anulus exists before birth, hydramnios is frequently present.[16] However, half of the patients with anular pancreas do not have symptoms until adulthood,[17] when they present with signs of duodenal obstruction. Currently, the procedures of choice to treat duodenal obstruction caused by anular pancreas are duodenoduodenostomy, first proposed by Gross and Chisholm,[18] or duodenojejunostomy.

### Pancreatic Gallbladder

In 1926, Boyden[19] described gallbladder duplications in cats in which the accessory organ arose from the ventral pancreatic bud instead of from the cystic primordium. He suggested that some duplications in humans might be of this type. Wrenn and Favara[20] reported the presence of a human pancreatic gallbladder. This was confirmed by Boyden.[21] Pancreatic tissue in the wall of an otherwise normal gallbladder[22] does not indicate origin from the ventral pancreatic primordium.[23]

### Ectopic Pancreas, Heterotopic Pancreatic Tissue, and Accessory Pancreas

It is not unusual to have pancreatic tissue in the stomach

### TABLE 21-3. Congenital Anomalies of the Pancreas

| | |
|---|---|
| Aplasia-hypoplasia | Pancreatic gallbladder |
| Hyperplasia-hypertrophy | Cystic fibrosis |
| Dysplasia | Pancreatic cysts |
| Variations and anomalies of the ducts—pancreas divisum | Rotational anomalies |
| | Ectopic pancreatic tissue |
| Anular pancreas | Vascular anomalies |
| | Intraperitoneal pancreas |

*Source:* Modified from Skandalakis LJ, Rowe JS Jr, Gray SW, Skandalakis JE. Surgical embryology and anatomy of the pancreas. Surg Clin North Am 73(4): 661-697, 1993; with permission.

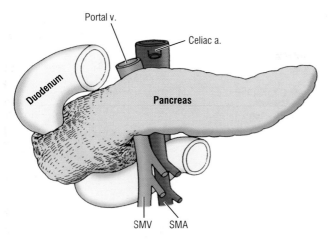

**FIG 21-2.** Anular pancreas; duodenum under anulus is usually stenosed. SMV, superior mesenteric vein; SMA, superior mesenteric artery. (Modified from Skandalakis JE, Gray SW, Rowe JS Jr, Skandalakis LJ. Anatomical complications of pancreatic surgery. Contemp Surg 1979;15(5):17-50; with permission.)

(Fig. 21-3), duodenal wall or ileal wall, Meckel's diverticulum, or at the umbilicus. Less common sites are the colon,[24] appendix,[25] gallbladder,[26] omentum or mesentery,[27] and in anomalous bronchoesophageal fistula.[28]

Most ectopic pancreatic tissue is functional. Islet tissue is often present in gastric and duodenal heterotopia, but it is usually absent in accessory pancreatic tissue elsewhere in the body.

Accessory duodenal pancreas may occur as lobules of normal pancreas in the submucosa sequestered beneath the muscularis externa. In other cases, pancreatized Brunner's glands might be considered to be a potential anlage. Development of accessory pancreatic tissue is usually suppressed by the earlier maturing normal pancreas, but may occasionally escape from such suppression.

Feldman and Weinberg[29] found duodenal pancreatic tissue in 13.7 percent of 410 necropsy specimens. Pearson[30] estimated that heterotopic pancreatic tissue could be found in as many as 2 percent of autopsies if it were sought carefully. About 6 percent of Meckel's diverticula can be expected to contain pancreatic tissue.[31] Fékété et al. reported six cases of a pseudotumor with cystic dystrophy developing in heterotopic pancreas.[32]

Atypical metaplasia of pluripotential endodermal cells of the embryonic foregut may account for the presence of pancreatic tissue in the stomach, Meckel's diverticulum, and intestinal duplications. Asymptomatic ectopic pancreatic tissue in the intestine is increasingly recognized as a potential source of pyloric obstruction, disruption of normal peristalsis, production of peptic ulcer, or neoplasm. Ravitch[33] wrote

that the presence of an ulcerated nodule of ectopic pancreas in the stomach or duodenum may give rise to ulcer-like symptoms that are relieved by removal of the nodule. According to Rosai,[34] if a patient with heterotopic pancreas develops acute pancreatitis, the inflammatory process will also affect the heterotopic foci.

## *Intraperitoneal Pancreas*

Tuncel et al.[35] presented a case of intraperitoneal pancreas where the head and a part of the body of the pancreas were found intraperitoneally. They summarized their findings as follows.

> *The pancreas was covered by the peritoneum within the omental bursa except its tail. Additionally, the anterior layer of the hepatogastric ligament turned over the hepatoduodenal ligament and continued behind the head of the pancreas together with the peritoneum which formed the posterior wall of the epiploic foramen (Winslow). The peritoneum also covered a part of the posterior surface of the body and directed to the right, forming a recessus just behind the pancreas.*

## *Gastrinoma and Insulinoma*

In all honesty, we do not know whether the gastrinoma

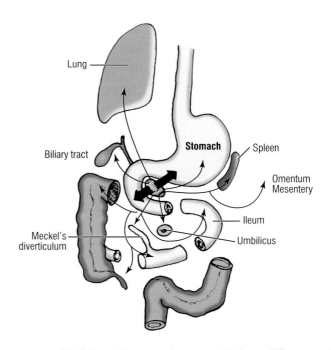

**FIG 21-3.** Chief sites of heterotopic pancreatic tissue. Fifty percent of these structures occur in the duodenum or pylorus. (Modified from Skandalakis JE, Gray SW. Embryology for Surgeons (2nd ed). Baltimore: Williams & Wilkins, 1994; with permission.)

is an embryologic phenomenon. We hope the reader will forgive us for mentioning this tumor and the insulinoma together with other "bona fide" congenital anomalies.

Gastrinoma, a benign or malignant tumor, is located primarily in the pancreas. It is responsible for the Zollinger-Ellison syndrome (ZES): acid and pepsin supersecretion by the parietal and chief cells of the mucosa of the fundus of the stomach. This syndrome is named for the two researchers who associated islet cell tumor, hormone hypersecretion, and the resulting severe clinical manifestations.[36] We agree with Stabile[37] that their work "served as the defining moment for the entire field of gastrointestinal endocrinology."

According to Stabile et al.,[38] most gastrinomas (90%) are anatomically located within the so-called gastrinoma triangle (Fig. 21-4). The boundaries of this triangle are the cystic duct, the border of the 2nd and 3rd portion of the duodenum, and the junction of the neck and body of the pancreas.

Passaro and colleagues,[39] fathers of the gastrinoma triangle, hypothesize that some gastrinomas are embryologically of ventral pancreatic bud stem origin. These authors postulate a very interesting conjecture that stem cells from the ventral bud disperse and are enveloped by lymphoid tissue and the duodenal wall. We agree with Townsend[40] that Passaro el al. "removed the mystery from the 'ectopic' gastrinomas," and add our encomiums to his.

According to Townsend and Thompson,[41] pancreatic

### TABLE 21-4. Pathology, Location, and Extent of Tumor in Patients with Zollinger-Ellison Syndrome

| Tumor Characteristics | % of Patients with Indicated Characteristic[a] | Range (%) |
|---|---|---|
| Extent of tumor | | |
|   No tumor found | 30 | 7-48 |
|   Localized tumor | 36 | 23-51 |
|   Metastatic tumor | 34 | 13-52 |
| Tumor location | | |
|   Pancreas | 42 | 21-65 |
|   Duodenum | 15 | 6-32 |
|   Other[b] | 2 | 0-18 |
|   Metastases only | 2 | 0-11 |
| Pathology | | |
|   Gastrinoma | 90 | 87-100 |
|     Malignant | | 60-90 |
|     Benign | | 10-39 |
|   Islet cell hyperplasia | 10[c] | 0-13 |

[a]Data from 12 studies (see source)
[b]Other locations include lymph nodes primarily, but also in the stomach, liver, mesentery, renal capsule, ovary
[c]In recent studies islet cell hyperplasia is felt not to be a cause of ZES

*Source:* Jensen RT, Gardner JD. Gastrinoma. In: Go VLW, DiMagno EP, Gardner JD, Lebenthal E, Reber HA, Scheele GA. The Pancreas: Biology, Pathobiology, and Disease, 2nd Ed. New York: Raven Press, 1993; with permission.

gastrinomas have an anatomic distribution in the head, body, and tail of 4:1:4. Fewer than 25% of patients have a single tumor. Two pancreatic areas are affected in 30% of patients, and 20% have tumors in all three areas.

Surgery is the procedure of choice for gastrinoma, benign or malignant, despite the occasional good result with careful conservative treatment. Table 21-4 presents the tumor characteristics of patients with ZES.

Norton et al.[42] stated that surgical resection of localized liver gastrinoma provides a cure rate similar to that of extrahepatic gastrinoma with excellent long-term survival.

Kisker et al.[43] advised intraoperative ultrasonography in association with pancreatic and duodenal exploration for localization of gastrinomas. They reported detection and excision of the tumor in 96% of their cases.

Proye et al.[44] advised including intraoperative gastrin measurement in the surgical treatment of gastrinoma.

REMEMBER: Occasionally, the student is confused by the differences between gastrinomas and insulinomas. We add a few comments about insulinomas to separate these two clinical entities, one perhaps congenital and the other acquired.

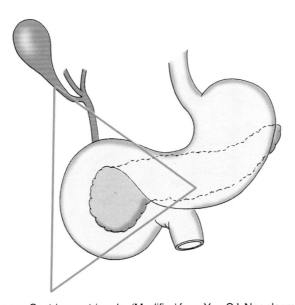

FIG. 21-4. Gastrinoma triangle. (Modified from Yeo CJ. Neoplasms of the endocrine pancreas. In: Greenfield LJ (ed). Surgery: Scientific Principles and Practice, 2nd Ed. Philadelphia: Lippincott-Raven, 1997, pp. 918-929; with permission.)

mas, glucagonomas, amphicrine tumors) (Table 21-5):

> Patients with duodenal gastrinoma with lymph node metasteses were curable, and cures were achieved occasionally after resection of liver metastases. Results of operation were similar for those with and without MEN I. MEN I and metastases were not contraindications to operation; instead, these patients should be operated on aggressively. Gastrinomas not found at operation were likely to be small duodenal gastrinomas. Gastrinomas can arise in a lymph node and can be cured by its removal. Parietal cell vagotomy is recommended after operation for gastrinomas in the event of residual tumor. With the exception of patients with MEN I or microadenomata, insulinomas were treated best by tumor enucleation. Otherwise, Whipple operation or distal pancreatectomy and enucleation of tumor in the remaining pancreas was indicated.

## Surgical Applications

- The embryologic and anatomic relationships between the pancreas, stomach, esophagus, duodenum, and spleen may have potential implications with respect to some surgical questions.

  The embryology of the stomach and related organs is such that the body and tail of the pancreas (derived from the dorsal pancreatic anlage), together with the spleen, lie in the dorsal mesogastrium. They share both a common blood supply (left gastric and splenic arteries) and a common lymphatic drainage with the proximal portion of the stomach.

### TABLE 21-5. Distribution of Neuroendocrine Tumors

| Tumor | n |
|---|---|
| Pancreatic gastrinoma | |
|   Without MEN I | 9 |
|   With MEN I | 3 |
| Duodenal and lymph node gastrinoma | 13 |
| Pancreatic and duodenal gastrinoma | 5 |
| Duodenal gastrinoma | 7 |
| Primary lymph node gastrinoma | 3 |
| Nonfunctioning neuroendocrine tumor | 16 |
| Neuroendocrine tumor not found | 11 |
| Insulinoma | 11 |
| Pancreatic amphicrine tumor | 2 |
| Glucagonoma | 1 |
| Somatostatinoma | 1 |

*Source:* Jordan PH Jr. A personal experience with pancreatic and duodenal neuroendocrine tumors. J Am Coll Surg 189:470-482, 1999; with permission.

---

## Editorial Comment

*The origin of gastrinomas found in periduodenal lymph nodes in the absence of an evident primary tumor has long been the subject of debate. The Passaro et al. theory (described above) of pancreatic stem cells being enveloped by lymphoid tissue is an explanation when no primary can be found. However, it should be noted that surgeons are becoming increasingly skillful at detecting primaries in the duodenum. Careful inspection of the duodenum with techniques such as transillumination and ultrasound are detecting many very small primaries. Previously these patients would have been suspected as having "lymph node primaries" rather than duodenal primaries. One wonders how many small primary gastrinomas are still undetected. (RSF Jr)*

Insulinoma syndrome, an overproduction of insulin, is caused by a β-cell tumor. Located at the islets of Langerhans, these small (less than 2 cm) tumors are solitary in 90% of cases.[7] Unlike gastrinomas, insulinomas are equally distributed in the head, body, and tail of the pancreas. Less than 10%[45] of insulinomas are malignant. After preoperative localization, surgery is the treatment of choice.

Kuzin et al.[46] advised the use of intraoperative ultrasonography, and selective celiac arteriography in combination with arterial stimulated venous sampling, for precise localization of organic hyperinsulinism. Boukhman et al.[47] found intraoperative ultrasonography more sensitive than preoperative ultrasonography or any other intraoperative localization study for localization of insulinomas.

We quote from Hashimoto and Walsh:[48]

> The diagnosis of an insulinoma does not require extensive localization studies before operation. The combination of surgical exploration and intraoperative ultrasonography identified more than 90% of insulinomas. When technically feasible, enucleation is curative and can be accomplished with low morbidity.

Simon et al.[49] described operative strategies for reoperation in patients with organic hyperinsulinism with diffuse or multiple disease (multiple tumors, MEN I syndrome [multiple endocrine neoplasia type I], and diffuse nodular hyperplasia).

Jordan[50] gave an excellent summary of his 35-year experience in treating pancreatic and duodenal neuroendocrine tumors (gastrinomas, insulinomas, somatostatino-

The head of the pancreas (derived from the ventral pancreatic anlage) lies in the mesoduodenum. The pancreatic head shares its blood supply (pancreaticoduodenal and gastroduodenal arteries) and lymphatic drainage with the duodenum, the distal CBD, and the distal stomach.

- Cancer of the proximal stomach can theoretically be treated effectively by en bloc resection of the distribution of the left gastric and splenic arteries (Fig. 21-5A). This includes the distal esophagus, the proximal two-thirds of the stomach and greater omentum, the spleen, and the body and tail of the pancreas.

- Similarly, cancer of the distal stomach can be treated by en bloc resection of the distribution of the common hepatic artery, sparing, of course, the artery itself (Fig. 21-5B). This resection includes the head of the pancreas, the distal stomach and greater omentum, the duodenum, and the distal bile duct.

- Visalli and Grimes[51] believe that the en bloc resections described above will check metastatic spread more effectively than will extirpation of peripheral lymph nodes only. Perhaps this will be the case in the future, but the procedure should be accompanied by lymphadenectomy. The reader is reminded of the high morbidity and mortality that accompany such procedures.

- Doglietto et al.[52] advocated pancreas-preserving total gastrectomy for cancer of the stomach due to its low incidence of postoperative complications and high survival rates.

- Duodenoduodenostomy is the best procedure for anular pancreas. Duodenojejunostomy also may be utilized. Both procedures avoid the formation of pancreatic fistula due to the presence of pancreatic ductules and an inability to relieve the stenosis due to mingling of the pancreatic tissues within the duodenal wall musculature.

- Ectopic or accessory pancreas should be removed to avoid future problems such as ulceration, bleeding, pancreatitis, intussusception, or even formation of benign or malignant neoplasms and other related problems.

- Chung et al.[53] reported duodenal ectopic pancreas complicated by chronic pancreatitis and pseudocyst formation. Allison et al.[54] reported ectopic pancreas in the gastric antrum with gastroduodenal prolapse. Salman et al.[55] reported ileocolic intussusception secondary to an ectopic pancreas located at the antimesenteric border of the terminal ileum. Kovari et al.[56] reported papillary cystic neoplasms in ectopic pancreas located in the omentum. Roshe et al.[57] presented a case of anaplastic carcinoma arising in ectopic pancreas located in the distal esophagus. Guillou et al.[58] reported ductal adenocarcinoma originating in an ectopic pancreas which was located in a hiatal hernia at the gastroesophageal junction.

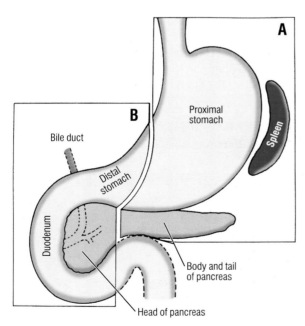

FIG. 21-5. Highly diagrammatic presentation for en bloc resections of **(A)** proximal stomach and related organs sharing a common blood supply and lymphatic drainage, and **(B)** distal stomach and related organs. (Modified from Skandalakis JE, Gray SW, Rowe JS Jr. Anatomical Complications in General Surgery. New York: McGraw-Hill, 1983; with permission.)

## SURGICAL ANATOMY

*The precise anatomy of the pancreas, its ducts, and its adjacent blood vessels achieves great importance in operating on the pancreas. Failure to be wary of the implications of surgical procedures on the pancreas is often followed by a string of complications that are serious at best and are not unlikely to be fatal. In this regard, the pancreas is one of the most treacherous organs to operate on.*

*R.J. Baker*[59]

### Topography and Relations

The pancreas is neither striking in appearance nor obvious in function. Its early history is hardly more than a list of the names of those who noticed it in their dissections before passing on to more interesting organs. It was only with demonstration of the digestive enzymes by Claude Bernard in 1850 that the pancreas became a complete

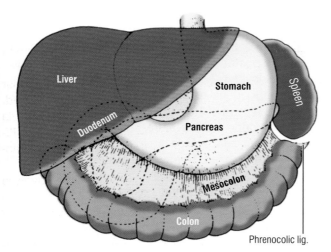

**FIG. 21-6.** Anterior relationships. (Modified from Skandalakis JE, Gray SW, Rowe JS Jr, Skandalakis LJ. Anatomical complications of pancreatic surgery. Contemp Surg 1979;15:17-50; with permission.)

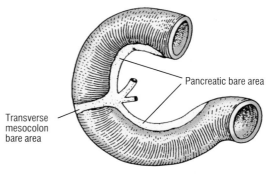

**FIG. 21-7.** Bare areas of duodenum. Pancreas is in intimate contact with the duodenum along the concave surface. Attachment of transverse mesocolon produces an additional bare area. (Modified from Skandalakis JE, Gray SW, Rowe JS Jr, Skandalakis LJ. Anatomical complications of pancreatic surgery. Contemp Surg 1979;15: 17-50; with permission.)

organ with an important function and thus an object worthy of study.

In spite of the apparent accessibility of the pancreas, several anatomic relations combine to make its surgical removal difficult. In 1898, Halstead was the first to successfully remove the head of the pancreas and a portion of the duodenum for ampullary cancer. Several surgeons, in the United States and elsewhere, subsequently developed two-stage operations for removal of the head of the pancreas. These efforts culminated in 1940 with the one-stage operation of Allen O. Whipple. A major factor in Whipple's success was the use of silk sutures, which tend to resist digestion by enzymes that destroy catgut sutures.

Sir Andrew Watt Kay[60] wrote in 1978, "For me, the tiger country is removal of the pancreas. The anatomy is very complex and one encounters anomalies."

The embryogenesis of the pancreas and its deep retroperitoneal anatomy are responsible for the tiger country. No other organ is so closely surrounded by so many anatomic entities, including the duodenum, stomach, spleen, left adrenal, transverse mesocolon and colon, left kidney, right ureter, and jejunum. Figures 21-6, 21-7, 21-8, and 21-9 show anterior and posterior relations of the pancreas.

The proximity of the pancreas to so many organs means it is prone to local invasion by carcinoma. Z'graggen et al.[61] reported metastasis to the pancreas from carcinoma of the kidney and lung. Isolated metastases may be amenable to palliation and even long term survival with resection. Similarly, pancreatic cancer is likely to invade other organs.

Two tables show important considerations in pancreatic cancer: organs directly invaded by pancreatic duct cancer (Table 21-6) and areas most likely to involve metastatic lesions from pancreatic cancer (Table 21-7).

## Location and Parts of the Pancreas

The pancreas lies transversely in the retroperitoneal sac, between the duodenum on the right and the spleen on the left. It is related to the omental bursa above, the transverse mesocolon anteriorly, and the greater sac below. For all practical purposes, the pancreas is a fixed organ.

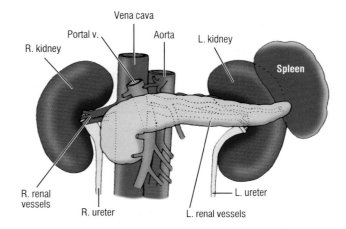

**FIG. 21-8.** Posterior relationships of the pancreas. (Modified from Skandalakis JE, Gray SW, Rowe JS Jr, Skandalakis LJ. Anatomical complications of pancreatic surgery. Contemp Surg 1979;15:17-50; with permission.)

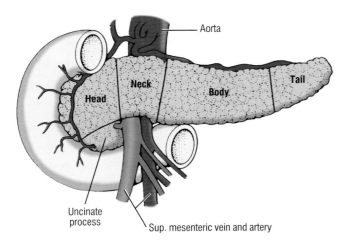

Aorta

Neck

Tail

Body

Head

Uncinate process

Sup. mesenteric vein and artery

FIG. 21-9. Five parts of pancreas. Line dividing body and tail is entirely arbitrary. (Modified from Skandalakis JE, Gray SW, Rowe JS Jr. Anatomical Complications in General Surgery. New York: McGraw-Hill, 1983; with permission.)

Busnardo et al.[62] studied the segmental anatomy of the human pancreas in 30 corrosion casts. Two anatomic segments were found (Figs. 21-10, 21-11), perhaps similar to the segmentation that can be found in the liver, spleen, kidneys, and other organs. The right segment (cephalocervical) and the left (corporocaudate) are separated from each other by a poorly vascularized area. They are connected by the main pancreatic duct and often, according to these authors, by a small artery.

The parts of the pancreas as traditionally accepted are discussed below and shown in Figure 21-9.

## Head

The head of the pancreas is flattened and has an anterior and a posterior surface. The anterior surface is adjacent to the pylorus and the transverse colon. The anterior pancreaticoduodenal arcade can be seen upon the ventral surface of the head of the pancreas, coursing roughly parallel with the duodenal curvature. The posterior pancreaticoduodenal vascular arcade is a major entity on the posterior surface of the head. This surface of the pancreatic head is close to the hilum and medial border of the right kidney, the right renal vessels and the inferior vena cava, the right crus of the diaphragm, and the right gonadal vein.

The head of the pancreas adheres to the duodenal loop. Osler offers a very poetic description of this junction: "The abdominal area of romance where the head of the pancreas lies folded in the arms of the duodenum."

The head the pancreas may be related to the third part of the common bile duct in a variety of ways.[63] Figures 21-12A and 21-12B show the most frequent conditions: the bile duct is partially covered by a tongue of pancreatic tissue (44 percent). In Figure 21-12C, the bile duct is completely covered (30 percent). The duct is uncovered on the posterior surface of the pancreas in 16.5 percent of cases (Fig. 21-12D). In 9 percent of cases, the third part of the common bile duct is covered by two tongues of pancreatic tissue (Fig. 21-12E).

## Uncinate Process

The uncinate ("hooklike") process is an extension of the head of the pancreas and is highly variable in size and

| | | Primary Site | | | | | |
|---|---|---|---|---|---|---|---|
| Anatomical Site Invaded | Total No. Patients | Head | | Body | | Tail | |
| | | No. | (%) | No. | (%) | No. | (%) |
| Duodenum | 30 | 24 | (67) | 6 | (24) | 0 | (0) |
| Stomach | 20 | 9 | (25) | 10 | (40) | 1 | (7) |
| Spleen | 8 | 0 | (0) | 3 | (12) | 5 | (36) |
| Left adrenal | 5 | 0 | (0) | 1 | (4) | 4 | (29) |
| Transverse colon | 6 | 1 | (3) | 3 | (12) | 2 | (14) |
| Left kidney | 2 | 0 | (0) | 1 | (4) | 1 | (7) |
| Jejunum | 3 | 1 | (3) | 1 | (4) | 1 | (7) |
| Ureter (right) | 1 | 1 | (3) | 0 | (0) | 0 | (0) |
| Total (%) | 75 | 36 | (48) | 25 | (33) | 14 | (19) |

**TABLE 21-6. Organ Directly Invaded (at Autopsy) by Pancreas Duct Cancer (75 Patients)**

*Source:* Cubilla AL, Fitzgerald PJ. Metastasis in pancreatic duct adenocarcinoma. In: Day SB, Meyers WPL, Stanley P, et al. (eds). Cancer Invasion and Metastasis: Biologic Mechanisms and Therapy. New York, Raven Press, 1977; with permission.

**TABLE 21-7. Sites of Metastases from Carcinoma of the Pancreas as Seen at Autopsy**

| Site of Metastasis | Location of Tumor | |
|---|---|---|
| | Head (%) | Body and Tail (%) |
| Regional nodes | 75 | 76 |
| Liver | 65 | 71 |
| Lungs | 30 | 14 |
| Peritoneum | 22 | 38 |
| Duodenum | 19 | 5 |
| Adrenals | 13 | 24 |
| Stomach | 11 | 5 |
| Gallbladder | 9 | 0 |
| Spleen | 6 | 14 |
| Kidney | 6 | 5 |
| Intestines | 4 | 5 |
| Mediastinal nodes | 4 | 5 |
| Other | 19 | 28 |
| No metastasis | 13 | 0 |

*Source:* Howard JM, Jordan JL Jr. Cancer of the pancreas. Curr Probl Cancer 2: 5-52, 1977; with permission.

cess is empiric.

- Division at the neck is equivalent to a 60 percent to 70 percent resection.
- Division at the proximal body to the left of the portal vein above and to the superior mesenteric vein below is a 50 percent to 60 percent resection.
- Even with an 80 percent pancreatectomy, good exocrine and endocrine activity are present.
- We cannot predict whether the physiology of the in situ remaining pancreas after pancreatectomy will be normal because we do not know how much pancreatic disease is present within the remaining part of the pancreas.

We have seen the ligament of the uncinate process where the process ends in the vicinity of the superior mesenteric vein. In such cases, the ligament is quite dense and attaches the process to the superior mesenteric artery. Pancreatitis or cancer makes the fixation even more adherent. An anomalous right hepatic artery may pass through the uncinate process. Because the aorta is behind the un-

shape. It passes downward and slightly to the left from the principal part of the head. It further continues behind the superior mesenteric vessels and in front of the aorta and inferior vena cava. In sagittal section, the uncinate process (Fig. 21-13) lies between the aorta and the superior mesenteric artery, with the left renal vein above and the duodenum below. If the junction of the superior mesenteric vein with the portal vein is low, the anterior surface of the uncinate process is related to the superior mesenteric vessels and the portal vein.

The uncinate process may be absent or may completely encircle the superior mesenteric vessels (Fig. 21-14). If the process is well developed, the neck of the pancreas must be sectioned from the front to avoid injury to the vessels. Short vessels from the superior mesenteric artery and vein supply the uncinate process and must be carefully ligated.

In an unpublished study by J.E. Skandalakis, dissection of the head of the pancreas was performed in 20 fresh cadavers. The uncinate process was observed in 18, and absent in 2. In most cases, the posterior surface of the uncinate process was in contact with the inferior vena cava and aorta and was crossed ventrally by the superior mesenteric vein and artery. Efforts to weigh the proximal and distal pancreas with or without the uncinate process did not provide any satisfactory data regarding the weight of the uncinate process.

REMEMBER:

- The extent of resection of the head or the uncinate pro-

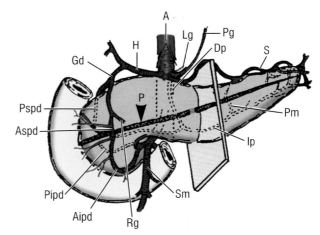

FIG. 21-10. Diagram of the arteries surrounding the human pancreas. The intersegmental plane has been drawn on the left of the superior mesenteric artery. The right and left pancreatic anatomicosurgical segments are united intraparenchymally only by the inferior pancreatic artery which corresponds, in this case, to the left terminal branch of the dorsal pancreatic artery. The pancreatic ducts are not shown in their entire extension until their termination in the major and minor duodenal papilla. A, Aorta; Lg, Left gastric artery; Pg, Posterior gastric artery; Dp, Dorsal pancreatic artery; S, Splenic artery; Pm, Pancreatica magna artery; Ip, Inferior pancreatic artery; Sm, Superior mesenteric artery; Rg, Right gastroepiploic (gastromental) artery; Aipd, Anterior inferior pancreaticoduodenal artery; Pipd, Posterior inferior pancreaticoduodenal artery; Aspd, Anterior superior pancreaticoduodenal artery; Pspd, Posterior superior pancreaticoduodenal artery; Gd, Gastroduodenal artery; H, Hepatic artery; P (arrow), Pancreatic duct. (Modified from Busnardo AC, DiDio LJA, Thomford NR. Anatomicosurgical segments of the human pancreas. Surg Radiol Anat 10:77-82, 1988; with permission.)

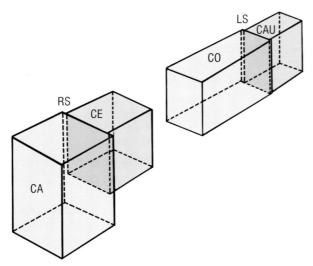

**FIG. 21-11.** Diagrams of the anatomicosurgical segments of the pancreas: RS, right (cephalocervical) and LS, left (corporocaudate). The right and left pancreatic segments are artificially separated at the level of the pauci-arterial area. CA, Caput (head); CE, Cervix; CO, Corpus; CAU, Cauda pancreatica. (Modified from Busnardo AC, DiDio LJA, Thomford NR. Anatomicosurgical segments of the human pancreas. Surg Radiol Anat 10:77-82, 1988; with permission.)

cinate process, pancreatic carcinoma can be inseparable from the aorta.

### Neck

The neck of the pancreas can be defined as the site of passage of the superior mesenteric vessels and the beginning of the portal vein dorsal to the pancreas. This pancreatic segment is 1.5 to 2.0 cm long, and it is partially covered anteriorly by the pylorus.

The gastroduodenal artery passes to the right of the neck and provides origin for the anterior superior pancreaticoduodenal artery. Posterior to the neck, the portal vein is formed by the confluence of the superior mesenteric and splenic veins. Near the inferior margin of the pancreatic neck, one can often see the terminations of the inferior pancreaticoduodenal vein and right gastroepiploic vein where they drain into the superior mesenteric or splenic veins or into the portal vein proper.

The inferior mesenteric vein drains, with essentially equal frequency, into the splenic vein, the superior mesenteric vein, or the site of formation of the portal vein. Careful elevation of the neck and ligation of any anterior tributaries, if present, are necessary. Bleeding can make it difficult to evaluate the structures lying beneath the neck.

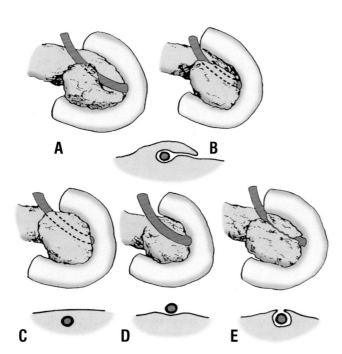

**FIG. 21-12.** Five variations of relation of third part of common bile duct to head of pancreas. (Data from Smanio T. Varying relations of the common bile duct with the posterior face of the pancreas in negroes and white persons. J Int Coll Surg 22:150, 1954; drawing modified from Skandalakis JE, Gray SW. Embryology for Surgeons (2nd ed). Baltimore: Williams & Wilkins, 1994; with permission.)

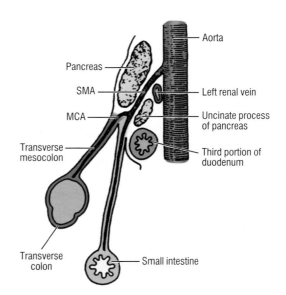

**FIG. 21-13.** Sagittal section through neck of pancreas. Uncinate process and third portion of duodenum lie posterior to superior mesenteric artery (SMA) and anterior to aorta. Middle colic artery (MCA) leaves SMA to travel in transverse mesocolon. (Modified from Akin JT, Gray SW, Skandalakis JE. Vascular compression of the duodenum: Presentation of ten cases and review of the literature. Surgery 1976;79:515-522; with permission.)

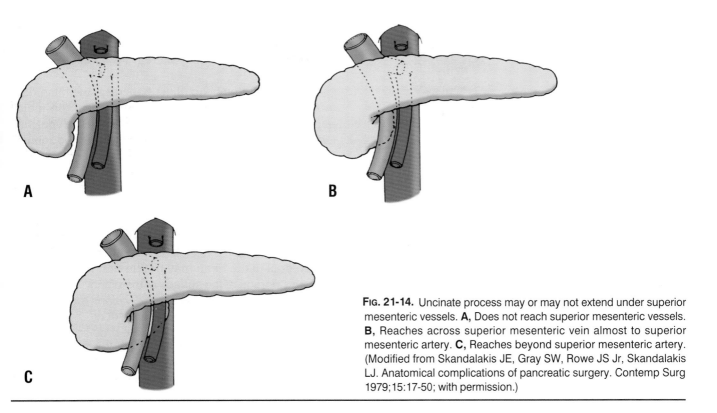

**A**

**B**

**C**

**FIG. 21-14.** Uncinate process may or may not extend under superior mesenteric vessels. **A,** Does not reach superior mesenteric vessels. **B,** Reaches across superior mesenteric vein almost to superior mesenteric artery. **C,** Reaches beyond superior mesenteric artery. (Modified from Skandalakis JE, Gray SW, Rowe JS Jr, Skandalakis LJ. Anatomical complications of pancreatic surgery. Contemp Surg 1979;15:17-50; with permission.)

The portal vein receives the posterior superior pancreaticoduodenal, right gastric, left gastric, and pyloric veins. It is fairly common for an anomalous vein to enter the anterior surface.

## Body

The anterior surface of the body of the pancreas is covered by the double layer of peritoneum of the omental bursa that separates the stomach from the pancreas. The omental tuberosity (tuber omentale) is a blunt upward projection from the body that contacts the lesser curvature of the stomach at the attachment of the lesser omentum. The body is also related to the transverse mesocolon. It divides into two leaves: the superior leaf covers the anterior surface; the inferior leaf passes inferior to the pancreas. The middle colic artery emerges from beneath the pancreas to travel between the leaves of the transverse mesocolon.

Posteriorly, the body of the pancreas is related to the aorta, the origin of the superior mesenteric artery, the left crus of the diaphragm, the left kidney and its vessels, the left adrenal gland, and the splenic vein. Small vessels from the pancreas enter the splenic vein and, during pancreatectomy, must be ligated in order to preserve the vein and the spleen.

## Tail

The tail of the pancreas is relatively mobile. Its tip reaches the hilum of the spleen in 50 percent of cases[64] (Fig. 21-15). Together with the splenic artery and the origin of the splenic vein, the tail is contained between two layers of the splenorenal ligament. If the reader will permit an analogy, the senior author of this chapter (JES) would characterize the pancreas as "playing footsie" with the spleen and behaving unfaithfully to the duodenum. As indicated earlier, Osler described the head of the pancreas as "folded in the arms of the duodenum."

The outer layer of the splenorenal ligament is the posterior layer of the gastrosplenic ligament. Careless division of this ligament may injure the short gastric vessels. The splenorenal ligament is almost avascular, but digital manipulation should stop at the pedicle. Commonly a caudate branch arises from the left gastroepiploic or an inferior splenic polar branch and passes to the tip of the tail of the pancreas. Anticipate this branch in the pancreaticosplenic ligament.

Baker[59] wrote the following comment about the relationship of the pancreas to the kidney.

*The relationship of the pancreas to the right and left kidneys is of more than passing interest when the pancreas is acutely inflamed. It is relatively common to find*

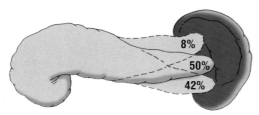

**FIG. 21-15.** Relations of tail of pancreas to splenic portas. (Modified from Skandalakis JE, Colborn GL, Pemberton LB, Skandalakis PN, Skandalakis LJ, Gray SW. The surgical anatomy of the spleen. Probl Gen Surg 1990;7:1-17; with permission.)

*that patients exhibit tenderness posteriorly in the left costovertebral angle (Murphy punch) as compared with the right and also often exhibit minor (trace to 1+) albuminuria during the acute phase. The reason for these findings is that the tail of the pancreas is contiguous with the superior pole of the left kidney. With an acute inflammatory process, there is exudation of activated enzymes, particularly trypsin, into the peripancreatic space, resulting in a modest but finite inflammatory change in the left kidney. This change results in the physical finding as well as the albuminuria, similar to interstitial nephritis on the left. The right kidney tends to be protected from the inflammatory enzymes because the inferior vena cava and duodenum are interposed between the head of the pancreas and the right kidney, making bathing of the right kidney by enzymes less likely than on the left. In operations for necrotizing pancreatitis, left perirenal fat is often necrotic and must be extensively debrided if the surgeon hopes to clean out most of the retroperitoneal peripancreatic necrotic tissue. Involvement of the right perirenal space is less likely to require extensive surgical debridement.*

### Pancreatic Ducts

The main pancreatic and accessory ducts lie anterior to the major pancreatic vessels. The *main pancreatic duct* arises in the tail of the pancreas. Through the tail and body of the pancreas, the duct lies midway between the superior and inferior margins, slightly more posterior than anterior.

The main duct crosses the vertebral column between the twelfth thoracic and second lumbar vertebrae. In more than one-half of persons, the crossing is at the first lumbar vertebra.

In the tail and body of the pancreas, from 15 to 20 short tributaries enter the duct at right angles; superior and inferior tributaries tend to alternate. In addition, the main duct may receive a tributary draining the uncinate process. In

some individuals, the accessory pancreatic duct empties into the main duct. Small tributary ducts in the head may open directly into the intrapancreatic portion of the common bile duct.

On reaching the head of the pancreas, the main duct turns caudad and posterior. At the level of the major papilla, the duct turns horizontally to join the caudal surface of the CBD and enters the wall of the duodenum, usually at the level of the second lumbar vertebra.

Frey[65] stated that if the head of the pancreas is 5 cm thick and the distance is 3 cm from the duodenum to the point on the main pancreatic duct at which the duct courses posteriorly and inferiorly, the distance from the junction of the central and dorsal duct to the ampulla of Vater is 6 cm (Fig. 21-16). He believes that the major pancreatic duct in the head may not be drained well by filleting this portion of the surface of the gland.

Baker[59] made the following observations regarding the precise location of the main pancreatic duct.

*One [anatomic] variation is the precise location of the main pancreatic duct of Wirsung. Characteristically, the main pancreatic duct is slightly superior to the midpoint of the pancreas from a superoinferior standpoint. The characteristic description has been that the main pancreatic duct is at the junction of the superior one third and the inferior two thirds of the pancreas when viewed from the front. The depth of the duct from the anterior surface of the pancreas is even more variable. It may be as close to the anterior surface as one-third of the distance from the anterior to the posterior surface, but not infrequently it is at the middle of the gland or, less commonly, is located toward the posterior surface. Surgeons who have attempted to aspirate pancreatic juice from a normal or slightly enlarged duct by inserting a needle through the anterior surface of the pancreas are usually frustrated by the failure to localize the duct unless intraoperative ultrasonography is used to assist in the localization. When pancreatic ductal obstruction occurs in the head or neck, the enlarged duct may be found if the surgeon's finger palpates over the anterior surface of the gland from the superior to the inferior aspect; the duct may be palpable as a groove or a "soft spot" in the midportion. This is a common finding in patients with carcinoma of the head of the pancreas and longstanding ductal hypertension, as well as in patients with single or multiple strictures of the pancreatic duct and ductal dilatation following or concomitant with chronic pancreatitis.*

The *accessory pancreatic duct* (of Santorini) may drain the anterosuperior portion of the head, either into the duo-

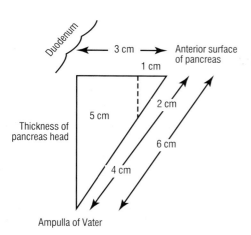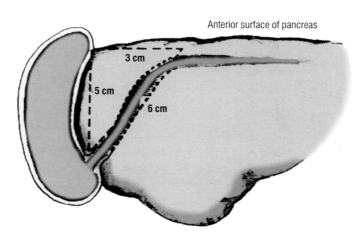

**FIG. 21-16.** After filleting, the anteroposterior segment of the major pancreatic duct in the head of the pancreas with dimensions shown will not be adequate for drainage from the anterior surface of the gland to the ampulla. (Modified from Frey CF. Partial and subtotal pancreatectomy for chronic pancreatitis. In: Nyhus LM, Baker RJ (eds). Mastery of Surgery, Vol II, 2nd ed. Boston: Little, Brown, 1992, pp. 1029-1049; with permission.)

denum at the minor papilla or into the main pancreatic duct (Fig. 21-1).

Because of the developmental origin of the two pancreatic ducts, several variations are encountered; most can be considered normal. The usual configuration is seen in Figure 21-17A. The accessory duct (Santorini) is smaller than the main pancreatic duct (of Wirsung) and opens into the duodenum on the minor papilla. Figures 21-17B, 21-17C, 21-17D and 21-17E show examples of progressive diminution in size of the accessory duct, and its absence. Figure 21-18, starting with the usual configuration, shows examples of prominence of the accessory duct and lessening caliber of the main duct. The relationships of the common bile duct, duct of Wirsung, and duct of Santorini are shown in Fig. 21-19.

In about 10 percent of individuals, there is no connection between the accessory duct and the main duct (Figs. 21-17D, 21-18C and 21-18D).[66] This fact is important to remember when contrast medium is injected into the main duct. There is no minor papilla in 30 percent[66] (Fig. 21-17B, 21-17C and 21-17E). In some individuals with a minor papilla, the terminal portion of the accessory duct is too small to permit the passage of any quantity of fluid. Three papillae have been seen[67,68] (Fig. 21-20A and 21-20D). A curious loop in the main pancreatic duct (Fig. 21-20B) was found in 3 of 76 specimens examined by Baldwin;[69] an identical example was reported by Rienhoff and Pickrell.[67]

Endoscopic retrograde cholangiopancreatography (ERCP) has made the determination of the length, diameter, and capacity of the pancreatic ductal system of considerable importance. Some published values are shown in Figs. 21-21 and 21-22.

The greatest diameter of the main pancreatic duct is in the head of the pancreas, just before the duct enters the duodenal wall. From this diameter, the duct gradually tapers toward the tail. Like the bile duct, the pancreatic duct is constricted in the wall of the duodenum.

The normal pancreatic ductal system is quite small. According to Baker,[59] as little as 1.0 to 2.5 ml contrast medium fills a normal pancreatic duct, so the hazards of injecting dye into the pancreatic duct must be recognized. Kasugai and colleagues[70] found that 2 to 3 ml of contrast medium would fill the main pancreatic duct in the living patient and 7 to 10 ml fills the branches and the smaller ducts. In autopsy specimens, Trapnell and Howard[71] found 0.5 to 1.0 ml sufficient to fill the ductal system.

Yamaguchi et al.[72] found that magnetic resonance cholangiopancreatography (MRCP), a non-invasive procedure, plays a complementary role to ERCP in diagnosis of pancreatic disorders. But MRCP has limitations in surgical application.

Since ERCP has become a valuable and frequently used diagnostic modality for numerous diseases of the pancreas and biliary tract, it is important to recognize the hazards of injecting dye into the pancreatic duct. Both volume of dye and pressure of injection are elements of concern.

If 5.0 ml or more of contrast medium is injected, the branches and smaller ducts will be visualized and sometimes ruptured, resulting in postendoscopic pancreatitis.[59] In such cases, the pancreatitis can be severe (necrotizing), with consequences that are always serious.

An experienced endoscopist injects dye into the pancreatic duct under very low pressure, sufficient to fill the duct but not to overdistend the delicate ductal system, and

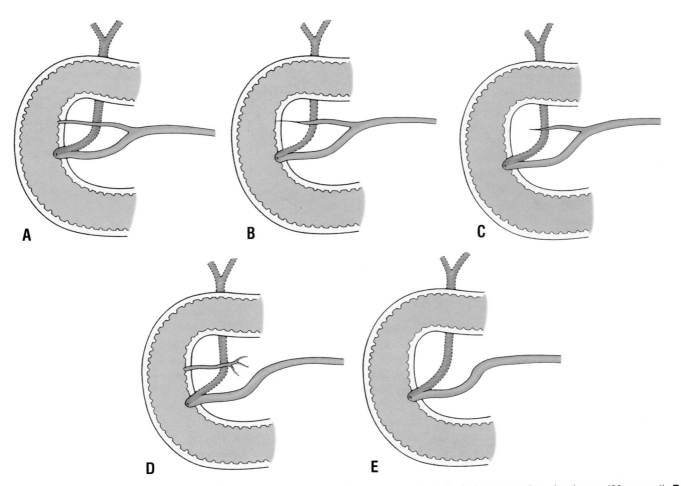

**FIG. 21-17.** Variations of pancreatic ducts. Degrees of suppression of accessory duct. **A,** Both ducts open into duodenum (60 percent). **B,** Accessory duct ends blindly in duodenal wall. **C,** Accessory duct ends blindly before reaching duodenum (30 percent). **D,** Accessory duct has no connection with main duct. **E,** Accessory duct absent. (Modified from Skandalakis JE, Gray SW, Rowe JS Jr, Skandalakis LJ. Anatomical complications of pancreatic surgery. Contemp Surg 1979; 15:17-50; with permission.)

limits the volume of dye infused. Patients with chronic pancreatitis often have large ducts and distal strictures, and the fibrosis of the gland makes the pancreas less susceptible to damage than a normal pancreas.

## Papilla of Vater and Ampulla of Vater

There is confusion in the literature regarding the true definitions of the terms *papilla* and *ampulla of Vater.* The so-called papilla of Vater, which should be called the *major duodenal papilla,* is a nipplelike formation and projection of the duodenal mucosa through which the distal end of the ampulla of Vater passes into the duodenum (Fig. 21-23A). The ampulla of Vater (hepatopancreatic), with its several formations, is the union of the pancreaticobiliary ducts.

## Major Duodenal Papilla

Although this structure bears the name of Abraham Vater (1720), it was first illustrated by Gottfreid Bidloo of The Hague in 1685, and perhaps should have been called the papilla of Bidloo.

The papilla is on the posteromedial wall of the second portion of the duodenum, 7 to 10 cm from the pylorus. Rarely, the papilla may be in the third portion of the duodenum.[73] On endoscopy, the papilla has been reported to lie to the right of the vertebral column at the level of the second lumbar vertebra in 75 percent[74] to 85 percent[75] of bodies examined. It has been reported to lie at the level of the third lumbar vertebra in 57 percent of autopsy specimens.[76]

Viewed from the mucosal surface of the duodenum, the papilla is found where a longitudinal mucosal fold or frenulum meets a transverse mucosal fold to form a T (Fig.

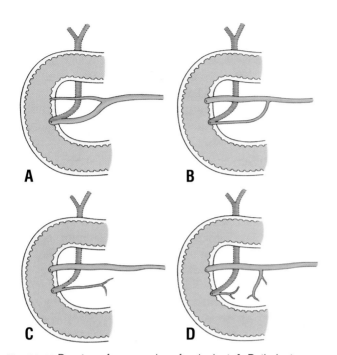

**FIG. 21-18.**Degrees of suppression of main duct. **A,** Both ducts open into duodenum. **B,** Main duct smaller than accessory duct. **C,** Main duct with no connection to larger accessory duct (10 percent). **D,** Main duct short or absent (10 percent). (Modified from Skandalakis JE, Gray SW, Rowe JS Jr, Skandalakis LJ. Anatomical complications of pancreatic surgery. Contemp Surg 1979;15:17-50; with permission.)

21-24). No such arrangement marks the site of the minor papilla.

The papilla of Vater may not be obvious. Too much traction may erase the folds, or it may be covered by one of the transverse folds. Dowdy et al.[77] stated that the papilla was "prominent" and easily found in 60 percent of their specimens. During the operation, if the T is not apparent and the papilla cannot be palpated, the CBD must be probed from above. A duodenal diverticulum near the papilla may confuse the surgeon or the endoscopist.

**Ampulla (of Vater)**

The ampulla is a dilatation of the common pancreaticobiliary channel adjacent to the major duodenal papilla and below the junction of the two ducts (Fig. 21-23A). If a septum extends as far as the duodenal orifice, the ampulla as such does not exist (Fig. 21-23B and 21-23C).

Michels[78] collected the findings of 25 investigators in 2500 specimens and concluded that an ampulla was present in 64 percent. An ampulla was said to be present if the edge of the septum between the two ducts did not reach the tip of the papilla. Actual measurements of the distance between septal edge and papillary tip range from 1 to 14 mm, 75 percent being 5 mm or less, according to Rienhoff and Pickrell.[67]

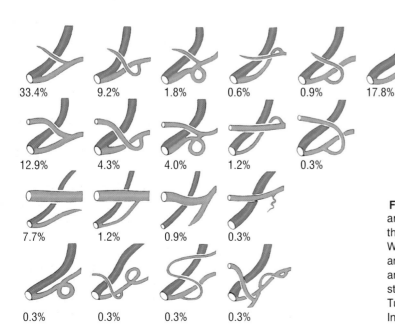

33.4%  9.2%  1.8%  0.6%  0.9%  17.8%

12.9%  4.3%  4.0%  1.2%  0.3%

7.7%  1.2%  0.9%  0.3%

0.3%  0.3%  0.3%  0.3%

**FIG. 21-19.**Relations of common bile duct, duct of Wirsung, and duct of Santorini to each other and duodenum. Upper thickest duct is common bile duct; smaller duct is duct of Wirsung; smallest duct is duct of Santorini. The white circular area indicates where the duct enters the duodenum. In rows 2 and 3, duct of Santorini is a major pancreatic duct. Injection studies of M. Stolte. (Modified from Cubilla AL, Fitzgerald PJ. Tumors of the Exocrine Pancreas. Washington: Armed Forces Institute of Pathology, 1984; with permission.)

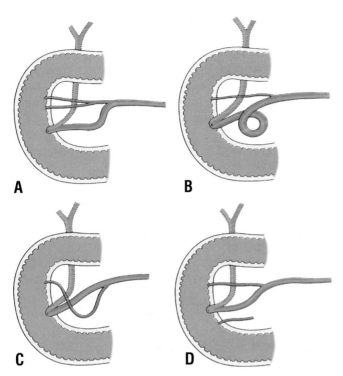

FIG. 21-20. Rare variations of pancreatic ducts. **A,** Duplication of accessory duct. **B,** Loop in main duct. **C,** Anomalous course of accessory duct. **D,** Triple pancreatic ducts. (Modified from Skandalakis JE, Gray SW, Rowe JS Jr, Skandalakis LJ. Anatomical complications of pancreatic surgery. Contemp Surg 1979;15:17-50; with permission.)

supply of the distal CBD and the pancreatic duct; these two anatomic entities participate with the duodenal wall to form the vaterian apparatus. Further information about the blood supply of the pancreas will be found later in this chapter under the heading "Vascular System."

What should we surgical anatomists advise the surgeon, laparoscopist, and gastroenterologist about the topography, length, and depth of the incision during sphincterotomy, sphincterostomy, or sphincteroplasty to avoid bleeding or duodenal perforation? The incision should be at 10 o'clock to 11 o'clock with an approximate length of 5 to 8 mm. Little is known about the best depth to make the incision to avoid bleeding.

*Arteries.* The senior author of this chapter, John E. Skandalakis, has done sphincterotomies and sphincteroplasties by the open method. He has always advised residents that the vessels responsible for bleeding are the retroduodenal artery and an anomalous right hepatic artery originating from the superior mesenteric artery (SMA). These two vessels are located between the distal CBD and the duodenum. Skandalakis agrees with Chassin[79] that during the open method the area behind the ampulla should be palpated to determine whether there is pulsation. If so, an anomalous artery is present.

**Posterior Superior Pancreaticoduodenal Artery.** Skandalakis' personal feeling and intuition is that the primary responsibility for the arterial blood supply of the ampulla of Vater is fulfilled by the posterior superior pancreat-

**AMPULLA CLASSIFICATION.** The following classification of Michels[78] is the most useful.

- *Type 1* (Figs. 21-23A and 21-23B). The pancreatic duct opens into the CBD at a variable distance from the opening in the major duodenal papilla. The common channel may or may not be dilated (85 percent).
- *Type 2* (Fig. 21-23C). The pancreatic and bile ducts open near one another, but separately, on the major duodenal papilla (5 percent).
- *Type 3.* The pancreatic and bile ducts open into the duodenum at separate points (9 percent).

A true ampulla with dilatation is present in about 75 percent of individuals of type 1 and is absent in types 2 and 3.

**BLOOD SUPPLY OF AMPULLA OF VATER** (Figs. 21-25, 21-26). What do we know about the arterial and venous networks of the ampulla? There are papers in the literature that mention some of the participating arteries and veins, but the topography of the vascular network has not been defined clearly enough to help operators avoid postoperative bleeding. Most of these writers report the blood

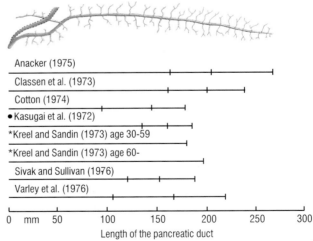

| | | | | | |
|---|---|---|---|---|---|
| Anacker (1975) | | | | | |
| Classen et al. (1973) | | | | | |
| Cotton (1974) | | | | | |
| ●Kasugai et al. (1972) | | | | | |
| *Kreel and Sandin (1973) age 30-59 | | | | | |
| *Kreel and Sandin (1973) age 60- | | | | | |
| Sivak and Sullivan (1976) | | | | | |
| Varley et al. (1976) | | | | | |

0    mm    50         100        150        200        250        300
Length of the pancreatic duct

\* Autopsy specimens
● Standard deviation

FIG. 21-21. Length of main pancreatic duct as reported by several authors; averages and extremes indicated. (Modified from Skandalakis JE, Gray SW, Rowe JS Jr, Skandalakis LJ. Anatomical complications of pancreatic surgery. Contemp Surg 1979;15:17-50; with permission.)

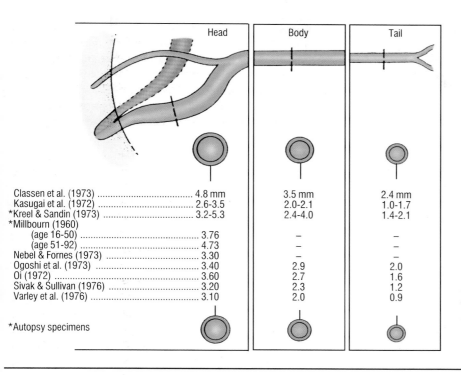

| | Head | Body | Tail |
|---|---|---|---|
| Classen et al. (1973) | 4.8 mm | 3.5 mm | 2.4 mm |
| Kasugai et al. (1972) | 2.6-3.5 | 2.0-2.1 | 1.0-1.7 |
| *Kreel & Sandin (1973) | 3.2-5.3 | 2.4-4.0 | 1.4-2.1 |
| *Millbourn (1960) | | | |
| (age 16-50) | 3.76 | – | – |
| (age 51-92) | 4.73 | – | – |
| Nebel & Fornes (1973) | 3.30 | – | – |
| Ogoshi et al. (1973) | 3.40 | 2.9 | 2.0 |
| Oi (1972) | 3.60 | 2.7 | 1.6 |
| Sivak & Sullivan (1976) | 3.20 | 2.3 | 1.2 |
| Varley et al. (1976) | 3.10 | 2.0 | 0.9 |

*Autopsy specimens

FIG. 21-22. Diameter of the main pancreatic duct as reported by several authors. (Modified from Skandalakis JE, Gray SW, Rowe JS Jr, Skandalakis LJ. Anatomical complications of pancreatic surgery. Contemp Surg 1979;15: 17-50; with permission.)

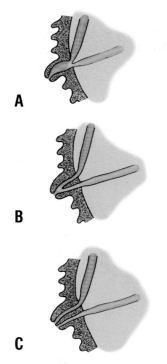

FIG. 21-23. Variations in relation of common bile duct and main pancreatic duct at duodenal papilla. **A,** Minimal absorption of ducts into duodenal wall during embryonic development. Ampulla present. **B,** Partial absorption of common channel. No true ampulla present. **C,** Maximum absorption of ducts into duodenum. Separate orifices on papilla, no ampulla. (Modified from Skandalakis JE, Gray SW, Rowe JS Jr, Skandalakis LJ. Anatomical complications of pancreatic surgery. Contemp Surg 1979;15:17-50; with permission.)

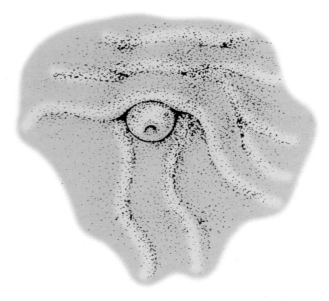

FIG. 21-24. T arrangement of duodenal mucosal folds indicates site of major duodenal papilla. Mucosal fold may cover orifice of papilla in some cases. Major papilla is rarely this obvious. This was beautifully illustrated in a plate by Santorini in 1775, and reproduced by Livingston in 1932. (Modified from Skandalakis JE, Gray SW, Rowe JS Jr, Skandalakis LJ. Anatomical complications of pancreatic surgery. Contemp Surg 1979; 15:17-50; with permission.)

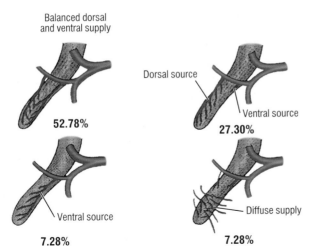

Balanced dorsal
and ventral supply

Dorsal source

52.78%

Ventral source

27.30%

Ventral source

7.28%

Diffuse supply

7.28%

FIG. 21-25. Frequency distribution of vascular supply of ampulla of Vater. (Modified from Stolte M, Wiessner V, Schaffner O, Koch H. [Vascularization of the papilla vateri and bleeding risk of papillotomy]. Leber Magen Darm 1980;10:293-301; with permission.)

icoduodenal arterial branch of the gastroduodenal artery (PSPD). The PSPD arises ventrally from the gastroduodenal artery and passes in a graceful, downward spiral around the retroduodenal segment of the CBD to reach the posterior surface of the pancreatic head. In most cases, it anastomoses with the posterior branch of the inferior pancreaticoduodenal branch of the SMA, very close to the ampulla of Vater. It may give origin to a supraduodenal branch to the duodenal bulb and also to the retroduodenal artery.

**Retroduodenal Artery.** The so-called retroduodenal artery is a branch of the gastroduodenal artery or, variably, of the PSPD. It is located very near the superior border of the duodenum and anterior to the lower CBD (in a transverse or slightly oblique way). Arising from the retroduodenal artery are ascending branches that travel upward along the CBD.

From the cystic and right hepatic arteries, descending branches travel downward and partially supply the arterial blood of the lower CBD. Some branches of the retroduodenal artery, which ascend and anastomose with the descending branches at the lower part of the common bile duct, also contribute to the lower CBD blood supply. The so-called 3 and 9 o'clock vessels mentioned by Northover and Terblanche[80] are another product of the anastomosing ascending and descending branches from the retroduodenal and right hepatic and cystic arteries.

Stolte et al.[81] studied vascular supply to the ampulla of Vater (Fig. 21-25). The four major types listed below comprised 52 of their 55 cases (94.64%):

- Equally strong ventral and dorsal branches of posterior duodenal artery (retroduodenal artery) (52.78%) (Fig. 21-26)

- Dominant dorsal branch (27.30%)
- Dominant ventral branch (7.28%)
- No dominant branch (arterial plexus of papilla composed of several vessels entering from sides) (7.28%)
- Rare variations (5.36%).

**Retroportal Artery.** The retroportal artery may spring from the SMA or directly from the celiac axis.[82] It joins the retroduodenal artery, and in 20% of cases, it joins the right hepatic artery behind the common bile duct.

Northover and Terblanche[80] reported that in almost 50 percent of cases, the retroportal artery originated from the celiac axis and its major branches. In almost 50 percent, it arose from the superior mesenteric artery and its major branches. In extremely rare cases it sprang from an aberrant right hepatic artery which arose from the SMA.

**Arterial Network.** How close is the anastomosis between the posterior superior and posterior inferior pancreaticoduodenal (PIPD) arteries to the ampulla of Vater? We have never done injection studies, so our knowledge depends on our sixth sense and the available literature. The caliber and branching patterns of the anastomosing vessels is often such that it is difficult to be certain of the identity and origin of the vessels exposed.

The possible arterial network of the ampullary apparatus should be carefully evaluated by the blood supply of the distal common bile duct, pancreatic head, proximal

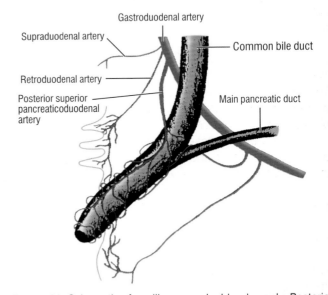

Gastroduodenal artery

Supraduodenal artery

Common bile duct

Retroduodenal artery

Posterior superior pancreaticoduodenal artery

Main pancreatic duct

FIG. 21-26. Schematic of papillary vascular blood supply. Posterior superior pancreaticoduodenal artery crosses bile duct and gives rise to dorsal and ventral branches. These join to form arterial plexus of papillae. (Modified from Stolte M, Wiessner V, Schaffner O, Koch H. [Vascularization of the papilla vateri and bleeding risk of papillotomy] Leber Magen Darm 1980;10:293-301; with permission.)

pancreas, and first, second, and third parts of the duodenum.

The classical anatomy of the area tells us that the blood supply of the second part of the duodenum and the head of the pancreas originates from several arteries that spring from the celiac axis and the SMA. This can be explained easily in view of the fact that the foregut (celiac trunk) and midgut (superior mesenteric artery) participate in the embryogenesis of the duodenum and pancreas.

The pancreaticoduodenal arcades, which are located anterior and posterior to the pancreatic head, are accepted as the chief blood supply of the pancreatic head and the second part of the duodenum. A small unnamed branch from the dorsal pancreatic artery may join the PSPD artery. We do not believe this type of connection is significant in the majority of cases.

Using kocherization of the pancreatic head, one can observe the pathway of the PSPD artery. This pathway is variable, but the artery is always close to the pancreaticobiliary junction.

Perhaps we will have some answers if we accept the notion that the arterial blood of the supraduodenal CBD is supplied by the vaterian system, or that it participates in the blood supply of the vaterian network.

Northover and Terblanche[80] studied the arterial blood supply of the bile duct. They reported that the retroduodenal, retroportal, gastroduodenal, and other arteries supplied the supraduodenal CBD in 60.1% of the cases. They found that the right and left hepatic, cystic, and other arteries were responsible for 38%. A small number (1.9%) came from the common hepatic artery.

The several small, nameless vessels associated with both borders of the CBD were referred to by Northover and Terblanche[80] as the 3 o'clock and 9 o'clock arteries. Therefore, both retroduodenal and retroportal arteries supply the distal part of the CBD, forming arterial and capillary plexuses around its wall.

Deltenre et al.[83] assessed the distance of the retroduodenal artery from the duodenal surface by identifying the arterial blood flow in 23 out of 26 patients prior to endoscopic sphincterotomy using ultrasonic Doppler probe. They limited the papillotomy length to less than the depth of the arterial sound (12.7 mm instead of 15 mm), and observed minimal capillary bleeding.

Kimura and Nagai[84] reported on duodenal preservation after resection of the pancreatic head. They stated that after the anterior superior pancreaticoduodenal artery (ASPD) departs from the gastroduodenal artery, it travels downward to a point 1.5 cm below the ampulla of Vater. At that point it turns toward the posterior aspect of the pancreas to anastomose with the anterior inferior pancreaticoduodenal artery (AIPD). They wrote that an arcade

is formed between the PSPD artery and the PIPD artery in 88 percent of cases.

In our experience, the exact site of anastomosis between the ASPD and AIPD arteries varies. It depends in part upon the topography of the pancreatic head and uncinate process and in part upon the manner of origin of the AIPD and PIPD arteries. Whether independently or in combination, they take origin from the superior mesenteric artery.

*Veins.* Biazotto[85] reported that three venous networks are associated with the papilla:

- The deep network resides in the mucous membrane of the intramural bile duct and in the hepatopancreatic ampulla.
- The intermediate network is in the deep region of the chorion of the papilla.
- The superficial network is in the duodenal submucous membrane covering the papilla.

Biazotto[85] stated that bleeding during papillotomies is insignificant because the thick veins lie in the body and at the base of the papilla. The location in the apex of the papilla of the many small veins draining into the duodenal submucous membrane also helps explain the diffuse and low intensity bleeding.

Kimura and Nagai[84] did not find any arcade formation by the ASPD and AIPD veins. They stated that arcade formation between the PSPD and PIPD veins is not always apparent, noting that these veins become quite small near the papilla of Vater.

According to Kimura and Nagai,[84] the PSPD vein crosses anterior to the CBD near the upper edge of the pancreatic head and travels toward the papilla of Vater along the right side of the bile duct. They described the anatomy of the veins of the head of the pancreas as a "complex variety of patterns." According to the same authors, the arterial and venous pancreaticoduodenal network is situated on a membrane on the posterior of the pancreas. They advised preserving this network and avoiding injury to it.

In another publication, Kimura et al.[86] reported the following crucial points for duodenal preservation.

- Kocherization will not cause any problem. After removing the connective tissue membrane behind the pancreatic head, the PSPD vein appears across the posterior surface of the CBD near the papilla of Vater. The PSPD vein is responsible for the venous drainage of the papilla of Vater and duodenum.
- The artery travelling toward the papilla of Vater and along the right side of the CBD provides important blood supply for the papillae.
- The connective tissue membrane on the posterior aspect of the pancreatic head should be kept intact be-

cause all the arterial and venous network is attached to the membrane.

*Summary.* Because of the limited quantity of published literature describing the blood supply of the ampulla of Vater, we asked Dr. Kimura to summarize his findings. He was kind enough to provide the following information, which we present verbatim (personal communication to John E. Skandalakis, October 31, 1996).

*When investigating the vascular system of the head of the pancreas, using the autopsy cases, the artery toward the papilla of Vater can be easily detected. This artery can also be grossly detected at the operation.*

*After departing from the PSPD artery, this artery runs along the just right side of the CBD toward the papilla of Vater. The angiography demonstrates this artery clearly, especially in the right oblique position of patients. No such big artery toward the papilla was found. Therefore we can easily imagine that this artery is very important for the blood supply of the papilla of Vater, although some of the branches from arteries of the arcades toward the duodenal wall might be also responsible for that.*

*With regard to the anastomosis of arcades between the ASPD-AIPD and the PSPD-PIPD, we could not find any anastomosis with naked eyes. Branches from each arcade might supply blood to the pancreas and the duodenum directly and individually.*

*The posterior surface of the pancreas is covered with the connective tissue membrane. When this connective tissue membrane is removed, the PSPD vein is detected. After departing from the portal vein, the PSPD vein runs across the posterior surface of the CBD, and reaches the duodenal wall near the papilla of Vater.*

*The PIPD vein departs from the upper jejunal vein (J1), and runs horizontally behind the superior mesenteric vein (SMV) toward the right on the connective tissue membrane of the head of the pancreas. It runs toward the papilla of Vater.*

*The venous draining of the papilla of Vater and duodenum would be done by these veins. Congestion of the papilla of Vater and surrounding duodenal wall would be avoided by preserving these veins.*

### *"Sphincter of Boyden"*

As it is currently understood, the "sphincter of Boyden" (Fig. 21-27) includes several sphincters of smooth muscle fiber surrounding the intramural part of the common bile duct, the main pancreatic duct, and the ampulla, if present. This muscle complex has a separate embryonic origin from

the duodenal musculature, and it functions separately.

While Boyden[87] and others properly describe the anatomy of this area, the terminology is unsettled. We suggest naming the entire sphincter complex the sphincter of Boyden in recognition of his contribution to the anatomy of this region.

The total length of the sphincteric complex may be as little as 6 mm or as great as 30 mm, depending on the obliquity of the path taken by the biliary and pancreatic ducts through the duodenal wall. In some instances, the sphincter may extend beyond the duodenal wall into the pancreatic portion of the bile duct. It is important to be aware of this fact when sphincterotomy is done.

Flati et al.[88] studied the biliopancreatic ducts and sphincteric apparatus of 49 specimens and reported the following findings:

1. Circular muscle fibers were found on the choledochus duct side up to 13.6 mm from the papillary pore, with more rarefied fibers present up to 20.5 mm.
2. Muscle fibers 7.3 mm from the papillary pore were noticed at the pancreatic duct with a sphincterlike formation 2-3 mm above the papillary pore.
3. There was no evidence suggesting the presence of upper, middle, and lower biliary sphincters.
4. The shape of the Wirsung-choledochus junction could be categorized as follows:

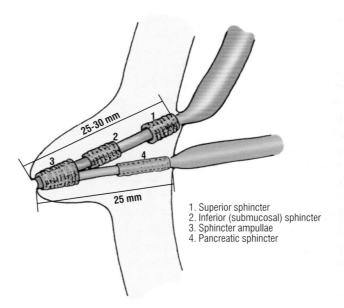

1. Superior sphincter
2. Inferior (submucosal) sphincter
3. Sphincter ampullae
4. Pancreatic sphincter

**Fig. 21-27.** Four entities composing sphincter of Boyden. (Measurements from White TT. Surgical anatomy of the pancreas. In: Carey LC (ed). The Pancreas. St. Louis: CV Mosby Co, 1973; drawing modified from Skandalakis JE, Gray SW, Rowe JS Jr, Skandalakis LJ. Anatomical complications of pancreatic surgery. Contemp Surg 1979;15:17-50; with permission.)

– Y type (with short or long common channel): 61.2%
– U type (virtually absent common channel): 22.4%
– V type (separate orifices of the Wirsung and chole-
dochus ducts within the same papilla): 14.3%
– II type (one papilla for the choledochus and one for the
Wirsung duct): 2.1%

5. The duct of Santorini with a normal papilla was present
in 16% of specimens.

Flati et al.[88] conclude that "these data along with other interesting observations on antireflux mechanisms (Santorini's valves) and on the ductal space orientation appear to be useful guidelines for a physiopathological understanding of bilio-pancreatic diseases and for any therapeutic procedure on these structures."

Perhaps these authors are right. But we, for sentimental reasons and because we believe in its scientific validity, will continue to teach the concept of our late, respected friend, Dr. Boyden.

The motility of the "sphincter of Oddi" (defined by Oddi in 1887 as a sphincter of the hepatopancreatic ampulla) is the subject of multiple debates. Shibata et al.[89] found possible dysfunction of the sphincter of Oddi secondary to proximal duodenal transection, but not gastric transection.

Based on canine studies, Marks et al.[90] recommend Botox injection into the sphincter of Oddi as a beneficial alternative to biliary stenting for reduction of common bile duct pressures and the treatment of biliary leaks and fistulae.

## Minor Duodenal Papilla

The minor duodenal papilla sits about 2 cm cranial and slightly anterior to the major papilla. It is smaller than the major duodenal papilla and its site lacks the characteristic mucosal folds that mark the site of the major papilla. Baldwin[69] found the minor papilla present in all of a series of 100 specimens. More recently, in a sample of the same size, Dowdy and associates[77] could find no minor papilla in 18 specimens. Some papillae may be difficult to identify even if present.

An excellent landmark for locating the minor papilla is the gastroduodenal artery, which is situated anterior to the accessory pancreatic duct (Santorini) and the minor papilla. During gastrectomy, duodenal dissection should end proximal to or at this artery. It becomes especially important in the few patients in whom the accessory duct carries the major drainage of the pancreas.

De Prates et al.[91] report that the muscular and elastic fibers of the minor papilla are arranged so that the contraction of its smooth muscle fibers opens the papillary orifice and permits pancreatic juice to flow. These authors stated that this papillary network (the sphincter of Helly) is not a typical anatomic sphincter.

## Surgical Applications

• When distal partial pancreatectomy is performed, the presence or absence of the uncinate process tends to determine how much of the pancreas is removed. A well-developed uncinate process usually belongs to a pancreas with a small head. If the uncinate process is present, a 60 percent to 65 percent pancreatectomy is done. If the uncinate process is absent, 70 percent to 80 percent of the pancreas is removed.

• The cephalocervical and corporocaudate segments of the pancreas can be used for transplantation.[62]

# Vascular System

The vascular system of the pancreas is complex and nontypical, with several different patterns. We will first present our analysis based on the excellent work of Van Damme.[92] Then we will present an analysis of the pancreatic blood supply by Bertelli and colleagues.[93-96] We hope the reader will benefit from both of the slightly differing presentations, remembering Sir Andrew Watt Kay's admonition about the "tiger country" of the pancreas.[60]

Consideration of the blood supply of the ampulla of Vater, which has preceded this, is not repeated here.

## Arterial Supply (Based on Van Damme)

Van Damme[92] states: "The most important pancreatic artery is the splenic artery" (Figs. 21-28 and 21-29). The pancreas is supplied with blood from branches arising from the celiac trunk and from the superior mesenteric artery (Figs. 21-28 and 21-29). Variations are common, and differing textbook illustrations are all "correct" for at least some patients. Toni et al.[97] report satisfactory sensitivity of the angiographic approach for evaluating the topography and anastomosis of pancreatic arteries.

The head of the pancreas and the concave surface of the duodenum are supplied by two pancreaticoduodenal arterial arcades. These are always present. The arcades are formed by a pair (anterior and posterior) of superior arteries from the gastroduodenal branch of the celiac trunk that join a second pair of inferior arteries from the superior mesenteric artery. These vascular arcades lie upon the surface of the pancreas but also supply the duodenal wall. They are the chief obstacles to complete pancreatectomy without duodenectomy.

At the neck, the dorsal pancreatic artery (Fig. 21-28) usually arises from the splenic artery, near its origin from the celiac trunk. A right branch of the dorsal pancreatic artery supplies the head of the pancreas and usually joins

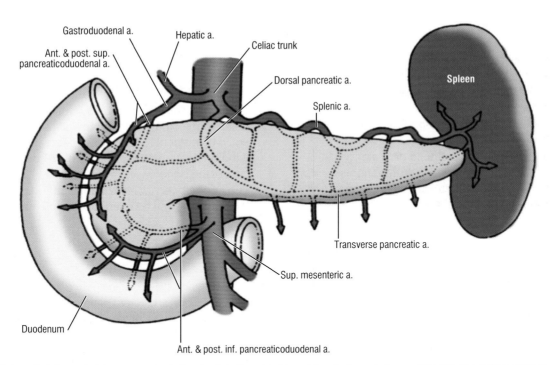

**FIG. 21-28.** Major arterial supply to pancreas (anterior view). Left and right gastric arteries not shown. (Modified from Skandalakis JE, Gray SW, Rowe JS Jr, Skandalakis LJ. Anatomical complications of pancreatic surgery. Contemp Surg 1979;15:17-50; with permission.)

the posterior arcade. It may also anastomose with the ASPD artery. One or two left branches pass through the body and tail of the pancreas, often making connections with branches of the splenic artery and, at the tip of the tail, with the splenic or the left gastroepiploic artery. The

left and right branches of the dorsal pancreatic artery characteristically lie within a groove on the inferior margin of the pancreas. Here they form the transverse, or inferior, pancreatic artery. All major arteries lie posterior to the ducts.

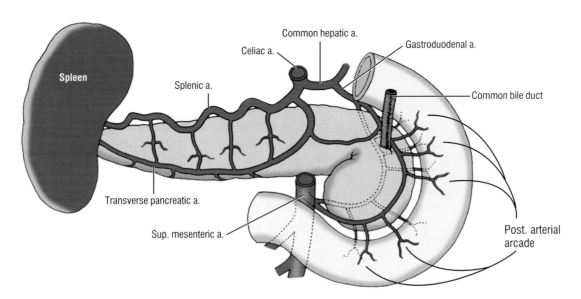

**FIG. 21-29.** Major arterial supply to pancreas (posterior view). Left and right gastric arteries not shown. (Modified from Skandalakis JE, Gray SW, Rowe JS Jr, Skandalakis LJ. Anatomical complications of pancreatic surgery. Contemp Surg 1979;15:17-50; with permission.)

## Pancreatic Arcades (Figs. 21-28, 21-29, 21-30)

**ANTERIOR ARCADE.** The gastroduodenal artery arises as one of the two terminal branches of the common hepatic artery branch of the celiac trunk. Shortly after it arises from the common hepatic artery branch, the gastroduodenal artery gives origin to the supraduodenal, retroduodenal, and posterior superior pancreaticoduodenal (PSPD) arteries. The supraduodenal and retroduodenal arteries arise, variably, as branches of the PSPD artery. The gastroduodenal artery ends by dividing into the right gastroepiploic and anterior superior pancreaticoduodenal (ASPD) arteries.

The ASPD artery lies on the anterior surface of the head of the pancreas, where it contributes eight to ten branches to the anterior surface of the pancreas and the duodenum. The main stem ends by anastomosing richly with the anterior inferior pancreaticoduodenal artery (AIPD) at the lower margin of the head of the pancreas.

Mellière[98] found four instances in which the anastomosis between superior and inferior vessels appeared to be absent, but he believed this to be the result of transient spasm.

The AIPD artery arises from the SMA at or above the inferior margin of the pancreatic neck. It may form a common trunk with the posterior inferior artery. One or both vessels may arise from the first or second jejunal branches of the SMA. Even more striking are instances in which a posterior inferior artery arises from an aberrant right hepatic artery springing from the SMA. Ligation of the jejunal branch endangers the blood supply to the fourth part of the duodenum.

The supraduodenal artery regularly crosses the bile duct after arising from its gastroduodenal or other source and may supply blood to the bile duct. It and the retroduodenal artery provide arterial supply to the first part of the duodenum. Either or both of these arteries can arise separately or as branches of the PSPD artery.

The PSPD artery arises from the gastroduodenal artery. It then takes a long, spiraling course in a clockwise direction around the CBD to reach the posterior aspect of the head of the pancreas. The terminal part of the PSPD artery's course is visible only when the pancreas is turned upward to expose its posterior surface (Fig. 21-29). This also exposes its interconnections with the PIPD artery. Branches may anastomose with other branches of the gastroduodenal artery or with the transverse (inferior pancreatic) artery. Duodenal branches supply the anterior and posterior surfaces of the second part of the duodenum.

**POSTERIOR ARCADE.** The course of the posterior arcade (Fig. 21-29) is farther from the duodenum than is that of the anterior arcade. It passes posterior to the intrapancreatic portion of the CBD.

The posterior arcade, like the anterior, may be doubled or tripled, with the extra arcades joining the PIPD artery or the SMA. The posterior arcade may also anastomose with an aberrant right hepatic artery (Fig. 21-31C) from the SMA, either separately or together with the anterior arcade.

### Branches of the Splenic Artery

The splenic artery (Figs. 21-28 and 21-29) courses to the left along the posterior surface of the body and tail of the pancreas, looping above and below the superior margin of the organ. This pathway may become more tortuous as the patient ages.

Ozan and Önderoglu[99] reported the case of a partially intrapancreatic splenic artery in a large pancreas. There were two pancreatic ducts and the uncinate process was absent.

If the posterior gastric artery is not present,[100] the first major branch of the splenic artery is the dorsal pancreatic artery. The dorsal pancreatic artery usually joins one of the posterosuperior arcades after giving off the inferior (transverse) pancreatic artery to the left. The dorsal pancreatic artery arises rather commonly from the celiac trunk or from the common hepatic artery.

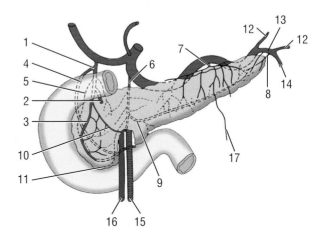

**FIG. 21-30.** Arteries of the pancreas. 1, Gastroduodenal artery; 2, Right gastroepiploic artery; 3, Anterior pancreaticoduodenal arcade; 4, Posterior pancreaticoduodenal arcade; 5, Intermediary pancreaticoduodenal arcade; 6, Artery for the neck; 7, Artery for the body; 8, Arteries for the tail; 9, Transverse pancreatic artery; 10, Prepancreatic arcade; 11, Branch for the uncinate process; 12, Superior and inferior splenic branch; 13, Spleno-gastroepiploic trunk; 14, Left gastroepiploic artery; 15, Superior mesenteric artery; 16, Superior mesenteric vein; 17, Epiploic branch. (Modified from Van Damme JP, Van der Schueren G, Bonte J. Vascularisation du pancréas: Proposition de nomenclature PNA et angioarchitecture des ilots. C R Assoc Anat 1968;139:1184-1192; with permission.)

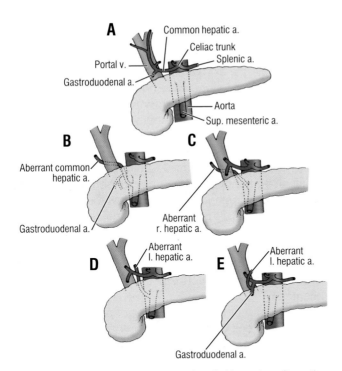

FIG. 21-31. Variations of hepatic arteries. **A,** Normal configuration. Common hepatic artery arises from celiac trunk. **B,** Aberrant common hepatic artery arises from superior mesenteric artery. **C,** Aberrant right hepatic artery arises from superior mesenteric artery. **D,** Aberrant left hepatic artery arises from superior mesenteric artery. **E,** Aberrant left hepatic artery arises from gastroduodenal artery. (Modified from Skandalakis JE, Gray SW, Rowe JS Jr, Skandalakis LJ. Anatomical complications of pancreatic surgery. Contemp Surg 1979;15:17-50; with permission.)

The origin of the inferior pancreatic artery varies. It may be doubled or absent. It may or may not freely anastomose with the splenic artery in the body and tail of the pancreas (Fig. 21-32). The inferior artery often joins the gastroduodenal artery or the ASPD artery to the right. If there are no anastomoses, thrombosis of the inferior pancreatic artery may produce emboli, infarction, and necrosis of the tail and perhaps partially of the distal body of the pancreas.

### Great Pancreatic Artery

The great pancreatic artery of Von Haller (pancreatica magna) (shown in Fig. 21-40A in following discussion by Bertelli) arises from the splenic artery and reaches the pancreas near the junction of the body and tail. This artery commonly anastomoses with the inferior pancreatic artery.

### Caudal Pancreatic Artery

The caudal pancreatic artery (shown in Fig. 21-40B in following discussion by Bertelli) arises from the distal seg-

ment of the splenic artery, the left gastroepiploic artery, or from a splenic branch at the hilum of the spleen. It anastomoses with branches of the great pancreatic and other pancreatic arteries. The caudal pancreatic artery supplies blood to accessory splenic tissue when it is present at the hilum.

Van Damme studied the pancreatic arteries extensively, paying particular attention to some of the important, unnamed arteries that supply the neck, body, and tail of the pancreas, as well as the transverse pancreatic artery. The following four paragraphs about these arteries are taken verbatim from Van Damme's work.[92]

***The Large Artery for the Neck.*** *Because the neck of the pancreas is lodged between the celiac and the superior mesenteric arteries, it is evident that the artery for the neck arises from the divisional branches of the celiac trunk (splenic or hepatic artery) or from the superior mesenteric artery. This important pancreatic artery runs behind the neck of the pancreas, where it divides into a right and a left branch. The right branch turns to the anterior surface of the head to anastomose with the gastroduodenal or right gastroepiploic artery*

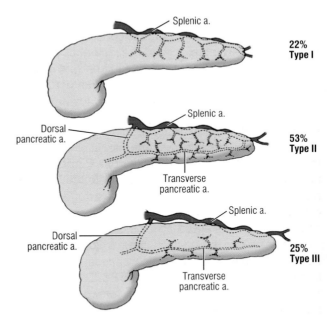

Fig 21-32. Diagram of possible configurations of blood supply to distal pancreas. Type I, Blood supply from splenic artery only. Type II, Blood supply from splenic and transverse (inferior) pancreatic arteries with anastomosis in tail of pancreas. Type III, Blood supply from splenic and transverse pancreatic arteries without distal anastomosis. This type is susceptible to infarction from emboli in transverse artery. (Modified from Skandalakis JE, Gray SW, Rowe JS Jr, Skandalakis LJ. Anatomical complications of pancreatic surgery. Contemp Surg 1979;15:17-50; with permission.)

*(prepancreatic artery, 76% of specimens); the left branch takes part in the formation of the transverse pancreatic artery.*

**The Medium-Sized Artery for the Body.** *The artery for the body (in 37% of specimens there is more than one) arises from the splenic artery. It is a typical vessel but less voluminous than the artery for the neck. When it reaches the upper border of the pancreas, it divides into several comb-shaped branches that are perpendicular to the gland and that anastomose with the transverse pancreatic vessel.*

**The Smaller Arteries for the Tail.** *The arteries for the tail (in 68% of specimens there is more than one) arise from the splenic artery (21%) and from its divisions (the left gastroepiploic artery in 20%, the splenogastroepiploic trunk in 50%, the superior or inferior splenic branches in 9%). They enter the pancreas immediately and anastomose richly with the artery for the body and with the transverse pancreatic artery. Some of these branches for the tail have a recurrent course. These small vessels, especially the recurrent ones, can be injured during splenectomy and may cause postsplenectomy pancreatitis.*

**The Transverse Pancreatic Artery.** *This collateral vessel runs within the pancreas and usually is formed by the artery for the neck. It can be more or less important. It may continue into the prepancreatic arcade,[101] which runs superficially upon the head of the pancreas and connects the anterior arcade or the gastroduodenal artery with the artery for the neck after turning around the uncinate process.*

## Anomalous Hepatic Arteries

The common hepatic artery (Fig. 21-31A) is usually a main branch of the celiac trunk, which arises cranial to the pancreas. The surgeon must always look for a possible anomalous hepatic artery before proceeding with a pancreatic resection. These aberrant arteries may be accessory to, or may replace, normal hepatic arteries.

In from 2.0 to 4.5 percent of persons, an anomalous common hepatic artery arises from the SMA.[102,103] It is related to the head or neck of the pancreas. Occasionally, it passes through the head (Fig. 21-31B) and subsequently passes behind the portal vein. Almost all of the duodenum's blood supply comes from the SMA.

The more frequent anomalous right hepatic artery also arises from the SMA. Its course is unpredictable, but it is related to the head and neck of the pancreas. Such an artery may pass behind the CBD or behind the portal vein (Fig. 21-31C). An aberrant right hepatic artery was present in 26 percent of bodies examined by Michels.[103] It may give off the inferior pancreaticoduodenal arteries.

An anomalous left hepatic artery presents a problem in operations on the pancreas only when it arises from the right side of the superior mesenteric artery (Fig. 21-31D) or from the gastroduodenal artery (Fig. 21-31E). Michels found an anomalous left hepatic artery in 27 percent of specimens, arising most commonly from the left gastric artery.[103]

## Anomalous Middle Colic Artery

A middle colic artery (Fig. 21-33) may pass through the head of the pancreas or between the head and the duodenum. It may arise from the superior mesenteric, dorsal pancreatic, or inferior pancreaticoduodenal arteries.

## Venous Drainage (Based on Van Damme)

In general, the veins of the pancreas parallel the arteries and lie superficial to them. Both lie posterior to the ducts in the body and tail of the pancreas. The drainage is to the portal vein, splenic vein, and superior and inferior mesenteric veins (Figs. 21-34 and 21-35).

### Veins of the Head of the Pancreas

Four pancreaticoduodenal veins form venous arcades draining the head of the pancreas and the duodenum. The ASPD vein joins the right gastroepiploic vein. The right gastroepiploic receives a colic vein and forms a short gastrocolic vein. This becomes a tributary to the superior mesenteric vein (SMV). The PSPD vein enters the portal vein above the superior margin of the pancreas. The anterior and posterior inferior pancreaticoduodenal veins enter the SMV together or separately. Other small, unnamed veins in the head and neck of the pancreas drain independently into the SMV and the right side of the portal vein.

White[104] stated that pancreatic tributaries do not enter the anterior surface of the portal or superior mesenteric veins. This reduces the risk of bleeding when incising the neck of the pancreas. Silen,[66] however, warned that in some patients the superior pancreatoduodenal vein and the gastrocolic vein may enter the portal vein and the SMV anteriorly.

We quote from a personal communication (Helge Baden to John E. Skandalakis, November 23, 1988) on the pancreatic veins:

> [Y]ou mention "a short gastrocolic vein" which Hollinshead[105] calls the gastrocolic trunk.
>
> This is a very important structure in pancreatic surgery. It should be identified and divided before preceding cephalad on the anterior aspect of the superior mesenteric vein. The anterior and posterior inferior pancreaticoduodenal vein...usually enter together,

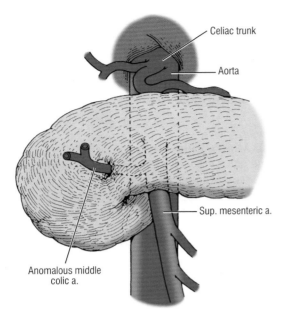

**FIG. 21-33.** Anomalous middle colic artery passing through head of pancreas. (Modified from Skandalakis JE, Gray SW, Rowe JS Jr, Skandalakis LJ. Anatomical complications of pancreatic surgery. Contemp Surg 1979; 15:17-50; with permission.)

---

*forming a big vein, that enters on the dorsal aspect of the superior mesenteric vein, and the surgeon may get into trouble freeing the superior mesenteric vein, if he is not aware of this.*

*I have never during more than 100 Whipple procedures seen pancreatic veins enter the anterior side of the superior mesenteric vein/portal vein.*

### Veins of the Neck, Body, and Tail of the Pancreas

The veins of the left portion of the pancreas form two large venous channels, the splenic vein above and the transverse (inferior) pancreatic vein below. A smaller superior pancreatic vein can sometimes be identified.

The splenic vein receives from 3 to 13 short pancreatic tributaries.[106] In a few instances one such tributary entered the left gastroepiploic vein in the tail of the pancreas. The inferior mesenteric vein (IMV) terminates in the splenic vein in about 38 percent of individuals, and the left gastric vein has a similar ending in 17 percent. The inferior pancreatic vein may enter the left side of the SMV, the IMV, or occasionally the splenic or the gastrocolic veins.

### Portal Vein

The hepatic portal vein (Figs. 21-34 and 21-35) is formed behind the neck of the pancreas by the union of the superior mesenteric and splenic veins. The inferior mesenteric vein entered at this junction in about one third of specimens examined by Douglass and associates.[106] In another third, the IMV joined the splenic vein close to the junction. In the remainder, it joined the SMV.

The portal vein lies behind the pancreas and in front of the inferior vena cava, with the CBD on the right and the common hepatic artery on the left. In the absence of disease, the portal vein and the SMV can be separated easily from the posterior surface of the pancreas.

In a dissection study of 23 cadavers,[107] the left gastric (coronary) vein entered the portal vein in 17 cadavers and the splenic vein in 6 cadavers. When drainage flowed to the portal vein, the left gastric vein lay in the hepatogastric ligament.

Rarely the portal vein may lie anterior to the pancreas

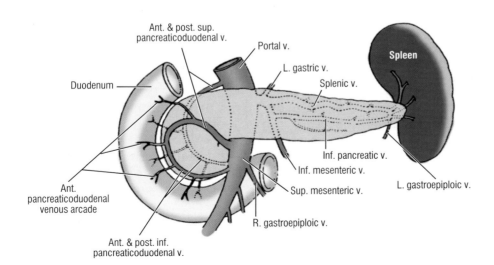

**FIG. 21-34.** Venous drainage of pancreas (anterior view). (Modified from Skandalakis JE, Gray SW, Rowe JS Jr, Skandalakis LJ. Anatomical complications of pancreatic surgery. Contemp Surg 1979;15: 17-50; with permission.)

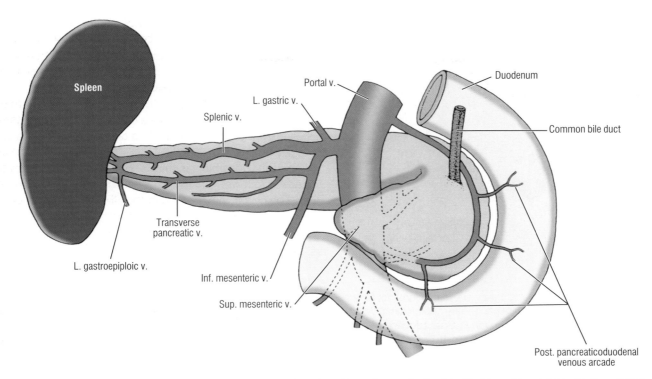

**FIG. 21-35.** Venous drainage of pancreas (posterior view) and tributaries of hepatic portal vein. (Modified from Skandalakis JE, Gray SW, Rowe JS Jr, Skandalakis LJ. Anatomical complications of pancreatic surgery. Contemp Surg 1979;15:17-50; with permission.)

and the duodenum. This represents persistence of the pre-duodenal rather than the postduodenal plexus of the embryonic vitelline veins (Fig. 21-36). Inadvertent section of this vessel could be fatal. It is often associated with anular pancreas, malrotation, and biliary tract anomalies. A preduodenal portal vein is rare in patients of any age, and extremely rare in adults. But even though there are only 11 cases reported by Ishizaki et al.,[108] the surgeon should be aware of this anomaly.

## Surgical Applications

- The right branch of the dorsal pancreatic artery anastomoses with the PSPD artery. This branch does not provide enough blood for survival of the head and duodenum after the arcades are ligated.
- The PSPD artery is the main supply for the ampulla through the epicholedochal plexus.
- Injury may occur to the ASPD artery during the Puestow side-to-side pancreaticojejunostomy.
- The superior and inferior pancreaticoduodenal arteries should not be ligated until the neck of the pancreas can be elevated from the underlying vessels. Premature ligation could cause necrosis of the head of the pancreas and duodenum.

- Angiography should be considered before surgery. Lo et al.[109] reported localization rates prior to surgery for

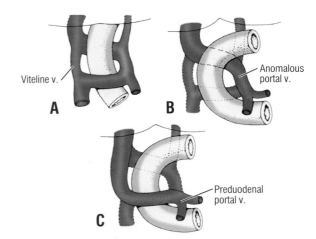

**FIG. 21-36.** Diagram of embryonic origin of preduodenal portal vein. **A,** Embryonic extrahepatic communications between vitelline veins. **B,** Normal development. Persisting superior communicating vein forms part of normal, retroduodenal portal vein. **C,** Anomalous persisting inferior communicating vein forms part of abnormal preduodenal portal vein. (Modified from Skandalakis JE, Gray SW, Rowe JS Jr, Skandalakis LJ. Anatomical complications of pancreatic surgery. Contemp Surg 1979;15:17-50; with permission.)

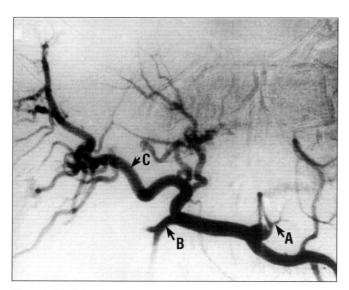

**FIG. 21-37.** Selective celiac angiogram showing segments of vascular tree. Note opacification of hepatic artery and proximal duodenal artery. **A,** Narrowing of celiac artery; **B,** Gastroduodenal artery; **C,** Hepatic artery. (From Koshi T, Govil S, Koshi R. Problem in diagnostic imaging: pancreaticoduodenal arcade in splanchnic arterial stenosis. Clin Anat 1998; 11:206-208; with permission.)

pancreatic insulinomas using ultrasonography (33%), computed tomography (44%) and angiography (52%). Intraoperative ultrasonography (IOUS) had the highest rate of accurate detection. Huai et al.[110] found that IOUS also delineated spatial relationships of neighboring anatomic entities such as the splenic and superior mesenteric vessels, portal vein, CBD, and pancreatic duct, aiding successful resection and avoiding blind pancreatectomy.

- Noncommunication between the splenic and transverse pancreatic arteries is possible. It can result in possible infarction at the area of the tail.
- Ligation of the splenic artery does not require splenectomy; ligation of the splenic vein does.
- Collateral circulation can develop as a result of stenosis of the superior mesenteric artery or celiac artery. Koshi et al.[111] found abnormal blood flow through the pancreaticoduodenal arcade during angiographic examination (Figs. 21-37 and 21-38).
- Ligation of both pancreaticoduodenal arterial arcades results in duodenal ischemia and necrosis.
- Two cadavers used in our first-year dissection lab had huge pancreatic carcinomas. We noticed that mesenteric arteries and veins were not obstructed and collateral circulation was not present. This may have been because these unfortunate individuals died at an age before obstruction of the vessels would normally occur.

- The veins of the pancreatic parenchyma are located between the ducts above and the arteries below.
- Pancreatic veins enter the lateral side of the portal vein or superior mesenteric vein from the pancreas to the right side of the portal vein. Be careful.
- The surgeon must avoid traction upon the head of the pancreas and carefully ligate veins in the area.
- There are usually no branches on the anterior surface of the portal vein.
- The four possible vascular anomalies of the portal vein are as follows.
  - The portal vein may lie anterior to the pancreas and duodenum (Fig. 21-39A).
  - The portal vein may empty into the superior vena cava.
  - A pulmonary vein may join the portal vein (Fig. 21-39B).
  - The portal vein may have congenital strictures (Fig. 21-39C).
- As part of a resident's training, it is advisable to arteriographically visualize the branches of the celiac axis and superior mesenteric artery which are related to the pancreas. We recommend this in addition to the other diagnostic tools often replacing selective arteriography. Justification for this expensive modality is the typical resident's woeful lack of knowledge of anatomy due to the

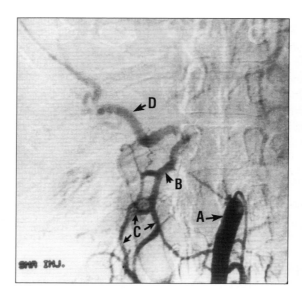

**FIG. 21-38.** Selective superior mesenteric angiogram showing segments of vascular tree. Note retrograde opacification of hepatic artery via pancreaticoduodenal arcade and gastroduodenal artery. **A,** Superior mesenteric artery; **B,** Gastroduodenal artery; **C,** Pancreaticoduodenal arcade; **D,** Hepatic artery. (From Koshi T, Govil S, Koshi R. Problem in diagnostic imaging: pancreaticoduodenal arcade in splanchnic arterial stenosis. Clin Anat 1998;11:206-208; with permission.)

extremely poor teaching of this discipline of basic science in the United States, and perhaps all over the world.

## *Arterial Blood Supply (by Bertelli and Colleagues)*

The arterial blood supply of the pancreas is provided mainly by the celiac and superior mesenteric arteries. From these arteries and/or from their major branches, eight main arteries arise with various patterns of origin and supply the pancreas:

- PSPD: posterior superior pancreaticoduodenal artery
- ASPD: anterior superior pancreaticoduodenal artery
- AIPD: anterior inferior pancreaticoduodenal artery
- PIPD: posterior inferior pancreaticoduodenal artery
- DP: dorsal pancreatic artery
- PM: pancreatica magna artery
- TP: transverse pancreatic artery
- CP: caudal pancreatic artery

The most common arrangements of these arteries are illustrated in Fig. 21-40. Many other arrangements are possible due to the variations in number, incidence, sites of origin and, sometimes, even course of pancreatic arteries. This marked irregularity, particularly in the distal segment of the pancreas (body/tail), leads to difficulty in interpreting the patterns of arterial vascularization and to strikingly divergent statistical analyses.

In this overview, we cite almost all the statistical surveys available in the anatomic literature (except that from "in vivo" angiographic studies) since, at the moment, it is impossible to ascertain which, among them, has been compiled most correctly. Our purpose is not to generate fruitless doubts in the reader's mind. On the contrary, we wish to strongly emphasize how tricky it is to delineate the pancreatic arterial network. It is doubtful that any definite anatomic conclusion can be drawn yet.

We present a detailed portrait of each artery involved in the blood supply of the pancreas. We will follow topographic criteria in our exposition, dividing the description into three parts corresponding to the head, the neck/ body, and the tail of the pancreas.

### **Head of the Pancreas** (Figs. 21-40, 21-41)

The head of the pancreas receives blood mainly from the hepatic artery, via the gastroduodenal artery, and from the superior mesenteric artery via the inferior pancreaticoduodenal (IPD) artery. The gastroduodenal artery supplies the PSPD and the ASPD arteries to the head of the pancreas, sometimes through a common superior pancreaticoduodenal (SPD) artery. The IPD artery divides into the PIPD and the AIPD arteries which, anastomosing with the two SPD arteries, form two pancreaticoduodenal (PD) arcades, namely the anterior and the posterior PD arcades.

A detailed description of this complex of PD arteries and their frequent variations can be found in a series of recent articles.[93,94,95,96,112] Here, we will summarize some notions of major interest to the surgeon.

**POSTERIOR SUPERIOR PANCREATICODUODENAL (PSPD) ARTERY.** The PSPD artery has been previously referred to as the retroduodenal artery.[113-116] This name can cause confusion, since "retroduodenal" has also been used for a distinct group of small arteries that arise a little above the terminal division of the gastroduodenal artery to supply the first and second portions of the duodenum.[117-120]

The PSPD artery is considered a constant.[98,121,122,123] In some cases, its calibre is so small as to be hardly detectable by routine angiography. The PSPD artery can also be as large as 3 mm.[115,121,123]

In about 70-80% of cases the PSPD artery arises within the first 2 cm of the gastroduodenal artery,[121,124,125] usually from its posterior aspect, as the first collateral branch. In general, the PSPD artery has a spiral, descending course

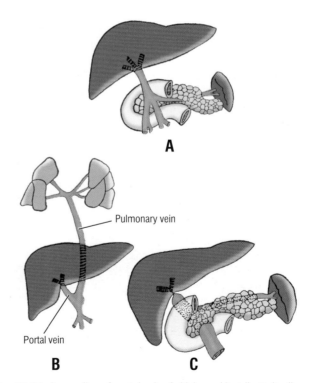

**FIG. 21-39.** Anomalies of portal vein. **A,** Vein and its tributaries lie anterior to pancreas and duodenum. **B,** Pulmonary vein joins portal vein. **C,** Congenital stricture of portal vein. (Modified from Mc Gregor AL, Du Plessis DJ. A Synopsis of Surgical Anatomy (10th ed). Baltimore: Williams & Wilkins, 1969; with permission.)

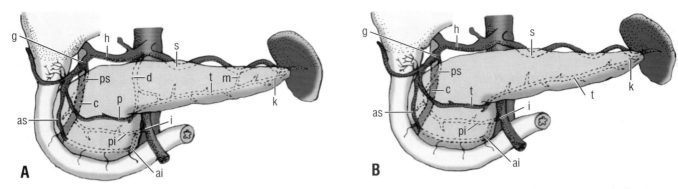

**FIG. 21-40.** Most common patterns of pancreatic arterial blood supply. h, common hepatic artery; g, gastroduodenal artery; s, splenic artery; as, anterior superior pancreaticoduodenal (ASPD) artery; ps, posterior superior pancreaticoduodenal (PSPD) artery; pi, posterior inferior pancreaticoduodenal (PIPD) artery; ai, anterior inferior pancreaticoduodenal (AIPD) artery; d, dorsal pancreatic (DP) artery; p, prepancreatic arcade; t, transverse pancreatic (TP) artery ("short type" in **A**, "long-type" in **B**); m, pancreatica magna (PM) artery; k, caudal pancreatic (CP) artery; c, choledochus; i, inferior pancreaticoduodenal artery. (Courtesy Dr. Eugenio Bertelli.)

that surrounds the choledochus: it runs transversely from left to right in front of the CBD, turns around its right lateral side, then again crosses the choledochus, from right to left (this time posteriorly), to anastomose with the PIPD artery. Several variations can occur, especially when the artery arises from other sources.

The PSPD artery can arise, in more than 20% of cases, from "non-conventional" sources, mainly the hepatic artery or its branches, regardless of their origin. These sites and the frequency of their occurrence have been noted by various investigators:

- common hepatic artery (3%)[115,125,126]
- right hepatic artery (2-3%)[114,121,122,125]
- an accessory right hepatic artery stemming from the

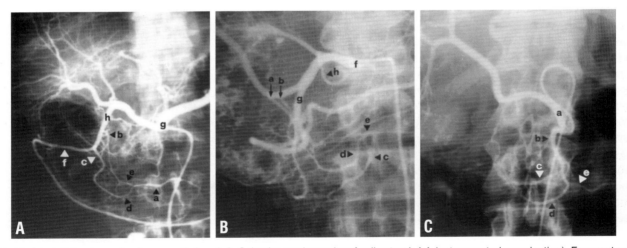

**Fig 21-41.** Arterial blood supply of pancreatic head. **A,** Selective angiography of celiac trunk **(g)** (anteroposterior projection). Frequent pattern of arterial vascularization: two SPD arteries arise from gastroduodenal artery **(h)**. Two IPD arteries originate from division of common IPD artery **(a)**. PSPD artery **(b)**; ASPD artery **(c)**; AIPD artery **(d)**; PIPD artery **(e)**; right gastroepiploic artery **(f)**. **B,** Selective angiography of common hepatic artery **(f)** (anteroposterior projection). Rare variation of origin of SPD arteries which stem separately from the right hepatic artery. PSPD artery **(a)**; ASPD artery **(b)**; AIPD artery **(c)**; PIPD artery **(d)**; IPD artery **(e)**; right gastroepiploic artery **(g)**; right gastric artery **(h)**. **C,** Selective angiography of accessory right hepatic artery arising from superior mesenteric artery **(a)** (anteroposterior projection). Variation of origin of two IPD arteries. The AIPD **(d)** and PIPD **(c)** arteries originate separately from common trunk **(b)** with jejunal artery **(e)**. SPD, superior pancreaticoduodenal; IPD, inferior pancreaticoduodenal; PSPD, posterior superior pancreaticoduodenal; ASPD, anterior superior pancreaticoduodenal; AIPD, anterior inferior pancreaticoduodenal; PIPD, posterior inferior pancreaticoduodenal; IPD, inferior pancreaticoduodenal. (Courtesy Dr. Eugenio Bertelli.)

superior mesenteric artery (3-8%)[94,113,114,125,126,127]
- common hepatic artery arising from the superior mesenteric artery (3%)[125]
- proper hepatic artery (2-8%)[94,121,124]
- superior mesenteric artery (3-5%)[94,125]
- SPD artery (5-7%)[93,124,125]
- DP artery (1%)[114]
- left hepatic artery (infrequent)[94,128]

Among the many possible collateral branches of the PSPD artery, we recall those of surgical interest:
- cystic artery (1%)[115]
- superficial cystic artery (3%)[115]
- right gastric artery (1%)[114]
- retroduodenal artery[117,120]
- accessory right hepatic artery[115,128]

**ANTERIOR SUPERIOR PANCREATICODUODENAL (ASPD) ARTERY.** The ASPD artery is an almost constant artery,[119,129] usually larger than the PSPD artery. In more than 90% of cases it arises from the gastroduodenal artery[122,124] as one of its terminal branches, behind the inferior edge of the first duodenal portion. In almost all other cases (5-7%) the ASPD artery originates from the SPD artery,[93,124,125] or exceptionally from other sources.[93,116,121,122]

Running downward, the ASPD artery can lie either in front of the duodenum or on the surface of the pancreatic head.[130] Sometimes it is buried in the parenchyma of the gland.[118] At the level of the duodenal papilla, the artery occasionally can be separated from the choledochus by only 1 mm of pancreatic parenchyma.[130] Upon reaching the lower flexure of the duodenum, the ASPD artery usually turns backward and courses over the posterior surface of the uncinate process,[115,118,122,125,127,131] where it anastomoses with the AIPD artery. In a minority of cases, the artery may remain on the anterior aspect of Winslow's process.[117,118,122]

Some collateral branches of surgical interest have been sporadically reported:
- TP artery (8-10%)[93,126,127]
- retroduodenal artery[93,120]
- cystic artery[121]
- right root of the prepancreatic arcade (see below)

**INFERIOR PANCREATICODUODENAL (IPD) ARTERY.** The AIPD and the PIPD arteries originate from the bifurcation of the IPD artery in 60-70% of cases.[115,119]

The IPD artery arises directly from the superior mesenteric artery[95] as its first right collateral branch. When an accessory right hepatic artery is present, the IPD artery is the second right collateral branch.[123] The incidence of such a pattern of origin has not been clearly determined; it has been reported as ranging from 4% to 47% of cases, de-

pending on the authors.[121,124,125,126,132,133]

The level at which the IPD artery arises from the superior mesenteric artery is variable, corresponding more frequently to the inferior edge of the neck of the pancreas.[118,121] An origin behind the pancreas is not uncommon.[95,118,119]

In other cases, the IPD artery arises through a common trunk with the first jejunal artery.[95] This trunk is referred to as the pancreaticoduodenojejunal (PDJ) trunk. Its occurrence has been reported in about 20% to 64% of cases.[121,124,125,126,132,133,134] Any statistical analysis could be affected by the interpretation that each investigator gave to the name "PDJ trunk." According to these authors, in fact, the term "PDJ trunk" could also refer to the common trunks composed of the first jejunal artery and just one of the IPD arteries, or by the first jejunal artery and both IPD arteries stemming without forming a common IPD artery.

Less frequent sites of origin for the IPD artery:
- accessory right hepatic artery arising from the superior mesenteric artery (1%)[95,98,115,123]
- through a common trunk with the DP artery (6-8%)[98,121,125]
- through a common trunk with the 2nd jejunal artery (2%)[125]
- through a common trunk with the first 2 or 3 jejunal arteries[95,117]
- middle colic artery[115,119]

The course of the first portion of the IPD artery varies according to the site of origin. It runs downward when arising behind the pancreas. When arising through common trunks with the jejunal arteries, it goes transversely from left to right, crossing the superior mesenteric artery posteriorly.[98,117,126,133] Regardless of its origination, the IPD artery crosses behind the superior mesenteric vein and is in contact with the posterior face of the uncinate process,[121] where it divides into the AIPD and the PIPD arteries.

Some important collateral branches of the IPD artery can be:
- jejunal arteries[121,123,133]
- right gastroepiploic artery[115]
- an anastomotic branch with the first jejunal artery[116]

**ANTERIOR INFERIOR PANCREATICODUODENAL (AIPD) ARTERY.** The AIPD artery is usually the smallest of the PD arteries.[133,135] It is almost always constant.[124]

In the majority of cases, the AIPD artery arises from the division of the IPD artery. Alternate sources are common:
- a common trunk with the first jejunal and the PIPD arteries (do not confuse with the PDJ trunk) (17-30%)[96,122,132,134]
- first jejunal artery (5-30%)[96,121,122,124,126,132,133]
- superior mesenteric artery (5-16%)[96,122,124,126,127,133]
- second jejunal artery (2-6%)[121,133]
- DP artery (infrequent)[126]

- an accessory right hepatic artery (infrequent)[121,126]
- middle colic artery (infrequent)[121]

When arising from a site situated on the left of the superior mesenteric artery, the AIPD artery crosses the superior mesenteric vessels posteriorly. The AIPD artery usually runs behind the uncinate process,[122] but it may be prepancreatic,[122,133] subpancreatic,[133] or even intrapancreatic.[133] In 90% of cases, it ends by anastomosing with the ASPD artery.[124]

### POSTERIOR INFERIOR PANCREATICODUODENAL (PIPD) ARTERY.
The PIPD artery is an almost constant artery which originates mainly from the IPD artery. Less frequently, it arises from:

- a common trunk with the first jejunal artery and the AIPD artery (do not confuse with the PDJ trunk) (17-30%)[96,122,132,133]
- superior mesenteric artery (8-25%)[121,122,124,126,127,132,133]
- first jejunal artery (3-16%)[121,122,124,126,132]
- an accessory right hepatic artery (2-7%)[121,124,126,132,133]
- DP artery (2-8%)[124,126,132]
- a common trunk with the TP artery (rare)[132,133]
- second jejunal artery (rare)[124]

The course of the PIPD artery is generally short. When the PIPD artery arises from the first jejunal artery or from the PDJ trunk, it may be longer, since it has to cross behind the superior mesenteric vessels.[126] On the whole, the PIPD artery has a course parallel to the AIPD artery, which is situated 2-3 cm below.[96]

### PREPANCREATIC (KIRK'S) ARCADE.
The head of the pancreas is supplied also by the right branch of the DP artery. This branch crosses the anterior surface of the head in an intermediate position. It forms the prepancreatic (Kirk's) arcade,[93,115,126] joining with a small artery coming from the gastroduodenal, right gastroepiploic or, less frequently, ASPD arteries. This arcade has been reported in 75% to 93% of cases.[125,126,135,136]

### VARIATIONS.
In relation to the head of the pancreas, two major variations of the pattern of arterial vascularization should be remembered:

- DP artery
  - In about 20% of cases, the DP artery may arise from the common hepatic artery. Therefore, its first portion can be found behind the head of the pancreas.
- TP artery
  - The TP artery, usually the left branch of the DP artery, may cross the anterior surface of the pancreatic head in about 30% of cases. It arises from the gastroduodenal,[115,116,126,137] ASPD,[115,118,126,127,137,138] or right gastroepiploic arteries.[114,115,127,138]

- The TP artery may also arise from an accessory right[94] or proper (Fig. 21-42) hepatic artery coming from the superior mesenteric artery, or from the IPD artery.[137]

REMEMBER: In all these variations, the TP artery, crossing the usual line of Whipple resection, may represent a vascular hazard, especially when it acquires dominance (see below).

### Neck and Body of the Pancreas
(Figs. 21-40, 21-42, 21-43)

The neck and body of the pancreas are supplied by 3 to 7 minor branches of the splenic artery,[134] and by the DP, PM, and TP arteries.

### DORSAL PANCREATIC (DP) ARTERY.
The DP artery was first described by Haller[128] who referred to it as "arteria pancreatica suprema." Subsequently, it has been called by many different names, thus creating confusion. We recall those frequently used:

- "superior pancreatic artery"[118,121,127]
- "middle pancreatic artery"[123,139]
- "isthmic pancreatic artery"[123,134]
- "arteria pancreatica magna"[117,123,124,134,139]
- "arteria colli pancreatis"[125,140]

In the absence of pathological collateral circulations, the DP artery is certainly the largest vessel of the pancreas; its calibre can be as large as 1 cm.[118] The DP artery is present in 80-98% of cases.[98,126,127,139,141,142]

The DP artery may arise from four main sources. Various investigators have found quite different incidences for each pattern of origin:

- first portion of the splenic artery (22-80%)[98,117,123,125,126,127,134,137,139,143]
- celiac trunk (3-33%)[98,117,121,123,125,126,127,134,137,139,143]
- first portion of the common hepatic artery (12-25%)[98,117,123,125,126,127,134,137,139]
- superior mesenteric artery (6-25%)[117,123,125,126,127,137,139,143]

Less frequently reported patterns of origin of the DP artery are from:

- an accessory right hepatic artery arising from the superior mesenteric artery[125,134,137]
- a common trunk with the IPD artery[98,115,121,125]
- gastroduodenal artery[121,125,127,137,144]
- aorta[128,138]
- left inferior phrenic artery[138]
- right gastric artery[134]
- left gastric artery[117,128]
- PSPD artery[127]
- middle colic artery[115,137,138]
- proper hepatic artery[97]

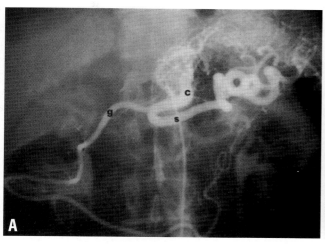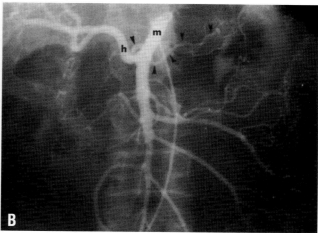

**FIG. 21-42.** Arterial blood supply of pancreatic body shows patient with dominant "short-type" TP artery. **A,** Selective angiography of **(c)** celiac trunk (anteroposterior projection). Note very limited blood supply to pancreas coming from **(g)** gastroduodenal and **(s)** splenic arteries. **B,** Selective angiography of **(m)** superior mesenteric artery (anteroposterior projection). The **(h)** proper hepatic artery stems from superior mesenteric artery and gives off a large dominant TP artery (arrowheads). TP, transverse pancreatic. (Courtesy Dr. Eugenio Bertelli.)

The course of the DP artery is rather constant since the origin is almost always situated close to the division of the celiac trunk.[117,137] When the DP artery has a high origin (hepatic, celiac, or splenic arteries), it goes downward with a course that slightly bends to the left when arising from the common hepatic artery, or to the right when arising from the splenic artery.[117]

In general, the DP artery, situated on the left of the portal vein, crosses the terminal segment of the splenic vein posteriorly.[101,115,117,118,138] When arising from the superior mesenteric artery, however, the DP artery divides into its terminal branches after a very short course directed upward.[115]

The site of division is rather constant. It is situated close to the lower border of the pancreas, at the junction between the neck and the body, near the corner formed by the splenic and superior mesenteric veins.[117,139]

The DP artery divides as an inverted T into two terminal branches which run transversely in opposite directions.[118,125,126,131,143] The right terminal branch runs behind the superior mesenteric vein[131,139] and forms the prepancreatic arcade[93] (see above); less frequently, it may resolve into minute branches for the ventral surface of the pancreatic head.[131] The left terminal branch of the DP artery is the TP artery (see below).

Some collateral branches of the DP artery have been reported occasionally. We mention those of surgical interest:

middle colic artery[115,117,118,125,126,137,138]

accessory right hepatic artery[138,145]

right colic artery[138]

left colic artery[98,138,146]

- IPD artery[115]
- PSPD artery[114,115,125,126]
- AIPD artery[124,125,126]
- PIPD artery[96,124,125,126,131,132]
- jejunal arteries[98]

**PANCREATIC MAGNA (PM) ARTERY.** The PM artery[126,147] is also known as "arteria corporis pancreatis"[125,140] or "great

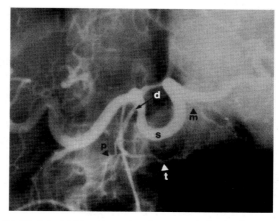

**FIG. 21-43.** Arterial blood supply of pancreatic body. Selective angiography of celiac trunk (anteroposterior projection). Frequent pattern of arterial vascularization: **(d)**, DP artery takes origin from **(s)** splenic artery soon after arising from celiac artery. DP artery divides into a right branch **(p)** prepancreatic arcade, and left branch **(t)** TP artery. TP artery anastomoses distally with **(m)** PM artery. DP, dorsal pancreatic; TP, transverse pancreatic; PM, pancreatica magna. (Courtesy Dr. Eugenio Bertelli.)

pancreatic artery."[144] Its incidence ranges between 64 and 98%.[126,140,141,142] Its calibre averages 2 mm.[140]

The PM artery is a branch of the splenic artery. Typically the PM artery arises from the middle third of the splenic artery, or at the junction between the middle and distal thirds.[116,126] Less frequently, the PM artery has been reported as originating from the proximal[142] or distal[142] third of the splenic artery, or from the left gastroepiploic artery.[140] Exceptionally, it arises from the superior mesenteric artery[144] or from the hepatic artery.[144]

The PM artery can be double (33-54%)[140,142] or triple (3%).[140]

As soon as it arises, the PM artery enters the substance of the pancreas[126] and passes behind the pancreatic duct.[116] The PM artery anastomoses with the TP artery in 90% of cases, with the DP artery in 20% of cases, and with the CP artery in 20% of cases. Multiple anastomoses are possible.[142]

**TRANSVERSE PANCREATIC (TP) ARTERY.** The TP artery is also called the "inferior pancreatic artery."[126,127,135] It is an almost constant artery, present in about 90% of cases.[127,141,142] It can be very thin, but in many cases its calibre can be as large as 3 to 4 mm.[98] Usually, the TP artery is detectable angiographically as a single vessel.[97,116] Numerical variations have been reported in a minority of cases.[97,129,134,142]

According to the site of origin, we can distinguish between "long-type" and "short-type" TP arteries. The TP artery is "long-type" in about 30% of cases. The distinction is important because the "short-type" supplies only the body/tail of the pancreas, whereas the "long-type" supplies the head as well.

The "long-type" TP artery may originate from the:
- gastroduodenal artery (2-5%)[98,126,129]
- ASPD artery (10-14%)[126,127]
- right gastroepiploic artery (3-14%)[114,127]
- common hepatic artery[97,144]

The "short-type" TP artery may arise from the:
- DP artery (37-84%)[98,126,127]
- superior mesenteric artery (1-33%)[98,126,127,129]
- IPD artery (6%)[129,134]
- aorta (3%)[134]
- PM artery (1%)[126]

The "short-type" may also arise from a proper hepatic artery coming from the superior mesenteric artery (Fig. 21-42B).

The "short-type" TP artery runs along the inferior edge of the pancreas toward the tail.[115,123,134,138] It is frequently embedded a few millimeters under the surface of its dorsal aspect.[101,118,126,143] In other individuals, the "short-type" TP artery runs superficially for a variable tract before sinking into the substance of the pancreas.[117,127]

The "long-type" TP artery crosses the anterior surface of the pancreatic head, runs superficial to the superior mesenteric vein,[127] and then follows the same course of the "short-type."

The TP artery may join with:
- a branch of the PM artery[115,126,137,138] (70% of cases)[142]
- CP arteries[115,117,126,137,138] (90% of cases)[142]
- left gastroepiploic artery[131]

In some cases the TP artery can bifurcate at the level of the neck of the pancreas; the superior branch can go to the left and upward.[101,148]

The TP artery represents the only connection between two arterial systems that are otherwise independent: the one supplying the head of the pancreas, and the other supplying the body. In other cases, when the TP artery is "short-type," this connection is guaranteed by the prepancreatic arcade.

**ARTERIAL DOMINANCE.** The DP, PM, and TP arteries, along with other minor branches of the splenic artery, supply the neck, body, and sometimes even the tail of the pancreas. It is important to emphasize that each of these arteries may acquire dominance in supplying its segment of pancreas. In other words, in some cases, just one artery can supply the entire distal part of the pancreas.

The concept of a dominant TP artery (Fig. 21-42) has been previously noted.[98] More recently, a dominant DP artery[149] as well as a dominant PM artery[149] have been demonstrated. However, a single artery supplying the distal segment of the pancreas has often been reported,[150,151] and should not be considered extraordinary.

### Tail of the Pancreas (Fig. 21-40)

The tail of the pancreas is supplied by one or more CP arteries and/or by the distal extremities of the arteries of the body.[152] CP arteries have been reported to occur in 66% to 95% of cases,[117,126,134,141,152] but are considered constant by many investigators.[140,142] In many cases (32-36%) the CP artery is single.[140,142] Two CP arteries are detectable in 46% of cases,[140,142] 3 CP arteries in 8-20% of cases,[140,142] and 4 CP arteries in 2% of cases.[142]

The CP arteries arise from:
- a common trunk formed by the left gastroepiploic artery and the inferior splenic branch (50%)[125]
- splenic artery (21%)[125]
- left gastroepiploic artery (20%)[125]
- inferior or superior splenic branches (9%)[125]

The CP arteries run downward or transversely to the right depending on the site of origin. In most cases, they enter the gland from the anterior face of the tail.[117] Anastomosis is usually with the TP artery, less frequently with the PM or DP artery.[142] In 33% of cases, the CP arteries are the sole source of blood for the tail of the pancreas with no apparent anastomosis with the arteries of the pancreatic body.[152]

### Some Considerations

If we imagine the pancreas as a stage where the play "Arterial Blood Supply of the Pancreas" is performed, we should consider the arteries as the actors of the play. The plot twist of this play is that the actors play extemporaneously. The spectator (the surgeon) can never be sure about a number of facts: the importance of the role played by each actor (dominance of an artery), the number of actors in the cast (at times all the arteries are present, other times just a few of them supply the pancreas), and the entrances and exits on the set (big variation of the source of each artery). Actors playing roles in other scenarios (i.e. liver, colon) may cross the pancreatic stage as well. There is only one plot device that keeps our play from turning into a tragedy: preoperative angiography.

## *Venous Drainage (By Bertelli and Colleagues)*

The venous drainage of the head of the pancreas is arranged mainly in two venous arcades. The venous arcades follow, on a more superficial plane, the course of the homonymous arterial arcades.[136]

The anterior PD venous arcade is formed by the ASPD and AIPD veins. The ASPD vein empties into the right gastroepiploic vein[118,127,136,153] that, in its turn, drains into the superior mesenteric vein through the gastrocolic trunk.[127,136] The AIPD vein follows the artery behind the uncinate process and the superior mesenteric vessels, and joins the uppermost jejunal vein,[127] usually via a common trunk with the PIPD vein. Less frequently, the AIPD vein drains directly into the superior mesenteric vein.[127,153]

The posterior PD venous arcade is formed by the PSPD and the PIPD veins. The PSPD vein is considered the largest venous trunk of the pancreatic head.[129] The PSPD vein follows the same course as the artery but, in 40% of cases, when it reaches the superior edge of the pancreas,[127,136] it leaves the PSPD artery and crosses behind the choledochus[123,147] before joining the right side of the portal vein.[118,127,153,154] The PIPD vein may join the AIPD vein, or may end directly into the superior mesenteric vein.[154]

In addition to the anterior and posterior PD arcades, two further vessels take part in the venous drainage of the pancreatic head: an inferior venous arcade joining the IPD veins[154] and the anteromedial PD vein.[122]

According to Olsen and Woodburne,[153] the anteromedial PD vein occurs only occasionally. It originates from the confluence of two or more branches coming from the second portion of the duodenum.[147] The anteromedial PD vein crosses the head of the pancreas transversely in an intermediate position.[122,147] It empties into the superior mesenteric vein or, less frequently, into the right gastroepiploic vein.[147]

To summarize: the neck, the body, and the tail of the pancreas are drained by a number of veins that usually follow the same course as the homonymous arteries:

- A system of small superior pancreatic veins (from 3 to 13) empties into the splenic vein.[147,149,153]
- In 34-50% of cases,[149,154] the TP vein originates from the splenic vein,[147] and joins the inferior mesenteric vein,[136,149,153,154] the superior mesenteric vein,[136,153] or the splenic vein itself.[136,149,153] The TP vein, also known as the inferior pancreatic vein,[149,153,154] may be as large as 10 mm.
- A DP vein,[147] a PM vein, and one or more CP veins are usually detectable close to the corresponding arteries.

## *Lymphatic Drainage*

As the position of the pancreas might predict, lymphatic drainage is centrifugal to the surrounding nodes. No standard terminology for those nodes exists, although Evans and Ochsner[155] propose one. None of the efforts to demarcate specific drainage areas of the pancreas have gained wide acceptance. Studies of Cubilla et al.[156] provide the basis for most recent works.

### Editorial Comment

*Dr. Bertelli appears to be recommending preoperative angiography prior to any pancreatic resection. I don't believe this is standard practice. Imaging techniques will continue to evolve, but currently the techniques for evaluating suspected tumors of the exocrine pancreas are ultrasonography, computed tomographic (CT) scanning, and endoscopic retrograde cholangiopancreatography (ERCP). Variations in arterial anatomy are then recognized and dealt with at the time of any resection. Wider acceptance of helical CT scanning for evaluation of the pancreas would as a byproduct provide the information on the vascular anatomy recommended by Dr. Bertelli. (RSF Jr)*

The lymphatic vessels of the pancreas arise in a rich, perilobular, interanastomosing network (Fig. 21-44A). Channels course along the surface of the gland and in the interlobular spaces with the blood vessels. These lymphatics drain into five main collecting trunks and five lymph node groups: superior nodes, inferior nodes, anterior nodes, posterior nodes, and splenic nodes (Fig. 21-44B). The following paragraphs discuss these nodes.

### Superior Nodes

The collecting trunks of this group of nodes arise from the anterior and posterior superior half of the pancreas. Most end in the suprapancreatic lymph nodes located along the superior border of the pancreas. The names of

the nodes typically reflect the areas drained, such as the superior head and the superior body. Some lymphatics occasionally terminate in the nodes of the gastropancreatic fold or in the lymph nodes of the hepatic chain.

### Inferior Nodes

These collecting trunks drain the anterior and posterior lower half of the head and body of the pancreas. They lead into the inferior pancreatic group of lymph nodes, most of which are located along the inferior border of the head and body of the pancreas. Further, they may extend into the superior mesenteric and left lateroaortic lymph nodes. Although infrequent, a collecting trunk may terminate directly in a lumbar trunk.

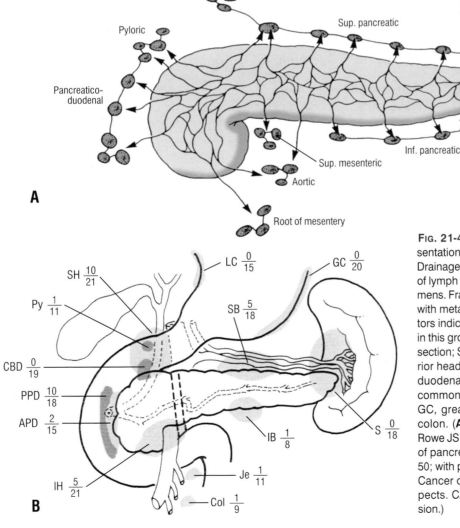

FIG. 21-44. **A,** Highly diagrammatic theoretical presentation of possible lymphatic drainage of pancreas. Drainage to nearest margin of pancreas. **B,** Distribution of lymph nodes in 21 pancreatectomy resection specimens. Fraction numerators indicate number of patients with metastasis in that lymph node group. Denominators indicate number of patients in which lymph nodes in this group were examined. Stippled line, Whipple resection; SH, superior head; SB, superior body; IH, inferior head; IB, inferior body; APD, anterior pancreatoduodenal; PPD, posterior pancreatoduodenal; CBD, common bile duct; Py, pylorus; LC, lesser curvature; GC, greater curvature; S, splenic; J, jejunum; Col, colon. (**A,** Modified from Skandalakis JE, Gray SW, Rowe JS Jr, Skandalakis LJ. Anatomical complications of pancreatic surgery. Contemp Surg 1979;15(6):17-50; with permission. **B,** From Cubilla AL, Fitzgerald PJ. Cancer of the exocrine pancreas: the pathologic aspects. CA Cancer J Clin 1985;35:2-18; with permission.)

## Anterior Nodes

Two collecting trunks run along the anterior surface of the superior and inferior portions of the head of the pancreas. They extend to the infrapyloric and anterior pancreatoduodenal lymph nodes. They may extend also to some of the mesenteric lymph nodes at the root of the mesentery of the transverse colon.

## Posterior Nodes

The posterior nodes follow the posterior surface of the superior and inferior portions of the head of the pancreas. They drain into the posterior pancreaticoduodenal lymph nodes, common bile duct lymph nodes, right lateroaortic lymph nodes, and some nodes at the origin of the superior mesenteric artery. Most lymphatics of the common bile duct and ampulla of Vater also end in the posterior pancreaticoduodenal group of lymph nodes.

## Splenic Nodes

These lymphatics originate from the tail of the pancreas. They drain into those at the hilum of the spleen, splenophrenic ligament, and inferior and superior lymph nodes of the tail of the pancreas. A few lymphatic channels, however, end in the lymph nodes superior and inferior to the body of the pancreas.

## Surgical Applications

We continue to learn more about pancreatic lymphatics. The following paragraphs describe some of this new information.

- Deki and Sato[157] state that the lymphatics of the anterior surface of the head and neck of the pancreas are associated with the common hepatic group and with the superior mesenteric nodal group. All terminate at a lymph node situated to the right of the origins of the celiac trunk and the superior mesenteric artery. Lymphatics of the posterior surface of the head terminate in a node located behind the previously described node. The lymphatics of the left half of the pancreas terminate in a node to the left of the celiac trunk and superior mesenteric artery. Both the right and left nodes drain into the abdominal aortic nodes.
- The lymphatics of the head and body of the pancreas do not drain toward the tail of the pancreas or the splenic nodes. Rarely, however, the lymph vessels from the tail of the pancreas can terminate in the superior body and inferior body subgroups of nodes.
- Donatini and Hidden[158] studied the routes of lymphatic drainage from the pancreas using injection into several pancreatic segments, followed by dissection. They concluded that dye injected into the body and tail followed the splenic and inferior pancreatic pathways, terminat-

ing first to the left interceliacomesenteric node and then to the suprarenal and infrarenal lymph nodes. From the head of the pancreas, dye followed one of three routes.
 - The lymphatics of the anterior and posterior aspects of the head followed the superior mesenteric route and reached the right interceliacomesenteric node and then terminated bilaterally in the suprarenal and infrarenal nodes.
 - The anterosuperior segment of the head followed two routes. The gastroduodenal joined the right interceliacomesenteric node. An inferior route terminated by flowing backward in direction to the isthmus.
 - The drainage of the posterosuperior segment of the head followed the CBD and hepatic artery, reaching the pericholedochal nodes and hepatic pedicular nodes and occasionally the right interceliacomesenteric node.
- Donatini and Hidden[158] consider the right interoceliacomesenteric node the principal relay station for the head of the pancreas.
- No lymphatic communications exist between the pancreas and the lymph nodes of the greater and lesser curvatures of the stomach.
- Lymph moves from the pancreas to the duodenum, not from the duodenum to the pancreas.
- Based on studies of the lymphatic network of the guinea pig, Bertelli et al.[159] concluded the following: "All lymph vessels in the pancreas are absorbing lymph vessels, characterized by a very thin endothelial wall, anchoring filaments and the absence of a definitive basal membrane."
- According to Cubilla et al.,[156] a total pancreatectomy may involve removing 70 nodes. The Whipple partial pancreatectomy may involve removing 33 nodes. It is the opinion of the authors of this chapter that 15-20 is a good harvest.
- Examination of surgical specimens removed during regional pancreatectomy in patients with pancreatic and peripancreatic cancers revealed both the number of lymph nodes present in each of the nodal drainage areas and the presence of metastatic disease in them.[156] The average number of lymph nodes present in each lymph node group is shown in Table 21-8.
- Pissas[160] wrote that the value of radical surgery is diminished by the very rapid passage of lymph into the thoracic duct.
- Delcore et al.[161] reported that 56 percent of patients undergoing curative resection for pancreatic carcinoma were found to have lymph node metastases.
- It is well known that pancreatic cancer disseminates rapidly because of the retroperitoneal position of the pancreas and its rich lymphatic and venous drainage.

**TABLE 21-8. Anatomic Distribution of Peripancreatic Lymph Nodes in Resected Specimens**

| Lymph Node | | Av. No. of Lymph Nodes Present | | |
| Group | Subgroup | Regional | Total | Whipple |
| --- | --- | --- | --- | --- |
| Superior | Gastric | 7 | 6 | 7 |
| | Superior head | 17 | 9 | 10 |
| | Superior body | 13 | 10 | 2 |
| Inferior | Inferior head | – | 1 | – |
| | Inferior body | 1 | – | – |
| | Mid colic | 1 | – | – |
| Anterior | Pyloric | – | 1 | 2 |
| | Pancreaticoduodenal | 3 | 2 | 4 |
| | Mesenteric (jejunal) | 3 | – | – |
| Posterior | Pancreaticoduodenal | 4 | 4 | 3 |
| | Common bile duct | 2 | 2 | 1 |
| Splenic | Tail of pancreas-spleen | 10 | 3 | – |

*Source:* Cubilla AL, Fortner J, Fitzgerald PJ. Lymph node involvement in carcinoma of the head of the pancreas area. Cancer 41:880-887, 1978; with permission.

- Mukaiya et al.[162] stated that excessive lymph node dissection in advanced cases of ductal adenocarcinoma of the head of the pancreas does not necessarily lead to a favorable prognosis. They found that patients who undergo a radical operation with adequate lymph node dissection have longer survival periods.
- Nakao et al.[163] presented a histopathologic examination of lymph nodes with metastasis from 139 specimens with cancer of the head of the pancreas (Fig. 21-45 and Tables 21-9, 21-10). Nakao et al. advised that wide dissection of lymph nodes, including paraaortic nodes, is necessary in patients with carcinoma of the pancreatic head.
- Vossen et al.[164] reported that pancreatic tumors in children are rare, the tumor pattern and biologic behavior is not the same as in adults, and complete surgical excision is the treatment of choice.
- Sho et al.[165] reported that intraductal papillary mucinous pancreatic tumors (IPMT) have high recurrence at the pancreatic remnant even after curative resection. The results of their study suggest that IPMT is a multicentric phenomenon and advise avoiding incomplete resection.
- Nakagohri et al.[166] found that intraductal papillary mucinous tumors, a localized malignancy, had a favorable prognosis after surgical treatment. They recommend curative pancreatectomy.
- We quote from Kobari et al.:[167]

    *Intraductal papillary mucinous tumors may be comprised of 2 clinically distinct subtypes: MDTs [main duct tumors] and BDTs [branch duct tumors]. Initially, although distal pancreatectomy can be recommended for most MDTs, the need for cancer-free margins in this more aggressive type may necessitate total pancreatectomy. Pylorus-preserving pancreatoduodenectomies are recommended for most BDTs, but, because these tumors are more often adenomas, a good prognosis can be expected.*

- The enigmatic malignancy of the pancreatic head still produces problems for the patient and the surgeon.
- We appreciate the emphatic statement of Warshaw[168] on the diagnosis of pancreatic cancer, "If I think there is a mass, I want to be sure I have a high-quality *contrast* CT scan in hand as my principal imaging modality."

**Editorial Comment**

*I do not believe that the tendency for carcinoma of the pancreas to metastasize is simply because of its extraperitoneal location and its rich lymphatic and venous drainage. Access to the vascular system (lymphatic and/or venous) is clearly necessary for vascular dissemination but pancreatic exocrine adenocarcinomas appear to have an unusually efficient biological capacity to metastasize. (RSF Jr)*

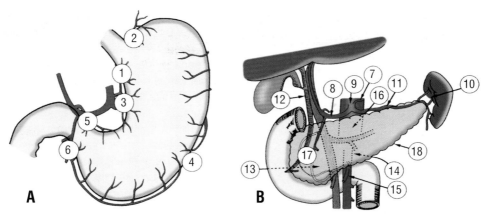

**Fig 21-45.** Nomenclature of **(A)** perigastric lymph nodes in patients with carcinoma of the head of the pancreas and **(B)** lymph nodes in carcinoma of the head of the pancreas region. 1, right cardiac lymph nodes; 2, left cardiac lymph nodes; 3, lesser curvature lymph nodes; 4, greater curvature lymph nodes; 5, suprapyloric lymph nodes; 6, infrapyloric lymph nodes; 7, lymph nodes around the left gastric artery; 8, lymph nodes around the common hepatic artery; 9, lymph nodes around the celiac trunk; 10, lymph nodes at the hilum of the spleen; 11, lymph nodes along the splenic artery; 12, lymph nodes of the hepatoduodenal ligament; 13, posterior pancreaticoduodenal lymph nodes; 14, lymph nodes around the superior mesenteric artery; 15, lymph nodes along the middle colic artery; 16, para-aortic lymph nodes; 17, anterior pancreticoduodenal lymph nodes; 18, inferior pancreatic body lymph nodes. (Modified from Nakao A, Harada A, Nonami T, Kaneko T, Murakami H, Inoue S, Takeuchi Y, Takagi H. Lymph node metastases in carcinoma of the head of the pancreas region. Br J Surg 1995;82:399-402; with permission.)

## Nerve Supply

Innervation of the pancreas occurs by the sympathetic division of the autonomic nervous system (Fig. 21-46) through the splanchnic nerves and by the parasympathetic division through the vagus nerve. The nerves generally follow blood vessels to their destinations. Perhaps together they constitute the "pancreatic nerve" of Holst.[169]

### *Efferent and Afferent Fibers*

Both the sympathetic and parasympathetic divisions provide efferent (motor) fibers to the wall of the blood vessels, the pancreatic duct, and pancreatic acini. Further, both contain visceral afferent (pain) fibers. The distribution of these in the pancreas, however, is not well understood.

### *Sympathetic Nerve Path*

Preganglionic sympathetic innervation is from the greater and lesser thoracic splanchnic nerves. The former is composed of preganglionic efferent fibers from the 5th to the 9th or 10th thoracic segments. The latter is composed of fibers from the 9th and 10th or the 10th and 11th segments. Some fibers may be contributed by the least splanchnic nerve.

The sympathetic nerves pierce the diaphragmatic crura

to reach the celiac and superior mesenteric ganglia. Postganglionic fibers arising from neurons in these ganglia accompany branches of the celiac and superior mesenteric arteries to reach the pancreas.

Some afferent fibers cross over the midline in the celiac plexus. The celiac ganglion contains cell bodies of efferent fibers for the pancreas. Cell bodies of afferent fibers are in the dorsal root ganglia at the same spinal nerve levels as

| TABLE 21-9. Operative Procedures for Carcinoma of the Head of the Pancreas Region | | |
|---|---|---|
| | No. of Total Pancreatectomies | No. of Pancreatoduodenectomies |
| Carcinoma of the head of the pancreas (n = 90) | 48 (48) | 42 (41) |
| Carcinoma of the distal bile duct (n = 22) | 1 (1) | 21 (2) |
| Carcinoma of the papilla of Vater (n = 27) | 1 (1) | 26 (2) |

Values in parentheses indicate the number of portal vein resections.

*Source:* Nakao A, Harada A, Nonami T, Kaneko T, Murakami H, Inoue S, Takeuchi Y, Takagi H. Lymph node metastases in carcinoma of the head of the pancreas region. Br J Surg 82:399-402, 1995; with permission.

**TABLE 21-10. Lymph Node Involvement in Patients with Carcinoma of the Head of the Pancreas Region**

| Lymph Nodes | Carcinoma of the Head of the Pancreas (n=90) | Carcinoma of the Distal Bile Duct (n=22) | Carcinoma of the Papilla of Vater (n=27) |
|---|---|---|---|
| 1 | 0 | 0 | 0 |
| 2 | 0 | 0 | 0 |
| 3 | 0 | 0 | 0 |
| 4 | 0 | 0 | 1 (4) |
| 5 | 0 | 0 | 0 |
| 6 | 13 (14) | 0 | 0 |
| 7 | 0 | 0 | 0 |
| 8 | 12 (13) | 1 (4) | 0 |
| 9 | 2 (2) | 1 (4) | 0 |
| 10 | 1 (1) | 0 | 0 |
| 11 | 16 (18) | 0 | 0 |
| 12 | 17 (19) | 5 (23) | 1 (4) |
| 13 | 46 (51) | 3 (14) | 11 (41) |
| 14 | 21 (23) | 2 (9) | 3 (11) |
| 15 | 0 | 0 | 0 |
| 16 | 23 (26) | 2 (9) | 0 |
| 17 | 35 (39) | 1 (4) | 6 (22) |
| 18 | 3 (3) | 1 (4) | 0 |

Values in parentheses represent percentages.

*Source:* Nakao A, Harada A, Nonami T, Kaneko T, Murakami H, Inoue S, Takeuchi Y, Takagi H. Lymph node metastases in carcinoma of the head of the pancreas region. Br J Surg 82:399-402, 1995; with permission.

those that contribute the preganglionic sympathetic fibers.

Interconnections of the afferent fibers from the pancreas with other sensory fibers from the body wall are presumably responsible for referral of pancreatic pain to the surface of the abdominal wall. Pain fibers from the pancreas pass cranially within the greater thoracic splanchnic nerve. They leave it by way of white communicating rami and enter the midthoracic spinal nerves. These neurons have their cell bodies within the dorsal root ganglia of those nerves.

## Parasympathetic Nerve Path

Parasympathetic innervation is by way of the celiac division of the posterior vagal trunk. The efferent fibers are preganglionic axons from cell bodies in the dorsal motor nucleus of the vagus nerve in the brain.

The preganglionic vagal fibers synapse with terminal ganglion cells within the pancreas. The postganglionic fibers terminate at pancreatic islet cells. Almost 90 percent of the fibers carried by the vagus nerve are sensory in function, having to do with stretch, chemoreceptors, osmoreceptors, and thermoreceptors.[170,171]

Grundy[172] states that fewer than 10 percent of the fibers carried by the vagus are autonomic efferents. The remaining fibers are sensory. These afferent fibers are processes of sensory neurons located in the sensory ganglia of the right vagus nerve at the jugular foramen of the skull. Vagal fibers pass through the esophageal hiatus of the diaphragm, usually as anterior and posterior trunks.

The posterior trunk divides into a posterior gastric and celiac division near the lesser curvature of the stomach.[107] The neuronal processes of the celiac division of the posterior vagus traverse the nerve plexuses at the origins of the celiac and superior mesenteric arteries and accompany the branches of these arteries to reach the organs supplied by them. None of the fibers carried by the vagus synapse within the celiac ganglia.

## Pain

Anatomically, it is not easy to explain the severe, excruciating pain of pancreatic disease. The etiology of pain

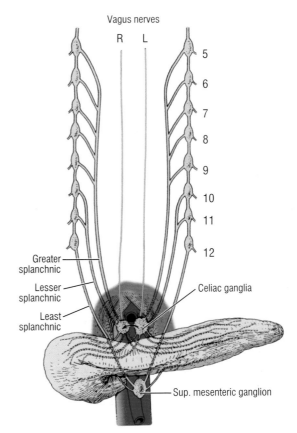

**FIG. 21-46.** Autonomic nerve supply to pancreas. (Modified from Skandalakis JE, Gray SW, Rowe JS Jr, Skandalakis LJ. Anatomical complications of pancreatic surgery. Contemp Surg 1979;15:17-50, with permission.)

secondary to pancreatic cancer is enigmatic and not easily understood. Drapiewski[173] believes the nerves are invaded by the tumor in 84 percent of cases. Bockman and colleagues[174] believe that the perineurium is damaged. Frey[65] and Bockman et al.[174] contend that inflammatory cells frequently concentrate around the nerves and the ganglia in patients with chronic pancreatitis.

Ductal hypertension, also, is responsible for the production of pain. Widdison et al.[175] speculate on a compartment syndrome due to increased tissue and ductal pressure.

Bockman[176] assumes that there are multiple paths for the genesis of pancreatic pain. He states that pain does not always occur with invasion of nerves by cancer or with distention of the pancreatic ducts.

### *Surgical Applications*

Both sympathetic and parasympathetic pancreatic networks of patients with pancreatitis or pancreatic carcinoma can be treated by sympathectomy and vagotomy. The hope is always that division of the pathways of pain will relieve the terrible suffering of these unfortunate individuals.

According to Howard,[177] sympathectomy has not proven a good procedure for palliation. However, Mallet-Guy,[178,179] the father of left splanchnicectomy, reported good or perfect results in 83 percent of his patients. Stone and Chauvin[180] found that pancreatic denervation (left transthoracic splanchnicectomy and bilateral vagotomy) gives reasonable control of incapacitating pain of chronic alcoholic pancreatitis. Cuschieri et al.[181] advise bilateral endoscopic splanchnicectomy through a posterior thorascopic approach for the relief of intractable pain in patients with advanced pancreatic cancer. Thorascopic splanchnicectomy for palliation of inoperable pancreatic carcinoma is also reported by various workers.[182,183]

We quote from Skandalakis et al.[184] about the use of vagotomy for treatment of severe pain secondary to pancreatic cancer or pancreatitis.

> *It is not clear whether afferent fibers of the vagus are involved in pancreatic pain. Vagotomy alone does not relieve the pain of pancreatitis,[185] but Merendino[186] believes that bilateral truncal vagotomy may provide relief from the pain of an inoperable carcinoma. This view has not won complete acceptance.*

Flanigan and Kraft[187] advised injection of 40 ml of 5% phenol in almond oil or 75% alcohol into the celiac plexus and splanchnic nerves. This chemical splanchnicectomy relieves pancreatic pain. Gardner and Solomon[188] also recommended chemical splanchnicectomy to control pain secondary to unresectable carcinoma of the pancreas.

Hegedus[189] reported that radiography-guided celiac ganglion block together with enzymatic substitution is useful for the relief of pancreatic pain.

## HISTOLOGY AND PHYSIOLOGY

For all practical purposes, the pancreas consists of the islets of Langerhans and the acinar cells, the former fulfilling the endocrine function and the latter the exocrine function. The pancreas is poorly "encapsulated" by a very thin connective tissue (if the word "encapsulated" is permissible), since in the posterior wall of the pancreas there is no peritoneum.

### Endocrine Function

The islets of Langerhans form small networks of cells that secrete hormones that control and regulate glucose. The islets of Langerhans constitute only 2 percent of the pancreatic mass. They consist of several types of cells: A (alpha), B (beta), D (delta), and F or PP (pancreatic polypeptide). Each type has a different physiological destiny: A secretes glucagon; B secretes insulin; D secretes somatostatin (inhibitor of insulin and glucagon); F secretes pancreatic polypeptide (inhibitor of pancreatic exocrine secretion).

It is well known that some bodybuilders use insulin to improve athletic performance. These athletes unfortunately ignore the health risks of insulin use.[190]

The distribution of the types of cells throughout the pancreas varies. For example, B and D cells are evenly distributed, while islets in the uncinate process are rich in F cells and poor in A cells. Islets in the body and tail are rich in A cells and poor in F cells.[191]

From the portion of the ventral diverticulum of the duodenum — which gives rise to the terminal portion of the main pancreatic duct (of Wirsung), the uncinate process, and part of the head of the pancreas — no islets (of Langerhans) are present in the pancreatic parenchyma.

### Exocrine Function

The exocrine pancreas is formed by acinar cells, ducts, and ductules. Together they constitute 80 percent to 90 percent of the pancreatic mass. An acinus is a collection of acinar cells responsible for the secretion of enzymes of digestion, pancreatic fluids, and electrolytes. All secretions of the acini drain through the ductal network into the duodenum through the major and minor duodenal papillae.

It is well known that vagal stimulation augments the exocrine secretion of the pancreas. Perhaps the sympathetic nervous system inhibits the exocrine secretion.

The pancreas secretes 500 to 800 mL/d of an alkaline fluid that contains bicarbonate and digestive enzymes such as amylase, lipase, and trypsinogen.[192]

## Surgical Applications

- Resection of the head of the pancreas for cancer by pancreaticoduodenectomy theoretically removes the cancer, but according to Seymour et al.,[193] also removes 95 percent of the PP cells because most of these cells are located in the uncinate process. Because of the even distribution of B and D cells throughout the pancreas, subtotal pancreaticoduodenectomy will not disturb the secretion of insulin and somatostatin. Since B cells are responsible for the synthesis of insulin, 80 percent of the islet mass[194] must be destroyed, surgically or otherwise, before diabetes will be obvious.
- Repeated episodes of chronic and acute pancreatitis will partially or totally destroy the ductular draining network. This produces not only pancreatic exocrine insufficiency but also pancreatic cysts and pain.
- Yamaguchi et al.[195] recommend the use of red litmus paper to detect pancreatoenterostomy leakage of alkaline pancreatic juice.
- Sato et al.[196] reported that there is a correlation between preoperative exocrine function and pancreatic juice secretion and leakage after pancreaticojejunostomy. Greater pancreatic juice production occurred in patients who had exhibited normal preoperative exocrine pancreatic function than in those with low pancreatic juice production. Greater pancreatic juice production also correlated with risk of pancreatic juice leakage.
- Sho et al.[197] demonstrated that evaluation of the function of the pancreatic remnant after pancreaticoduodenectomy is feasible with secretin-stimulated magnetic resonance cholangiopancreatography.

## PANCREATITIS

Laboratory findings and etiological factors of acute pancreatitis presented by Ranson[198] are shown in Table 21-11 and Table 21-12 respectively.

The etiologic factors of pancreatitis are multiple:

- Alcohol-induced (most common)
- Postoperative
- Endoscopic retrograde cholangiopancreatography- and endoscopic sphincterotomy-induced
- Infectious disease

Lad et al.[199] reported recurrent pancreatitis secondary to a duodenal duplication cyst.

We recommend the excellent text by Berger and colleagues[200] to the interested student.

## Extravasations of Pancreatic Fluid

The track of pathological peripancreatic fluid collections (Figs. 21-47 to 21-50), as in pancreatitis, depends on the involved part of the organ. However, the chest and peritoneal cavity are not immune. Occasionally the scrotum is involved. Primarily, the spaces around the kidneys are the first to be occupied by pancreatic fluid. To understand the pathways of the fluid, the extraperitoneal

**TABLE 21-11. Routine Laboratory Findings in 100 Patients with Acute Pancreatitis Versus those in 100 Patients with Other Acute Abdominal Emergencies**

| Laboratory Test | Acute Pancreatitis (%) | Other (%) |
|---|---|---|
| Serum amylase (Somogyi units/dl) | | |
| >500 | 59 | 1 |
| 200-500 | 36 | 4 |
| <200 | 5 | 95 |
| Hematocrit (%) | | |
| >45 | 31 | 23 |
| <45 | 69 | 77 |
| White blood cell count (cells/mm³) | | |
| >12,000 | 41 | 53 |
| <12,000 | 59 | 47 |
| Blood glucose (mg/dl) | | |
| >300 | 7 | 0 |
| 200-300 | 9 | 7 |
| Diabetics excluded: <200 | 84 | 93 |
| Serum calcium (mg/dl) | | |
| >9 | 76 | 67 |
| 8-9 | 15 | 31 |
| <8 | 9 | 2 |
| Serum LDH (IU/L) | | |
| >225 | 48 | 24 |
| <225 | 52 | 76 |
| Serum GOT (Sigma-Frankel units/dl) | | |
| >100 | 37 | 8 |
| <100 | 63 | 92 |

*Source:* Ranson JHC. Diagnostic standards for acute pancreatitis. World J Surg 21:136-142, 1997; with permission.

### TABLE 21-12. Etiologic Factors of Acute Pancreatitis

Metabolic
    Alcohol abuse
    Hyperlipoproteinemia
    Hypercalcemia
    Drugs
    Genetic
    Scorpion venom
Mechanical
    Cholelithiasis
    Postoperative (gastric, biliary)
    Pancreas divisum
    Posttraumatic
    Retrograde pancreatography
    Pancreatic duct obstruction: pancreatic tumor, *Ascaris*
      infestation
    Pancreatic ductal bleeding
    Duodenal obstruction
Vascular
    Postoperative (cardiopulmonary bypass)
    Periarteritis nodosa
    Atheroembolism
Infection
    Mumps
    Coxsackie B
    Cytomegalovirus
    *Cryptococcus*

*Source:* Ranson JHC. Diagnostic standards for acute pancreatitis. World J Surg 21:136-142, 1997; with permission.

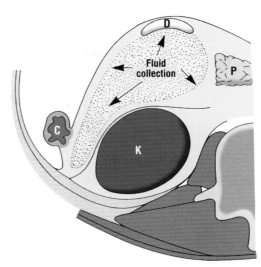

**Fig 21-47.** Fluid collection in right anterior pararenal compartment with viscus displacement. P, pancreas; C, colon; K, kidney; D, duodenum. (Modified from Meyers MA. The extraperitoneal spaces: normal and pathologic anatomy. In: Meyers MA. Dynamic Radiology of the Abdomen (4th ed). New York: Springer-Verlag, 1994. Original drawing appeared in Meyers MA, Whalen JP, Peelle K. Radiologic features of extraperitoneal effusions: an anatomic approach. Radiology 1972; 104:249-257; with permission.)

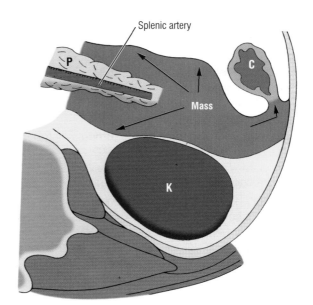

**FIG. 21-48.** Anterior pararenal hemorrhage from ruptured calcified splenic artery aneurysm (arrows). Extension from ruptured splenic artery into anterior pararenal space and into phrenicocolic ligament. C, colon; P, pancreas; K, kidney. (Modified from Meyers MA. The extraperitoneal spaces: normal and pathologic anatomy. In: Meyers MA. Dynamic Radiology of the Abdomen (4th ed). New York: Springer-Verlag, 1994. Original drawing appeared in Meyers MA, Whalen JP, Peelle K. Radiologic features of extraperitoneal effusions: an anatomic approach. Radiology 1972;104:249-257; with permission.)

spaces should be studied. These are described below.

### *Extraperitoneal Spaces and the Pancreas*

The posterior parietal peritoneum and the transversalis fascia are the anterior and posterior boundaries, respectively, of the retroperitoneal space. This space extends from the pelvic brim inferiorly to the diaphragm superiorly. Among the major structures it encompasses are the adrenal glands, kidneys, ureters, portions of the duodenum, pancreas, inferior vena cava, aorta, portal vein, and ascending and descending colon. In a horizontal cross section, the space is somewhat C-shaped due to the curvature of the lumbar spine. As a result, some retroperitoneal structures (pancreas and duodenal loop) lie anterior to others (spleen, kidneys, and posterior aspect of the liver).

Meyers[201] divides the extraperitoneal region into three compartments according to their demarcation by well-defined fascial planes (Figs. 21-51 to 21-53). The anterior and posterior layers of Gerota's fascia are central to the division of the extraperitoneal region. The kidney and the

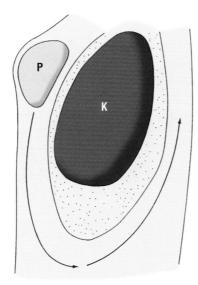

**FIG. 21-49.** Pancreatic extravasation with extension down anterior pararenal space, then upward into posterior pararenal compartment. Sagittal diagram illustrates fluid collection in left anterior pararenal space from pancreas, and continuity under and around cone of renal fascia into posterior pararenal compartment. P, pancreas; K, kidney. (Modified from Meyers MA. Acute extraperitoneal infection. Semin Roentgenol 1973;8:445-464; with permission.)

perirenal fat are enveloped by this dense sheath. The fusion of its two layers behind the ascending or descending colon forms a single lateroconal fascia. This continues around the flank to blend with the peritoneal reflection and to form the paracolic gutter.

Meyers named these three compartments, listed here and discussed in the paragraphs below.

- Anterior pararenal space. This space extends from the posterior parietal peritoneum to the anterior renal fascia. It is confined laterally by the lateroconal fascia.
- Perirenal space. Within this space, the kidney and perirenal fat reside within the confines of Gerota's fascia.
- Posterior pararenal space. This area extends from the posterior renal fascia to the transversalis fascia. It is a thin layer of fat lateral to the lateroconal fascia, also known as the preperitoneal fat.

### Anterior Pararenal Space

The anterior pararenal space includes the ascending and descending colon, the duodenal loop, and the pancreas, which are the extraperitoneal portions of the alimentary tract. This space is continuous across the midline. It is important to understand this anatomy when considering the pathways that pancreatic extravasations can take.

### Perirenal Space

Although debate continues on the issue, it is often said that the perirenal space has no continuity across the midline. This is due to fusion at two locations. The posterior fascial layers fuse with the psoas or quadratus lumborum fascia medially. The renal fascia fuse with the dense mass of connective tissue surrounding the great vessels in the root of the mesentery and behind the pancreas and duodenum anteriorly. If continuity of the perirenal spaces is present, as seen in the passage of extravasating fluids or blood across the midline, it usually appears at the level of the hila and inferior poles of the kidneys.

### Posterior Pararenal Space

The fusion of the transversalis fascia medially with the muscle fascia demarcates the posterior pararenal space. Thus, the margin of the psoas muscle limits and parallels the

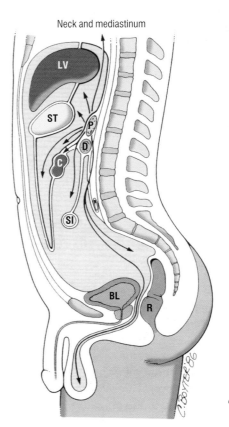

**FIG. 21-50.** Pathways of pancreatic extravasations to neck, mediastinum, lesser sac, root of small bowel mesentery, mesentery of transverse colon, pouch of Douglas, and scrotum through a patent tunica vaginalis. Lv, liver; ST, stomach; P, pancreas, D, duodenum; C, colon; SI, small intestine; BL, bladder; R, rectum. (Modified from Skandalakis LJ, Skandalakis JE, Gray SW. Anatomy of the pancreas. In: Glazer G, Ranson JHC (eds). Acute Pancreatitis. London: Baillière Tindall, 1988, pp. 51-99; with permission.)

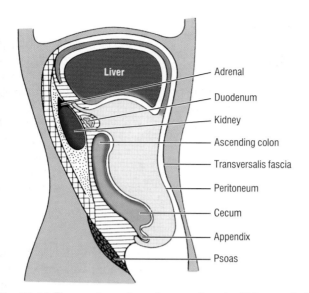

FIG. 21-51. Three extraperitoneal compartments. Stripes, anterior pararenal space; stipples, perirenal space; cross-hatches, posterior pararenal space. (Modified from Meyers MA. Radiologic features of the spread and localization of extraperitoneal gas and their relationship to its source: An anatomical approach. Radiology 1974;111: 17-26; with permission.)

space. No organs are contained within this space. Potential communication with the preperitoneal fat of the anterior lateral abdominal wall, however, is possible.

## Anatomy of Pancreatitis

Having reviewed the anatomy of the retroperitoneum, one can begin to understand the pathways that pancreatic extravasations can take. Eventually these extravasations arrest and form a pseudocyst, or subsequently an abscess. Knowledge of the extraperitoneal structures and planes can help us understand how adjacent structures contribute to the wall of the pseudocyst or abscess.

Different portions of the pancreas drain and localize to different areas. Drainage from the head of the pancreas is downward and to the right. The fluid can then come into contact with the ascending colon when traveling in the anterior pararenal space. Extravasations from the tail of the pancreas travel to the left in the anterior pararenal space, encountering the left colon, spleen, and left kidney.

Pancreatic extravasations can travel from any portion of the pancreas craniad to the neck, mediastinum, or lesser sac, into the root of the small bowel mesentery, and transperitoneally to settle into the most dependent portion of the peritoneal cavity. If a patent tunica vaginalis exists, this extravasation can present as a hydrocele in the male. This fluid can then extend below the level of the lateroconal fascia, gain access to the preperitoneal flank fat, and continue externally to the peritoneum.

With severe pancreatitis, the extravasations can travel through fascial planes to the posterior pararenal space from the anterior pararenal space without contaminating the perirenal compartment. Pancreatic extravasations can

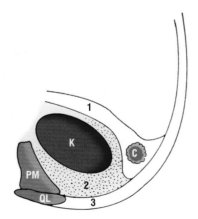

FIG. 21-52. Three extraperitoneal spaces. 1, anterior pararenal space; 2, perirenal space; 3; posterior pararenal space; QL, quadratus lumborum muscle; C, colon; K, kidney; PM, psoas major muscle. (Modified from Meyers MA. The extraperitoneal spaces: normal and pathologic anatomy. In Meyers MA. Dynamic Radiology of the Abdomen (4th ed). New York: Springer-Verlag, 1994; with permission.)

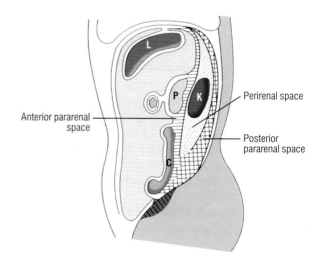

FIG. 21-53. Relationships and structures of three extraperitoneal spaces on left. Sigmoid colon in continuity with posterior and anterior pararenal compartments. L, liver; P, pancreas; K, kidney; C, colon. (Modified from Meyers MA. Acute extraperitoneal infection. Semin Roentgenol 1973;8:445-464; with permission.)

travel down the anterior pararenal space, rise posterior to the cone of the renal fascia, and thus reside within the posterior pararenal space. This displaces the kidney and colon anteriorly. This pathway provides an explanation for the classical signs of extensive pancreatitis, such as the subcutaneous discoloration known as Grey Turner's sign or Cullen's sign.

After the pancreatic extravasation enters the posterior pararenal space, it can violate the transversalis fascia. It can travel up to the chest or mediastinum. Though the transversalis fascia is known as "the girdle of the abdomen," there are some areas where it is attenuated and therefore weak. As the transversalis fascia ascends toward the diaphragm, it becomes thinner, especially where it blends with the diaphragm. Fibers of transversalis fascia can actually become lost in the area of fat external to Gerota's fascia covering the posterior surface of the kidneys. The transversalis fascia can become attenuated in this area posterior to the kidney. It is here, also, that fluid in the posterior pararenal space can gain access to the plane outside the transversalis fascia.

A study by Nakamura et al.[202] found that pancreaticobiliary maljunction (PBM), an anomaly commonly associated with congenital dilatation of the bile duct (CDBD), may be a possible cause of recurrent pancreatitis. Reflux of pancreatic juice into the bile duct is possible through the PBM. This study suggested involvement of activated phospholipase A2 in the pathogenesis of choledochal cyst-associated pancreatitis. Sugiyama et al.[203] reported that magnetic resonance cholangiopancreatography is an accurate method for the diagnosis of anomalous pancreaticobiliary junction.

## Retroperitoneal Dissection Secondary to Pancreatic Inflammatory Disease

Pancreatic inflammation at the height of the attack does not respect fascial planes, although residual exudate may be confined to definite spaces. If pancreatic fluid violates the retroperitoneal spaces, it may rupture into a hollow viscus such as the duodenum or transverse colon or it may rupture into the peritoneal cavity.

The continuity of the retroperitoneal spaces allows extension of pancreatic fluid into the thorax above and the scrotum below, as well as into the left retroperitoneal space, perihepatic and peripancreatic spaces, transverse mesocolon, and gastrocolic omentum[204,205] (Fig. 21-54). Jaffe and colleagues[206] reported 12 cases with dissection into the mediastinum, six through the aortic hiatus, and six through the esophageal hiatus.

Schoenberg et al.[207] defined "pancreatic abscess" as a

localized collection of pus surrounded by a capsule or a pseudocapsule. "Septic (infected) necrosis" is a diffuse bacterial inflammatory process of necrotic pancreatic and peripancreatic tissues. Surgery is the treatment of choice for both conditions. However, for culture-positive peripancreatic fluid collections or abscesses Baril and colleagues[208] recommended percutaneous catheter drainage as the initial treatment, with surgical intervention reserved for patients in whom treatment fails.

We quote from Seifert et al.[209]:

*Standard management of infected peripancreatic necrosis consists of open surgical debridement and lavage - a traumatic intervention with substantial mor-*

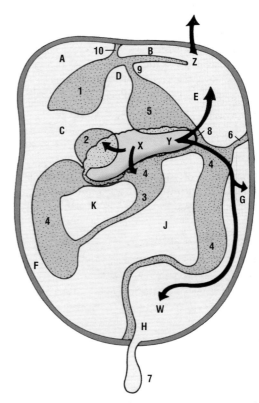

FIG. 21-54. Spaces and peritoneal reflections of abdomen. *Spaces:* A, right subphrenic; B, left subphrenic; C, right subhepatic; D, lesser sac; E, perisplenic; F, right paracolic; G, left paracolic; H, pelvic; J, left infracolic; K, right infracolic. *Reflections:* 1, coronary ligaments and bare area; 2, duodenum; 3, small intestine; 4, colon; 5, stomach; 6, phrenicocolic ligament; 7, scrotum; 8, gastrosplenic ligament; 9, hepatogastric ligament; 10, falciform ligament. *Possible pathways of pancreatic drainage:* W, left paracolic space to scrotum; X, perforation into duodenum or colon; Y, perforation into perisplenic or left paracolic spaces; Z, perforation through diaphragm to pleura and lung. (Modified from Skandalakis JE, Gray SW, Rowe JS Jr. Anatomical Complications in General Surgery. New York: McGraw-Hill, 1983; with permission.)

*bidity and mortality. [A]n alternative and novel approach with minimum invasiveness...[is] fenestration of the gastric wall and debridement of infected necrosis by direct retroperitoneal endoscopy...this strategy led to rapid clinical improvement and no serious complications. Transgastric endoscopic therapy may be a less traumatic alternative to surgery and should be further assessed in prospective studies.*

Beger et al.[210] reported the determinants of the natural course of acute pancreatitis.
- Pancreatic parenchymal necrosis
- Extrapancreatic retroperitoneal fatty tissue necrosis
- Biologically-active compounds in pancreatic ascites
- Infection or necrosis

Two subgroups of patients with necrotizing pancreatitis have been identified by Sakorafas et al.[211] The group with totally necrotic pancreatic parenchyma and peripancreatic tissues had a poor prognosis. The second group, with peripancreatic necrosis only and with viable pancreatic parenchyma, had a better prognosis.

A standard treatment protocol for managing biliary pancreatitis used by Liu et al.[212] is shown in Figure 21-55. Uomo et al.[213] concluded that severe biliary pancreatitis in patients with sterile necrosis frequently produces loss of integrity of the main pancreatic duct, and this should not be considered an absolute indication for surgical intervention.

Stolte and Waltschew[214] studied the relation of chronic pancreatitis and the papilla of Vater. They reported the following:
1. Chronic pancreatitis is often associated with inflammatory changes of the papilla of Vater.
2. Benign stenosis of the papilla may be caused by heterotopic pancreas or by peripapillary duodenal wall cysts.
3. Benign stenosis is located at the pre-papillary part of the pancreatic duct.
4. The function of the papilla is enigmatic.

Do Stolte and Waltschew mean ampulla of Vater or papilla?

Bosscha et al.[215] advised open management of the abdomen and planned reoperation for the treatment of patients with fulminant acute pancreatitis.

Chronic pancreatitis in childhood is a rare but potentially debilitating disorder. Weber and Keller[216] advocate distal pancreatectomy and pancreaticojejunostomy to treat this condition. DuBay and colleagues[217] favor the modified Puestow procedure (longitudinal pancreaticojejunostomy), and state that direct pancreatic duct localization during the procedure carries a lower morbidity rate than localization via distal pancreatectomy.

Apoptotic cell death of renal tubules takes place in severe acute pancreatitis and thus might be one of the

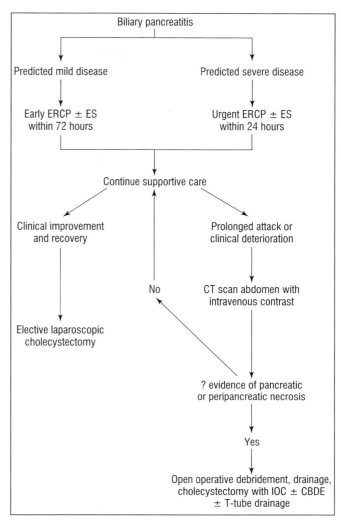

FIG. 21-55. Treatment protocol for biliary pancreatitis. ERCP, endoscopic retrograde cholangiopancreatography; ES, endoscopic sphincterotomy; CT, computed tomography; IOC, intraoperative cholangiogram; CBDE, common bile duct exploration. (From Liu CL, Lo CM, Fan ST. Acute biliary pancreatitis: diagnosis and management. World J Surg 1997;21:149-154; with permission.)

mechanisms of renal failure, according to Takase et al.[218]

## SURGERY

### Exploration of the Pancreas

The entire pancreas must be methodically evaluated. It can be approached by dividing the hepatogastric omentum or the gastrocolic omentum. Under usual circumstances, the gastrocolic omentum is incised widely and provides good exposure of the entire pancreas. If this exposure proves to be inadequate, the hepatogastric omenta can be divided also, and upward traction can be applied to the stomach.

Kocherization of the duodenum is necessary for palpation of the head of the pancreas. The hepatic flexure of the colon is mobilized, then the peritoneum is incised lateral to the second part of the duodenum. After completing this step, the left index and middle fingers are placed posterior to the duodenum and the head of the pancreas, with the left thumb anterior. The surgeon can now palpate the head of the pancreas as well as the pancreatic portion of the common bile duct. Lymph nodes can sometimes be felt at the distal portion of the CBD, near the upper part of the posterior surface of the head of the pancreas.

The left index finger can continue the exploration posterior to the neck of the pancreas. Occasionally, both index fingers can be used (Fig. 21-56). The surgeon's left hand approaches the neck from above, the left index finger posterior to the neck. The right hand proceeds from below, the right index finger posterior to the neck.

One criterion for resection for cancer is the ability to separate the neck of the pancreas from the underlying superior mesenteric and portal veins. Silen[66] rejects this maneuver because of possible avulsion of a posterosuperior pancreatoduodenal vein that may enter the superior mesenteric vein on its anterior surface.

Papadimitriou et al.[219] presented a modificaton of pancreaticoduodenectomy for the treatment of carcinoma of the pancreas and stated the following:

> Careful detachment of the posterior surface of the pancreas from the anterior surface of the portal vein and performance of pancreaticojejunal anastomosis to a defunctionalized jejunal loop results in lower mortality and morbidity rates, thus making pancreatoduodenectomy a safe procedure.

The uncinate process is the most difficult part of the pancreas to explore and evaluate because of its close relation to the superior mesenteric artery and vein.

The following paragraphs report research findings regarding surgical methods and prognosis. Preliminary abdominal exploratory maneuvers are discussed in the chapter on the peritoneum and omenta. Here we are concerned with specific approaches to the pancreas after the abdomen has been opened. Pancreatic carcinoma is discussed following this section.

There are at least six possible routes for abdominal exploration. Each route has particular advantages and disadvantages:[220]

- Through the gastrocolic ligament: route used by most surgeons.
- Through the hepatogastric omentum: useful in patients with exceptionally ptotic stomachs.
- By detaching the greater omentum from the transverse colon: time consuming, but better visualization of the entire lesser sac.
- Through the mesocolon: limited exposure of the pancreas, and risks injury to the middle colic blood vessels.
- Kocher maneuver: good exposure of the posterior surface of the head of the pancreas.
- Mobilization of the splenic flexure inferiorly and the spleen and tail of the pancreas: appropriate when partial pancreatectomy and splenectomy are seriously contemplated.

### Evaluating Resectability

We believe the most appropriate way to evaluate the re-

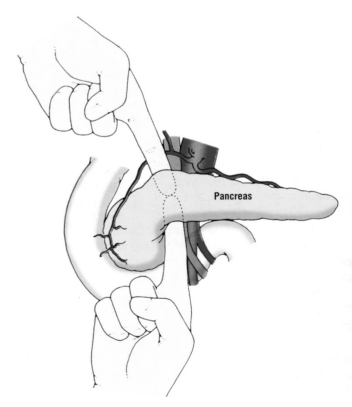

FIG. 21-56. Exploration of pancreas. Surgeon's fingers shown passing behind neck of pancreas, which should separate easily from underlying blood vessels. (Modified from Skandalakis JE, Gray SW, Rowe JS Jr, Skandalakis LJ. Anatomical complications of pancreatic surgery. Contemp Surg 1979; 15:17-50; with permission.)

sectability of a cancerous pancreas is to evaluate the area least likely to be invaded by the neoplasm and proceed to areas most likely to be invaded. Our criteria for resectability are as follows:

- The surgeon must perform good general exploration of the abdomen with special attention to the pancreas.
- Attention must be given to specific areas of lymph node drainage that are accessible without further incision, i.e., the pyloric and pancreatoduodenal nodes and the nodes at the root of the mesentery (Fig. 21-44A).
- Further investigation of lymph nodes is necessary. This requires some incision of the hepatogastric omenta and a Kocher maneuver. Pancreatoduodenal, celiac, and left gastric nodes, together with nodes of the superior and inferior pancreatic borders, should be inspected.
- Once the diagnosis of cancer has been determined and the previously outlined exploration has indicated a resectable lesion, the following final steps should be undertaken before the start of the actual resection.
  - Further exploration of the area of the ligament of Treitz to ensure mobility of the fourth part of the duodenum and the first portion of the jejunum.
  - Evaluation of the posterior surface of the head of the pancreas and the distal common bile duct. Ensure there is no fixation to underlying structures, including the inferior vena cava.
  - Gentle examination of the uncinate process and elevation of the neck of the pancreas with one or two fingers. Ensure they are not fixed to the superior mesenteric vessels or to the portal vein (see Fig. 21-56). Cattell and Warren[221] recommend incision of the hepatogastric ligament with division of the right gastric and gastroduodenal arteries to ensure adequate evaluation of possible fixation in this region.
  - Final review of the local anatomy to identify any previously undetected vascular anomalies. Any available angiograms should be studied.

Recently, Merchant et al.[222] found that positive peritoneal cytology is very specific in predicting when a pancreatic carcinoma is not resectable.

In their classic paper published in 1979, Hermann and Cooperman[223] wrote that localized masses in the head of the pancreas should be resected, even in the absence of histologic proof of malignancy. They suggested that "the smallest tumors, and perhaps those with the most favorable outcome, may never be resected for lack of histologic proof of the diagnosis."

Commenting on a more radical operation, Roder et al.[224] reported that portal vein resection did not prolong survival in patients with carcinoma of the head of the pancreas or of the distal common bile duct. The authors considered the prognosis "dismal" for such patients. Nakao and Kaneko[225]

recommend intravascular ultrasonography to rule out invasion of the portal vein by pancreatic carcinoma.

Farouk et al.[226] reported excision of the papilla of Vater for benign and malignant processes. In all cases, pathology had been suggested by endoscopic biopsy.

Sauvanet et al.[227] stated that a combination of endoscopic sphincterotomy and endoscopic ultrasonography prior to surgery are not accurate to distinguish benignancy from malignancy. Therefore, local excision of the tumor is not safe.

Howard et al.[228] found that helical CT scanning prior to surgery is the best diagnostic test to determine tumor resectability. According to these authors, endoscopic ultrasonography underestimates resectability, and selective angiography is no longer helpful for evaluation of periampullary tumors.

Sohn et al.[229] reported that in 33% of patients with periampullary adenocarcinoma at The Johns Hopkins Medical Institutions, the tumors were not resectable. Surgical palliation, with operative mortality of 3.1% and morbidity of 22%, produced excellent long-term results.

Kasahara et al.[230] suggested careful papillo-choledochectomy as an alternative to pancreaticoduodenectomy to treat periampullary cancer.

Ryu et al.[231] advised that segmental duodenal resection, including what the authors call the papilla of Vater, for focal cancer in adenoma and anastomosis of the jejunum to the duodenum, common bile duct, and pancreatic duct, is a safe and effective procedure. (There is confusion in the literature regarding the terms *ampulla* and *papilla*. A papilla is a nipplelike process. The duodenal papilla, for all practical purposes, is the mucosal exit of the ampulla, permitting excretions from the pancreaticobiliary system to enter the duodenum. An ampulla is a dilation of a canal or a duct. Near its exit at the duodenal papilla the common pancreaticobiliary channel is dilated, forming the ampulla of Vater.)

Martignoni et al.[232] reported that preoperative biliary instrumentation and biliary drainage do not affect early or late surgical outcome in patients undergoing pancreaticoduodenectomy.

## Pancreatic Carcinoma

Despite all the modern diagnostic procedures, an early diagnosis of pancreatic cancer is still a rare phenomenon. The senior author of this chapter (JES) has performed a very small number of duodenopancreatectomies, but a great number of palliative procedures. However, one of the other authors of this chapter (LJS), the product of the current era of surgery, has performed more Whipple duodenopancreatectomies than palliative procedures such as choledochoduodenostomies.

In a study of 7,145 patients,[233] cancer of the pancreas was located in the head in 73.2 percent, in the body in 19.9 percent, and in the tail in 6.8 percent. Pancreatic carcinoma is a terrible disease whose cause is not known. We know something from demographic and epidemiological studies, but not enough to explain the etiology of primary pancreatic cancer.

Gudjonsson,[234] using data collected 1972-1982, found that fewer than 1% of patients survive for more than five years. Sperti et al.[235] and Ihse[236] characterized long-term survival after surgical removal of pancreatic carcinoma as "poor" and "dismal."

However, Tan et al.[237] wrote that there is no reason for a nihilistic approach to pancreatic carcinoma. The median 5-year survival rate for resection alone is achievable in 15-25 percent of patients. A combined modality treatment approach may improve on that rate.

We quote from Tsiotos et al., who separate actual from actuarial survival (Table 21-13):[238]

*Although pancreatectomy is still performed in fewer than 20% of all patients with pancreatic cancer, and 99% of all patients who develop pancreatic cancer eventually die of their disease, significant improvements have been made. Pancreatectomy is now safer, with major morbidity occurring in about 20% and operative deaths in less than 5%. After curative resection, the five year actual survival is realistically about 10%, with median survivals of 12 to 18 months. In smaller subgroups with favorable pathologic characteristics (neoplasms <2 cm without nodal or perineural invasion), the prognosis appears to be significantly better, with the 5-year survival about 20%. Further improvements in survival should be sought at the areas of earlier diagnosis and novel treatments designed to prevent locoregional recurrences; the actual role of extended resections will be determined by current, ongoing prospective, randomized trials.*

Hirata et al.[239] presented 1001 cases of pancreatic resection for invasive ductal carcinoma. They report that extensive lymph node dissection does not necessarily produce a favorable prognosis. In commenting on these findings, Traverso[248] emphasized the difference between Japanese anatomic staging and Western clinical staging. Gouma et al.[241] reported that there are no results which confirm that palliative resection should be performed routinely for pancreatic cancer.

Harrison et al.[242] recommended pancreaticoduodenectomy to treat isolated metastatic or locally advanced nonperiampullary tumors. Edwards et al.[243] described pancreaticoduodenectomy with en bloc colectomy as curative procedures for primary malignancies of the duodenum.

Crawford[244] reported cytologic diagnosis of solid and papillary epithelial pancreatic neoplasm. This tumor, which

**TABLE 21-13. Survival Data after Pancreatectomy for Pancreatic Cancer in Recent Publications (Since 1990)**

| Study | Time Period | Year of Publication | No. of Patients | 5-Year Actuarial Survival (%) | 5-Year Actual Survival (%) | Median Survival (Months) |
|---|---|---|---|---|---|---|
| Nitecki (4) | 1981-1991 | 1995 | 174[a] | 7 | | 18 |
| Trede (5) | 1972-1984 | 1990 | 44 | | 25 | |
| Yeo (6) | 1970-1994 | 1995 | 201 | 26 | 13 | 18 |
| Mosca (14) | 1980-1994 | 1997 | 105 | 10 | | 15 |
| Connoly (26) | 1946-1983 | 1987 | 89 | | 3 | |
| Wade (29) | 1987-1991 | 1995 | 252 | 9 | | 15 |
| Janes (31) | 1983-1985 | 1996 | 758[a] | 17 | | |
| Conlon (32) | 1983-1989 | 1996 | 118[a] | | 10 | 14.3 |
| Tsao (33) | 1979-1992 | 1994 | 27 | 7 | | |
| Bramhall (34) | 1977-1986 | 1995 | 145[a] | 10 | | |
| Sperti (38) | 1970-1992 | 1997 | 113 | | 6 | |
| Griffin (39) | 1977-1987 | 1990 | 36[a] | 17 | | 11.5 |
| Fortner (40) | 1979-1991 | 1996 | 56 | | 14 | |
| Niederhuber (41) | 1985-1986, 1991 | 1995 | 2160[a] | 12 | | |
| Enayati (42) | 1987-1995 | 1997 | 37[a] | 35 | "Few" | |
| Klempnauer (43) | 1971-1993 | 1995 | 170[a] | | 7 | |
| Roder (44) | 1982-1990 | 1992 | 53 | 6 | | 12 |

[a]Studies including tumors of the body/tail requiring distal pancreatectomy.

*Source:* Tsiotos GG, Farnell MB, Sarr MG. Are the results of pancreatectomy for pancreatic cancer improving? World J Surg 23:913-919, 1999; with permission.

## Editorial Comment

*I believe that pancreaticoduodenectomy for attempted cure of selected patients with adenocarcinoma of the head of exocrine pancreas is appropriate, provided the procedure can be done with a relatively low mortality rate. When I first reviewed this subject in the 1960s the average published operative mortality from major centers was 35%! When tumors of the endocrine pancreas were excluded, five year survivals for ductal adenocarcinoma were rare, and there were some well documented five-year survivals for patients treated with bypass procedures after biopsy confirmation of adenocarcinoma of the exocrine pancreas. With in-hospital mortality rates of 35% after "curative" resections and institutional comparison data showing that the average survival time for those patients treated by radical operations was shorter than that after operations done as palliative measures, some highly skilled surgeons of the previous era concluded that patients with resectable adenocarcinomas of the head of the exocrine pancreas were better served by bypass procedures.[251]*

*Earlier diagnosis, improved operative techniques, and the availabilty of intensive care units, when needed, has led to much lower operative mortality rates at highly specialized centers. A small portion of the patients with adenocarcinoma of the head of the pancreas are rewarded with long-term survival after pancreaticoduodenectomy. When complication rates and mortality rates are low such resections are reasonable palliative procedures for the many patients who are not cured. But I would emphasize the need to have low operative morbidity and mortality to have a marginal gain in such patients. Several recent geographically based studies have demonstrated that the relatively good results at specialized centers are not universal. Low volume hospitals had pancreaticoduodenectomy mortality rates of 12% to 14% and minimal volume hospitals had 22% mortality rates.[252,253] (RSF Jr)*

typically is found in young women, does not metastasize, and is amenable to cure.

John et al.[245] found laparoscopic ultrasonography indispensable for detecting occult intraperitoneal metastases and pancreatic malignancies.

DiFronzo et al.[246] stated that the procedure of choice for unresectable carcinoma of the pancreas is choledochoduodenostomy, which provides relief of jaundice and causes little morbidity.

Clavien and Selzner[247] advised partial resection of the duodenum and pancreatic head for selected patients with duodenal and pancreatic pathological entities that do not require complete pancreatic head resection. Di Carlo et al.[248] stated that the treatment of choice for cancer of the pancreatic head is the pylorus-preserving pancreaticoduodenectomy.

Hiraoka and Kanemitsu[249] recommended intraoperative radiotherapy and extended pancreatic resection for local pancreatic carcinoma. They advocated hepatic resection with metastasis to the liver. Yeo and Cameron[250] supported adjuvant chemoradiation therapy for resected patients with pancreatic carcinoma.

REMEMBER:

- Cancer of the pancreas is a disease of acquired and inherited mutations in cancer-causing genes.[254]

- There is no "correct" staging approach for the patient with pancreatic cancer. Nonetheless, Conlon's study[255] at Memorial Sloan Kettering Cancer Center found that pancreatic resections were performed in 77% of cases between 1993 and 1997 in comparison to 35% for the years 1983 to 1992. In most cases laparoscopic staging is used in combination with CT imaging, resulting in a decrease in unnecessary laparotomy but increased resection in cases where surgery is beneficial.

- Yeo[256] reported the following topographic locations of pancreatic pathology:

| | |
|---|---|
| Pancreatic cancer | 43% |
| Ampullary cancer | 11% |
| Duodenal cancer | 4% |
| Chronic pancreatitis | 11% |
| Neuroendocrine tumors | 5% |

The same author also reported the following from the Johns Hopkins experience:

*The tumor-specific 10-year actuarial survival rates were: pancreatic, 5%; ampullary, 25%; distal bile duct, 21%; and duodenal, 59%. Particularly for patients with pancreatic adenocarcinoma, 5-year survival is not equated with cure because patients succumb to recurrent disease more than 5 years following resection.*

- Sarr wrote (personal communication, 1999, between M.G. Sarr and J.E. Skandalakis) that ductal adenocarcinoma of the body and tail of the pancreas accounts for 15-20% of all pancreatic cancers. He stated also that because a pancreatic tumor could be other than adenocarcinoma, a nihilistic approach would not be appropriate; the approach should be aggressive and realistic. The five-year survival was less than 10% at the Mayo Clinic, where Sarr practices.

- Böttger and Junginger[257] stated that pancreaticoduodenectomy should be performed for any pancreatic tumor even without histologic confirmation.

- Balcom and colleagues[258] noted a trend of older patients undergoing pancreatic resection for malignant and benign conditions, with an increasing frequency of operations being performed for cystic tumors and fewer for chronic pancreatitis.

- Beger et al.[259] concluded the following:

  In patients with villous adenoma of the ampulla, ampullectomy was an adequate surgical treatment. In patients with a low-risk cancer in stages pTis and PT1 N0 M0, G1 or G2, a local resection with ampullectomy including local lymph node dissection is justified. An oncological resection of cancer of the ampulla by means of a pylorus-preserving partial pancreatoduodenectomy or the Kausch-Whipple resection is the surgical procedure of choice; the 3- and 5-year survival rates were 72% and 52%, respectively, in patients with R0 resections.

- We quote Treitschke et al.[260]:

  Villous adenoma is the most common tumor of the papilla of Vater, and transition from adenoma to carcinoma is now generally accepted as proven. It is thus essential for an adenoma to be removed... Ampullectomy provides an adequate surgical treatment of benign adenoma of the ampulla of Vater...If the histological findings as to benignity are unclear, resection of the head of the pancreas with preservation of the pylorus by an experienced surgeon is indicated.

- Schwarz et al.[261] advised that in patients with pancreatic carcinoma, splenectomy should be avoided unless required due to tumor proximity or invasion to the spleen.

- Horvath and Chabot[262] advocated that all patients able to tolerate surgery who have been diagnosed with a cystic pancreatic neoplasm undergo an aggressive surgical approach.

## Pancreatic Resection

### Total Pancreatectomy (Pancreatoduodenectomy)

Total pancreatectomy involves resection of the entire pancreas, as well as the distal stomach, duodenum, proximal jejunum, distal CBD, and spleen. It preserves the portal vein, the superior mesenteric artery and vein, the middle colic artery, and anomalous hepatic arteries. There are several modifications of the procedure.

Karpoff et al.[263] offer this concise summary:

Total pancreatectomy can be performed safely with low mortality; survival is predicted by the underlying pathologic findings: patients undergoing total pancreatectomy for adenocarcinoma have a uniformly poor outcome. Those undergoing total pancreatectomy for benign disease or nonadenocarcinoma variants can have long-term survival. In patients who require total pancreatectomy for ductal carcinoma, the survival is so poor as to bring into question the value of the operation.

In editorial remarks about the National Cancer Data Base, Brennan[264] reemphasized the lethality of pancreatic adenocarcinoma.

Trede[265] stated, "Whipple's duodenopancreatectomies remain the gold standard of surgical treatments for adenocarcinoma of the head of the pancreas." Sung et al.[266] found that "Whipple's pancreatoduodenectomy offers not only a superior palliation but also the hope of cure." Böttger et al.[267] agreed with Sung and colleagues. They advised that even with elderly patients, the procedure of choice for ampullary carcinoma is radical resection.

But Madura et al.[268] suggested that in patients with adenosquamous carcinoma of the pancreas, aggressive therapy should be tempered by the recognition that few patients with this disease live more than one year.

We quote from Moosa[269]:

Although the Whipple resection remains the first and best option for cancer of the head of the gland and periampullary region, total pancreatectomy should still be considered in rare specific instances for patients with long-standing diabetes who require insulin, such as (1) when there is obvious tumor growth along the main pancreatic duct or when multicentricity is suspected clinically; (2) when the pancreatic remnant is atrophic, soft, and friable and does not hold sutures; and (3) when a post operative pancreatojejunal leak cannot be controlled and reexploration necessitates a complete pancreatectomy.

### Whipple Procedure (Partial Pancreatoduodenectomy)

Partial pancreatoduodenectomy differs from a total procedure in that the body and tail of the pancreas are preserved (Fig. 21-57). The Whipple procedure has been called proximal resection, but that term is ambiguous. The

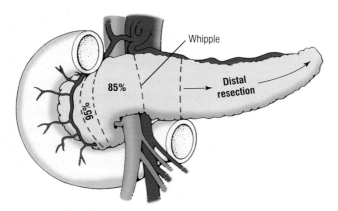

**FIG. 21-57.** Partial pancreatectomy: 95 percent pancreatectomy; 85 percent pancreatectomy; Whipple procedure; distal pancreatectomy. (Modified from Skandalakis JE, Gray SW, Rowe JS Jr. Anatomical Complications in General Surgery. New York: McGraw-Hill, 1983; with permission.)

head of the pancreas is proximal in the developmental sense, but it is distal in terms of secretory flow in the pancreatic ducts.

Traverso and Longmire[270] describe a pancreato-duodenectomy in which the pylorus and the first part of the duodenum, together with their blood supply, are preserved. The tail of the pancreas is preserved by a pancreaticojejunostomy, biliary function by a choledochojejunostomy, and continuity of the gut by a duodenojejunostomy. Van Berge Henegouwen et al.[271] reported that pylorus-preserving pancreaticoduodenectomy (PPPD) is as safe a procedure as classic pancreaticoduodenectomy. Mosca et al.[272] found that PPPD was as successful as the Whipple procedure, with nearly identical long term survival.

Takao et al.[273] reported that pylorus-preserving pancreaticoduodectomy is an acceptable procedure in comparison to Whipple procedure for the treatment of periampullary cancer, having practically the same long-term survival and recurrence. PPPD has been advised by other authors as well.[274-276]

Tamura et al.[277] reported that in cancer patients with pylorus-preserving pancreaticoduodenectomy and extensive resection of the portal vein, a splenic-inferior mesenteric venous anastomosis prevents gastric congestion.

Beger et al.[278] also emphasized the preservation of the endocrine pancreatic function after doing a duodenum-preserving surgery for pancreatitis. Another study by Beger et al.[279] reported that ampullectomy (removal of papilla and ampulla of Vater) has a mortality of 0.4% and morbidity less than 10%.

Pancreas-sparing duodenectomy or duodenum-sparing pancreatectomy for benign diseases are new proce-dures that are not in use by the majority of surgeons. Nagakawa et al.[280] presented two cases with total resection of the pancreatic head and preservation of the duodenum, bile duct, and papilla. After careful study of the vasculature of the pancreatic head (anterior and posterior pancreaticoduodenal arcades), the following were ligated: right gastroepiploic artery and vein, anterior superior pancreaticoduodenal artery, several vessels running into the portal vein from the proximal portion of the pancreas, and the posterior inferior pancreaticoduodenal artery. Eddes et al.[281] stated that neither endocrine nor exocrine function of the pancreas are negatively influenced by duodenum-preserving pancreatic head resection.

Sugiyama et al.[282] recommended ultrasonography for detection of pancreatobiliary carcinomas as well as for detection of invasion of the portal vein.

Takahashi et al.[283] advised that the branches of the uncinate process to the accessory pancreatic duct should be studied carefully for an accurate diagnosis of the pancreatic head region.

Furukawa et al.,[284] using CT arteriography, found that the pancreatic head can be separated into two segments, each of which can be removed due to separate blood supplies (Fig. 21-58). The blood supply for the right cephalic side springs from the celiac artery. The blood supply for the left caudal side (uncinate process) is derived from the superior mesenteric artery.

Takano et al.[285] reported that pancreaticogastrostomy after pancreaticoduodenectomy is safer than pancreaticojejunostomy, especially with regard to the incidence of pancreatic fistula.

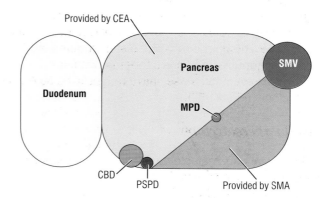

**FIG. 21-58.** Schema of blood supply to the peripancreatic region. SMV, Superior mesenteric vein; PSPD, Posterior superior pancreaticoduodenal artery; CEA, Celiac axis; MPD, Main pancreatic duct; CBD, Common bile duct; SMA, Superior mesenteric artery; SMV, Superior mesenteric vein. (Modified from Furukawa H, Iwata R, Moriyama N, Kosuge T. Blood supply to the pancreatic head, bile duct, and duodenum. Arch Surg 1999;134: 1086-1090; with permission.)

## Ninety-Five Percent Pancreatectomy

Partial pancreatectomy and 95% pancreatectomy (which was first described by Barrett and Bowers[286] and popularized by Fry and Child[287] for chronic pancreatitis) are used instead of total pancreatectomy whenever possible because of the high mortality associated with total pancreatectomy.

In 1979, in a monograph about the surgical anatomy of the pancreas that was published in *Contemporary Surgery,* Skandalakis et al.[136] wrote:

> *Embryologically, anatomically and surgically these three anatomical entities [pancreas, duodenum, common bile duct] form an inseparable unit. Their relations and blood supplies make it impossible for the surgeon to remove completely the head of the pancreas without removing the duodenum and the distal part of the common bile duct. Here embryology and anatomy conspire to produce some of the most difficult surgery of the abdominal cavity. The only alternative procedure, the so-called 95% pancreatectomy, leaves a rim of pancreas along the medial border of the duodenum to preserve the duodenal blood supply.*

Fry and Child[287] had presented their work on 95% distal pancreatectomy in *Annals of Surgery* in 1965. The senior author of this chapter, JES, had several conversations about 95% distal pancreatectomy with Dr. Child in Atlanta. He remembers him emphasizing the importance of carefully preserving the blood supply of the duodenum. This technique was popularized with several publications about duodenal perservation by Beger et al.[288-292]

A 95% pancreatectomy preserves a margin of pancreatic tissue along the concave border of the duodenum, together with the four pancreatoduodenal arteries and their arcades.[293] The duodenum, the distal stomach, and the proximal jejunum are spared, together with about 5% of the pancreas. A more conservative variant is the 85% pancreatectomy (Fig. 21-57).

## Distal Pancreatectomy

In a distal pancreatectomy, the pancreas is transected at the neck and the body. The tail and, usually, the spleen are removed (Fig. 21-57). The removal of the spleen is either to facilitate pancreatic resection[294] or because of inflammatory fixation of the splenic vessels to the pancreas.[295] In children, every effort should be made to preserve the spleen in pancreatic surgery.[296]

Sawyer and Frey[297] indicated that for a select group of patients with chronic pancreatitis, namely, those with severe pain, ducts less than 5 mm in diameter, and whose disease is confined to the body or the tail of the pancreas, a 50% to 60% distal pancreatectomy may be the best operation.

According to White and colleagues,[298] chronic pancreatitis may be treated with spleen-preserving pancreatectomy, with 80% of patients exhibiting complete pain relief. They caution that when the splenic artery and vein cannot be preserved, there is minimal risk of splenic complications needing further treatment, but splenectomy is avoided for the majority of patients.

Benoist et al.[299] stated that for benign pancreatic disease, distal pancreatectomy with splenectomy has a lower morbidity rate than spleen-preserving distal pancreatectomy, and was considered the best procedure.

Kau et al.[300] reported that the carbohydrate antigen 19-9 (CA 19-9) provides more diagnostic, resectability, and prognostic values than the carcinoembryonic antigen (CEA) in cases of periampullary carcinoma.

Mason[301] reported that pancreatogastrostomy following pancreaticoduodenectomy for carcinoma of the pancreas is a good, safe procedure with anastomotic leakage rate of 4% in 733 cases.

Siech et al.[302] reported that the treatment of choice for all pancreatic cysts and intraductal papillary mucinous pancreatic tumors is surgical resection.

Huguier and Mason[303] reported that resection, if feasible, gives the best survival rates irrespective of tumor size or spread in groups of carefully selected patients with cancer of the exocrine pancreas.

Lo et al.[304] advised distal subtotal pancreatectomy and enucleation of any tumor of the pancreatic head for insulinomas in multiple endocrine neoplasia type 1 (MEN-I) patients.

Doherty et al.[305] advised aggressive screening programs for identification and initiation of treament of malignant MEN-I. Skogseid et al.[306] recommended OctreoScan testing (Indium-111-penteoctreotide scan detection) for patients with multiple endocrine neoplasia type I, since conventional pancreatic imaging was not helpful. In cases other than limited disease, OctreoScan testing found true positives more often than any other method (75%).

Park et al.[307] reported that most islet-cell tumors of the pancreatic head can be removed with enucleation and not with pancreaticoduodenectomy. However, if the lesion is located close to the pancreatic duct, pancreaticoduodenectomy is the procedure indicated.

## Segmental Pancreatectomy

Is segmental pancreatectomy a useful procedure? Most likely, yes.

Warshaw et al.[308] evaluated resection in the body of the

pancreas. We strongly advise that the pancreatic surgeon read this beautiful paper. In commenting on this procedure, Lillemoe[309] supported midpancreatic resection in selected patients for "making the operation fit the disease." To summarize, the operation consists of:

- Segmental resection of middle segment with tumor
- Closure of the cephalic stump
- Roux-en-Y jejunal loop mucosa-to-mucosa anastomosis of remaining body and tail of pancreas

In contrast, Borghi et al.[310] advocated extended resections over segmental pancreatectomy in patients with pancreatic cancer. They cited close embryologic relations of both pancreatic buds with lymphatic and nerve networks and a possible relation to metastasis.

Espat et al.[311] of Memorial Sloan-Kettering Cancer Center report the following in regard to patients with laparoscopically staged unresectable pancreatic adenocarcinoma:

1. Their study did not support the practice of routine prophylactic bypass procedures.
2. They advised biliary bypass only for patients with obstructive jaundice who fail endoscopic stent placement.
3. They advocated that gastroenterostomy be reserved for patients with confirmed gastric outlet obstruction.

## Controversy

The controversy between total and partial pancreatectomy continues. One wonders why we should not always strive for total pancreatectomy, considering the anatomy of the pancreas. Perhaps it is because it does not increase survival!

Anatomic points to consider:
- Absence of a capsule in which to place firm sutures
- Intimate relations with the duodenum, CBD, and large blood vessels
- Residual tumor left in about one-third of patients undergoing the Whipple partial pancreatectomy[312]

## Drainage

### *Drainage for Chronic Pancreatitis: Pancreaticojejunostomy (Puestow Procedure)*

A pancreaticojejunostomy (Fig. 21-59A) requires a longitudinal incision of the pancreas and the pancreatic ducts. This incision opens and drains all pockets of accumulated secretions. The spleen is removed and the tail and body of the pancreas are mobilized. The pancreas, thus prepared, is inserted into a defunctionalized limb of jejunum that has

been brought through the transverse mesocolon. The jejunal stoma is sutured to the pancreas and the pancreatic duct. The blood supply is not impaired.[313]

An alternate method for a pancreas too broad to fit into the jejunum is to incise the pancreatic ducts without mobilizing the pancreas or removing the spleen. The defunctionalized limb of jejunum is anastomosed side-to-side to the incised pancreas (Fig. 21-59B). This gives adequate drainage if all obstructed pockets of the pancreatic duct are opened.

### *Internal Drainage of Pancreatic Pseudocysts*

The treatment of pancreatic pseudocyst is controversial. Fusaro and Davis[314] discuss the use of simple

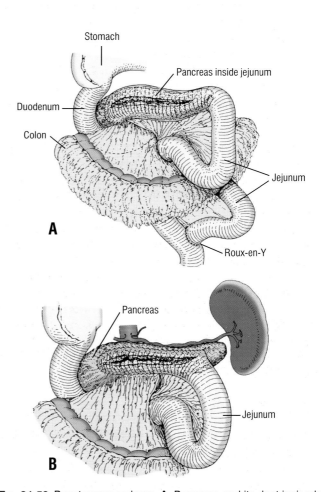

**FIG. 21-59.** Puestow procedures. **A,** Pancreas and its duct incised; entire pancreas is placed in a defunctionalized limb of jejunum; spleen is removed; end-to-side jejunojejunostomy completes operation. **B,** Pancreas may be too broad to fit into jejunum. (Modified from Skandalakis JE, Gray SW, Rowe JS Jr. Anatomical Complications in General Surgery. New York: McGraw-Hill, 1983; with permission.)

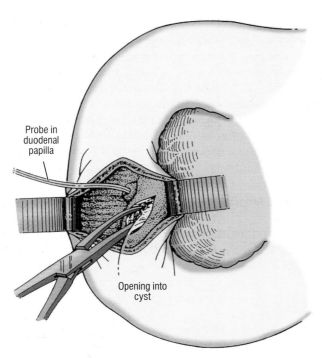

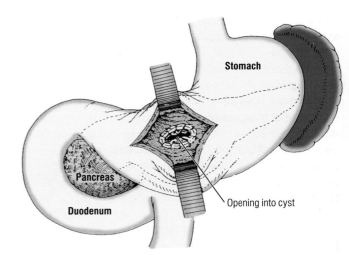

**FIG. 21-61.** Cystogastrostomy. (Modified from Skandalakis JE, Gray SW, Rowe JS Jr. *Anatomical Complications in General Surgery.* New York: McGraw-Hill, 1983; with permission.)

**FIG. 21-60.** Cystoduodenostomy. (From Skandalakis JE, Gray SW, Rowe JS Jr. *Anatomical Complications in General Surgery.* New York: Mc Graw-Hill, 1983; with permission.)

catheter drains, Roux-en-Y cystojejunostomy, and distal pancreatectomy.

The location of the pseudocyst determines the selection of the drainage site.[315] The following paragraphs describe the treatment of pseudocysts.

**Cystoduodenostomy**

If the pseudocyst is in the head of the pancreas, it may be drained into the duodenum (Fig. 21-60). A probe is placed in the duodenal papilla to identify and protect the pancreatic duct. The pancreatic cyst is incised through the duodenal wall and the opening is sutured.

**Cystogastrostomy**

If the pseudocyst is adherent to or displaces the posterior wall of the stomach, it may be drained into the stomach (Fig. 21-61). The anterior wall of the stomach is opened and the pancreatic cyst is incised through the posterior wall. The stomach wall and the cyst are sutured to provide drainage.

Trías et al.[316] performed laparoscopic cystogastrostomy for treatment of pancreatic pseudocyst.

**Cystojejunostomy**

If the pseudocyst is not close to the duodenum or the

stomach, it may be drained into the jejunum (Fig. 21-62). The jejunal loop is raised and sutured to the pancreatic cyst to drain the cyst.

Vitale et al.[317] concluded that endoscopic drainage of pancreatic pseudocysts provides adequate treatment, and can be a valid option in selected patients before standard surgical treatment is utilized. Spivak et al.[318] reported that operative management of pancreatic pseudocysts may be

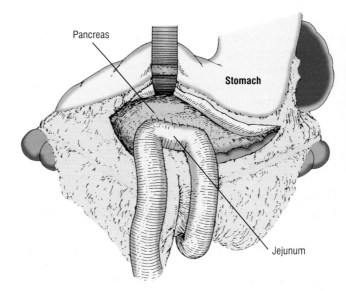

**FIG. 21-62.** Cystojejunostomy. (Modified from Skandalakis JE, Gray SW, Rowe JS Jr. *Anatomical Complications in General Surgery.* New York: McGraw-Hill, 1983; with permission.)

more successful than computed tomographic guided external drainage, currently very popular in many medical centers.

### Stenting

Patients with a history of pancreatitis who exhibit signs of bile duct obstruction and pain, both of which resolve rapidly, should be examined for spontaneous pancreatic pseudocyst. According to Boulanger et al.,[319] this rare complication of biliary fistula can be treated nonoperatively by endoscopic stenting of both the biliary tract and the fistula.

## Pancreas and Laparoscopy

Laparoscopic procedures for pancreatic diseases began appearing in the literature in the mid-1990s. Hunter,[320] one of the best laparoscopists, wrote the following in *World Journal of Surgery:*

> *It is perhaps surprising that I did not suggest in this "epilogue" that new procedures just over the horizon will again revolutionize minimally invasive surgery. It should be clear to the reader that every procedure that is usually performed through a laparotomy has been performed via laparoscopic access. This revolution will not be complete until we can objectively and reproducibly assess the value of each minimally invasive procedure and until we provide better uniform and reproducible training in endoscopic skills so these "herculean" procedures remain not in the domain of a few advanced laparoscopists but may be safely performed by most surgeons taking care of that organ system or disease group.*

Park et al.[321] reported the following:

1. For palliation in patients with pancreatic carcinoma, laparoscopic cholecystoenterostomy is technically straightforward, but has a higher rate of failure and complications than choledochoenterostomy (CDE). CDE requires advanced laparoscopic skills that preclude it from widespread adoption. Park et al. state their belief that a new CDE technique will be developed soon that will be technically feasible and practical.

2. Laparoscopic distal pancreatic resection, but not laparoscopic pancreaticoduodenectomy, benefits the patient with pancreatic cancer.

Laparoscopic pancreatic surgery for internal drainage of pancreatic pseudocysts and enucleation of benign insulinomas has had positive early reported outcomes, but experience is limited.[322]

## ANATOMIC COMPLICATIONS

## Complications of Exploration and Evaluation

### *Vascular Injury*

The left gastric artery and vein may be injured by incision of the hepatogastric ligament. The middle colic artery may be injured by incision of the gastrocolic ligament. Bleeding from pancreatoduodenal arcades may result from an overenthusiastic Kocher maneuver.

Berney et al.[323] stated that if the celiac axis is occluded due to atheromatous disease or arcuate ligament compression, temporary clamping of the gastroduodenal artery in some cases produces obvious ischemia. The above authors indicated that such occlusion in patients undergoing pancreatoduodenectomy rarely leads to significant problems. They also advised that trial clamping of the gastroduodenal artery is necessary to decide about the need for revascularization.

### *Organ Injury*

The hepatic division of the anterior vagal trunk runs within the hepatogastric ligament and might be injured by incision of the ligament. The celiac ganglion should be identified and distinguished from lymph nodes removed for biopsy.

### *Inadequate Procedure*

Failure to recognize metastatic lymph nodes can be a problem.

## Complications of Diagnostic Procedures

Several diagnostic procedures that go beyond simple inspection may be necessary for diagnosis. These procedures and their possible complications are listed in Table 21-14.

Suits et al.[324] reported that endoscopic ultrasound-guided fine needle aspiration is highly accurate in the diagnosis of pancreatic masses.

Is percutaneous core biopsy an attractive alternative to the diagnostic laparotomy, as stated by Karlson et al.[325]? Moossa,[326] in an invited commentary on a paper by Tillou et al., was not convinced, and wrote "...one cannot escape the impression that routine preoperative biopsy of pancreatic

**TABLE 21-14. Complications of Some Diagnostic Procedures**

| Procedure | Complications |
|---|---|
| 1. Arteriography | Hemorrhage |
| 2. Percutaneous transhepatic cholangiography | Hemorrhage<br>Bile peritonitis<br>Cholangitis |
| 3. Transpancreatic or transduodenal pancreatography | Pancreatitis |
| 4. Endoscopic retrograde cholangiopancreatography (ERCP) | Transient hyperamylasemia and hyperamylasuria (Classen et al., 1973)<br>Pancreatitis<br>Drug reactions<br>Pancreatic sepsis and pseudocyst abscess<br>Cholangitis (Bilbao et al., 1976)<br>Instrumental injury |
| 5. Percutaneous core biopsy | Sampling error<br>False negative results<br>Viscus perforation<br>Dissemination of cancer by seeding of the needle tract |

*Source:* Modified from Skandalakis JE, Gray SW, Rowe JS Jr, Skandalakis LJ. Anatomical complications of pancreatic surgery. Contemp Surg 15: 21-50, 1979; with permission.

masses is a triumph of technology over reason." Moossa cited problems including sampling error, false negative findings, anatomic complications such as abscesses and fistulas resulting from colon perforation, dissemination of cancer by seeding of the needle tract, and interpretative errors by even the most accomplished pathologists.

Based on a study by Brandt et al.,[327] Karlson et al.[325] wrote, "Percutaneous passes through the stomach, spleen, colon, and small intestine previously have been accompanied by absence of complications in pancreatic biopsy." This may be so, but we are in agreement with Moossa.[326]

## Complications of Endoscopic Sphincterotomy

Lo et al.[328] reported successful endoscopic sphincterotomy in 689 patients. Of these, complications (primarily associated with bleeding) occurred in 50 cases (7.1%), and 13 patients required emergency surgery.

We quote from Howard et al.[329] on complications of en-doscopic sphincterotomy (ES):

> ES perforation has 3 distinct types: guidewire, peri-ampullary, and duodenal. Guidewire perforations are recognized early and resolve with medical treatment. Periampullary perforations diagnosed early respond to aggressive endoscopic drainage and medical treatment. Postsphincterotomy perforations diagnosed late (particularly duodenal) require surgical drainage, which carries a high morbidity and mortality rate.

Stapfer et al.[330] classified duodenal perforation injuries into four types by anatomic location:

I   Lateral or medial wall (large injuries caused by endoscope requiring immediate surgery)

II   Sphincter of Oddi (more discrete and less likely to require surgery)

III   Distal bile duct near an obstructing entity (related to wire or basket instrumentation; manage with close surveillance)

IV   Retroperitoneal air alone (no surgical intervention)

They stated that late recognition of duodenal perforation and nonsurgical treatment failures have a high complication and mortality rate.

## Complications of Pancreatic Resection

### *Vascular Injury*

#### Arteries

The surgeon should always determine whether an anomalous hepatic artery is present before proceeding with resection. If it is present, it should be preserved.

ABERRANT COMMON HEPATIC ARTERY. Accidental ligation of the aberrant common hepatic artery will not only result in hepatic ischemia and perhaps rare necrosis, but will jeopardize the duodenum as well.

ABERRANT RIGHT HEPATIC ARTERY. The aberrant right hepatic artery occurs more frequently than the aberrant common hepatic artery. Since it is the only artery supplying the right lobe of the liver (or, to be more anatomically correct, the right half ot the liver), to avoid ischemia and necrosis, the aberrant right hepatic artery should not be ligated.

ABERRANT LEFT HEPATIC ARTERY. An aberrant left hepatic artery presents a problem in pancreatic surgery only when it arises from the right side of the superior mesenteric artery or from the gastroduodenal artery.

**MIDDLE COLIC ARTERY.** Accidental ligation of the middle colic artery may compromise the blood supply of the transverse colon.

**INFERIOR PANCREATODUODENAL ARTERY.** While there is a common origin of the inferior pancreatoduodenal artery and the proximal jejunal arteries, ligation of the common trunk may compromise the viability of the proximal jejunum.[220]

**GASTRODUODENAL ARTERY.** Ligation of the gastroduodenal artery may result in ischemia. Section will result in hemorrhage.

### Veins

Small veins from the neck of the pancreas occasionally drain into the anterior surfaces of the superior mesenteric or portal veins. These are a potential source of hemorrhage.[220]

**PORTAL VEIN.** Hemorrhage from unsuspected tumor infiltration of the wall of the portal vein is a possible complication of pancreatoduodenectomy.[331] The existence of this complication must be confirmed or excluded during the evaluation procedure before starting a pancreatoduodenectomy.

**OTHER VESSELS SUBJECT TO INJURY.** Other vessels subject to injury are the superior mesenteric artery or vein,[332] splenic artery or vein,[293] inferior vena cava, and renal artery or vein.

### *Organ Injury*

In addition to the organs directly involved in total pancreatoduodenectomy, the cisterna chyli is vulnerable to injury, resulting in chylous ascites. The cisterna chyli lies beneath the pancreas and to the right of the superior mesenteric vessels at the level of the disk between the 12th thoracic and 2nd lumbar vertebrae. If sectioned accidentally, it must be ligated.[333]

Leakage of pancreatoenterostomy is a serious common complication of pancreatic resection. Yamaguchi et al.[195] stated that red litmus paper can detect nondrained, transected pancreatic ductules on the cut surface of the pancreas. They can then be transfixed and closed with sutures.

To avoid dehiscence of pancreaticojejunostomy, Hamanaka and Suzuki[334] cover the pancreatic stump with jejunal submucosa using a purse-string suture on the mucosal edge of the jejunum.

According to Büchler et al.,[335] pancreatic fistula no longer seems to be a major problem after pancreatic head resection and rarely necessitates surgical treatment.

### *Inadequate Procedure*

Any partial pancreatectomy must be considered inadequate if portions of the tumor remain in the unresected pancreatic tissue. Other complications related to inadequate procedure are listed in Table 21-15.

| TABLE 21-15. Anatomic Complications of Pancreatic Resection | |
|---|---|
| **Procedure** | **Complications** |
| 1. Pancreatoenteric anastomosis (the least secure anastomosis) | Leakage or disruption with:<br>a. Abscess or peritonitis<br>b. Ileus<br>c. Pancreatic fistula<br>d. Wound infection and dehiscence<br>e. Bleeding from erosion of large vessels (Gadacz et al., 1978)<br>f. Ductal fibrosis, obstruction, and pancreatitis |
| 2. Biliary-enteric anastomosis (the most secure anastomosis) | Leakage or disruption with:<br>a. Abscess or bile peritonitis<br>b. Biliary obstruction<br>c. Biliary fistula<br>d. Obstruction at the anastomotic site<br>e. Ascending or descending cholangitis |
| 3. Inadequate gastric resection | Gastrojejunal ulceration (anastomotic ulcer) |
| 4. General | Operating room hemorrhage from major vessels:<br>a. Portal vein<br>b. Hepatic artery, normal or aberrant<br>c. Superior mesenteric artery or vein<br>d. Splenic artery or vein<br>e. Inferior vena cava<br>f. Renal arteries or veins<br>g. Middle colic artery<br>Acute postoperative pancreatitis with:<br>a. Ductal obstruction<br>b. Direct injury to pancreas with leakage from pancreatic parenchyma<br>c. Interference with blood supply or drainage |

*Source:* Skandalakis JE, Gray SW, Rowe JS Jr, Skandalakis LJ. Anatomical complications of pancreatic surgery. Contemp Surg 15:21-50, 1979; with permission.

# Complications of Procedures Related to Pancreatitis

## *Pancreaticojejunostomy (Puestow Procedure)*

### Vascular Injury

Because the major vessels to the pancreas are not ligated, there should be few complications of major hemorrhage or ischemia. Sutures at the jejunal stoma must be placed so they avoid the main pancreatoduodenal arteries and veins. Injury may occur to the ASPD artery during the Puestow side-to-side pancreaticojejunostomy. Be careful with the middle colic artery.

### Organ Injury

The spleen, if preserved, is subject to injury.

### Inadequate Procedure

Failure to incise all dilated pockets of the pancreatic ducts may result in unrelieved pain after operation and require reoperation.[313]

## *Pancreatic Pseudocyst Drainage*

We have generally considered the anatomy of pathologic processes to be beyond the scope of this book. Inflammatory pancreatic disease, however, so closely mimics iatrogenic complications that both conditions must be considered together. Some of these complications are shown in Table 21-16.

For bleeding pseudocysts of the pancreas secondary to pancreatitis, Gambiez and colleagues[326] advised arterial embolization of the affected artery (splenic, gastroduodenal, etc). In a separate study, Gambiez et al.[327] advocate endoscopic retroperitoneal drainage of peripancreatic necrotic collections.

## *Retroperitoneal Dissection Secondary to Pancreatic Inflammatory Disease*

### Vascular Injury

Bleeding associated with pancreatitis may be from gastritis, duodenal ulcer, or esophageal varices. Erosion of major arteries and veins is the greatest danger. Gadacz and coworkers[328] reviewed the literature (44 cases) and added 9 cases of their own.

The splenic artery is by far the most vulnerable vessel. The gastroduodenal artery is the second most frequently injured.[293,339] Among 22 cases of preoperative hemorrhage reported by Gledhill,[340] the splenic artery was the source of

## TABLE 21-16. Complications of Surgical Procedures

| Procedure | Complications |
|---|---|
| 1. Internal drainage of pancreatic cyst | |
|    a. Cystogastrostomy | Hemorrhage |
| | Pancreatic necrosis |
|    b. Cystoduodenostomy | Injury to common bile duct |
| | Injury to pancreatic duct |
| | Hemorrhage |
|    c. Cystojejunostomy | Hemorrhage |
|      (Roux-en-Y preferred) | Reflux from too short defunctionalized limb or too small stoma |

*Comment:* The site selected for internal drainage depends upon the location of the cyst. The lowest portion of the cyst must be able to drain by gravity into the anastomotic viscus chosen. Thus the operation must be planned to satisfy the need of the particular patient.

| Procedure | Complications |
|---|---|
| 2. External drainage of pancreatic cyst | Complications minimal |
| | Peritonitis |

*Comment:* External drainage is outdated and is unpleasant for the patient. We have had to use it only twice. In a poor risk patient with multiple problems, external drainage of a pancreatic cyst should not be considered a sign of timidity but rather evidence of mature surgical judgment.

| Procedure | Complications |
|---|---|
| 3. Excision of cyst | Duodenal fistula |
| | Hemorrhage |
| | Recurrence of cyst |
| | Injury to common bile duct |

*Comment:* Because the cyst is usually fixed firmly to surrounding organs, excision is not often recommended. It is the ideal operation where the cyst is in the body or tail and can be removed by itself. Only about 13 percent (Collins, 1950) are of this type. The mortality following excision is 8.7 percent (Warren et al., 1958).

| Procedure | Complications |
|---|---|
| 4. Sphincterotomy and sphincteroplasty | Operating room complications: duodenal perforation, acute pancreatitis, postoperative hemorrhage, postoperative fibrosis and stenosis of ampulla, incomplete division of sphincter |
| | Endoscopic complications: injury to the bile duct (Classen and Safrany, 1975), acute pancreatitis |
| 5. Pancreaticoduodenostomy and pancreaticojejunostomy | Anastomotic leak |
| | Hemorrhage |
| | Inadequate stoma |
| | Injury to ducts with leakage and obstruction |
| | Pancreatic necrosis from injury to vessel |

*Source:* Skandalakis JE, Gray SW, Rowe JS Jr, Skandalakis LJ. Anatomical complications of pancreatic surgery. Contemp Surg 15:21-50, 1979; with permission.

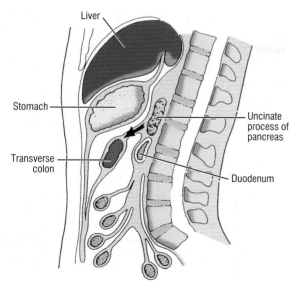

FIG. 21-63. Relation of uncinate process of pancreas to transverse colon. Arrow indicates path pancreatic fluid may take to colon. (Modified from Skandalakis JE, Gray SW, Rowe JS Jr. Anatomical Complications in General Surgery. New York: McGraw-Hill, 1983; with permission.)

bleeding in nine, the gastroduodenal artery in three. Eckhauser and colleagues[341] noted five cases of gastrointestinal bleeding secondary to aneurysmal degeneration of the gastroduodenal artery. There were three other cases in which the pancreatoduodenal artery was implicated. All were sequelae of acute or chronic pancreatitis.

### Organ Injury

The organ most frequently affected by pancreatitis is the transverse colon, by reason of proximity (Fig. 21-63). Colonic complications include pseudo-obstruction owing to colonic spasm,[342] ischemic obstruction,[343] fistula formation,[344] and gastrointestinal bleeding.

Other sites of injury, iatrogenic or from pancreatic juice, are the duodenum, CBD, and spleen. Splenic invasion by pancreatic pseudocysts leading to splenic rupture and hemorrhage is uncommon. However, it may be more common than findings indicate, because it may go unrecognized.[339]

### Inadequate Procedure

Lack of knowledge of the best drainage route may result in failure to drain the pseudocyst. Lack of appreciation of the magnitude of peritoneal extension of the inflammatory process may result in failure to properly drain the fluid collection and perhaps to further the existing inflammation.

## PANCREATIC TRANSPLANTATION

### Anatomy of Pancreatic Transplantation

Most pancreas transplants are performed with kidney transplantation. Sudan et al.[345] stated that simultaneous kidney-pancreas transplantation is a safe and effective treatment for advanced diabetic nephropathy associated with stable metabolic function, decreased cholesterol, improved hypertension control, and improved rehabilitation with low morbidity and mortality after the first year. We strongly advise consulting the chapter by Chauvin and Kittur in Cameron's excellent book, *Current Surgical Therapy*, sixth edition[346] for further information on simultaneous pancreas-kidney (SPK) transplantation.

### *Organ Procurement from Donor*

1. Make a long midline incision from the sternal notch to the symphysis pubis (sternotomy and celiotomy).
2. Isolate the distal aorta and inferior vena cava. Control with vascular tape.
3. Enter the lesser sac through the gastrosplenic ligament by dividing and ligating the short gastric vessels.
4. Mobilize the spleen by incising the splenorenal ligament.
5. Rotate the pancreas and spleen medially.
6. Ligate and divide the inferior mesenteric vein.
7. Prepare and control the aortic segment just above the celiac axis by division of the diaphragmatic crura.
8. Isolate the origins of the celiac axis and superior mesenteric artery.
9. Identify and protect the left renal vessels.
10. Ligate the left adrenal and left gonadal veins.
11. Perform extensive duodenal kocherization.
12. Identify the distal common bile duct and ligate 1 cm to 2 cm from the pancreatic parenchyma.
13. Prepare and isolate the portal vein.
14. Mobilize the colon by dividing the gastrocolic and hepatocolic ligaments.
15. Ligate the mesentery of the small bowel with multiple nonabsorbable sutures.
16. Divide the gastropyloric junction using a TA-55 stapler.
17. Divide the small bowel distal to the ligament of Treitz using a GIA stapler.
18. Remove the small and large bowel from the peritoneal cavity.
19. The portal vein can be divided and the liver and pancreas can be removed en bloc.
20. Remove the donor iliac vessels (iliac Y graft) (Fig. 21-64) to be used for reconstruction of the splenic and superior mesenteric artery.

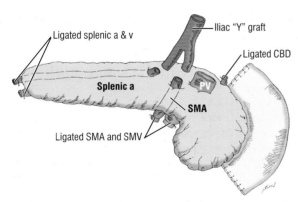

FIG. 21-64. Donor pancreas prepared by splenectomy and ligation of splenic and superior mesenteric arteries (SMA) and veins (SMV). Duodenal stump secured with Lembert nonabsorbable suture. CBD, common bile duct; PV, portal vein. (Modified from Chauvin KD, Kittur DS. Pancreas transplantation. In Cameron JL. Current Surgical Therapy (6th ed). St. Louis: Mosby, 1998, pp. 539-543; with permission).

21. Perform duodenal resection leaving a 10 cm to 12 cm duodenal segment.
22. Perform splenectomy.

## Organ Implantation to Recipient

1. Make a midline incision.

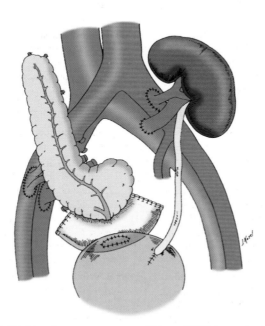

FIG. 21-65. Simultaneous pancreas-kidney (SPK) transplantation utilizing ureteroneocystostomy. (Modified from Chauvin KD, Kittur DS. Pancreas transplantation. In Cameron JL. Current Surgical Therapy (6th ed). St. Louis: Mosby, 1998, pp. 539-543; with permission).

2. Graft the pancreas to the right iliac vessels.
3. Mobilize the right and left colon.
4. Expose the common, external, and internal iliac arteries.
5. Carefully prepare the right iliac vein by dividing and ligating all its posterior tributaries.
6. Anastomose the portal vein to the right iliac vein lateral to the iliac arteries.
7. Anastomose the reconstructed Y-graft and the common iliac artery.
8. Using your procedure of choice, anastomose the duodenum of the transplanted pancreas (exocrine secretion) to the urinary bladder (Fig. 21-65) or to a loop of small bowel, or perhaps ligate the pancreatic duct.

Stratta et al.[347] reported that pancreas transplantation with portal venous delivery of insulin and enteric drainage of exocrine secretions can be performed with short-term results comparable to those of the more common procedures employing systemic venous delivery of insulin and bladder drainage of secretions.

Hricik et al.[348] compared the prevalence and severity of hypertension in simultaneous pancreas-kidney transplantation patients and those receiving kidneys alone. They found that the beneficial effect of the pancreas transplant was limited to bladder-drained patients, and that blood

### TABLE 21-17. Surgical Complications (Nonurologic) after Simultaneous Pancreas-Kidney Transplantation in 237 Recipients

| Complications | No. | % |
|---|---|---|
| Non-transplant related | | |
|   Small bowel obstruction | 11 | 4.6 |
|   Reoperation for intra-abdominal bleeding | 11 | 4.6 |
|   Wound infection | 11 | 4.6 |
|   Wound dehiscence | 10 | 4.2 |
|   Incisional hernia | 5 | 2.1 |
|   Negative laparotomy | 4 | 1.7 |
|   Intra-abdominal abscess drainage | | |
|     Operative | 5 | 2.1 |
|     Percutaneous | 3 | 1.3 |
|   Enterocutaneous fistula repair | 1 | 0.4 |
|   Fasciitis | 1 | 0.4 |
| Transplant related | | |
|   Lymphocele drainage | 3 | 1.5 |
|   Graft thrombosis | | |
|     Pancreas only | 3 | 1.3 |
|     Pancreas-kidney | 4 | 1.7 |
|   Renal artery stenosis | 1 | 0.4 |
|   Iliac artery stenosis | 1 | 0.4 |

Source: Chauvin KD, Kittur DS. Pancreas transplantation. In: Cameron JL. Current Surgical Therapy (6th ed). St. Louis: Mosby, 1998, pp. 539-543; with permission.

**TABLE 21-18. Urologic Complications Related to Pancreas Transplant**

| Complications | No. | % |
|---|---|---|
| Hematuria | 35 | 14.8 |
| Bladder/duodenal segment leak | 35 | 14.8 |
| Reflux pancreatitis | 24 | 10.1 |
| Recurrent urinary tract infection | 24 | 10.1 |
| Urethritis | 7 | 2.9 |
| Urethral stricture/disruption | 7 | 2.9 |

*Source:* Chauvin KD, Kittur DS. Pancreas transplantation. In: Cameron JL. Current Surgical Therapy (6th ed). St. Louis: Mosby, 1998, pp. 539-543; with permission.

pressure did not increase after conversion from bladder to enteric drainage.

The increased popularity of pancreas transplants has led to a growing number of potential candidates for re-transplants after the initial graft has been lost to technical failure or rejection. Humar and colleagues[349] stated that while retransplants can be performed with a minimal increase in surgical complications, graft survival is slightly inferior and patients require more aggressive monitoring for rejection.

## Anatomic Complications of Simultaneous Pancreas-Kidney Transplantation and Pancreas Transplantation

To illuminate urologic and nonurologic surgical complications of transplantation, we present two tables from the work of Chauvin and Kittur[346] (Tables 21-17 & 21-18).

Multiple nephrogenic adenomas of the bladder were reported in a patient three years after a simultaneous kidney-pancreas transplant. Pancreatic drainage was successfully converted from the bladder to the small bowel.[350]

## PANCREATIC TRAUMA

Pancreatic injury is an infrequent occurrence. Takashima and colleagues[351] presented a classification of blunt pancreatic duct injuries discovered at pancreatography and their treatment:

- Class 1. Radiographically normal ducts; no surgery required
- Class 2a. Ductal branch damage without leakage; no surgery required
- Class 2b. Ductal branch damage with minimal leakage; drainage laparotomy
- Class 3. Main duct injuries; laparotomy

## REFERENCES

1. Longmire WP Jr. Foreword. In: Trede M, Carter DC. Surgery of the Pancreas. Edinburgh: Churchill Livingstone, 1993, p. ix.
2. Polak M, Bouchareb-Banaei L, Scharfmann R, Czernichow P. Early pattern of differentiation in the human pancreas. Diabetes 2000;49:225-232.
3. Debas HT. Molecular insights into the development of the pancreas. Am J Surg 1997;174:227-231.
4. Suda K, Mogaki M, Matsumoto Y. Gross dissection and immuno-histochemical studies on branch fusion type of ventral and dorsal pancreatic ducts: A case report. Surg Radiol Anat 13:333-337, 1991.
5. Skandalakis JE, Gray SW. Embryology for Surgeons, 2nd ed. Baltimore: Willliams & Wilkins, 1994.
6. Leung YK, Lebenthal E. Gastrointestinal peptides. In: Lebenthal E (ed). Human Gastrointestinal Development. New York: Raven, 1989.
7. Trede M, Carter DC (eds). Surgery of the Pancreas. Edinburgh: Churchill Livingstone, 1993.
8. Cotton P. Congenital anomaly of pancreas divisum as cause of obstructive pain and pancreatitis. Gut 21:105, 1980.
9. Richter J, Schapiro R, Mulley A, Warshaw A. Association of pancreas divisum and pancreatitis, and its treatment by sphincteroplasty of the accessory ampulla. Gastroenterology 81:1104, 1981.
10. Gregg J, Monaco A, McDermott W. Pancreas divisum: results of surgical intervention. Am J Surg 145:488, 1983.
11. Boerma D, Huibregtse K, Gulik TM, Rauws EA, Obertop H, Gouma DJ. Long-term outcome of endoscopic stent placement for chronic pancreatitis associated with pancreas divisum. Endoscopy 2000;32:452-456.
12. Ertan A. Long-term results after endoscopic pancreatic stent placement without pancreatic papillotomy in acute recurrent pancreatitis due to pancreas divisum. Gastrointest Endosc 2000;52:9-14 and 134-137.
13. Neblett WW III, O'Neill JA Jr. Surgical management of recurrent pancreatitis in children with pancreas divisum. Ann Surg 2000; 231:899-908.
14. Kamisawa T, Tabata I, Isawa T, Ishiwata J, Fukayama M, Koike M. Annular pancreas associated with carcinoma in the dorsal part of pancreas divisum. Int J Pancreatol 1995;17:207-211.
15. Nobukawa B, Otaka M, Suda K, Fujii H, Matsumoto Y, Miyano T. An annular pancreas derived from paired ventral pancreata, supporting Baldwin's hypothesis. Pancreas 2000;20:408-410.
16. Hayes DM, Greaney EM Jr, Hill JT. Annular pancreas as a cause of acute neonatal duodenal obstruction. Ann Surg 153:103, 1961.
17. Lloyd-Jones W, Mountain JC, Warren KW. Annular pancreas in the adult. Ann Surg 176:163, 1972.
18. Gross RE, Chisholm TC. Annular pancreas producing duodenal obstruction. Ann Surg 119:759, 1944.
19. Boyden EA. The accessory gallbladder. An embryological and comparative study of aberrant biliary vesicles occurring in man and domestic mammals. Am J Anat 38:177, 1926.

20. Wrenn EL, Favara BE. Duodenal duplication (or pancreatic bladder) presenting as double gallbladder. Surgery 69:858, 1971.

21. Boyden EA. Discussion. Wrenn EL, Favara BE. Duodenal duplication (or pancreatic bladder) presenting as double gallbladder. Surgery 69:858, 1971.

22. Garcia Ferris G, Raul Juan J. Pancreas aberrante en la pared vesicular con perforacion aguda. Prensa Med Argent 58:1829, 1971.

23. Harlaftis N, Gray SW, Skandalakis JE. Multiple gallbladders. Surg Gynecol Obstet 145:928, 1977.

24. Burne JC. Pancreatic and gastric heterotopia in a diverticulum of the transverse colon. J Pathol Bacteria 75:470, 1958.

25. Collins DC. A study of 50,000 specimens of the human vermiform appendix. Surg Gynecol Obstet 101:437, 1955.

26. Horanyi J, Fusy F. Nebenleber in der Gallenblasenwand. Zentralbl Chir 88:768, 1963.

27. Warthin AS. Two cases of accessory pancreas (omentum and stomach). The Physician Surgeon (Detroit) 26:337, 1904.

28. Beskin CA. Intralobar enteric sequestration of the lung containing aberrant pancreas. J Thorac Cardiovasc Surg 41:314, 1961.

29. Feldman M, Weinberg T. Aberrant pancreas; cause of duodenal syndrome. JAMA 148:893, 1952.

30. Pearson S. Aberrant pancreas. Review of the literature and report of three cases, one of which produced common and pancreatic duct obstruction. Arch Surg 63:168, 1951.

31. Curd H. Histologic study of Meckel's diverticulum with special reference to heterotopic tissues. Arch Surg 32:506, 1936.

32. Fékété F, Noun R, Sauvanet A, Fléjou JF, Bernades P, Belghiti J. Pseudotumor developing in heterotopic pancreas. World J Surg 20:295-298, 1996.

33. Ravitch MM. Anomalies of the pancreas. In: Carey LC (ed). The Pancreas. St. Louis, CV Mosby, 1973.

34. Rosai J. Ackerman's Surgical Pathology (8th ed). St. Louis: Mosby, 1996.

35. Tuncel M, Erbil M, Bayramoglu A, Abbasoglu O. A case of intraperitoneal pancreas. Surg Radiol Anat 17:343-346, 1995.

36. Zollinger RM, Ellison EH. Primary peptic ulcerations of the jejunum associated with islet cell tumors of the pancreas. Ann Surg 1955;142:709-728.

37. Stabile BE. Gastrinoma before Zollinger and Ellison. Am J Surg 1997;174:232-236.

38. Stabile BE, Morrow DJ, Passaro E Jr. The gastrinoma triangle: operative implications. Am J Surg 1984;147:25-31.

39. Passaro E Jr, Howard TJ, Sawacki MP, Watt PC, Stabile BE. The origin of sporadic gastrinomas within the gastrinoma triangle: a theory. Arch Surg 1998;133:13-17.

40. Townsend CM Jr. Invited commentary. Passaro E Jr, Howard TJ, Sawacki MP, Watt PC, Stabile BE. The origin of sporadic gastrinomas within the gastrinoma triangle: a theory. Arch Surg 1998; 133:13-17.

41. Townsend CM Jr, Thompson JC. Neoplasms of the endocrine pancreas. In: Greenfield LJ (ed). Surgery: Scientific Principles and Practice (2nd ed). Philadelphia: JB Lippincott, 1993, pp. 833-842.

42. Norton JA, Doherty GM, Fraker DL, Alexander HR, Doppman JL, Verzon DJ, Gibril F, Jensen RT. Surgical treatment of localized gastrinoma within the liver: A prospective study. Surgery 1998; 124:1145-1152.

43. Kisker O, Bastian D, Bartsch D, Nies C, Rothmund M. Localization, malignant potential, and surgical management of gastrinomas. World J Surg 22:651-658, 1998.

44. Proye C, Pattou F, Carnaille B, Paris JC, d'Herbomez M, Marchandise X. Intraoperative gastrin measurements during surgical management of patients with gastrinomas: experience with 20 cases. World J Surg 22:643-650, 1998.

45. Norton JA, Doherty GM, Fraker DL. Surgery for endocrine tumors of the pancreas. In: Go VLW, DiMagno EP, Gardner JD, Lebenthal E, Reber HA, Scheele GA (eds). The Pancreas: Biology, Pathobiology, and Disease (2nd ed). New York: Raven Press, 1993, p. 1020.

46. Kuzin NM, Egorov AV, Kondrashin SA, Lotov AN, Kuznetzov NS, Majorova JB. Preoperative and intraoperative topographic diagnosis of insulinomas. World J Surg 1998;22:593-598.

47. Boukhman MP, Karam JM, Shaver J, Siperstein AE, DeLorimier AA, Clark OH. Localization of insulomas. Arch Surg 1999;134: 818-823.

48. Hashimoto LA, Walsh RM. Preoperative localization of insulinomas is not necessary. J Am Coll Surg 1999;189:368-373.

49. Simon D, Starke A, Goretzki PE, Roeher HD. Reoperative surgery for organic hyperinsulinism: indications and operative strategy. World J Surg 1998;22:666-672.

50. Jordan PH Jr. A personal experience with pancreatic and duodenal neuroendocrine tumors. J Am Coll Surg 1999;189:470-482.

51. Visalli JA, Grimes OF. An embryologic and anatomic approach to the treatment of gastric cancer. Surg Gynecol Obstet 103:401, 1956.

52. Doglietto GB, Pacelli F, Caprino P, Bossola M, Di Stasi C. Pancreas-preserving total gastrectomy for gastric cancer. Arch Surg 2000;135:89-94.

53. Chung JP, Lee SI, Kim KW, Chi HS, Jeong HJ, Moon YM, Kang JK, Park IS. Duodenal ectopic pancreas complicated by chronic pancreatitis and pseudocyst formation — a case report. J Korean Med Sci 9(4):351-356, 1994.

54. Allison JW, Johnson JF III, Barr LL, Warner BW, Stevenson RJ. Induction of gastroduodenal prolapse by antral heterotopic pancreas. Pediatr Radiol 25(1):50-51, 1995.

55. Salman B, Besbas N, Coskun T, Yilmazbayhan D, Sarialioglu F. Intussusception due to ectopic pancreatic tissue in a nine-month-old child. Turk J Pediatr 34(4):255-258, 1992.

56. Kovari E, Jaray B, Pulay I. Papillary cystic neoplasms in the ectopic pancreas [Hungarian]. Orv Hetil 137(17):923-925, 1996.

57. Roshe J, Del Buono E, Domenico D, Colturi TJ. Anaplastic carcinoma arising in ectopic pancreas located in the distal esophagus. J Clin Gastroenterol 22(3):242-244, 1996.

58. Guillou L, Nordback P, Gerber C, Schneider RP. Ductal adenocarcinoma arising in a heterotopic pancreas situated in a hiatal hernia. Arch Pathol Lab Med 118(5):568-571, 1994.

59. Baker RJ. Editor's Comment. Skandalakis LJ, Rowe JS Jr, Gray SW, Skandalakis JE. Surgical anatomy of the pancreas. In: Nyhus LM, Baker RJ. Mastery of Surgery (2nd ed). Boston: Little, Brown, 1992, pp. 995-1009.

60. Kay AW. Reflections of Sir Andrew Watt Kay. Contemp Surg 1978;13:71.

61. Z'graggen K, Fernández-del Castillo C, Rattner DW, Sigala H, Warshaw AL. Metastases to the pancreas and their surgical extirpation. Arch Surg 1998;133:413-417.

62. Busnardo AC, DiDio LJA, Thomford NR. Anatomicosurgical segments of the human pancreas. Surg Radiol Anat 10:77-82, 1988.

63. Smanio T. Varying relations of the common bile duct with the

posterior face of the pancreas in negroes and white persons. J Int Coll Surg 22:150, 1954.

64. Skandalakis JE, Colborn GL, Pemberton LB, Skandalakis TN, Skandalakis LJ, Gray SW. The surgical anatomy of the spleen. Probl Gen Surg 7:1, 1990.

65. Frey CF. Partial and subtotal pancreatectomy for chronic pancreatitis. In: Nyhus LM, Baker RJ (eds). Mastery of Surgery, Vol II (2nd ed). Boston: Little, Brown, 1992, pp. 1029-1049.

66. Silen W. Surgical anatomy of the pancreas. Surg Clin North Am 44:1253, 1964.

67. Rienhoff WF Jr, Pickrell KL. Pancreatitis: an anatomic study of pancreatic and extrahepatic biliary systems. Arch Surg 51:205, 1945.

68. Berman LG, Prior JT, Abramow SM, Ziegler DD. A study of the pancreatic duct system in man by the use of vinyl acetate casts of postmortem preparations. Surg Gynecol Obstet 110:391, 1960.

69. Baldwin WM. The pancreatic ducts in man, together with a study of the microscopical structure of the minor duodenal papilla. Anat Rec 5:197, 1911.

70. Kasugai T, Kuno N, Kobayashi S, Hattori K. Endoscopic pancreatocholangiography. Gastroenterology 63:217, 1972.

71. Trapnell JE, Howard JM. Transduodenal pancreatography: An improved technique. Surgery 60:1112, 1966.

72. Yamaguchi K, Chijiiwa K, Shimizu S, Yokohata K, Morisaki T, Tanaka M. Comparison of endoscopic retrograde and magnetic resonance cholangiopancreatography in the surgical diagnosis of pancreatic disease. Am J Surg 1998;175:203-208.

73. Wood MacD. Anomalous location of the papilla of Vater. Am J Surg 111:265, 1966.

74. Varley PF, Rohrmann CA, Silvis SE, Vennes JA. The normal endoscopic pancreatogram. Radiology 118:295, 1976.

75. Cotton PB. The normal endoscopic pancreatogram. Endoscopy 6:65, 1974.

76. Kreel L, Sandin B. Changes in pancreatic morphology associated with aging. Gut 14:962, 1973.

77. Dowdy GS Jr, Waldron GW, Brown WG. Surgical anatomy of the pancreaticobiliary ductal system. Arch Surg 84:229, 1962.

78. Michels NA. Blood Supply and Anatomy of the Upper Abdominal Organs. Philadelphia: Lippincott, 1955.

79. Chassin JL. Operative Strategy in General Surgery (2nd ed). New York: Springer-Verlag, 1994, p. 550.

80. Northover JMA, Terblanche J. A new look at the arterial supply of the bile duct in man and its surgical implications. Br J Surg 66:379-384, 1979.

81. Stolte M, Wiessner V, Schaffner O, Koch H. Vascularization of the papilla vateri and bleeding risk of papillotomy [German]. Leber Magen Darm 10(6):293-301, 1980.

82. Williams PL. Gray's Anatomy (38th ed). New York: Churchill Livingstone, 1995, pp. 1550-1551.

83. Deltenre et al. as cited in Staritz M, Meyer Zum Büschenfelde KH. Endoscopic measurements of intravascular pressure and flow in blood vessels of the gastrointestinal tract. Clin Gastroenterol 15 (2):235-247, 1986.

84. Kimura W, Nagai H. Study of surgical anatomy for duodenum-preserving resection of the head of the pancreas. Ann Surg 221(4): 359-363, 1995.

85. Biazotto W. The fine venous architecture of the major duodenal papilla in human beings. Anat Anz (Jena) 171:105-108, 1990.

86. Kimura W, Morikane K, Futakawa N, Shinkai H, Han I, Inoue T, Muto T, Nagai H. A new method of duodenum-preserving subtotal resection of the head of the pancreas based on the surgical anatomy. Hepato-Gastroenterology 43:463-472, 1996.

87. Boyden EA. The anatomy of the choledochoduodenal junction in man. Surg Gynecol Obstet 1957;104:641.

88. Flati G, Flati D, Porowska B, Ventura T, Catarci M, Carboni M. Surgical anatomy of the papilla of Vater and biliopancreatic ducts. Am Surg 60:712-718, 1994.

89. Shibata C, Sasaki I, Naito H, Ohtani N, Sato S, Ise H, Matsuno S. Duodenal but not gastric transection disturbs motility of the sphincter of Oddi in the dog. World J Surg 1997;21:191-194.

90. Marks JM, Bower AL, Goormastic M, Malycky JL, Ponsky JL. A comparison of common bile duct pressures after botulinum toxin injection into the sphincter of Oddi versus biliary stenting in a canine model. Am J Surg 2001;181:60-64.

91. Barbato De Prates NEV, Smanio T, Domingos M de M, Ferraz De Carvalho CA. "Sphincter" of the minor papilla of the human duodenum. Clin Anat 9:34-40, 1996.

92. Van Damme J-P J. Behavioral anatomy of the abdominal arteries. Surg Clin North Am 73(4):699-725, 1993.

93. Bertelli E, Di Gregorio F, Bertelli L, Mosca S. The arterial blood supply of the pancreas: a review. I. The superior pancreaticoduodenal and the anterior superior pancreaticoduodenal arteries. An anatomical and radiological study. Surg Radiol Anat 1995; 17:97-106.

94. Bertelli E, Bertelli L, Di Gregorio F, Civeli L, Mosca S. The arterial blood supply of the pancreas: a review. II. The posterior superior pancreaticoduodenal artery. An anatomical and radiological study. Surg Radiol Anat 1996;18:1-9.

95. Bertelli E, Di Gregorio F, Bertelli L, Civeli L, Mosca S. The arterial blood supply of the pancreas: a review. III. The inferior pancreaticoduodenal artery. An anatomical and radiological study. Surg Radiol Anat 1996;18:67-74.

96. Bertelli E, Bertelli L, Di Gregorio F, Orazioli D, Bastianini A. The arterial blood supply of the pancreas: a review. IV. The anterior inferior pancreaticoduodenal artery, the posterior inferior pancreaticoduodenal artery and minor sources of blood supply for the head of the pancreas. An anatomical review and a radiological study. Surg Radiol Anat 1997;19:203-212.

97. Toni R, Favero L, Mosca S, Ricci S, Roversi R, Vezzadini P. Quantitative clinical anatomy of the pancreatic arteries studied by selective celiac angiography. Surg Radiol Anat 1988;10:53-60.

98. Mellière D. Variations des artères hépatiques et du carrefour pancréatique. J Chir (Paris) 1968;95:5-42.

99. Ozan H, Önderoglu S. Intrapancreatic course of the splenic artery with combined pancreatic anomalies. Surg Radiol Anat 1997;19:409-411.

100. Berens AS, Aluisio FV, Colborn GL, Gray SW, Skandalakis JE. The incidence and significance of the posterior gastric artery in human anatomy. J Med Assoc Ga 1991;80:425-428.

101. Kirk E. Untersuchungen über die grössere und feinere topographische Verteilung der Arterien, Venen und Ausführungsgänge in der menschlichen Bauchspeicheldrüse. Z Anat Entwicktungsgesch 1931;94:822-875.

102. Thompson IM. On the arteries and ducts in the hepatic pedicle. A study in statistical human anatomy. Univ Calif Publ Anat 1:55, 1953.

103. Michels NA. The hepatic, cystic, and retroduodenal arteries and their relations to the biliary ducts. Ann Surg 133:503, 1951.

**PANCREAS**

CHAPTER **21**

104. White TT. Surgical anatomy of the pancreas. In: Carey LC (ed). The Pancreas. St. Louis: CV Mosby, 1973.

105. Hollinshead WH. Anatomy for Surgeons. Volume 2. The Thorax, Abdomen, and Pelvis. New York: Hoeber-Harper, 1956.

106. Douglass TC, Lounsbury BF, Cutter WW, Wetzel N. An experimental study of healing in the common bile duct. Surg Gynecol Obstet 91:301, 1950.

107. Skandalakis JE, Gray SW, Rowe JS, Skandalakis LJ. Anatomical complications of pancreatic surgery, Part 2. Contemp Surg 15:21-50, 1979.

108. Ishizaki Y, Tanaka M, Okuyama T. Surgical implications of preduodenal portal vein in the adult. Arch Surg 129:773-775, 1994.

109. Lo CY, Lam KY, Kung AWC, Lam KSL, Tung PHM, Fan ST. Pancreatic insulomas: a 15-year experience. Arch Surg 1997;132:926-930.

110. Huai JC, Zhang W, Niu HO, Su ZX, McNamara JJ, Machi J. Localization and surgical treatment of pancreatic insulinomas guided by intraoperative ultrasound. Am J Surg 1998;175:18-21.

111. Koshi T, Govil S, Koshi R. Problem in diagnostic imaging: pancreaticoduodenal arcade in splanchnic arterial stenosis. Clin Anat 1998;11:206-208.

112. Bertelli E, Di Gregorio F, Mosca S, Bastianini A. The arterial blood supply of the pancreas: a review. V. The dorsal pancreatic artery. An anatomic review and a radiologic study. Surg Radiol Anat 20:445-452, 1998.

113. Edwards LF. The retroduodenal artery. Anat Rec 1941;81:351-355.

114. Michels NA. Blood supply of the stomach. Anat Rec 1952; 112:361.

115. Michels NA. The anatomic variations of the arterial pancreaticoduodenal arcades: their import in regional resection involving the gallbladder, bile ducts, liver, pancreas and parts of the small and large intestines. J Int Coll Surg 1962;37:13-40.

116. Nebesar RA, Kornblith PL, Pollard JJ, Michels NA. Coeliac and Superior Mesenteric Arteries. A Correlation of Angiograms and Dissections. Boston: Little Brown, 1969.

117. Evrard HL. Les artères du duodénum et du pancréas [thesis]. Paris, 1932, these #640.

118. Pierson JM. The arterial blood supply of the pancreas. Surg Gynecol Obstet 1943;77:426-432.

119. Shapiro AL, Robillard GL. Morphology and variations of the duodenal vasculature. Arch Surg 1946;52:571-602.

120. Voisin MM, Devambez L. Contribution a l'étude de la vascularisation artérielle du bulbe duodénal. C R Assoc Anat 1949; 36:691-696.

121. Kosinski C. Quelques observations sur les rameaux du tronc cœliaque et des artères mésentériques chez l'homme. C R Assoc Anat 1928;23:241-260.

122. Petren T. Die Arterien und Venen des Duodenums und des Pankreaskopfes beim Menschen. Z Ges Anat 1929;90:234-277.

123. Rio Branco da Silva P. Essai sur l'Anatomie et la Médecine Opératoire du Tronc Cœliaque et de ses Branches de l'Artère Hépatique en Particulier. Paris: Steinheil, 1912.

124. Calas F, Martin R, Bouchet Y, Polliak D. Les artères de la tête du pancréas. C R Assoc Anat 1955;89:362-367.

125. Van Damme JP, Van der Schueren G, Bonte J. Vascularisation du pancréas: proposition de nomenclature PNA et angioarchitecture des ilots. C R Assoc Anat 1967;137:1184-1189.

126. Woodburne RT, Olsen LL. The arteries of the pancreas. Anat Rec 1951;111:255-270.

127. Falconer CWA, Griffiths E. The anatomy of the blood-vessels in the region of the pancreas. Br J Surg 1950;37:334-344.

128. Haller Von A. Iconae anatomicarum. Vol. 2. Gottingae: Vandenhoeck, 1745.

129. Couinaud C, Huguet C. La greffe du duodéno-pancréas chez l'homme. I^{re} partie: étude anatomique. J Chir 1966;92:293-312.

130. Farisse J, Cannoni M, Gau M, Miliani P, Niel J, Richelme H. Sur les artères de la papille duodénale. C R Assoc Anat 1966;134:384-395.

131. Pitzorno M. Morfologia delle arterie del pancreas. Arch Ital Anat Embriol 1920;18:1-48.

132. Martin R, Couppié G. Étude des variations des branches du tronc artériel pancréatico-duodéno-jéjunal. Arch Anat Path 1963;11:A29-A32.

133. Meyer P. Étude du tronc artériel pancréatico-duodéno-jéjunal. C R Assoc Anat 1953;40:99-119.

134. Delagrange AB, Barbin JY. Contribution a l'étude de la vascularisation artériélle du pancréas. C R Assoc Anat 1966;135:297-306.

135. Donatini B. A systematic study of the vascularization of the pancreas. Surg Radiol Anat 1990;12:173-180.

136. Skandalakis JE, Gray SW, Rowe JS, Skandalakis LJ. Surgical anatomy of the pancreas. Contemp Surg 1979;15;17-40.

137. Michels NA. Blood supply of pancreas. Anat Rec 1951;109:326.

138. Michels NA. Variations in blood supply of liver, gallbladder, stomach, duodenum, and pancreas. J Int Coll Surg 1945;8: 502-504.

139. Del Campo JC. Circulación del duodeno. Anales Facultad Med Montevideo 1931;16:1-27.

140. Van Damme JPJ, Bonte J. Systematization of the arteries in the splenic hilus. Acta Anat 1986;125:217-224.

141. Bolognese A, Di Giorgio A, Stipa V. Arterial vascularization of the pancreas; anatomical findings by means of vascular injection of plastic material. Surg Ital 1979;9:346-351.

142. Toni R, Favero L, Bolzani R, Roversi R, Vezzadini P. Further observations on the anatomical variation in the arteries of the human pancreas. IRCS Med Sci 1985;13:605-606.

143. Vergoz M. Artère pancréatique principale. Bull Mem Soc Anat Paris 1921;18:97-99.

144. Thomford NR, Chandnani PC, Taha AM, Chablani VN, Busnardo AC. Anatomic characteristics of the pancreatic arteries: radiologic observations and their clinical significance. Am J Surg 1986;151:690-693.

145. Gordon DH, Martin EC, Kim YH, Kutcher R. Accessory blood supply to the liver from the dorsal pancreatic artery: an unusual anatomic variant. Cardiovasc Radiol 1978;1:199-201.

146. Inoue K, Yamaai T, Odajima G. A rare case of anastomosis between the dorsal pancreatic and the inferior mesenteric arteries. Okajimas Folia Anat Jpn 1986;63:45-46.

147. Peri G, Veralli E, Trivellini G. La vascolarizzazione del pancreas. Arch It Chir 1969;95:287-300.

148. Moretti S. Studio anatomo-radiologico del circolo arterioso pancreatico. Radiol Med 1965;51:1-16.

149. Stingl J, Boruvka V, Breštáková M, Ruzbarský V, Vaněk I. Vascularization of the body and tail of the pancreas. Folia Morphol (Praha) 1985;33:338-347.

150. Ross B, Fox M. Blood supply of the distal part of the human pancreas. Transplantation 1981;31:134-136.

151. Martin R, Bouchet Y, Couppié G. Considération sur l'artère splénique et ses branches pancréatique. C R Assoc Anat 1961;113:513-529.

152. Ebner I, Anderhuber F. Arterielle Gefässversorgung der Cauda pancreatis unter besonderer Berücksichtigung der cauda-corporealen Gefässbeziehungen. Acta Anat 1985;121:115-123.

153. Olsen L, Woodburne RT. The vascular relations of the pancreas. Surg Gynec Obstet 1954;99:713-719.

154. Calas F, Couppié G, Martin R, Bouchet Y. Étude des affluents et de la formation de la veine porte. C R Assoc Anat 1959;99:254-271.

155. Evans BP, Ochsner A. Gross anatomy of the lymphatics of the human pancreas. Surgery 36:177, 1954.

156. Cubilla AL, Fortner J, Fitzgerald PJ. Lymph node involvement in carcinoma of the head of the pancreas area. Cancer 41:880, 1978.

157. Deki H, Sato T. An anatomic study of the peripancreatic lymphatics. Surg Radiol Anat 10:121-135, 1988.

158. Donatini B, Hidden G. Routes of lymphatic drainage from the pancreas: A suggested segmentation. Surg Radiol Anat 14:35-42, 1992.

159. Bertelli E. Regoli M, Comparini L. Histotopographic and ultrastructural study on the lymphatic network of the pancreas in the guinea pig. Acta Anat 1993;147:233-239.

160. Pissas A. Clinical and surgical anatomy studies of the lymphatic circulation of the pancreas. [French]. Bull Mem Acad R Med Belg 145(8-9):351-364, 1990.

161. Delcore R, Rodriguez FJ, Forster J, Hermreck AS, Thomas JH. Significance of lymph node metastases in patients with pancreatic cancer undergoing curative resection. Am J Surg 172:463-469, 1996.

162. Mukaiya M, Hirata K, Satoh T, Kimura M, Yamashiro K, Ura H, Oikawa I, Denno R. Lack of survival benefit of extended lymph node dissection for ductal adenocarcinoma of the head of the pancreas: retrospective multi-institutional analysis in Japan. World J Surg 1998;22:248-253.

163. Nakao A, Harada A, Nonami T, Kaneko T, Murakami H, Inoue S, Takeuchi Y, Takagi H. Lymph node metastases in carcinoma of the head of the pancreas region. Br J Surg 1995;82:399-402.

164. Vossen S, Goretzki PE, Goebel U, Willnow U. Therapeutic management of rare malignant pancreatic tumors in children. World J Surg 1998;22:879-882.

165. Sho M, Nakajima Y, Kanehiro H, Hisanaga M, Nishio K, Nagao M, Ikeda N, Kanokogi H, Yamada T, Nakano H. Pattern of recurrence after resection for intraductal papillary mucinous tumors of the pancreas. World J Surg 1998;22:874-878.

166. Nakagohri T, Kenmochi T, Kainuma O, Tokoro Y, Asano T. Intraductal papillary mucinous tumors of the pancreas. Am J Surg 1999;178:344-347.

167. Kobari M, Egawa S, Shibuya K, Shimamura H, Sunamura M, Takeda K, Matsuno S, Furukawa T. Intraductal papillary mucinous tumors of the pancreas comprise 2 clinical subtypes. Arch Surg 1999;134:1131-1136.

168. Lillemoe KD, Conlon KC, Evans DB, Warshaw AL. Symposium: Ductal adenocarcinoma of the pancreas. Contemp Surg 2001;57:68-76.

169. Holst JJ. Neural regulation of pancreatic exocrine function. In: Go VLW, DiMagno EP, Gardner JD, Lebenthal E, Reber HA, Scheele GA (eds). The Pancreas (2nd ed). New York: Raven Press, 1993, pp. 381-402.

170. Camilleri M. Autonomic regulation of gastrointestinal motility. In: Low PA (ed). Clinical Autonomic Disorders (2nd ed). Boston: Little, Brown, 1997, pp. 135-146.

171. Cooke HJ. Role of the "little brain" in the gut in water and elec-

trolyte homeostasis. FASEB J 3:127-138, 1989.

172. Grundy D. Vagal control of gastrointestinal function. Baillieres Clin Gastroenterol 2:23-43, 1988.

173. Drapiewski JF. Carcinoma of the pancreas: a study of neoplastic invasion of nerves and its possible clinical significance. Am J Clin Pathol 14;549-556, 1944.

174. Bockman DE, Buchler M, Malfertheiner P, Beger HG. Analysis of nerves in chronic pancreatitis. Gastroenterology 94:1459-1469, 1988.

175. Widdison AL, Alvarez C, Karanjia ND, Reber HA. Experimental evidence of beneficial effects of ductal decompression in chronic pancreatitis. Endoscopy 23:151-154, 1991.

176. Bockman DE. Anatomy of the pancreas. In: Go VLW, DiMagno EP, Gardner JD, Lebenthal E, Reber HA, Scheele GA (eds). The Pancreas (2nd ed). New York: Raven Press, 1993, pp. 1-8.

177. Howard JM. Treatment of relapsing and chronic pancreatitis. In: Howard JM, Jordan GL (eds). Surgical Diseases of the Pancreas. Philadelphia: JB Lippincott, 1960, pp. 223-248.

178. Mallet-Guy P, DeBeaujeu MJ. Left splanchnicectomy in the treatment of chronic relapsing pancreatitis; personal follow-up of 52 patients. Lyon Chir 1952;47:531.

179. Mallet-Guy P. Surgical treatment of chronic relapsing pancreatitis. Arch Surg 1955;70:609.

180. Stone HH, Chauvin EJ. Pancreatic denervation for pain relief in chronic alcohol associated pancreatitis. Br J Surg 1990;77:303-305.

181. Cuschieri A, Shimi SM, Crosthwaite G, Joypaul V. Bilateral endoscopic splanchnicectomy through a posterior thoracoscopic approach. J R Coll Surg Edinb 1994;39:44-47.

182. Cierpka K, Koella C, Schaub N, Huber A. [Thorascopic splanchnicectomy for pain management in inoperable pancreatic carcinoma]. Schweiz Med Wochenschr 1997;127:1251.

183. Pietrabissa A, Vistoli F, Carobbi A, Boggi U, Bisà M, Mosca F. Thoracoscopic splanchnicectomy for pain relief in unresectable pancreatic cancer. Arch Surg 2000;135:332-335.

184. Skandalakis JE, Gray SW, Rowe JS Jr. Anatomical Complications in General Surgery. New York: Mc Graw-Hill, 1983, p. 162.

185. Rack FJ, Elkins CW. Experiences with vagotomy and sympathectomy in the treatment of chronic recurrent pancreatitis. Arch Surg 1950;61:937.

186. Merendino KA. Vagotomy for the relief of pain secondary to pancreatic cancer [editorial]. Am J Surg 1964;108:1.

187. Flanigan DP, Kraft RO. Continuing experience with palliative chemical splanchnicectomy. Arch Surg 1978;113:509-511.

188. Gardner AMN, Solomon G. Relief of the pain of unresectable carcinoma of pancreas by chemical splanchnicectomy during laparotomy. Ann R Coll Surg Engl 1984;66:409-411.

189. Hegedus V. Relief of pancreatic pain by radiography-guided block. AJR Am J Roentgenol 1979;133:1101-1103.

190. Rich JD, Dickinson BP, Merriman NA, Thule PM. Insulin use by bodybuilders. JAMA 1998;279:1613.

191. Stefan Y, Orci L, Malaisse-Legae F, Perrelet A, Patel Y, Unger RH. Quantitation of endocrine cell content in the pancreas of nondiabetic and diabetic humans. Diabetes 31:694, 1982.

192. Andersen DK, Brunicardi C. Pancreatic anatomy and physiology. In: Greenfield LJ. Surgery: Scientific Principles and Practice (2nd ed). Philadelphia: Lippincott-Raven, 1997, pp. 857-874.

193. Seymour NE, Brunicardi FC, Chaiken RL. Reversal of abnormal glucose production after pancreatic resection by pancreatic poly-

peptide administration in man. Surgery 1988;104:119.

194. Leahy JL, Bonner-Weir S, Weir GC. Abnormal glucose regulation of insulin secretion in models of reduced B-cell mass. Diabetes 33:667, 1984.

195. Yamaguchi K, Chijiiwa K, Shimizu S, Yokohata K, Tanaka M. Litmus paper helps detect potential pancreatoenterostomy leakage. Am J Surg 1998;175:227-228.

196. Sato N, Yamaguchi K, Yokohata K, Shimizu S, Morisaki T, Mizumoto K, Chijiiwa K, Tanaka M. Preoperative exocrine pancreatic function predicts risk of leakage of pancreaticojejunostomy. Surgery 1998;124:871-876.

197. Sho M, Nakajima Y, Kanehiro H, Hisanaga M, Nishio K, Nagao M, Tatekawa Y, Ikeda N, Kanokogi H, Yamada T, Hirohashi S, Hirohashi R, Uchida H, Nakano H. A new evaluation of pancreatic function after pancreatoduodenectomy using secretin magnetic resonance cholangiopancreatography. Am J Surg 1998;176:279-82.

198. Ranson JHC. Diagnostic standards for acute pancreatitis. World J Surg 1997;21:136-142.

199. Lad RJ, Fitzgerald P, Jacobson K. An unusual cause of recurrent pancreatitis: duodenal duplication cyst. Can J Gastroenterol 2000;14:341-345.

200. Berger HG, Warshaw AL, Büchler MW, Carr-Locke DL, Neoptolemos JP, Russell C, Sarr MG (eds). The Pancreas. Oxford UK: Blackwell Science, 1998.

201. Meyers MA. Dynamic Radiology of the Abdomen. Normal and Pathologic Anatomy (4th ed). New York: Springer-Verlag, 1994.

202. Nakamura T, Okada A, Higaki J, Tojo H, Okamoto M. Pancreaticobiliary maljunction-associated pancreatitis: An experimental study on the activation of pancreatic phospholipase $A_2$. World J Surg 20:543-550, 1996.

203. Sugiyama M, Baba M, Atomi Y, Hanaoka H, Mizutani Y, Hachiya J. Diagnosis of anomalous pancreaticobiliary junction: value of magnetic resonance cholangiopancreatography. Surgery 1998;123:391-397.

204. Steedman RA, Doering R, Carter R. Surgical aspects of pancreatic abscess. Surg Gynecol Obstet 125:757, 1967.

205. Hubbard TB, Eilber FR, Oldroyd JJ. Retroperitoneal extension of necrotizing pancreatitis. Surg Gynecol Obstet 134:927, 1972.

206. Jaffe BM, Ferguson TB, Holtz S, Shields JB. Mediastinal pancreatic pseudocysts. Am J Surg 124:600, 1972.

207. Schoenberg MH, Rau B, Berger HG. [Diagnosis and therapy of primary pancreatic abscesses]. Chirurg 1995;66:588-596.

208. Baril NB, Ralls PW, Wren SM, Selby RR, Radin R, Parekh D, Jabbour N, Stain SC. Does an infected peripancreatic fluid collection or abscess mandate operation? Ann Surg 2000;231:361-367.

209. Seifert H, Wehrmann T, Schmitt T, Zeuzem S, Caspary WF. Retroperitoneal endoscopic debridement for infected peripancreatic necrosis. Lancet 2000;356:653-655.

210. Beger HG, Rau B, Mayer J, Pralle U. Natural course of acute pancreatitis. World J Surg 1997;21:130-135.

211. Sakorafas GH, Tsiotos GG, Sarr MG. Extrapancreatic necrotizing pancreatitis with viable pancreas: a previously under-appreciated entity. J Am Coll Surg 1999;188:643-648.

212. Liu CL, Lo CM, Fan ST. Acute biliary pancreatitis: diagnosis and management. World J Surg 1997;21:149-154.

213. Uomo G, Molino D, Visconti M, Ragozzino A, Manes G, Rabitti PG. The incidence of main pancreatic duct disruption in severe biliary pancreatitis. Am J Surg 1998;176:49-52.

214. Stolte M, Waltschew A. The papilla of Vater and chronic pancreatitis. Hepato-Gastroenterology 1986;33:163-169.

215. Bosscha K, Hulstaert PF, Hennipman A, Visser MR, Gooszen HG, van Vroonhoven TJMV, v d Werken C. Fulminant acute pancreatitis and infected necrosis: results of open management of the abdomen and "planned" reoperations. J Am Coll Surg 1998;187:255-262.

216. Weber TR, Keller MS. Operative management of chronic pancreatitis in children. Arch Surg 2001;136:550-555.

217. DuBay D, Sandler A, Kimura K, Bishop W, Eimen M, Soper R. The modified Puestow procedure for complicated hereditary pancreatitis in children. J Ped Surg 2000;35:343-348.

218. Takase K, Takeyama Y, Nishikawa J, Ueda T, Hoir Y, Yamamoto M, Kuroda Y. Apoptotic cell death of renal tubules in experimental severe acute pancreatitis. Surgery 1999;125:411-420.

219. Papadimitriou JD, Fotopoulos AC, Smyrniotis B, Prahalias AA, Kostopanagiotou G, Papadimitriou LJ. Subtotal pancreatoduodenectomy: Use of a defunctionalized loop for pancreatic stump drainage. Arch Surg 1999;134:135-139.

220. Howard JM, Jordan GL Jr. Surgical Diseases of the Pancreas. Philadelphia: Lippincott, 1960.

221. Cattell RB, Warren KW. Surgery of the Pancreas. Philadelphia: Saunders, 1953.

222. Merchant NB, Conlon KC, Saigo P, Dougherty E, Brennan MF. Positive peritoneal cytology predicts unresectability of pancreatic adenocarcinoma. J Am Coll Surg 1999;188:421-426.

223. Hermann RE, Cooperman AM. Current concepts in cancer. N Engl J Med 301:482, 1979.

224. Roder JD, Stein HJ, Siewert R. Carcinoma of the periampullary region: Who benefits from portal vein resection? Am J Surg 171:170-175, 1996.

225. Nakao A, Kaneko Y. Intravascular ultrasonography for assessment of portal vein invasion by pancreatic carcinoma. World J Surg 1999;23:892-895.

226. Farouk M, Niotis M, Branum GD, Cotton PB, Meyers WC. Indications for and the technique of local resection of tumors of the papilla of Vater. Arch Surg 1991;126:650-652.

227. Sauvanet A, Chapuis O, Hammel P, Fléjou JF, Ponsot P, Bernardes P, Belghiti J. Are endoscopic procedures able to predict the benignity of ampullary tumors? Am J Surg 1997;174:355-358.

228. Howard TJ, Chin AC, Streib EW, Kopecky KK, Wiebke EA. Value of helical computed tomography, angiography, and endoscopic ultrasound in determining resectability of periampullary carcinoma. Am J Surg 1997;174:237-241.

229. Sohn TA, Lillemoe KD, Cameron JL, Huang JJ, Pitt HA, Yeo CJ. Surgical palliation of unresectable periampullary adenocarcinoma in the 1990s. J Am Coll Surg 1999;188:658-669.

230. Kasahara K, Saito K, Kondo Y, Yasuda T, Yasuda Y, Nakada M, Nagai H, Kanazawa K. Papillo-choledochectomy in the operative management of mucosal neoplasms of the periampullary region. HPB Surg 1993;6:211-217.

231. Ryu M, Kinoshita T, Konishi M, Kawano N, Arai Y, Tanizaki H, Cho MN. Segmental resection of the duodenum including the papilla of Vater for focal cancer in adenoma. Hepato-Gastroenterology 1996;43:835-838.

232. Martignoni ME, Wagner M, Krähenbühl L, Redaelli CA, Friess H, Büchler MW. Effect of preoperative biliary drainage on surgical outcome after pancreaticoduodenectomy. Am J Surg 2001;181:52-59.

233. Macdonald JS, Gunderson LL, Cohn I Jr. Cancer of the pancreas. In: DeVita VT Jr, Hellman S, Rosenberg SA (eds). Cancer: Principles & Practice of Oncology. Philadelphia: JB Lippincott, 1982, p. 564.

234. Gudjonsson B. Cancer of the pancreas: 50 years of surgery. Cancer 1987;60:2284-2303.

235. Sperti C, Pasquali C, Piccoli A, Pedrazzoli S. Recurrence after resection for ductal adenocarcinoma of the pancreas. World J Surg 1997;21:195-200.

236. Ihse I. Invited commentary. Sperti C, Pasquali C, Piccoli A, Pedrazzoli S. Recurrence after resection for ductal adenocarcinoma of the pancreas. World J Surg 1997;21:200.

237. Tan HP, Smith J, Garberoglio CA. Pancreatic adenocarcinoma: an update. J Am Coll Surg 183:164-184, 1996.

238. Tsiotos GG, Farnell MB, Sarr MG. Are the results of pancreatectomy for pancreatic cancer improving? World J Surg 1999;23:913-919.

239. Hirata K, Sato T, Mukaiya M, Yamashiro K, Kimura M, Sasaki K, Denno R. Results of 1001 pancreatic resections for invasive ductal adenocarcinoma of the pancreas. Arch Surg 1997;132:771-776.

240. Traverso LW. Invited commentary. Hirata K, Sato T, Mukaiya M, Yamashiro K, Kimura M, Sasaki K, Denno R. Results of 1001 pancreatic resections for invasive ductal adenocarcinoma of the pancreas. Arch Surg 1997;132:777.

241. Gouma DJ, Nieveen van Dijkum EJM, van Geenen RCI, van Gulik TM, Obertop H. Are there indications for palliative resection in pancreatic cancer? World J Surg 1999;23:954-959.

242. Harrison LE, Merchant N, Cohen AM, Brennan MF. Pancreaticoduodenectomy for non periampullary primary tumors. Am J Surg 1997;174:393-395.

243. Edwards MJ, Nakagawa K, McMasters KM. En bloc pancreaticoduodenectomy and colectomy for duodenal neoplasms. South Med J 1997;90:733-735.

244. Crawford BE. Solid and papillary epithelial neoplasm of the pancreas, diagnosis by cytology. South Med J 1998;91:973-976.

245. John TG, Wright A, Allan PL, Redhead DN, Paterson-Brown S, Carter DC, Garden OJ. Laparoscopy with laparoscopic ultrasonography in the TNM staging of pancreatic carcinoma. World J Surg 1999;23:870-881.

246. DiFronzo LA, Egrari S, O'Connell TX. Choledochoduodenostomy for palliation in unresectable pancreatic cancer. Arch Surg 1998;133:820-825.

247. Clavien P-A, Selzner M. End-to-end pancreaticoduodenostomy: an alternative reconstruction for partial resection of the head of the pancreas. J Am Coll Surg 1998;187:330-332.

248. Di Carlo V, Zerbi A, Balzano G, Corso V. Pylorus-preserving pancreaticoduodenectomy versus conventional Whipple operation. World J Surg 1999;23:920-925.

249. Hiraoka T, Kanemitsu K. Value of extended resection and intraoperative radiotherapy for resectable pancreatic cancer. World J Surg 1999;23:930-936.

250. Yeo CJ, Cameron JL. Improving results of pancreaticoduodenectomy for pancreatic cancer. World J Surg 1999;23:907-912.

251. Crile G Jr. The advantages of bypass operations over radical pancreatoduodenectomy in the treatment of pancreatic carcinoma. Surg Gynec Obstet 130:1049-1053.

252. Lieberman MD, Kilburn H, Lindsey M, Brennan MF. Relation of perioperative deaths to hospital volume among patients undergoing pancreatic resection for malignancy. Ann Surg 222:638-645, 1995.

253. Gordon TA, Bowman HM, Tielsch JM, Bass EB, Burleyson GP, Cameron JL. Statewide regionalization of pancreaticoduodenectomy and its effect on in-hospital mortality. Ann Surg 228:71-78, 1998.

254. Hruban RH. The molecular biology of pancreatic cancer. In: Yeo CJ (moderator). Pancreatic cancer: 1998 update. J Am Coll Surg 1998;187:429-442.

255. Conlon KC. Staging: current status. In: Yeo CJ (moderator). Pancreatic cancer: 1998 update. J Am Coll Surg 1998;187:429-442.

256. Yeo CJ. Pancreaticoduodenectomy: techniques and outcome. In: "Pancreatic cancer: 1998 update," Yeo CJ (moderator). J Am Coll Surg 1998;187:429-442.

257. Böttner TC, Junginger T. Treatment of tumors of the pancreatic head with suspected but unproved malignancy: is a nihilistic approach justified? World J Surg 1999;23:158-163.

258. Balcom JH IV, Rattner DW, Warshaw AL, Chang Y, Fernandez-del Castillo C. Ten-year experience with 733 pancreatic resections. Arch Surg 2001;136:391-398.

259. Beger HG, Treitschke F, Gansauge F, Harada N, Hiki N, Mattfeldt T. Tumor of the ampulla of Vater: Experience with local or radical resection in 171 consecutively treated patients. Arch Surg 1999;134:526-532.

260. Treitschke F, Berger HG, Meessen D, Schoenberg MH. [Benign tumors of the Vater's papilla]. Dtsch Med Wochenschr 2000;125:1030-1034.

261. Schwarz RE, Harrison LE, Conlon KC, Klimstra DS, Brennan MF. The impact of splenectomy on outcomes after resection of pancreatic adenocarcinoma. J Am Coll Surg 1999;188:516-521.

262. Horvath KD, Chabot JA. An aggressive resectional approach to cystic neoplasms of the pancreas. Am J Surg 1999;178:269-274.

263. Karpoff HM, Klimstra DS, Brennan MF, Conlon KC. Results of total pancreatectomy for adenocarcinoma of the pancreas. Arch Surg 2001;136:44-47.

264. Brennan MF. Pancreatic cancer: "True, false, or just a start?" J Am Coll Surg 1999;189:129-130.

265. Trede M. Invited commentary. Ihse I, Anderson H, Andrén-Sandberg A. Total pancreatectomy for cancer of the pancreas: Is it appropriate? World J Surg 1996;20:288-294.

266. Sung JP, Stewart RD, O'Hara VS, Westhpal KF, Wilkinson JE, Hill J. A study of forty-nine consecutive Whipple resections for periampullary adenocarcinoma. Am J Surg 1997;174:6-10.

267. Böttger TC, Boddin J, Heintz A, Junginger T. Clinicopathologic study for the assessment of resection for ampullary carcinoma. World J Surg 1997;21:379-383.

268. Madura JA, Jarman BT, Doherty MG, Yum M-N, Howard TJ. Adenosquamous carcinoma of the pancreas. Arch Surg 1999;134:599-603.

269. Moosa AR. Invited critique. Karpoff HM, Klimstra DS, Brennan MF, Conlon KC. Results of total pancreatectomy for adenocarcinoma of the pancreas. Arch Surg 2001;136:44-47.

270. Traverso LW, Longmire WP. Preservation of the pylorus in pancreaticoduodenectomy: A follow-up evaluation. Ann Surg 192:306, 1980.

271. Van Berge Henegouwen MI, van Gulik TM, DeWit LT, Allema JH, Rauws EAJ, Obertop H, Gouma DJ. Delayed gastric emptying after standard pancreaticoduodenectomy versus pylorus-preserving pancreaticoduodenectomy: an analysis of 200 consecutive patients. J Am Coll Surg 1997;185:373-379.

272. Mosca F, Guilianotti PC, Balestracci T, Di Candio G, Pietrabissa A, Sbrana F, Rossi G. Long-term survival in pancreatic cancer: pylorus-preserving versus Whipple pancreaticoduodenectomy. Surgery 1997;122:553-566.

273. Takao S, Aikou T, Shichi H, Uchikura K, Kubo M, Imamura H, Maenohara S. Comparison of relapse and long-term survival between pylorus-preserving and Whipple pancreaticoduodenectomy in periampullary cancer. Am J Surg 1998;176:467-470.

274. Belli L, Riolo F, Romani, Baticci F, Rossetti O, Puttini M. Pylorus preserving pancreatoduodenectomy versus Whipple procedure for adenocarcinoma of the head of the pancreas. HPB Surg 1989;1:195-200.

275. Sharp KW, Ross CB, Halter SA, Morrison JG, Richards WO, Williams LF, Sawyers JL. Pancreatoduodenectomy with pyloric preservation for carcinoma of the pancreas: a cautionary note. Surgery 1989;105:645-653.

276. Morel P, Mathey P, Corboud H, Huber O, Egeli RA, Rohner A. Pylorus-preserving duodenopancreatectomy: long-term complications and comparison with the Whipple procedure. World J Surg 1990;14:642-647.

277. Tamura K, Sumi S, Koike M, Yano S, Nagami H, Nio Y. A splenic-inferior mesenteric venous anastomosis prevents gastric congestion following pylorus preserving pancreatoduodenectomy with extensive portal vein resection for cancer of the head of the pancreas. Int Surg 1997;82: 155-159.

278. Beger HG, Schoenberg MH, Link KH, Safi F, Berger D. Duodenum-preserving pancreatic head resection: a standard method in chronic pancreatitis. Chirurg 1997;68:874-880.

279. Beger HG, Staib L, Schoenberg MH. Ampullectomy for adenoma of the papilla and ampulla of Vater. Langenbecks Arch Surg 1998; 383:190-193.

280. Nagakawa T, Ohta T, Kayahara M, Ueno K. Total resection of the head of the pancreas preserving the duodenum, bile duct, and papilla with end-to-end anastomosis of the pancreatic duct. Am J Surg 173:210-212, 1997.

281. Eddes EH, Masclee AAM, Gooszen HG, Frölich M, Lamers CBHW. Effect of duodenum-preserving resection of the head of the pancreas on endocrine and exocrine pancreatic function in patients with chronic pancreatitis. Am J Surg 1997;174:387-392.

282. Sugiyama M, Hagi H, Atomi Y. Reappraisal of intraoperative ultrasonography for pancreatobiliary carcinomas: assessment of malignant portal venous invasion. Surgery 1999;125:160-165.

283. Takahashi S, Akita K, Goseki N, Sato T. Spatial arrangement of the pancreatic ducts in the head of the pancreas with special reference to the branches of the uncinate process. Surgery 1999; 125:178-185.

284. Furukawa H, Iwata R, Moriyama N, Kosuge T. Blood supply to the pancreatic head, bile duct, and duodenum. Arch Surg 1999; 134:1086-1090.

285. Takano S, Ito Y, Watanabe Y, Yokoyama T, Kubota N, Iwai S. Pancreaticojejunostomy versus pancreaticogastrostomy in reconstruction following pancreaticoduodenectomy. Br J Surg 2000; 87:423-427.

286. Barrett O, Bowers WF. Total pancreatectomy for chronic relapsing pancreatitis and calcinosis of the pancreas. US Armed Forces Med J 8:1037, 1957.

287. Fry WJ, Child CG III. Ninety five percent distal pancreatectomy for chronic pancreatitis. Ann Surg 162:543-549, 1965.

288. Beger HG, Witte C, Kraas E, Bittner R. Erfahrung mit einer das Duodenum erhaltenden Pankreaskopfresektion bei chronischer Pankreatitis. Chirurg 1980;51:303.

289. Beger HG, Krautzberger W, Bittner R, et al. Duodenum-preserving resection of the head of the pancreas in patients with severe chronic pancreatitis. Surgery 1985;97:467-473.

290. Beger HG. Die duodenumerhaltende Pankreaskopfresektion bei chronischer Pankreatitis. Langenbecks Arch Chir 1987;372:357-362.

291. Beger HG, Büchler M, Bittner RR, Oettinger W, Roscher R. Duodenum-preserving resection of the head of the pancreas in severe chronic pancreatitis. Ann Surg 1989;209:273-278.

292. Beger HG, Büchler M. Duodenum-preserving resection of the head of the pancreas in chronic pancreatitis with inflammatory mass in the head. World J Surg 1990;14:83-87.

293. Frey CF. Pancreatic pseudocyst — Operative strategy. Ann Surg 188: 652, 1978.

294. Yellin AE, Vecchione TR, Donovan AJ. Distal pancreatectomy for pancreatic trauma. Am J Surg 124:135, 1972.

295. Puestow CB, Gillesby WJ. Retrograde surgical drainage of pancreas for chronic relapsing pancreatitis. Arch Surg 76:898, 1958.

296. Morgenstern L, Shandling B, Burrington JD. Symposium: Splenectomy or splenic salvage? Contemp Surg 16:79, 1980.

297. Sawyer R, Frey CF. Is there still a role for distal pancreatectomy in surgery for chronic pancreatitis? Am J Surg 1994;168:6-9.

298. White SA, Sutton CD, Weymass-Holden S, Berry DP, Pollard C, Rees Y, Dennison AR. The feasibility of spleen-preserving pancreatectomy for end-stage chronic pancreatitis. Am J Surg 2000;179:294-297.

299. Benoist S, Dugué L, Sauvanet A, Valverde A, Mauvais F, Paye F, Farges O, Belghiti J. Is there a role of preservation of the spleen in distal pancreatectomy? J Am Coll Surg 1999;188:255-260.

300. Kau S-Y, Shyr Y-M, Su C-H, Wu C-W, Lui W-Y. Diagnostic and prognostic values of CA 19-9 and CEA in periampullary cancers. J Am Coll Surg 1999;188:415-420.

301. Mason GR. Pancreatogastrostomy as reconstruction for pancreatoduodenectomy: Review. World J Surg 1999;23:221-226.

302. Siech M, Tripp K, Schmidt-Rohlfing B, Mattfeldt T, Görich J, Beger HG. Intraductal papillary mucinous tumor of the pancreas. Am J Surg 1999;177:117-120.

303. Huguier M, Mason NP. Treatment of cancer of the exocrine pancreas. Am J Surg 1999;177:257-265.

304. Lo CY, Lam KY, Fan ST. Surgical strategy for insulinomas in multiple endocrine neoplasia type 1. Am J Surg 1998;175:305-307.

305. Doherty GM, Olson JA, Frisella MM, Lairmore TC, Wells SA, Norton JA. Lethality of multiple endocrine neoplasia Type I. World J Surg 1998;22:581-587.

306. Skogseid B, Öberg K, Äkerström G, Eriksson B, Westlin J-E, Janson ET, Eklöf H, Elvin A, Juhlin C, Rastad J. Limited tumor involvement found at multiple endocrine neoplasia type I pancreatic exploration: can it be predicted by preoperative tumor localization? World J Surg 1998;22:673-678.

307. Park BJ, Alexander HR, Libutti SK, Huang J, Royalty D, Skarulis MC, Jensen RT, Gorden P, Doppman JL, Shawker TH, Fraker DL, Norton JA, Bartlett DL. Operative management of islet-cell tumors arising in the head of the pancreas. Surgery 1998; 124, 1056-1062.

308. Warshaw AL, Rattner DW, Fernández-del Castillo C, Z'graggen K. Middle segment pancreatectomy: a novel technique for conserving pancreatic tissue. Arch Surg 1998;133:327-331.

309. Lillemoe KD. Invited commentary. Warshaw AL, Rattner DW

Fernández-del Castillo C, Z'graggen K. Middle segment pancreat-ectomy: a novel technique for conserving pancreatic tissue. Arch Surg 1998;133:327-331.

310. Borghi F, Gattolin A, Garbossa D, Bogliatto F, Garavoglia M, Levi AC. Embryologic bases of extended radical resection in pan-creatic cancer. Arch Surg 1998;133:297-301.

311. Espat NJ, Brennan MF, Conlon KC. Patients with laparoscopically staged unresectable pancreatic adnocarcinoma do not require sub-sequent surgical biliary or gastric bypass. J Am Coll Surg 1999;188:649-657.

312. Knight RW, Scarborough JP, Goss JC. Adenocarcinoma of the pancreas. Arch Surg 113:1401, 1978.

313. Puestow CB, Gillesby WJ. Longitudinal pancreaticojejunostomy for chronic pancreatitis. Surg Proc 3:2, 1966.

314. Fusaro J, Davis JM. Case initiates discussion of 3 contoversial is-sues for surgical treatment of pancreatic pseudocysts. Contemp Surg 1999;54:162-164.

315. Cooperman AM, Hoerr SO. Surgery of the Pancreas: A Text and Atlas. St. Louis: Mosby, 1978.

316. Trías M, Targarona EM, Balagué C, Cifuentes A, Taurá P. Intraluminal stapled laparoscopic cystogastrostomy for treatment of pancreatic pseudocyst. Br J Surg 1995;82:403.

317. Vitale GC, Lawhon JC, Larson GM, Harrell DJ, Reed DN Jr, MacLeod S. Endoscopic drainage of the pancreatic pseudocyst. Surgery 1999;126:612-623.

318. Spivak H, Galloway JR, Amerson JR, Fink AS, Branum GD, Redvanly RD, Richardson WS, Mauren SJ, Waring JP, Hunter JG. Management of pancreatic psuedocysts. J Am Coll Surg 1998;186:507-511.

319. Boulanger S, Volpe CM, Allah A, Lindfield V, Doerr R. Pan-creatic pseudocyst with biliary fistula: treatment with endoscopic internal drainage. South Med J 2001;94:347-349.

320. Hunter JG. Minimally invasive surgery: the next frontier. World J Surg 23:422-424, 1999.

321. Park A, Schwartz R, Tandan V, Anvari M. Laparoscopic pan-creatic surgery. Am J Surg 1999;177:158-163.

322. Cuschieri A. Minimally invasive surgery: hepatobiliary-pancreatic and foregut. Endoscopy 2000;32:331-344.

323. Berney T, Pretre R, Chassot G, Morel P. The role of revascular-ization in celiac occlusion and pancreatoduodenectomy. Am J Surg 1998;176:352-356.

324. Suits J, Frazee R, Erickson RA. Endoscopic ultrasound and fine needle aspiration for the evaluation of pancreatic masses. Arch Surg 1999;134:639-643.

325. Karlson BM, Forsman CA, Wilander E, Skogseid B, Lindgren PG, Jacobson G, Rastad J. Efficiency of percutaneous core biopsy in pancreatic tumor diagnosis. Surgery 120(1):75-79, 1996.

326. Moosa AR. Invited commentary. Tillou A, Schwartz MR, Jordan PH Jr. Percutaneous needle biopsy of the pancreas: When should it be performed? World J Surg 1996;20:283-287.

327. Brandt KR, Charboneau JW, Stephens DH, Welch TJ, Goellner JR. CT and US guided biopsy of the pancreas. Radiology 187:99-104, 1993.

328. Lo C-Y, Lai ECS, Lo C-M, Mok FPT, Chu K-M, Liu C-L, Fan S-T. Endoscopic sphincterotomy: 7-year experience. World J Surg 21(1):67-71, 1997.

329. Howard TJ, Tan T, Lehman GA, Sherman S, Madura JA, Fogel E, Swack ML, Kopecky KK. Classification and management of per-forations complicating endoscopic sphincterotomy. Surgery

1999;126:658-665.

330. Stapfer M, Selby RR, Stain SC, Kathouda N, Parekh D, Jabbour N, Garry D. Management of duodenal perforation after endo-scopic retrograde cholangiopancreatography and sphincterotomy. Ann Surg 2000;232:191-198.

331. Spratt JS. Improving trends with pancreatoduodenectomy. Am J Surg 131:239, 1976.

332. Mergenthaler FW, Harris MN. Superior mesenteric vein throm-bosis complicating pancreatoduodenectomy: Successful treatment by thrombectomy. Ann Surg 167:106, 1968.

333. Walker WM. Chylous ascites following pancreatoduodenectomy. Arch Surg 95:640, 1967.

334. Hamanaka Y, Suzuki T. Modified dunking pancreatojejunostomy for a soft pancreas. Br J Surg 1995;82:404-405.

335. Büchler MW, Friess H, Wagner M, Kulli C, Wagener V, Z'Graggen K. Pancreatic fistula after pancreatic head resection. Br J Surg 2000;87:883-889.

336. Gambiez LP, Ernst OJ, Merlier OA, Porte HL, Chambon JPM, Quandalle PA. Arterial embolization for bleeding pseudocysts complicating chronic pancreatitis. Arch Surg 1997;132:1016-1021.

337. Gambiez LP, Denimal FA, Porte HL, Saudemont A, Chambon JPM, Quandalle PA. Retroperitoneal approach and endoscopic management of peripancreatic necrosis collections. Arch Surg 1998; 133:66-72.

338. Gadacz TR, Trunkey D, Kiefter RF. Visceral vessel erosion asso-ciated with pancreatitis: Case reports and a review of the liter-ature. Arch Surg 113:1438, 1978.

339. Shafiroff BB, Berkowtis D, Li JK, Fletcher P. Splenic erosion and hemorrhage secondary to pancreatic pseudocyst. Am J Gastro-enterol 68:145, 1977.

340. Gledhill T. Erosion of the splenic artery after pancreatic cysto-gastrostomy. J R Coll Surg Edinb 23:373, 1978.

341. Eckhauser FE, Stanley JC, Zelenock GB, Borlaza GS, Freier DT, Lindenauer SM. Gastroduodenal and pancreaticoduodenal artery aneurysms: A complication of pancreatitis causing spontaneous gastrointestinal hemorrhage. Surgery 88:335, 1980.

342. Kraft AR, Saletta JD. Acute alcoholic pancreatitis: Current con-cepts and controversies. Surg Annu 8:145, 1976.

343. Mair WS, McMahon MJ, Goligher JC. Stenosis of the colon in acute pancreatitis. Gut 17:692, 1976.

344. Berne TV, Edmondson HA. Colonic fistulization due to pancrea-titis. Am J Surg 111:359, 1966.

345. Sudan D, Sudan R, Stratta R. Long term outcome of simultaneous kidney-pancreas transplantation: analysis of 61 patients with more than 5 years follow-up. Transplantation 2000;69:550-555.

346. Chauvin KD, Kittur DS. Pancreas transplantation. In: Cameron JL. Current Surgical Therapy (6th ed). St. Louis: Mosby, 1998, pp. 539-543.

347. Stratta RJ, Gaber AO, Shokouh-Amiri MH, Reddy KS, Egidi MF, Grewal HP, Gaber LW. A prospective comparison of systemic-bladder versus portal enteric drainage in vascularized pancreas transplantation. Surgery 2000;127:217-226.

348. Hricik DE, Chareandee C, Knauss TC, Schulak JA. Hypertension after pancreas-kidney transplantation: role of bladder versus en-teric pancreatic drainage. Transplantation 2000;70:494-496.

349. Humar A, Kandaswamy R, Drangstveit MB, Parr E, Gruessner AG, Sutherland DE. Surgical risks and outcome of pancreas re-transplants. Surgery 2000;127:634-640.

350. Whang M, Katz L, Ongcapin E, Geffner S, Fiedman G,

Mulgaonkar S, Kaplan B. Nephrogenic adenomas occurring in a patient with simultaneous kidney-pancreas transplant. Urology (Online) 2000;55:949.

351. Takashima T, Hirata M, Kataoka Y, Asari Y, Sato K, Ohwada T, Kakita A. Pancreaticographic classification of pancreatic ductal injuries caused by blunt injury to the pancreas. J Trauma Inj Infect Crit Care 2000;745-752.

# Chapter 22

# Spleen

PANAJIOTIS N. SKANDALAKIS, LEE J. SKANDALAKIS,
ANDREW N. KINGSNORTH, GENE L. COLBORN, THOMAS A. WEIDMAN,
GEORGE F. HATCH III, RICHARD C. LAUER, JOHN E. SKANDALAKIS

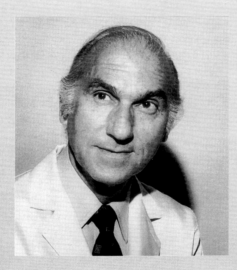

**Leon Morgenstern (1919--)** introduced segmental splenic resection in the United States.

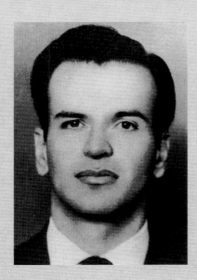

**M. Campos Christo (1920--)** revived the partial splenectomy as a viable alternative to total splenectomy.

*It is the position of the liver on the right side of the body that is the main cause for the formation of the spleen; the existence of which thus becomes to a certain extent a matter of necessity in all animals, though not a very stringent necessity.*

*Aristotle[1]*

## HISTORY

The anatomic and surgical history of the spleen is shown in Table 22-1.

## EMBRYOGENESIS OF THE SPLEEN

### Normal Development

The mesoderm is responsible for the genesis of the spleen, the largest of the lymphatic organs. Around the fifth week of gestation, mesenchymal cells between the leaflets of the dorsal mesogastrium and the cells of the coelomic epithelium of the dorsal mesentery form the early spleen. The dorsal mesogastrium (Fig. 22-1), which supports the embryonic stomach, expands around the fifth to sixth weeks to form the greater omentum.

The spleen remains within the mesenteric expansion but does not follow the downward formation of the omentum. In other words, the spleen is located between the leaves of the dorsal mesogastrium, and occupies this location in adult life (Fig. 22-2). All these embryogenic mechanisms take place on the left side of the dorsal mesogastrium, at the left upper quadrant, which will be the permanent home of the spleen. The organ's origin is neither midline nor bilateral.

The left side of the dorsal mesogastrium gives rise to the splenic ligaments (Fig. 22-3). With the possible rotation of the stomach, the left surface of the mesogastrium becomes fused to the peritoneum over the left kidney. The splenic artery is found posterior to the lesser sac and anterior to the left kidney. It is enveloped by the splenorenal ligament, which is the posterior portion of the dorsal meso-

gastrium. Mesenchymal cells differentiate to form both the capsule and a connective tissue framework.

At 10 to 20 days, differentiation to true epithelium with visible basement membrane is evident. Clefts of mesenchymal origin (sinusoids without endothelial lining) are present at 29 to 30 days; they show evidence of communication with the capillaries. The spleen assumes its characteristic shape in the early fetal period; fetal lobulation normally disappears late in the prenatal period.

Around the 13th week, surface immunoglobulin-bearing B cells and erythrocyte rosette-forming T cells emerge. Immunoglobulins A and, perhaps, E are not synthesized during fetal life, but IgM and IgG antibodies are synthesized during the third trimester. The spleen cannot be considered a giant lymph node, since there is no connection of the splenic lymphatics with other lymph vessels.

Splenic lobules form around the central arteries in the first weeks of the second trimester. The red pulp develops at the periphery of the lobules. There is also an accumulation of lymphocytes, monocytes, and macrophages during the second trimester; this is the white pulp, which forms around the central arteries.

### Congenital Anomalies

#### *Asplenia*

Asplenia may be associated with several other congenital anomalies. Asplenia is autosomal recessive, while splenic hypoplasia is autosomal dominant.

#### *Polysplenia*

Polysplenia may be associated with several other congenital anomalies. It is distinct from accessory spleen, in which the normal spleen is present but is joined by one,

## TABLE 22-1. Anatomic and Surgical History of the Spleen

| | | |
|---|---|---|
| Hua To (115-205 A.D.) | | Performed possible splenectomies in China |
| Jewish Talmud (2ⁿᵈ - 6ᵗʰ Centuries) | | Described the spleen ("techol") as the seat of laughter while providing analysis of its associated pathologies |
| Maimonides (1135-1204) | | Described the blood-purifying properties of the spleen |
| Zaccarelli | 1549 | Performed one of the earliest splenectomies (many have argued that it was an ovariectomy instead) |
| Ballonii | 1578 | Told of a splenectomy performed by an unknown barber surgeon. In his report he asked, "Este igitur splenatam necessarius" (Is the spleen so necessary for life). |
| Rosetti | 1590 | First successful partial splenectomy |
| van Leeuwenhoeck (1632-1723) | | Studied the spleen arguing that it played a role in the purification of the blood |
| Read | 1638 | Reported on a splenectomized dog with a six-week survival period. In his paper he argued, "...the spleen may be excised without harm." |
| Clark | 1673 | Removed a portion of the spleen after his patient's unsuccessful suicide attempt |
| Matthias | 1678 | Performed the first successful splenectomy for trauma |
| Fantoni of Turin | ca. 1700 | As reported by Grebezius he operated on the exposed spleen of a girl abused by her mother |
| Ferguson | 1734 | Performed a partial splenectomy |
| Hewson | 1777 | Cautiously speculated that the spleen formed erythrocytes |
| Assolant | 1802 | Ligated branches of the terminal division of the splenic artery in dogs, noting the segmental distribution of the splenic blood supply |
| O'Brien | 1816 | Performed the first splenectomy for trauma (knife wound) in the United States |
| Quittenbaum | 1826 | Deliberately performed splenectomy. His patient died six hours later from shock. |
| deGray | 1844 | Provided a case report of splenectomy to the French Academy of Surgeons. He noted that the patient recovered as expected but died thirteen years later of pneumonia (possibly the earliest reported case of Overwhelming Post-Splenectomy Infection [OPSI]). |
| Bryant | 1866 | Performed a splenectomy on a 20-year-old leukemia patient |
| Evans | 1866 | Reported delayed rupture of the spleen |
| Péan | 1867 | Performed the first segmental resection of the spleen on a 20-year-old woman suffering from a splenic tumor (she was originally thought to have an ovarian cyst) |
| Deeble | 1889 | Removed ³/₄ of the spleen to treat a gunshot wound |
| Billroth | 1891 | Reported an incidental autopsy finding of the spleen where, "[f]rom the appearance of the rent and the small quantity of blood effused, we conclude that the injury might have healed completely." In this statement he ushered in the possibility of non-surgical management of splenic trauma. |
| James | 1892 | Sutured both the spleen and the diaphragm to treat a gunshot wound |
| Riegner | 1892 | Successfully removed a transected spleen for blunt trauma in a 14-year-old construction worker who had fallen off a scaffold and hit a board. On the justification of splenectomy for trauma he argued: "If the situation is so desperate and bleeding so extensive that we cannot think about the possibility of saving the patient through compression ...ligate the specific vessels and remove the spleen." |
| Zikoff | 1895 | Successfully sutured a lacerated spleen |
| Pitts and Ballance | 1896 | Reported a delayed splenic rupture with a five-day latent period |
| Jordan | 1898 | Reported partial splenectomy in dogs |
| Funaioli | 1901 | Offered a description of partial splenectomy and splenic hemostasis using segmental arterial ligation in dogs |
| Berger | 1902 | Used tamponade of the spleen as an alternative to splenectomy |
| Baudet | 1907 | Provided detailed descriptions of delayed splenic rupture latency, known now as the latent period of Baudet |

## TABLE 22-1 *(cont'd)*. Anatomic and Surgical History of the Spleen

| | | |
|---|---|---|
| Gibbon | 1908 | Argued, "...if the spleen were not so easily removed, fewer splenectomies for rupture would be reported, since the majority of these cases of hemorrhage can be controlled by judicious packing." |
| W. Mayo | 1910 | Reported on a splenectomized patient treated for severe pneumonia |
| Pearce | 1918 | Published his classic book *The Spleen and Anaemia* stating that splenectomy was indicated for Banti's diseases, pernicious anemia, hemolytic jaundice, Gaucher's disease, trauma, cysts, tuberculosis, syphilis, and wandering spleen |
| Morris and Bullock | 1919 | Performed classic experiments observing an 80% mortality in splenectomized rats given plague bacillus. In the control group the mortality rate was 35%. |
| Volkmann | 1923 | Argued that partial splenectomy is feasible in humans |
| Henschen | 1928 | Confirmed the segmental anatomy of the spleen in a review of several studies |
| Dretzka | 1930 | Reported on a series of 27 patients with rupture of the spleen treated with splenorrhaphy |
| McIndoe | 1932 | Offered his classical study on the concept of delayed splenic rupture |
| Ballance, Baudet, McIndoe, Zabinski | 1943 | Reported that the incidence of delayed splenic rupture is between 15-30%, noting a two-year latency in some |
| Gruber, Redner, and Kogut | 1951 | Provided the first report of post-splenectomy sepsis in infants |
| King and Shumacker | 1952 | Observed severe sepsis in five patients with congenital spherocytosis |
| Smith | 1957 | Reported the first severe infections following splenectomy for traumatic rupture |
| Campos Christo | 1962 | Revived the partial splenectomy as a viable alternative to total splenectomy |
| Coler | 1963 | Provided the first reported deaths of splenectomized children succumbing to overwhelming post-splenectomy sepsis |
| Ellis and Smith | 1966 | Reviewed immunologic properties of spleen |
| Bodon and Verzosa | 1967 | Challenged the necessity for splenectomy in all cases of incidental splenic injury |
| Najjar et al. | 1970 1973 | Discovered "tuftsin," a splenic peptide associated with immunity |
| Douglas and Simpson Simpson et al. | 1971 1977 | Provided a scheme for observation and nonoperative treatment in children with suspected splenic injury |
| Dixon et al. | 1980 | Divided spleen anatomically into three-dimensional cones. Advocated conservative treatment of vascular injury to the most external zone, and segmental ligation for deeper injury. |
| Delany et al. | 1982 1985 | Used enveloping mesh to tamponade parenchymal bleeding |
| Carroll et al. Cuschieri et al. Delaitre and Magignieu Thibault et al. | 1992 | Reported successful laparoscopic splenectomy |
| Liu et al. | 1996 | Provided anatomic segmental classification based on arterial patterns |

*History table compiled by David A. McClusky III and John E. Skandalakis.*

**References**

Coon WW. The spleen and splenectomy. Surg Gynecol Obstet 1991;173:403-414.

Justicz AG, Skandalakis PN, Skandalakis LJ. Management of splenic trauma in adults. Probl Gen Surg 1990;7:128-141.

McClusky DA III, Skandalakis LJ, Colborn GL, Skandalakis JE. Tribute to a triad: History of splenic anatomy, physiology, and surgery. Part 1. World J Surg 1999;23:311-325.

McClusky DA III, Skandalakis LJ, Colborn GL, Skandalakis JE. Tribute to a triad: History of splenic anatomy, physiology, and surgery. Part 2. World J Surg 1999;23:514-526.

McDermott WV. Liver, biliary tract, pancreas, and spleen. In: Warren R. Surgery. Philadelphia, WB Saunders, p. 867.

Morgenstern L. The surgical inviolability of the spleen: Historical evolution of a concept. In: International Congress of the History of Medicine, 23rd, 1972: Proceedings. London: Wellcome Institute of the History of Medicine, 1974.

Pearce RM, Krumbhaar EB, Frazier CH. The Spleen and Anaemia: Experimental and Clinical Studies. Philadelphia: JB Lippincott, 1918, pp. 3-10.

Sherman R. Perspectives in Management of Trauma to the Spleen: 1979 Presidential Address, American Association for the Surgery of Trauma. J Trauma 1980;20:1-13.

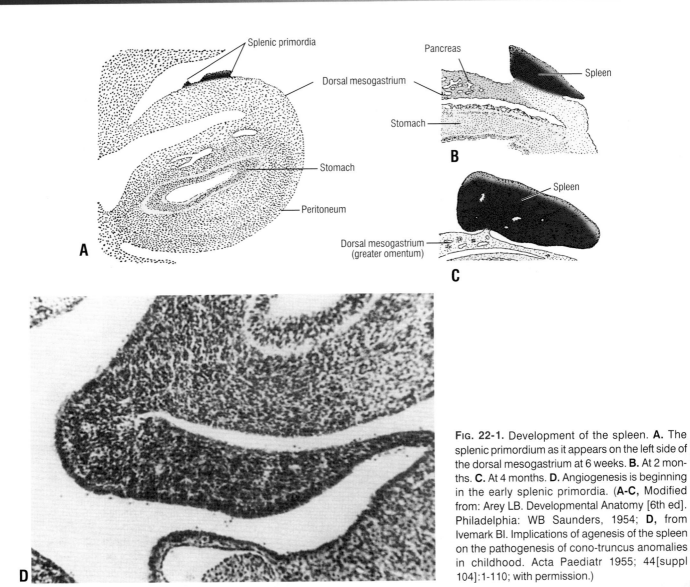

FIG. 22-1. Development of the spleen. **A.** The splenic primordium as it appears on the left side of the dorsal mesogastrium at 6 weeks. **B.** At 2 months. **C.** At 4 months. **D.** Angiogenesis is beginning in the early splenic primordia. (**A-C,** Modified from: Arey LB. Developmental Anatomy [6th ed]. Philadelphia: WB Saunders, 1954; **D,** from Ivemark BI. Implications of agenesis of the spleen on the pathogenesis of cono-truncus anomalies in childhood. Acta Paediatr 1955; 44[suppl 104]:1-110; with permission.)

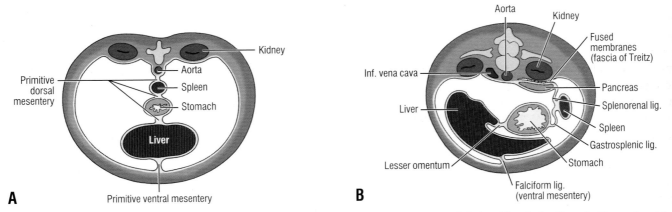

FIG. 22-2. Peritoneal reflections of the spleen develop from the primitive dorsal mesentery. **A.** Relationships during the primitive embryonic stage. **B.** Relationships in the adult. (Modified from Skandalakis JE, Gray SW, Rowe JS Jr. Anatomical Complications in General Surgery. New York: McGraw-Hill, 1983; with permission.)

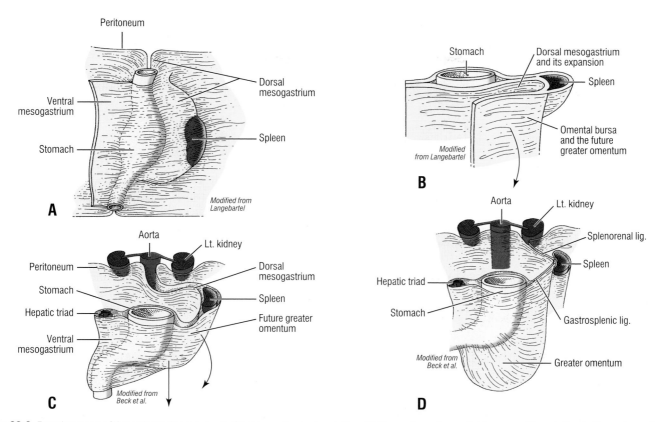

FIG. 22-3. Development of the splenic ligaments. **A.** Gastric and splenic rotation. **B.** Formation of omental bursa and its relation to the spleen. **C.** Beginning of formation of the greater omentum and its relationship to spleen. **D.** Formation of two major splenic ligaments. (Modified from Allen KB, Gay BB Jr, Skandalakis JE. Wandering spleen: anatomic and radiologic considerations. South Med J 1992;85:976-984; with permission.)

two, or more splenic nodules of small size that are completely separated from the main organ.

## Wandering Spleen

Although the etiology of wandering spleen may be multifactorial, the most compelling evidence points toward an error in the embryologic development of the spleen's primary supporting ligaments (Fig. 22-4). The ligaments may be abnormal (too long, too short, too wide, too narrow, abnormally fused) or absent. Laxity of these ligaments and abnormal length of the splenic vessels can result in excessive splenic mobility and therefore, in the phenomenon of ptotic (wandering) spleen.

Six ligaments (gastrosplenic, splenorenal, splenophrenic, splenocolic, and pancreatosplenic ligaments, and presplenic fold) are directly associated with the spleen. Two others (pancreaticocolic and phrenicocolic) are indirectly associated with the spleen. Most of the literature holds the gastrosplenic, splenorenal, and phrenicocolic ligaments responsible for ptosis of the spleen. Allen et al.[2] suggested

that from an anatomic standpoint, the other ligaments (especially the splenocolic ligament) also participate in the development of ptosis of the spleen (Fig. 22-5).

Due to its abnormal fixation, the wandering spleen is susceptible to infarction as a result of twisting about its elongated vascular pedicle.[3] Clinically the wandering spleen, whether infarcted or not, can present as either an acute or a chronic process: it can appear as an asymptomatic mass, a mass with pain, or an acute abdomen.[4] In the pediatric population, Desai et al.[3] recommend surgical splenopexy as definitive treatment except in cases of infarction. However, splenectomy should be done if there is no evidence of blood flow to the spleen.[3]

Wandering spleen is a rare clinical diagnosis, particularly in the pediatric population.[5] In a review of 97 cases of wandering spleen with torsion of the pedicle, Abell[6] found only one patient under 10 years of age. A review of the literature by Allen and Andrews[7] yielded only 35 cases in children younger than 10. Wandering spleen that produced small-bowel obstruction in a neonate was reported by Gosselin and Chou.[8] Spector and Chappell[9] reported

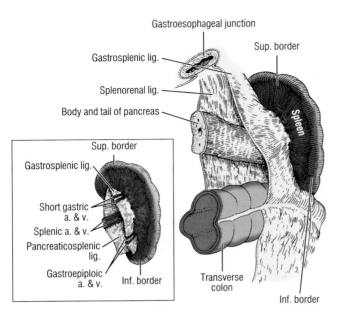

FIG 22-4. Peritoneal attachments of the spleen. *Inset:* Hilum of the spleen, showing the short gastric and gastroepiploic vessels in the gastrosplenic ligament. (Modified from Skandalakis JE, Gray SW, Rowe JS Jr. Anatomical Complications in General Surgery. New York: McGraw-Hill, 1983; with permission.)

wandering spleen associated with gastric volvulus in a 5-year-old, in whom "normal ligamentous connections between the stomach, spleen, and posterior abdominal wall were absent. Developmental anomalies that result in wandering spleen may lead to hypermobility of the stomach and a predisposition to gastric volvulus. In such patients, prophylactic gastropexy should be considered."

## *Splenogonadal Fusion*

Splenic tissue is known to fuse with male and female gonads, as well as with the pancreas and liver. The latter two organs are derived from the caudal foregut, with which the development of the spleen is physically closely related although it is not a foregut derivative. In males splenogonadal fusion is indicated by the presence of splenic tissue in the left scrotum. As rare as the condition is, it is occasionally associated with two other rare defects: ectromelia and micrognathia. Splenogonadal fusion with limb deficiency and micrognathia was reported by Moore et al.[10]

The literature contains differing classifications of splenogonadal fusion. Putschar and Manion[11] termed the condition *continuous* when there is a cord of splenic tissue or a

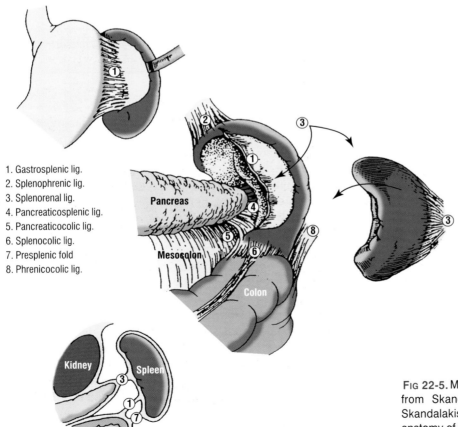

1. Gastrosplenic lig.
2. Splenophrenic lig.
3. Splenorenal lig.
4. Pancreaticosplenic lig.
5. Pancreaticocolic lig.
6. Splenocolic lig.
7. Presplenic fold
8. Phrenicocolic lig.

FIG 22-5. Major and minor splenic ligaments. (Modified from Skandalakis JE, Colborn GL, Pemberton LB, Skandalakis PN, Skandalakis LJ, Gray SW. The surgical anatomy of the spleen. Probl Gen Surg 1990; 7:1-17; with permission.)

fibrous formation between the main spleen and the go-nadal-mesonephric structures, and *discontinuous* when discrete masses of splenic tissue are found fused to these structures. Le Roux and Heddle[12] proposed that "contin-uous splenogonadal fusion with or without limb defects and micrognathia constitutes one syndrome... discontin-uous splenogonadal fusion amounts to no more than a rare variant of an accessory spleen." The authors of this chapter agree.

To correct splenogonadal fusion, surgery is the treat-ment of choice and is performed as follows in males:

1. Sever the band connecting the spleen with the left scrotum if obstruction is present
2. Remove the nodule with or without orchidectomy
3. Repair coexisting left indirect hernia

Splenogonadal fusion is far less common in women than in men. According to Gouw et al.,[13] of 84 reported cases of splenogonadal fusion only 6 were females. Nonetheless, the phenomenon of splenic pregnancy has been reported. Alcaly et al.[14] believes that primary splenic pregnancy is the rarest form of extrauterine pregnancy. There are fewer than 10 cases in the literature.[15-17]

Can mesonephric tissue produce splenic tissue (a very bizarre ectopia)? The authors do not know.

## *Splenic Cysts*

Congenital splenic cysts are lined with epithelium. In 1970 Talerman and Hart[18] reported several hundred ep-ithelial cysts. Most of these cases involved children and young adults. Panossian et al.[19] reported an epidermoid cyst of the spleen as a generalized peritonitis. The authors reviewed 159 cases, adding one of their own and advising splenectomy and an antibiotic regimen, including cover-age for *Salmonella* infection.

## *Accessory Spleens*

Accessory spleens are found in one fifth to one third of autopsies.[20] Seventy-five percent of accessory spleens are located at the hilum (splenic porta). Although it may be possible for several accessory spleens to be found at the hilum, rarely is accessory splenic tissue found in more than two locations.[21]

The following is an analysis of 602 males whose ac-cessory spleens were discovered at autopsy[22,23]:

|  | *Number of cases* |
|---|---|
| One accessory spleen | 519 |
| Two accessory spleens | 65 |
| Three accessory spleens | 13 |
| Four accessory spleens | 3 |
| Five accessory spleens | 2 |

Curtis and Movitz[21] reported a case with 10 accessory spleens. Abu-Hijleh[24] reported 11 accessory spleens in a cadaver, with diameters from 0.5 cm to 6.0 cm. The lo-cations of the accessory spleens in the splenic area were as follows: 2 at the hilum, 5 at the gastrosplenic ligament, and 4 at the splenorenal ligament.

We quote from Habib et al.[25]:

> *Accessory spleens are not infrequent and occur in 11 to 44 per cent of the population with a greater inci-dence in those with hematological disease. They may remain clinically silent or result in a number of patho-logic processes. Abscess of an accessory spleen is rare but must be considered in the differential diagno-sis of fever of unknown origin or sepsis in select groups of patients. Computerized tomography is the imaging modality of choice and may also be used in the per-cutaneous drainage of select cases. Laparoscopic splenectomy in the hands of the experienced laparoen-doscopic surgeon is a viable treatment option.*

Wekerle et al.[26] reported intrahepatic splenic tissue in a patient with recurrent idiopathic thrombocytopenic pur-pura.

## *Splenosis*

Splenic tissue in the peritoneal cavity may be produced by autotransplantation secondary to injury. Although the majority of cases are asymptomatic, there have been iso-lated reports in the literature of splenosis producing intesti-nal obstruction from adhesions, pain resulting from tor-sion, and stomach masses simulating carcinoma.[27] Metwally and Ravo[28] stated that the theory that splenosis is beneficial for a patient with an infection is controversial.

# SURGICAL ANATOMY OF THE SPLEEN

## Topography and Relations

The spleen is located in the left upper quadrant of the abdomen in a niche formed by the diaphragm above it (posterolateral). The stomach is located medially (antero-medial), the left kidney and left adrenal gland posteriorly (posteromedial), the phrenicocolic ligament below, and the chest wall (the ninth to eleventh left ribs) laterally. The tail of the pancreas in most cases is related to the splenic hilum. The spleen is concealed at the left hypochondrium. It is not palpable under normal conditions.

The spleen is associated with the posterior portions of

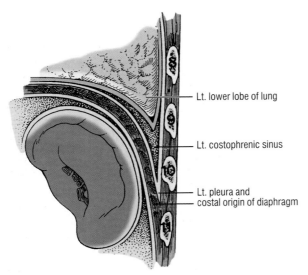

FIG 22-6. Location of the spleen. (Modified from Skandalakis JE, Colborn GL, Pemberton LB, Skandalakis PN, Skandalakis LJ, Gray SW. The surgical anatomy of the spleen. Probl Gen Surg 1990; 7:1-17; with permission.)

the left ninth, tenth, and eleventh ribs. It is separated from them by the diaphragm and the costodiaphragmatic recess (Fig. 22-6). The spleen is oriented obliquely. Its upper end is situated some 5 cm from the dorsal midline, approximating the level of the spinous processes of the tenth and eleventh thoracic vertebrae. The lower end lies just behind the midaxillary line. The long axis of the organ roughly parallels the course of the tenth rib. On roentgenograms, the spleen is typically about 5 cm wide and 14 cm long. The spleen descends about 2 to 5 cm with deep inspiration.[29]

If one divides the spleen into three parts, the upper third is related to the lower lobe of the left lung, the middle third to the left costodiaphragmatic recess, and the lower third to the left pleura and costal origin of the diaphragm.

### Size of the Spleen

The spleen can be very small or very large. The extremes are 1 ounce and 20 pounds, as reported by Gould and Pyle.[30] Spleens of extreme size may be healthy or diseased.

The size of the spleen can change readily, enlarging with increases in blood pressure. The size increases after meals; conversely, its size decreases during exercise or immediately postmortem. The lymphoid tissue of the spleen, like lymphoid tissue elsewhere in the body, undergoes diminution sometime after the patient reaches the age of 10 years.[31] There is some involution of the organ as a whole after the age of 60 years.

Under normal conditions, the long axis of the organ runs parallel to the tenth rib. With splenomegaly, the spleen is palpable below the left costal margin, with its long axis extending down and forward along the tenth rib.[32,33]

Harris's odd numbers 1, 3, 5, 7, 9, and 11 (as reported by Last[33]) help one memorize certain average dimensions of the spleen:

- The spleen measures 1 × 3 × 5 inches (2.5 × 7.5 × 12.5 cm)
- The spleen weighs 7 oz (220 g)
- The spleen relates to left ribs 9 through 11

### Shape of the Spleen

According to Michels,[34] the spleen has three forms. It is wedge-shaped in 44% of specimens, tetrahedral in 42%, and triangular in 14% (Fig. 22-7).

A more useful system, also suggested by Michels,[34] notes two forms of the spleen (Fig. 22-8). The first (30%) is a compact type of spleen with almost even borders and a narrow hilum in which the arterial branches are few and

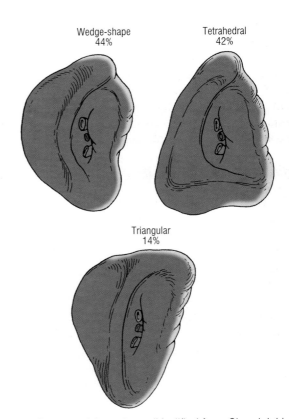

FIG 22-7. Shapes of the spleen. (Modified from Skandalakis JE, Colborn GL, Pemberton LB, Skandalakis PN, Skandalakis LJ, Gray SW. The surgical anatomy of the spleen. Probl Gen Surg 1990; 7:1-17; with permission.)

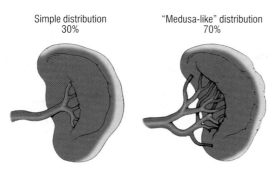

Simple distribution
30%

"Medusa-like" distribution
70%

**FIG 22-8.** Classification of spleen shape based on general arterial distribution. (Adapted and modified from Skandalakis JE, Colborn GL, Pemberton LB, Skandalakis PN, Skandalakis LJ, Gray SW. The surgical anatomy of the spleen. Probl Gen Surg 1990; 7:1-17; with permission.)

large. The second (70%) is a distributed type, with notched borders and a large hilum, in which the arterial branches are small and numerous.

In an enlarged spleen the notched anterior border, when present, can be palpated. Michels[34] advised surgeons that spleens with notched borders have multiple (more than two) arteries entering the medial surface. Polar arteries are common in this type of spleen. Consequently, a spleen with a notched anterior border is difficult to remove. However, in our small number of dissections in the laboratory and in our splenectomies in the operating room, we have observed these differences of vascular distribution on both notched and unnotched spleens. Therefore, an unnotched spleen does not necessarily indicate a limited vascular distribution.

## *Surfaces and Borders of the Spleen*

For all practical purposes, the spleen has two surfaces: parietal and visceral. The convex parietal surface is related to the diaphragm; the concave visceral surface is related to the surfaces of the stomach, kidney, colon, and tail of the pancreas. On the concave hilar surface, the entrance and exit of the splenic vessels at the splenic portas in most specimens form the letter S, which is evident if one connects the upper polar, hilar, and lower polar vessels.

The spleen has two borders (Fig. 22-9): the superior (anterior) and the inferior (posterior). The superior border separates the gastric area from the diaphragmatic area, and the inferior border separates the renal area from the diaphragmatic area.

## *Surgical Applications*

• A patient with fractures of the left ninth to eleventh ribs

should be observed closely. Such a patient is a candidate for an underlying splenic rupture. In a child, however, the spleen may rupture without rib fractures. We have seen spontaneous rupture of the pediatric spleen in the presence of diseases such as malaria, kala azar, and mononucleosis.

• Morrell et al.[35] reported a thirty-year trend in the growth of splenorrhaphy and observation instead of splenectomy for splenic injury treatment. In a study of trauma patients with blunt splenic injury, Goodley et al.[36] found that nonoperative management was ineffective for older patients.

• In a patient with empyema, a thoracic surgeon inadvertently placed a left thoracotomy tube through the left hemidiaphragm and into the upper pole of the spleen. Bleeding and a left subdiaphragmatic abscess ensued. With splenectomy, drainage, and large doses of antibiotics, the patient survived (JES, unpublished results).

• In a series of articles, Moody[37] and Moody et al.[38,39] stated that the lower splenic pole is variable in position. It can relate to the upper half of the first lumbar vertebra or, more inferiorly, to the upper half of the fifth lumbar vertebra. Most frequently, it is related to the upper third of the third lumbar vertebra.

• In splenomegaly, the spleen is always located in front of the splenic flexure of the colon. Adhesions are almost always present and are sometimes vascular. Often, an enlarged spleen has extensive adhesions to the colon. In elective splenectomies, intestinal preparation is essential if splenomegaly is present. The size of the spleen will dictate the type of incision (see "Incision" in this chapter). Remember what Arthur H. Keeney[40] stated: "Pray before surgery, but remember God will not alter a faulty incision."

• A notched spleen has multiple arteries that should be

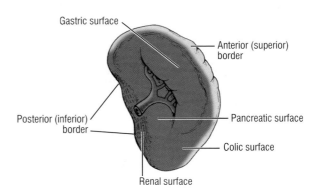

Gastric surface

Anterior (superior) border

Posterior (inferior) border

Pancreatic surface

Colic surface

Renal surface

**FIG 22-9.** Splenic borders. (Modified from Skandalakis JE, Colborn GL, Pemberton LB, Skandalakis PN, Skandalakis LJ, Gray SW. The surgical anatomy of the spleen. Probl Gen Surg 1990; 7:1-17; with permission.)

carefully ligated, one-by-one, close to the splenic porta (hilum). But remember, an unnotched spleen could also have an extreme vascular distribution.

- The concave visceral surface should be handled with care. The small, short gastric veins retract instantly and therefore, require meticulous individual ligation. The tail of the pancreas should be separated from the spleen with great care to avoid pancreatic injury. If present, the pancreaticosplenic ligament should be ligated.
- The posterior splenic border is related to the renal and diaphragmatic areas; separation of tissues should be toward the diaphragm to avoid injury to the renal capsule.
- The convex parietal surface of the spleen is related to the diaphragm. It is avascular in most cases, but it would be wise to ligate the splenophrenic ligament, whether it is short or long.
- By applying knowledge of the simple guidelines to the surgical anatomy of the spleen as described above, the surgeon can examine the shape, surfaces, and borders of the spleen and perhaps better anticipate potential troubles that may arise during splenectomy. If the surgeon is careful and proceeds slowly, he or she can avoid bleeding from the spleen, from the greater curvature of the stomach, and perhaps from the capsule of the left kidney.

### Segmental Anatomy

Knowledge of the anatomic phenomenon of splenic segmentation is imperative for segmental resection. Kyber[41] may have been the first to suggest splenic segmentation. Skandalakis et al.[42] reported, however, that there is no consistent segmental arterial anatomy. Furthermore, the existence of arterial collaterals prevents stan-

dardized anatomic partial splenectomy based on blood supply. Remember that the segmentation of the spleen can be explained embryologically: the organ is formed by the fusion of vascularized, isolated mesenchymal aggregates.

Segmentation of the spleen appears to be variable (as is its description in the literature). Gupta et al.[43] reported that the spleens examined had two lobes (superior and inferior) or three lobes (superior, middle, and inferior). In a study of 66 full-term newborn infants, Mandarim-Lacerda et al.[44] found two lobar branches in a majority of splenic specimens (Fig. 22-10); the other specimens had either three or four lobar branches. In a study of 850 spleens Liu et al.[45] found that there are two lobar arteries in most splenic specimens; the other specimens had three, one, or four lobar arteries (Fig. 22-11). These data are compiled into a single table for the purposes of comparison (Table 22-2). (See "Branches of the splenic artery" below for more discussion of this topic.)

The number of segments or segmental arteries varies considerably also (Fig. 22-12, Fig. 22-13). Liu and colleagues[45] reported finding three to eight segmental arteries in a subgroup of specimens. In the same study, 83% of the

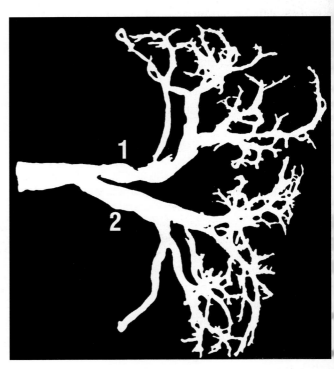

**FIG 22-10.** Cast of the spleen with a bifurcated splenic artery. 1, superior segment, 2, inferior segment. (From Mandarim-Lacerda CA, Sampaio FJB, Passos MARF. Segmentation vasculaire de la rate chez le nouveau-ne. J Chir (Paris) 1983; 120:471-73; with permission.)

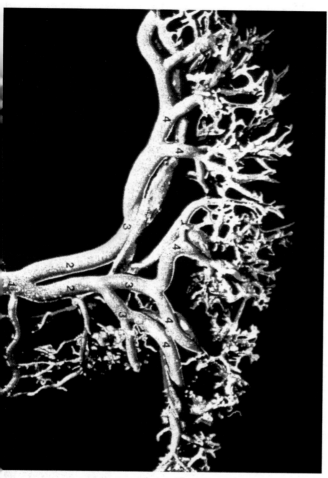

FIG 22-11. Vasculature of splenic hilum and intraspleen. 1. Common splenic artery; 2. Lobar arteries; 3. Segmental arteries; 4. Submental arteries. Relatively avascular planes between lobes or segments are observed. (From Liu DL, Xia S, Xu W, Qifa Y, Gao Y, Qian J. Anatomy of vasculature of 850 spleen specimens and its application in partial splenectomy. Surgery 1996;119:27-33; with permission.)

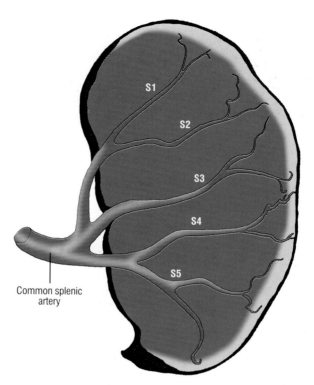

FIG 22-12. Arrangement of intrasplenic vasculature manifests transverse pattern of arterial supply to lobes or segments. Spleen is defined as having three to five segments. Anatomically, they are named in sequence of segment 1 to segment 5 from superior pole to inferior pole (S1-S5). (Modified from Liu DL, Xia S, Xu W, Qifa Y, Gao Y, Qian J. Anatomy of vasculature of 850 spleen specimens and its application in partial splenectomy. Surgery 1996;119:27-33; with permission.)

spleens examined had polar arteries (Table 22-3). Redmond et al.[46] found three to seven segments among

**TABLE 22-2. Distribution of "Lobes," "Lobar Branches," and "Lobar Arteries" in Splenic Specimens from Three Studies**

|  | 1 | 2 | 3 | 4 |
|---|---|---|---|---|
| Gupta et al. ("lobes") |  | 84% | 16% |  |
| Mandarim-Lacerda et al. ("lobar branches")* |  | 68.2% | 10.6% | 4.5% |
| Liu et al. ("lobar arteries") | 0.8% | 86% | 12.2% | 1% |

*Remaining 16.7% of specimens had intersegmental anastomoses

**References**

Gupta CD, Gupta SC, Aorara AK, Singh P. Vascular segments in the human spleen. J Anat 1976; 121:613-616.

Mandarim-Lacerda CA, Sampaio FJ, Passos MA. Segmentation vasculaire de la rate chez le nouveau-ne: support anatomique pour la resection partielle. J Chir (Paris) 1983; 120:471.

Liu DL, Xia S, Xu W, Qifa Y, Gao Y, Qian J. Anatomy of vasculature of 850 spleen specimens and its application in partial splenectomy. Surgery 1996; 119:27-33.

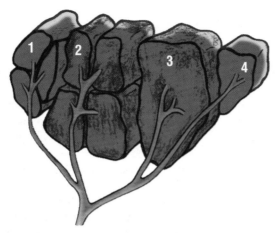

FIG 22-13. Diagram illustrating segments and subsegments. 1, polar subsegment; 2, central subsegment; 3, central segment; 4 polar segment. (Modified from Redmond HP, Redmond JM, Rooney BP, Duignan JP, Bouchier-Hayes DJ. Surgical anatomy of the human spleen. Br J Surg 1989, 76:198-201; with permission.)

**TABLE 22-3. Distribution of Polar Arteries in 280 Splenic Specimens**

| No. of Spleen Specimens | SPA (%) | IPA (%) | SIPA (%) |
|---|---|---|---|
| 280 | 31.3 | 38.8 | 13.3 |

SPA, Superior polar artery; IPA, inferior polar artery; SIPA, superior and inferior polar arteries.

*Source:* Liu DL, Xia S, Xu W, Qifa Y, Gao Y, Qian J. Anatomy of vasculature of 850 spleen specimens and its application in partial splenectomy. Surgery 1996; 119:27-33; with permission.

their specimens (Fig. 22-14), and Voboril[47] reported finding as many as 10 splenic segments. The vasculature of each segment appears to be largely independent of that of its neighboring segments.

There is confusion in the literature about the terms splenic *lobe, pole,* and *segment.* Extrasplenic bifurcation of the splenic artery will produce two lobes, superior and inferior. However, further bifurcation or trifurcation often occurs and this gives rise to the vasculature of segments and poles. We propose that the term *segments* be used when referring to splenic parts separated by avascular planes, elsewhere called lobes. In surgery we speak of splenic segmentectomy and not about lobectomy or polectomy.

The planes separating segments or subsegments are usually obliquely situated with respect to the long axis, and often do not traverse the full thickness of the spleen from the visceral to the parietal surface.[48]

Segmentation can also be observed with respect to the venous drainage of the spleen. Dreyer and Budtz-Olson[49] reported venous segmentation of the spleen. Dawson et al.[48] found that 71% of spleens had two lobes and 29% had three. In half of the specimens the lobes were further subdivided into two segments. The avascular lines of separation of the lobes followed those of the arteries. In more than half of the specimens, the lines of lobar separation could be equated with marginal notching of the splenic border. The veins emanating from the lobes were individually accessible at the hilum. Examination of doubly injected (arterial and venous vessels) specimens confirmed that neither the arterial nor the venous supply to the lobes or segments crossed to adjacent parenchyma.

Garcia-Porrero and Lemes,[50] using radiopaque injection media, found anastomoses between splenic arterial branches, especially between secondary branches, in about 30.5% of specimens. This low frequency of intrasplenic anastomoses was noted also by Mandarim-Lacerda et al.,[44] who reported that 16.7% of specimens from full-term infants had intersegmental anastomoses (Fig. 22-15). They concluded that segmental splenic resection is possible in infants as well as adults.

Dixon et al.[51] stated that intrasplenic vessels are lobar, segmented, and generally without intersegmental communication (Fig. 22-16). They conceived of the spleen as being divided into three-dimensional zones referred to as hilar, intermediate, and peripheral. Each zone requires a special technique for hemostasis. They advised conservative treatment such as the application of microfibrillar collagen to the exposed surface for the peripheral zone (arteriole and venous injury), and ligation for the intermediate and hilar zones (to take care of trabecular and segmental vessels).

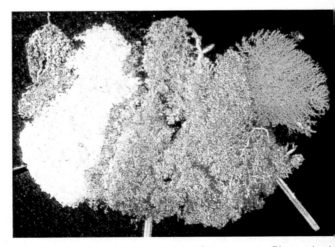

FIG 22-14. Cast of a spleen containing five segments. Blue and yellow, polar; white, green and red, central. Note the avascular planes between the segments. (From Redmond HP, Redmond JM, Rooney BP, Duignan JP, Bouchier-Hayes DJ. Surgical anatomy of the human spleen. Br J Surg 1989, 76:198-201; with permission.)

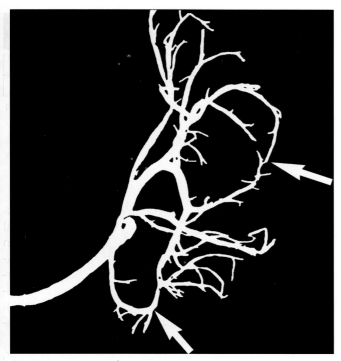

FIG 22-15. Cast of a spleen containing anastomoses between the inferior and superior segments. (From Mandarim-Lacerda CA, Sampaio FJB, Passos MARF. Segmentation vasculaire de la rate chez le nouveau-ne. J Chir (Paris) 1983; 120:471-73; with permission.)

## Spaces of the Left Upper Quadrant

The left suprahepatic space is bounded medially by the falciform ligament and superiorly by the left anterior coronary ligament and the left triangular ligament. Inferiorly, the space opens into the general peritoneal cavity.

The left infrahepatic space is subdivided into anterior and posterior spaces by the hepatogastric ligament, the stomach, and the gastrocolic ligament. The anterior space is the perigastric space; the posterior space is the lesser sac. The healthy spleen is closely related to the lesser sac, which is almost closed by the splenorenal and gastrosplenic ligaments.

In splenomegaly, the long axis of the spleen is directed down and forward, following the orientation of the tenth rib. It is parallel with the greater curvature of the stomach, and extends toward the umbilicus, in front of the left transverse colon and the splenic flexure. This oblique splenic axis is usual. Rarely, the axis is vertical or even transverse. These patterns further complicate the understanding of the perisplenic space.

The surfaces, borders, and topographic anatomy of the spleen all help radiologists to more accurately view and interpret the anatomy and condition of the spleen.

## Peritoneum and Ligaments of the Spleen

The right and left layers of the greater omentum separate to enclose the spleen almost completely, except at the hilum, providing its serosal covering, or capsule (see Figs. 22-2, 22-3 and 22-17). The capsule formed by the visceral peritoneum is as friable as the spleen itself and as easily injured (see Fig. 22-4).

The peritoneal layers that enclose and suspend the spleen form the two chief ligaments of the spleen, the gastrosplenic ligament and the splenorenal ligament. These are portions of the embryonic dorsal mesentery, or mesogastrium, the leaves of which separate to surround the spleen. These two ligaments form the splenic pedicle (Fig. 22-18).

In addition to the two chief ligaments, there are several minor splenic ligaments and other topographically related ligaments, the names of which indicate their connections. These are the splenophrenic ligament, splenocolic ligament, pancreaticosplenic ligament, presplenic fold, phrenicocolic ligament, and pancreaticocolic ligament (see Fig. 22-5).

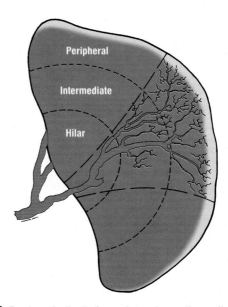

FIG 22-16. Regions indicated are shaped as a three-dimensional cone described by the length of a radius originating at the point of entrance of the major artery into the spleen. All regions contain penicilli, venules, and sinuses with addition of larger vessels as the hilum is approached. (Modified from Dixon JA, Miller F, McCloskey D, Siddoway J. Anatomy and techniques in segmental splenectomy. Surg Gynecol Obstet 1980;150:518; with permission.)

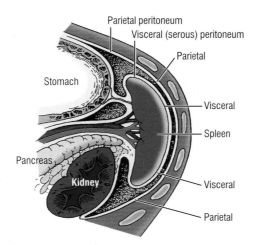

FIG 22-17. Sagittal view of peritoneum covering the spleen. (Modified from Skandalakis JE, Colborn GL, Pemberton LB, Skandalakis PN, Skandalakis LJ, Gray SW. The surgical anatomy of the spleen. Probl Gen Surg 1990; 7:1-17; with permission.)

## Gastrosplenic Ligament

The portion of the dorsal mesentery between the stomach and the spleen is the gastrosplenic ligament. Whitesell[52] suggested that the ligament is best thought of as a triangle (Fig. 22-19). The two sides are the upper portion of the greater curvature of the stomach and the medial border of the spleen. At the apex of this triangle, the superior pole of the spleen lies close to the stomach and may be fixed to it. At the base of the triangle, the inferior pole of the spleen lies 5 to 7 cm from the stomach. The more cranial part of the gastrosplenic ligament contains the short gastric arteries, and the more caudal part contains the left gastroepiploic vessels.

At the apex of the triangle just described, the leaves of the mesentery are reflected to the posterior body wall and the inferior surface of the diaphragm as the splenophrenic ligament. Perhaps the splenophrenic ligament is a reflection of the gastrosplenic ligament to the diaphragm. Remember the presence of this entity during surgery of the spleen. In 80% of bodies examined, Whitesell[52] found smooth muscle fibers within the gastrosplenic ligament in its passage from the cardia of the stomach to the superior pole of the spleen. The muscle was well developed in some specimens and attenuated in others. Division of these muscle fibers mobilizes the superior pole of the spleen.

## Splenorenal Ligament

The splenorenal ligament is the posterior portion of the primitive dorsal mesogastrium. It envelops the splenic

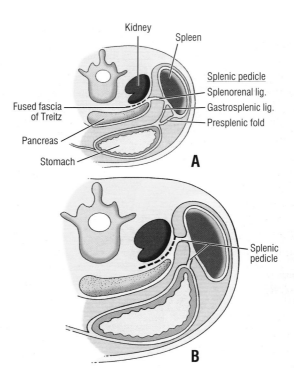

FIG 22-18. The splenic pedicle. A. Long pedicle with a presplenic fold. B. Short pedicle. (Modified from Skandalakis JE, Gray SW, Rowe JS. Anatomical Complications in General Surgery. New York: McGraw-Hill, 1983; 178; with permission.)

vessels and the tail of the pancreas. Incision of the peritoneal layer of this ligament, together with mobilization of the tail of the pancreas, reestablishes the primitive condition. It is curious that the existence of the splenorenal ligament is often overlooked. In ten operating room reports selected at random, there was no mention made of the liga-

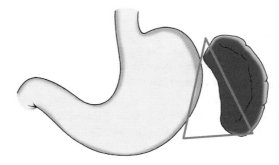

FIG 22-19. The gastrosplenic ligament connects the stomach and spleen. The two organs may be in contact superiorly, and the ligament is short. Inferiorly, the two organs are 5 to 7 cm apart and the ligament is longer. (Modified from Skandalakis JE, Gray SW, Rowe JS. Anatomical Complications in General Surgery. New York: McGraw-Hill, 1983; 177; with permission.)

ment, even though it obviously was encountered in the course of surgery.[53]

The outer layer of the gastrosplenic ligament forms the posterior layer of the splenorenal ligament. Therefore, careless division of the former can injure the short gastric vessels. Bleeding from these vessels may be the result of too-enthusiastic deep posterior excavation by the index and middle fingers of an operator seeking to mobilize and retract the spleen to the right.

The splenic pedicle can be narrow or wide, depending on the extent to which the primitive dorsal mesogastrium was absorbed into the body wall (see Fig. 22-18). The degree of effective mobilization of the spleen depends not on the splenorenal ligament, but on the length of the splenic vessels after incision of the ligament. A short splenic artery can make it impossible to deliver the spleen out of the abdomen. Gently pushing the tail of the pancreas away from the hilum of the spleen can increase splenic mobility.

Rosen et al.[54] reported that the length of the splenorenal ligament ranges from 2.5 to 5.5 cm. The relations between the pancreatic tail and the splenic porta (hilum) are as follows:
- 24.0% tail did not penetrate the ligament
- 32.0% tail was within the ligament and did not reach the porta
- 29.7% tail reached the porta
- 13.0% tail passed over the hilum and penetrated the gastrosplenic ligament

The above authors classified the variations of the splenorenal ligament and the tail of the pancreas into four groups:
- Type I: short ligament enveloped the tail
- Type II: short ligament not penetrated by the tail
- Type III: long ligament enveloped the tail
- Type IV: long ligament not penetrated by the tail.

## Splenophrenic Ligament

The splenophrenic ligament (see Fig. 22-5) may be said to be the reflection of the leaves of the mesentery to both the posterior body wall and to the inferior surface of the diaphragm at the area of the upper pole of the spleen close to the stomach. According to O'Rahilly,[55] it is not known if the splenophrenic ligament gives rise to the splenorenal ligament from its lower part. It may be that the splenophrenic ligament is a reflection of the gastrosplenic ligament to the diaphragm.

Seufert and Mitrou[56] suggest that the splenophrenic ligament contains the tail of the pancreas and all the splenic vessels. We believe that normally the splenorenal ligament

is their home. If, however, the splenophrenic ligament reaches the hilum, then it may contain the tail of the pancreas and all the splenic vessels, including the root of the left gastroepiploic artery. The surgeon should remember the splenophrenic ligament during splenic surgery. It is usually avascular, but it should be inspected for possible bleeding after section.

## Splenocolic Ligament

The splenocolic ligament (see Fig. 22-5, Fig. 22-20) is a remnant of the extreme left end of the transverse mesocolon. The mesocolon develops a secondary attachment to the spleen during embryonic fixation of the colon to the body wall. Because it is a secondary attachment, one would expect it to contain no large blood vessels. However, tortuous or aberrant inferior polar vessels of the spleen or a left gastroepiploic artery can lie close enough to be injured by careless incision of the ligament, possibly resulting in massive bleeding.[34]

## Pancreaticosplenic Ligament

The pancreaticosplenic ligament (see Fig. 22-5, Fig. 22-20) is said to be present when the tail of the pancreas does not touch the spleen. This cordlike formation is usually thin.

## Presplenic Fold

Henry[57] called attention to a peritoneal fold anterior to the gastrosplenic ligament (see Figs. 22-5, 22-18). The fold is usually free on its lateral border, but in a large, diseased spleen, it may be attached. Such a fold may be derived from the anterior limb of the inverted-Y arrangement of some hili.[58] The presplenic fold often contains the left gastroepiploic vessels. Excessive traction during upper abdominal operations can result in a tear in the splenic capsule, which will require conservative procedures for splenic salvage.

## Phrenicocolic Ligament

The phrenicocolic ligament (see Figs. 22-5, 22-20) develops at the region of the junction of the midgut and the hindgut, after the descending colon has become retroperitoneal. It is the rudimentary left end of the transverse mesocolon. Smooth muscle cells migrate into the ligament from the mesocolic taeniae. The ligament fixes the splenic flexure in place. Moreover, the development of the upper abdominal organs results in a descent of the spleen and contact of the caudal pole of the spleen with the liga-

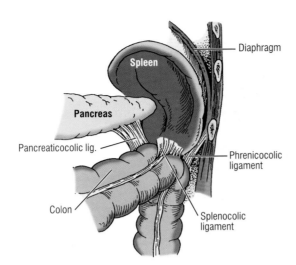

FIG 22-20. Relation of the pancreaticocolic, phrenicocolic, and splenocolic ligaments to the spleen. (Modified from Skandalakis JE, Colborn GL, Pemberton LB, Skandalakis PN, Skandalakis LJ, Gray SW. The surgical anatomy of the spleen. Probl Gen Surg 1990; 7:1-17; with permission.)

ment. As the spleen continues to grow, the phrenicocolic ligament is deformed, forming a pocket for the spleen.[59]

The phrenicocolic ligament extends between the splenic flexure and the diaphragm. It is not an intrinsic ligament of the spleen, but the spleen rests upon it. It is the "splenic floor," but it is not connected to the spleen.

The surgeon should remember that the phrenicocolic ligament acts as a barricade at the left paracolic gutter. It is responsible, in most instances, for prohibiting blood from a ruptured splenic artery, or from the spleen itself, from traveling downward. Such blood collects at the anterior pararenal space retroperitoneally, or around the spleen at the left upper quadrant by displacing the colon laterally.

It is a mistake to call the phrenicocolic ligament the left phrenicocolic ligament because there is no right phrenicocolic ligament. There is but one phrenicocolic ligament, and it is on the left side.[60]

### Pancreaticocolic Ligament

The pancreaticocolic ligament (see Figs. 22-5, 22-20) is the upper extension of the transverse mesocolon.

There is a degree of ambiguity about the three "colic" ligaments: the pancreaticocolic, the splenocolic, and the phrenicocolic. Do these peritoneal folds belong to the transverse mesocolon? Most likely, the answer is yes.

### Other Peritoneal Folds

One of the authors of this chapter, John Skandalakis,

has seen several unnamed peritoneal folds in the laboratory as well as in the operating room. Morgenstern[61] was right when he stated that clear descriptions of these are absent from anatomic textbooks. The fold that is most constant and that Skandalakis observed several times is an avascular peritoneal fold from the left upper portion of the omentum to the medial part of the lower segment of the spleen, and especially to the lower pole of the spleen (Fig 22-21). Morgenstern called this the "criminal fold," since careless traction may traumatize the spleen. Skandalakis calls this the *spleno-omental "criminal" fold of Morgenstern.* Rarely, Skandalakis has observed separate ligamentous bands interconnecting the summit of the convex surface of the spleen with the diaphragm. Obviously, rough handling of such an organ could lead readily to rupture of the capsule.

There has been controversy as to whether another avascular fold, the sustentaculum lienis (Fig. 22-22), supports the spleen. It is rarely seen in open surgery, but Poulin and Thibault[62] wrote that it is readily seen through the laparoscope, and they described it as follows:

> The phrenicocolic ligament courses from the diaphragm to the splenic flexure of the colon; its superior end is referred to as the phrenosplenic ligament.[63] The attachment of the lower pole on the internal side is called the splenocolic ligament. Between these two, a horizontal shelf is formed on which rests the inferior pole of the spleen. It is often moulded into a sac that opens cranially and is called the sustentaculum lienis, acting as a brassière to the inferior pole of the spleen.

### Surgical Applications

- The short gastric vessels and the left gastroepiploic vessels should be ligated individually. The gastrosplenic ligament should be incised between clamps.
- The splenorenal ligament is itself avascular, but it envelops the splenic vessels and the tail of the pancreas. Incision and finger excavation to mobilize the organ should be done with care.
- Traction upon the splenophrenic ligament, if the ligament is short, can result in bleeding of the spleen, due to a tear of the capsule. Do not apply more traction than is necessary.
- The splenocolic ligament, in close relation to the lower polar vessels of the spleen and the left gastroepiploic vessels, should be incised between clamps.
- The presplenic fold is close to the left gastroepiploic vessels. Excessive traction can result in bleeding.
- The pancreaticosplenic ligament, if present and long enough, should be incised between clamps. If this liga-

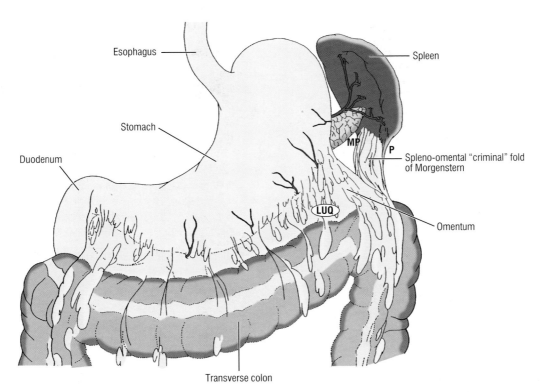

**FIG 22-21.** Highly diagrammatic presentation of the spleno-omental "criminal" fold of Morgenstern from the left upper quadrant (LUQ) of the omentum to the medial part (MP) of the lower splenic segment and lower pole (P).

ment is absent or short, careful separation of the pancreatic tail from the spleen is necessary to avoid pancreatic or splenic injury.

- If the phrenicocolic ligament is short or fused, injury of the lower pole of the spleen or the splenic flexure of the colon is unlikely, but possible.
- Careless traction of a short or fused pancreaticocolic ligament can also lead to colonic or pancreatic injury.
- Remember that the Morgenstern fold should be divided carefully to avoid splenic capsular avulsion.

## Splenic Mobility

### Key Structures Affecting Splenic Mobility

The mobility of the spleen depends on the degree of laxity of both the splenic ligaments and the splenic blood vessels. We believe that only four of the ligaments can affect the position of the spleen in most cases. These are the gastrosplenic, splenorenal, splenocolic, and phrenicocolic ligaments (Fig. 22-22).

The limitation of movement of the spleen due to the gastrosplenic ligament depends on the mobility of the sto-

mach. If the left kidney is fixed in its normal position without other abnormalities, the splenorenal ligament may play a small role. It is well known to radiologists that the left transverse colon and the splenic flexure are not displaced by renal tumors, and it is well known to clinicians that colonic resonance is present in that area. It appears that the restraint to the spleen provided by the splenocolic ligament depends on the mobility of the transverse colon and the splenic flexure. A low splenic flexure contributes to mobility of the spleen. The phrenicocolic ligament limits the downward movement of the spleen. The remaining ligaments appear to have little effect on the movement of the spleen.

Adkins[64] stated that splenoptosis (wandering spleen) can be congenital or acquired. The congenital type is the result of a long splenic pedicle, and the acquired type is a sequela to splenomegaly and a relaxed abdominal wall.

The following questions arise regarding the mobility of the spleen:

- When does ptosis become ectopia (i.e., displacement or malposition)?
- Is ptosis a normal variation?
- Is ectopia a pathologic entity involving several organs secondary to a named pathologic condition?

Radiologists suggest that the following conditions af-

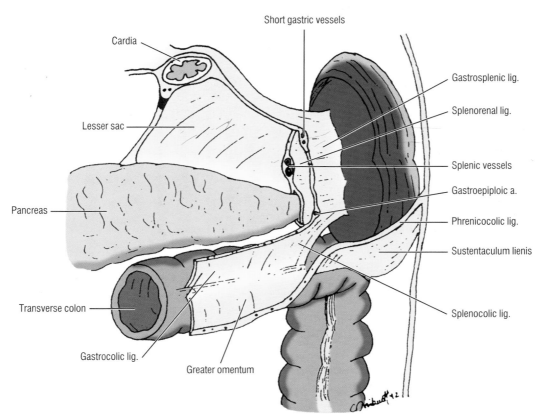

**FIG 22-22.** Suspensory ligaments of the spleen. (Modified from Poulin EC, Thibault C. The anatomic basis for laparoscopic splenectomy. Can J Surg 1993;36:484; with permission.)

fect the position and movement of abdominal organs:[29]
- Posture (gravity)
- Respiratory movements
- Tonus of the abdominal wall and the diaphragm
- Degree of distention of the viscera
- Tonus of the organ
- Intrinsic movements of the viscera
- Pressure of adjacent viscera

If one compares the liver with the spleen, one finds that hepatoptosis does not exist. The liver is fixed by the inferior vena cava and hepatic veins, the upper porta, and the falciform and coronary ligaments. The fixation of the spleen to the left upper quadrant is most likely the result of the combined tethering action of several ligaments, not the result of vessels passing into or leaving the spleen.[64]

Taveras[65] wrote (Fig. 22-23):

*[T]he spine, aorta, and the vena cava are probably the only structures which do not shift with change in position of the body. From the viewpoint of the cephalic end of the subject, all of the movable organs rotate in a counterclockwise direction when the body is turned on its left side, and vice versa when it is turned*

*on its right side. Gravity tends to displace movable structures towards the earth.*

### *Complications Resulting from Adjacent Visceral Pathology*

The reader should remember that the peritoneal covering of the splenic vessels, which is in continuity with the splenic capsule, can be violated by pancreatic fluid during acute pancreatitis. It can also produce an intrasplenic pancreatic pseudocyst with splenic rupture and hemorrhage. McMahon et al.[66] reported one instance of such an event and collected 19 others that had been reported previously.

The route and sequelae of pancreatic pseudocyst complicated by splenic involvement may be described as follows:
- Secretion by the pancreas
- Violation of the peritoneal coverage of the splenic vessels and the splenic portas
- Intrasplenic collection of pancreatic fluid
- Rupture of the splenic capsule
- Bleeding

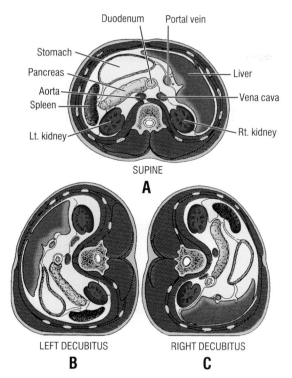

Duodenum    Portal vein

Stomach

Pancreas                                    Liver

Aorta

Spleen                                      Vena cava

Lt. kidney                                  Rt. kidney

SUPINE

**A**

LEFT DECUBITUS          RIGHT DECUBITUS

**B**                    **C**

**FIG 22-23.** Schematic drawing of horizontal sections viewed from the head illustrates Taveras'[65] concept of the mobility of organs caused by change in position. **A.** With the patient in the supine position, the liver and spleen remain in a posterior position. **B.** With the patient in the left lateral decubitus position, the right kidney and descending duodenum drop forward and the left lobe of the liver extends anteriorly toward the stomach, causing a prominent indentation on the anterior surface of the stomach. **C.** With the patient in the right lateral decubitus position, the left kidney and spleen and tail of the pancreas extend forward. The descending duodenum drops laterally and posteriorly, effacing the inferior vena cava. The left lobe of the liver does not indent the anterior surface of the stomach as prominently as in the left decubitus position. (Modified from Whalen JP. Radiology of the Abdomen. Baltimore: Lea & Febiger, 1976; with permission.)

- Collection of blood and pancreatic fluid in the left upper quadrant
- Pancreatic bloody ascites if there is no left upper quadrant localization
- Possible involvement of the perirenal and pararenal spaces with the aggregation of bloody fluid

# Vascular System

## *Arterial Supply*

### Splenic Artery

In most people, the splenic artery is a branch of the celiac trunk, arising together with the common hepatic and left gastric arteries. The most common form of the celiac trunk is tripodal. According to Michels,[67] the tripodal form occurs in 82% of individuals. Van Damme and Bonte[68] report that this form occurs in 86% of individuals. When the above-mentioned arteries or other upper abdominal arteries arise from atypical sources, the tripodal arrangement may be replaced by a dipodal or a tetrapodal pattern of branching.

**COURSE AND FORM OF THE SPLENIC ARTERY.** In the majority of cases, subsequent to its origin from the celiac trunk the splenic artery courses leftward in close relation to the upper border of the pancreas (Fig. 22-24). Occasionally its course may be in front of or completely behind the pancreas. Very rarely it may be partially or totally within the pancreatic parenchyma. The splenic artery's termination in the splenic porta is unpredictable owing to its number of branches to the spleen or neighboring organs, such as the left kidney, stomach, and omentum.

The splenic artery varies in length from 8 to 32 cm and in diameter from 0.5 to 1.2 cm. It is noteworthy that the distance from the aorta to the spleen is only about 10 cm yet, in the extreme, the splenic artery can attain a length of 50 cm.

No definitive answer has been found to explain the peculiar degree of tortuosity present in the splenic artery that is seen in most individuals. Its amount of tortuosity does seem to be related to the age of individuals, but not to the presence of vascular disease affecting the vessel.[69]

The convolution characteristic of the splenic artery is not seen in animals such as the dog or the pig. However, this feature has been noted in infrahuman primates, including rhesus monkeys and baboons, although to a lesser degree than in humans.[70]

Waizer et al.[71] reported that in nine out of 26 cadavers, the splenic artery made a loop to the right immediately after its origin from the celiac trunk. It appeared at the border of the lesser omentum. Therefore, it was vulnerable to iatrogenic injury during procedures on supracolic organs.

On its way to the spleen, the splenic artery forms the splenic peritoneal fold. It then ends in the splenorenal ligament, forming a peculiar tree whose pattern of branching seems different in every case. Thereafter, its branches reach and enter the splenic porta.

**BRANCHES OF THE SPLENIC ARTERY.** Skandalakis et al.[53] studied the splenic artery and its branches in toto, paying the most attention to the two distal segments - the prepancreatic and prehilar. Michels'[67] four-part segmental arterial anatomy (suprapancreatic, pancreatic, prepancreatic, and prehilar) classification system was used. Angiography revealed unpredictable variations, with differences in the number and

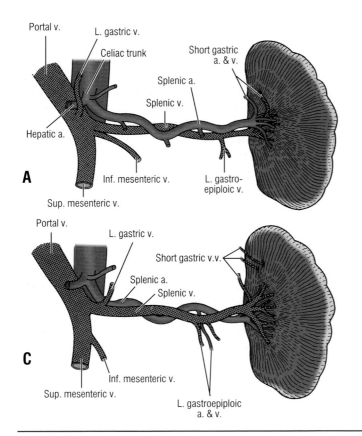

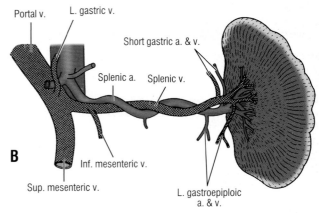

FIG 22-24. Relation of splenic artery and splenic vein. **A.** Vein posterior to artery (this is the usual pattern). **B.** Vein both anterior and posterior to artery. **C.** Vein anterior to artery (this is the least common configuration). (Modified from Skandalakis JE, Gray SW, Rowe JS Jr. Anatomical Complications in General Surgery. New York: McGraw-Hill, 1983; with permission.)

pattern of origin of arterial branches, and in the length, width, tortuosity, and course of the splenic artery with regard to the pancreas (above the upper border, in front or behind, or partially or totally within the pancreatic parenchyma).

There is considerable agreement that the splenic artery most commonly divides into two major branches (80-94% of the time[72]) and less commonly into three principal branches. Subsequent branching of these primary vessels three or more times results in a widely varying number of branches, which ultimately gain access to the hilum of the spleen. Garcia-Porrero and Lemes[50] observed that the number of branches varied from 5 to 20, with an average of 11. Michels[65] determined the extremes in numbers of terminal branches to be between 3 and 38.[43,50,73,74]

Differences in interpretation of the data related to numbers of branches of the splenic artery are the result of a number of factors, including the way in which one chooses to describe or number polar branches. There also seems to be a difference between male and female patients in the branching pattern of the splenic artery. In a study of 181 spleens from victims of accidental death, Garcia-Porrero and Lemes[50] noted trifurcation of the splenic artery in 16.7% of female patients but only about 4% in male

patients. They also observed a superior polar artery in 29.3% of specimens, in comparison with an inferior polar segmental artery in 44.8% of specimens. These terminal branches arise from the pancreatic, the prepancreatic, or the prehilar segments of the splenic artery.[67] In contrast, Michels[67] found a superior polar artery 65% of the time, and an inferior polar artery or arteries 82% of the time. The segmental origin of splenic arterial branches, according to Michels, is presented in Table 22-4.

Skandalakis et al.[53] dissected the splenic artery to learn about common patterns of the distal branches – those related to splenectomies. After dissecting 29 cadavers, no consistent pattern of branching could be observed. They found that 27 arteries arose from a hepatosplenogastric trunk (the normal form of the celiac artery), one arose from the common hepatic artery (hepatosplenic trunk), and one took origin from the left gastric artery (gastrosplenic trunk). Michels[67] was correct when he stated that the patterns are never the same.

The splenic artery passes retroperitoneally under the posterior wall of the omental bursa, close to the upper posterior surface of the body and tail of the pancreas. In its course, it loops like a snake above and below the superior margin of the organ. According to Michels,[67] the splenic

**TABLE 22-4. Segmental Origin of Splenic Arterial Branches**

The suprapancreatic segment (The atypical branches are shown in *italics.*)
  *Left inferior phrenic a.*
  Dorsal pancreatic a.
  Superior polar a.
  *Posterior cardioesophageal a.*
  *Accessory gastric or hepatic a.*
  *Inferior mesenteric a.*
  Posterior (dorsal) gastric a.
The pancreatic segment
  Great pancreatic a. (frequent)
  Superior polar a. (infrequent)
  Left gastroepiploic a. (rare)
  Posterior cardioesophageal a. (rare)
  One or more short gastric aa.
    Accessory left gastric a.
    Posterior gastric a.
The prepancreatic segment
  70% of the time, the terminal divisions begin here
  Inconstant branching patterns with several combinations, such as:
    Upper arterial trunk
    Middle arterial trunk
    Lower arterial trunk
    Left gastroepiploic a.
    Caudal pancreatic a.
    Superior polar a.
    Inferior polar a.
The prehilar segment
  More branching if the branching started in the pancreatic segment
  30% of the time, terminal branching starts here, not in the pancreatic segment
    In the 30%, the branches enter the spleen into a limited hilum

*Source:* Modified from Skandalakis JE, Colborn GL, Pemberton LB, Skandalakis TN, Skandalakis LJ, Gray SW. The surgical anatomy of the spleen. Prob Gen Surg 7(1):1-17, 1990; with permission.

**Reference**
Michels NA. The variational anatomy of the spleen and the splenic artery. Am J Anat 1942; 70:21.

artery appears more tortuous with the increasing age of the individual, there being little tortuosity in the artery of infants. Michels also called attention to the paradox of a large splenic artery supplying a relatively small organ, the spleen, in contrast to the narrower hepatic artery, which serves an organ five times larger. Sylvester et al.[69] cautiously agreed with Michels in analyzing cadaveric and angiographic data of splenic artery tortuosity.

We strongly advise the interested student to study the work of Van Damme and Bonte.[73]

**SHORT GASTRIC ARTERIES.** In 29 cadaveric dissections,[53] all the short gastric arteries arose from the proper splenic branches of the splenic artery. Helm[75] wrote that their common origin is from the left gastroepiploic artery or from proper splenic branches. Michels[67] found an average range of between two and four short gastric arteries and as many as nine such branches. Four to six short gastric arteries were found in each of our specimens, and they were considered to be end arteries, not anastomosing at the greater curvature of the stomach. In the series by Skandalakis et al.,[53] there was a total of 145 short gastric arteries in 29 cadavers.

Because the left gastroepiploic artery does not reach the greater curvature of the stomach until the approximate midpoint of that curvature, the short gastric arteries are of special importance in supplying the more proximal part. The short gastric arteries anastomose with the cardiac branches of the left gastric artery. According to Keramidas,[76] the short gastric arteries provide the collateral circulation of the spleen. Farag et al.[77] stated that the short gastric arteries provide sufficient circulation to sustain just the upper third of a normal-sized spleen following removal of the lower two-thirds of the spleen.

**LEFT GASTROEPIPLOIC ARTERY.** According to Michels,[67] the left gastroepiploic artery arises from the splenic trunk 72% of the time, from the inferior terminal splenic branch or its branches 22% of the time, and, rarely, from the middle splenic trunk or the superior terminal branch. In the series of Skandalakis et al.,[53] the left gastroepiploic arose from the distal splenic trunk in 18 cadavers and from terminal branches entering the lower part of the hilum (including the lower polar artery) in ten cadavers. In one specimen, the left gastroepiploic artery originated from the caudal pancreatic artery (or, conversely, the caudal pancreatic artery originated from the left gastroepiploic artery); nonetheless, the arteries were branches of the pancreatic part of the splenic artery.

**OTHER BRANCHES OF THE SPLENIC ARTERY.** There are named and small unnamed branches of the splenic artery. Among the named branches to the pancreas are the posterior gastric artery, dorsal pancreatic artery, transverse pancreatic artery, great pancreatic artery (pancreatica magna), and caudal pancreatic artery.

*Posterior Gastric Artery.* The posterior gastric (dorsal gastric) artery is a branch to the dorsum of the fundus of the stomach and the upper part of the body of the stomach. The reported incidence of the posterior gastric artery ranges from 4% to 99%, according to a table by Berens et al.[78] that included studies from 1729 to 1991 (Table 22-5). This artery arises from the main stem of the splenic artery before its terminal bi- or trifurcation at the splenic hilum.

Often, it appears nearly at the midpoint of the length of the splenic artery, ascending nearly vertically to reach the deep side of the proximal part of the stomach.

The posterior gastric artery is, characteristically, the sole branch to arise from the splenic artery and passes in a cephalic direction before the appearance of the hilar or polar branches. It may create a slight fold in the peritoneum of the posterior wall of the lesser omental bursa as it passes upward toward the stomach. Van Damme and Bonte[68] pointed out that this artery can be confused with a gastric artery originating from a posterior polar branch of the splenic artery. They cited the incidence of the posterior gastric artery as 36%,[79] similar to the 1985 findings of Trubel et al.[80]

*Dorsal Pancreatic Artery.* The dorsal pancreatic artery is the "supreme pancreatic artery" described by Kirk.[81] It lies posterior to the splenic vein and is about 1.5 mm in diameter. Michels[67] considered it the most variable of the celiacomesenteric vessels. According to Lippert and Pabst,[82]

---

**TABLE 22-5. Reported Incidence of Posterior Gastric Artery**

| Year | Authors | Incidence | Breakdown |
|------|---------|-----------|-----------|
| 1729 | Walther | N/A | N/A |
| 1745 | Haller | N/A | Origin-Midportion |
| 1796 | Sommerring | "Sometimes" | N/A |
| 1873 | Hyrtl | "Inconsistent" | N/A |
| 1901 | Haberer | "In most cases" | N/A |
| 1904 | Rossi and Cova | 65.8% | 2.5 cm from celiac |
| 1907 | Leriche and Villemin | 12.7% | Origin-Distal |
| 1910 | Piquand | 99.0% | Origin-Distal |
| 1912 | Rio-Branco | 50.0% | Origin-Proximal |
| 1915 | Helm | 16.0% | Origin-Proximal |
| 1928 | Adachi | 21.6% | 3-5 cm from celiac |
| 1931 | Testut and Latarjet | N/A | N/A |
| 1932 | Versari | 66.0% | N/A |
| 1952 | Franchi and Stuart | N/A | N/A |
| 1955 | Michels | N/A | N/A |
| 1957 | Weisz and Bianco | 48.0% | N/A |
| 1959 | Chiarugi | 66.0% | 2.5 cm from celiac |
| 1962 | Aboltin | 77.1% | N/A |
| 1963 | Tanigawa | Adults 36.0% Fetuses 67.8% | 2.2-13.1 cm from celiac axis |
| 1963 | Couinaud | N/A | N/A |
| 1967 | Delteil et al. | 64.3% | N/A |
| 1967 | Kupic et al. | 36.8% | N/A |
| 1968 | Levasseur & Couinaud | 50.0% | N/A |
| 1972 | Laude et al. | 4.0% | N/A |
| 1977 | Ruzicka and Rankin | N/A | N/A |
| 1978 | Suzuki et al. | 62.3% | 18.4% Proximal third 47.8% Middle third 34.2% Distal third |
| 1980 | DiDio et al. | 46.0% | N/A |
| 1983 | Wald and Polk | 88.0% | N/A |
| 1985 | Trubel et al. | 37.5% | 33% had splenic branch |
| 1986 | Van Damme and Bonte | 36% | N/A |
| 1988 | Trubel et al. | 27.7% (stomachial supply only) | |
| 1990 | Yu and Whang | 84.0% | 13% Proximal third 78% Middle third 9% Distal third |
| 1990 | Kaneko | Fetuses 16.0% | N/A |
| 1991 | Berens | 48% | Proximal third (3 cm) |

*Source:* Modified from Berens AS, Aluisio FV, Colborn GL, Gray SW, Skandalakis JE. The incidence and significance of the posterior gastric artery in human anatomy. J Med Assoc Ga 80(8):425-428, 1991; with permission.

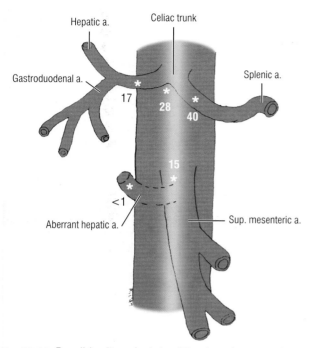

thrombosis of the artery can produce infarction and limited necrosis of the body and tail of the pancreas.[84] The transverse pancreatic artery may be large enough that it could be mistaken for the splenic artery; however, the fact that it normally lies in a groove on the inferior border of the pancreas should preclude this mistake in identification.

*Great Pancreatic Artery.* One of the largest branches of the splenic artery, the great pancreatic artery (arteria pancreatica magna of Von Haller) (Fig. 22-27), is the chief blood supply of the distal body and tail of the pancreas. If this artery is singular, it usually arises from the midportion of the splenic artery.[67] Van Damme and Bonte[68] described in detail the confusion involved in the naming of the arteries which supply the body of the pancreas.

*Caudal Pancreatic Artery.* According to Van Damme and Bonte,[68] one (32%), two (46%), or more (22%) caudal pancreatic arteries arise from the terminal part of the splenic artery, or, variably, from the left gastroepiploic artery or a splenic branch at the hilum of the spleen. The caudate branch anastomoses with branches of the great pancreatic and transverse pancreatic arteries. When it is present at the hilum of the spleen, the caudal pancreatic artery can supply blood to accessory splenic tissue. It often courses within the pancreaticosplenic ligament to reach the pancreatic tail or spleen.

**FIG 22-25.** Possible sites of origin of the dorsal pancreatic artery (percentages from Lippert and Pabst[82]). More than half of these arteries arise from the proximal splenic artery or the celiac trunk. (Modified from Lippert H, Pabst R. Arterial Variations in Man. Munich: J.F. Bergmann Verlag, 1985, pp. 41-45; with permission).

the dorsal pancreatic artery (Fig. 22-25) originates from the splenic artery in 40% of specimens, but it may arise from other arteries including the celiac trunk (28%), common hepatic artery (17%), superior mesenteric artery (15%), or an aberrant hepatic artery (<1%). Occasionally it can be derived from the middle colic, accessory middle colic, or gastroduodenal artery. Details can be found in the chapter on the pancreas.

The dorsal pancreatic artery provides origin to the transverse pancreatic artery (also known as the inferior pancreatic artery) to the left. It commonly has a branch to the right, which anastomoses with arteries on the ventral surface of the head of the pancreas. Such a branch provides supply to the head and uncinate process. When the dorsal pancreatic artery arises from a branch to the colon, the main stem continues in the transverse mesocolon. In some cases, a dorsal pancreatic artery may give off an epiploic branch. Arteriography is essential for determining the origin and course of the dorsal pancreatic artery.

*Transverse Pancreatic Artery.* The transverse (inferior) pancreatic artery (Fig. 22-26) is the left branch of the dorsal pancreatic artery supplying the body and tail of the pancreas. The artery may be single, double, or absent; it may anastomose with the splenic arteries or not.[83] If it does not,

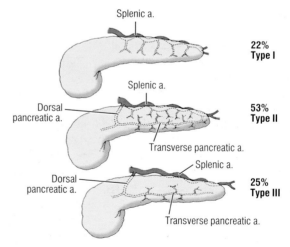

**FIG 22-26.** Possible configurations of the blood supply to the distal pancreas. Type I, blood supply from the splenic artery only. Type II, blood supply from the splenic and transverse pancreatic arteries with anastomosis in the tail of the pancreas. Type III, blood supply from splenic and transverse pancreatic arteries without distal anastomoses. This type is susceptible to infarction from emboli in the transverse artery. (Modified from Skandalakis JE, Colborn GL, Pemberton LB, Skandalakis PN, Skandalakis LJ, Gray SW. The surgical anatomy of the spleen. Prob Gen Surg 1990; 7:1-17; with permission.)

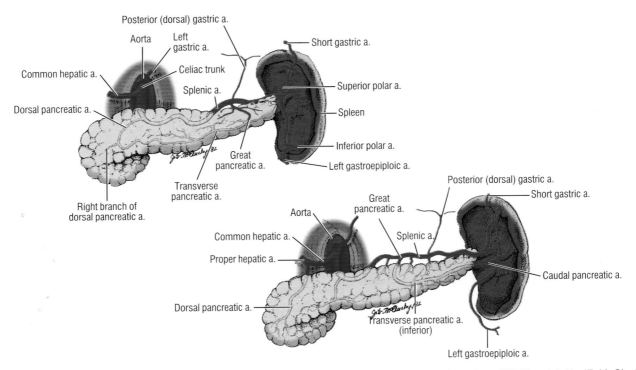

FIG 22-27. Highly diagrammatic illustration of two variations of the great pancreatic artery. (Modified from Gray SW, Skandalakis JE, McClusky DA. Atlas of Surgical Anatomy for General Surgeons. Baltimore: Williams & Wilkins, 1985; with permission.)

## Collateral Circulation

The splenic artery is not the only artery to supply the spleen with blood. The additional blood supply comes from the inferior or transverse pancreatic artery (especially when it arises from the gastroduodenal), other pancreatic arteries, the short gastric arteries, or the left gastroepiploic artery. In 50 patients with schistosomal portal hypertension who were candidates for partial or total splenectomy, Petroianu and Petroianu[85] observed that the number of splenogastric (short gastric) arteries varied from one to as many as 13. In 32 cases, the upper splenic pole remained viable even after division of both the splenic artery and the splenic vein, presumably because of the anastomoses present between the gastric and splenic parenchymal vessels.

Romero-Torres[86] stated that the true blood supply of the spleen consists of the splenic artery, the short gastric vessels, and the left gastroepiploic artery. Because of the organization and anastomoses of the several arteries, he recommended that a distal pancreatectomy be performed without splenectomy and that ligation of the splenic artery is not necessary in portal hypertension if "disconnection" (ligation) of the portal-azygous system takes place (Fig. 22-28). Romero-Torres also ligates the left gastric artery and vein and the vasa brevia.

## *Venous Drainage*

The splenic vein (Fig. 22-29) originates from several veins that leave the hilum of the spleen and join to form the major vessel at variable distances from the hilum. Polar tributaries are not uncommon. The splenic vein is of large caliber, but does not possess the tortuosity of the splenic artery. The vein passes through the splenorenal ligament with the artery and the tail of the pancreas, deep to the pancreas. The splenic vein receives tributaries from the pancreas, often indenting its dorsal surface, in a position inferior to the splenic artery. Deep to the region of the neck of the pancreas, the splenic vein joins the superior mesenteric vein to form the portal vein (see Fig. 22-24). Woodburne[87] stated that in 60% of cases the splenic vein receives the inferior mesenteric vein before the formation of the portal vein.

Skandalakis et al.[53] studied the splenic vein in 27 dissections and found that the vein was formed by three trunks in 16 cases, and four trunks in eight cases. In the remaining three cases, three trunks plus the left gastroepiploic vein formed the splenic vein. Douglass et al.[88] also studied the anatomy of the splenic vein. Their findings can be summarized in Figure 22-29. The patterns are highly variable, and, as with the arteries, no one arrangement of veins duplicated

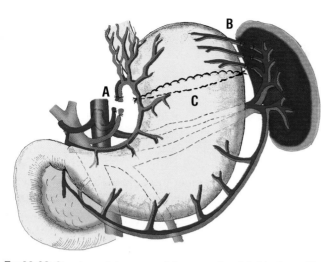

**FIG 22-28.** Simple portal-azygous "disconnection." A, Ligature of the left gastric vessels. B, Coagulation (or clipping) and cutting of the vasa brevia. C, Continuous locking suture of the anterior and posterior walls of the stomach. (With permission of R. Romero-Torres; modified.)

the next. Considerable variation was found in the points of exit of the veins from the spleen, their point of confluence for the formation of the main splenic vein, and their entrance into other veins at the hilum or outside it.

The student of splenic anatomy should remember that *very rarely* do the short gastric veins enter the upper part of the spleen directly from the greater curvature of the stomach. More commonly, the short gastric veins cross the gastrosplenic ligament en route to the splenic vein or one of its tributaries.[89]

The relationship of the splenic vein to the splenic artery in their course together is subject to some variations (see Fig. 22-24). In 75 consecutive autopsies, Gerber et al.[90] found three anatomic arrangements:

- The vein lay entirely posterior to the artery in 54% of individuals
- The vein was wrapped around the artery, in part posterior to it and in part anterior to it in 44% of individuals
- The vein lay entirely anterior to the artery in 2% of individuals

## *Surgical Applications*

- If the spleen has not been mobilized, ligation of the splenic arteries is permissible. The spleen remains viable if the collateral circulation is intact (polar arteries, short gastric arteries, and left gastroepiploic arteries). If the color of the spleen is changed, however, and there is evidence of ischemia, a splenectomy should be performed. In general,

ligation of the splenic artery should be done only if absolutely necessary (i.e., during splenectomy).

- Proximal double and distal ligation of the artery is advisable.
- Ligation of the splenic vein alone should be avoided.
- Total splenectomy is indicated with splenic vein thrombosis.
- As a rule, ligation of the artery should precede ligation of the vein.
- The tortuous splenic artery should be ligated with care, avoiding pancreatic and splenic vein injury. The elevated segments of the splenic artery facilitate ligation of the artery without anatomic complications.
- The terminal arterial and venous branches should be isolated and ligated close to the splenic portas to avoid bleeding, because the origin and ultimate termination of these vessels are unpredictable.
- Because the origins of the splenic branches also are unpredictable, the use of a preoperative arteriogram is essential in determining the point of ligation of the splenic artery. Because collateral circulation is available, there is no question that the spleen can tolerate ligation of the splenic artery. Therefore, the spleen can be saved if necessary. Surgeons should remember that ligation of the splenic artery near its origin can produce hyperamylasemia resulting from deterioration of the pancreatic blood supply.[56] Preoperative splenic arterial occlusion as an adjunct to high-risk splenectomy has been advised by Fujitani et al.[91] According to *Gray's Anatomy*,[89] there are no anastomoses between the smaller branches of the

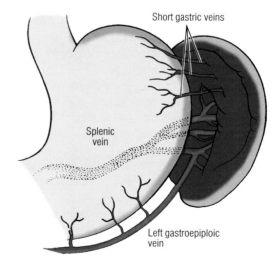

**FIG 22-29.** Anatomy of the splenic vein. (Modified from Skandalakis JE, Colborn GL, Pemberton LB, Skandalakis PN, Skandalakis LJ, Gray SW. The surgical anatomy of the spleen. Probl Gen Surg 1990; 7:1-17; with permission.)

splenic arteries, so that obstruction leads to infarction of the spleen. Dumont and Lefleur[92] suggested that there is increased splenic arterial flow in patients with isolated obstruction of the splenic vein.

- For all practical purposes, the main splenic arteries are the terminal branches of the splenic artery. They are responsible for the arterial blood supply of the organ. They originate either from the superior and inferior terminal arteries or from other terminal branches. The superior and inferior polar arteries should be considered part of the main splenic artery. They penetrate the splenic parenchyma above and below the portas and usually originate from the prehilar segment. The superior polar artery is almost always present.

- According to Guyton and Hall,[93] 60 percent of all the blood in the circulatory system is usually within the veins, making the venous system the blood reservoir for the circulatory system. When necessary, the spleen can release as much as 100 ml of blood into the circulation from both of its storage areas (venous sinuses and pulp).

- Lankisch[94] found a 95 percent incidence of splenic vein thrombosis in patients whose pancreatitis was complicated by splenomegaly in association with gastric and esophageal varices.

- Partial splenectomy is now feasible due to increased understanding of the arterial and venous segmentation of the organ. The arteries and veins serve essentially as end vessels. Because of the immunologic importance of the spleen, awareness of this aspect of surgical anatomy has been an important development. Dawson et al.[48] verified the segmentation of the spleen. They demonstrated that the spleen is divided most commonly into two or three lobes, each of which possesses one or two segments. The avascular planes between lobes pass perpendicularly to the long axis of the organ, although the intersegmental avascular planes are more variable. Dawson et al. emphasized that the venous segmentation is as predictable as the arterial segmentation. In more than half of their cases, the intersegmental planes of the spleen were indicated by notches in the margin of the organ.

- In addition to the two or three hilar branches of the splenic artery, a separate superior polar branch (in about 30% of spleens) and an inferior polar branch (in about 45%) were observed by Garcia-Porrero and Lemes.[50] They demonstrated the segmental nature of the vascular supply in most spleens, and observed anastomotic bridges between segmental branches and between these and polar branches in about 20% of cases.

Orozco et al.[95] reported that splenectomy is not routinely necessary in devascularization procedures for bleeding esophageal or gastric varices.

Firstenberg et al.[96] reported successful treatment of delayed splenic rupture by embolization of the splenic artery.

## *Lymphatic Drainage*

The lymphatic vessels of the spleen arise from the splenic capsule and some of the larger splenic trabeculae. One of the peculiarities of this enigmatic organ is the lack of provision for lymphatics for the splenic pulp. In the classification of the various groups of lymph nodes and lymphatic vessels draining the spleen, as described by Rouviere,[97] the splenic chain (Fig. 22-30) includes suprapancreatic nodes, infrapancreatic nodes, and afferent and efferent lymph vessels. Weiss et al.[98] reported that pancreatic tumors divide the splenic nodes into two groups: the nodes of the splenic hilum and the nodes of the tail of the pancreas. The lymph nodes described above just happen to be located in the splenic neighborhood. Their primary function is that of draining the lymph of the stomach rather than that of the spleen.

The splenopancreatic lymph glands are located along the splenic artery. This is the largest group of splenic lymph nodes. However, a small number can be found in the area of the short gastric vessels. The local lymph nodes that receive lymph from the spleen also receive lymphatic drainage from the stomach and the pancreas.

REMEMBER:

- The spleen comprises one quarter of the lymphoid mass of the body.
- The sum of the body's lymphoid tissue and the lymphocytes in the bone marrow correspond to 1 percent of the weight of the body. As a mass, it is approximately one-half the weight of the liver.[99]

The dilemma often facing the surgeon is whether the spleen ought to be removed when the splenic lymph nodes are involved in disease. We do not yet have a definitive answer. Boles et al.[100] advised partial splenectomy for staging Hodgkin's disease. Dearth et al.[101] in-

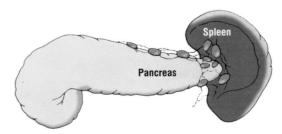

FIG 22-30. Lymphatic drainage of the spleen. (Modified from Skandalakis JE, Colborn GL, Pemberton LB, Skandalakis PN, Skandalakis LJ, Gray SW. The surgical anatomy of the spleen. Probl Gen Surg 1990; 7:1-17; with permission.)

dicated that although "occult splenic involvement by Hodgkin's disease cannot be confidently excluded by ...partial splenectomy," retaining a splenic remnant offers some protection against postoperative sepsis, which is often fatal in children. In the event that total splenectomy is performed, antibiotics and active immunization against pneumococci definitely lessen the risk of postsplenectomy sepsis.

## Splenic Innervation

The nerve supply to the spleen arises from the more medial and anterior portions of the celiac plexus (Fig. 22-31). Visceral nerve fibers from this plexus accompany the splenic vessels into the hilum. Allen[31] stated that fibers from the right vagus nerve or the posterior vagal trunk also pass to the spleen. However, this configuration has been questioned by others, based on the results of nerve degeneration studies after vagotomy performed on cats.[102] Some myelinated fibers, few and probably sensory in function, can be identified histologically in a ratio of about 1:20 to unmyelinated autonomic fibers. These sensory fibers terminate in the spinal cord at the level of the sixth to eighth thoracic vertebrae. From these same levels, preganglionic sympathetic neurons arise in the intermediolateral cell column, passing within the greater thoracic splanchnic nerve to the celiac ganglion and to extensions of the ganglion along the splenic artery. In some mammals, the postganglionic sympathetic autonomic fibers terminate upon smooth muscle of the capsule, trabeculae, arteries, and veins.[103] In humans, however, the autonomic fibers appear to travel together with the branches of the splenic arteries.[89]

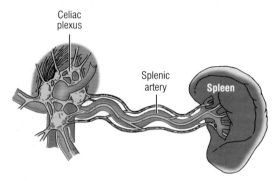

**FIG 22-31.** Splenic innervation. (Modified from Skandalakis JE, Colborn GL, Pemberton LB, Skandalakis PN, Skandalakis LJ, Gray SW. The surgical anatomy of the spleen. Probl Gen Surg 1990; 7:1-17; with permission.)

## HISTOLOGY AND PHYSIOLOGY

The spleen is composed of 75-85 percent red pulp and approximately 20 percent white pulp. Some arterioles apparently open directly into sinusoids as a closed circulation; others open into meshwork as part of an open circulation. In open circulation, which processes 80-90 percent of splenic blood flow, the blood passes through splenic capillaries into the splenic red pulp. Splenic macrophages in the intercellular gaps of the red pulp phagocytize damaged red blood cells and particulate matter. In closed circulation, blood cells pass through the capillaries directly into venous sinusoids.

The spleen is relatively small in size, but it is the largest lymphatic organ in the body. According to Seufert and Mitrou,[56] it comprises about 0.1% of the body's weight and receives 300 mL/min of blood (approximately 6% of the cardiac output) per minute, which corresponds to approximately 3 mL/min per gram of splenic tissue. The spleen contains only 1% of the total red blood cell mass, which corresponds to 25 ml of red blood cells. As each red blood cell passes through the spleen, its destruction, if it is old or defective, is assured. Even the escape of a normal red blood cell is occasionally difficult.

We quote from Chadburn[104]:

> [T]he spleen is able to maintain the integrity of the blood and respond to circulating antigens. However, this can be a double-edged sword in the case of patients suffering from autoimmune diseases such as immune thrombocytopenic purpura since the spleen can be the site of both antibody production and circulating cell destruction.

The spleen serves four functions: blood storage, hematopoiesis, filtration, and immunologic response. We have not found a more complete and elegant description of the filtration process than that of Wolf and Neiman[105] (Table 22-6).

In addition to the four known functions, the spleen probably has other unknown roles. In contemplating this unfathomable organ, one of the authors of this chapter (JES) is reminded of Winston Churchill's[106] characterization of Russia: "...a riddle wrapped in a mystery inside an enigma."

## SURGERY OF THE SPLEEN

### Twelve Principles of Splenic Surgery

The surgical procedures of the spleen include total

**TABLE 22-6.**

Filtration
A. Culling—erythrocyte (or other blood cell) destruction
   1. Physiologic (as red blood cells age)
   2. Pathologic
      a. Associated with blood cell abnormalities
      b. Associated with primary splenic changes
B. Pitting ("facelifting" of erythrocytes)
   1. Removal of cytoplasmic inclusions*
   2. Remodeling of cell membranes
C. Erythroclasis—destruction of abnormal red blood cells with liberation into circulation of erythrocyte fragments*
D. Removal of other particulate material (e.g., bacteria, colloidal particles)*

*Editorial note:* These functions were mentioned by Galen.

*Source:* Modified from: Wolf BC, Neiman RS. Disorders of the Spleen. Philadelphia: Saunders, 1989 (Table 2-1); with permission.

open splenectomy, partial splenectomy, laparoscopic splenectomy, splenic repair, splenic fixation, splenic detorsion and splenopexy, distal pancreatectomy with splenic preservation, treatment of splenic artery aneurysm, staging laparotomy, transplantation, incision and draining of parasitic or nonparasitic cysts, and removal of accessory spleens.

Surgery of the spleen is the surgery of its ligaments, vessels, and segments. Twelve principles of splenic surgery should be followed strictly, without deviation. We do not claim that the collection of rules presented here is complete, but we believe that if a surgeon follows these procedures, anatomic complications will be avoided and treatment will be successful.

**1. Know surgical anatomy.** A surgeon should know not only the unpredictable vascular supply of the spleen but also the various ligaments associated with the spleen and its neighboring organs, as well as their relations to the vessels that they envelop. The ligaments may or may not be avascular, but routine clamping and ligation of them are signs of good and sound surgical judgment.

Knowledge of the segmental anatomy of the spleen and its relation to the vascular system helps a surgeon perform a partial splenectomy.

It is important to know, for example, that the splenic lymph nodes are above and below the pancreatic tail. In metastatic disease, the lymph nodes should be removed, and splenectomy may be required as well.

**2. Know clinical and surgical pathology.** Cooperation with a hematologist and a pathologist is essential. The anatomy of the peripheral blood, normal or abnormal, and the surgical pathologic characteristics of the specimen or specimens help the surgeon, and later the oncologist and radiation therapist, treat the patient.

**3. Know surgical procedures.** No one procedure is adequate for all patients. The surgeon should be knowledgeable about all surgical techniques.

**4. Perform a physical examination.** A physical examination should include the detection of metabolic problems, tests for collagen deficiency disease, tests for allergic reactions and susceptibility to anesthesia, and a hematologic consultation.

**5. Assess the diseased spleen.** The key person here is the internist or the hematologist. The surgeon performs the procedure requested by the hematologist.

**6. Know how to treat a ruptured spleen.** The Luna and Dellinger[107] flow-chart is helpful (Fig. 22-32).

**7. Perform adequate preoperative preparations.** Polk[108] proposed a simple preoperative checklist (Table 22-7). We consider this to be one of the best of such lists available.

**8. Adhere to operating room rules.** One should not break dress code or fail to use sterile techniques. Good hemostasis should be obtained and kept. The surgeon should make a well-informed decision about a drain and select appropriate suture and wrapping material in case of ruptured spleen.

**9. Place the patient in a convenient position.**

**10. Choose an incision.** The type of incision is up to the surgeon, who must know the anatomy pertinent to opening and closing an incision.

**11. Assess congenital anomalies and variations.**

**12. Provide optimal postoperative care.**

## Splenectomy

### Total Open Splenectomy

Total open splenectomy (the removal of the spleen in toto) can be performed by an anterior approach or a posterior approach (Fig. 22-33). In the anterior approach, the surgeon first incises the gastrocolic ligament, allowing entry to the lesser sac, and then ligates the splenic artery. In the posterior approach, the surgeon ligates the splenic artery after incising the posterior layer of the splenorenal ligament and mobilizing the spleen to the right, thereby working within the greater peritoneal cavity. The aim of both approaches is the ligation of the splenic pedicle.

A mass ligation of the splenic pedicle after incision of the posterior part of the splenorenal ligament includes the following structures: the presplenic fold, gastrosplenic ligament, splenic artery, and the incised portion of the splenorenal ligament.[109]

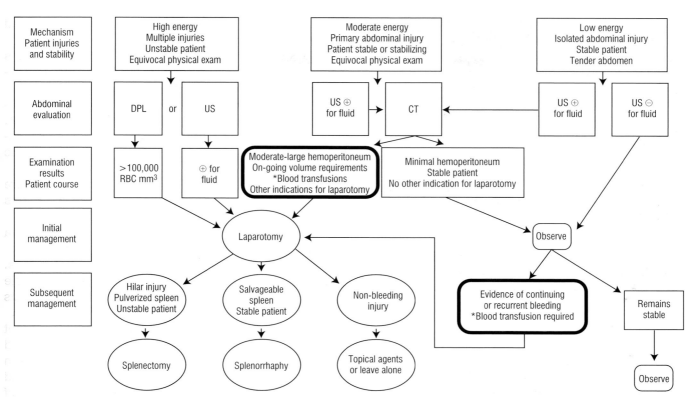

**Fig 22-32.** Flow chart for decisions in the management of splenic injuries. Asterisk (*) indicates transfusions required for abdominal injury. DPL, diagnostic peritoneal lavage; RBC, red blood cell count; CT, computed tomography; US, ultrasonography. (Modified by DV Feliciano from Luna GK, Dellinger EP. Nonoperative observation therapy for splenic injuries: a safe therapeutic option? Am J Surg 1987;153:463; with permission.)

## Editorial Comment

*Splenectomy patients are at risk for overwhelming postsplenectomy infection from encapsulated bacteria. In decreasing order of frequency, the most common organisms are* **Streptococcus pneumoniae, Neisseria meningitidis, Hemophilus influenzae, Escherichia coli,** *and* **Staphylococcus** *and* **Streptococcus.** *Patients can go from apparent good health to death is less than 24 hours. To protect against overwhelming postsplenectomy infection the goal is to preserve as much splenic tissue as possible, but the minimum amount of splenic tissue needed to protect against serious infection is probably 30% to 50% of the normal splenic mass.*

*Immunization with polyvalent pneumococcal vaccines as well as vaccines against* **Hemophilus influenzae** *type B and* **Neisseria meningitidis** *is appropriate. Prior to elective splenectomy immunizations should ideally be given two or more weeks preoperatively, as immunizations are less successful in splenectomized patients. I have avoided giving immunizations in the days*

*immediately before splenectomy as there are data from the experimental laboratory indicating that giving animals the antigen one day prior to splenectomy induces anergy and inhibits the ability to make antibodies when subsequently challenged with the antigen. Immunizations two or more weeks prior to elective splenectomy are probably best; immunizations after splenectomy are second best. There is at least a theoretical possibility that immunizations immediately prior to splenectomy may be harmful.*

*All patients should be counseled about the risk of infection and advised to seek medical attention at the first signs of illness or the development of a fever. Such patients should also carry identification that they are splenectomized. I believe it is appropriate for splenectomized patients to have a supply of an antibiotic against gram positive organisms. If necessary the antibiotic can be taken immediately after telephone consultation with their physician. (RSF Jr)*

### TABLE 22-7. Sample Preoperative Checklist

Operative permit—appropriately signed and witnessed
Dietary considerations
 For abdominal operation, liquid diet and laxatives to ensure
  clean, collapsed bowel
 Nothing by mouth at least 6 hr. before operation
Review of life-support systems
 Vital signs recorded often enough to establish normal
 Pulmonary system—chest films; other studies as indicated
 Cardiac function—electrocardiogram; other studies as
  indicated
 Renal function—urinalysis; blood urea nitrogen and possibly
  creatinine determinations
Adequate hydration up to time of operation—especially to com-
 pensate for laxatives and fasting
Area of operation washed with appropriate germicidal detergent
 and shaved, clipped, or cleansed with depilatory agent
Blood transfusions prepared as anticipated
Order that patient should void on call to operating room
Preoperative medications—vagolytic and sedative drugs
Special medications—digitalis, insulin, and so forth

*Source:* Polk HC Jr. Principles of preoperative preparation of the surgical
patient. In: Sabiston DC Jr (ed). Textbook of Surgery (15th ed).
Philadelphia: WB Saunders, 1997, p. 116. Modified from Houston MC,
Ratcliff DG, Hays JT, Gluck FW. Preoperative medical consultation and
evaluation of surgical risk. South Med J 80:1385, 1987; with permission.

In an anterior approach to the splenic artery at the pedicle (Fig. 22-34), if there is a well-developed presplenic fold,
six sheets of peritoneum, fat, lymph nodes, and pancreas
fused into a single mass may be encountered.[57] The lesser
sac, as well as the space between the presplenic fold and
the gastrosplenic ligament, may be obliterated. In the anterior approach, the surgeon incises three peritoneal layers
(two layers of the gastrosplenic ligament and the one layer
comprising the anterior leaflet of the splenorenal ligament)
(Fig. 22-35A). Ligation of the splenic artery and short gastric vessels by the anterior approach is indicated in Figure
22-35B and ligation of the splenic vein and its branches is
shown in Figure 22-35C. In the posterior approach (see
Fig. 22-34), only one layer, the anterior layer of the
splenorenal ligament, is incised (Fig. 22-36).

Selection of an anterior or posterior approach is up to
the surgeon, who should have a good understanding of
the indications for splenectomy, the nature of the particular
disease of the spleen, and thorough knowledge of splenic
anatomy.

## *Partial Open Splenectomy*

The following information about partial splenectomy

### Editorial Comment

*Mass ligation of the splenic pedicle would indeed
include the structures mentioned above. Such ligations
might also include a portion of the tail of the spleen.
When mass ligations were performed in the past, there
were occasional reports of fistulization between the artery and the vein. Most surgeons would now advocate
visualization and individual ligation of the vessels.
(RSF Jr)*

comes from a personal communication to John E. Skandalakis from Steven R. Shackford, M.D., on November 21,
1997.

*Partial splenectomy (as opposed to total splen-
ectomy) requires a mature judgment and technical skill.
Judgment must be exercised in knowing when to preserve the spleen and when to excise it. Generally, this
decision is based upon the age of the patient, the condition of the patient, and the condition of the spleen.*

*With regard to the age of the patient, every attempt
should be made to preserve the spleen in the pediatric*

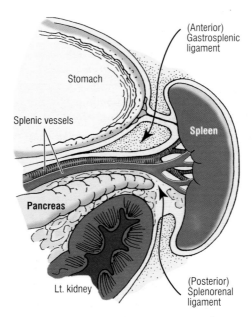

**FIG 22-33.** The anterior and posterior approaches to total splenectomy. (Modified from Pemberton LB, Skandalakis LJ. Indications for
and technique of total splenectomy. Probl Gen Surg 1990;7:85-102;
with permission.)

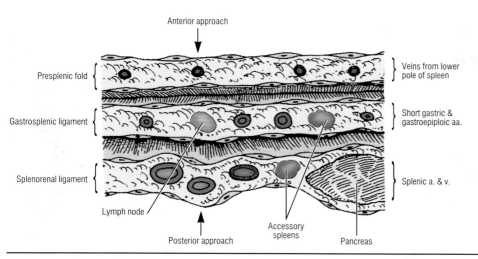

FIG 22-34. Diagrammatic section through the splenic pedicle containing presplenic fold, gastrosplenic ligament, and spleno-renal ligament. Vessels, fat, lymph nodes, accessory spleens, and the tail of the pancreas are all present. (Modified from Skandalakis JE, Gray SW, Rowe JS Jr. Anatomical Complications in General Surgery. New York: McGraw-Hill, 1983, p.182; with permission.)

*population, in whom exposure to encapsulated organisms may be quite limited. In the older population (greater than age 30) splenic preservation becomes less necessary and less important. In those cases, splenic preservation will be determined primarily by the condition of the spleen (grade of injury) and the condition of the patient (hemodynamic and metabolic stability).*

*Two points deserve emphasis. First, complete mobilization of the spleen is absolutely necessary. This means freeing the spleen of all retroperitoneal, diaphragmatic, and colonic attachments. In addition, all of the short gastrics should be divided. This will allow complete mobilization of the spleen and allow the surgeon to completely examine the spleen for all*

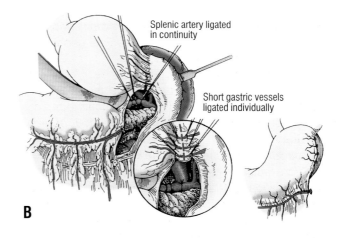

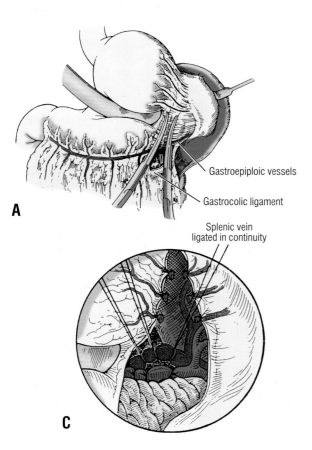

FIG 22-35. Splenectomy by the anterior approach. **A,** Anterior approach and access to the lesser sac. **B,** Ligation of the splenic artery and the short gastric arteries and vein. **C,** Ligation of the splenic vein. (Modified from Pemberton LB, Skandalakis LJ. Indications for and technique of total splenectomy. Probl Gen Surg 1990;7:85-102; with permission.)

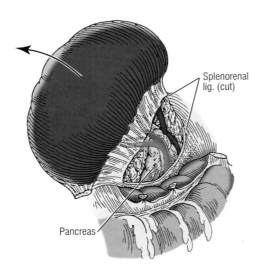

**FIG 22-36.** Splenectomy by the posterior approach. (Modified from Pemberton LB, Skandalakis LJ. Indications for and technique of total splenectomy. Probl Gen Surg 1990;7:85-102; with permission.)

*types of injury. Second, in the pediatric population the splenic capsule is relatively thick compared to the splenic capsule found in older patients. This is because, in children, the myoepithelial capsule is retained. As the spleen enlarges and matures, the myoepithelial elements "thin out." As a result, the capsule in the pediatric patient is more "forgiving" and holds sutures much better than that of the older population.*

Morgenstern[110] stated:

*Partial splenectomy is a feasible method of preserving immunologic function in the traumatized spleen. At least one-third and preferably one-half of viable spleen should be preserved in suitable patients. Essential steps in the technique include an adequate incision, temporary splenic artery occlusion, atraumatic mobilization of the spleen, selective ligation of segmental vasculature, and controlled intrasplenic dissection, with individual ligation or clipping of the intraparenchymal vessels. Variations on this technique include the use of an absorbable mesh for coaptation of multiple fragments and the use of an ultrasonic surgical aspirator for dissection of the intrasplenic vessels. Drains are not recommended unless there is concomitant pancreatic injury. The technique is also feasible for resection of splenic cysts and may be applicable to disorders such as Gaucher's disease and schistosomiasis.*

Morgenstern advised the following:[110]
- Administration of polyvalent antipneumococcal vaccine before surgery, plus a broad-spectrum antibiotic adminis-

tered in three doses — one prior to surgery and two after
- For a segmental (partial) splenectomy, the best incision is left upper quadrant (LUQ). However, a midline incision is acceptable if there is a possibility of multiple intraabdominal injuries.
- Temporary occlusion of the splenic artery
- Preparation and isolation of segmental splenic arteries and veins and ligation of the vessels that supply the segment to be removed
- A check of the color, size, and consistency of the segment to be preserved
- Separation by noncircumferential incision of the viable segment from the splenic part to be removed. The surgeon should proceed with careful intrasplenic dissection and ligation of bleeding vessels, using miniclips or regular hemoclips.
- If there are deep lacerations in the splenic remnant, an absorbable polyglycolic mesh should be used as a wrap
- Replacement of the splenic segment in the LUQ
- Observation of the segment for 5 to 10 minutes for color and bleeding
- Usage of drains is required if pancreatic injury is suspected; in other cases drains are used at the discretion of the surgeon

## *Laparoscopic Splenectomy*

Poulin and Thibault[62] advised that the surgeon acquire thorough knowledge of the standard anatomy and possible variations of the following anatomic entities before performing laparoscopic splenectomy:
- Length of the splenic artery
- Number of arterial branches entering the medial splenic surface (see Fig. 22-8, Fig. 22-37)
- Ligaments of the spleen (Fig. 22-5)
- Relation of the pancreatic tail and the spleen (Fig 22-38).

Brunt et al.[111] suggested that laparoscopic splenectomy should become the procedure of choice for the removal of a normal or near-normal sized spleen. They stated that the laparoscopic operation is not only safe, but also has advantages when compared to open procedures. Waldhausen and Tapper[112] found that laparoscopic splenectomy can be performed safely in children, and advocated it because it permits faster return to normal activities. Decker et al.[113] stated, based on a small study sample, that laparoscopic splenectomy may be as beneficial for patients with malignant processes as for those with benign hematologic conditions. According to Katkhouda et al.,[114] "laparoscopic splenectomy is feasible for the surgeon, teachable for the resident, and beneficial to the patient."

Park et al.[115] stated that "[c]ompared with OS (open splenectomy), the lateral approach to LS (laparoscopic

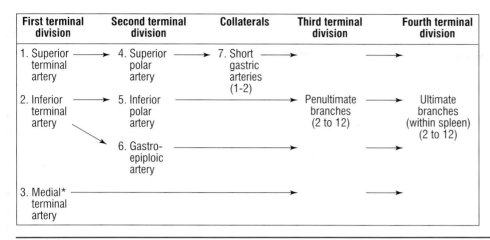

| First terminal division | Second terminal division | Collaterals | Third terminal division | Fourth terminal division |
|---|---|---|---|---|
| 1. Superior terminal artery | 4. Superior polar artery | 7. Short gastric arteries (1-2) | | |
| 2. Inferior terminal artery | 5. Inferior polar artery | | Penultimate branches (2 to 12) | Ultimate branches (within spleen) (2 to 12) |
| | 6. Gastro-epiploic artery | | | |
| 3. Medial* terminal artery | | | | |

FIG 22-37. General scheme of splenic artery branches. Asterisk (*) indicates present in only 20 percent of cases. (From Poulin EC, Thibault C. The anatomic basis for laparoscopic splenectomy. Can J Surg 1993;36:484; with permission.)

splenectomy) takes longer to perform but results in reduced blood loss, shorter postoperative stay, and fewer complications. Mean weighted cost of LS is lower than OS at the study institutions."

We highly recommended that the interested student read the beautiful description of laparoscopic splenectomy by Phillips et al.[116]

## *Considerations in Splenectomy*

In at least three diseases — sickle-cell anemia, cold antibody immune hemolytic anemia, and glucose-6-phosphate deficiency — splenectomy is of little or no benefit to the patient, and therefore rarely indicated.

Al-Salem[117] reported that splenectomy in children with massive splenomegaly is a safe and effective procedure if the perioperative management is good.

Because performing a splenectomy or adding it to another abdominal operation has a high operative morbidity (15-50%) and mortality (6-27%), surgeons have tried to devise operative methods to minimize or prevent complications.[118,119] The operative anatomy of splenectomy is summarized in Table 22-8.

The main goal of performing a splenectomy, regardless of the size of the spleen, is to remove the spleen rapidly and safely. This part of the operation should result in minimal blood loss, clean removal of the entire spleen, and minimal injury to the adjacent structures. In addition, the surgeon wants to try to avoid the most common complications of splenectomy: atelectasis, subphrenic abscess, and postoperative hemorrhage from the splenic bed.

After rupture of the spleen, the surgeon should evaluate the organ and decide if it is salvageable. Consideration should be given to partial splenectomy or splenorrhaphy (Fig. 22-39). One should also evaluate the possibility of applying topical items, hemostatic agents, or splenic mesh

wrap (Fig. 22-40). Autotransplantation should also be contemplated to preserve the spleen and retain immunological function (Fig. 22-41).

Powell et al.[120] stated that successful nonoperative treatment of blunt splenic trauma in children can be accomplished in more than 90% of patients, though it has not been as successful with adults. This is because in addition to different splenic anatomy, the mechanism of injury also differs in children.

Autotransplantation of splenic tissue within the peritoneal cavity can also follow injury. Multiple splenic fragments of small size produce splenosis. Splenosis can be an asymptomatic benign process, although it is occasionally symptomatic. Metwally and Ravo[28] stated that it is generally agreed that patients who have undergone partial splenectomy survive bacterial challenge better than those receiving autotransplantation of much larger volumes of spleen.

Studies by Weber et al.[121] showed that when in situ preservation of the spleen is not possible by other techniques, splenic autotransplantation into the greater omentum should be considered, especially in the pediatric patient.

There are three different types of splenectomy. The first

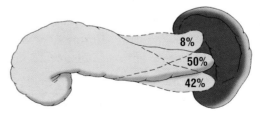

FIG 22-38. Relations of the tail of the pancreas to the spleen. (Modified from Skandalakis JE, Colborn GL, Pemberton LB, Skandalakis PN, Skandalakis LJ, Gray SW. The surgical anatomy of the spleen. Probl Gen Surg 1990; 7:1-17; with permission.)

| TABLE 22-8. The Technical Steps in Performing a Splenectomy | | |
|---|---|---|
| **For Trauma** | **For Hematologic Disorders** | **Staging Procedure** |
| Incision | Incision | Incision |
| Mobilizing the spleen | Arterial ligation | Detailed exploratory laparotomy (lymph nodes) |
| Vascular ligation | Mobilizing the spleen | Wedge and needle biopsies of both lobes of liver |
| Dividing the hilum | Dividing the hilum | Total splenectomy |
| Hemostasis | Hemostasis | Retroperitoneal exploration |
| Drains | Accessory spleen | Biopsy of iliac crest marrow |
| Closure | Drains | Search for accessory spleens |
| | Closure | Translocation of ovaries |
| | | Application of metal clips |

*Source:* Pemberton LB, Skandalakis LJ. Indications for the technique of total splenectomy. Probl Gen Surg 7(1):85-102, 1990; with permission.

type is the rapid, safe excision of a normal- or almost normal-sized spleen. This type of operation includes most splenectomies done for such diagnoses as external trauma and intraoperative trauma, and many hematologic diseases.

The second type of splenectomy is excision of a massively enlarged spleen. These spleens frequently extend down to the iliac crest and occasionally to the pelvic cavity. Their sheer weight and size make them difficult to move or lift without rupturing the capsule or the attachments. This type of splenectomy requires patience and some special technical maneuvers.

The third type of splenectomy is staging splenectomy for Hodgkin's disease. The operation for staging has many different components and represents a special type of splenectomy. The components of the operation for the

staging of Hodgkin's disease are presented in the last part of this section.

## Incisions

The midline incision (Fig. 22-42) is the incision of choice for most indications, such as trauma, hypersplenism with coagulation problems, staging laparotomy for Hodgkin's disease, and massive splenomegaly. The midline incision has several important advantages in splenectomy. First, with a large enough incision and adequate exposure of the left upper quadrant, the surgeon can safely remove the spleen, no matter what size it is. Second, the incision is quick and easy to make, and results in little loss of blood. Third, this incision allows the surgeon to explore the entire abdomen and to deal with any other associated problems, such as gallstones, lacerated liver, and splenosis, and to

### Editorial Comment

*I am skeptical about the value of autotransplantation, particularly using a large remnant as pictured in Fig. 22-41. Non-vascularized transplants receive their oxygen and nutrients by diffusion until they develop a blood supply and most of such a large remnant would necrose. Smaller splenic fragments placed in the omentum have been shown to persist as implants by liver-spleen scans, but the animal and human studies that I am aware of have not been convincing that these implants provide normal splenic function. It has been reported that splenic autotransplants have not eliminated the increased rate of postsplenectomy infection. (RSF Jr)*

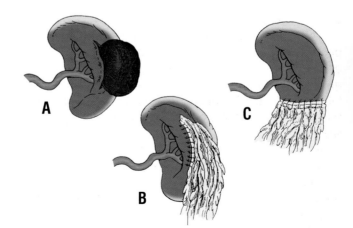

**FIG 22-39. A,** Splenic rupture with hematoma. **B,** Splenorrhaphy with omental fixation. **C,** Partial splenectomy with omental fixation. (Modified from Pemberton LB, Skandalakis LJ. Indications for and technique of total splenectomy. Probl Gen Surg 1990;7:85-102; with permission.)

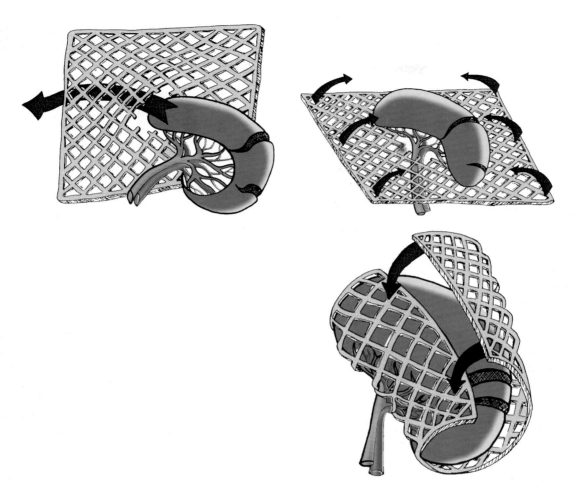

**FIG 22-40.** Splenic mesh wrap. *Top left,* Passage of injured spleen through hole in center of mesh. *Top right,* Wrapping spleen in mesh. *Bottom,* Sewing opposite edges of mesh to each other to create tamponade. (Modified from Lange DA, Zaret P, Merlotti GJ, Robin AP, Sheaff C, Barrett JA. The use of absorbable mesh in splenic trauma. J Trauma 1988;28:269-275; with permission.)

perform multiple biopsies, if necessary.

The left subcostal incision, also, can give adequate exposure for a splenectomy. It is appropriate for a mass in a normal-sized spleen or even a spleen that is twice the normal size, or when no other abdominal procedures are contemplated.[122] But because these indications occur infrequently, most splenectomies are performed through a midline incision.

No difference in postoperative complications has been observed between midline and subcostal incisions, so the surgeon should choose the incision that gives the best exposure for the operation planned[123] and with which he or she is most familiar.

Occasionally, a thoracoabdominal incision may make removal of a massive spleen with many adhesions safe and easy.[124] The risks of increased morbidity and mortality from this incision must be compared with the benefits of improved exposure and control. The thoracoabdominal inci-

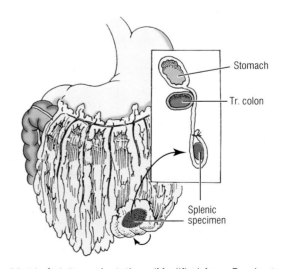

**FIG 22-41.** Autotransplantation. (Modified from Pemberton LB, Skandalakis LJ. Indications for and technique of total splenectomy. Probl Gen Surg 1990; 7:85-102; with permission.)

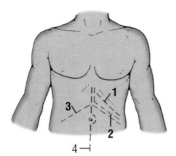

1. Subcostal
2. Kehr subcostal
3. Bilateral subcostal
4. Midline

FIG 22-42. Incision for total splenectomy. (Modified from Pemberton LB, Skandalakis LJ. Indications for and technique of total splenectomy. Probl Gen Surg 1990;7:85-102; with permission.)

sion is an operation that can be considered for use in splenectomy in a few selected patients.

### Drains

The use of drains is controversial. Advice ranges from always using drains to never using drains.[118,125] Drains are used in patients having splenectomy to prevent a left subphrenic collection and an abscess formation. The risk of a subphrenic infection developing is greatly increased when the gastrointestinal tract is opened, the indication for splenectomy is hypersplenism, or the patient has a pancreatic injury or a malignant disease. When one of these conditions is present, the patient may be a candidate for a drain. Carmichael et al.[126] supported selective splenic bed drainage.

Although some are better than others, most drains accomplish their purpose of removing an accumulation of blood, lymph, or pancreatic fluid from the subphrenic space. The main problem with placing drains in the splenic bed is the possibility of an ascending infection inoculating the splenic bed and producing an abscess. Thus, the drain could cause, rather than prevent, a subphrenic abscess.

The three main types of drains available are the Penrose, the open sump suction, and the closed suction drains. The advantage of the Penrose is that it provides very good drainage. Its disadvantage is that there is no way to apply suction to the drain, so bacteria and fluid can ascend as well as descend. The advantage of open and closed suction drains is decreased risk of infection, but their disadvantage is that the lumina of the drainage tubes can become occluded with coagulated blood and other matter, thus limiting drainage.

Ellison and Fabri[127] reported a 4.2% incidence of subphrenic abscesses in 1,944 splenectomies. They reviewed five studies of the use of drains (Penrose or open suction) after splenectomy and found an incidence of 6.5% to

48% of subphrenic infections in patients with drains compared with 0.4% to 12% in patients without drains. These authors concluded that drains should be avoided when possible; if drainage is needed, a closed-suction system should be used and removed as soon as feasible.

Two studies investigated the efficacy of using closed-suction drains to prevent subphrenic collection and infection. In a prospective, randomized, controlled study, Pachter et al.[128] compared 23 patients with no drains and 30 patients with Jackson-Pratt closed-suction drains. All drains were removed within 48 hours, except for those in two patients with persistent drainage who had 48 more hours (4 days total) of the drainage. Neither drained nor undrained patients developed subphrenic infection.

The duration of the use of drains is an important part of their safe implementation after splenectomy. Ugochukwu and Irving[125] reported the use of closed-suction drains in 282 consecutive splenectomies in which the drains were removed in 3 to 5 days. The incidence of subphrenic infection in this large group of patients with drains was 0.71%.

Scanlon[129] wrote that intraabdominal dead space following splenectomy "usually is filled by the small intestine, and, to a certain extent, by the colon and the stomach." He indicated that when residual air persists it is replaced by serum, which can become infected. He suggested that the presence of fluid in the dead space posed a greater risk of infection than did a drain.

Olsen and Beaudoin[130] reported that prophylactic drainage increases the incidence of subphrenic abscess. Jordan[131] did not recommend routine drainage. Maingot[132] believed that drainage is unnecessary. McNair[133] avoided the use of drains. Fabri et al.[134] did a retrospective study of splenectomy, citing authors who drained the splenic bed along with others who believed that drainage

### Editorial Comment

*It has been my general policy to avoid the use of drains after splenectomy. If drainage is to be used for a specific reason, it should be a closed suction type of drainage. Scanlon's[129] statement that the dead space following removal of the spleen is usually filled by the small intestine is not consistent with my experience. It is my impression that it is the stomach and colon that shift into the space formerly occupied by the spleen. (RSF Jr)*

has become a matter of election; Fabri and colleagues used no drainage. Chassin[135] advises drainage if there is injury to the pancreas or if there is incomplete hemostasis.

## Surgery for Splenic Artery Aneurysms

The most common visceral artery aneurysms are those of the splenic artery;[136] they may be multiple.[137,138] They occur most frequently in the distal splenic artery.[139] Multiparous women constitute a well-recognized risk group; the mechanism of this association is uncertain.[140] Portal hypertension is reportedly also associated with an increased risk of aneurysm formation[140-142] (probably secondary to increased splenic flow).[143] Since most splenic aneurysms are asymptomatic, they are often identified only at the discovery of a calcified lesion in the left upper quadrant.[141] Majeski[144] advised that if calcifications are present in the left upper quadrant, diagnostic imaging procedures will help differentiate the diagnosis of splenic artery aneurysm from a calcified tortuous splenic artery.

Sometimes splenic aneurysms present with left upper quadrant pain; a small percentage proceed to rupture. Of those that rupture, 25 percent exhibit a double-rupture phenomenon: bleeding occurs first in the lesser sac (where it is temporarily contained) before free rupture into the peritoneal cavity.[139,142,145] According to Lumsden et al.,[136] patients with symptomatic or expanding aneurysms should undergo resection.

Pregnant women are at particular risk of aneurysm rupture.[146] They should have resection, ideally in midtrimester. Those planning pregnancy should have aneurysm repair before their pregnancy. Patients with small aneurysms (<2.5 cm) may be observed carefully.[147] Should intervention be necessary, there are a variety of options. Surgically, the best option is aneurysm resection. However, if it is fixed to the pancreas, ligation alone may suffice. For distal aneurysms, splenectomy or distal pancreatectomy and splenectomy may be necessary. Splenic artery embolization is feasible, particularly if surgery is contraindicated.

De Perrot et al.[148] reported that of 8 patients presenting with rupture of splenic artery aneurysm between 1977 and 1996, 7 survived. They stated that an aneurysm of the splenic artery may rupture at any age, and aggressive surgery is the procedure of choice.

The true incidence of splenic artery aneurysms is difficult to ascertain; estimates range from 0.098% to 10.4% of the population.[147,149,150] However, splenic artery aneurysms are more common than generally suspected. Autopsy studies have demonstrated that 10% of elderly patients have a splenic artery aneurysm.[149,150] Other researchers, using postmortem injection of the splenic artery, observed a 7.5% incidence of aneurysm formation.[151] Retrospective reviews of patients who had celiac angiography demonstrated an incidence of 5 to 13%.[143,151] Splenic artery aneurysms were found to occur in 9% of patients with portal hypertension having splenic arteriography.[152] However, in an unselected series of 28,500 autopsies, a 0.16% incidence of splenic artery aneurysms was observed;[141] this latter figure probably most accurately reflects the incidence in the general population.

The type of procedure to be performed in treating a splenic arterial aneurysm is largely dictated by the site of the aneurysm (Fig. 22-43). Those situated away from the celiac axis, not embedded in the pancreas, and not at the splenic hilum, should be excised, and the splenic artery ligated doubly (proximal and distal ligation). For aneurysms deeply embedded within the pancreas, the feeding vessels should be ligated and the devascularized aneurysmal sac left in situ. Aneurysms occurring in the splenic hilum require a concomitant splenectomy. Occasionally, when an aneurysm is partially embedded in the distal pancreas, a distal pancreatectomy and splenectomy may be warranted.

With an increased awareness of postsplenectomy sepsis, some authors strongly advocate splenic conservation, with proximal and distal ligation of the splenic artery, when technically feasible.[153] Although this approach is appealing, there is good evidence that interruption of the splenic artery with preservation of the spleen may still compromise splenic function. Consequently, the risk of postsplenectomy sepsis may persist.[154] Excision of an aneurysm with reanastomosis of the splenic artery has also been reported in a patient in whom the aneurysm developed after a distal splenorenal shunt.[155]

Embolization (Fig. 22-44) has been proposed for patients at high risk. This technique is in fairly widespread use for the treatment of bleeding pseudoaneurysms.[156,157]

## Indications for Splenic Surgery

One of a surgeon's primary responsibilities is to know the reasons for operating, meaning that the surgeon must understand the benefits a patient will derive from a splenectomy. The four main indications or reasons for performing a splenectomy are hemorrhage, hypersplenism, Hodgkin's disease staging, and hodgepodge (this word was chosen for lack of a better word beginning with "h" to complete the mnemonic device). When a surgeon decides to operate, these items are the determining factors in making that decision. Thus surgeons do not operate on diseases of the spleen but on special circumstances during

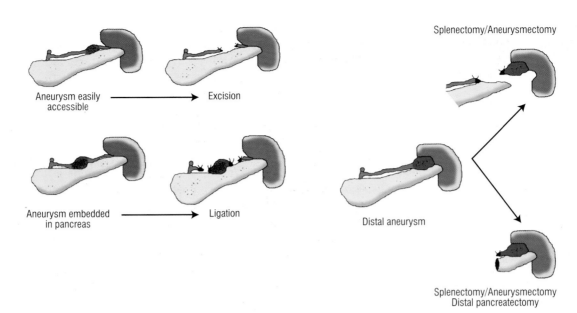

Splenectomy/Aneurysmectomy

Aneurysm easily
accessible                →        Excision

Aneurysm embedded
in pancreas              →        Ligation

Distal aneurysm

Splenectomy/Aneurysmectomy
Distal pancreatectomy

**FIG 22-43.** Type of procedure performed is dictated largely by the site of the aneurysm. *Top left,* When feasible, the aneurysm should be excised and the splenic artery ligated. *Bottom left,* If the aneurysmal sac is embedded within the pancreas, then proximal and distal ligation of the artery should be performed. *Right.* Distal aneurysms may be treated by excision with either the spleen or a concomitant distal pancreatectomy. (Modified from Lumsden AB, Riley JD, Skandalakis JE. Splenic artery aneurysms. Probl Gen Surg 1990;7:113-121; with permission.)

those diseases that appear to be best treated by an operation.[124,158,159]

### Hemorrhage

The primary disorder that causes splenic hemorrhage is trauma. Trauma can be classified into two main categories: external and internal (Table 22-9).

External trauma is the most common disorder of the spleen, and is divided into either blunt or penetrating injuries. The spleen is more commonly injured by blunt trauma than any other abdominal organ.[160] Usually, the blunt trauma causes a left upper quadrant injury with rib fractures or contusions of the left flank or lower left chest. A chest roentgenogram may show these injuries as an elevated diaphragm, rib fractures, or pleural effusion.[161] The well-protected posterior position of the spleen causes blunt trauma with high energy to split or fragment the solid spleen.

One useful diagnostic test for hemorrhage is peritoneal lavage, which reveals intraabdominal blood. Other tests involve detection of the injured spleen itself. They include computed tomography (CT), ultrasonography, or arteriography. Andrews[162] found ultrasound useful for noninvasive examination of the spleen and identification of splenic injury, hemangioma, accessory spleens, splenomegaly, focal solid or cystic masses, calcifications, thicken-

ing of the cystic wall, and splenic infarction. Penetrating trauma injures the spleen much less frequently because of the small size of the organ and its protected location.

Nonoperative management of blunt splenic injury has emerged as the most common method of splenic con-

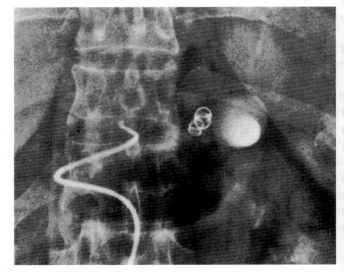

**FIG 22-44.** Selected aneurysms may be successfully embolized with Gianturco coils. (From Lumsden AB, Riley JD, Skandalakis JE. Splenic artery aneurysms. Probl Gen Surg 1990;7:113-121; with permission.)

**TABLE 22-9. The Traumatic Indications for Splenectomy in Hemorrhage**

| |
|---|
| External trauma |
| Blunt |
| Penetrating |
| Internal trauma |
| Operative |
| Spontaneous |

*Source:* Pemberton LB, Skandalakis LJ. Indications for and technique of total splenectomy. Probl Gen Surg 7(1):85-102, 1990; with permission.

ervation. According to Krause et al.,[163] hemodynamically table patients age 55 years and older who do not require ignificant blood transfusion and have no other associated bdominal injuries meet the criteria for nonoperative management. Velmahos et al.[164] found that patients who reuired a transfusion of more than one unit of blood or ustained a severe blunt injury were likely to need surgery fter a period of nonoperative management, and recomended that they be closely monitored.

Using a large database from 27 trauma centers, eitzman et al.[165] reported that "38.5% of adults with blunt plenic injury went directly to laparotomy. Ultimately, 4.8% of patients were successfully managed nonoperatively; the failure rate of planned observation was 10.8%, ith 60.9% of failures occurring in the first 24 hours. uccessful nonoperative management was associated ith higher blood pressure and hematocrit, and less evere injury based on the Injury Severity Score, Glasgow oma Scale, grade of splenic injury, and quantity of emoperitoneum."

Nonoperative management is also the treatment of hoice for traumatic injury of the spleen in newborns, a re condition.[166]

Splenic injury can occur from a knife or gunshot wound the left upper quadrant, the left flank, or the left lower nest. Any penetrating injury below the level of the nipple nteriorly, or the tip of the scapula posteriorly, can injure pleen. Penetrating splenic trauma usually injures one or ore adjacent organs, such as the stomach, colon, kidney, aphragm, or pancreas.[167] Because almost all of these enetrating injuries are explored, the surgeon is the one reonsible for identifying other associated injuries and eating them in the operating room.

Internal trauma accounts for 10% to 30% of splenic inries and splenectomies. It is caused most often by intraerative splenic injury, or, infrequently, by spontaneous pture of an enlarged spleen.[127,168] Although intraerative splenic injury complicates 2% of abdominal opations, it occurs mostly during operations on abdominal organs of the left upper quadrant.[127]

The most common form of left upper quadrant intraoperative splenic injury comes from traction on the greater omentum and avulsion of its attachment to the inferior pole of the spleen. One can avoid this intraoperative complication either by ligating and dividing this attachment, or by retracting only the omentum and the stomach or the left transverse colon toward the patient's left foot.

The other form of internal trauma is spontaneous rupture of the spleen, which is quite unlikely with a normal spleen. Patients with spontaneous rupture have abnormal spleens and no history of trauma. The two most common causes are malaria and infectious mononucleosis.[124] Some other diagnoses that have accompanied spontaneous splenic rupture are sarcoidosis, leukemia, and congestive splenomegaly. Celebrezze et al.[169] reported spontaneous splenic rupture secondary to splenic peliosis (blood-filled cystic structures).

Splenosis develops frequently following traumatic splenic rupture, and should be considered in the differential diagnosis of previously splenectomized patients who present with occult gastrointestinal bleeding or unexplained masses.[170]

De Vuysere et al.[171] reported a case of intrahepatic splenosis:

> [T]he diagnosis of intrahepatic splenosis occurring after previous splenic trauma and splenectomy was suggested by a constellation of MRI findings. The diagnosis was confirmed by histologic examination. Knowledge of these MRI characteristics may avoid the use of surgical interventions to arrive at the correct diagnosis of these rare liver lesions.

The nontraumatic indications for splenectomy are shown in Table 22-10.

## Hypersplenism

One of the main functions of the spleen is to remove the damaged blood elements, and diseases of the spleen can cause an acceleration in this removal.[124] If rapid destruction and removal involves one of the three elements — red blood cells, white blood cells, or platelets — the result is anemia, leukopenia, or thrombocytopenia, respectively. If this accelerated destruction involves all three blood elements, the process results in pancytopenia.

Hypersplenism is, in effect, an exaggeration of the normal splenic physiologic state. The syndrome is characterized by splenic enlargement, a decrease in circulating levels of one or more of the blood lines, and a compensatory increase in bone marrow activity in response to the defi-

**TABLE 22-10. The Nontraumatic Indications for Splenectomy**

| |
|---|
| Hypersplenism |
|     Congenital anemias |
|     Hemolytic anemias |
|     Leukemia or lymphoma |
|     Other nonspecific diseases |
| Hodgkin staging |
|     Diagnostic laparotomy |
| Hodgepodge (1-2% of operations) |
|     Abscess |
|     Cyst |
|     Tumor |

*Source:* Pemberton LB, Skandalakis LJ. Indications for and technique of total splenectomy. Probl Gen Surg 7(1):85-102, 1990; with permission.

ciency in the circulating blood elements. As a result of these defects there is increased cell turnover of the affected cell lines. In order for the diagnosis of hypersplenism to be considered correct there must be some degree of improvement following splenectomy.

Hypersplenism is classified as either primary or secondary. Primary hypersplenism is a diagnosis of exclusion, where identification of exaggerated splenic function is made without an apparent etiology. It is important to note that true primary hypersplenism is an exceedingly rare entity usually found in women. Diagnosis can be made only after an extensive search for other causes. Secondary hypersplenism refers to cases in which the disorder is found in association with a specific disease process. Diseases commonly associated with secondary hypersplenism are listed in Table 22-11.

Splenomegaly is sometimes confused with hypersplenism. Splenomegaly simply refers to the enlargement of the spleen from any cause. Hypersplenism refers to an excessive removal of the blood elements resulting in some form of cytopenia. Furthermore, these two splenic disorders usually occur separately. Most patients with hypersplenism do not have splenomegaly (more than 90%). Fewer than 10% of patients with splenomegaly have hypersplenism.[124]

Some patients with massive splenomegaly have hypersplenism as part of the indication for splenectomy.[172] Almost all patients with splenomegaly who require surgery have either hypersplenism, splenic infarction, or splenic rupture as the precipitating indication for a splenectomy. Splenomegaly by itself seldom appears to be an appropriate indication for splenectomy.

Cytopenia (hyperfunction of the spleen's removal of any of the blood elements) is an indication for splenectomy. The four main categories of diseases that cause these cytopenias are the congenital anemias, the hemolytic anemias, white blood cell malignancies, and miscellaneous disorders.

Spherocytosis and elliptocytosis are congenital diseases that produce round and ovoid red blood cells, respectively. The shape of these cells makes it difficult for them to pass through the splenic filter. Because the red blood cells pass through the spleen about 1,000 times per day, the splenic cords and sinuses have many opportunities to trap and destroy the cells with these abnormal shapes.[124] Splenectomy removes the splenic filter that destroys the cells, and improves the red blood cell survival rate.

Idiopathic thrombocytopenic purpura (ITP) is thought to involve an immune mechanism that causes premature platelet destruction and low platelet counts.[124] Its signs are bleeding into the skin, such as purpura or ecchymosis, and bleeding into the gastrointestinal, urinary, or genital tract. ITP occurs mostly in women, and may follow an upper respiratory infection. Initial treatment is with steroids. If steroids fail or the disease recurs, a splenectomy is indicated and produces a favorable response 85% to 95% of the time.[124]

**TABLE 22-11. Diseases Associated with Secondary Hypersplenism**

| |
|---|
| Congestive splenomegaly |
|     Cirrhosis |
|     Splenic vein thrombosis |
|     Portal hypertension |
| Neoplastic |
|     Metastatic carcinoma |
|     Lymphoma |
|     Leukemia |
| Chronic inflammatory |
|     Sarcoidosis |
|     Systemic lupus erythematosus |
|     Felty's syndrome |
| Infiltrative |
|     Amyloidosis |
|     Gaucher's disease |
|     Niemann-Pick disease |
| Infectious |
|     Tuberculosis |
|     Mononucleosis |
|     Malaria |
| Chronic hemolytic diseases |
|     Spherocytosis |
|     Thalassemia |
|     Elliptocytosis |
| Myeloproliferative disorders |
|     Myelofibrosis with myeloid metaplasia |

*Source:* Modified from Way LW. Current Surgical Diagnosis and Treatment 11th ed. Norwalk, Conn: Appleton & Lange, 1994; with permission.

Removal of accessory spleens must also be done. ITP accounts for about 20% of the hematologic diseases treated by splenectomy.[119,173]

Schwartz[174] evaluated the role of splenectomy in hematologic disorders. He stated that for hereditary spherocytosis, splenectomy is curative; for ITP, splenectomy is therapeutic. Winde et al.[175] emphasized that splenectomy is the treatment of choice for idiopathic thrombocytopenic purpura. In contrast, Bussel[176] reviewed splenectomy-sparing treatment for chronic ITP, and suggested a measured tolerance for lower platelet counts before recommending intervention. Bell[177] added further cautions:

> [S]plenectomy as a treatment for ITP has a fairly favorable initial response rate of 60% to 80%. Few studies that have followed such patients for extended periods, however, show a durable response, and there is no question that the longer the follow-up period for ITP patients who have undergone splenectomy, the lower the success rate.

White blood cell malignancies, namely lymphoma and leukemia, can produce hypersplenism in the course of these chronic diseases. Patients with lymphocytic lymphoma and chronic lymphocytic leukemia have splenic infiltration that causes splenomegaly, slow transit time of blood elements, and pancytopenia.[124] Positive chromium-labeled red blood cell studies confirm splenic sequestration. A splenectomy can ameliorate the pancytopenia in these patients.

Cusack et al.[178] reported that if splenectomy in chronic lymphocytic leukemia is performed early in patients with Hb ≤10 g/dL or plt ≤50 × 109/L, the survival rate of these patients is significantly improved.

## Hodgkin's Disease Staging

Since 1971, laparotomy has been recommended for more accurate staging of Hodgkin's lymphoma. This has allowed treatment to be optimized for early- as well as late-stage disease. Taylor et al.[179] reported on 825 patients with Hodgkin's disease who had a staging laparotomy. They found that 356 (43%) patients had a change in their clinical staging as a result of this operation: an increase in 296 patients (36%) and a decrease in 60 patients (7%). Even though the study was retrospective, they concluded that the improvements in survival and the freedom from progression that resulted from the accurate staging and more precise therapy justified the continued use of staging laparotomy. Furthermore, they concluded that splenectomy must remain an essential part of staging laparotomy because the spleen was the only tissue that contained Hodgkin's disease in 50%, or 160, of the 321 patients who had positive findings.[179]

With the development of better imaging technology, reliance on the staging laparotomy has diminished. Although staging laparotomy is performed much less commonly, in select patients, such as those who are not candidates for chemotherapy, this procedure may still be quite useful. Baccarani et al.[180] stated that laparoscopic staging of Hodgkin's disease is, from an oncologic standpoint, equivalent and functionally superior to open staging laparotomy.

Recently, both Klasa et al.[181] and Santoro et al.[182] have reported complete remission in 95-98% of patients with stage I-II disease. Given the risks associated with splenectomy and the fact that it will be difficult to improve on these data, many are advocating that the treatment of Hodgkin's disease be based on clinical staging, i.e., physical exam, CT and magnetic resonance imaging, and bone marrow aspiration.

If a staging laparotomy is to be performed, understanding the stages of Hodgkin's disease is helpful in this exploratory surgery to define the anatomic sites of involvement. The four stages of Hodgkin's disease and clinical modifiers are listed in Table 22-12.[183] A staging laparotomy should be preceded by the following: history, physical examination, complete blood count, urinalysis, blood chemistries, bone marrow aspiration, chest roentgenogram, CT or magnetic resonance imaging of the abdomen, and sometimes lymphangiography.

**TABLE 22-12. Ann Arbor Staging System for Hodgkin's Disease**

| Stage | |
|---|---|
| Stage I | Single lymph node region or extralymphoid size |
| Stage II | Two or more lymph node areas or one extralymphoid site with one lymph node area; but all are on one side of the diaphragm |
| Stage III | Multiple lymph node sites on both sides of the diaphragm. With localized extralymphoid sites, this is IIIE; with splenic involvement, IIIS; and with both, IIIES. |
| Stage IV | Diffuse involvement of extralymphoid organs, with or without adenopathy |
| **Clinical Modifiers** | |
| A | No systemic symptoms |
| B | Temperature above 38°C, night sweats, or weight loss |

*Source:* Meyer AA. Spleen. In: Greenfield LJ, Mulholland M, Oldham KT, Zelenock GB, Lillemoe KD (eds). Surgery: Scientific Principles and Practices, 2nd ed. Philadelphia: Lippincott-Raven, 1997, p. 1274; with permission).

Staging procedures for Hodgkin's disease and limited non-Hodgkin's lymphoma include the following (Fig. 22-45):

- Detailed exploratory laparotomy
- Examination of nodes, and wedge and needle biopsies of both lobes of the liver
- Total splenectomy with splenic lymph node biopsy
- Retroperitoneal exploration of the celiac axis, hepato-duodenopancreatic lymph nodes, periaortic lymph nodes, inferior vena caval lymph nodes, iliac lymph nodes, and mesenteric lymph nodes of the small and large intestines for lymph node biopsies
- Biopsy of iliac crest marrow
- Search for accessory spleens
- Oophoropexy (ovarian translocation) in young women
- Placement of metal clips at the splenic pedicle, the areas where biopsies have been done on lymph nodes, the areas of lymph nodes on which biopsies have not been performed, and at the site of ovarian translocation

Because a staging laparotomy is done for diagnosis, the correct handling of these fresh specimens usually requires the presence of a pathologist in the operating room.[184] Touch preparations of the lymph nodes and spleen should be made. Tissues should be placed in a special fixative solution for electron microscope examination. Slides of bone marrow specimens should be made. The pathologist can then choose any other tissue preparation for future examination. The proper handling of these tissues completes the staging laparotomy for Hodgkin's disease.

### Hodgepodge

This last category includes a miscellaneous group of disorders. Splenic abscesses, cysts, and tumors produce a mass within the spleen. Their removal and definitive treatment usually requires a splenectomy.

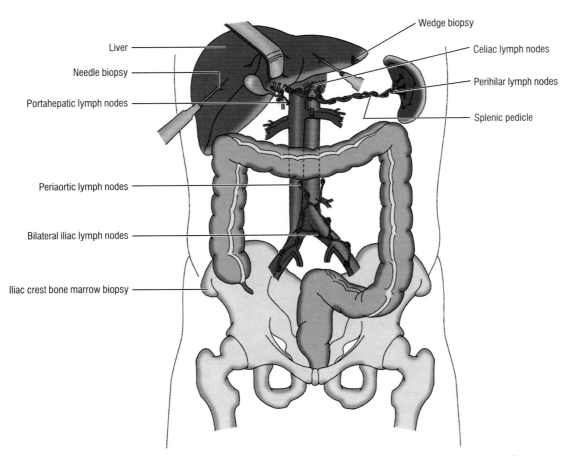

FIG 22-45. The tissues to be removed or to undergo biopsy in a staging laparotomy for Hodgkin's disease. Splenectomy, liver biopsy, and lymph node sampling in the specific sites are shown. Bone marrow biopsy can be done if necessary. (Modified from Meyer AA. Spleen. In: Greenfield LJ, Mulholland M, Oldham KT, Zelenock GB, Lillemoe KD (eds.) Surgery: Scientific Principles and Practices, 2nd ed. Philadelphia: Lippincott-Raven, 1997, p. 1275; with permission.)

## Splenic Abscesses

Isolated splenic abscess is a rare condition, with fewer than 400 cases being reported from the beginning of the century until 1986.[185-187] However, over the last 15 years this uncommon clinical entity has been increasingly identified as the cause of intraabdominal sepsis in a wide variety of clinical situations, particularly in immunosuppressed patients. In a study of 287 cases reported in the literature between 1987 and 1995, Ooi and Leong[187] found that immunosuppressed states were present in 33.5% of the cases. Acquired immune deficiency syndrome and intravenous drug use accounted for half of the immunosuppressed cases. The authors reported *Staphylococcus, Salmonella,* and *Escherichia coli* to be the organisms most commonly identified by culture.

Early diagnosis is the key to effective treatment of splenic abscesses. Ultrasonography and computerized tomography are diagnostic. Splenectomy is the treatment of choice. Percutaneous drainage, however, is a possible alternative in selected or debilitated patients.[188,189] Ooi and Leong[187] report that US- or CT-guided percutaneous aspiration and catheter drainage have demonstrated sufficient success rates (75%)[190,191] to be considered first-line therapy in certain situations such as uncomplicated solitary lesions, critically ill patients, and pediatric patients in whom splenic conservation is important.

Phillips et al.[192] advised that the diagnosis of splenic abscess should be considered in patients using intravenous drugs who are suffering fever and abdominal pain.

## Splenic Cysts

Cysts of the spleen are rare, but more common than primary tumors. Worldwide, the most common splenic cysts are parasitic, the majority of which are echinococcal. Even in countries where echinococcus is endemic, however, hydatid disease of the spleen is a rare clinical entity.[193] The spleen ranks third, behind the liver and the lung, as the most commonly involved organ in hydatid disease.[193-196]

In North America, nonparasitic cysts are found much more frequently than parasitic cysts. Sirinek and Evans[184] reported that nonparasitic splenic cysts usually occur in persons between the ages of 10 and 40 years. These cysts include the following (in decreasing order of frequency): pseudocysts, hemangiomas, epidermoid cysts, and dermoid cysts. Because most splenic cysts are unilocular (80%), CT scan is the preferred method of detecting these rare lesions. With the exception of small nonparasitic cysts, for which observation may be sufficient, splenectomy is usually the treatment of choice for all types of splenic cysts, parasitic or nonparasitic.

Atraumatic rupture of the spleen due to ceroid histiocytosis was reported by Wilson et al.[197]

## Splenic Tumors

Primary tumors of the spleen are very rare entities.[122] The treatment of choice for splenic tumors is splenectomy.

The most common splenic tumors are not from lymphoid tissue but are vascular neoplasms: hemangioma, hemangioendothelioma, lymphangioma, and hamartoma. The other primary tumors are various malignant tumors (Table 22-13). Although the majority of primary splenic tumors are vascular in origin, primary splenic lymphoma and primary tumors of other origin have been reported. Salgado et al.[198] reported cases of B-type large-cell primary splenic lymphoma with massive involvement of the red pulp. Rosso et al.[199] reported three cases of splenic marginal zone cell lymphoma arising from the white pulp of the spleen, but without splenomegaly or bone marrow and lymph node involvement. Usually this disease produces massive splenomegaly with bone marrow and lymph node involvement. Westra et al.[200] reported a malignant mixed (epithelial

### TABLE 22-13. Malignant Splenic Lesions

I. Lymphoproliferative disorders
    Non-Hodgkin's lymphoma
    Hodgkin's disease
    Chronic lymphocytic leukemia
    Hairy cell leukemia
    Acute lymphoblastic leukemia
    Waldenström's macroglobulinemia
    Plasmacytoma
II. Myeloproliferative disorders
    Chronic myelogenous leukemia
    Myelofibrosis (agnogenic myeloid metaplasia)
    Polycythemia vera
    Essential thrombocythemia
III. Vascular tumors
    *Benign*
      Hemangioma
      Hamartoma
      Lymphangioma
    *Malignant*
      Hemangiosarcoma
      Lymphangiosarcoma
IV. Metastatic tumors
    Breast, lung, melanoma, cervix, etc.
V. Others
    Lipoma
    Malignant fibrous histiocytoma
    Fibrosarcoma
    Leiomyosarcoma
    Malignant teratoma
    Kaposi's sarcoma

*Source:* Giles FJ, Lim SW. Malignant splenic lesions. In: Hiatt JR, Phillips EH, Morgenstern L (eds). Surgical Diseases of the Spleen. Berlin: Springer, 1997; with permission.

and stromal elements) primary tumor of the spleen, perhaps of extrauterine mullerian origin. Brune et al.[201] reported splenic lymphoma with villous lymphocytes. This is a distinct entity, separate from other B-cell lymphoproliferative disorders.

Clinically, metastasis to the spleen is a rare phenomenon even though it is found fairly frequently by careful examination at autopsy.[202] If, indeed, metastasis occurs, it is probably hematogenous or resulting from invasion of the spleen by neighboring organs such as the stomach, pancreas, colon, left kidney, or by malignant tumors of the retroperitoneal space. We have seen only one instance of metastatic carcinoma to the spleen in patients hospitalized with carcinoma. The subject of metastasis to the spleen will be addressed in depth later in this chapter.

## Specific Notes on Surgical Anatomy

- The splenorenal ligament has small veins that can cause problems.
- The perisplenic adhesions are vascular.
- The terminal splenic vessels are fragile and easily torn or perforated.
- The splenic capsule, also, is friable.
- Dissection of the splenic artery close to the celiac artery, through the gastrocolic omentum, can be done if the spleen is large or has moderate splenomegaly and adhesions. However, one must not forget the superfragile splenic vein; it can coil around the artery and produce a sudden large loss of blood.
- With huge spleens (such as those secondary to malaria or kala azar) with heavy and vascular multiple adhesions, the artery can be ligated along the upper pancreatic border after the gastrocolic ligament is opened.
- A healthy ruptured spleen can be delivered easily from the abdomen.
- A large, diseased spleen requires careful dissection of the prehilar area and ligation of the vessels.
- In thrombocytopenic purpura, the abdomen should be explored after the spleen is removed.
- In ITP, the splenic artery should be ligated as soon as possible.
- In the presence of hemolytic anemia, transfusions should not be given before the operation. Platelets should be transfused after splenic artery ligation.
- Short gastric arteries and veins should be transfixed, and the greater curvature of the stomach should be inverted to avoid bleeding and gastric necrosis. In the period immediately after splenectomy, a roentgenographic gastrointestinal series should be taken, and the image of the deformity of the greater curvature should be saved for future comparison.
- If the splenic artery requires ligation proximally, it should also be ligated distally, as close to the hilum as feasible.
- The pancreatic tail should be handled gently, particularly where it is usually vulnerable: at the hilum, posterior to the pedicle.
- The renocolosplenic area should be handled gently to avoid renal or colonic injury or bleeding from the spleen.
- If the splenic pedicle is ligated en masse, the hilar vessels should be religated. The pedicle should be ligated twice.
- An autologous splenic capsule should be used over the raw splenic surface; the graft should be secured with fine sutures.[203]
- The pancreas should be separated from the spleen by division of the splenic artery and the splenic vein distal to the tip of the pancreas. The spleen can survive on the short gastric vessels, which should be carefully preserved. Warshaw[204] applied the technique successfully in 22 of 25 consecutive patients.
- The technique selected for ligation of the splenic vessels for splenectomy depends on the length of the splenic pedicle, the close relation of the pedicle and the hilum of the spleen to the tail of the pancreas, the presence of splenic adhesions, and the size of the spleen.
- Because the splenic pedicle is formed by the splenorenal ligament, gastrosplenic ligament, and presplenic fold, the length of the pedicle depends on the length of these anatomic entities, including the distal branches of the splenic artery (see Fig. 22-5). Also, the splenic pedicle may be narrow or wide, depending on the extent to which the primitive dorsal mesogastrium was absorbed into the body wall. The degree of effective mobilization of the spleen depends ultimately not on the splenorenal ligament, but on the length of the splenic vessels after inci-

### Editorial Comment

*While I agree with transfixing in ligating the short gastric vessels on the greater curvature of the stomach, I have not found it necessary to invert the greater curvature of the stomach to avoid bleeding and/or gastric necrosis. I would imbricate the greater curvature only if I thought there had been an injury to the gastric wall. It has not been my policy to routinely obtain a roentgenographic gastric contrast study after splenectomy. (RSF Jr)*

sion of the ligament. Short splenic vessels may make it impossible to deliver the spleen out of the abdomen. Gently pushing the tail of the pancreas away from the hilum of the spleen may increase splenic mobility. Occasionally, the tail of the pancreas does not touch the spleen, but the tail and the spleen are bridged by the pancreatosplenic ligament. Careful division of this ligament in splenectomy avoids intraoperative bleeding or postoperative pancreatitis.

The hilum of the spleen and the tail of the pancreas touch one another in about one-third of individuals,[63] and are within 1 cm of each other in about half of the population.[52] In 50% of individuals, the closest approach of the pancreas is at the middle of the spleen.[52] In 42%, the closest approach is near the inferior pole.[52]

The major artery limiting mobilization of the pancreas away from the spleen is the great pancreatic artery, which usually arises from the second or third segment of the splenic artery. In addition, if there are caudal pancreatic arteries arising from terminal branches of the splenic artery, they can be ruptured if the tail of the pancreas is too vigorously mobilized. Whitesell[52] stated that the tail of the pancreas can be dissected back 3.5 to 5.0 cm. Phelan et al.[205] suggested 2 to 3 cm as the limit to be expected.

- When there is splenomegaly, heavy adhesions may be present between the spleen and the diaphragm (above and laterally), the stomach (medially), and the splenic flexure (below). In many cases, the spleen is fixed with the anterolateral peritoneum of the abdominal wall. These adhesions can contain large neoplastic vessels, which can produce tremendous bleeding if not ligated and secured before their division.

- If a patient has a hemorrhagic disorder, a nasogastric tube should not be passed until the patient is in the operating room. Then the anesthesiologist should pass it under direct vision.

- In elective splenectomy with a large spleen, intravenous preoperative antibiotics and occlusion of the splenic artery are advisable. The latter should be per-

formed by a radiologist just before the incision is made. With such a procedure, the surgeon is committing to a total splenectomy.

- If a blood transfusion becomes necessary for a successful splenorrhaphy, then splenectomy without transfusion is the safer treatment.[206]

- Otsuji and colleagues[207] reported that splenectomy during total gastrectomy for gastric cancer did not have an effect on the survival rate. The simultaneous splenectomy itself was correlated with postoperative complications.

- Cocanour et al.[208] reported that significant numbers of delayed (>48 hours) complications occur with nonoperative management of adult splenic injury. Without attempting to define the controversial management of blunt splenic injury, these authors advised very close followup of patients with splenic trauma.

## ANATOMIC COMPLICATIONS OF SPLENIC SURGERY

The anatomic complications of splenic surgery are summarized in Table 22-14.

## Total Splenectomy

### *Vascular Injury*

**Hemorrhage and Ischemia**

Hemorrhage following splenectomy results from either surgical error or the presence of hemolytic disease that produces pathologic bleeding. Martin and Cooper[209] found hemorrhage to have been mentioned in 2.8 percent of 777 splenectomies performed by 11 authors.

Vascularization of the several splenic ligaments increases with portal hypertension. Therefore, careful division and ligation between clamps is essential.

**Surgical Considerations for Hemostasis**

Based on the vascular anatomy described earlier, we can determine the origins of bleeding following ligation of the splenic artery and removal of the spleen. There are two major sources of such bleeding: (1) bleeding from polar arteries arising proximal to the ligation (a superior polar artery may arise from the third segment of the splenic artery), and (2) retrograde bleeding from splenic arteries distal to the ligation (short gastric, caudal pancreatic, and

**TABLE 22-14. Summary of Anatomic Complications of Some Splenic Procedures**

| Procedure | Vascular Injury | Organ Injury | Inadequate Procedure |
|---|---|---|---|
| Total splenectomy | Hemorrhage from polar arteries; retrograde from branch of splenic artery. Ischemia to greater curvature. | Diaphragm, tail of pancreas, stomach, transverse colon, left kidney, etc. | Preservation of accessory spleen in splenectomy for hemolytic disease |
| Partial splenectomy | As above; hemorrhage from splenic remnant | As above; rupture of splenic capsule | Unlikely |
| Laparoscopic splenectomy | As above | As above | As in total and partial |
| Splenic repair | Bleeding | As above but very rare | Unlikely |
| Splenopexy | Bleeding | As above but very rare | Ptosis after repair |
| Splenic detorsion and splenopexy | Total or partial infarction | As above but very rare | Unlikely if viability of spleen is obvious |
| Distal pancreatectomy with splenic preservation | Bleeding and splenic infarction | Pancreas | Unlikely |
| Splenic artery aneurysm | Bleeding | Pancreas | Not ligating the feeding artery after proximal and distal ligation |
| Staging laparotomy | Bleeding | | By not performing multiple biopsies, oophoropexy, etc. |
| Transplantation | Infarction and necrosis | None | Unlikely |
| Incision and drainage | Bleeding | None | Contamination of the abdominal cavity |

left gastroepiploic arteries may arise from terminal branches of the splenic artery beyond the point of ligation). Such vessels must be identified and ligated separately. Where possible, the ligation should be distal to the origin of the left gastroepiploic artery. The short gastric veins are another source of bleeding.

The splenic artery may be ligated without removing the spleen; the short gastric arteries are the collateral circulation of the spleen.[76,210,211,212] If the splenic vein is injured, the spleen must be removed or the vein must be anastomosed to another vein.

## *Organ Injury*

### Diaphragm

Martin and Cooper[209] mentioned trauma to the diaphragm.

If diaphragmatic injury involves the entire thickness of the diaphragm, the defect should be repaired with through-and-through interrupted nonabsorble sutures.

### Pancreas

The close proximity of the tail of the pancreas to the spleen may result in pancreatic injury during splenectomy.

The insult may involve pancreatic ducts, pancreatic vessels, and severe injury to the tail of the pancreas. Injury of ducts and/or vessels should be treated by ligation. Resection of the pancreatic tail is necessary when it is severely injured. Closed drainage is recommended.

There were 14 injuries to the pancreas (2.2 percent) among 632 splenectomies in four series.[213-216]

### Stomach

Injury to the stomach or ischemia of the gastric remnant may accompany splenectomy and the sacrifice of the short gastric arteries.[217] With gastric injury superficial to or through the total thickness of the gastric wall, gastrorrhaphy and inversion is the procedure of choice.

Harrison et al.[218] reported 18 cases of gastrocutaneous fistula following splenectomy. They listed five conditions that predispose to the formation of gastric fistula after splenectomy:

- Abrasions or denudation of the serosal covering of the greater curvature of the stomach, which often results from a technically difficult splenectomy
- Interruption of a reflection of gastric muscle fibers into the gastrosplenic ligament at the attachment to the stomach wall[52]
- Decreased vascularity, especially in elderly patients with

arteriosclerosis of the gastric vessels
- An organizing hematoma with inflammatory reaction in the gastrosplenic omentum adjacent to the gastric wall secondary to rupture of the spleen
- Severe trauma with multiple injuries or any conditions predisposing to stress ulcerations

### Colon

The distal transverse colon, the splenic flexure, and the proximal descending colon may be injured during splenic artery surgery. The segments related to the spleen via the splenocolic and phrenicocolic ligaments are the most vulnerable. There is occasional involvement of the pancreaticocolic ligament, dependent on the ligament's width and the spleen's size. Gentle treatment and ligation of these ligaments will avoid colon injury.

Colonic wall repair in two layers is the procedure of choice.

### Kidney, Ureter, Adrenal, and Retroperitoneal Space

Occasionally, a megaspleen is heavily fixed to organs of the left retroperitoneal space, namely the left adrenal gland, the left kidney, and the left ureter. The ureteric part involved is again related to the size of the spleen. While these are very rare injuries, the wise surgeon will not forget their potential.

Bleeding must be controlled. If the ureter is injured, the surgeon should proceed with the anastomosis of his or her choice.

Splenectomy complicating nephrectomy was reported by Cooper et al.[219] To our knowledge, nephrectomy complicating splenectomy has not been reported, but it is a possibility.

### Other Organs

The authors have occasionally seen patients with severe adhesions of loops of small bowel as well as adhesions to the left ovary and tube from splenomegaly secondary to malaria and kala azar. In these cases, total splenectomy plus small bowel resection and left salpingo-oophorectomy were performed.

## Partial Splenectomy

The anatomic complications of partial splenectomy are similar to those of total splenectomy. In addition, there is the possibility of bleeding from the preserved splenic remnant. Excessive traction on the presplenic fold containing the left gastroepiploic vessels may tear the splenic capsule. Infarction of the splenic remnant is possible. Partial splenectomy is preferable to total splenectomy when it is

possible because it decreases the likelihood of postsplenectomy sepsis.

The authors witnessed a case of iatrogenic splenosis. This can occur with or without other complications such as intestinal obstruction or hematologic problems.

## Laparoscopic Splenectomy

For all practical purposes, the anatomic complications of laparoscopic splenectomy are those of total and partial splenectomy. In view of its efficacy and reduction in morbidity and mortality, the laparoscopic approach to splenctomy is now regarded by many authors as being preferable to open splenectomy for hematologic disease.[220,221] Glasgow and Mulvihill[222] stated that laparoscopic splenectomy is evolving and may become the procedure of choice for the treatment of splenic disorders.

In a case-controlled study of patients undergoing elective splenectomies in immune thrombocytopenia purpura, hairy cell leukemia, and staging for Hodgkin's disease, Diaz et al.[221] reported that laparoscopic splenectomy resulted in shorter hospitalization (2.3 vs 8.8 days with open splenectomy) and fewer postoperative complications.

Targarona et al.[223] stated that laparoscopic splenectomy is a promising procedure in the management of hematologic disorders, but it is absolutely essential to avoid parenchymal rupture and cell spillage as well as to avoid leaving accessory spleens, which can lead to the failure of surgical treatment.

Lozano-Salazar et al.[224] reported that laparoscopic splenectomy in the treatment of immune thrombocytopenic purpura (ITP) is comparable to open splenectomy in terms of safety and efficacy, and is associated with a shorter hospital stay. Tanoue et al.,[225] reported that for treatment of ITP, laparoscopic splenectomy is an alternative modality. Fass et al.[226] concurred that it was a safe and effective treatment for elderly patients. Katkhouda and Mavor[227] stated, "Laparoscopic splenectomy for selected hematologic disorders should replace open splenectomy as the technique of choice and prompt earlier consideration of surgery when it is indicated."

A study by Rescorla et al.[228] found that in comparison to open splenectomy in children with hematologic disorders, laparoscopic splenectomy resulted in longer operative times, less narcotic administration, shorter length of stay, and lower total hospital charge.

Based on a retrospective chart review, Terrosu et al.[229] concluded that laparoscopic splenectomy by experienced laparoscopic surgeons is feasible, effective, safe, and offered several advantages over open surgery.

Splenic laceration may occur during laparoscopic

surgery, with distortion and stretching of small vascular adhesions between the spleen and abdominal wall. Chang et al.[230] reported a case of splenic laceration complicating salpingoplasty.

## METASTASIS AND THE SPLEEN

Various studies have shown that metastatic carcinoma of the spleen is a rare occurrence.[231-233] In routine autopsy series, involvement has been found in 0.3 to 9% of patients with cancer.[234,235] Berge[202] studied 7,165 postmortem cases of primary carcinomatous tumors, of which 4,404 (61.5%) were found to have spread to one or more organs; only 312 cases (7.1%) metastasized to the spleen.

When splenic metastasis is found, it usually reflects late disseminated disease.[235-237] Harmon and Dacorso[237] found splenic metastases in 50% of postmortem patients with evidence of metastasis to organs in both the thoracic and abdominal cavities. Berge[238] reported finding microscopic evidence of splenic metastasis in 70% of all subjects who had metastases in six or more organs.

Marymont and Gross[236] reported that 30-67% of all splenic metastases arise from primary carcinoma of the breast and lungs. Breitbart and Harris[239] reported metastatic breast carcinoma to the spleen. Reports of metastases from the skin (melanoma),[202,240] ovary,[202,235] and endometrium,[241,242] and also in lymphoma,[237,243] have been well documented in the literature. Murthy et al.[244] reported a very unusual case of metastasis from esophageal carcinoma.

From postmortem examination on 312 patients with splenic involvement, Berge[238] reported microscopic metastasis from adenocarcinoma of the colon and rectum in 4.4% and 1.6% of the cases, respectively. Interestingly, isolated splenic involvement (without visceral or nodal metastasis) with regard to colonic and rectal carcinoma is exceedingly rare. With the addition of one case report from our own experience,[245] review of the English literature produced only seven proven cases of colorectal adenocarcinoma with metastatic disease limited to the spleen.[233,243,245,246,247,248,249]

An ileal carcinoid tumor with splenic metastasis was reported by Falk and Stutte.[250] Sharpe et al.[251] reported on a patient with hairy-cell leukemia found to have metastatic adenocarcinoma in the spleen.

One of the few tumors that will metastasize to the spleen is melanoma.[252-254] Its most common diagnosis usually occurs as an incidental finding of a liver-spleen scan, an abdominal CT scan, or a laparotomy. Metastatic melanoma may be a rare cause of splenomegaly. Up to 88% of patients with splenic metastases have concomitant liver or pancreatic metastases.[255]

## Hypotheses for Splenic Resistance to Metastasis

Splenic metastases from solid, nonreticular neoplasms are rare compared with the incidence of spread to the lymph nodes, liver, and lungs.[256] Since the spleen represents one-fourth of the reticuloendothelial system, this apparent paradox warrants explanation. We agree with Hull et al.[257] that the influence of a functional spleen on induction and growth of cancer remains unexplained. Nonetheless, anatomic, histologic, and functional explanations of this phenomenon have been proposed.[258]

### *Anatomic Basis for Splenic Resistance*

In 1922, Sappington[259] thought that the sharp angle that exists at the origin of the splenic artery from the celiac artery limits tumor metastasis. This sharp angle would theoretically impede larger tumor emboli from reaching the spleen.

### *Histologic Bases for Splenic Resistance*

There are two histologic theories regarding the relationship between cancer and the spleen. The contraction theory advanced by Kettle,[260] and later by Herbut and Gabriel,[261] stated that the rhythmic contractions provided by the sinusoidal splenic architecture prevent implantation of malignant cells on vascular endothelial cells.

The second theory, presented by Warren and Davis,[235] is that in addition to the limitations from the contractions, the scarcity of lymphatic vessels extending into the intrasplenic parenchyma also limits splenic metastases. They considered this scarcity to be of even greater significance than the contractions. This is an attractive argument because today we believe that the splenic parenchyma and capsule have a paucity of lymphatic vessels. The matter is still controversial. Sporadic metastases of epithelial and nonepithelial tumors to the spleen have been reported from time to time in the literature.

### *Functional Theory of Splenic Resistance*

While anatomic and histologic theories offer intriguing possibilities, the spleen's functional capacity with regard to its immunologic surveillance and antitumorigenic properties seems most likely to be responsible for the rarity of splenic metastases. Hull et al.[257] attributed the ability of the spleen to protect rats from the induction of malignant colonic tumors induced by 1,2-dimethylhydrazine (DMH) to the preservation of immunologic surveillance in the host.

The possibility of production by the spleen of antineoplastic substances inhibiting tumor growth has been reported by Pollard[262] and also by Woglam.[263] Miller and Milton[232] demonstrated experimentally that tumor cells implanted within mice grow at a significantly slower rate in the spleen than in the liver. Small and Trainin[264] illustrated the antigenic response to splenic inoculation with tumor cells in mice. These specific tumor-inhibitory cells, identified as inhibitory T-cells, are thought to play a key role in the inhibition of splenic metastases.

The spleen's inhibitory effect may simply prevent microscopic metastases from maturing into macroscopic metastases with clinical significance. In an autopsy series, Warren and Davis[235] noted that only 42 of 1140 subjects studied without regard to tumor type had histologic evidence of splenic metastases; macroscopic tumor involvement was present in only 22 of those 42.

Numerous studies suggest that the spleen has an antitumorigenic effect on the host. Sato et al.[265] found that growth of colonic tumors in mice was enhanced after splenectomy. Wanebo et al.[266] recently reported their results from a study that reviewed and analyzed the effect of splenectomy on survival in patients having curative gastrectomy for stomach cancer. The authors found that the 5-year survival rate was 20.9% in patients having elective splenectomy versus 31% in patients who did not receive splenectomy (P <0.0001). Davis et al.[267] suggested that splenectomy should be considered a probable factor in the decreased survival of patients operated on for regional colorectal cancer. Arwari, in a discussion of Davis' findings,[267] asked this question: "If colon cancer is metastatic to the splenic hilar nodes and invades the pancreatic capsule, should en bloc dissection including the pancreatic tail take place while leaving the spleen alone?" Davis's answer was to "save the spleen, if possible."[267]

There is some evidence that the spleen may not be protective against malignant tumor growth in animal models. Meyer et al.[268] reported decreased tumor growth in rats whose spleens had been removed. Ferrer[269] found the rate of growth of sarcoma to be reduced in rats without spleens.

Description of the natural history of carcinoma metastatic to the spleen is incomplete because the event is so rare. This rarity may be due to anatomic, histologic, and functional characteristics of the spleen. Although no long-term follow-up data are available, splenectomy for isolated metastasis is clearly indicated, especially when no other evidence of metastatic disease is detectable.

The spleen is an enigmatic organ that still does not unveil its secrets to us. The authors recommend that all primary or metastatic tumors of the spleen be reported, so that in the future, medical science may be able to answer some of today's questions.

Skandalakis et al.[258] posed the following questions about this spleen-cancer phenomenon. There are many other unanswered questions:

- What is the relationship between cancer and the spleen?
- Why is the spleen so rarely a primary or a metastatic site?
- What is the survival rate among patients with cancer metastatic to other areas after splenectomy?
- Is splenectomy itself carcinogenic?
- Are all the effects of radiation and immunosuppression following splenectomy known?
- Does normal splenic function influence the growth of malignant tumors?

## DISEASE AND THE SPLEEN

## Association of the Spleen with Diseases of the Liver

The liver and the spleen are fellow travelers in certain well-known diseases, and also in some extremely rare conditions.

There is a notable tendency for splenomegaly to be associated with hepatomegaly.[258] This is not always the case, but enlargement of both organs is a common phenomenon in hepatosplenic disorders. The spleen is extremely sensitive to elevation of vascular pressure. Because of the anatomic vascular relations of the two organs, splenic changes such as splenomegaly can take place secondary to hepatic changes such as portal hypertension associated with certain pathologic processes of the liver. The involvement of the spleen with diseases of the liver, such as Budd-Chiari syndrome, is also well known. Diagnostic procedures such as venography and splenoportography, and therapeutic procedures such as placement of splenorenal shunts (Fig. 22-46), have been developed.

Thoracic transposition of the spleen, or splenopneumopexy, has been employed for the treatment of portal hypertension. Surgery consists of mobilization of the spleen, left diaphragmotomy, splenic displacement into the left thoracic cavity, partial removal of the splenic capsule, partial abrasion of the surface of the left lower lobe, and suturing the prepared areas of the spleen and lung. It is doubtful that this procedure produces neovascular venous connections between the two systems that are sufficiently large to decompress the liver.

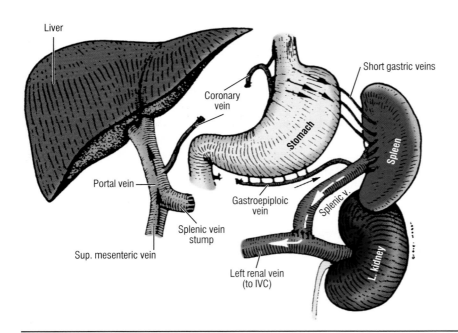

FIG 22-46. Diagrammatic illustration of the selective distal splenorenal shunt. (Modified from Salam AA, Warren WD. Anatomic basis of the surgical treatment of portal hypertension. Surg Cllin North Am 1974;54:1247-1257; with permission.)

Salvage of the spleen in splenomegaly resulting from cirrhosis has also been urged. In their studies of splenic conservation, Ying-jian et al.[158] observed that the splenic artery divided into two major branches in 46 of 61 patients and three branches in 15. External lobulation of the spleen could be predicted on the basis of hilar branching patterns. Partial splenectomy was used to treat portal hypertension with associated splenomegaly. Drainage was maintained for 24 to 36 hours. The remaining portion of the spleen was effective in lessening the incidence of fever after splenectomy. The residual spleen was still within normal limits of size one year after the operation. Bleeding from the salvaged spleen was controlled with an omental graft.

## Association of the Spleen with Diseases of the Pancreas

Pancreatitis and pancreatic carcinoma are the most common causes of occlusion of the splenic vessels. Ku et al.[159] described three phases in the clinical course of the disease:

- The splenic vein is partially occluded; gastric varices and splenomegaly are absent
- The splenic vein is completely occluded; the splenic artery is patent; gastric varices and splenomegaly are present
- In the vanishing phase, the effects of arterial occlusion are superimposed on those of venous occlusion; gastric

varices disappear and the enlarged spleen shrinks

We quote from Mercie et al.[270]:

Splenic venous thrombosis is a frequent complication occurring in the course of pancreatic cancer. It is easily diagnosed using abdominal computerized tomography. Arterial thrombosis is rarely observed.

Chronic pancreatitis can lead to splenic rupture, which is secondary to peptic digestion of the splenic parenchyma with the formation of an intrasplenic pseudocyst.[271,272] Hemorrhagic pleural effusion may follow such a catastrophe.[273,274] How can this transdiaphragmatic voyage of blood from the spleen be explained? Perhaps the several openings of the diaphragm, which are weak areas, are responsible. These openings are the three large openings for the inferior vena cava, the esophagus, and the aorta and the nine small openings for structures such as the greater and lesser thoracic splanchnic nerves and the hemiazygous vein. The well-known communications by lymphatics between the peritoneal and pleural cavities may be responsible as well. Involvement of mediastinal lymph nodes from intraabdominal disease may also be a cause. Intrathoracic disease, such as pulmonary carcinoma or tuberculosis, may metastasize to the adrenal glands. We agree with Nath and Warshaw[275] that the subject is open to speculation.

Extravascular inflammation of the splenic artery and its branches secondary to erosion from chronic pancreatitis with the formation of micropseudoaneurysms or macro-

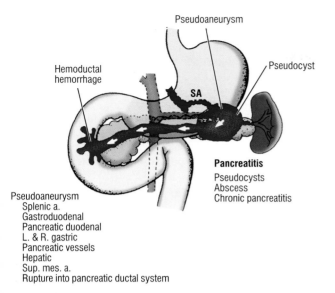

**Pseudoaneurysm**

Pseudoaneurysm
  Splenic a.
  Gastroduodenal
  Pancreatic duodenal
  L. & R. gastric
  Pancreatic vessels
  Hepatic
  Sup. mes. a.
  Rupture into pancreatic ductal system

**Pancreatitis**
Pseudocysts
Abscess
Chronic pancreatitis

**FIG 22-47.** Pseudoaneurysms resulting from pancreatitis may cause hemorrhage by rupture either into the pancreatic ductal system or directly into the stomach or duodenum. SA, splenic artery. (Modified from Frey CF, Eckhauser F, Stanley JC. Hemorrhage. In: Bradley EL (ed). Complications of Pancreatitis. Philadelphia: WB Saunders, 1982; with permission.)

pseudoaneurysms was described by Frey et al.[276] According to Frey and colleagues, splenic artery pseudoaneurysms resulting from pancreatitis constitute less than 5% of all splenic artery aneurysms, most of them located at vessel bifurcations. These pseudoaneurysms may cause bleeding by rupture (Fig. 22-47). The association of splenic and portal venous thrombosis (Fig. 22-48) with chronic pancreatitis, with or without the formation of pancreatic abscess, is also well known. Nishiyama et al.[277] presented splenic vein thrombosis secondary to pancreatitis; one of his three cases had an abscess. Bradley[278] reported on 11 cases of splenic thrombosis secondary to pancreatitis with bleeding but without abscess formation.

## Spleen and AIDS

In an excellent paper on human immunodeficiency virus-related immune thrombocytopenia, Ferguson[279] reported the following:

> Infection by human immunodeficiency virus (HIV) may result in immune thrombocytopenia. The etiology of this immune thrombocytopenia (ITP) is not entirely clear, but treatment is similar to that of classic ITP. However, response to steroids is unpredictable and short-lived. Splenectomy provides immediate resolu-

tion of thrombocytopenia in the majority of cases and does not appear to increase the incidence of opportunistic infections.

Tsoukas et al.[280] stated that the absence of a spleen during the asymptomatic phase of HIV infection seems to have a beneficial effect on HIV disease progression.

## Unusual Disease Processes

The following is a list of some very rare eponymous syndromes or diseases that we call splenic curiosities:

- Magocchi's syndrome: Symmetric skin hemangiomas with hemangiomas of spleen, liver, and other organs
- Omenn's disease: Familial reticuloendotheliosis with eosinophilia, splenomegaly, and hepatomegaly
- Tangier disease (Tangier is an island in Chesapeake Bay): storage disease with splenomegaly, hepatomegaly, lymphadenopathy, and hypercholesterolemia
- Savitsky, Hyman, and Hyman disease: a disease associated with unidentified reticuloendothelial cell storage with splenomegaly and hepatomegaly
- Chediak-Higashi syndrome (Caesar syndrome): oculocutaneous albinism, anomaly of the granules of leukocytes, lipid metabolism, and splenohepatomegaly
- Prasad syndrome: dwarfism, hypogonadism, iron-deficiency anemia, and splenohepatomegaly
- Sicca syndrome: Hashimoto thyroiditis, generalized lymphadenopathy, splenohepatomegaly, nonthrombocytopenic purpura, leukopenia, lymphopenia, hypergammaglobulinemia, and circulating tissue antibodies

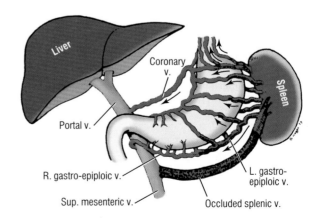

**FIG 22-48.** Diagrammatic representation of collateral circulation characteristic of isolated occlusion of the splenic vein. (Modified from Salam AA, Warren WD. Anatomic basis of the surgical treatment of portal hypertension. Surg Clin North Am 1974;54: 1252; with permission.)

all occuring together with enlargement of the salivary glands

• Dacie syndrome: a congenital anomaly associated with pancytopenia and nontropical idiopathic splenomegaly.

# REFERENCES

1. Ogle W (translator). Aristotle on the Parts of Animals. London: Kegan Paul, Trench & Co, 1882, Book III, Chapter 7 (p. 77).

2. Allen KB, Gay BB Jr, Skandalakis JE. Wandering spleen: anatomic and radiologic considerations. South Med J 1992;85: 976-984.

3. Desai DC, Hebra A, Davidoff AM, Schnaufer L. Wandering spleen: a challenging diagnosis. South Med J 90:439-443, 1997.

4. Buchner M, Baker MS. The wandering spleen. Surg Gynecol Obstet 175:373-387, 1992.

5. Allen KB. Wandering spleen. Probl Gen Surg 1990;7:122-127.

6. Abell I. Wandering spleen with torsion of the pedicle. Ann Surg 1933;98:722-735.

7. Allen KB, Andrews G. Pediatric wandering spleen, the case for splenopexy: review of 35 reported cases in the literature. J Pediatr Surg 1989;24:432-435.

8. Gosselin C, Chou S. Wandering spleen producing small-bowel obstruction in a neonate. Pediatr Surg Int 9:583-584, 1994.

9. Spector JM, Chappell J. Gastric volvulus associated with wandering spleen in a child. J Pediatr Surg 2000;35:641-642.

10. Moore PJ, Hawkins EP, Galliani CA, Guerry-Force ML. Spleno-gonadal fusion with limb deficiency and micrognathia. South Med J 90(11):1152-1155, 1997.

11. Putschar WGJ, Manion WC. Splenic-gonadal fusion. Am J Pathol 1956;32:15-33.

12. Le Roux PJ, Heddle RM. Splenogonadal fusion: is the accepted classification system accurate? BJU Int 2000;85:114-115.

13. Gouw AS, Elema JD, Bink-Boelkens MT, de Jongh HJ, ten Kate LP. The spectrum of splenogonadal fusion: case report and review of 84 reported cases. Eur J Pediatr 1985;144:316-323.

14. Alcalay J, Reif RM, Bogokowsky H. Primary splenic pregnancy [Hebrew]. Harefuah 100(12):577, 1981.

15. Kushner DH, Dobrzynski FA. Abdominal pregnancy with placenta attached to the spleen. Am J Obstet Gynecol 52:160-161, 1946.

16. Repin AV. Abdominal pregnancy of 28 weeks with implantation of the fertilized ovum at the hilum of the spleen [Russian]. Akush Ginekol 2:107-108, 1962.

17. Caruso V, Hall WHJ. Primary abdominal pregnancy in the spleen: a case report. Pathology 16:93-94, 1984.

18. Talerman A, Hart S. Epithelial cysts of the spleen. Br J Surg 1970; 57:201-204.

19. Panossian DH, Wang N, Reeves CD, Weeks DA. Epidermoid cyst of the spleen presenting as a generalized peritonitis. Am Surg 1990;56:295-298.

20. Neiman RS, Orazi A. Disorders of the Spleen, 2nd Ed. Philadelphia: WB Saunders, 1999, p. 18.

21. Curtis GM, Movitz D. The surgical significance of the accessory spleen. Ann Surg 1946; 123:276-298.

22. Halpert B, Gyorkey F. Lesions observed in accessory spleens of 311 patients. Am J Clin Pathol 1959;32:165-168.

23. Halpert B, Alden ZA. Accessory spleens in or at the tail of the pancreas. Arch Pathol 1964;77:652-654.

24. Abu-Hijleh MF. Multiple accessory spleens: case report and literature review. Clin Anat 1993;6:232-239.

25. Habib FA, Kolachalam RB, Swason K. Abscess of an accessory spleen. Am Surg 2000;66:215-218.

26. Wekerle T, Eichinger S, Maier A, Wrba F, Möschl P. Intrahepatic splenic tissue in a patient with recurrent idiopathic thrombocytopenic purpura. Surgery 123:596-599, 1998.

27. Fleming CR, Dickson ER, Harrison EG. Splenosis: autotransplantation of splenic tissue. Am J Med 61:414, 1976.

28. Metwally N, Ravo B. Splenosis: a review. Contemp Surg 1991; 39:33.

29. Hamilton WJ, Simon G, Hamilton SGI. Surface and Radiological Anatomy. Baltimore: Williams and Wilkins Co, 1976.

30. Gould GM, Pyle WL. Anomalies and Curiosities of Medicine (2nd ed). New York: Bell Publishing Co, 1956, p. 657.

31. Allen L. The lymphatic system and the spleen. In: Anson BJ (ed). Morris's Human Anatomy (12th ed). New York: McGraw-Hill, 1966, p. 907.

32. Healey JE Jr. A Synopsis of Clinical Anatomy. Philadelphia: WB Saunders, 1969, p. 162.

33. Last RJ. Anatomy: Regional and Applied (5th ed). Baltimore: Williams & Wilkins, 1972, p. 470.

34. Michels NA. Blood Supply and Anatomy of the Upper Abdominal Organs, with a Descriptive Atlas. Philadelphia: JB Lippincott, 1955.

35. Morrell DG, Chang FC, Helmer SD. Changing trends in the management of splenic injury. Am J Surg 1995;170:686-690.

36. Goodley CD, Warren RL, Sheridan RL, McCabe CJ. Nonoperative management of blunt splenic injury in adults: age over 55 years as a powerful indicator for failure. J Am Coll Surg 1996;183: 133-139.

37. Moody RO. The position of the abdominal viscera in healthy young British and American adults. J Anat 1927;61:223.

38. Moody RO, Chamberlain WE, Van Nuys RG. Visceral anatomy of healthy adults. Am J Anat 1926;37:273.

39. Moody RO, Van Nuys RG. Some results of a study of roentgenograms of the abdominal viscera. AJR 1928;20:348.

40. Strauss MB (ed). Familiar Medical Quotations. Boston: Little, Brown and Co, 1968, p. 598.

41. Kyber E. Uber die Milz des Menschen und einiger Saugetiere. Arch Mikrosk Anat Entw Mech 1870;6:540-570.

42. Skandalakis PN, Colborn GL, Skandalakis LJ, Richardson DD, Mitchell WE Jr, Skandalakis JE. The surgical anatomy of the spleen. Surg Clin North Am 1993;73:747-768.

43. Gupta CD, Gupta SC, Aorara AK, Singh P. Vascular segments in the human spleen. J Anat 1976; 121:613-616.

44. Mandarim-Lacerda CA, Sampaio FJ, Passos MA. Segmentation vasculaire de la rate chez le nouveau-ne: support anatomique pour la resection partielle. J Chir (Paris) 1983; 120:471.

45. Liu DL, Xia S, Xu W, Qifa Y, Gao Y, Qian J. Anatomy of vasculature of 850 spleen specimens and its application in partial splenectomy. Surgery 1996;119:27-33.

46. Redmond HP, Redmond JM, Rooney BP. Surgical anatomy of the human spleen. Br J Surg 1989; 76:198-201.

47. Voboril Z. On the question of segmentation of the human spleen. Folia Morphol 1982; 30:295-314.

48. Dawson DL, Molina JE, Scott-Conner CEH. Venous segmentation of the human spleen. Am Surg 1986;52:253.

49. Dreyer B, Budtz-Olson OE. Splenic venography: demonstration of the portal circulation with diodone. Lancet 1952;1:530.

50. Garcia-Porrero JA, Lemes A. Arterial segmentation and sub-segmentation in the human spleen. Acta Anat 1988;131:276.

51. Dixon JA, Miller F, McCloskey D, Siddoway J. Anatomy and techniques in segmental splenectomy. Surg Gynecol Obstet 1980; 150:516.

52. Whitesell FB. A clinical and surgical anatomic study of rupture of the spleen due to blunt trauma. Surg Gynecol Obstet 1960;110: 750.

53. Skandalakis JE, Colborn GL, Pemberton LB, Skandalakis PN, Skandalakis LJ, Gray SW. The surgical anatomy of the spleen. Probl Gen Surg 1990;7:1-17.

54. Rosen A, Nathan H, Luciansky E, Sayfan J. The lienorenal ligament and the tail of the pancreas: a surgical anatomical study. Pancreas 1988;3:104-107.

55. O'Rahilly R. Gardner-Gray-O'Rahilly Anatomy: A Regional Study of Human Structure (5th ed). Philadelphia: WB Saunders, 1986, pp. 414-415.

56. Seufert RM, Mitrou PS. Surgery of the spleen. Reber HA (trans). New York: Thieme, 1986.

57. Henry AK. The removal of large spleens. Br J Surg 1940;107:464.

58. Lord MD, Gourevitch A. The peritoneal anatomy of the spleen, with special references to the operation of partial gastrectomy. Br J Surg 1965;52:202.

59. VanderZypen E, Revez E. Investigation of development, structure and function of the phrenicocolic and duodenal suspensory ligaments. Acta Anat (Basel) 1984;119:142.

60. Skandalakis JE, Colborn GL, Skandalakis LJ. Benign anatomical mistakes: myths or enigmas? Am Surg 15(1):88-89, 1999.

61. Morgenstern L. Splenic repair and partial splenectomy. In: Nyhus LM, Baker RJ (eds). Mastery of Surgery (2nd ed). Boston: Little, Brown, 1992, pp. 1102-1112.

62. Poulin EC, Thibault C. The anatomic basis for laparoscopic splenectomy. Can J Surg 1993;36:484.

63. Baronofsky ID, Walton W, Noble JF. Occult injury to the pancreas following splenectomy. Surgery 1951;29:852.

64. Adkins EH. Ptosed spleen with torsion of pedicle. Ann Surg 1938; 107:832.

65. Taveras JM. Golden's Diagnostic Roentgenology. Baltimore, Williams & Wilkins, 1964.

66. McMahon WG, Norwood SH, Silva JS. Pancreatic pseudocyst with splenic involvement: an uncommon complication of pancreatitis. South Med J 1988;81:910.

67. Michels NA. The variational anatomy of the spleen and the splenic artery. Am J Anat 1942;70:21.

68. Van Damme JPJ, Bonte J. The blood supply of the stomach. Acta Anat 1988;131:89-96.

69. Sylvester PA, Stewart R, Ellis H. Tortuosity of the human splenic artery. Clin Anat 1995;8:214-218.

70. Borley NR, McFarlane JM, Ellis H. A comparative study of the tortuosity of the splenic artery. Clin Anat 1995;8:219-221.

71. Waizer A, Baniel J, Zin Y, Dintsman M. Clinical implications of anatomic variations of the splenic artery. Surg Gynecol Obstet 1989; 168:57.

72. Treutner KH, Klosterhalfen B, Winkeltau G, Moench S, Schumpelick V. Vascular anatomy of the spleen: the basis for organ-preserving surgery. Clin Anat 1993;6:1-8.

73. Van Damme JPJ, Bonte J. Systemization of the arteries in the splenic hilus. Acta Anat 1986;125:217.

74. Katritsis E, Parashos A, Papadopoulos N. Arterial segmentation of the human spleen by post-mortem angiograms and corrosion casts. Angiology 1982;33:720.

75. Helm HM. The gastric vasa brevia. Anat Rec 1915;9:637.

76. Keramidas DC. The ligation of the splenic artery in the treatment of traumatic rupture of the spleen. Surgery 1979;85:530-533.

77. Farag A, Shoukry A, Nasr SE. A new option for splenic preservation in normal sized spleen based on preserved histology and phagocytic function of the upper pole using upper short gastric vessels. Am J Surg 1994;168:257-261.

78. Berens AS, Aluisio FV, Colborn GL, Gray SW, Skandalakis JE. The incidence and significance of the posterior gastric artery in human anatomy. J Med Assoc Ga 1991;8:425-428.

79. Van Damme JPJ, Bonte J. Arteria splenica and the blood supply of the spleen. Probl Gen Surg 1990;7:18-27.

80. Trubel W, Turkof E, Rokitansky A, Firbas W. Incidence, anatomy and territories supplied by the posterior gastric artery. Acta Anat 1985;124:26-30.

81. Kirk E. Untersuchungen uber die grossere und feinere topographische Verteilung der Arterien, Venen und Ausfuhrungsgange in der menschlichen Bauchspeicheldruse. Ztschr Ges Anat 1931; 94:822.

82. Lippert H, Pabst R. Arterial Variations in Man. Munich: J.F. Bergmann Verlag, 1985, pp. 41-45.

83. Mellière D. Variations des artères hépatiques et du carrefour pancréatique. J Chir (Paris) 98:5-42, 1968.

84. Jonsell G, Boutelier P. Observations during treatment of acute necrotizing pancreatitis with surgical ablation. Surg Gynecol Obstet 148:385, 1979.

85. Petroianu A, Petroianu S. Anatomy of splenogastric vessels in patients with schistosomal portal hypertension. Clin Anat 1994; 7:80-83.

86. Romero-Torres R. The true splenic blood supply and its surgical applications. Hepato-Gastroenterology 45:885-888, 1998.

87. Woodburne RT. Essentials of Human Anatomy. New York: Oxford University Press, 1969, p. 430.

88. Douglass BE, Baggenstoss AH, Hollinshead WH. The anatomy of the portal vein and its tributaries. Surg Gynecol Obstet 1950;91: 562.

89. Williams PL (ed). Gray's Anatomy (38th ed). New York: Churchill Livingstone, 1995, p. 1603.

90. Gerber AB, Lev M, Goldberg SL. The surgical anatomy of the splenic vein. Am J Surg 1951;82:339.

91. Fujitani RM, Johs SM, Cobb SR, Mehringer CM, White RA, Klein SR. Preoperative splenic artery occlusion as an adjunct for high risk splenectomy. Am Surg 1988;54:602.

92. Dumont AE, Le Fleur RS. Significance of an enlarged splenic artery in patients with splenic vein thrombosis. Am Surg 1988;54: 613.

93. Guyton AC. Textbook of Medical Physiology, Arthur C. Guyton, John E. Hall (9th ed). Philadelphia: WB Saunders, 1996.

94. Lankisch PG. The spleen in inflammatory pancreatic disease. Gastroenterology 1990;88:509.

95. Orozco H, Mercado MA, Martinez R, Tielve M, Chan C, Vasquez M, Zenteno-Guichard G, Pantoja JP. Is splenectomy necessary in devascularization procedures for treatment of bleeding portal hypertension? Arch Surg 133:36-38, 1998.

96. Firstenberg MS, Plaisier B, Newman JS, Malangoni MA. Successful treatment of delayed splenic rupture with splenic artery embolization. Surgery 123:584-586, 1998.

97. Rouviere H. Anatomy of the Human Lymphatic System. Ann Arbor MI: Edwards Brothers, 1938.

98. Weiss L, Gilbert HA, Ballon SC (eds). Lymphatic System Metastasis. Boston: GK Hall Medical Publishers, 1980.

99. Drinker CK, Yoffey JM. Lymphatics, Lymph, and Lymphatic Tissue. Cambridge, Mass: Harvard University Press, 1941, p 12.

100. Boles ET Jr, Haase GM, Hamoudi AB. Partial splenectomy in staging laparotomy for Hodgkin's disease: an alternative approach. J Pediatr Surg 1978;13:581-586.

101. Dearth JC, Gilchrist GS, Telander RL. Partial splenectomy for staging Hodgkin's disease: risk of false-negative results. N Engl J Med 1978;299:345-346.

102. Utterback RA. Innervation of the spleen. J Comp Neurol 1944; 81: 55.

103. Crosby ED, Humphrey T, Lauer EW. Correlative Anatomy of the Nervous System. New York: Macmillan and Co., 1962.

104. Chadburn A. The spleen: anatomy and anatomical function. Semin Hematol 2000;37 (Suppl 1) 13-21.

105. Wolf BC, Neiman RS. Disorders of the spleen. Philadelphia: WB Saunders, 1989.

106. Churchill W. Radio speech (October 1, 1939). Cited in Rawson H, Miner M. The New International Dictionary of Quotations. New York: EP Dutton, 1986, p. 188.

107. Luna GK, Dellinger EP. Nonoperative observation therapy for splenic injuries: a safe therapeutic option? Am J Surg 1987;153: 463.

108. Polk HC Jr. Principles of preoperative preparation of the surgical patient. In: Sabiston DC Jr (ed). Textbook of Surgery (13th ed). Philadelphia: WB Saunders, 1986, pp. 87-98.

109. Dunphy JE. Splenectomy for trauma. Am J Surg 1946;71:450.

110. Morgenstern L. Technique of partial splenectomy. Prob Gen Surg 1990;7:103-112.

111. Brunt LM, Langer JC, Quasebarth MA, Whitman ED. Comparative analysis of laparoscopic versus open splenectomy. Am J Surg 1996;172:596-601.

112. Waldhausen JHT, Tapper D. Is pediatric splenectomy safe and cost-effective? Arch Surg 132:822-824, 1997.

113. Decker G, Millat B, Guillon F, Atger J, Linon M. Laparoscopic splenectomy for benign and malignant hematologic diseases: 35 consecutive cases. World J Surg 22:62-68, 1998.

114. Katkhouda N, Waldrep DJ, Feinstein D, Soliman H, Stain SC, Ortega AE, Mouiel J. Unresolved issues in laparoscopic splenectomy. Am J Surg 1996;172:585-590.

115. Park A, Marcaccio M, Sternbach M, Witzke D, Fitzgerald P. Laparoscopic vs open splenectomy. Arch Surg 134:1263-1269, 1999.

116. Phillips EH, Korman JE, Friedman R. Laparoscopic splenectomy. In: Hiatt JR, Phillips EH, Morgenstern L (eds). Surgical Diseases of the Spleen. New York: Springer-Verlag, 1997, pp. 211-232.

117. Al-Salem AH. Is splenectomy for massive splenomegaly safe in children? Am J Surg 178:42-45, 1999.

118. Tractow WD, Fabri PJ, Carey LC. Changing indications for splenectomy: 30 years experience. Arch Surg 1980;115:447.

119. Musser G, Lazar G, Hocking W, Busuttil RW. Splenectomy for hematologic disease: the UCLA experience with 306 patients. Ann Surg 1984;200:40.

120. Powell M, Courcoulas A, Gardner M, Lynch J, Harbrecht BG, Udekwu AO, Billiar TR, Federle M, Ferris J, Meza MP, Peitzman AB. Management of blunt splenic trauma: significant differences between adults and children. Surgery 122(4):654-660, 1997.

121. Weber T, Hanisch E, Baum RP, Seufert RM. Late results of heterotopic autotransplantation of splenic tissue into the greater omentum. World J Surg 22:883-889, 1998.

122. Morgenstern L, Rosenberg BA, Geller SA. Tumors of the spleen. World J Surg 1985;9:468.

123. Hiatt JR, Allins A, Kong LR. Open splenectomy. In: Hiatt JR, Phillips EH, Morgenstern L (eds.) Surgical Diseases of the Spleen. New York: Springer-Verlag, 1997, pp. 197-210.

124. Mitchell A, Morris PJ. Surgery of the spleen. Clin Haematol 1983; 12:565.

125. Ugochukwu AI, Irving M. Intraperitoneal low pressure suction drainage following splenectomy. Br J Surg 1985;72:247.

126. Carmichael J, Thomas WO, Dillard D, Luterman A, Ferrara JJ. Indications for placement of drains in the splenic fossa. Am Surg 1990;56:313-318.

127. Ellison EC, Fabri DJ. Complications of splenectomy: etiology, prevention and management. Surg Clin North Am 1983;63:1313.

128. Pachter HL, Hofstetter SR, Spencer FC. Evolving concepts in splenic surgery. Am Surg 1981;194:262.

129. Scanlon EF. The intraabdominal dead space and abscess formation. Surg Gynecol Obstet 1978;146:789.

130. Olsen WR, Beaudoin DE. Wound drainage after splenectomy: indications and complications. Am J Surg 1969;117:615.

131. Jordan GL Jr. Complications of splenectomy. In: Hardes JD (ed). Complications in Surgery and Their Management. Philadelphia: WB Saunders, 1981.

132. Maingot R. Abdominal Operations (6th ed). New York: Appleton-Century-Crofts, 1974.

133. McNair TJ (ed). Hamilton Bailey's Emergency Surgery (9th ed). Baltimore: Williams & Wilkins, 1972.

134. Fabri PJ, Metz EN, Nick WV, Zollinger RM. A quarter century with splenectomy. Arch Surg 1974;108:569.

135. Chassin JL. Operative Strategy in General Surgery: An Expositive Atlas. New York: Springer-Verlag, 1984.

136. Lumsden AB, Riley JD, Skandalakis JE. Splenic artery aneurysms. Probl Gen Surg 1990;7:113-121.

137. Rogers DM, Thompson JE, Garrett WV, Talkington CM, Patmen RD. Mesenteric vascular problems: a twenty six year experience. Ann Surg 195:554, 1982.

138. Busuttil RW, Brin BJ. The diagnosis and management of visceral artery aneurysms. Surgery 88:619, 1980.

139. Spittel JA, Fairbairn JF, Kincaid OW, Remine WH. Aneurysm of the splenic artery. JAMA 175:452, 1961.

140. Stanley JC, Fry WJ. Pathogenesis and clinical significance of splenic artery aneurysms. Surgery 76:898, 1974.

141. DeVries JE, Schattenkerk ME, Malt RA. Complications of splenic artery aneurysm other than intraperitoneal rupture. Surgery 91: 200, 1980.

142. O'Grady JP, Day EJ, Toole AL, Paust JC. Splenic artery aneurysm rupture in pregnancy: a review and case report. Obstet Gynecol 50:627, 1977.

143. Boijsen E, Efsing HO. Aneurysm of the splenic artery. Acta Radiol 8:29, 1969.

144. Majeski J. Splenic artery tortuosity simulating a splenic artery aneurysm. South Med J 91(10):949-950, 1998.

145. McFarlane JR, Thorbjarnarson B. Rupture of the splenic artery during pregnancy. Am J Obstet Gynecol 95:1025, 1966.

146. Vassalotti SB, Schaller JA. Spontaneous rupture of splenic artery aneurysm in pregnancy: report of first known antepartum rupture with maternal and fetal survival. Obstet Gynecol 30:264, 1967.

147. Stanley JC, Wakefield TW, Graham LM. Whitehouse WM, Zelenock GB, Lindenhauer SM. Clinical importance and management of splanchnic artery aneurysms. J Vasc Surg 3:836, 1986.

148. de Perrot M, Bühler L, Deléaval J, Borisch B, Mentha G, Morel P. Management of true aneurysms of the splenic artery. Am J Surg 175:466-468, 1998.

149. Bedford PD, Lodge B. Aneurysm of the splenic artery. Gut 1960; 1:312.

150. Ferrari L. The recognition and incidence of splenic artery aneurysms. Australas Radiol 1972;16:126

151. Kreel L. The recognition and incidence of splenic artery aneurysms. Australas Radiol 1974;18:415.

152. Puttini M, Aseni P, Brambilla G, Belli L. Splenic artery aneurysms in portal hypertension. J Cardiovasc Surg 1982;23:490.

153. Taylor JL, Woodward DAK. Splenic conservation and the management of splenic artery aneurysms. Ann R Coll Surg Engl 1987; 69:179.

154. Horton J, Ogden ME, Williams S, Coln D. The importance of splenic blood flow in clearing pneumococcal organisms. Ann Surg 1982;95:172.

155. Gonzalez EM, Garcia-Blanch G, Blanco JMS, Garcia IG, Ocana AG. Treatment of splenic artery aneurysm after distal splenorenal shunt: a case report. Jpn J Surg 1981;11:377.

156. Mandel SR, Jaques PF, Mauro MA, Sanofsky S. Nonoperative management of peripancreatic arterial aneurysms. Ann Surg 1987; 205:126.

157. Baker KS, Tisnado J, Cho SR, Beachley MC. Splanchnic artery aneurysms and pseudoaneurysms: transcatheter embolization. Radiology 1987;163:135.

158. Ying-jian A, Qing-you L. Subtotal splenectomy in cirrhotic patients. Chin Med 99:191, 1986.

159. Ku Y, Kawa Y, Fujiwara S, Nishiyama H, Tanaka Y, Okumura S, Ohyanagi H, Saitoh Y. Hemodynamic study of occlusion of the splenic vein caused by carcinoma of the pancreas. Surg Gynecol Obstet 168(1):17-24, 1989.

160. Miller TA, Rowlands BJ (eds). Physiologic Basis of Modern Surgical Care. St. Louis: CV Mosby, 1988.

161. Blaisdell FW, Trunkey DD (eds). Trauma Management. Vol 1: Abdominal trauma. New York: Thieme-Stratton, 1982.

162. Andrews MA. Ultrasound of the spleen. World J Surg 2000;24:183-187.

163. Krause KR, Howells GA, Bair HA, Glover JL, Madrazo BL, Wasvary HJ, Bendick PJ. Nonoperative management of blunt splenic injury in adults 55 years and older: a twenty-year experience. Am Surg 2000;66:636-640.

164. Velmahos GC, Chan LS, Kamel E, Murray JA, Yassa N, Kahaku D, Berne TV, Demetriades D. Nonoperative management of splenic injuries: have we gone too far? Arch Surg 2000;135:674-681.

165. Peitzman AB, Heil B, Rivera L, Federle MB, Harbrecht BG, Clancy KD, Croce M, Enderson BL, Morris JA, Shatz D, Meredith JW, Ochoa JB, Fakhry SM, Cushman JG, Minei JP, McCarthy M, Luchette FA, Townsend R, Tinkoff G, Block EFJ, Ross S, Frykberg ER, Bell RM, Davis F III, Weireter L, Shapiro MB,

Kealey GP, Rogers F, Jones LM, Cone JB, Dunham CM, McAuley CE. Blunt splenic injury in adults: multi-institutional study of the Eastern Association for the Surgery of Trauma. J Trauma 2000;4 9:177-189.

166. Bickler S, Ramachandran V, Gittes GK, Alonso M, Snyder CL. Nonoperative management of newborn splenic injury: a case report. J Pediatr Surg 2000;35:500-501.

167. Skandalakis JE, Gray SW, Rowe JS Jr. Anatomical Complications in General Surgery. New York: McGraw-Hill, 1983.

168. Danforth DN, Thorbjarnarson B. Incidental splenectomy: a review of the literature and the New York hospital experience. Am Surg 1976;183:124.

169. Celebrezze JP Jr, Cottrell DJ, Williams GB. Spontaneous splenic rupture due to isolated splenic peliosis. South Med J 91(8):763-764, 1998.

170. Sikov WM, Schiffman FJ, Weaver M, Dyckman J, Shulman R, Torgan P. Splenosis presenting as occult gastrointestinal bleeding. Am J Hematol 2000;65:56-61.

171. De Vuysere S, Van Steenbergen W, Aerts R, Van Hauwaert H, Van Beckevoort D, Van Hoe L. Intrahepatic splenosis: imaging features. Abdom Imaging 2000:25:187-189.

172. Goldstone J. Splenectomy for massive splenomegaly. Am J Surg 1978;135:385.

173. Schwartz SJ. Splenectomy for thrombocytopenia. World J Surg 1985;9:416.

174. Schwartz SI. Role of splenectomy in hematologic disorders. World J Surg 1996;20:1156-1159.

175. Winde G, Schmid KW, Lügering N, Fischer R, Brandt B, Berns T, Bünte H. Results and prognostic factors of splenectomy in idiopathic thrombocytopenic purpura. J Am Coll Surg 183:565-574, 1996.

176. Bussel JB. Splenectomy-sparing strategies for the treatment and long-term maintenance of chronic idiopathic (immune) thrombocytopenic purpura. Semin Hematol 2000;37(Suppl 1):1-4.

177. Bell WR Jr. Long-term outcome of splenectomy for idiopathic thrombocytopenic purpura. Semin Hematol 2000;37(Suppl 1):22-25.

178. Cusack JC, Seymour JF, Lerner S, Keating MJ, Pollock RE. Role of splenectomy in chronic lymphocytic leukemia. J Am Coll Surg 185:237-243, 1997.

179. Taylor MA, Kaplan HS, Nelsen RS. Staging laparotomy with splenectomy for Hodgkin's disease: the Stanford experience. World J Surg 1985;9:449.

180. Baccarani U, Carroll BJ, Hiatt JR, Donini A, Terrosu G, Decker R, Chandra M, Bresadola F, Phillips EH. Comparison of laparoscopic and open staging in Hodgkin disease. Arch Surg 133: 517-522, 1998.

181. Klasa RJ, Connors J, Hoskins P, et al. Early stage Hodgkin's disease: impact of brief chemotherapy together with radiotherapy without staging laparotomy. Proc Am Soc Clin Oncol 13:372, 1994.

182. Santoro A, Bonfante V, Viviani S, et al. Subtotal nodal versus involved field irradiation after 4 cycles of ABVD in early stage Hodgkin's disease. Proc Am Soc Clin Oncol 15:415, 1996.

183. Meyer AA. Spleen. In: Greenfield LJ, Mulholland MW, Oldham KT, Zelenock GB, Lillemoe KD (eds.). Surgery: Scientific Principles and Practice (2nd ed). Philadelphia: Lippincott-Raven, 1997, pp. 1262-81.

184. Sirinek KR, Evans WE. Non-parasitic splenic cysts: case report of an epidermoid cyst and review of the literature. Am J Surg 1973; 126:8.

185. Chun CH, Raff MJ, Contreras L. Splenic abscess. Medicine 59: 50-65, 1980.

186. Nelken N, Ignatius J, Skinner M, Christensen N. Changing clinical spectrum of splenic abscess. A mullticenter study and review of the literature. Am J Surg 154:27-34, 1987.

187. Ooi LP, Leong SS. Splenic abscesses from 1987 to 1995. Am J Surg 174:87-93, 1997.

188. Gadacz JR. Splenic abscess. World J Surg 1985;9:410.

189. Lerner RM, Spataro RF. Splenic abscess: percutaneous drainage. Radiology 1984;153:643.

190. Quinn SF, Van Sonnenberg E, Casola G. Interventional radiology in the spleen. Radiology 161:289-291, 1986.

191. Gleich S, Wolin DA, Herbsman H. A review of percutaneous drainage in splenic abscess. Surg Gynecol Obstet 167:211-216, 1988.

192. Phillips GS, Radosevich MD, Lipsett PA. Splenic abscess. Arch Surg 132:1331-1336, 1997.

193. Safioleas M, Misiakos E, Manti C. Surgical treatment for splenic hydatidosis. World J Surg 21:374-378, 1997.

194. Uriarte C, Pomares N, Martin M, et al. Splenic hydatidosis. Am J Trop Med Hyg 44:420, 1991.

195. Moumen M, El Alaoui M, Mokhtari M, El Fares F. Pour un traitement conservateur du kyste hydatique de la rate. J Chir 128: 260, 1991.

196. Berrada S, Ridai M, Mokhtari M. Kystes hydatiques de la rate: splenectomies ou chirurgie conservatrice? Ann Chir 45:434, 1991.

197. Wilson CI, Cabello-Inchausti B, Sendzischew H, Robinson MJ. Ceroid histiocytosis: an unusual cause of splenic rupture. South Med J 2001;94:237-239.

198. Salgado C, Feliu E, Monserrat E, Villamor N, Ordi J, Aguilar JL, Vives-Corrons JL, Rozman C. B-type large-cell primary splenic lymphoma with massive involvement of the red pulp. Acta Haematol 1993;89:46-49.

199. Rosso R, Neiman RS, Paulli M, Boveri E, Kindl S, Magrini U, Barosi G. Splenic marginal zone cell lymphoma: report of an indolent variant without massive splenomegaly presumably representing an early phase of the disease. Human Pathol 1995;26: 39-46.

200. Westra WH, Anderson BO, Klimstra DS. Carcinosarcoma of the spleen: an extragenital malignant mixed mullerian tumor? Am J Surg Pathol 1994;18:309-315.

201. Brune MB, Cain DL, Cardwell EM, Janckila AJ. Splenic lymphoma with villous lymphocytes: diagnosis by flow cytometry and immunocytochemistry. South Med J 1995;88:1260-1263.

202. Berge T. Splenic metastases. Frequencies and patterns. Acta Pathol Microbiol Scand (A) 82:499-506, 1974.

203. Brown DA, Mukherjer D. Partial splenectomy with autologous capsule graft. Surg Gynecol Obstet 1988;166:555.

204. Warshaw AL. Conservation of the spleen with distal pancreatectomy. Arch Surg 1988;123:550.

205. Phelan JT, Grace JT, Wayne AL, Moore GE. A technique of splenectomy. Surg Gynecol Obstet 1963;116:501.

206. Beal SL, Spisso JM. The risk of splenorrhaphy. Arch Surg 1988; 123:1158.

207. Otsuji E, Yamaguchi T, Sawai K, Ohara M, Takahashi T. End results of simultaneous splenectomy in patients undergoing total gastrectomy for gastric carcinoma. Surgery 1996;120:40-44.

208. Cocanour CS, Moore FA, Ware DN, Marvin RG, Clark JM, Duke JH. Delayed complications of nonoperative management of blunt adult splenic trauma. Arch Surg 133:619-625, 1998.

209. Martin JC, Cooper MN. Complications of splenectomy. South Surg 1950;16:1047.

210. Shackleford RT. Surgery of the Abdominal Tract. Philadelphia: Saunders, 1955.

211. Dalton ML, West RL. Fate of dearterialized spleen. Arch Surg 1965;91:541.

212. Piedad OH, Wels PB. Retrograde distal pancreatectomy. Am J Surg 1972;124:431.

213. Schmeiden V, Sebening W. Surgery of the pancreas with especial consideration of acute pancreatic necrosis. Surg Gynecol Obstet 1928;46:735.

214. Daoud F, Fischer D, Hafner CD. Complications following splenectomy with special emphasis on drainage. Arch Surg 1966;92: 32.

215. Hodam RP. The risk of splenectomy: a review of 10 cases. Am J Surg 1970;119:709.

216. Kassum D, Thomas EJ. Morbidity and mortality of incidental splenectomy. Can J Surg 1977;20:209.

217. Graves HA, Nelson A, Byrd BF. Gastrocutaneous fistula as a postoperative complication. Ann Surg 1970;171:656.

218. Harrison BF, Glanges E, Sparkman RS. Gastric fistula following splenectomy: its cause and prevention. Ann Surg 1977;185:210.

219. Cooper CS, Cohen MB, Donovan JF Jr. Splenectomy complicating left nephrectomy. J Urol 1996;155:30-36.

220. Sabiston DC. Textbook of Surgery: The Biological Basis of Modern Surgical Practice, 15th Ed. Philadelphia: WB Saunders Co, 1997.

221. Diaz J, Eisenstat M, Chung R. A case-controlled study of laparoscopic splenectomy. Am J Surg 173:348-350, 1997.

222. Glasgow RE, Mulvihill SJ. Laparoscopic splenectomy. World J Surg 1999;23:384-88.

223. Targarona EM, Espert JJ, Balaguè C, Sugrañes G, Ayuso C, Lomeña F, Bosch F, Trias M. Residual splenic function after laparoscopic splenectomy: a clinical concern. Arch Surg 133:56-60, 1998.

224. Lozano-Salazar RR, Herrera MF, Vargas-Voráckouvá F, López-Karpovitch X. Laparoscopic versus open splenectomy for immune thrombocytopenic purpura. Am J Surg 176:366-369, 1998.

225. Tanoue K, Makoto H, Morita M, Migoh S, Tsugawa K, Yagi S, Ohta M, Sugimachi K. Results of laparoscopic splenectomy for immune thrombocytopenic purpura. Am J Surg 1999;177:222-226.

226. Fass SM, Hui TT, Lefor A, Maestroni U, Phillips EH. Safety of laparoscopic splenectomy in elderly patients with idiopathic thrombocytopenic purpura. Am Surg 2000;66:844-847.

227. Katkhouda N, Mavor E. Laparoscopic splenectomy. Surg Clin North Am 2000;80:1285-1297.

228. Rescorla FJ, Breitfeld PP, West KW, Williams D, Engum SA, Grosfeld JL. A case controlled comparison of open and laparoscopic splenectomy in children. Surgery 124:670-676, 1998.

229. Terrosu G, Donini A, Baccarani U, Vianello V, Anania G, Zala F, Pasgualucci A, Bresadola F. Laparoscopic versus open splenectomy in the management of splenomegaly: our preliminary experience. Surgery 124:839-843, 1998.

230. Chang MY, Shiau CS, Chang CL, Hou HC, Chiang CH, Hsieh TT, Soong YK. Spleen laceration, a rare complication of laparoscopy. J Am Assn Gynecol Laparosc 2000;7:269-272.

231. McWorter JE, Cloud JW. Malignant tumors and their metastasis. Ann Surg 1930;92:434-443.

232. Miller JN, Milton GW. An experimental comparison between tumor growth in the spleen and liver. J Pathol 1965;90:515-519.

233. Slavin JD, Mathews J, Spencer RP. Splenectomy for splenic metastasis from carcinoma of the colon. Clin Nucl Med 1986;11: 491-492.

234. Hirst AE Jr, Bullock WK. Metastatic carcinoma of the spleen. Am J Med Sci 223:414-417, 1952.

235. Warren S, Davis H. Studies on tumor metastasis: V. The metastases of carcinoma to the spleen. Am J Cancer 21:517-533, 1934.

236. Marymont JH, Gross H. Patterns of metastatic cancer in the spleen. Am J Clin Pathol 1963;10:58-63.

237. Harmon JW, Dacorso P. Spread of carcinoma to the spleen. Arch Pathol 1975;45:179-186.

238. Berge T. Metastasis of carcinoma with special reference to the spleen. Acta Pathol Microbiol Scand Suppl 188:1128, 1967.

239. Breitbart AS, Harris MN. Isolated metastatic breast carcinoma to the spleen. Contemp Surg 1991;38:42.

240. Schoket E, Dembrow VD. Splenic metastases from melanoma of the nasal mucosa. Am J Surg 16:949-953, 1963.

241. Jorgensen LN, Chrintz H. Solitary metastatic endometrial carcinoma of the spleen. Acta Obstet Gynecol Scand 679:91-92, 1988.

242. Klein B, Stein M, Kuten A. Splenomegaly and solitary spleen metastasis in solid tumors. Cancer 60:100-102, 1987.

243. Waller RM, Fajman WA. An unusual case of an isolated, focal splenic defect demonstrated by liver-spleen scintigraphy. Clin Nucl Med 7:5-7, 1982.

244. Murthy SK, Prabhakaran PS, Rao SR, et al. Unusual splenic metastases from oesophageal cancer. Indian J Cancer 28:81-83, 1991.

245. Capizzi PJ, Allen KB, Amerson JR, Skandalakis JE. Isolated splenic metastasis from rectal carcinoma. South Med J 85:1003-1005, 1992.

246. Mainprize KS, Berry AR. Case report: solitary splenic metastasis from colorectal carcinoma. Br J Surg 84:70, 1997.

247. Indudura R, Vogt D, Levin HS, Church J. Isolated splenic metastasis from colon cancer. South Med J 90:633-636, 1997.

248. Dunbar WH, Beahrs OH, Morlock CG. Solitary splenic metastasis incidental to rectal carcinoma: report of a case. Mayo Clin Proc 44:40-45, 1969.

249. Thomas ST, Fitzgerald JB, Pollock RE, et al. Isolated splenic metastases from colon carcinoma. Eur J Surg Oncol 19:485-490, 1993.

250. Falk S, Stutte HJ. Splenic metastasis in an ileal carcinoid tumor. Pathol Res Pract 1989;185:238-244.

251. Sharpe RW, Rector JT, Rushin JM, Garvin DF, Cotelingam JD. Splenic metastasis in hairy cell leukemia. Cancer 1993;71:2222-2226.

252. Das Gupta T, Brasfield R. Metastatic melanoma: a clinicopathologic study. Cancer 1964;17:1323.

253. Meyer JE, Stolbach L. Pretreatment radiographic evaluation of patients with malignant melanoma. Cancer 1978;42:125.

254. Amer MH, Al-Sarraf M, Vaitkevicius VK. Clinical presentation, natural history and prognostic factors in advanced melanoma. Surg Gynecol Obstet 1979;149:687.

255. Balch CM, Houghton AN, Peters LJ. Cutaneous melanoma. In: DeVita VT Jr, Hellman S, Rosenberg SA. Cancer: Principles & Practice of Oncology (4th ed). Philadelphia: JB Lippincott, 1993.

256. Brown BC. Pathology of the spleen. Probl Gen Surg 1990;7:48-68.

257. Hull CC, Galloway P, Gordon N, Gerson SL, Hawkins N, Stellato TA. Splenectomy and the indication of murine colon cancer. Arch Surg 1988;123:462.

258. Skandalakis LJ, Gray SW, Skandalakis JE. Splenic realities and curiosities. Probl Gen Surg 1990;7:28-32.

259. Sappington SW. Carcinoma of the spleen. JAMA 1922;78:953-955.

260. Kettle EH. Carcinomatous metastases in the spleen. J Pathol Bacteriol 1913;17:40-46.

261. Herbut PA, Gabriel FR. Secondary cancer of the spleen. Arch Pathol 1942;33:917.

262. Pollard BR. Role of the spleen in resistance to experimental tumors. Texas Rep Biol Med 1953;11:48.

263. Woglam WH. Immunity to transplantable tumors. Cancer Rev 1929; 4:129.

264. Small AG, Trainin N. Kinetics of the response of spleen cells from tumor-bearing animals in an in vivo tumor neutralization assay. Int J Cancer 1976;18:813-819.

265. Sato M, Michaelides MC, Wallack MK. Effect of splenectomy on the growth of murine colon tumors. J Surg Oncol 1983;22:73.

266. Wanebo HJ, Kennedy BJ, Winchester DP, Stewart AK, Fremgen AM. Role of splenectomy in gastric cancer surgery: adverse effect of elective splenectomy on longterm survival. J Am Coll Surg 185: 172-176, 1997.

267. Davis CJ, Ilstrup DM, Pemberton JH. Influence of splenectomy on survival rate of patients with colorectal cancer. Am J Surg 1988; 155:173.

268. Meyer JD, Argyzis BF, Meyer JA. Splenectomy suppression cell activity and survival in tumor bearing rats. J Surg Res 1980;29: 527.

269. Ferrer ZF. Enhancement of the growth of sarcoma 180 in splenectomized and sham operated AKR mice. Transplantation 1968;6:160.

270. Mercie P, Faure I, Viallard JF, Demeaux H, Dilhuydy MS, Leng B, Pellegrin JL. [Splenic vascular occlusion in the course of pancreatic cancer]. Rev Mal Intern 2000;21:628-631.

271. Warshaw AL, Chesney TM, Evans GW, McCarthy HF. Intrasplenic dissection by pancreatic pseudocyst. N Engl J Med 1972; 287:72.

272. Okuda K, Taguchi T, Ishihara K, Konno A. Intrasplenic pseudocyst of the pancreas. J Clin Gastroenterol 1981;3:37.

273. Byrd BF, Couch OA Jr. Pancreatitis with rupture of spleen and hemorrhagic pleural effusion. JAMA 1955;157:1112.

274. Catanzaro FP, Abiri M, Allegra S. Spontaneous rupture of spleen and pleural effusion complicating pancreatitis. RI Med J 1968; 51:328.

275. Nath BJ, Warshaw AL. Pulmonary insufficiency. In: Bradley EL (ed). Complications of Pancreatitis. Philadelphia: WB Saunders, 1982.

276. Frey CF, Eckhauser F, Stanley JC. Hemorrhage. In: Bradley EL (ed). Complications of Pancreatitis. Philadelphia: WB Saunders, 1982.

277. Nishiyama T, Iwao N, Myose H, Okamoto T, Fujitomi Y, Chinen M, Komichi Y, Kobayashi T. Splenic vein thrombosis as a consequence of chronic pancreatitis: a study of three cases. Am J Gastroenterol 1986;81:1193-8.

278. Bradley EL. The natural history of splenic vein thrombosis due to chronic pancreatitis: indications for surgery. Int J Pancreatol 1987;2:87-92.

279. Ferguson CM. Human immunodeficiency virus-related immune thrombocytopenia. Probl Gen Surg 7(1):149-150, 1990.

280. Tsoukas CM, Bernard NF, Abrahamowicz M, Strawczynski H, Growe G, Card RT, Gold P. Effect of splenectomy on slowing human immunodeficiency virus disease progression. Arch Surg 133:25-31, 1998.

# Chapter 23

# Kidneys and Ureters

JOHN E. SKANDALAKIS, GENE L. COLBORN, THOMAS A. WEIDMAN,
ROBERT A. BADALAMENT, THOMAS S. PARROTT,
NIALL T.M. GALLOWAY, WILLIAM M. SCALJON

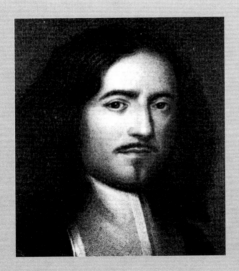

**Marcello Malpighi (1628-1694)** discovered and described the capillaries.

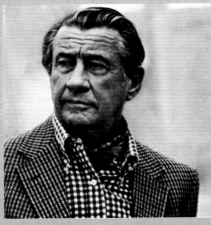

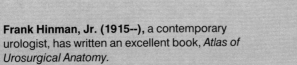

**Frank Hinman, Jr. (1915--),** a contemporary urologist, has written an excellent book, *Atlas of Urosurgical Anatomy.*

# *Introduction to the Urogenital System*

The detailed surgical anatomy of the anatomic entities most immediately associated with the urogenital system will be found in the chapters on the kidneys/ureters, urinary bladder, male genital system, and female genital system.

But the study of surgical anatomy of the urogenital system is also related to the following areas:
- Retroperitoneal spaces
- Adrenals
- Anterolateral abdominal wall and inguinal canal
- Posterior abdominal wall
- Thoracic wall
- Pelvic diaphragm
- Urogenital diaphragm
- Lateral pelvic wall
- Perineum

Knowledge of the anatomy of the urogenital system is necessary not only for urologists and gynecologists, but also for general surgeons, radiologists, and transplant surgeons. In addition to being familiar with the anatomic entities, it is important that such medical professionals also understand the embryogenesis, anomalies, and variations of these anatomic entities.

*Surgery of the upper urinary tract and the retroperitoneal spaces is a constant invitation to potentially serious bleeding. An adequate well-organized exposure of the pathologic condition involved, detailed knowledge of the regional anatomy and its variations, careful gentle dissection of the major vessels, and a calm disposition of the surgeon are the critical factors in preventing intraoperative hemorrhage.*

*Zinman and Libertino*[1]

## HISTORY

The anatomic and surgical history of the kidney and ureter is found in Table 23-1.

## EMBRYOGENESIS OF THE KIDNEYS AND URETERS

### Normal Development

Three excretory organs (pronephroi, mesonephroi, and metanephroi) develop from the intermediate mesoderm[2,3] (Figs. 23-1, 23-2). However, since pronephroi are never functional in human embryos and degenerate on days 24 or 25, we will present only the concepts of mesonephroi and metanephroi.

The mesonephroi ("interim or temporary kidneys") (Fig. 23-3) appear late in the 4th week (day 24 or 25) just caudal to the pronephroi. The mesonephroi have a brief functional period from the late embryonic to the early fetal period (weeks 6 to 10), during which they produce very dilute urine. The mesonephroi take over a portion of the pronephric duct in the thoracic and upper lumbar regions, making it the mesonephric (or Wolffian) duct (Figs. 23-1

**TABLE 23-1. Anatomic and Surgical History of the Kidney and Ureter**

| | | |
|---|---|---|
| Hippocrates (470-373 BC) | | Prohibited renal surgery; felt it was too dangerous. Only nephritic abscesses could be opened. |
| Aretaeus (2nd-3rd century) | | Described the kidneys; considered them to be true glands |
| Berenger (1470-1530) | | Studied renal vasculature |
| Cardan of Milan | 1510 | Removed 18 renal stones while draining renal abscess |
| Vesalius (1514-1564) | | Contributed to the early understanding of renal anatomy |
| Zambeccari Rounhyzer Blancard | 1670 1672 1690 | Performed animal experiments showing one kidney was enough to sustain life. Advocated nephrectomy for persistent renal colic. |
| de Marchetti | (ca. 1680) | Utilized open surgical removal of kidney stones |
| Bowman | 1832 | Described the relation of the glomerulus to the tubule |
| Henle (1809-1885) | | Discovered the loop of Henle |
| Ludwig | 1844 | Suggested that urine formation begins with filtration of protein-free fluid in the glomeruli |
| Simon | 1851 1869 | Performed first planned ureterosigmoidostomy Performed first planned nephrectomy (for urethral vaginal fistula) in which patient survived |
| Morris | 1880 | Performed first nephrolithotomy |
| Czerny | 1880 | Performed first pyelolithotomy |
| Hyrtl | 1882 | Described the avascular plane between anterior and posterior vascular segments |
| Wells | 1884 | Performed first partial nephrectomy |
| Witzel | 1896 | Described ureteric reimplantation using tunneling of the ureter |
| Robson | 1898 | First suggested use of x-rays to localize stones |
| Brodel | 1901 | Confirmed Hyrtl's work. Published and illustrated his studies on the intrinsic blood supply of the kidney. |
| Lower | 1913 | Advocated pyelolithotomy for stones in the renal pelvis |
| Judd | 1919 | Recommended nephroureterectomy for transitional cell carcinoma of the kidney |
| Braasch; Carman | 1919 | Used interoperative fluoroscopy to localize stones |
| Demmings | 1928 | Described incision through avascular plane |
| Hunt | 1929 | Recommended nephroureterectomy with en bloc removal of a cuff of bladder for transitional cell carcinoma of the kidney |
| Young | 1929 | Reported first endoscopy of ureter. Inserted cystoscope in the dilated ureter of boy with posterior urethral valves. |
| Boari | 1932 | Utilized bladder flap to replace distal ureter |
| Foley | 1937 | Introduced Y-V plasty for ureteropelvic junction (UPJ) obstruction |
| Kolff & Berk | 1942 | Introduced the artificial kidney into clinical medicine |
| Davis | 1943 | Described intubated uterostomy |
| Anderson & Hynes | 1949 | Introduced dismembered pyeloplasty for UPJ obstruction |
| Bricker | 1950 | Popularized ureteroileal conduits |
| Hume | 1951-1953 | Performed nine cadaveric kidney transplants |
| Stewart | 1952 | Pioneered partial nephrectomy |
| Hutch | 1952 | Noted relationship between vesicoureteric reflux and pyelonephritis |
| Harrison & Murray Merrill et al. | 1954 1956 | Performed successful human kidney transplantation in identical twins (Harrison and Murray later transplanted cadaveric kidneys) |
| Jameson, McKinney, & Rushton | 1957 | Introduced ureterocalicostomy |

## TABLE 23-1 (cont'd). Anatomic and Surgical History of the Kidney and Ureter

| Politano, Leadbetter | 1958 | Described technique for ureteroneocystostomy involving initial intravesical dissection, with the ureter passed extravesically and then brought back through a new, more superiorly located position in the bladder |
|---|---|---|
| Paquin | 1959 | Described combined extravesical and intravesical approaches to ureteroneocystostomy |
| Lich, Gregoir | 1961 | Described extravesical ureteric reimplantation procedure |
| Robson | 1963 | Defined survival for patients with renal cell cancer treated by radical nephrectomy. Described modern classification system for renal cell cancer. |
| Hardy Woodruff et al. | 1963 1966 | Early successful autotransplantations of the kidney |
| Smith, Boyce | 1967 | Pioneered anatrophic nephrolithotomy |
| Glenn & Anderson | 1967 | Described most popular ureteric advancement technique |
| Cohen | 1977 | Described technique of crosstrigonal advancement |
| Goodman | 1977 | Reported on endoscopic inspection of lower ureter |
| Perez-Castro Ellendt Martinez-Pineiro | 1980 | Performed ureteroscopy to level of renal pelvis |
| Chaussey | 1980 | Published first report on extracorporeal shock wave lithotripsy (ESWL) |
| Ploeg | 1990 | Report of improved preservation of kidney, permitting longer cold ischemia times and more complex resections and reconstructions |

*History table compiled by David A. McClusky III and John E. Skandalakis.*

**References**

Dimopoulos C, Gialas A, Likourinas M, Androutsos G, Kostakopoulos A. Hippocrates: founder and pioneer of urology. Br J Urol 1980;52:73-74.
Ek A, Bradley WE. History of cystometry. Urology 1983;23:335-350.
Ellis H. Famous Operations. Media PA: Harwal, 1984.
Haeger K. The Illustrated History of Surgery. London: Starke, 1989.
Hardy JD. High ureteral injuries: management by autotransplantation of the kidney. JAMA 1963;184:97-101.
Mettler CC. History of Medicine. Philadelphia: Blakinston Co., 1947.
Ploeg RJ. Kidney preservation with the UW and Euro-Collins solutions: a preliminary report of a clinical comparison. Transplantation 1990;49:281-284.
Wells S. Successful removal of two solid circumferential tumors. Br Med J 1884;1:758.
Woodhead DM. Urology: past, present, future. Int Surg 1968;49:534-543.
Woodruff MFA, Doig A, Donald KW, Nolan B. Renal autotransplantation. Lancet 1966;1:433.

and 23-2). The mesonephric tubules form excretory units: the medial end forms Bowman's capsule; lateral branches from the aorta form capillaries that become glomeruli which fit into Bowman's capsule, thus forming renal corpuscles. The tubules open into mesonephric ducts. Some tubules persist in males to become ductuli efferentia which open into the mesonephric (Wolffian) ducts to become ductuli deferentia.

The metanephroi ("hind kidneys") (Fig. 23-4) are the final developmental stage. The metanephric diverticulum (ureteric bud) arises on day 35 from the caudal part of the mesonephric duct. This entity is destined to give rise to the collecting apparatus of the urinary system which consists of 1-3 million collecting tubules, minor and major calices, the renal pelvis, and ureters. The metanephrogenic blastema (metanephric mesoderm) forms from the caudal portion of the intermediate mesoderm and gives rise to the nephrons

(800,000 to 1,000,000 in each kidney). Blastema tissue capping each arched collecting tubule differentiates into the nephron. Glomeruli form and are enveloped by Bowman's capsule to form the renal corpuscle. The proximal convoluted tubule, loop of Henle, and distal convoluted tubule form the remainder of the nephron. The distal convoluted tubule opens into the arched collecting duct. To start with, the ureter has a lumen which later occludes and which subsequently recanalizes.

When the kidneys ascend from the pelvis to their permanent location in the upper lumbar region (Fig. 23-5), they come into apposition with the adrenal glands, which develop in situ. During ascent, the kidneys rotate medially so that the hilum, which initially faced anteriorly, now faces medially. The segmental vessels supplying the kidney are added cranially and lost caudally[4] during ascent.

Approximately 25 percent of adult kidneys have two to

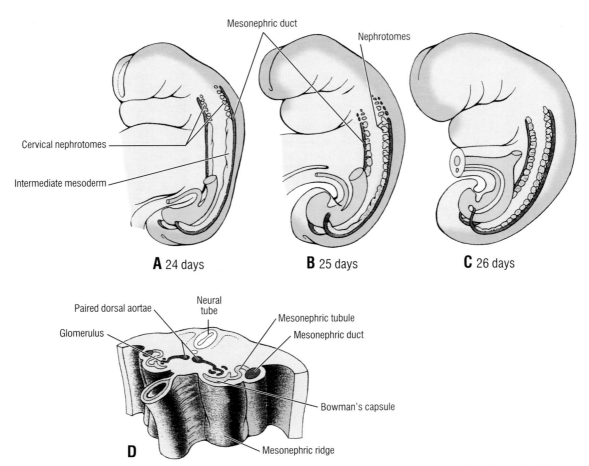

**FIG. 23-1.** Development of the cervical nephrotomes and mesonephros. **A.** A pair of cervical nephrotomes forms in each of five to seven cervical segments, but these quickly degenerate during the 4th week. The mesonephric ducts first appear on day 24. **B, C.** Mesonephric nephrotomes and tubules form in craniocaudal sequence throughout the thoracic and lumbar regions. The more cranial pairs regress as caudal pairs form, and the definitive mesonephroi contain about 20 pairs confined to the first three lumbar segments. **D.** The mesonephroi contain functional nephric units consisting of glomeruli, Bowman's capsules, mesonephric tubules, and mesonephric ducts. (Modified from Larsen WJ. Essentials of Human Embryology. New York: Churchill Livingstone, 1998; with permission.)

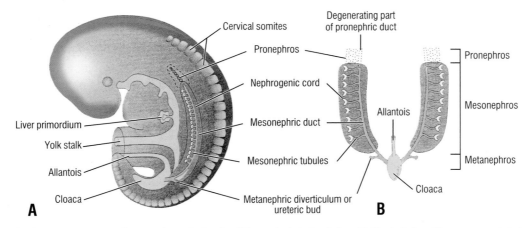

**FIG. 23-2.** The three sets of excretory systems in an embryo during the fifth week. **A.** Lateral view. **B.** Ventral view. The mesonephric tubules have been pulled laterally; their normal position is shown in **A**. (Modified from Moore KL, Persaud TVN. The Developing Human. Clinically Oriented Embryology (6th ed). Philadelphia: WB Saunders, 1998; with permission.)

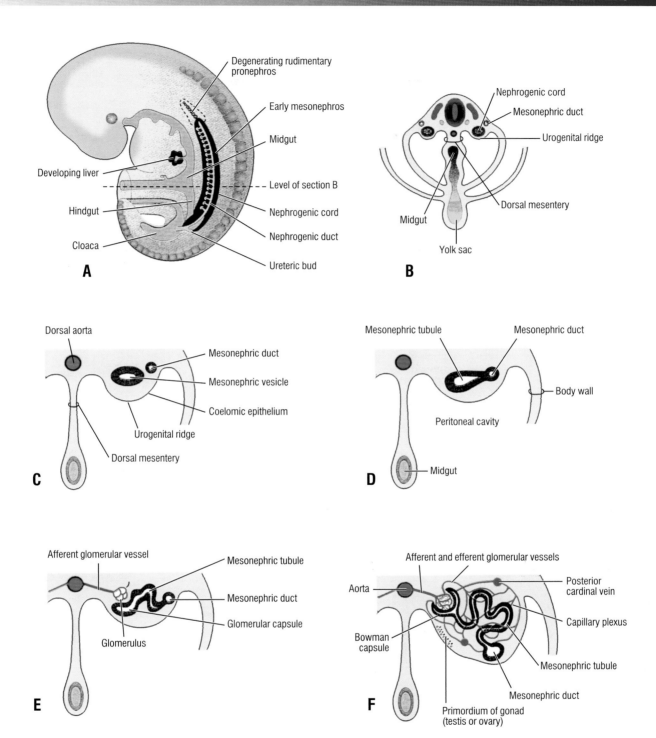

Fɪɢ. 23-3. **A.** Lateral view of a five-week embryo showing the extent of the mesonephros and the primordium of the metanephros or permanent kidney. **B.** Transverse section of the embryo showing the nephrogenic cords from which the mesonephric tubules develop. **C-F.** Transverse sections showing successive stages in the development of a mesonephric tubule between the fifth and eleventh weeks. Note that the mesenchymal cell cluster in the nephrogenic cord develops a lumen, thereby forming a mesonephric vesicle. The vesicle soon becomes an S-shaped mesonephric tubule and extends laterally to join the pronephric duct, now renamed the mesonephric duct. The expanded medial end of the mesonephric tubule is invaginated by blood vessels to form a glomerular capsule (Bowman's capsule). The cluster of capillaries projecting into this capsule is known as a glomerulus. (Modified from Moore KL, Persaud TVN. The Developing Human. Clinically Oriented Embryology (6th ed). Philadelphia: WB Saunders, 1998; with permission.)

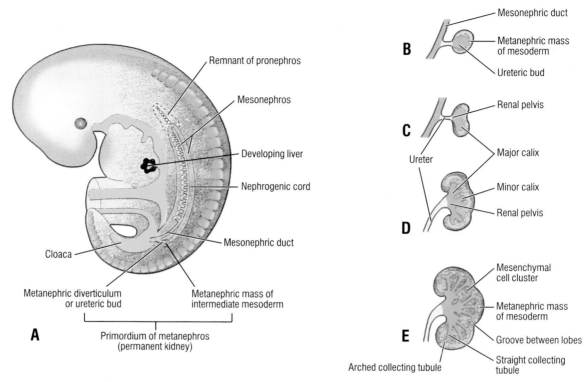

**FIG. 23-4. A.** Lateral view of a five-week embryo, showing the primordium of the metanephros or permanent kidney. **B-E.** Successive stages in the development of the metanephric diverticulum or ureteric bud (fifth to eight weeks). Observe the development of the ureter, renal pelvis, calices, and collecting tubules. The renal lobes, illustrated in **E**, are still visible in the kidneys of a 28-week fetus. (Modified from Moore KL, Persaud TVN. The Developing Human. Clinically Oriented Embryology (6th ed). Philadelphia: WB Saunders, 1998; with permission.)

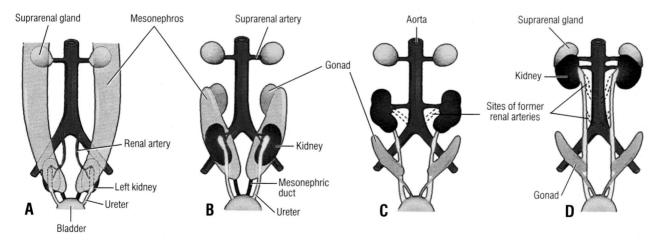

**FIG. 23-5. A-D.** Ventral views of the abdominopelvic region of embryos and fetuses (sixth to ninth weeks), showing medial rotation and 'ascent' of the kidneys from the pelvis to the abdomen. **A, B.** Observe also the size regression of the metanephroi. **C, D.** Note that as the kidneys 'ascend,' they are supplied by arteries at successively higher levels and that the hilum of the kidney (where the vessels and nerves enter) is eventually directed anteromedially. (Modified from Moore KL, Persaud TVN. The Developing Human. Clinically Oriented Embryology (6th ed). Philadelphia: WB Saunders, 1998; with permission.)

four arteries. Accessory renal arteries usually arise from the aorta; they may be superior or inferior to the main renal artery, and are end arteries. Accessory arteries usually form at the superior or inferior poles of the kidney. The inferior accessory artery may pass anteriorly to the ureter, sometimes compressing it and causing blockage; this is hydronephrosis, a common form of ureteropelvic junction obstruction.[5] The right inferior accessory artery may cross anteriorly to both the ureter and the inferior vena cava. Supernumerary arteries are twice as common as supernumerary veins.

The ureteric bud is responsible for the genesis of the ureters. The bud, a diverticulum of the mesonephric duct, is located close to the cloaca, just above the duct's entrance into the cloaca. The bud grows into the mesodermal metanephrogenic mass, and its cranial end becomes the renal pelvis. The stalk of the ureteric bud becomes the ureter, which enters into the urinary bladder.

## Congenital Anomalies

Congenital anomalies of the kidney and ureter are seen in Figure 23-6.

Renal agenesis is caused by failure of the ureteric bud to develop or by early degeneration of the bud. Unilateral renal agenesis occurs in 1 in 1000 newborns (Fig. 23-6A). The condition is twice as common in males. Usually, the left kidney is absent, and the other kidney undergoes compensatory hypertrophy. With a unilateral functioning kidney, compensatory renal hypertrophy is detectable in utero and may occur as early as 22 weeks gestation.[6] Bilateral renal agenesis, which is incompatible with life, occurs in 1 in 3000 births. It presents with oligohydramnios, Potter's facies, hypertelorism, epicanthic folds, low-set ears, and limb defects.

Non-rotation or abnormal rotation of the kidneys (Fig. 23-6C) is another congenital anomaly. Non-rotation results in the hilum facing anteriorly. With excessive rotation, the hilum faces posteriorly; it may face laterally if rotation occurs in the wrong direction. Abnormalities of rotation are often associated with ectopic kidneys.

Ectopic kidneys may be unilateral or bilateral. Most are located inferior to their normal location, with the hilum facing anteriorly. Most ectopic kidneys lie in the pelvis; some are found in the lower abdomen (Fig. 23-6B). Pelvic kidneys often fuse to form pancake (discoid) kidneys (Fig. 23-6E). In crossed renal ectopia, one kidney has crossed to the contralateral side (Fig. 23-6D). The blood supply of ectopic kidneys is often from multiple arteries which arise from nearby arteries such as the internal iliac, the external iliac, and/or the aorta.

Campbell[7] reported 22 cases of renal ectopia with only one intrathoracic finding. Kubricht et al.[8] reported such a case with renal cell carcinoma. Their patient had a thin membrane of diaphragm covering the kidney, thus making it subdiaphragmatic while being intrathoracic in position (diaphragmatic eventration). The embryogenesis of such an anomaly is enigmatic.

Horseshoe kidney occurs in 1 in 500 births. There is a seven percent incidence of horseshoe kidney in individuals with Turner's syndrome; children with this condition are 2 to 8 times more likely to have Wilms' tumors. In horseshoe kidney, the caudal poles fuse across the midline. Usually the horseshoe lies in the hypogastrium anterior to the lower lumbar vertebrae because of the failure of ascent which occurs when the kidney is 'hung up' on the inferior mesenteric artery. Horseshoe kidney is usually symptomless.

Various duplications of the urinary tract may occur. Supernumerary kidney is rare; it is probably due to two ureteric primordia forming on one side (Fig. 23-6F). The location of division of the ureteric bud determines the extent of duplication. One possibility is a divided kidney with bifid ureter (Fig. 23-6B). Occasionally the division may result in a double kidney with bifid ureter or separate ureters.

The discovery of complete ureteric duplication warrants careful imaging studies for detection of fetal renal abnormalities. According to Peng and Chen,[9] upper pole nephroureterectomy is performed on a child with a nonfunctioning moiety, and ureteropyelostomy or ureteric reimplantation is utilized for functioning segments.

Ectopic ureteric orifices are defined as openings located anywhere other than at the bladder. In males, the usual opening is into the neck of the bladder or prostatic urethra; unusual places include the ductus deferens, seminal vesicle or prostatic utricle. In females the ectopic opening is at the bladder neck, urethra, vagina, or vaginal vestibule. In males with ectopic urethra, incontinence is not seen because the ectopic ureter enters into the genitourinary system (bladder neck, prostatic urethra, seminal vesicle) above the external sphincter. In females with ectopic ureter, incontinence from the urethra or vagina is common because the ectopic opening is below the external sphincter. Cloacal outlet obstruction may occur with an ectopic ureter.[10]

Primary obstructive megaureter is the result of an adynamic segment of the distal ureter due to derangement of ureteral musculature.[11] The condition may be bilateral or unilateral, with presentation in later years. Bapat et al.[12] reported that endoureterotomy is a safe and effective treatment.

Ectopic ureteric orifices result from the ureter not being incorporated into the posterior part of the bladder. The ureter is carried caudally with the mesonephric duct to

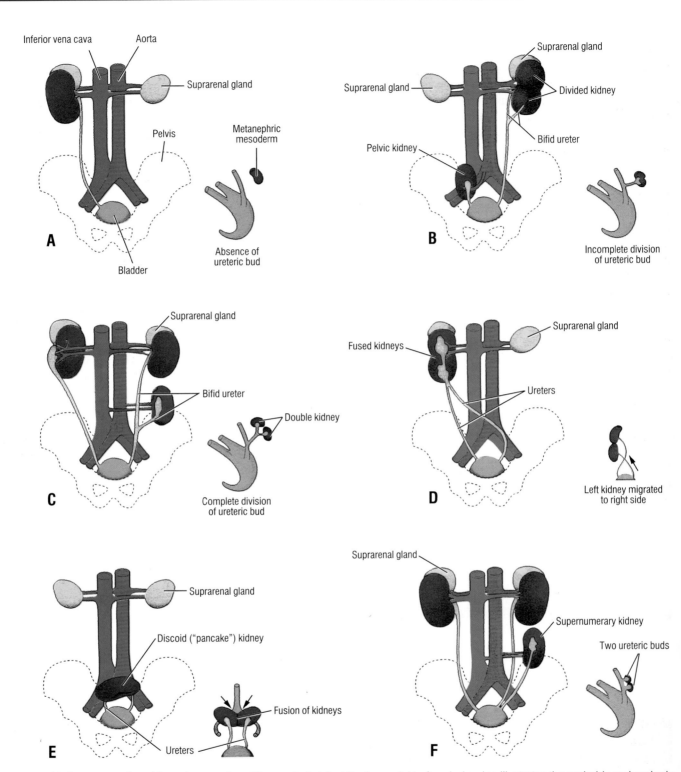

FIG. 23-6. Various anomalies of the urinary system. The small sketch at the lower right of each drawing illustrates the probable embryologic basis of the anomaly. **A.** Unilateral renal agenesis. **B.** Right side, pelvic kidney; left side, divided kidney with a bifid ureter. **C.** Right side, mal-rotation of the kidney; left side, bifid ureter and double kidney. **D.** Crossed renal ectopia. The left kidney crossed to the right side and fused with the right kidney. **E.** 'Pancake' or discoid kidney resulting from fusion of the kidneys while they were in the pelvis. **F.** Supernumerary left kidney resulting from the development of two ureteric buds. (Modified from Moore KL, Persaud TVN. The Developing Human. Clinically Oriented Embryology (6th ed). Philadelphia: WB Saunders, 1998; with permission.)

open into the lower part of the vesical portion of the urogenital sinus which becomes the urethra in females and the prostatic urethra in males. When two ureters form, the one from the upper pole of the kidney opens more caudally into the bladder or prostatic urethra; this phenomenon is known as the Weigert-Meyer rule.

Shindo et al.[13] report a retrocaval ureter and a preaortic iliac vein confluence on a patient with an infrarenal aortic aneurysm.

Fetal obstructive uropathy is characterized by obstruction of the urethra, renal anomalies, ureterovesical dilatation, oligohydramnios, cryptorchidism, and abdominal muscle wall changes. The renal anomalies might be related to the gestational age at which the injury occurred and to the duration of the obstruction.[14]

Cystic diseases of the kidney[5] fall under two broad categories: genetic and non-genetic.

Autosomal recessive (infantile) polycystic disease occurs in 1 in 40,000 births. It is associated with biliary duct ectasia or hepatic fibrosis and always appears in infancy or childhood. It follows an essentially ominous clinical course, with progressive uremia in infants and portal hypertension in older children. Infantile polycystic disease is characterized histologically by multiple diffuse small cysts and marked collecting tubule ectasia.

Autosomal dominant (adult) polycystic disease occurs at a rate of 1 in 400 to 1000. It is associated with cysts of the liver and other organs. While the condition may appear in infancy or childhood it more commonly becomes apparent in the 4th decade, with azotemia. Successful minimally invasive surgery for nephrolithiasis associated with autosomal dominant polycystic kidney disease was reported by Ng et al.[15] Adult polycystic disease is characterized histologically by diffuse cysts of varying size and large kidneys. Rarely, renal cell carcinoma may occur in adults with polycystic kidney disease. Hemal and colleagues[16] advocate noninvasive diagnosis (ultrasound or contrast-enhanced CT) and radical nephrectomy for these patients.

Other genetic cystic diseases of the kidney include

- Juvenile nephronopthisis-medullary cystic disease complex (recessive-dominant)
- Congenital nephrosis (recessive)
- Familial hypoplastic glomerulocystic kidney disease (dominant)
- Cysts associated with multiple malformation syndromes. A current theory is that cysts are wide dilations of parts of nephrons, especially in the loops of Henle.

Non-genetic cystic diseases of the kidney include multicystic kidney, multilocular cyst, simple cyst, and medullary sponge kidney (sponge kidney disease). The occurrence of multiple unilateral renal cysts in two children with no family history or associated renal cystic disease syndromes was reported by Dugougeat et al.,[17] who suggest the possibility that this might represent a distinct clinical entity.

A family in which the father and his two daughters had ureteroceles involving the upper half of a duplex system suggests a genetic background for ureteroceles, according to Aubert and colleagues.[18]

# *Kidneys*

## SURGICAL ANATOMY OF THE KIDNEYS

### General Topographic Features

The kidneys are paired, bean-shaped organs located on either side of the vertebral column in the perirenal compartment of the retroperitoneal space between the anterior and posterior leaflets of the renal fascia (Gerota's fascia). A stroma of adipose tissue (thick or thin) covers all their surfaces.

Renal size in pediatric patients varies with age. A reasonable nomogram using ultrasound measurements, in which the kidney size is shown to vary with age, is presented in Table 23-2.

The adult kidney has a length of 10-14 cm, width of 5-7

| TABLE 23-2. Renal Size in Pediatric Patients Using Ultrasound Measurements | | |
|---|---|---|
| Age | Size (cm) | Standard Deviation (cm) |
| Birth | 4.5 | 3.8-5.3 |
| 1 year | 6.2 | 5-7.7 |
| 2 | 7 | 5.9-8.0 |
| 3 | 7.4 | 6.3-8.3 |
| 4 | 7.6 | 6.6-8.6 |
| 5 | 7.8 | 6.8-9.0 |
| 6 | 8 | 6.7-9.1 |
| 7 | 8 | 6.8-9.2 |
| 8 | 8.4 | 7.0-10.0 |
| 9 | 9 | 7.2-10.8 |
| 10 | 9.1 | 7.4-10.7 |
| 11 | 9.3 | 8.0-10.6 |
| 12 | 10 | 8.4-11.2 |
| 13 | 10 | 8.3-11.4 |
| 14 | 10 | 8.4-11.1 |
| 15 | 10.2 | 9.0-11.4 |

*Source:* Thomas S. Parrott, M.D.; with permission.

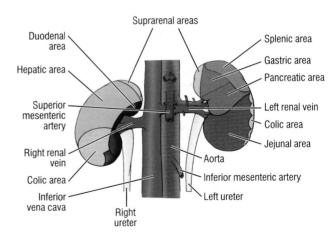

FIG. 23-7. The anterior surface of the kidney showing the areas related to neighboring viscera.

cm, and thickness of 2.5-3.0 cm. Its approximate weight is 135 g in women and 150 g in men.

Each kidney has two surfaces (anterior and posterior), two borders (lateral and medial), and two poles (superior and inferior); each kidney also has its own relations with several other anatomic entities. The kidney is related anteriorly to the abdominal viscera and posteriorly to the osteomuscular area. The right kidney lies at a lower level in comparison with the left, a phenomenon that permits the right lower pole to be palpable.

When the patient is in the recumbent position, the kidneys may extend from T12 to L3, but in the erect position both may extend from L1 to L4. In addition to changing with alterations in posture, the kidneys may move upward and downward approximately 1-7 cm with respiration, according to O'Rahilly.[19] The above numbers represent, if the term is permissible, the "physiologic" movements of the kidney, not the ptotic (nephroptotic, mobile, floating) kidney.

## Relations

### Anterior Surfaces

The anterior surfaces of the kidneys are covered by the following anatomic entities:
- Perirenal fat
- Gerota's fascia
- Pararenal fat

- Parietal posterior peritoneum (partially)

The anterior surface of the right kidney is related to (Fig. 23-7, Fig. 23-8):
- Right adrenal gland
- Liver
- Second part of duodenum
- Inferior vena cava
- Ureter
- Ascending colon
- Hepatic flexure of the colon

The anterior surface of the left kidney is related to:
- Left adrenal gland
- Pancreas
- Splenic vessels
- Stomach
- Spleen

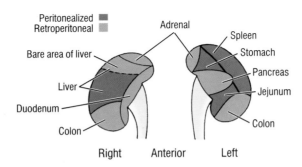

FIG. 23-8. Anterior relations of the kidneys to the abdominal organs. (Modified from Kabalin JN. Surgical anatomy of the retroperitoneum, kidneys, and ureters. In: Walsh PC, Retik AB, Vaughan ED Jr, Wein AJ (eds). Campbell's Urology (7th ed). Philadelphia: WB Saunders, 1998; with permission.)

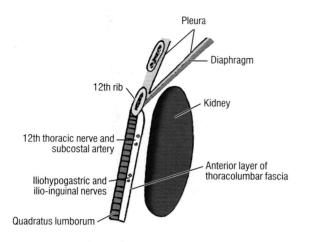

**FIG. 23-9.** Schematic representation of the posterior relations of the kidney. (Modified from Decker GAG, Du Plessis DJ. Lee McGregor's Synopsis of Surgical Anatomy (12th ed). Bristol UK: Wright, 1986; with permission.)

- Duodenojejunal flexure
- Ligament of Treitz
- Inferior mesenteric vein
- Descending colon
- Splenic flexure of the colon
- Loops of jejunum

**Posterior Surfaces**

The posterior surfaces (Figs. 23-9, 23-10, 23-11) of the kidneys are related to:

- Psoas muscles
- Transversus abdominis muscles
- Quadratus lumborum muscles
- Diaphragm
- 12th thoracic nerves
- Iliohypogastric nerves
- Ilioinguinal nerves
- Subcostal vessels
- Anterior layer of thoracolumbar (lumbodorsal) fascia
- Transversalis fascia
- Pararenal fat
- 11th and 12th ribs
- Pleurae
- Posterior layer of Gerota's fascia
- Perirenal fat
- Medial and lateral arcuate ligaments of the diaphragm

The posterior surface of the right kidney is related to the 12th rib, with the superior pole extending upward into the 11th intercostal space; the posterior surface of the left kidney is related to the 11th and 12th ribs.

**Lateral Border**

The lateral border of the kidney is related to the perirenal fat, Gerota's fascia, and pararenal fat. From a surgical standpoint, the lateral renal border is not important.

**Medial Border**

In the medial border of each kidney there is a vertical fissure called the renal porta or hilum. The renal arteries

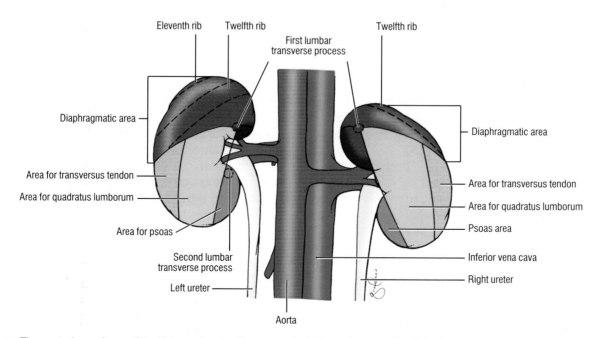

**FIG. 23-10.** The posterior surfaces of the kidney, showing the areas of relation to the posterior abdominal wall.

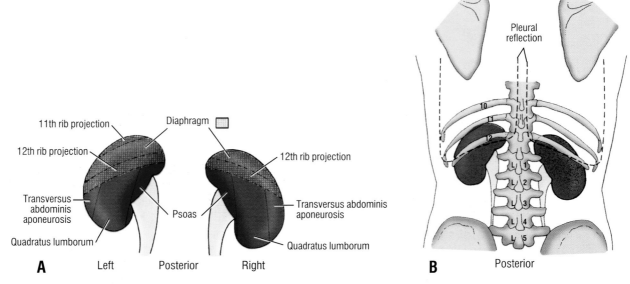

FIG. 23-11. Anatomic relations of the kidneys. **A.** Posterior relations to the muscles of the posterior body wall and ribs. **B.** Relations to the pleural reflections and skeleton posteriorly. (Modified from Kabalin JN. Surgical anatomy of the retroperitoneum, kidneys, and ureters. In: Walsh PC, Retik AB, Vaughan ED Jr, Wein AJ (eds). Campbell's Urology (7th ed). Philadelphia: WB Saunders, 1998; with permission.)

and nerves enter through the renal hilum, while the veins, lymphatics, and proximal ureter exit through it. For all practical purposes the concavity of the hilum is continuous with a deep declivity in the medial border of the kidney, the so-called renal sinus. This recess is lined by the tissues of the renal capsule and envelops the renal vessels and the renal pelvis, according to Narath.[20]

Within the renal sinus is the renal pelvis, a funnel-shaped sac formed by the widely expanded portion of the proximal ureter and by the junctions of the major calices. It is entirely arbitrary whether to consider the pelvis part of the kidney (e.g., 'renal pelvis') or part of the ureter (e.g., 'ureteric pelvis'). Current usage in which 'renal pelvis' is the norm is not untidy, and has universal acceptance. Using the philosophy that would call it the 'ureteric pelvis,' why not call infundibuli 'ureteric infundibuli' and calices 'ureteric calices'?

The term 'intrarenal pelvis' denotes a pelvis that is almost covered or completely covered by renal parenchyma. This term is in general use among reconstructive renal surgeons. Such terminology is helpful in describing that entity in which technical difficulty in exposure of the obstructed 'renal pelvis' may occur at the time of pyeloplasty.

The renal pelvis bifurcates or trifurcates within the sinus producing two or three major calices. Each of the major calices again subdivides into 7 to 14 minor calices which receive the collecting tubules (approximately 500). Fine and Keen[21] reported that occasionally no formation of major calices takes place.

The renal pelvis most commonly lies posterior to the renal vessels. Occasionally it may be situated between or in front of the vessels. In some instances the renal pelvis is small, lacks an extrarenal portion, and is located entirely within the renal parenchyma.

The upper pole of each kidney is related to its associated adrenal gland, separated from it only by a thin diaphragm of connective tissue originating from the fascia of Gerota, which totally envelops each adrenal (Fig 23-12). The right and left adrenal glands are located superomedially at the front of the upper part of each kidney.

Davie[22] reported that in 6 out of 1500 necropsies the adrenals were fixed with the upper pole of the kidney in such a way that a nephrectomy would necessarily include the adrenal glands. This knowledge is critical for a surgeon undertaking laparoscopic adrenalectomy. The laparoscopic operation can be undertaken safely, though, according to the report of Prinz[23] comparing laparoscopic adrenalectomy with open adrenalectomy. The lower pole is occasionally located close to the lumbar triangle.

REMEMBER:
- The pleura and the diaphragm separate the kidney from the 12th rib (see Fig. 23-9).
- The inner half of the 12th rib is related to the pleura.
- The pleura (for all practical purposes) has a horizontal pathway related to the length of the 12th rib (Fig. 23-13).
- The anterior surface of the right kidney (which is related

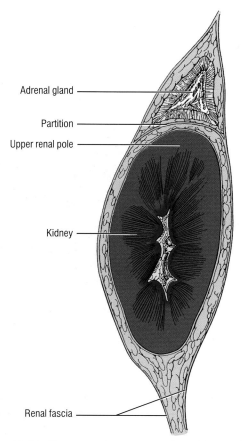

FIG. 23-12. Highly diagrammatic representation of the renal fascia. The partition, a type of diaphragm, separates the adrenal from the upper renal pole.

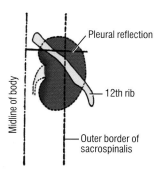

FIG. 23-13. Showing certain important posterior relationships of the kidney. (Modified from Decker GAG, Du Plessis DJ. Lee McGregor's Synopsis of Surgical Anatomy (12th ed). Bristol UK: Wright, 1986; with permission.)

to the liver and loops of small bowel) is the only area of the organ covered by peritoneum. The anterior surface of the left kidney (which is related to the stomach, spleen and loops of small bowel) is also covered by peritoneum.

- The upper part of the upper pole of the right kidney is associated with the peritoneum which forms the hepatorenal pouch of Morison. This is bounded as follows (Fig. 23-14):
  – Above, by the posterior layer of the coronary ligament
  – Anteriorly, by the inferior surface of the liver
  – Posteriorly, by the peritoneum lining the inferior surface of the diaphragm
- Occasionally, the upper pole of the kidney close to the vertebrocostal angle is separated from the pleura only by a layer of connective tissue (which may be thin or thick).
- The anterior pararenal space contains comparatively less fat than the posterior pararenal space, where the adipose tissue stroma is rich.
- According to some authors the renal fascia does not invest each kidney completely, since at the region of the lower

pole the anterior and posterior laminae of the fascia do not fuse (see Fig. 23-12); others believe the opposite.
- We quote the cadaveric studies of Wolfram-Gabel et al.[24] on closure of the renal space:

> On each side, the kidney and the suprarenal gland are disposed in a space that is closed on all sides. The anterior and posterior layers of the renal fascia fuse at the upper pole of the space to become continuous with the inferior fascia of the diaphragm. Likewise, they merge at the lower pole and at the lateral border of the space to become continuous with the fasciae of the parietal muscles. At the medial border of the space, the two layers merge to continue medially with the peri-aortocaval connective tissue; they penetrate the hilum and beneath it enclose the ureter.

## Position of the Kidneys

Factors which are responsible for the position of the kidney include:
- Renal fascia (upper part)
- Peri- and paranephric fat
- Intraperitoneal viscera

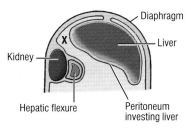

FIG. 23-14. The hepatorenal or Morison's pouch (X). (Modified from Decker GAG, Du Plessis DJ. Lee McGregor's Synopsis of Surgical Anatomy (12th ed). Bristol UK: Wright, 1986; with permission.)

• Intraabdominal pressure

Nephroptosis (mobile or floating kidney) is acquired; it should not be confused with the ectopic kidney. Renal ectopia is a congenital phenomenon related to placement, form, and orientation of the kidney.

The pathway of nephroptosis is downward. We believe this is due to lack of adequate fusion of the anterior and posterior laminae of the renal fascia in the vicinity of the lower pole of the kidney.

The right kidney is more mobile than the left. The ideal treatment of nephroptosis is nephropexy, either by nephrorrhaphy or one of several other methods.

We are happy to present verbatim an excellent letter which was published in the *Western Journal of Medicine*.[25] We agree with the conclusions of the author, Jane M. Hightower, M.D., and we are grateful to her and to the journal for permission to reprint it.

### Dietl's Crisis Revisited — The Enigma of Nephroptosis

*To The Editor: I would like to report a new twist on an old condition. I am a 32-year-old female physician who is athletic and thin. In January 1993 I began having intermittent abdominal pain that radiated to my back and groin. This was accompanied by a protruding mass on my right side adjacent to the lateral rectus muscle. I went to a surgeon who diagnosed a spigelian hernia. This quarter-sized defect was repaired without difficulty using mesh. After the procedure, I still had a painful mass protruding into the area of repair that was mobile in a vertical plane of about 12 cm. I then went back for a laparoscopic evaluation, but no abnormal masses were seen. After an ultrasonogram, computed tomographic (CT) scan, and intravenous pyelogram, we realized that my kidney was the culprit. The inferior pole was pushing against my abdomen where it had previously herniated. It was highly mobile and at times rotated by 90 degrees on its axis. The CT scan revealed hydronephrosis of my right ureter when lying prone. In an effort to avoid another operation and to get some relief from the pain, I learned how to manipulate the kidney by pushing it up and posteriorly, trying to hold it under my ribs. Between seeing patients, I would lie supine on the floor. When I stood up, my blood pressure would go from 90/60 to 150/90 mm of mercury. Eventually, I had the aberration fixed and have not had problems since.*

*The results of a literature search left me disillusioned; this condition, once known as Dietl's crisis and which mostly affects women, had been greatly misunderstood.[26] Some surgeons operated on asymptomatic ptotic kidneys in women who actually had other causes of pain.[27] The surgical techniques used in the past were*

*also known to cause complications[27,28] which led to the idea that repair was futile. McWhinnie and Hamilton took this idea further by concluding that "The predominance of female patients might suggest that this syndrome was the early equivalent of later forms of nonorganic pain," and that "like other ineffective treatments for imaginary disease, surgery for the movable kidney simply faded away."[29] As a result of earlier misfortunes of diagnosis and treatment, this anatomic variant, which occurs in 20% of women and 2% to 7% of men,[28,30] is not mentioned in our current texts.*

*Abnormal renal mobility should be investigated and treated when secondary complications or severe symptoms occur.[27,28,30,31] Information about this condition should be placed back into our kidney and urologic texts to help us diagnose and treat this common anatomic variant, which can cause real, not imaginary, symptoms.*

## Vascular Supply of the Kidneys

### Arterial Supply

The anatomic nomenclature describing renal arteries other than the main ones – the left and right renal arteries – is confusing and controversial. In fact, sometimes the term "main" is used for clarification. More details regarding this problem will follow.

The paired (right and left) renal arteries originate from the lateral wall of the aorta just below the origin of the superior mesenteric artery at the level of the intervertebral disc between the L1 and L2 vertebrae. However, the origin of the longer right renal artery (Fig. 23-15) is more posterior in comparison to the left. Rarely, the right renal artery originates from the posterior wall and travels posterior to the inferior vena cava to reach the right kidney. Remember that arising from each renal artery prior to its trifurcation are two small arteries that must not be molested: the inferior suprarenal artery and the artery for the renal pelvis and proximal ureter.

Studying 30 adult abdominal aorta specimens dissected from cadavers, Ozan et al.[32] reported the origin of the renal arteries from the aorta. The ostium of the right renal artery was more cranial than the ostium of the left renal artery (53.3%). However, the ostia of both right and left renal arteries were at the same level in three cases (10%). Locations of the ostia of the renal arteries were usually on the lateral and anterolateral regions of the aortic wall.

Each artery reaching the hilum divides into anterior and posterior divisions in relation to the renal pelvis (Fig. 23-16). Furthermore, the five branches of each renal artery partici-

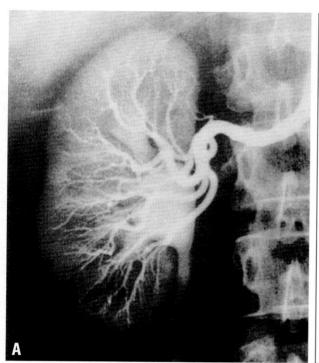 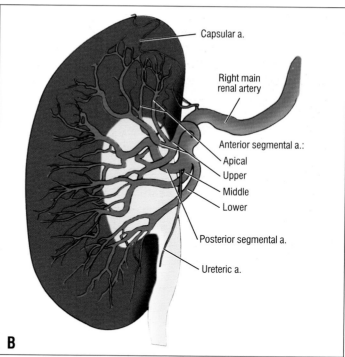

FIG. 23-15. Segmental branches of the right renal artery demonstrated by renal angiogram **(A)** and corresponding diagram **(B)**. (Modified from Kabalin JN. Surgical anatomy of the retroperitoneum, kidneys, and ureters. In: Walsh PC, Retik AB, Vaughan ED Jr, Wein AJ (eds). Campbell's Urology (7th ed). Philadelphia: WB Saunders, 1998; with permission.)

pate in the formation of four renal segments: (1) apical (superior), (2) anterior (subdivided into superior and inferior), (3) posterior, and (4) basilar (inferior) (Figs. 23-17, 23-18).

The arteries of each segment, which are end arteries without any collateral circulation, are as follows:
• Apical branch
• Basilar branch
• Artery for the superior portion of the anterior segment
• Artery for the inferior portion of the anterior segment
• Artery for the posterior segment

Different authors give different names to the segments, as is obvious when comparing Fig. 23-19 with Fig. 23-16. Also, different authors refer to the segmental arteries by different names, such as "suprahilar" instead of "apical." Graves stated that aberrant renal arteries are normal segmental arteries and not accessory arteries.[33,34]

The anterior division has branches that supply the apical, basilar, superior, and inferior portions of the anterior segment. The posterior division supplies the posterior segment of the kidney.

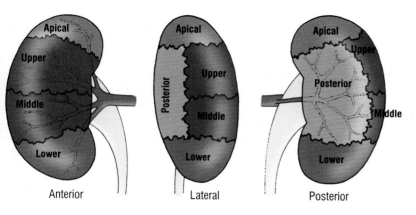

FIG. 23-16. Typical segmental circulation of the right kidney, shown diagrammatically. Note that the posterior segmental artery is usually the first branch of the main renal artery, and extends behind the renal pelvis. (Modified from Kabalin JN. Surgical anatomy of the retroperitoneum, kidneys, and ureters. In: Walsh PC, Retik AB, Vaughan ED Jr, Wein AJ (eds). Campbell's Urology (7th ed). Philadelphia: WB Saunders, 1998; with permission.)

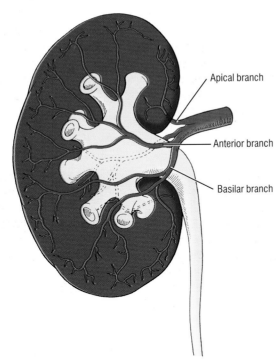

**Right Kidney – Anterior Surface**

FIG. 23-17. The intrarenal course and relation to the anterior calices of the apical, basilar, and anterior segmental arteries. Note the short length of the apical branch. The posterior branch is shown by a broken line.

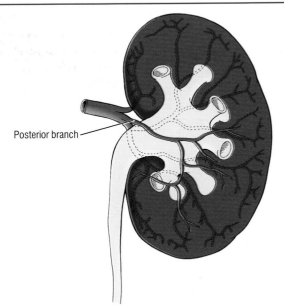

**Right Kidney – Posterior Surface**

FIG. 23-18. The branch of the renal artery supplying the posterior segment of the kidney passes along the posterior surface of the renal pelvis and then divides into smaller branches that course between the posterior calices. The apical, basilar, and anterior branches are shown by broken lines.

REMEMBER:
- The very short apical artery supplies the anterior and posterior surfaces of the apical segment.
- The basilar artery provides blood for the anterior and posterior surfaces of the basilar segment.
- The anterior segment is supplied by two branches: one for its superior part and another for its inferior part.
- The blood supply of the posterior segment is provided by a single artery.
- The renal arteries are end arteries without collateral circulation.

The "avascular" line or plane (also known as Brödel's line) (Figs. 23-20, 23-21) is the most avascular area of the kidney. It is located slightly behind the convex border at the posterior half of the kidney at the junction of the area supplied by the anterior and posterior divisions of the renal artery. This is approximately 2/3 of the way along a line from the hilum to the lateral margin of the kidney. Incision in this area will permit removal of a stone within the renal calices with minimal damage.

According to Banowsky,[35] unilateral multiple renal arteries occur in approximately 23 percent of the population. Another 10 percent have bilateral multiple arteries. Multiple renal arteries are more common on the left side.

Banowsky[35] differentiates between multiple and accessory renal arteries. He states that multiple renal arteries supply one renal segment and accessory arteries supply only part of the segment. He emphasizes that it is advisable to ligate only the accessory arteries.

Singh et al.[36] stated that accessory renal arteries are

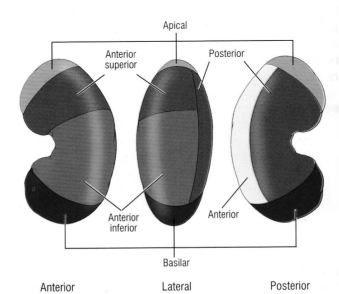

FIG. 23-19. The vascular segments of the left kidney, as shown in the anterior, lateral, and posterior projections.

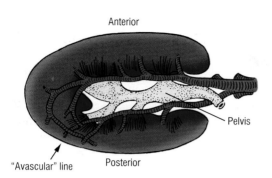

FIG. 23-20. Schema of the anterior and posterior branches of the renal artery, in a horizontal section of the kidney. The "avascular" line is the region of overlap between the anterior and posterior branches, situated posterolaterally rather than laterally because of the wider distribution of the anterior branches. (Modified from Hollinshead WH. Anatomy for Surgeons. New York: Hoeber, 1956; with permission.)

more common on the left side, occurring in as many as 30-35% of cases and usually entering the upper or lower pole of the kidney (Fig. 23-22). Such an accessory artery of the lower pole may produce ureteric obstruction with secondary hydronephrosis.

A study by Satyapal et al.[37] refers to "additional" renal arteries and offers this definition:

> *An additional renal artery, other than the main renal artery, is one which arises from the aorta and terminates in the kidney.*

They add that "additional renal arteries" have been described as "accessory," "aberrant," "anomalous," "supernumerary," "supplementary," "multiple," "accessory aortic hilar," "aortic superior polar," "aortic inferior polar," "upper polar," and "lower polar." They comment on the need for standardization of the nomenclature to facilitate accurate reporting of the incidence of the entities they choose to refer to as "additional."

The above-mentioned study by Satyapal et al.[37] presented these findings:

> *Single additional renal arteries were more common on the left side (27.6%) than the right side (18.6%). Second additional renal arteries occurred with similar incidences on either side (right, 4.7%; left, 4.4%). The lengths (cm) and diameters (cm) of first and second additional renal arteries were 4.5, 0.4 and 3.8, 0.3 (right) and 4.9, 0.3, and 3.7, 0.3 (left), respectively.*

Ligation of an accessory renal artery can result in the production of an area of infarction of variable size, though often small. Renovascular hypertension may occur as a sequela of the ischemia.

Every surgeon performing renal surgery should be fa-

miliar with the segmental anatomy of the kidney. Such knowledge can save lives. A case in point can be provided by one of the authors of this chapter (JES). A patient with bilateral renal malignancy required radical nephrectomy on the left side. Twelve years after surgery the patient was still alive and well, with only two segments of the right kidney remaining in situ.

## Venous Drainage

The kidney is drained by several veins which together form the renal vein (Fig. 23-23). The left renal vein is longer than the right. It receives blood from the left adrenal, the left gonad, and the body wall, including the diaphragm. The left adrenal vein enters the renal vein superiorly; the left gonadal vein enters inferiorly. Usually one or two lumbar veins empty into the posterior wall of the left renal vein.

Temporary or permanent occlusion of the left renal vein close to its entrance into the inferior vena cava can usually be done with impunity. Unlike the left renal vein, the short right renal vein contains a thin valve which is not good material for suture. Therefore, in addition to excising the right renal vein, the surgeon should excise a small cuff of the medial wall of the inferior vena cava where the right renal vein enters. Multiple renal veins are not common and left renal vein duplication is rare.

Aluisio et al.[38] studied the normal and anomalous anatomy of the left renal vein and its tributaries in 20 cadavers. They reported the following:
- Other than the left suprarenal (adrenal) and left gonadal veins, the left renal vein had no additional tributaries
- Study of the left suprarenal and left gonadal veins revealed no direct connections to the inferior vena cava
- Anomalies of the left renal venous drainage system:

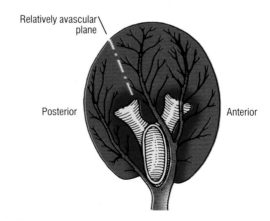

FIG. 23-21. Avascular plane of kidney. (Modified from Decker GAG, Du Plessis DJ. Lee McGregor's Synopsis of Surgical Anatomy (12th ed). Bristol UK: Wright, 1986; with permission.)

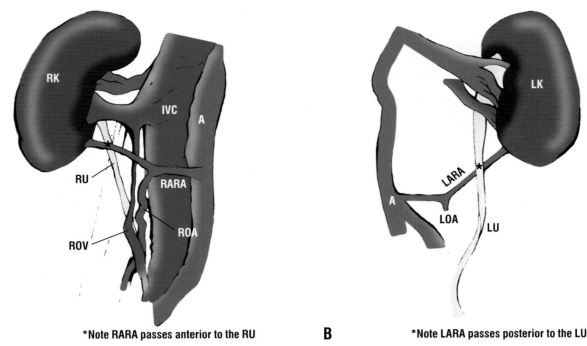

**A**      *Note RARA passes anterior to the RU      **B**      *Note LARA passes posterior to the LU

FIG. 23-22. Schematic drawings of accessory renal arteries. **A.** Right kidney. **B.** Left kidney. RK, right kidney; LK, left kidney; RU, right ureter; LU, left ureter; ROA, right ovarian artery; LOA, proximal part of the left ovarian artery; ROV, right ovarian vein; A, aorta; IVC, inferior vena cava; RARA, right accessory renal artery; LARA, left accessory renal artery. (Modified from Singh G, Ng YK, Bay BH. Bilateral accessory renal arteries associated with some anomalies of the ovarian arteries:a case study. Clin Anat 1998;11:417-420; with permission.)

– Anomaly of the left renal vein itself manifested as a supernumerary left renal vein
– Bifurcation of the gonadal vein
– Bifurcation of the suprarenal vein
– Inferior phrenic vein draining into the left renal vein distal to the superior mesenteric artery
– Lumbar vein drainage into the left renal vein that may represent either an anomaly or a normal variation

Aluisio et al.[38] found no evidence of a systemic collateral flow system for drainage of the left kidney following left renal vein division.

Satyapal et al.[39] presented the following left renal vein variations (*Note*: A renal collar is the renal venous channel coursing both anteriorly and posteriorly to the abdominal aorta) (Fig. 23-24, Fig. 23-25, Fig. 23-26, Fig. 23-27):

- Renal collars: 0.3%
- Retroaortic vein: 0.5%
- Additional veins: 0.4%
- Posterior primary tributary: 23.2% (16.7%, Type IB; 6.5%, Type IIB)

A retroaortic left renal vein connected directly to the azygos system and the third lumbar vein was reported by Yoshinaga et al.[40] The anomaly coursed dorsal to the abdominal aorta and opened into the IVC at the upper level of the third lumbar vertebra. It also received the posterior

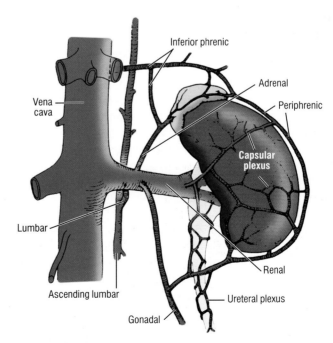

FIG. 23-23. Venous drainage of the left kidney, showing potentially extensive venous collateral circulation. (Modified from Kabalin JN. Surgical anatomy of the retroperitoneum, kidneys, and ureters. In: Walsh PC, Retik AB, Vaughan ED Jr, Wein AJ (eds). Campbell's Urology (7th ed). Philadelphia: WB Saunders, 1998; with permission.)

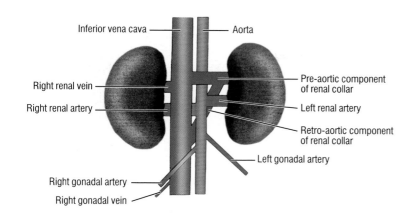

FIG. 23-24. Schematic drawing of renal collar. (Modified from Satyapal KS, Kalideen JM, Haffejee AA, Singh B, Robbs JV. Left renal vein variations. Surg Radiol Anat 1999;21:77-81; with permission.)

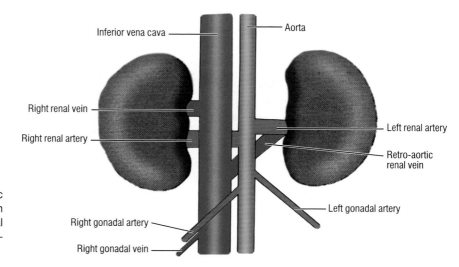

FIG. 23-25. Schematic drawing of retroaortic vein. (Modified from Satyapal KS, Kalideen JM, Haffejee AA, Singh B, Robbs JV. Left renal vein variations. Surg Radiol Anat 1999;21:77-81; with permission.)

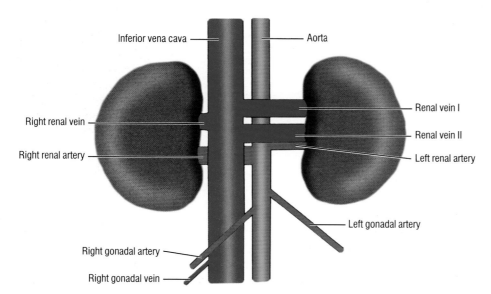

FIG. 23-26. Schematic drawing of additional renal vein. (Modified from Satyapal KS, Kalideen JM, Haffejee AA, Singh B, Robbs JV. Left renal vein variations. Surg Radiol Anat 1999; 21: 77-81; with permission.)

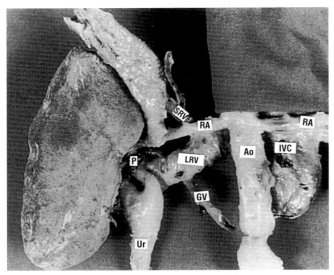

FIG. 23-27. Posterior view of plastinated left kidney demonstrating Type IB renal venous drainage. LRV, left renal vein; IVC, inferior vena cava; GV, gonadal vein; SRV, suprarenal vein; P, posterior primary tributary; Ao, aorta; RA, renal artery; Ur, ureter. (Modified from Satyapal KS, Kalideen JM, Haffejee AA, Singh B, Robbs JV. Left renal vein variations. Surg Radiol Anat 1999;21:77-81; with permission.)

REMEMBER:
- The renal veins intercommunicate with each other.
- Temporary occlusion or permanent ligation of the left renal vein can be done with impunity if this procedure is done close to the inferior vena cava.

## Lymphatics

The renal lymphatic network is very rich. The renal lymphatics follow the blood vessels and form large lymphatic trunks. The trunks exit through the renal sinus where they receive communicating lymphatics from the renal capsule and perinephric fat. Lymphatics from the renal pelvis and upper ureter communicate with others at the renal hilum. Two or three lymph nodes close to the renal vein accept the lymph and then drain to the para-aortic lymph nodes.

The lymphatics of the right kidney (Fig. 23-29) drain into lymph nodes located between the inferior vena cava and the aorta, lateral paracaval nodes, and anterior and posterior inferior vena caval lymph nodes. They also drain upward toward the right diaphragm, and downward to the common iliac lymph nodes. Other pathways are into the thoracic duct or crossing the midline into the left lateral aortic lymph nodes.

The lymphatics of the left kidney (Fig. 23-30) drain into the lateral paraaortic lymph nodes and anterior and posterior aortic lymph nodes. They also travel upward to the di-

suprarenal and posterior inferior phrenic veins.

The renal vasculature may be appreciated by Figure 23-28.

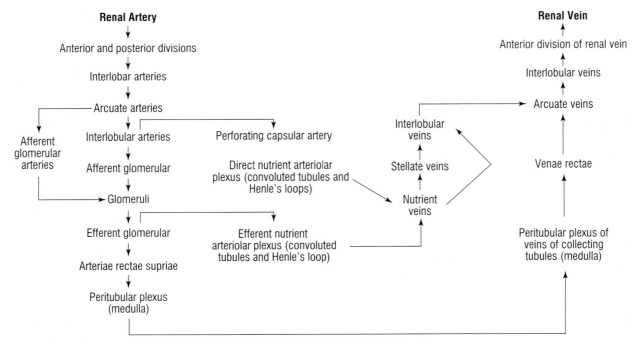

FIG. 23-28. The renal vasculature. (From Hinman F Jr. Atlas of Urosurgical Anatomy. Philadelphia: WB Saunders, 1993; with permission.)

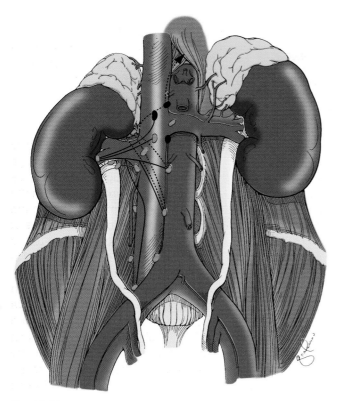

FIG. 23-29. Regional lymphatic drainage of the right kidney. Green nodes, anterior; black nodes, posterior. Solid lines, anterior lymphatic channels; dashed lines, posterior lymphatic channels. Arrow leads to thoracic duct.

aphragm and downward to lymph nodes associated with the inferior mesenteric artery. According to Kabalin,[41] malignancy of the left kidney does not metastasize to the nodes between the inferior vena cava and aorta except in advanced disease.

## Innervation

The kidneys characteristically exhibit a very rich network of neural elements that originate at the celiac ganglion, aorticorenal ganglion, celiac plexus, and intermesenteric plexuses. These elements intermingle, form plexuses, and follow the renal artery.

Thoracic nerves T10 to L1 participate in the innervation of the kidney. They receive pain fibers from the renal pelvis and proximal ureter that enter the spinal cord at those levels of the spinal nerves. The renal nerves have a vasomotor function.

The right and left vagus nerves participate in the formation of the renal plexus. The renal plexus gives branches to the ureteric and gonadal plexuses.

REMEMBER
- Avoid injury to the 11th and 12th intercostal nerves, not only to avoid postoperative paresthesias and neuralgias, but also to avoid postoperative bulging from partial paralysis of the muscles involved.[42]
- Close the incision anatomically. Be sure not to entrap the lower intercostal nerves.
- Avoid the phrenic nerve during opening of the diaphragm.
- Partial anesthesia will develop in the gluteal area (about 20 × 10 cm) with transection of the T12 nerve.

## HISTOLOGY AND PHYSIOLOGY

A detailed presentation of the histology and physiology of the kidney is beyond the scope of this chapter. We hope that the interested reader will augment this basic presentation through study of standard texts on renal histology and physiology.

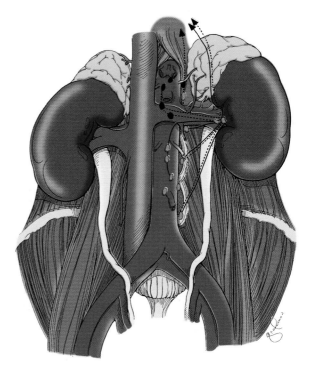

FIG. 23-30. Regional lymphatic drainage of the left kidney. Green nodes, anterior; black nodes, posterior. Solid lines, anterior lymphatic channels; dashed lines, posterior lymphatic channels. Arrows lead to thoracic duct.

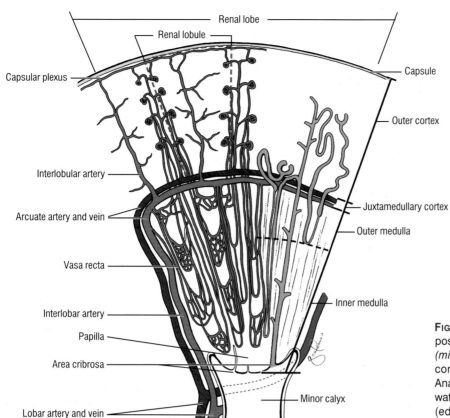

FIG. 23-31. The major blood vessels *(left)*, the position of cortical and juxtamedullary nephrons *(middle),* and the major structures in the renal cortex and medulla *(right).* (After Redman JF. Anatomy of the genitourinary system. In: Gillenwater JY, Grayhack JT, Howards SS, Duckett JW (eds). Adult and Pediatric Urology, 2nd ed. St. Louis: Mosby Year Book, 1991, Fig. 1-40.)

## Renal Structure

The renal parenchyma is formed by the cortex and the medulla (Figs. 23-31, 23-32).

The renal cortex consists of:
- Renal (malpighian) corpuscles, each one consisting of a glomerulus and its capsule
- Convoluted tubules
- Loop of Henle partially connecting the convoluted tubules

The renal medulla consists of:
- Collecting and partially secretory tubules
- Part of the loop of Henle
- Renal pyramids. Their apices (the renal papillae) are cupped with minor calices.

The renal cortex covers the pyramids peripherally. It also extends between the pyramids to the renal sinus.[43] The renal vessels enter and exit in these areas of cortex between the pyramids. For all practical purposes, the medulla consists of the renal pyramids.

The renal capsule consists of connective tissue. In the absence of underlying pathologic processes, it may be stripped with ease.

A renal lobe is formed by a pyramid covered by overlying renal capsule. The number of lobes is variable. Each renal lobe is subdivided into lobules. Each lobule has a central medullary ray and a surrounding stroma of cortical tissue.

## Nephron and Pathway of Urine

It is not within the scope of this chapter to discuss the embryologic, anatomic, and histologic entities of nephrons (about which many authors agree to disagree).

Listed below are the parts of the nephron, as well as the path of urine flow:
- Renal corpuscle (glomerulus, Bowman's glomerular capsule)
- Proximal convoluted tubule
- Proximal straight tubule
- Loop of Henle

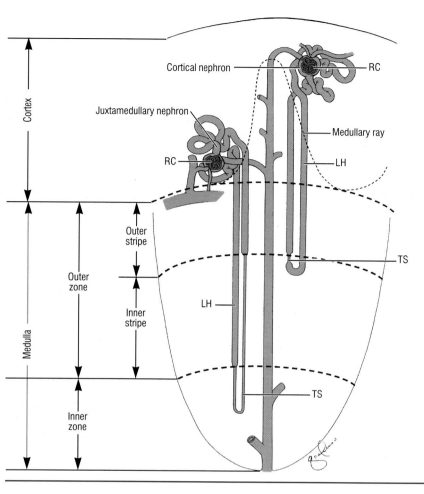

FIG. 23-32. The nephron with short loop of Henle (LH) and thin segment (TS). RC, renal corpuscle. (After Redman JF. Anatomy of the genitourinary system. In: Gillenwater JY, Grayhack JT, Howards SS, Duckett JW (eds). Adult and Pediatric Urology, 2nd ed. St. Louis: Mosby Year Book, 1991, Fig. 1-41.)

- Distal convoluted tubule
- Collecting tubules

Table 23-3 gives the subdivisions of the nephron and collecting duct system.

Each kidney contains approximately 1 million nephrons. Each nephron is formed by the glomerulus or renal corpuscle (glomerulus and glomerular capsule) and the uriniferous tubule.

The glomerulus is a rich vascular network enveloped by an epithelial sac (Bowman's capsule). The physiologic destiny of the glomerulus is to form plasma ultrafiltrate and transmit the plasma to the Bowman's capsule, which in turn transmits it to the uriniferous tubule and then to the pelvicaliceal system as urine.[44]

Modification of urine takes place within the uriniferous tubule. According to Venkatachalam and Kriz,[44] the uriniferous tubule is "made up of many anatomically and cytologically distinct segments," each performing a different function.

## SURGERY OF THE KIDNEY

Renal surgery includes:
- Nephrotomy
- Nephrostomy
- Segmental resection (partial nephrectomy)
- Pediatric partial nephrectomy
- Simple nephrectomy
- Radical nephrectomy (right, left)
- Calicorrhaphy
- Calicoplasty
- Surgery for trauma
- Renal transplantation

Only the six procedures that are performed most frequently will be presented here.

Surgeons should use the correct incisions for the procedures they will perform; they should be familiar with all approaches, including transperitoneal and retroperitoneal

**TABLE 23-3. Subdivisions of the Nephron and Collecting Duct System**

I. Nephron
   A. Renal corpuscle
      1. Glomerulus (the most frequently used term to refer to the entire renal corpuscle)
      2. Bowman's capsule
   B. Tubule
      1. Proximal tubule
         a. Convoluted part
         b. Straight part (pars recta) or descending thick limb of Henle's loop
      2. Intermediate tubule
         a. Descending part or thin descending limb of Henle's loop
         b. Ascending part or thin ascending limb of Henle's loop
      3. Distal tubule
         a. Straight part or thick ascending limb of Henle's loop, subdivided into a medullary and a cortical part; the latter contains in its terminal portion the macula densa
         b. Convoluted part
II. Collecting duct system
   A. Connecting tubule (including the arcades in most species)
   B. Collecting duct
      1. Cortical collecting duct
      2. Outer medullary collecting duct subdivided into an outer- and inner-stripe portion
      3. Inner medullary collecting duct subdivided into a basal, middle, and papillary portion

*Source:* Venkatachalam MA, Kriz W. Anatomy. In: Jennette JC, Olson JL, Schwartz MM, Silva FG. Heptinstall's Pathology of the Kidney, 5th ed. Philadelphia: Lippincott-Raven, 1998; with permission.

(Table 23-4). While surgeons will use the incision with which they are most comfortable, renal or ureteric pathology will dictate the most logical approach to help avoid anatomic complications. A poorly chosen incision can be catastrophic.

Surgeons must also be very familiar with the structures of the anterior abdominal wall (Figs. 23-33 - 23-35) and the posterior abdominal wall (Figs. 23-36 - 23-40), including the respiratory, pelvic, and urogenital diaphragms.

## Surgical Approaches to the Kidney and Ureter Through the Posterolateral Wall

There are many surgical approaches to the kidney and ureter. Of course, knowledge of anatomy of the posterior, lateral, and anterior abdominal wall is essential. Here we re-emphasize careful study of the anatomy of the postero-lateral body wall.

For purposes of description, the muscles of the posterolateral wall can be divided into four layers: outer, middle, inner, and innermost.

The outer layer (Fig. 23-41A & B) consists of:
- Latissimus dorsi muscle
- External oblique muscle (posterior part)
- Serratus posterior inferior muscle
- External intercostal muscles
- Posterior lamina of thoracolumbar fascia

The middle layer (Fig. 23-42) contains
- Sacrospinalis muscle
- Internal oblique muscle
- Internal intercostal muscles
- Middle lamina of thoracolumbar fascia

The composition of the inner layer (Figs. 23-43, 23-44) includes:
- Quadratus lumborum muscle
- Psoas major and minor muscles
- Innermost intercostal muscles
- Transversus abdominis muscle (partial)

The innermost layer (Figs. 23-45, 23-46, 23-47) is made up of:
- Psoas major muscle
- Psoas minor muscle
- Diaphragm

REMEMBER
- If you decide to resect the 11th or 12th rib, use a subperiosteal incision. Push the periosteal instrument down toward the umbilicus at the upper side of the rib, and push up and posteriorly on the downside of the rib. Remember the phrase "above forward, below backward."[45]
- An anterior transperitoneal approach to the renal pedicle has excellent exposure. A posterior transperitoneal approach has limited exposure.
- Remember that the lumbar fascia has three laminae (Fig. 23-45): posterior, middle, and anterior. The posterior lamina covers the sacrospinalis muscle and is the most superficial layer. The middle lamina is between the sacrospinalis and quadratus lumborum muscles. The anterior lamina covers the sacrospinalis and quadratus lumborum muscles. These three laminae unite close to the lateral borders of the quadratus lumborum and sacrospinalis. Incision of the fascia between the latissimus dorsi and sacrospinalis muscles as well as between the internal oblique and quadratus lumborum muscles will reach the transversalis fascia and posterior lamina of Gerota's fascia.

## TABLE 23-4. Approaches to the Kidney

| Anatomic Area | Incision |
|---|---|
| Flank | Subcostal (right or left) (Fig. 1)<br>11th rib (right or left) (Fig. 2)<br>With extension to the anterior lateral (right or left) abdominal wall (Fig. 3) |
| Anterior abdominal | Subcostal, unilateral (Fig. 4)<br>Bilateral subcostal "chevron" (Fig. 5)<br>Extraperitoneal (Fig. 6)<br>11th rib transperitoneal (right or left) (Fig. 7)<br>Midline upper (Fig. 8)<br>Midline lower (Fig. 9)<br>Midline long (xiphoid/pubis) (Fig. 10)<br>Modified Gibson (right or left) (Fig. 11) |
| Combination (flank and anterior abdominal) | Thoracoabdominal (right or left) (Fig. 12) |
| Posterior | Over the 12th rib (right or left) (Fig. 13)<br>Dorsal lumbotomy (Fig. 14) |
| Laparoscopic<br>   Transperitoneal<br><br><br>   Retroperitoneal | <br>Two 12 mm trocars in the midclavicular line, one approximately 4 cm below the level of the umbilicus and the other 2 cm below the costal margin (Fig. 15). All secondary trocars placed under direct vision.<br>Three ports along the inferior border of the 12th rib: a 12 mm port just posterior to the tip of the rib (superior lumbar triangle); a 12 mm port two finger breadths posterior to the first 12 mm port; a 5 mm port two finger breadths anterior to the first 12 mm port. Also, a 12 mm port at the inferior lumbar triangle (Fig. 16) |

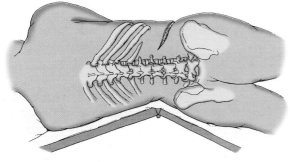

**1.** Subcostal flank incision.

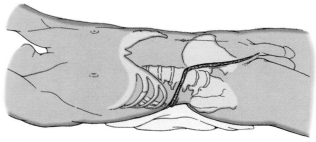

**3.** Flank incision with extension to the anterior lateral abdominal wall.

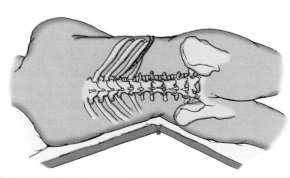

**2.** Flank incision at the 11th rib.

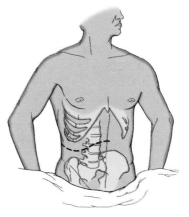

**4.** Unilateral subcostal incision of anterior abdominal area.

*(Table continues on the following page)*

**TABLE 23-4** *(cont'd)*. Approaches to the Kidney

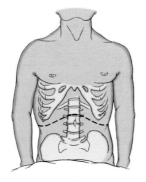

**5.** Bilateral subcostal "chevron" incision of anterior abdominal area.

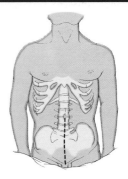

**9.** Midline lower incision of anterior abdominal area.

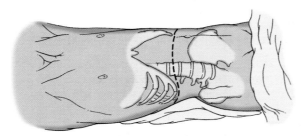

**6.** Extraperitoneal incision of anterior abdominal area.

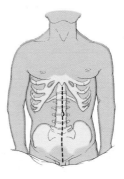

**10.** Midline long (xiphoid/pubis) incision of anterior abdominal area.

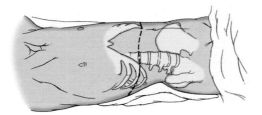

**7.** Eleventh rib transperitoneal incision of anterior abdominal area.

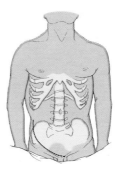

**11.** Modified Gibson incision of the anterior abdominal area.

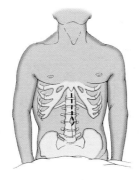

**8.** Midline upper incision of anterior abdominal area.

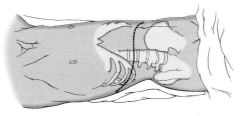

**12.** Thoracoabdominal incision of flank and anterior abdominal area.

*(Table continues on the following page)*

**TABLE 23-4 *(cont'd).* Approaches to the Kidney**

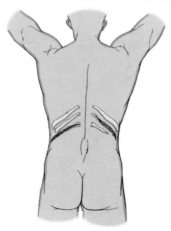

**13.** Incision over the 12th rib in posterior area.

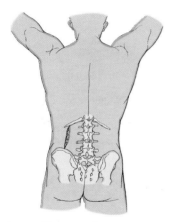

**14.** Dorsal lumbotomy of the posterior area.

*Note: Figures 1-14 in Table 23-4 are based on Montague DK. Surgical incisions. In: Novick AC, Streem SB, Pontes JE (eds). Stewart's Operative Urology, 2nd ed, Vol 1. Baltimore: Williams & Wilkins, 1989, pp. 15-40.*

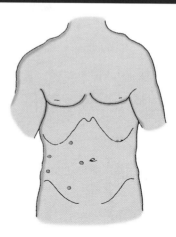

**15.** Trocar sites for laparoscopic nephrectomy. (Modified from Phillips EH, Rosenthal RJ (eds). Operative Strategies in Laparoscopic Surgery. New York: Springer, 1995; with permission.)

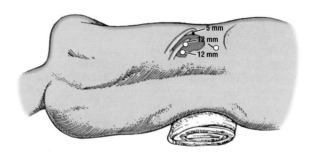

**16.** Port placement for retroperitoneal laparoscopic nephrectomy. (Modified from Pearle MS, Nakada SY. Laparoscopic nephrectomy: retroperitoneal approach. Sem Laparosc Surg 1996;3:75-83; with permission.)

- The most common tumor of the ureter (more than 90%) is the urothelial transitional cell carcinoma.[46] The treatment of choice is nephroureterectomy. However in older patients with low grade malignancy a ureteroureterostomy may be sufficient.

## Partial Nephrectomy

The following are the steps of a partial nephrectomy:
1. Use the flank approach
2. Dissect the kidney
3. Isolate the vessels
4. Place a rubber dam and ice slush around the kidney

(Lasix or Mannitol can also be used)
5. Clamp the artery first, then the vein. The kidney will become pale and soft
6. Incise the affected area. Close the collecting system and segmental vessels. Always use absorbable suture
7. Close the defect. Release the clamps
8. If the defect cannot be closed by use of the renal capsule, a peritoneal graft or omentum can be used

## Pediatric Partial Nephrectomy

Pediatric partial nephrectomy is usually performed for

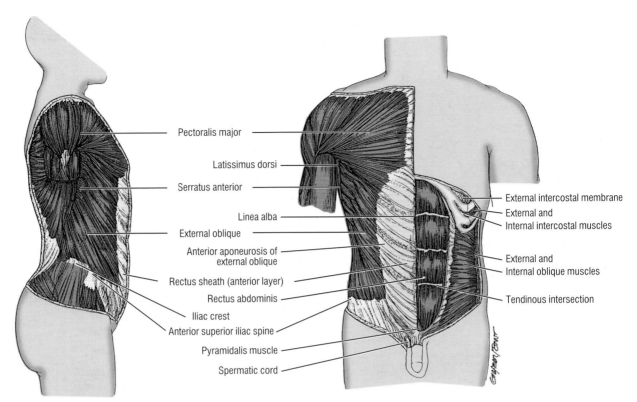

**FIG. 23-33.** Superficial musculature of the anterior abdominal and thoracic walls. (After Redman JF. Anatomy of the genitourinary system. In: Gillenwater JY, Grayhack JT, Howards SS, Duckett JW (eds). Adult and Pediatric Urology, 2nd ed. St. Louis: Mosby Year Book, 1991, Fig. 1-1.)

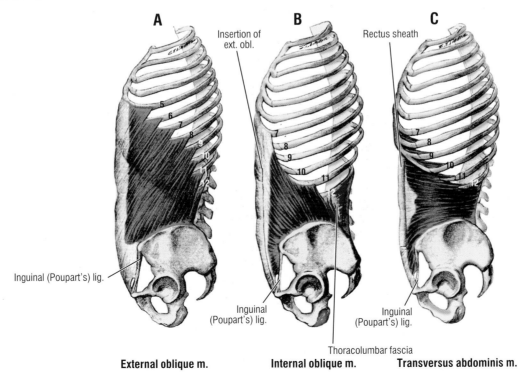

**FIG. 23-34. A.** The external oblique muscle. **B.** The internal oblique muscle. **C.** The transverse abdominis muscle. (Modified from Thorek P. Anatomy in Surgery (3rd ed). New York: Springer-Verlag, 1985; with permission.)

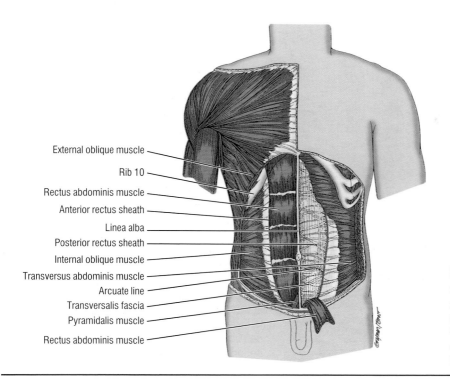

External oblique muscle

Rib 10

Rectus abdominis muscle

Anterior rectus sheath

Linea alba

Posterior rectus sheath

Internal oblique muscle

Transversus abdominis muscle

Arcuate line

Transversalis fascia

Pyramidalis muscle

Rectus abdominis muscle

**FIG. 23-35.** Relationships of internal oblique, transversus abdominis and rectus abdominis muscles. (After Redman JF. Anatomy of the genitourinary system. In: Gillenwater JY, Grayhack JT, Howards SS, Duckett JW (eds). Adult and Pediatric Urology, 2<sup>nd</sup> ed. St. Louis: Mosby Year Book, 1991, Fig. 1-3.)

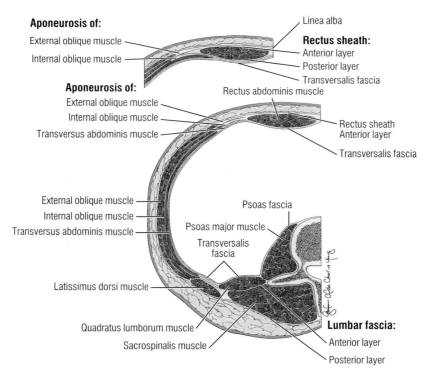

**Aponeurosis of:**

External oblique muscle

Internal oblique muscle

Linea alba

**Rectus sheath:**
Anterior layer
Posterior layer
Transversalis fascia

**Aponeurosis of:**

External oblique muscle

Internal oblique muscle

Transversus abdominis muscle

Rectus abdominis muscle

Rectus sheath
Anterior layer

Transversalis fascia

External oblique muscle

Internal oblique muscle

Transversus abdominis muscle

Psoas fascia

Psoas major muscle

Transversalis fascia

Latissimus dorsi muscle

Quadratus lumborum muscle

Sacrospinalis muscle

**Lumbar fascia:**
Anterior layer
Posterior layer

**FIG. 23-36.** Cross section in the lumbar region showing lamina of the lumbar (thoracolumbar) fascia and the musculature and fusion of the anterior abdominal wall below the arcuate line. Inset shows composition of rectus sheath above the arcuate line. (After drawing in Redman JF. Anatomy of the genitourinary system. In: Gillenwater JY, Grayhack JT, Howards SS, Duckett JW (eds). Adult and Pediatric Urology (3rd ed). St. Louis: Mosby Year Book, 1996; with permission.)

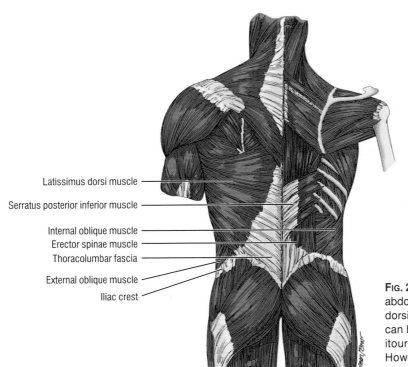

Latissimus dorsi muscle

Serratus posterior inferior muscle

Internal oblique muscle

Erector spinae muscle

Thoracolumbar fascia

External oblique muscle

Iliac crest

FIG. 23-37. *Left,* superficial musculature of the posterior abdominal wall. *Right,* with the removal of the latissimus dorsi and the external oblique, the intermediate group can be seen. (After Redman JF. Anatomy of the genitourinary system. In: Gillenwater JY, Grayhack JT, Howards SS, Duckett JW (eds). Adult and Pediatric Urology, 2nd ed. St. Louis: Mosby Year Book, 1991, Fig. 1-5.)

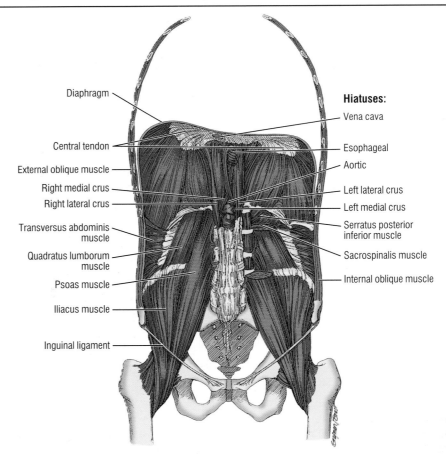

Diaphragm

Central tendon

External oblique muscle

Right medial crus

Right lateral crus

Transversus abdominis muscle

Quadratus lumborum muscle

Psoas muscle

Iliacus muscle

Inguinal ligament

**Hiatuses:**

Vena cava

Esophageal

Aortic

Left lateral crus

Left medial crus

Serratus posterior inferior muscle

Sacrospinalis muscle

Internal oblique muscle

FIG. 23-38. The diaphragm and posterior abdominal wall musculature. (After Redman JF. Anatomy of the genitourinary system. In: Gillenwater JY, Grayhack JT, Howards SS, Duckett JW (eds). Adult and Pediatric Urology, 2nd ed. St. Louis: Mosby Year Book, 1991, Fig. 1-6.)

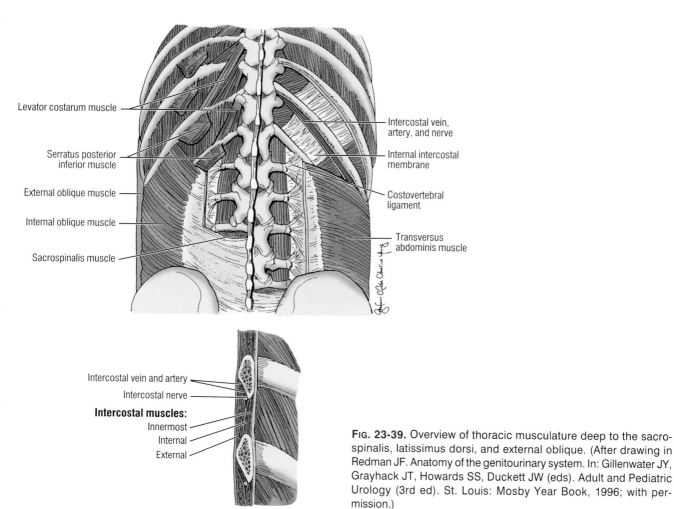

Levator costarum muscle

Serratus posterior
inferior muscle

External oblique muscle

Internal oblique muscle

Sacrospinalis muscle

Intercostal vein,
artery, and nerve

Internal intercostal
membrane

Costovertebral
ligament

Transversus
abdominis muscle

Intercostal vein and artery

Intercostal nerve

**Intercostal muscles:**
Innermost
Internal
External

**FIG. 23-39.** Overview of thoracic musculature deep to the sacrospinalis, latissimus dorsi, and external oblique. (After drawing in Redman JF. Anatomy of the genitourinary system. In: Gillenwater JY, Grayhack JT, Howards SS, Duckett JW (eds). Adult and Pediatric Urology (3rd ed). St. Louis: Mosby Year Book, 1996; with permission.)

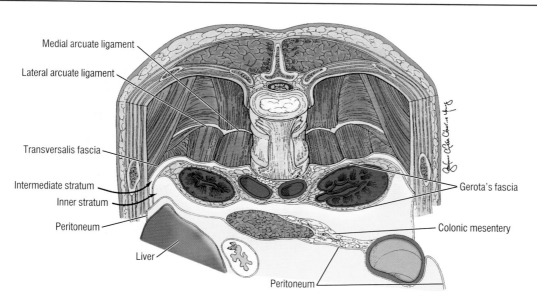

Medial arcuate ligament

Lateral arcuate ligament

Transversalis fascia

Intermediate stratum

Inner stratum

Peritoneum

Liver

Gerota's fascia

Colonic mesentery

Peritoneum

**FIG. 23-40.** Cross-sectional view of posterolateral abdominal wall and retroperitoneal connective tissue showing potential cleavage planes. After drawing in Redman JF. Anatomy of the genitourinary system. In: Gillenwater JY, Grayhack JT, Howards SS, Duckett JW (eds). Adult and Pediatric Urology (3rd ed). St. Louis: Mosby Year Book, 1996; with permission.

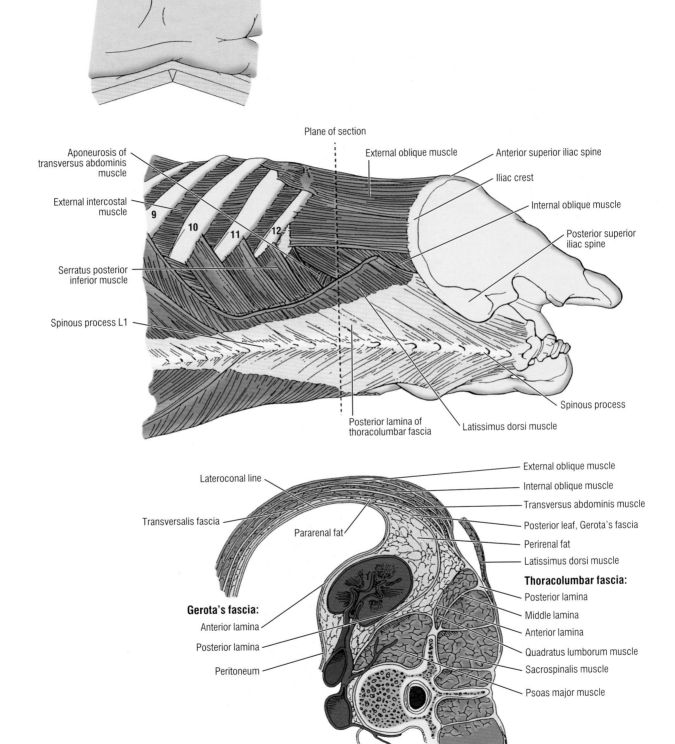

**FIG. 23-41.** Structures of the outer muscle layer. *Top:* Posterior view. Dashed line indicates the plane of section in illustration below. *Bottom:* Transverse section. (After Hinman F Jr. Atlas of Urosurgical Anatomy. Philadelphia: WB Saunders, 1993; Fig. 8.5A,B).

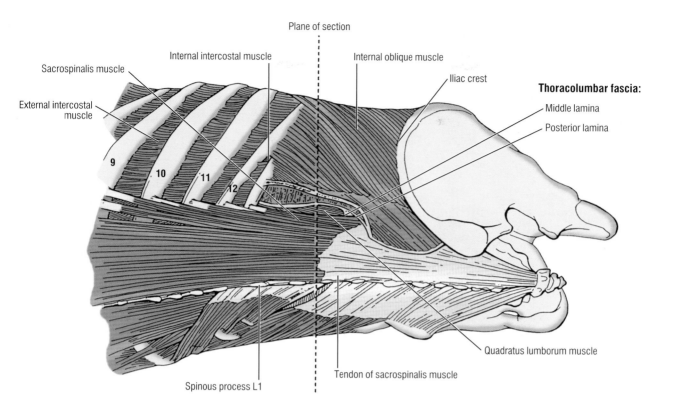

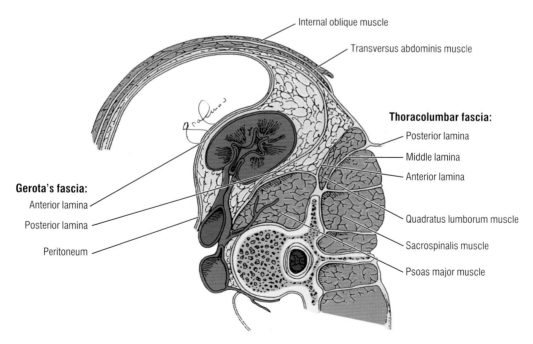

**FIG. 23-42.** Structures in the middle layer. *Top:* Posterolateral view. *Bottom:* Transverse section of the plane indicated in top illustration. (After Hinman F Jr. Atlas of Urosurgical Anatomy. Philadelphia: WB Saunders, 1993; Fig. 8.6A,B).

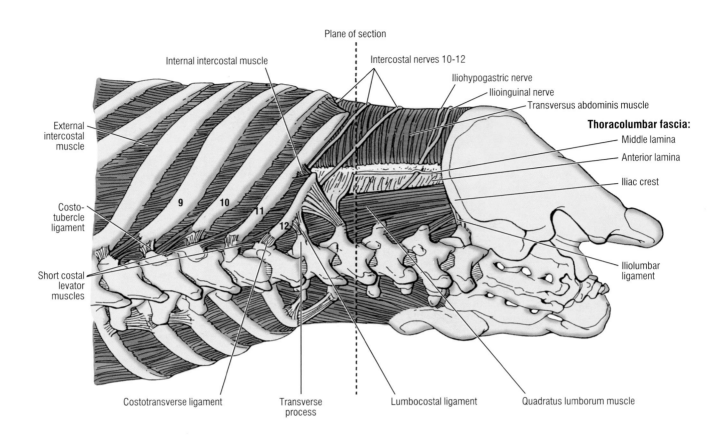

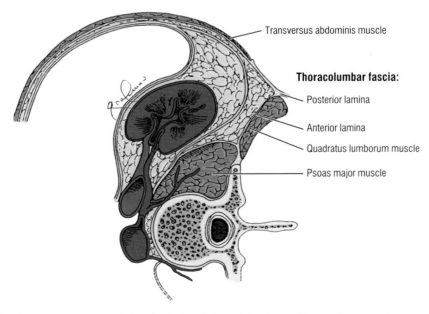

**FIG. 23-43.** Structures in the inner layer. *Top:* Sagittal cut at the level of the right kidney. *Bottom:* Cut in the transverse plane indicated in top illustration. (After Hinman F Jr. Atlas of Urosurgical Anatomy. Philadelphia: WB Saunders, 1993; Fig. 8.7A,B).

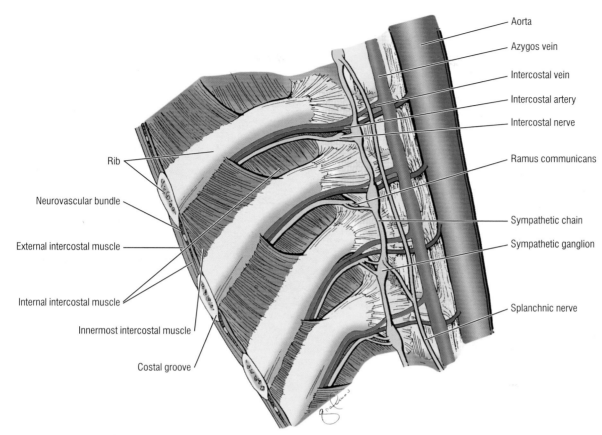

FIG. 23-44. Attachment of the intercostal muscles, viewed anteriorly. (After Hinman F Jr. Atlas of Urosurgical Anatomy. Philadelphia: WB Saunders, 1993; Fig. 8.8).

diseased upper pole renal tissue associated with ureteric duplication anomalies, such as those seen with ectopic ureter or ectopic ureterocele. While some surgeons prefer a more anterior approach to the kidney in children, others find that the classic flank approach works well in this population, and leaves a less noticeable scar.

It is rarely necessary to use cooling techniques in infants and children. Because of the distinct polar distribution of blood vessels, ligation of vessels prior to division of renal tissue limits blood loss, and clamping of major vessels is unnecessary.

The surgeon can usually find the proper plane for division of the renal parenchyma by mobilizing the upper pole ureter on its inferior aspect, directly into the renal sinus. Using blunt technique, the parenchyma is dissected away to the lower pole. Often a small amount of parenchyma, in addition to the overlying capsule, requires division.

## Simple Nephrectomy

Simple nephrectomy may be accomplished by the flank approach, subcapsular technique, or transperitoneal approach. It is indicated when there is no malignant process.

## Radical Nephrectomy

Radical nephrectomy is the procedure of choice for renal malignancy. Suspicious renal masses may present with clinical and/or radiological features which lead to difficulties in diagnosis. According to Burga et al.,[47] large renal masses are found to be malignant in approximately 85% of cases. Renal cell carcinoma is an aggressive malignant neoplasm with a usually fatal outcome, while renal oncocytoma has a characteristically benign course; both require resection.

By definition, radical nephrectomy is the removal of the kidney, adrenal, and upper (proximal) ureter by an extrafascial en bloc resection. This is carried out together with an extended lymphadenectomy from the diaphragm above to the area below the aortic bifurcation or, if necessary, down to the pelvic diaphragm.

The major renal vessels can be visualized anteriorly by separation of the peritoneum from the anterior lamina of

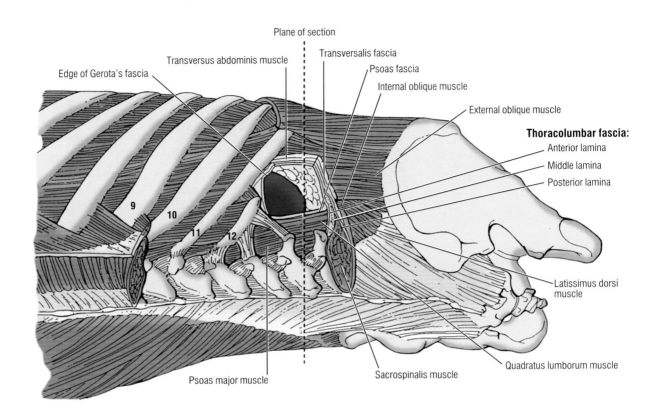

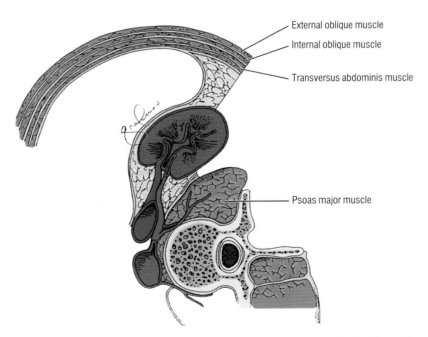

**FIG. 23-45.** Structures in the innermost layer. *Top:* Posterior view. *Bottom:* Transverse section at dashed line. (After Hinman F Jr. Atlas of Urosurgical Anatomy. Philadelphia: WB Saunders, 1993; Fig. 8.9A,B).

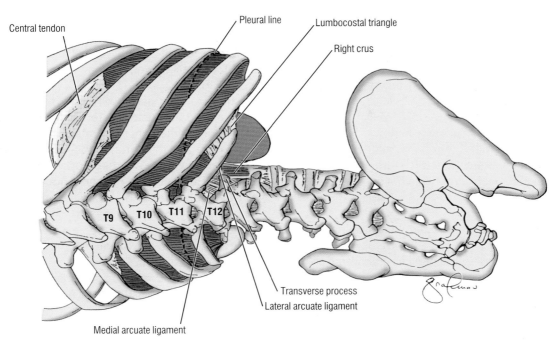

Central tendon
Pleural line
Lumbocostal triangle
Right crus
T9
T10
T11
T12
Transverse process
Lateral arcuate ligament
Medial arcuate ligament

**FIG. 23-46.** Diaphragm. (After Hinman F Jr. Atlas of Urosurgical Anatomy. Philadelphia: WB Saunders, 1993; Fig. 8.10).

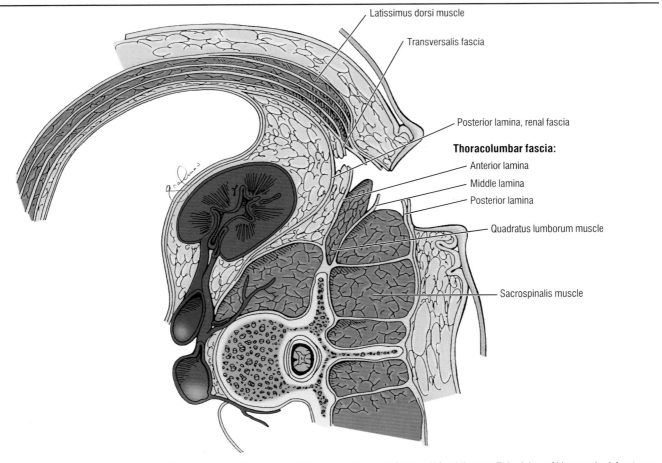

Latissimus dorsi muscle
Transversalis fascia
Posterior lamina, renal fascia
**Thoracolumbar fascia:**
Anterior lamina
Middle lamina
Posterior lamina
Quadratus lumborum muscle
Sacrospinalis muscle

**FIG. 23-47.** Posterior approach to the kidney through the lamina of the thoracolumbar fascia. (After Hinman F Jr. Atlas of Urosurgical Anatomy. Philadelphia: WB Saunders, 1993; Fig. 8.11).

Gerota's fascia and posteriorly by separation of the posterior lamina of Gerota's fascia from the transversalis fascia. In other words, the major renal vessels will be found within the anterior and posterior pararenal spaces, both of which may contain malignant cells that were spread by metastasis or direct extension of the tumor. A beautiful description of radical nephrectomy was written by Droller in 1990 in the journal *Urology*.[48]

Doublet et al.[49] reported retroperitoneal laparoscopic nephrectomy without surgical or postsurgical complications. Conversion to open surgery did not occur.

### Right Radical Nephrectomy

The following are the steps in a right radical nephrectomy:

1. Mobilization of ascending and proximal transverse colon
2. Kocherization of duodenum
3. Isolation and inspection of the inferior vena cava and right renal vein
4. Isolation of the right renal artery
5. Ligation of right renal artery to be followed by ligation of right renal vein
6. Careful exploration of the retroperitoneal space
7. Preparation and ligation of the right adrenal vein, inferior phrenic vein, and all vessels encountered
8. The lymph nodes around the inferior vena cava and between the inferior vena cava and aorta may be completely resected or biopsied.

REMEMBER: In most cases the right renal artery is located superior and posterior to the right renal vein. Be careful about a branch to the ureter and one to three branches to the suprarenal gland. The renal pelvis and upper ureter are located behind the right renal artery and vein. Remember, also, that the blood supply of the renal pelvis and the upper ureter can include contributions from the common iliac artery and the gonadal artery.

### Left Radical Nephrectomy

The following are the steps in a left radical nephrectomy:

1. Identify the renal pedicle (artery, vein, and ureter) as in right nephrectomy.
2. Protect the superior mesenteric artery. Its origin (Fig. 23-7) is just above the left renal vein, and it crosses the vein anteriorly. Posterior to the vein is the aorta.
3. Be careful with the distal pancreas, because the left renal artery has unpredictable posterior and inferior relations.

## Renal Trauma

The approach for renal trauma is as follows:

1. Make a midline incision (because of possible associated intraperitoneal injury).
2. Incise the root of the small bowel mesentery.
3. Reflect small bowel, cecum, and ascending colon cephalad.
4. If a hematoma is visible within Gerota's fascia, the surgeon should first control the renal vessels near their site of origin (or, for the right renal artery, between the inferior vena cava and the aorta). If the kidney is approached directly and Gerota's fascia is opened, the tamponade effect of Gerota's fascia will no longer be present. With a direct approach, bleeding is often profuse and nephrectomy is often the result.
5. If there is a pelvic fracture with evidence of hematoma, do not try to evacuate the hematoma prior to controlling the renal vasculature.

Severe blunt trauma may cause complete avulsion of the kidney into the chest through a ruptured diaphragm.[50]

## Renal Transplantation

An overview of organ replacement by Niklason and Langer[51] points out the significant role played by the kidneys. After the first successful dialysis of a uremic patient with a device called "the artificial kidney" was reported in 1944,[52] the kidney became the first anatomic entity to undergo successful transplantation in 1954. The first renal allograft was implanted in 1959.[53,54,55]

### *Surgical Anatomy of the Renal Donor*

The surgeon should be very familiar with not only the normal and abnormal anatomy of the renal vessels, but also the hepatic, pancreatic, and small bowel vasculature. Remember that 20 percent of kidneys have some vascular anomalies or variations. Pollak et al.[56] found a 49% rate of renovascular variants in cadaveric kidneys procured for transplantation.

Some anatomic problems of renal transplantation relate to the means available for lengthening arteries and veins and whether multiple vessels should be ligated or left alone. Occasionally, segmental aortic and inferior vena cava resection may be necessary to secure good renal vascularization.

Special attention must be given to the blood supply of the proximal ureter, which is very closely associated with the blood supply of the renal pelvis. We agree with Hinman[57] that it is absolutely necessary that the renal arteries not be dissected within the hilum and that the shortest necessary ureteric segment should be used, together with all possible perirenal and periureteric fat in this area.

A study by Sasaki et al.[58] of laparoscopic technique to perform live donor nephrectomy concluded that "[p]roper surgical training and patient selection can result in a safe donor operation that provides kidneys of excellent quality."

## *Procedure for Cadaveric Nephrectomy*

### Right Side

1. Incise at the peritoneal reflection at the right paracolic gutter
2. Elevate and reflect the right colon medially (cecum, ascending colon, hepatic flexure)
3. Kocherize the duodenum and reflect it medially
4. Carefully mobilize the inferior vena cava
5. Carefully clean the aorta
6. Locate the ureter medial to the right gonadal vessels
7. Be careful with the right gonadal vein
8. The anterior lamina of Gerota's fascia is in view. It is not well developed
9. Do not skeletonize the ureter, but preserve 2 cm of tissue surrounding the organ to protect its blood supply
10. Do not mobilize the ureteric segment from the renal pelvis to the lower renal pole
11. Divide the ureter close to the urinary bladder
12. Remove en bloc both kidneys. Include the posterior lamina of Gerota's fascia by separating it from the transversalis fascia

### Left Side

1. As on the right side, mobilize and reflect medially the left colon (distal transverse, splenic flexure, descending, and sigmoid) and mesocolon
2. Be careful of the inferior mesenteric vein
3. Be careful with the mobilization of the spleen and the pancreatic tail. Good knowledge of the splenic ligaments is essential
4. Remember that the peritoneum is adherent to the ureter
5. Expose the left crus of the diaphragm for good visualization of the aorta and its branches, such as the inferior phrenic artery (which is superior to the crus) and the first and second lumbar arteries arising from the posterior wall of the abdominal aorta
6. Preserve the periureteric tissue as on the right and divide the ureter close to the urinary bladder

## Laparoscopic Nephrectomy

Laparoscopic nephrectomy is a recent innovative approach in which the kidney can be removed by maceration or laparoscopic-assisted technique. For information on the topic, readers are referred to articles by Clayman et al.,[59] McDougall et al.,[60] Doehn et al.,[61] Sasaki et al.,[62] Shalhav et al.,[63] Yao and Poppas,[64] and Fabrizio et al.[65]

## ANATOMIC COMPLICATIONS OF RENAL SURGERY

Anatomic complications of renal surgery include the following:

- Diaphragmatic injury
- Pneumothorax secondary to diaphragmatic, pleural, and lower lobe lung injuries
- Bleeding secondary to adrenal injury
- Bleeding secondary to splenic injury
- Pancreatitis and bleeding secondary to pancreatic injury
- Bleeding and bile leak secondary to hepatic injury
- Peritonitis secondary to duodenal injury
- Peritonitis secondary to colonic injury
- Adrenal insufficiency (bilateral surgery)

## Diaphragmatic Injury

Diaphragmatic injury with or without pleural involvement is an extremely rare phenomenon. The injury occurs because occasionally the posterior lamina of the Gerota's fascia is heavily fixed to the diaphragm. A tear of the diaphragm can take place when tension is applied to the fascia. It is necessary to repair the tear with interrupted, nonabsorbable 0 sutures to avoid the possibility of later occurrence of an iatrogenic diaphragmatic hernia.

## Pneumothorax Secondary to Diaphragmatic, Pleural, and Lower Lobe Lung Injuries

- Any flank incision, with or without rib resection, can produce pneumothorax.
- The relation of the 12th rib to the transverse (horizontal) orientation of the pleural reflection should always be kept in mind.
- If the opened pleura is recognized in the operating room, it should be closed, using 3-0 absorbable sutures.
- A Robinson catheter with underwater seal should be used if it is necessary and if previous air aspiration is not satisfactory. Alternatively a chest tube can be placed.

## Bleeding Secondary to Adrenal Injury

Prevention of this very common injury is imperative. The adrenal gland is a very friable organ with very rich vascularization. Venous bleeding is the result of injury of the adrenal parenchyma or its draining veins, especially the right one (which is very short, emptying directly into the inferior vena cava). In the event of a caval tear due to adrenal vein avulsion, use 5-0 vascular continuous suture for closing the defect produced at the wall of the inferior vena cava. For injuries of the parenchyma, continuous absorbable sutures can be used or, if the other adrenal is in situ, partial adrenalectomy or total adrenalectomy can be considered.

## Bleeding Secondary to Splenic Injury

Splenic injuries can be prevented by careful mobilization of the spleen and good knowledge of the splenic ligaments. Be conservative and try to save the spleen, thus avoiding postsplenectomy infections. Even with severe lacerations try to avoid splenectomy, if possible, by performing a partial segmental splenectomy, as well as by using surgical Avitene (see the chapter on the spleen).

## Pancreatitis and Bleeding Secondary to Pancreatic Injury

Pancreatic injuries can result in bleeding or pancreatitis. Most often they occur during left kidney surgery by elevation of the tail and distal body of the pancreas. The Kocher maneuver for mobilization of the duodenum and the head of the pancreas can produce pancreatic injury, but this is rare.

If pancreatic injury is suspected, the use of a Jackson-Pratt suction drain is essential, with follow-up of serum amylase and perhaps radiologic imaging. If a pancreatic laceration is recognized in the operating room, close the pancreatic parenchyma using 4-0 nonabsorbable sutures and a Jackson-Pratt (J-P) drain.

Bleeding from the pancreas can be controlled by gently applying mosquito clamps and 5-0 nonabsorbable suture ligatures. Rest the GI tract by eliminating food by mouth, perhaps using parenteral hyperalimentation. The pancreatic leak will heal spontaneously.

Somatostatin may be useful.

## Bleeding and Bile Leak Secondary to Hepatic Injury

Prevent liver lacerations by being gentle and careful. Lacerations, whether superficial or deep, should be repaired using 3-0 absorbable interrupted sutures. With deep lacerations, we favor the J-P drain. Severe bleeding should be treated by ligation of the corresponding vessels (right or left hepatic artery, portal vein, or hepatic vein) and hepatic ducts (right and left). Injury to the common hepatic duct and common bile duct is rare.

## Peritonitis Secondary to Duodenal Injury

Close the laceration in two layers, using 4-0 nonabsorbable suture. Cover with a piece of omentum. If the laceration is long and closure is not satisfactory, duodenostomy will be very helpful, using a T-tube or Foley catheter. It may be possible to control duodenal hematoma by pressure; occasionally the hematoma should be opened and the bleeding vessel isolated and ligated.

If a perforated viscus is diagnosed after the patient leaves the operating room, exploratory laparotomy should be done immediately for correction.

## Peritonitis Secondary to Colonic Injury

Repair the injured colon in two layers with nonabsorbable 4-0 sutures. Injuries and openings of the mesentery should be repaired to avoid internal herniation. Recognition of mesenteric arterial or venous damage without obvious bleeding is the most difficult part. We like to observe these lesions for 10 minutes and act accordingly. The surgeon must evaluate whether reoperation, partial colectomy, or perhaps exteriorization is required.

## Acute Adrenal Insufficiency (Bilateral Surgery)

Acute adrenal insufficiency or acute addisonian crisis may occur among adult surgical patients in three situations: while taking chronic preoperative exogenous corticosteroids; development of bilateral adrenal hemorrhage while taking anticoagulants; and following surgical removal of all functioning adrenal glandular tissue. Chronic adrenal insufficiency is characterized by hypoglycemia, hyponatremia, hyperkalemia, hypotension, hyperpigmentation, fatigue and weakness, nausea and vomiting, and abdominal pain. Acute addisonian crisis is characterized by hypotension and fever and, if not promptly treated by corticosteroids, will result in death.

## Complications of Renal Transplantation

We quote Brown et al.[66]:

*The most frequent complications of renal transplantation include perinephric fluid collections; decreased renal function; and abnormalities of the vasculature, collecting system, and renal parenchyma. Perinephric fluid collections are common following transplantation, and their clinical significance depends on the type, location, size, and growth of the fluid collection,*

*features that are well-evaluated with US (ultrasound). Causes of diminished renal function include acute tubular necrosis, rejection, and toxicity from medications. Radionuclide imaging is the most useful modality for assessing renal function. Vascular complications of transplantation include occlusion or stenosis of the arterial or venous supply, arteriovenous fistulas, and pseudoaneurysms. Although the standard for evaluating these vascular complications is angiography, US is an excellent noninvasive method for screening. Other transplant complications such as abnormalities of the collecting system and renal parenchyma are well-evaluated with both radionuclide imaging and US.*

# *Ureters*

*Injury to the urinary tract is one of the major complications in gynecologic surgery... The only gynecologist who has not injured a ureter or bladder is one who has done little surgery.*

*Wharton*[41]

## SURGICAL ANATOMY OF THE URETERS

The right and left ureters are retroperitoneal muscular tubes which have a length of 25 to 34 cm; their upper half is abdominal and their lower half is pelvic.

## Abdominal Course

Each ureter starts at the renal pelvis close to the hilum, posterior to the renal vessels. It is surrounded by the perirenal fat. On its downward pathway, it is related to the tips of the transverse processes of the lumbar vertebrae and to the psoas major muscle (Fig. 23-48). The ureter crosses over the genitofemoral nerve, passes under the

gonadal vessels, and crosses the common iliac artery or the external iliac artery.

Observations on the abdominal course of the ureter:

- The right ureter is covered by the second portion of the duodenum
- The left ureter is adherent to the mesocolon
- The left ureter is very close to the inferior mesenteric artery, passing under it
- The abdominal part of the ureter is fused to the peritoneum
- The abdominal course of the ureter is the same in male and female
- The anatomic landmark of the left ureter is the intersigmoid fossa (Fig. 23-49). The ureter passes behind the fossa and therefore behind the sigmoid colon at the apex of the capital Greek lambda (Λ)

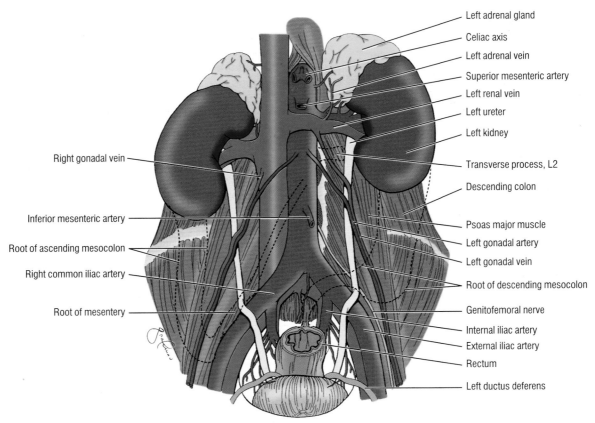

Fig. 23-48. Ureteric course in the abdomen. (After Hinman F Jr. Atlas of Urosurgical Anatomy. Philadelphia: WB Saunders, 1993; Fig. 12.43).

## Pelvic Course

The pelvic course begins after the ureter has passed anterior to the internal iliac artery and its anterior division. The pelvic ureter is not related to the peritoneum because it leaves the lateral pelvic wall at the level of the ischial spine. It follows a medial path toward the urinary bladder, at the base of and posterior to the broad ligament. In this area the ureter crosses over the uterine artery 1 cm, or per-

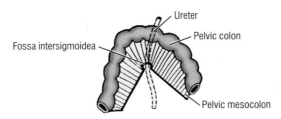

Fig. 23-49. The intersigmoid fossa lies in the apex of the Λ (capital Greek lambda) attachment of the pelvic mesocolon. The ureter is shown passing behind the fossa. (Modified from Decker GAG, Du Plessis DJ. Lee McGregor's Synopsis of Surgical Anatomy (12th ed). Bristol UK: Wright, 1986; with permission.)

haps slightly more, from the uterine cervix.
Observations on the pelvic course of the ureter:
In both male and female:
• The ureter is crossed anteriorly by the obliterated umbilical artery
• On the left, the ureter is located behind the sigmoid arteries
• Remember that the upper abdominal ureter should be mobilized laterally and the pelvic ureter medially during ureteric mobilization. At the middle segment, dissection of the periureteric tissue should be avoided

In the male
• The ductus deferens crosses the ureter anteriorly (Fig. 23-50)
• The ureter enters the bladder just above the apex of the seminal vesicle (Fig. 23-51)

In the female
• The uterine artery crosses the ureter anteriorly about 1-4 cm lateral to the cervix
• Before entering the urinary bladder, the ureter passes 1

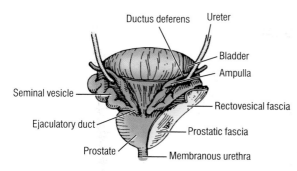

**FIG. 23-50.** The ductus passes anterior to the ureter to gain its medial side. (Modified from Decker GAG, Du Plessis DJ. Lee McGregor's Synopsis of Surgical Anatomy (12th ed). Bristol UK: Wright, 1986; with permission.)

cm above the lateral fornix of the vagina close to its anterior wall and about 1-4 cm lateral to the cervix (Fig. 23-52)

• The pelvic ureter is very vulnerable anterior to the bifurcation of the common iliac artery
• The pelvic ureter crosses the ovarian vessels and nerves posteriorly

Barksdale et al.[68] reported the position of the ureter in the female pelvis relative to several anatomic landmarks (Fig. 23-53). The mean distances are displayed in Table 23-5. The vertical distances were measured from the ureter to the pelvic floor at three points: at the levels of the ischial spine, the obturator canal, and the insertion of the arcus tendineus, obturator internus, or arcus tendineus levator ani in the pubic bone. Vertical measurements were taken also from the arcus tendineus to the pelvic floor at the levels of the ischial spine, the obturator canal, and from the point of insertion of the arcus to the pelvic floor.

The anatomic topographic ureteric pathway from above downward is as follows.

• The ureter rests anterior to the psoas muscle and is located lateral to the tip of the transverse processes of the lumbar vertebrae.
• It passes behind the gonadal vessels.
• The ureter crosses anterior to the common iliac vessels at the pelvic brim.
• The right ureter passes behind the:
  – duodenum
  – ascending colon and its mesentery
  – cecum
  – appendix
  – terminal ileum
• The left ureter is behind the descending colon and the sigmoid colon and its mesentery.
• In the pelvis the ureter is related to different anatomic entities depending on the person's sex.

– In the male pelvis the ureter is posterior to the ductus deferens and just proximal to the ureterovesical junction. It enters the wall of the bladder obliquely.
– In the female pelvis the ureter is located anterior to the internal iliac artery, and posterior to the ovary, under the broad ligament just behind the uterine vessels; it obliquely enters the wall of the bladder. (The phrase "water under the bridge," which represents the ureter passing beneath the uterine artery, is a helpful way to remember the relationship of these structures, and particularly important for avoiding ureteric injury in gynecologic surgery.)

## Characteristic Narrowings of the Ureters

Narrowing of the ureter occurs
• At the ureteropelvic junction
• At the pelvic brim (iliac vessels)
• At the intravesical course (ureterovesical junction)

When both ureters approach the urinary bladder they are approximately 5 cm apart. Their openings within the full bladder are also approximately 5 cm apart, but in an empty bladder the openings are only 2.5 cm apart.

According to Anson and McVay,[69] the intravesical course of the ureter measures about 0.5-1 cm with a diameter of 3-4 mm. It is the most contracted part of the ureter and a stone may be lodged at this point (Fig. 23-54). On vaginal examination this part of the ureter can be palpated, according to Ellis.[70]

## Ureteric Wall

The wall of the ureter is formed by five layers (Fig. 23-55):
• Retroperitoneal connective tissue sheath
• Adventitia
• Muscular coat
• Lamina propria
• Mucosa

The retroperitoneal connective tissue (ureteric) sheath is a very thin layer of connective tissue fixed to the posterior surface of the peritoneum.

The adventitia is formed by collagenous fibers. It is the home of the periureteric arterial plexus, in addition to fine, unmyelinated nerves. The adventitia is loosely attached to the muscularis.

REMEMBER:
• During ureteric mobilization, the adventitia as well as the ureteric vessels should be protected and preserved.
• The ideal procedure produces a watertight, tension-free,

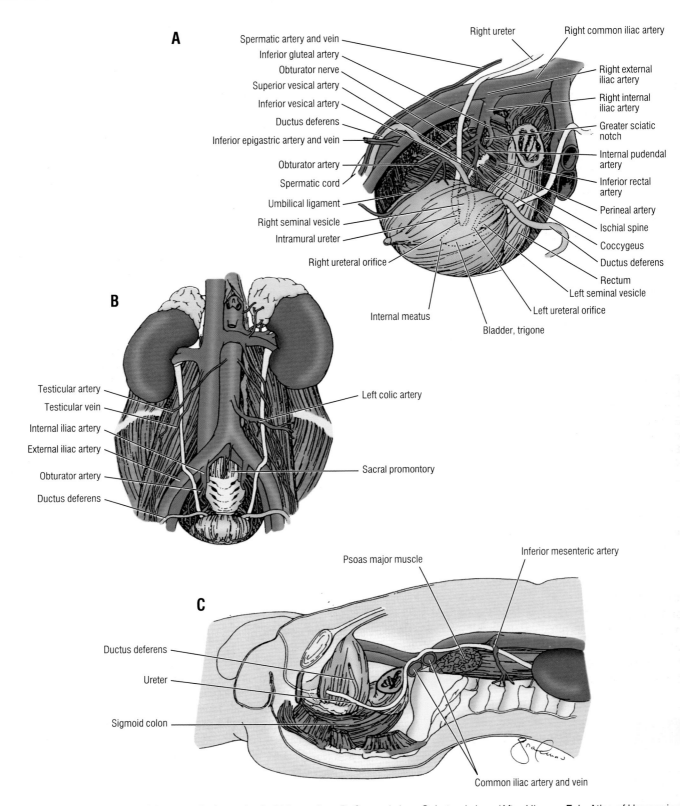

FIG. 23-51. Pelvic relations of the ureter in the male. **A.** Oblique view. **B.** Coronal view. **C.** Lateral view. (After Hinman F Jr. Atlas of Urosurgical Anatomy. Philadelphia: WB Saunders, 1993; Fig. 12.44A,B,C).

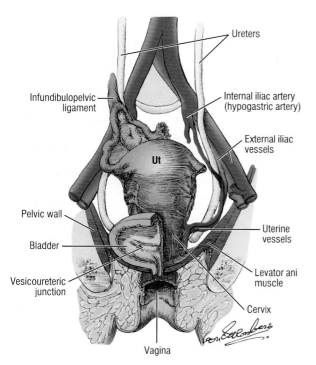

**FIG. 23-52.** Normal anatomy of the ureters and their relations to other pelvic organs encountered in gynecologic surgery. UT, uterus. (Modified from Wharton LR Jr. Surgery of benign adnexal disease: Endometriosis, residuals of inflammatory and granulomatous diseases, and ureteral injury. In: Ridley JH. Gynecologic Surgery: Errors, Safeguards, and Salvage (2nd ed). Baltimore: Williams & Wilkins, 1981; with permission.)

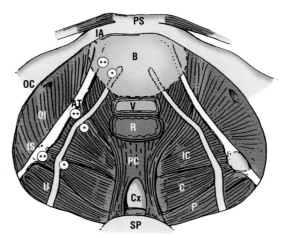

**FIG. 23-53.** Anatomic references to the ureter in relationship to other landmarks. AT, arcus tendineus. B, bladder. C, coccygeus muscle. Cx, coccyx. IA, pubic insertion of arcus tendineus. IC, iliococcygeus muscle. IS, ischial spine. OC, obturator canal. OI, obturator internus muscle. P, piriformis muscle. PC, pubococcygeus muscle. PS, pubic symphysis. R, rectum. SP, sacral promontory. V, vagina. U, ureter. *, location of measurement from ureter to base of pelvic cavity in a vertical plane. **, location of measurement from arcus tendineus to base of pelvic cavity in a vertical plane. (Modified from Barksdale PA, Brody SP, Garely AD, Elkins TE, Nolan TE, Gasser RF. Surgical landmarks of the ureter in the cadaveric female pelvis. Clin Anat 10:324-327, 1997; with permission.)

mucosa-to-mucosa anastomosis.

• Pathology dictates whether long or short segmental mobilization of the ureter is required.

The muscular coat is formed by three longitudinal layers: inner, middle, and outer. Smooth muscle cells are seen throughout, but there is more accumulation in the middle portion. The upper ureteric portion (the abdominal ureter) has a thin muscular network. The lower ureteric portion (the lower pelvic or juxtavesical ureter) has two layers of smooth muscle: an outer circular layer and an inner lon-

gitudinal layer. We suggest that the surgeon in the operating room consider this muscular layer not as three separate layers, but as a single layer.

The lamina propria acts as a submucosa (thin layer of fibrous tissue).

Mucosa is formed by transitional epithelium.

## Vascular Supply of the Ureters

### *Arteries*

The blood supply of the ureters is peculiar: it is both rich and poor. The overall supply is excellent, with a rich anastomotic network in the ureteric adventitia. But the

**TABLE 23-5. Mean Distances from the Ureter and from the Arcus Tendineus to the Pelvic Floor**

|  | Ureter to Pelvic Floor | Arcus Tendineus to Pelvic Floor |
|---|---|---|
| Ischial spine | 3.2 ± 0.1 cm | 1.9 ± 0.1 cm |
| Obturator canal | 3.2 ± 0.1 cm | 2.8 ± 0.1 cm |
| Insertion of arcus tendineus on pubic bone | 1.6 ± 0.1 cm | 3.2 ± 0.1 cm |

Source: Adapted from Barksdale PA, Brody SP, Garely AD, Elkins TE, Nolan TE, and Gasser RF. Surgical landmarks of the ureter in the cadaveric female pelvis. Clin Anat 1997;10:324-327; with permission.

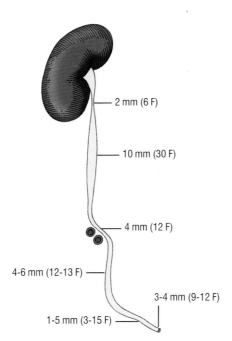

2 mm (6 F)

10 mm (30 F)

4 mm (12 F)

4-6 mm (12-13 F)

3-4 mm (9-12 F)

1-5 mm (3-15 F)

**FIG. 23-54.** The ureter, demonstrating variations in caliber including three anatomic narrowings — at the ureteropelvic junction, the iliac vessels (pelvic brim), and the ureterovesical junction (the intravesical course). Note also the anterior displacement of the ureter, which occurs over the iliac vessels, shown here diagrammatically. F, French calibration scale. (Modified from Kabalin JN. Surgical anatomy of the retroperitoneum, kidneys, and ureters. In: Walsh PC, Retik AB, Vaughan ED Jr, Wein AJ (eds). Campbell's Urology (7th ed). Philadelphia: WB Saunders, 1998; with permission.)

blood supply in the middle segment (between the lower renal pole and the pelvic brim) is poor in comparison to that of the proximal and distal segments (Fig. 23-56).

The arteries that are more commonly observed providing arterial supply to the ureter include the renal artery, the gonadal artery, and the common iliac and internal iliac arteries. However, vessels other than these usually contribute to the blood supply of the ureter from the renal pelvis to the urinary bladder (Fig. 23-57). These additional vessels include:

- Capsular arteries
- Adrenal arteries
- Aortic branches
- Umbilical artery
- Superior vesical artery
- Inferior vesical artery
- Uterine artery
- Middle rectal artery

In relation to its blood supply, the ureter can be divided into three parts: upper, middle, and lower:

- The upper part (from the renal pelvis to the lower pole) receives blood from the adrenal, capsular, renal, and go-

nadal arteries. The renal artery is the most important artery of this segment.

- The middle part (from the lower pole to the pelvic brim) receives branches of the gonadal artery, the aorta, and the common iliac artery.
- The lower part (from the pelvic brim to the urinary bladder) receives branches of the internal iliac (hypogastric), superior, and inferior vesical arteries.

According to Redman,[71] the richest arterial supply is to the pelvic ureter. The poorest arterial supply is to the abdominal portion; that is, from the lower pole of the kidney to the brim of the pelvis. In this area, the aorta and the common iliac give off only a few segmentally arranged lumbar rami. Therefore, mobilize laterally; leave the medial aspect intact if possible.

The rich anastomotic network of the ureter is formed by the "long arteries." These originate above from the renal artery and other arteries, sending descending branches, and below from the internal iliac artery and others, sending ascending branches which anastomose somewhere in the middle segment. The meeting place of all these vessels is the adventitia, where all branches intercommunicate.

The anastomoses of these vessels are so rich that ischemia is a rare phenomenon; the literature supports this. However, it is our opinion that in spite of the excellence of the ureteric blood supply, extensive mobilization should be resolutely avoided. It is best to clip or ligate ureteric bleeders rather than to cauterize them. Devascularization can undoubtedly produce ischemia, necrosis, urinary fistula, or stenosis with secondary ureteric obstruction.

Basing their findings on dissection of 100 ureters, Daniel and Shackman[72] reported the following:

- Only two ureters did not receive blood from the renal and vesical or uterine arteries, but received three arteries in the middle part arising from the aorta, internal spermatic, common, and internal iliacs.
- Ten received only peritoneal twigs, reaching them between the upper and lower ends.
- The blood supply of the middle ureteric portion consisted of a single artery in 64 of 88 cases, two arteries in 20 cases, and three arteries in 4 cases.

Daniel and Shackman[72] speculated that in perhaps 10 to 15 percent of cases, necrosis may occur if ureteric division takes place below the anastomosis between adjacent vessels. They advised division of the ureter 2 cm below a visible vessel or 2 cm below the common iliac arteries. They also recommended that skeletonization of the middle part should not exceed 2.5 cm.

Hinman[57] reported that division of any or all except the most proximal of the multiple arteries that anastomose along the length of the ureter does not produce ureteric ischemia. He also stated that separation of the ureter from

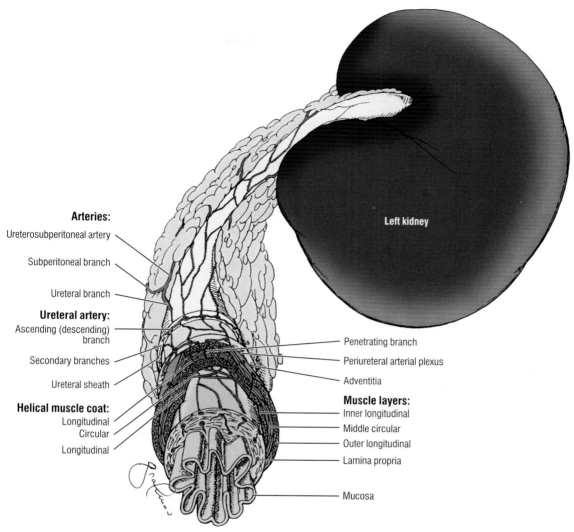

**Arteries:**
Ureterosubperitoneal artery
Subperitoneal branch
Ureteral branch
**Ureteral artery:**
Ascending (descending) branch
Secondary branches
Ureteral sheath
**Helical muscle coat:**
Longitudinal
Circular
Longitudinal

Left kidney

Penetrating branch
Periureteral arterial plexus
Adventitia
**Muscle layers:**
Inner longitudinal
Middle circular
Outer longitudinal
Lamina propria

Mucosa

**FIG. 23-55.** The ureteric wall.

the peritoneum by division of the arterial twigs may compromise ureteric blood supply, especially in the lower ureter. Hinman wrote that the vascular network permits division of the ureter, but interference with the arterial plexus jeopardizes the viability of the ureteric end. Other workers emphasize that the most practical suggestion is to disturb as little as possible the adventitia surrounding the ureter, because this provides great protection for the collateral vascular supply.

## Veins

The veins of the ureter originate in the submucosa (lamina propria) and spread out in the adventitia. In the upper part of the ureter they drain into the renal vein or the go-

nadal vein. At the lower end the ureteric veins drain into the venous network of the broad ligament and can produce varicosities.

## Lymphatics

According to Kabalin,[41] the lymphatics of the ureter follow the pathways of the arterial and venous networks. However, there are different drainage pathways for the various segments:
- The lymphatics of the upper ureter and renal pelvis drain to the ipsilateral renal lymphatics
- The lymphatics of the abdominal ureter differ by side
  - Right: Drains to right paracaval and interaortocaval nodes

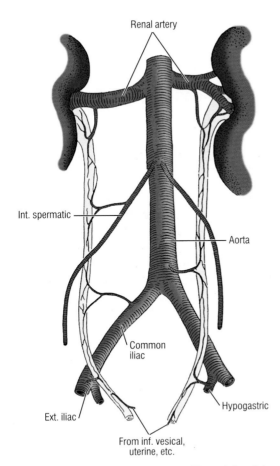

FIG. 23-56. Blood supply of the ureter. The origin of the various vessels is indicated, but tiny twigs from the peritoneum are not shown. (Modified from Hollinshead WH. Anatomy for Surgeons. New York: Hoeber, 1956; with permission.)

– Left: Drains to left paraaortic nodes
• The lower (pelvic) ureter drains to the common iliac and the internal and external iliac nodes

Ureteric tumors can be benign or malignant, primary or metastatic. The lymphatic pathway of metastatic disease of the ureter is shown in Fig. 23-58. The treatment for benign tumors is local excision; however, because these tumors are potentially malignant some authors advise radical treatment as in malignant tumors. Ureteroscopy allows the surgeon to obtain a tissue diagnosis preoperatively and, if the specimen is diagnosed as benign, the lesion can be excised endoscopically. The treatment for malignant tumors is total nephroureterectomy, including a cuff of the urinary bladder.

## Innervation

The ureter has three sources of nerve supply: superior, middle, and inferior. The superior supply originates from the renal and aortic plexuses; the middle originates from the superior hypogastric plexus; and the inferior originates from the pelvic plexus. The patterns of referred somatic pain from the proximal ureter are shown in Fig. 23-59. Pain fibers from the ureter are often carried principally to the level of spinal nerve L2. Thus, a cremasteric reflex may occur by way of referral of pain to the genitofemoral nerve (L1, L2), which supplies the cremasteric muscle.

According to Lapides,[73] ureteric contractions do not need any autonomic nerve stimulus. Pacemaking cells in the renal pelvis are apparently responsible for the peristaltic waves of ureteric contraction. As a matter of fact, autonomic ganglion cells are not clearly apparent, except near the very terminal part of the ureter.

REMEMBER:
• The ureteric wall does not have autonomic ganglia.
• The nervous system does not activate ureteric peristalsis;

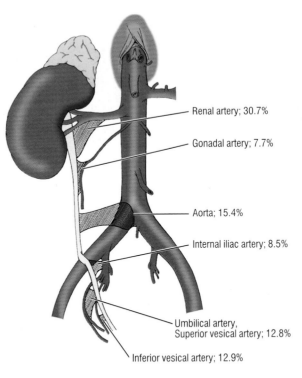

FIG. 23-57. Ureteric arteries (schematic). Sources of supply indicated, with percentage of vessels from each of the important contributory vessels, in 50 specimens. The combined percentages cover 88 percent of the vessels (remaining 12 percent include vessels derived from the capsular, suprarenal, uterine, and urethral arteries). (Data from McCormack LJ, Anson BJ. Arterial supply of ureter. Quart Bull Northwestern Univ Med School 1950;24:291-294.)

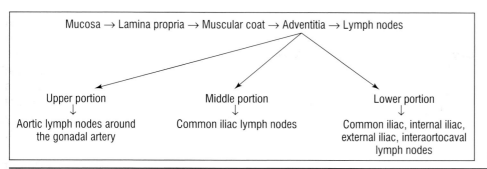

Mucosa → Lamina propria → Muscular coat → Adventitia → Lymph nodes

| Upper portion | Middle portion | Lower portion |
|---|---|---|
| ↓ | ↓ | ↓ |
| Aortic lymph nodes around the gonadal artery | Common iliac lymph nodes | Common iliac, internal iliac, external iliac, interaortocaval lymph nodes |

**FIG. 23-58.** The lymphatics of the ureter.

ureteric peristalsis is stimulated by urine stretching the ureteric muscular coat.

- Pain from a dilated ureter is distributed to the flank, inguinal area, and scrotum, all of which are supplied by T11, T12, L1, L2 nerves. The pain is carried upward by way of thoracic and lumbar splanchnic nerves, which also carry the sympathetic nerve supply transmitted by the autonomic nervous system.
- The action of parasympathetic fibers is enigmatic.
- Hinman[57] believes that the severe pain secondary to renal pelvic distention is not associated with ureteric spasm, but results from the distention itself.

# HISTOLOGY AND PHYSIOLOGY OF URETERS

The histology of the ureters has been covered pre-

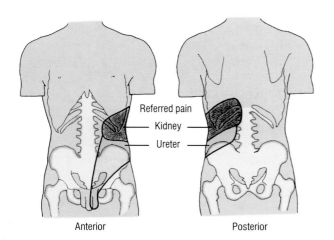

**FIG. 23-59.** Patterns of referred somatic pain from the upper urinary tract. (Modified from Kabalin JN. Surgical anatomy of the retroperitoneum, kidneys, and ureters. In: Walsh PC, Retik AB, Vaughan ED Jr, Wein AJ (eds). Campbell's Urology (7th ed). Philadelphia: WB Saunders, 1998; with permission.)

viously under the heading "Ureteric Wall."

The ureteric wall of smooth muscle, innervated by the autonomic system and its intramural plexus of neurons and nerves, is perhaps responsible for a peristaltic contraction that forces the urine downward to the urinary bladder. During micturition, backflow of urine from the bladder to the ureters is prevented by pressure of the bladder wall on the ureteric walls where they have penetrated the bladder obliquely.

Wemyss-Holden et al.[74] found that each ureter produces three contractions every minute; during diuresis the frequency increases.

Ureterorenal reflex is a decrease in urinary output from a kidney in response to pain or blockage of the ureter, most commonly by a stone. Severe pain may accompany the obstruction.

# SURGERY OF THE URETER

From a surgicoanatomic standpoint the ureter may be divided into three parts: upper, middle, and lower. The upper segment is from the ureteropelvic junction to the area of the upper sacrum; the middle part is at the sacral area; and the lower segment travels through the pelvis.

The approach for each third is different. The incision should be located such that the pathologically-involved segment has excellent exposure.

Some anatomy books divide the ureter into only two parts: upper abdominal and lower pelvic. Both of these segments are divided by the iliac vessels.

## Surgical Approaches

### Upper Ureteric Segment

The upper ureteric segment including the ureteropelvic junction may be approached with a flank or dorsal lumbar incision.

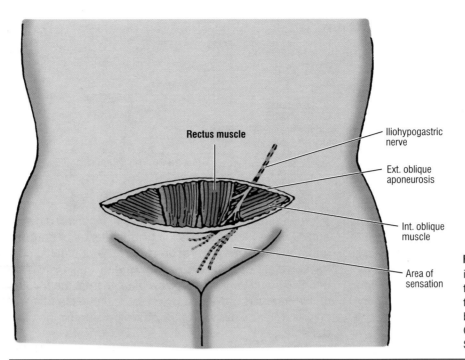

**FIG. 23-60.** Pfannenstiel transverse abdominal incision showing the iliohypogastric nerve between the internal oblique muscle and the external oblique aponeurosis just lateral to the border of the rectus muscle. (Modified from Grosz CR. Iliohypogastric nerve injury. Am J Surg 1981; 142:628; with permission.)

## Middle Ureteric Segment

A transperitoneal approach through a midline or paramedian incision will expose not only the middle segment but also the upper and lower segments. An extraperitoneal approach with the so-called Gibson incision gives excellent exposure to the middle segment.

This incision begins 2-3 cm medial to the anterior superior iliac spine and 2-3 cm above the inguinal ligament. It ends 2-3 cm above the pubic tubercle. The three flat muscles are incised parallel to their fibers. To expose the retroperitoneal space the transversalis fascia is opened and the peritoneum is pushed medially. This incision may be extended upward or medially if necessary.

## Lower Ureteric Segment

The lower ureteric segment may be exposed with several incisions including the:
- Lower anterior midline
- Gibson incision
- Pfannenstiel incision

The transverse Pfannenstiel incision is made horizontally just above the pubis. The anterior rectus sheaths and the linea alba are transected and reflected upward 8 to 10 cm. The rectus muscles are retracted laterally, and the transversalis fascia and the peritoneum may be cut in the midline. The iliohypogastric nerve must be identified and protected (Fig. 23-60).

The Pfannenstiel incision may be extended in the midline or laterally by dividing the tendinous attachment of the rectus muscle to the pubis. Lateral extension also may be attained by leaving the rectus muscle attached, but retracting it medially and splitting the muscles of the anterolateral wall. This usually requires ligation of the inferior epigastric vessels. Extension too far laterally may jeopardize the iliohypogastric and ilioinguinal nerves (Fig. 23-61).

## Ureteric Reconstruction

Franke and Smith[75] reported that the type of ureteric reconstruction selected is based on the length of the ureteric defects and the ureteric pathology (Table 23-6).

## Endoscopic Surgery of the Ureter

It is not within the scope of this chapter to present endoscopic ureteric surgery. The reader is strongly advised to read "Surgery of the Ureter" by Franke and Smith in *Campbell's Urology.*[75]

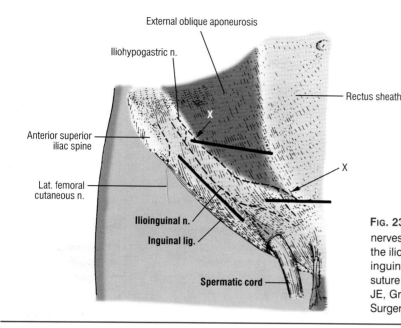

External oblique aponeurosis

Iliohypogastric n.

Rectus sheath

Anterior superior
iliac spine

Lat. femoral
cutaneous n.

**Ilioinguinal n.**

**Inguinal lig.**

**Spermatic cord**

FIG. 23-61. The courses of the iliohypogastric and ilioinguinal nerves. Transverse incisions carried too far laterally may cut (X) the iliohypogastric nerve. Inguinal incisions may injure the ilioinguinal nerve directly or it may be inadvertently included in a suture during closure of the incision. (Modified from Skandalakis JE, Gray SW, Rowe JS. Anatomical Complications in General Surgery. New York: McGraw-Hill, 1983; with permission.)

# ANATOMIC COMPLICATIONS OF URETERIC SURGERY

General surgeons, gynecologists, urologists, and vascular surgeons are involved with ureteric injuries during colectomies, hysterectomies, and retroperitoneal and vascular procedures.

The anatomic complications of ureteric injuries include:
- Bleeding
- Ligation
- Laceration or division
- Stripping
- Stenosis
- Fistula

Handle the ureter carefully because the ureteric wall can be molested or violated easily. Bleeding from the ureteric wall can be prevented by careful mobilization. If bleeding occurs, avoid using clamps or ligation, but use pressure with a sponge stick. If bleeding continues, use fine mosquito clamps and ligate carefully, using 6-0 nonabsorbable sutures. Insertion of a ureteric stent by ureterotomy or cystostomy is imperative in this case.

Laceration of the ureter can frequently be easily recognized in the operating room, either by identification of the lumen, or by urine leak, or both. If there is uncertainty as to whether there is a urine leak, indigo carmine will stain the urine. The injury should be repaired. Ligation without lacer-

ation is not recognized in the operating room in most cases; this is a postoperative problem. Laceration or division should be repaired in the operating room immediately by ureteroureterostomy using the technique with which the surgeon is familiar (spatulation, oblique anastomosis, right or left transureteroureterostomy with formation of retroperitoneal tunnel, reimplantation of the ureter into the bladder via psoas muscle [hitch, ileal ureter, etc.]) If it proves necessary to form an ileal conduit, the left ureter must be carefully placed so it is not twisted or kinked.

The most logical explanation for ureteric stenosis or late fistula formation is that the ureter was devascularized by stripping the periureteric sheath.

Wharton[67] listed the following errors in surgery of the

**TABLE 23-6. Categorization of the Usual Length of Ureteral Defect that can be Bridged with Various Surgical Techniques for Ureteral Reconstruction**

| Procedure | Ureteral Defect |
|---|---|
| Ureteroureterostomy | 2-3 cm |
| Ureteroneocystostomy alone | 4-5 cm |
| Ureteroneocystostomy with psoas hitch | 6-10 cm |
| Ureteroneocystostomy with Boari flap | 12-15 cm |
| Renal descensus | 5-8 cm |

*Source:* Franke JJ, Smith JA Jr. Surgery of the Ureter. In: Walsh PC, Retik AB, Vaughn ED, Wein AJ. Campbell's Urology, 7th Ed. Philadelphia: WB Saunders, 1998; with permission.

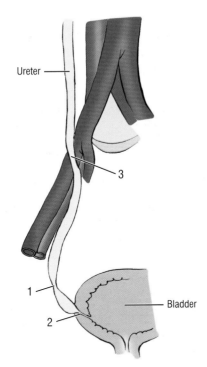

Ureter

3

1

2

Bladder

**FIG. 23-62.** Most common sites of ureteric injury in gynecologic surgery. (1) Pelvic wall lateral to uterine vessels; (2) Area of ureterovesical junction; (3) Base of infundibulopelvic ligament. (Modified from Wharton LR Jr. Surgery of benign adnexal disease: Endometriosis, residuals of inflammatory and granulomatous diseases, and ureteral injury. In: Ridley JH. Gynecologic Surgery: Errors, Safeguards, and Salvage (2nd ed). Baltimore: Williams & Wilkins, 1981; with permission.)

ureter as the most common:
- Failure to know the exact position of the ureter at all times during pelvic surgery or placing clamps and sutures without knowing the position of the ureter
- Failure to recognize ureteric injury immediately; incorrectly evaluating and repairing injury
- Failure to recognize urinary tract injury after operation
- Failure to insure adequate drainage for injury to the urinary tract
- Failure to perform ureteroureteric or ureterovesical anastomosis without tension on suture lines
- Failure to protect kidneys from damage when the ureter is injured
- Correcting the urinary tract injury at the wrong time
- Selection of the wrong procedure or technique to correct a urinary tract injury

Figs. 23-52 and 23-62 show the most common sites of ureteric injury in gynecologic surgery.

## REFERENCES

1. Zinman L, Libertino JA. Surgical hemostats in upper urinary tract and retroperitoneal surgery. In: Bern MM (ed). Urinary Tract Bleeding: Diagnosis and Control by Medical, Radiologic, and Surgical Techniques. New York: Futura, 1985, pp. 215-239.
2. Larsen WJ. Human Embryology (2nd ed). New York: Churchill Livingstone, 1997.
3. Moore KL, Persaud TVN. The Developing Human (5th ed). Philadelphia: WB Saunders, 1993.

## Editorial Comment

*The potential for complications is inherent in any surgical procedure. The wise surgeon will not simply accept Wharton's statement at the beginning of this section that the only surgeon to not injure a ureter is the surgeon who has done little surgery in the area of the ureters[67]. The wise surgeon will be alert to the variety of possible complications so as to decrease their frequency, but will also have an organized approach to recognition and treatment should a complication occur. Ureteral injuries are most commonly iatrogenic and the best time for successful repair is in the operating room at the time of the initial injury.*

*The ureter has a remarkable ability to regenerate its components and heal if provided the opportunity. The principles of repair are debridement of devitalized tissue followed by a tension-free anastomosis with a closure that is both watertight and nonconstricting. Many feel that a ureteral stent and retroperitoneal drainage are also appropriate.*

*For lower ureteral injuries reimplantation of the ureter into the bladder with an antireflux technique may be the procedure of choice. Midureteral injuries are repaired by ureteroureterostomy or by transureteroureterostomy. Injuries to the upper ureter are repaired by ureteroureterostomy. In rare circumstances the repair may be by autotransplantation of the kidney into the pelvis with reimplantation of the ureter into the bladder as is done in renal transplantation. (RSF Jr)*

4. Hamilton, WJ, Mossman, HW. Hamilton, Boyd and Mossman's Human Embryology (4th ed). Baltimore: Williams & Wilkins, 1972.

5. Kelalis PP, King LR, Belman AB. Clinical Pediatric Urology. Philadelphia: WB Saunders, 1992.

6. Hill LM, Nowak A, Hartle R, Tush B. Fetal compensatory renal hypertrophy with a unilateral functioning kidney. Ultrasound Obstet Gynecol 2000;15:191-193.

7. Campbell MF. Renal ectopy. J Urol 1930;24:187-189.

8. Kubricht WS III, Henderson RJ, Bundrick WS, Venable DD, Eastham JA. Renal cell carcinoma in an intrathoracic kidney: Radiographic findings and surgical considerations. South Med J 1999;92:628-629.

9. Peng HC, Chen HC. Surgical management of complete ureteric duplication abnormalities in children. Chin Med J 2000;63:182-188.

10. Dodson JL, Ferrer FA, Jackman SV, Blakesmore KJ, Docimo SG. Cloacal outlet obstruction with an ectopic ureter. Urology (Online) 2000;55:775.

11. Weiss RM, George NJR, O'Reilly PH. Comprehensive Urology. New York: Mosby, 2001.

12. Bapat S, Bapat M, Kirpekar D. Endoureterotomy for congenital primary obstructive megaureter: preliminary report. J Endourol 2000;14:263-267.

13. Shindo S, Kobayashi M, Kaga S, Hurukawa H, Kubota K, Kojima A, Iyori K, Ishimoto T, Kamiya K, Tada Y. Retrocaval ureter and preaortic iliac venous confluence in a patient with an abdominal aortic aneurysm. Surg Radiol Anat 1999;21:147-149.

14. Poucell-Hatton S, Huang M, Bannykh S, Benirschke K, Masliah E. Fetal obstructive uropathy: patterns of renal pathology. Pediatr Dev Pathol 2000;3:223-231.

15. Ng CS, Yost A, Streem SB. Nephrolithiasis associated with autosomal dominant polycystic kidney disease: contemporary urological management. J Urol 2000;163:726-729.

16. Hemal AK, Khaitan A, Singh I, Kumar M. Renal cell carcinoma in cases of adult polycystic kidney disease: changing diagnostic and therapeutic implications. Urol Int 2000;64:9-12.

17. Dugougeat F, Navarro O, Soares Souza AS, Geary D, Daneman A. Multiple unilateral renal cysts in two children. Pediatr Radiol 2000;30:346-348.

18. Aubert J, Irani J, Baumert H. Familial ureteral duplication and ureterocele: two sisters and their father. Eur Urol 2000;37:714-717.

19. O'Rahilly R. Gardner-Gray-O'Rahilly Anatomy (5th ed). Philadelphia: WB Saunders, 1986.

20. Narath PA. Renal Pelvis and Ureter. New York: Grune and Stratton, 1951.

21. Fine H, Keen EN. The arteries of the human kidney. J Anat 1966;100:881-894.

22. Davie TB. Renal-adrenal adherence. Br J Surg 1935;22:428.

23. Prinz RA. A comparison of laparoscopic and open adrenalectomies. Arch Surg 1995;130:489-494.

24. Wolfram-Gabel R, Kahn J, Rapp E. Is the renal space closed? Clin Anat 2000;13:168-176.

25. Hightower JM. Dietl's crisis revisited: the enigma of nephroptosis. West J Med 1995;162:471.

26. Lowsley OS, Kirwin TJ. Nephroptosis. In: Lowsley OS (ed). Clinical Urology. Baltimore: Williams & Wilkins, 1956, pp. 838-842.

27. Dodson AI. Nephroptosis and its treatment. In: Glenn JF (ed). Urologic Surgery. St. Louis: Mosby, 1970, pp. 124-132.

28. Rais O. Does the movable kidney require surgical treatment? Acta Chir Scand 1974;140:566-570.

29. McWhinnie DL, Hamilton DNH. The rise and fall of surgery for the 'floating' kidney. Br Med J [Clin Res] 1984;288:845-847.

30. Glikman L, Glicksman A, Pevsner J, Levin I. Abnormal renal mobility — An indication for surgical intervention. Urol Int 1989; 44:166-168.

31. Buser S, Hagmaier V, Locher JT, et al. Diagnostic relevance of urinary dehydrogenase determination in nephroptosis and for the indication to nephropexy. Curr Probl Clin Biochem 1979;9:44-55.

32. Ozan H, Alemdaroglu A, Sinav A, Gümüsalan Y. Location of the ostia of the renal arteries in the aorta. Surg Radiol Anat 19:245-247, 1997.

33. Graves FT. The anatomy of the intra-renal arteries in health and disease. Br J Surg 43(182):605-616, 1956.

34. Graves FT. The aberrant renal artery. Proceedings of the Royal Society of Medicine (London), pp. 368-370, 1957.

35. Banowsky LHW. Surgical anatomy. In: Novick AC (ed). Stewart's Operative Urology (2nd ed). Baltimore: Williams & Wilkins, 1989.

36. Singh G, Ng YK, Bay BH. Bilateral accessory renal arteries associated with some anomalies of the ovarian arteries: a case study. Clin Anat 1998;11:417-420.

37. Satyapal KS, Haffejee AA, Singh B, Ramsaroop L, Robbs JV, Kalideen JM. Additional renal arteries: incidence and morphometry. Surg Radiol Anat 2001;23:33-38.

38. Aluisio FV, Berens AS, Colborn GL, Scaljon WM, Skandalakis JE. Examination of collateral flow and anomalies of the left renal vein with clinical correlations. J Med Assoc Ga 1991;80:429-433.

39. Satyapal KS, Kalideen JM, Haffejee AA, Singh B, Robbs JV. Left renal vein variations. Surg Radiol Anat 21:77-81, 1999.

40. Yoshinaga K, Kawai K, Kodama K. An anatomical study of the retroaortic left renal vein. Okajimas Folia Anat Jpn 2000;77:47-52.

41. Kabalin JN. Surgical anatomy of the retroperitoneum, kidneys, and ureters. In: Walsh PC, Retik AB, Vaughan ED Jr, Wein AJ (eds). Campbell's Urology (7th ed). Philadelphia: WB Saunders, 1998.

42. Skandalakis JE, Gray SW, Rowe JS. Anatomical Complications in General Surgery. New York: McGraw-Hill, 1983.

43. Kabalin JN. Anatomy of the retroperitoneum and kidney. In: Walsh PC, Retik AB, Stamey TA, Vaughan ED Jr (eds). Campbell's Urology (6th ed). Philadelphia: WB Saunders, 1992.

44. Venkatachalam MA, Kriz W. Anatomy. In: Jennette JC, Olson JL, Schwartz MM, Silva FG. Heptinstall's Pathology of the Kidney, 5th ed. Philadelphia: Lippincott-Raven, 1998, pp. 3-66.

45. Smith RB. Complications of renal surgery. In: Smith RB, Ehrlich RM. Complications of Urologic Surgery. Philadelphia: WB Saunders, 1990.

46. Williams RD, Donovan JF. Urology. In: Way LW (ed). Current Surgical Diagnosis & Treatment, 9th Ed. Norwalk, CT: Appleton & Lange, 1991, p. 928.

47. Burga AM, Cohen EL, Unger P. Kidney neoplasms - can renal oncocytoma be distinguished from renal cell carcinoma? Contemp Surg 2001;57:64-68.

48. Droller MJ. Anatomic considerations in extraperitoneal approach to radical nephrectomy. Urology 1990;36(2):118-123.

49. Doublet JD, Barreto HS, Degremont AC, Gattegno B, Thibault P. Retroperitoneal nephrectomy: comparison of laparoscopy with open surgery. World J Surg 1996;20:713-716.

50. Cohen Z, Gabriel A, Mizrachi S, Kapuler V, Mares AJ. Traumatic avulsion of the kidney through a ruptured diaphragm in a boy. Pediatr Emerg Care 2000;16:180-181.

51. Niklason LE, Langer R. Prospects for organ and tissue replace-

ment. JAMA 2001;285:573-576.

52. Kolff WJ, Berk HT, ter Welle M, van der Ley AJ, van Dijk EC, van Noordwijk J. The artificial kidney: a dialyser with a great area. Acta Med Scand 1944;117:121-134.

53. Murray JE, Merrill JP, Harrison JH. Renal homotransplantation in identical twins. Surg Forum 1955;6:432-440.

54. Murray JE, Merrill JP, Dammin GJ. Study on transplantation immunity after total body irradiation: clinical and experimental investigation. Surgery 1960;48:272-285.

55. Murray JE, Tilney NL, Wilson RE. Renal transplantation: a twenty-five year experience. Ann Surg 1976;184;565-573.

56. Pollak R, Prusak BF, Mozes MF. Anatomic abnormalities of cadaver kidneys procured for purposes of transplantation. Am Surg 1986;52:233-235.

57. Hinman F Jr. Atlas of Urosurgical Anatomy. Philadelphia: WB Saunders, 1993.

58. Sasaki T, Finelli F, Barhyte D, Trollinger J, Light J. Is laparoscopic donor nephrectomy here to stay? Am J Surg 177:368-370, 1999.

59. Clayman RV, Kavoussi LR, McDougall EM, Soper NJ, Figenshau RS, Chandhoke PS, Albala DM. Laparoscopic nephrectomy: a review of 16 cases. Surg Laparosc Endosc 2:29, 1992.

60. McDougall EM, Clayman RV, Elashry O. Laparoscopic nephroureterectomy for upper tract transitional cell cancer: The Washington University experience. J Urol 154:975-980, 1995.

61. Doehn C, Fornara P, Fricke L, Jocham D. Comparison of laparoscopic and open nephroureterectomy for benign disease. J Urol 159(3):732-734, 1998.

62. Sasaki TM, Finelli F, Bugarin E, Fowlkes D, Trollinger J, Barhyte DY, Light JA. Is laparoscopic donor nephrectomy the new criterion standard? Arch Surg 2000;135:943-947.

63. Shalhav AL, Dunn MD, Portis AJ, Elbahnasy AM, McDougall EM, Clayman RV. Laparoscopic nephroureterectomy for upper tract transitional cell cancer: the Washington University experience. J Urol 2000;163:1100-1104.

64. Yao D, Poppas DP. A clinical series of laparoscopic nephrectomy, nephroureterectomy and heminephroureterectomy in the pediatric population. J Urol 2000;163;1531-1535.

65. Fabrizio MD, Kavoussi LR, Jackman S, Chan DY, Tseng E, Ratner LE. Laparoscopic nephrectomy for autotransplantation. Urology (Online) 2000;55:145.

66. Brown ED, Chen MY, Wolfman NT, Ott DJ, Watson NE Jr. Complications of renal transplantation: evaluation with US and radionuclide imaging. Radiographics 2000;20:607-622.

67. Wharton LR Jr. Surgery of benign adnexal disease: Endometriosis, residuals of inflammatory and granulomatous diseases, and ureteral injury. In: Ridley JH. Gynecologic Surgery: Errors, Safeguards, and Salvage. (2nd ed). Baltimore: Williams & Wilkins, 1981.

68. Barksdale PA, Brody SP, Garely AD, Elkins TE, Nolan TE, Gasser RF. Surgical landmarks of the ureter in the cadaveric female pelvis. Clin Anat 1997;10:324-327.

69. McVay CB. Anson & McVay Surgical Anatomy (6th ed). Philadelphia: WB Saunders, 1984.

70. Ellis H. Clinical Anatomy (6th ed). Oxford: Blackwell Scientific Publications, 1977.

71. Redman JF. Anatomy of the genitourinary system. In: Gillenwater JY, Grayhack JT, Howards SS, Duckett JW (eds). Adult and Pediatric Urology (3rd ed). St. Louis: Mosby Year Book, 1996.

72. Daniel O, Shackman R. The blood supply of the human ureter in relation to ureterocolic anastomosis. Br J Urol 1952;24:549-550.

73. Lapides J. The physiology of the intact human ureter. J Urol 1948;59:288.

74. Wemyss-Holden GD, Rose MR, Payne SR, Testa HJ. Non-invasive investigation of normal individual ureteric activity in man. Br J Urol 71:156-160, 1993.

75. Franke JJ, Smith JA Jr. Surgery of the ureter. In: Walsh PC, Retik AB, Vaughn ED, Wein AJ. Campbell's Urology, 7th Ed. Philadelphia: WB Saunders, 1998.

# Chapter *24*

# *Urinary Bladder*

JOHN E. SKANDALAKIS, GENE L. COLBORN, THOMAS A. WEIDMAN,
ROBERT A. BADALAMENT, THOMAS S. PARROTT,
NIALL T.M. GALLOWAY, PETROS MIRILAS, WILLIAM M. SCALJON

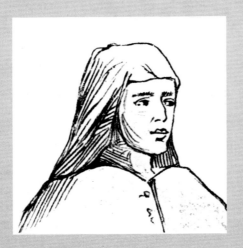

**Herophilus of Chalcedon** (ca. 335-280 B.C.) was the first person known to have performed post-mortem examinations. He is considered the "Father of Neuroanatomy."

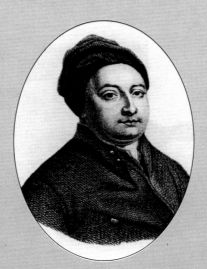

**William Cheselden (1688-1752)** was one of the foremost surgeons of England.

*As men draw near the common goal,*
*Can anything be sadder*
*Than he who, master of his soul,*
*Is servant to his bladder.*

***Anonymous***

## HISTORY

The anatomic and surgical history of the urinary bladder is shown in Table 24-1.

## EMBRYOGENESIS

### Normal Development

The cloaca, a cavity lined with endoderm, is an expansion of the terminal hindgut. It develops around the 4th or 5th week and receives the allantois and the mesonephric ducts. The urorectal septum, a transverse ridge between the allantois and hindgut, divides the cloaca into an anterior urogenital sinus and a posterior rectum.

The urogenital sinus is subdivided into three parts:[1,2]

- Vesical (cranial) portion or urinary bladder. Continuous with the allantois.
- Pelvic (middle) portion. Produces the prostatic and membranous portions of the urethra in the male and the membranous urethra in the female.
- Phallic (caudal) portion or definitive urogenital sinus. Separated from the exterior by the urogenital membranes. Forms the penile urethra in the male and the vestibule of the vagina in the female.

The allantois constricts and forms the urachus. This passes from the apical end of the bladder to the umbilicus, forming the median umbilical ligament.

The caudal ends of the mesonephric ducts and ureters form the trigone, a part of the bladder wall. Early in development, the mucosa of the trigone is of mesodermal origin. Later, endodermal epithelium forms the mucosa of the trigone and the bladder.

The bladder is located in the abdomen in infants and children. It enters the pelvis major at age six and enters the true pelvis after puberty.[3,4]

## Congenital Anomalies

Congenital anomalies of the bladder are shown in Table 24-2. We will briefly consider malformations of the urachus and exstrophy of the bladder.

Anomalies of the urachus include the presence of cysts, sinuses or fistulas, and patent urachus (Fig. 24-1). Persistence of the lumen is more frequent in the lower part of the urachus, near the bladder. The lumen is continuous with the bladder cavity in 50 percent of affected cases.[5] It can enlarge to form a urachal sinus or cyst, but rarely forms a fistula. The term "urachal diverticulum" is commonly used to describe urachal remnants connected to the bladder, with no connection to the skin/umbilicus.

Exstrophy of the bladder (Fig. 24-2) occurs in 1 in 10,000 to 40,000 births[4] and most frequently in males. The bladder opens out to the exterior in the lower abdomen, and the posterior wall of the bladder protrudes. This exposes the trigone and ureteric openings. Characteristics of exstrophy of the bladder include

- Epispadias
- Widely separated pubic bones
- Separated scrotum/labia majora
- Divided penis/clitoris
- Lack of muscle and scant connective tissue over the bladder
- Incomplete closure of lateral folds forming the anterior abdominal wall. This condition occurs because mesenchymal cells fail to migrate between the ectoderm of the abdominal wall and the cloaca during the fourth week.
- Shortened ureterovesical tunnels (frequently). These result in a high propensity for vesicoureteral reflux.

Since individual cases of complete duplication of the

## TABLE 24-1. Anatomic and Surgical History of the Bladder

| | | |
|---|---|---|
| Sushruta (ca. 600 BC) | | Described perineal approach for removal of bladder stone in *Sushruta Samhita* |
| Herophilus of Chalcedon (ca. 335-280 BC) | | Advocated use of the perineal approach for bladder surgery. Well known lithologist. |
| Colot | 1475 | Advocated suprapubic approach to bladder stones |
| Lacuna | 1551 | Gave first definitive report of a bladder tumor |
| Marian | 1552 | Apprentice of Franciscus de Romanis. Published description of the apparatus major, an operation in which a fluted probe was inserted into the urethra. The surgeon opened the bladder by cutting alongside the probe. |
| Franco | 1561 | First to remove stone by suprapubic approach |
| Covillard | 1639 | Reported first deliberate removal of a bladder tumor using perineal approach |
| Cheselden | 1728 | Premier lithotomist of his time. Reported brilliant results, with only 20 mortalities out of 213 patients. |
| Lieutaud | 1742 | First to give a clear description of the trigone of the bladder |
| John Hunter | 1757 | Compared renal and bladder calculi |
| Heister (1710-1779) | | Wrote textbooks illustrating urinary incontinence devices |
| Duncan | 1805 | Wrote first English language reference to an artificial bladder |
| Bozzini | 1807 | Developed first endoscope for looking into bladder |
| Amussat Civiale d'Etiolles | 1814 | Employed transurethral instruments to fragment bladder calculi |
| Simon | 1852 | First description of diverting urine into bowel in patient with bladder exstrophy |
| Henle (1809-1885) | | Discovered external sphincter of the bladder |
| Billroth | 1874 | Described removal of bladder tumor using suprapubic approach |
| Nitze | 1877 | Developed first cystoscope, which he employed to remove bladder stones in over 150 patients |
| Bigelow | 1878 | Introduced transurethral lithrotrites used in litholapaxy |
| Emmet | 1882 | Great master and teacher of plastic surgery of the bladder and perineum |
| Hartwig; Leiter | 1887 | Independently, each placed an Edison electric lamp on the end of a Nitze cystoscope |
| Bardenheuer | 1887 | Performed first total cystectomy |
| Albarran y Dominguez (1860-1912) | | Described the subtrigonal glands of the bladder |
| Kilvington | 1907 | Proposed urinary bladder reinnervation using crossover nerve surgery |
| Beer | 1908 | Performed endoscopic fulguration of bladder tumors |
| Frazier & Mills | 1912 | Reported first technically successful nerve root crossing procedure for urinary bladder innervation |
| Chiasserini | 1935 | Developed and performed reinnervation surgery through anastomosis |
| Marshall, Marchetti, & Krantz | 1949 | Described retropubic bladder suspension |
| Bricker | 1950 | Popularized ileal conduit cutaneous urinary diversion |
| Bogash | 1959 | First to use prosthetic bladder with ureteral valves |
| Peyrera | 1959 | Described needle suspension of bladder |
| Hopkinson & Lightwood | 1966 | Used an anal plug electrode to stimulate pelvic musculature for micturition |

**TABLE 24-1. Anatomic and Surgical History of the Bladder**

| Carlsson & Sundin | 1967 1980 | Attempted reconstruction of nerve pathways to the bladder in patients with spina bifida and paraplegia |
|---|---|---|
| Pollitano | 1973 | Injected Teflon paste periurethrally to control incontinence |
| Turnbull et al. Emmott et al. | 1975 1985 | Modified Bricker's ileal conduit with loop stoma |
| Kock et al. | 1978 | Used ileum in bladder replacement (hemi-Kock augmentation) |
| Hodges et al. | 1980 | Advocated transuretero-ureterostomy to bypass a diseased distal ureter |
| Mitrofanoff | 1980 | Performed appendicovesicostomy |
| Bloom et al. | 1982 | Advocated combining early cystectomy with radiation therapy for bladder cancer |
| Lutzeyer | 1984 | Inserted single-chambered silicone bladder in sheep |
| Rowland et al. | 1987 | Developed the Indiana pouch |
| Hall; Tolley et al. | 1996 | Combined radical transurethral resection of bladder tumors with systemic chemotherapy |
| Klevmark; Heslington | 1997 | Studied ambulatory urodynamics |

*History table compiled by David A. McClusky III and John E. Skandalakis.*

**References**

Coptcoat MJ, Oliver RTD. The role of surgery in the multimodality treatment of bladder cancer. In: Oliver RTD, Coptcoat MJ (eds). Bladder Cancer. Plainview NY: Cold Springs Harbor Laboratory Press, 1998, pp. 129-147.

Kaleli A, Ansell JS. The artificial bladder: a historical review. Urology 1984;24:423-428.

Kaufman JJ. History of surgical correction of male urinary incontinence. Urol Clin North Am 1978;5:265-278.

Mettler CC. History of Medicine. Mettler FA (ed.) Philadelphia: Blakiston, 1947.

Pyrah LN. John Hunter and after: renal calculi and cancer of the bladder. Ann R Coll Surg 1969;45:1-22.

Schmidt JE. Medical discoveries: Who and when. Springfield, IL: Charles C. Thomas, 1959.

Schmidt RA, Tanagho EA. Feasibility of controlled micturition through electric stimulation. Urol Int 1979;34:199-230.

Simon J. Ectopia vesicae (absence of the anterior walls of the bladder and pubic abdominal parietes); operation for directing the orifices of the ureter into the rectum; temporary success; subsequent death; autopsy. Lancet 1852;2:568.

Skinner EC, Boyd SD. Urinary diversion, augmentation procedures, and urinary unidiversion. In: Whitehead ED (ed). Atlas of Surgical Techniques in Urology. Philadelphia: Lippincott-Raven, 1998, pp. 57-124.

Vorstman B, Schlossber S, Kass L. Investigation on urinary bladder reinnervation: historical perspective and review. Urology 1987;30:89-96.

Wein AJ. Ambulatory bladder monitoring: is it an advance? J Urol 1998;160:2310-2311.

urogenital system in females are associated with different anomalies, corrective surgical procedures depend on multiple anatomic variables.[6]

## SURGICAL ANATOMY

### Topography

The age and sex of the individual and the amount of urine within the urinary bladder are responsible for the position, relations, shape, and size of this muscular, hollow, midline pelvic organ.

#### Age

The urinary bladder is abdominal at birth, positioned at the extraperitoneal area of the lower abdominal wall. Around the 5th or 6th year of age the bladder gradually descends into the area of the true (minor) pelvis, positioning between the pubic bones anteriorly and the vagina (in the female) or the rectum (in the male) posteriorly. For all practical purposes it is related to the pelvic diaphragm.

### *Empty and Full Bladder*

The normal capacity of the adult bladder is approximately 300 ml to 500 ml, although it normally accommodates 250 ml to 300 ml before micturition. The normal male first senses content of the bladder at 100 ml to 150 ml. Distension becomes distinctly uncomfortable in the male when the volume is at about 350 ml to 400 ml. As maximum capacity is approached, involuntary micturition occurs. In the female, the preceding numeric values are considerably less, because of the smaller size of the bladder and differ-

**TABLE 24-2. Anomalies of the Bladder and Urethra**

| Anomaly | Prenatal Age at Onset | First Appearance | Sex Most Affected | Relative Frequency | Remarks |
|---|---|---|---|---|---|
| Agenesis of the bladder | 3rd week? | At birth | Female? | Very rare | Other genitourinary tract anomalies usually present |
| Urachal anomalies: | | | | | |
|   Patent urachus | 9th week or later | In infancy | Male | Very rare | |
|   Umbilical sinus | 9th week or later | At any age | ? | Rare | Usually found only if infected |
|   Vesical sinus | 9th week or later | None | Equal | Common | |
|   Urachal cyst | 9th week or later | At maturity | Equal | Common | Small cysts may exist without symptoms |
| Duplication of the bladder: | | | | | |
|   Bilateral | 3rd week | At birth | Equal | Very rare | Usually with duplication of all hindgut derivatives |
|   Frontal | ? | In childhood | Female | Very rare | Redundancy of mucosa only |
|   Hourglass | ? | At any age | ? | Very rare | Questionably congenital |
| Diverticula of the bladder | 7th week | In infancy and childhood | ? | Rare | Not to be confused with acquired diverticula in adult males |
| Extrophy of the bladder | 5th week | Birth | Male | Very rare | Associated with epispadias |
| Ectopic ureter | 6th week | In childhood | Female | Common | Urinary incontinence in females; usually asymptomatic in males; often associated with double ureter |
| Ureterocele | 8th week | 1st year of life | Female | Common | Often associated with double ureter |
| Vesicoureteral reflux | ? | Males - at birth; females - at age 4 yr | Probably female | Common | Associated with urinary tract infection |
| Posterior urethral valves | ? | In childhood | Male | Common | |
| Aganglionic bladder | 9th week | In childhood | ? | Rare | With or without associated megacolon |
| Duplication of the urethra: | | | | | |
|   Female | ? | At birth | Female | Very rare | |
|   Male | 10-14 weeks | At birth | Male | Rare | Accessory urethra often hypospadiac |

*Source:* Skandalakis JE, Gray SW (eds). Embryology for Surgeons, 2nd Ed. Baltimore: Williams & Wilkins, 1994; with permission.

ences in the anatomy of the urinary system. In infants and children, the bladder capacity in ounces can be calculated by adding the number 2 to the age.

The empty bladder (Fig. 24-3) is within the pelvis, but the full bladder extends up to the periumbilical area. In both states the bladder is enveloped entirely by the vesical representation of the endopelvic fascia. This fascia consists of areolar, fibrous, and fatty tissues.

## Relations

For descriptive purposes we present the empty bladder as having four surfaces, four ducts, and four angles or junctions (Fig. 24-4).

*Surfaces*
- One superior
- Two inferolateral
- One inferoposterior

*Ducts*
- Two ureters
- One urachus
- One urethra

*Angles or junctions*
- One urachovesical junction (apex)

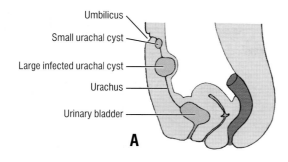

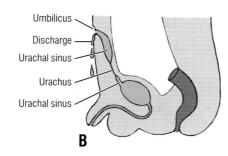

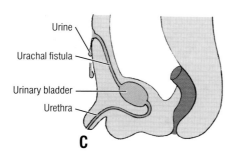

FIG. 24-1. Malformations of urachus. **A.** Urachal cysts. The most common site is in the superior end of the urachus just inferior to the umbilicus. **B.** Two types of urachal sinus ("urachal diverticulum") are illustrated; one is continuous with the bladder, the other opens at the umbilicus. **C.** Patent urachus or urachal fistula connecting the bladder and umbilicus. (Modified from Moore KL, Persaud TVN. The Developing Human (5th ed). Philadelphia: WB Saunders, 1993; with permission.)

- Two ureterovesical junctions
- One urethrovesical junction (neck)

Each angle is associated with one of the ducts:
- The anterior angle (apex) is related to the urachus (median umbilical fold)
- The posterolateral angles are related to both ureters
- The inferior angle (neck) is related to the urethra

The relations of the urinary bladder are detailed below.
- *Anterior.* These consist of the symphysis pubis and pubic bones, separated from the bladder by the space

of Retzius. The peritoneum covers the superior surface (dome) and the upper part of the inferoposterior surface (fundus). When the bladder is full, it lifts the suprapubic peritoneum away from the anterior abdominal wall.
- *Posterior.* These include the seminal vesicles, ductus deferens, rectovesical space, prostatic fascia, rectum (in males), and anterior vaginal wall and cervix (in females).
- *Lateral.* These are the pubic bone, obturator internus (right and left), and levator ani muscles (just above the obturator internus).
- *Base.* In the female the base of the urinary bladder is related to the anterior vaginal wall and to the cervix. Under normal conditions, the fundus and body of the anteverted and anteflexed uterus rest upon the base and the superior surface of the bladder.

The clinician subdivides the urinary bladder as follows.
- Base (posterior wall)
- Lateral walls
- Dome
- Apex
- Neck
- Trigone

REMEMBER:
- The apex is the meeting of the superior and inferolateral surfaces and the site of the beginning of the urachus.
- The vesical neck is the anterior midline meeting point of the right and left inferolateral surfaces. It is attached to the pelvic diaphragm by the fibromuscular pubovesical fascia which, in the female, is part of the pubovesico-cervical fascia.
- The body, or corpus, is the part of the urinary bladder between the fundus (posterior) and the apex (anterior).

*Prevesical Space of Retzius and Ligaments of the Bladder*

For all practical purposes, the space of Retzius, the so-called prevesical space, extends into both the abdomen and the pelvis, being a division of the entire extraperitoneal space. The space of Retzius is situated in front and to the sides of the urinary bladder. Its boundaries are listed below.
- *Anterior.* Symphysis pubis
- *Lateral.* Pubic bone, fascia of obturator internus muscle, superior fascia of levator ani muscle, lateral pubo-prostatic ligament
- *Medial.* Inferior lateral surface of bladder
- *Superior.* Peritoneum bridging the upper surface of the bladder and lateral pelvic wall
- *Posterior.* Vascular stalk of the internal iliac artery and

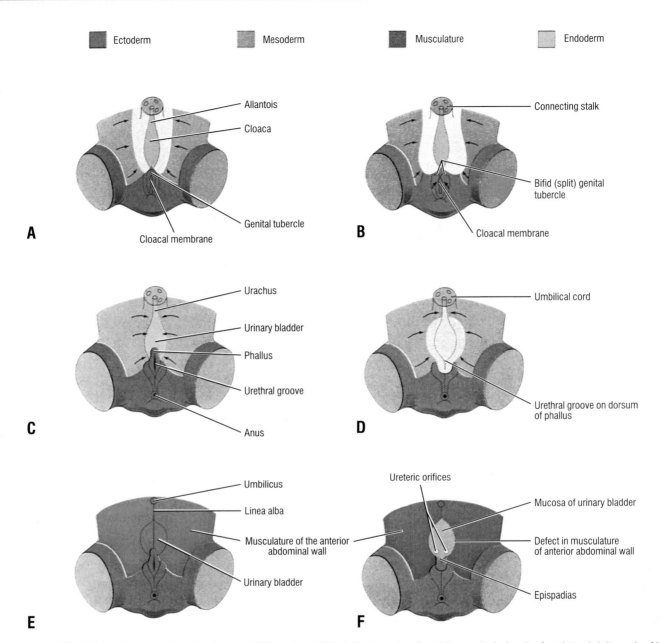

Ectoderm   Mesoderm   Musculature   Endoderm

Fig. 24-2. **A, C, E.** Normal stages in the development of the infraumbilical abdominal wall and the penis during the fourth to eighth weeks. Note that the mesoderm and later muscle reinforce the ectoderm of the developing anterior abdominal wall. **B, D, F.** Probable stages in the development of exstrophy of the bladder and epispadias. In **B** and **D,** note that the mesenchyme (embryonic connective tissue) fails to extend into the anterior abdominal wall anterior to the urinary bladder. Also note that the genital tubercle is located in a more caudal position than usual and that the urethral groove has formed on the dorsal surface of the penis. In **F,** the surface ectoderm and anterior wall of the bladder have ruptured, resulting in exposure of the posterior wall of the bladder. Note that the musculature of the anterior abdominal wall is present on each side of the defect. (From Moore KL, Persaud TVN. The Developing Human (6th ed). Philadelphia: WB Saunders, 1998; with permission.)

vein with their sheath. Sheath reaches posterolateral border of the bladder.

• *Inferior.* Puboprostatic or pubovesical ligaments, reflection of the superior fascia of levator ani muscle to the urinary bladder from the arcus tendineus fascia pelvis

Potentially, the space of Retzius is larger than the retropubic space. It extends upward and laterally to form a triangular space between the medial umbilical ligaments (the obliterated umbilical arteries), with its apex at the umbilicus and its base provided by the puboprostatic or pub-

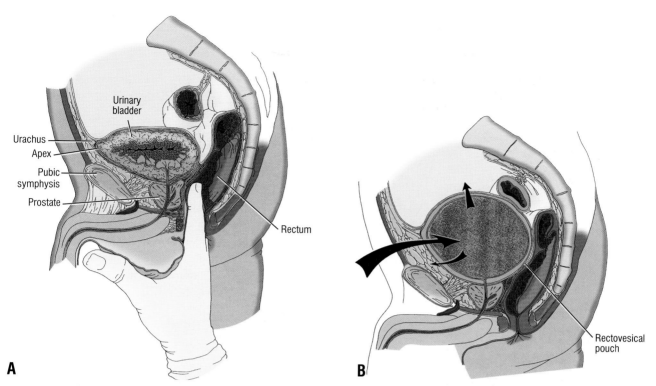

**A**   **B**

FIG. 24-3. **A.** The empty urinary bladder. The prostate is being palpated per rectum. **B.** The full urinary bladder. The peritoneum is stripped away from the anterior abdominal wall as the bladder fills; hence, access to a full bladder may be gained extraperitoneally. Rupture may be intraperitoneal or extraperitoneal. Large arrow indicates the direction of the trochar. The lower small arrow points to the extraperitoneal space; the upper small arrow points into the intraperitoneal space.

ovesical ligaments. The space is "a continuous bursa-like cleft in the areolar tissue at the sides and front of the bladder which allows the bladder to fill and empty without hindrance."[7]

The space of Retzius is bounded behind by the vesicoumbilical fascia, a mantle of mixed connective tissue that extends upward from the urinary bladder toward the umbilicus and posterolaterally as the lateral pillars of the bladder. The space of Retzius is continuous above with the space of Bogros, the potential space between the extraperitoneal connective tissue and the transversalis fascia.

Therefore the space anterior to the urinary bladder (Fig. 24-5) contains connective tissue which is divided into two areas by the umbilical prevesical fascia: 1) the retropubic space, which is anterior to the umbilical prevesical fascia and posterior to the lower abdominal wall and symphysis pubis, and 2) the perivesical or preperitoneal space, which is located between the prevesical fascia and the peritoneum that partially covers the urinary bladder.

The peritoneum of the bladder has several folds attaching it to the pelvic wall (Fig. 24-6). These overlie con-

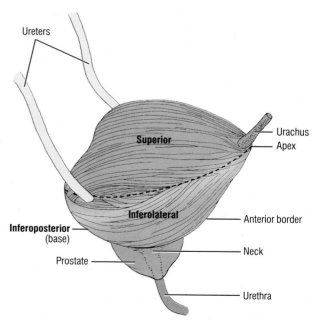

FIG. 24-4. The four surfaces, four ducts, and four angles of the urinary bladder.

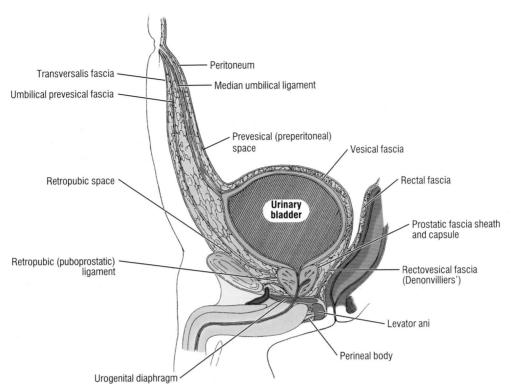

**FIG. 24-5.** Fascial spaces and laminae associated with the bladder, prostate, and rectum. The bladder is shown distended.

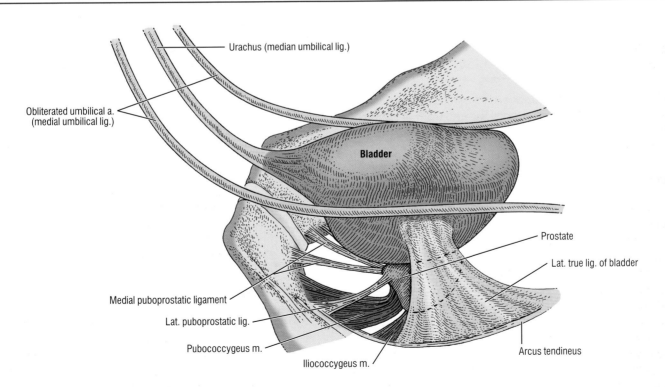

**FIG. 24-6.** Diagram of the bladder and some of its ligaments. (Modified from Skandalakis LJ, Gadacz TR, Mansberger AR Jr, Mitchell WE Jr, Colborn GL, Skandalakis JE. Modern Hernia Repair: The Embryological and Anatomical Basis of Surgery. New York: Parthenon, 1996; with permission.)

**TABLE 24-3. Ligaments of the Bladder**

| Ligament | Location |
| --- | --- |
| *True ligaments* | |
| Median umbilical ligament (urachus) (unpaired) | Dome of bladder to umbilicus |
| Lateral true ligament | Lateral wall of bladder to tendinous arch of pelvic fascia |
| Medial umbilical ligament (obliterated umbilical arteries) | Inguinal ligament |
| Medial puboprostatic ligament (male) | Pelvic wall to prostate gland |
| Lateral puboprostatic ligament | Pelvic wall to prostate gland |
| *False ligaments* | |
| Superior false ligament (unpaired) | Covers the urachus |
| Lateral false ligament | Bladder to wall of pelvis |
| Lateral superior ligament | Covers the medial umbilical ligament |
| Posterior ligament (sacrogenital fold) | Side of bladder, around rectum to anterior aspect of sacrum |

*Source:* Skandalakis LJ, Gadacz TR, Mansberger AR Jr, Mitchell WE Jr, Colborn GL, Skandalakis JE. Modern Hernia Repair: The Embryological and Anatomical Basis of Surgery. New York: Parthenon, 1996; with permission.

densations of connective tissue, nerves, and vessels which are referred to as the "ligaments" or "pillars" of the bladder.

The concept of "true" and "false" ligaments has been with us for over a century. It refers to their apparent strength ("true") or weakness ("false") as supports of the bladder. These terms are mostly of mnemonic value, and are listed in Table 24-3.

## *Retrovesical Space*

The boundaries of the retrovesical, or rectovesical, space in the male (Fig. 24-7A) are:
- *Anterior.* Posterior surface of the bladder with vesical fascia, seminal vesicles, ducti deferentes, terminal ureteric segments, lateral true ligament of the bladder
- *Superior.* Peritoneum and transverse fold of bladder
- *Posterior.* Anterior surface of the rectal ampulla with intervening prerectal fascia and rectovesical septum (fascial septum of Denonvilliers)
- *Inferior.* Rectourethral ligament, pelvic diaphragm
  Both the vesical and rectal fasciae are loose connective tissue. Between them lies a stronger fascia, the bilaminar fascia of Denonvilliers, with the so-called space of Proust between the two laminae. Thus the true retrovesical space

lies between the vesical fascia and the anterior layer of the rectovesical or rectoprostatic membrane (Denonvilliers' fascia) in the male.

The vesical plexuses are located posterolaterally on either side of the bladder. The retropubic space is located between the pubic bones and symphysis pubis anteriorly and the bladder and vesical plexus (in its hypogastric sheath) posteriorly and posterolaterally.

Between the fundus of the urinary bladder and the rectum lie the following anatomic entities enveloped by the visceral fasciae of the urinary bladder and the rectal ampulla (Figs. 24-7, 24-8):
- Seminal vesicles
- Terminal part of the bilateral ducti deferentes and their ampullae
- Base of the prostate gland

In the female the boundaries of the retrovesical space (Fig. 24-7B) are:
- *Anterior.* Posterior surface of the bladder with vesical fascia; the true lateral ligament of the bladder
- *Superior.* Peritoneum
- *Posterior.* Anterior surface of the vagina with anterior vaginal fascia or the pubocervical ligament
- *Inferior.* Reflection of the posterior vesical fascia and anterior vaginal fascia; pelvic and urogenital diaphragms or the pubocervical ligament; pelvic and urogenital diaphragms

Information about hernias of the prevesical and retrovesical spaces will be found in the chapter on the peritoneum, omenta, and internal hernias.

## *Fixation of the Bladder*

The following entities furnish the anatomic fixation of the bladder (see Fig. 24-6):
- Median umbilical ligament (urachus)
- Right and left medial umbilical ligaments (obliterated portions of the umbilical arteries)
- Medial puboprostatic ligament
- Lateral puboprostatic ligament
- Lateral ligament (pillar) of the bladder

## *Bladder Wall*

The wall of the urinary bladder is formed by four coats: serous, muscular, submucosal, and mucosal.
- *Serous coat.* Covers the bladder partially as the peritoneum. The fibrous stroma also covers those parts of the bladder not covered by peritoneum.
- *Muscular coat.* This is the well known detrusor muscle. It is composed of smooth muscle, arranged in whorls and

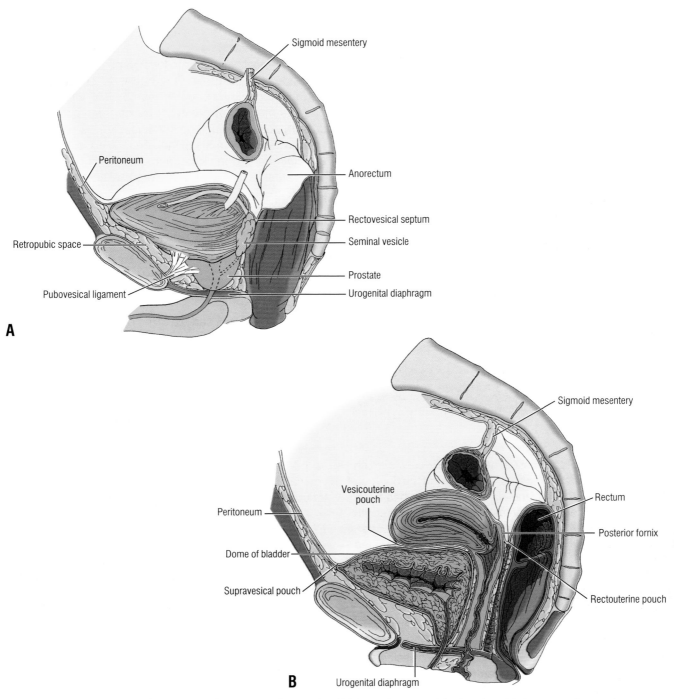

FIG. 24-7. **A.** The peritoneum of the male pelvis in paramedian section. **B.** The peritoneum of the female pelvis in paramedian section.

spirals in a single layer, except in the area of the trigone and neck where two or three layers (inner longitudinal, middle circular, outer longitudinal) are described (Fig. 24-9).

- *Layer of submucosa.* Demonstrable everywhere in the vesical wall except in the area of the trigone.

- *Mucosal coat.* This thick coat lining the interior of the bladder is formed by several layers of transitional epithelium.

This combination of muscular architecture is responsible for the formation of the four following anatomic entities.

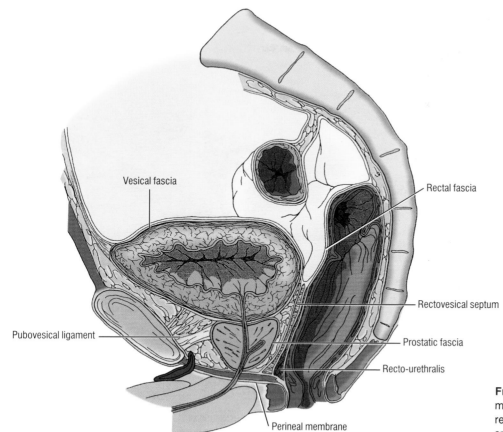

**FIG. 24-8.** The pelvic fascia of the male in median sagittal section. The rectourethralis consists of strands of smooth muscles.

Labels on figure: Vesical fascia, Rectal fascia, Rectovesical septum, Prostatic fascia, Recto-urethralis, Pubovesical ligament, Perineal membrane

---

- *Interureteric ridge* (or bar of Mercier) is formed between the right and left ureteric orifices at the interior of the urinary bladder, forming the base, or the upper boundary of the trigone of the bladder.
- *Uvula,* in men, is a projection into the posterior aspect of the internal urethral meatus at the apex of the vesical trigone, produced by the underlying trigone musculature and the median lobe of the prostate gland.
- *Pubovesical muscles* (right and left) are formed by muscular fibers arising anteriorly from the pubic bone.
- *Rectovesical muscles* (right and left) are formed by muscular fibers interconnecting the bladder and the rectum.

From a surgical standpoint, however, the muscle of the bladder is singular, and should be considered as such in the operating room. However, the reader should remember the structural and functional differences between the detrusor muscle and the musculature of the vesical trigone. According to Tanagho,[8] the bladder neck is formed by participation of the trigonal musculature, the detrusor muscle, and the urethral musculature.

Elbadawi[9] studied the pathology and pathophysiology of the detrusor in incontinence. Routine biopsy evaluation reveals its structural morphology (smooth muscle, interstitium, and intrinsic nerves).

The detrusor is an involuntary smooth muscle under the control of the parasympathetic nervous system. We agree with Malvern[10] that the musculature of the detrusor is "both embryologically and histochemically separate from that of the urethra." There is also an intrinsic innervation among the detrusor smooth muscle fibers.

Bates and colleagues[11] were the first to use the term "detrusor instability" when discussing the so-called "urgency syndrome." This condition presents with frequency of micturition, nocturia, urgency, and urge incontinence. Couillard and Webster[12] presented a table of etiological factors of this syndrome (Table 24-4).

According to Rivas and Chancellor,[13] urodynamic testing should be used for accurate evaluation of normal and abnormal functions of the urinary bladder and urethral sphincters.

### Anatomy of the Trigone

The trigone is a smooth area within the base of the blad-

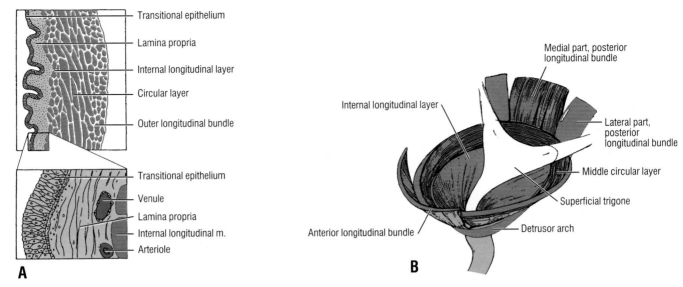

A

B

FIG. 24-9. Structure of the bladder wall. (Modified from Hinman F Jr. Atlas of Urosurgical Anatomy. Philadelphia: WB Saunders, 1993; with permission.)

der. It is bounded by three orifices: the right and left ureterovesical orifices and the internal urethral meatus at the neck of the bladder.

The trigone region is relatively indistensible. It is formed by two muscular layers — superficial and deep — located deep to the mucosa, as reported by Tanagho and Pugh.[14] This area is relatively smooth, even in the empty bladder (Fig. 24-10).

The superficial layer of the trigone is formed by longitudinal fibers of the intravesical ureter at the ureterovesical orifice that spread into the base of the urinary bladder. The final destination of some fibers is perhaps in the urethra or (in the male) in the ejaculatory ducts, contributing to the formation of the crista urethralis. In the female, however, the termination of these fibers is at the external meatus.

The deep layer of the vesical trigone, under the superficial trigone and above the detrusor muscle, is the continuation of the fibromuscular tissue around the terminal part of the ureters (sheath of Waldeyer). The bladder outlet is surrounded by the middle layer of the detrusor muscle deeply, and by the trigone superficially.

Tanagho,[8] the scholar of the subject, reported that the superficial trigone can be dissected from the deep trigone. The deep trigone can be separated from the detrusor muscle, at least in its upper half. He stated the following about the trigone, "The ureter has merely changed from a tubular to a sheet-like form. One may say that the ureter does not end at the ureteral orifice but continues uninterrupted as a flat sheet instead of a tubular structure."[8]

### Vesical Neck

The sphincteric apparatus of the vesical neck is formed by the middle circular layer of the detrusor and the anterior longitudinal bundles of the outer coat (Fig. 24-9B). However, according to Nergardh and Boreus[15] and Klück,[16] the nonstriated muscle of the neck is different from that of the detrusor. Therefore, the neck of the bladder probably acts as a separate functional entity. In the male, smooth muscle forms a complete circular collar around the preprostatic portion of the urethra. This is the internal or proximal sphincter.

In the female child, striated fibers completely surround the urethra, according to Oelrich.[17] In the adult, the sphincter muscle of the urethra is thickest on its ven-

| TABLE 24-4. Suggested Etiologic Factors in the Hyperactive Bladder |
|---|
| Neurologic disease — detrusor hyperreflexia |
| Detrusor instability |
|    Congenital |
|    Bladder outlet obstruction |
|    Aging |
|    Vesical neck patency, stress incontinence |
|    Urethral instability |
|    Psychosomatic |

*Source:* Couillard DR, Webster GD. Detrusor instability. Urol Clin North Am 1995; 22:593-612; with permission.

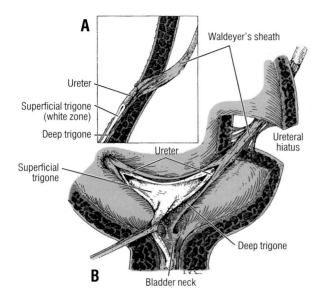

**A**

Waldeyer's sheath

Ureter

Superficial trigone
(white zone)

Deep trigone

Ureter

Ureteral
hiatus

Superficial
trigone

Deep trigone

**B**

Bladder neck

FIG. 24-10. The normal uterovesical junction and trigone. **A.** Section of the bladder wall perpendicular to the ureteral hiatus shows the oblique passage of the ureter through the detrusor and also shows the submucosal ureter with its detrusor backing. Waldeyer's sheath surrounds the prevesical ureter and extends inward to become the deep trigone. **B.** Waldeyer's sheath continues in the bladder as the deep trigone, which is fixed at the bladder neck. Smooth muscle of the ureter forms the superficial trigone and is anchored at the verumontanum. (Modified from Brooks JD. Anatomy of the lower urinary tract and male genitalia. In: Walsh PC, Retik AB, Vaughan ED Jr, Wein AJ (eds). Campbell's Urology (7th ed). Philadelphia: WB Saunders, 1998; with permission.)

tral aspect and thins as it passes to the dorsal side of the urethra. There appears to be a dorsal septum or raphe into which the fibers insert. A variable number of fibers cross the midline. Some muscle fibers run obliquely and some proximal fibers course vertically upward into the bladder musculature. This muscular coat is also infiltrated with smooth muscle fibers. Smooth muscle bundles from the bladder overlie the proximal part of the urethral sphincter.

REMEMBER:

• Striated muscle fibers form the external sphincter of the urethra. It is located within the urogenital diaphragm. Therefore it is distal to the internal sphincter, which is formed by a mixture of striated and smooth muscle in the proximal urethra.

Geppert et al.[18] reported that the obturator fascia and the internal obturator muscle may be used in a modified technique of cystourethropexy for the elevation of the vesical neck.

## Vascular Supply

### *Arteries*

The blood supply of the urinary bladder is very rich and the collateral circulation is excellent. The arteries of the bladder are the superior, middle and inferior vesical arteries. These originate from the anterior division of the internal iliac (hypogastric) artery. The obturator and inferior gluteal arteries may contribute small branches (Fig. 24-11). When present (40%), aberrant obturator arteries may contribute, variably (but in some cases by branches of significant caliber), to the vascular supply. In the female the uterine and vaginal arteries also participate in the arterial blood supply of this organ.

### *Veins*

A rich network of veins, located deep to the adventitia, surrounds the urinary bladder. The network is drained by several veins which empty into the internal iliac vein (Fig. 24-12). Variations are numerous.

Several plexuses drain into other venous networks in the space of Retzius. These networks include the plexus of Santorini (prostatovesical or pudendal plexus). This plexus receives tributaries from the perineum, particularly from the shaft of the clitoris or the penis, by way of the deep dorsal vein and the cavernous veins. These veins are not usually accompanied by arteries, except in the presence of aberrant deep or dorsal arteries of the penis/clitoris.

### *Lymphatics*

The bladder wall has three levels of lymphatic vessels: submucosal, muscular, and perivesical. All unite at the subadventitial area, then drain to the external iliac nodes through three lymphatic networks, depending on their site of origin in the bladder.

The lymphatics of the base, neck, and trigone travel upward, anterior to the insertion of the ureter, and terminate in the internal, external, and sacral nodes. The lymphatics of the anterior wall, together with prostatic lymphatics, terminate in the external iliac nodes. Remember, the obturator nodes are usually the "landing site" for the prostate (cancer, etc.), and are the most important clinically. The lymphatics of the posterior wall drain into the internal iliac nodes. In general, the lymphatic vessels follow the superior and inferior vesical arteries.

Carcinoma of the urinary bladder will metastasize to the obturator, external iliac, and occasionally the sacral nodes.

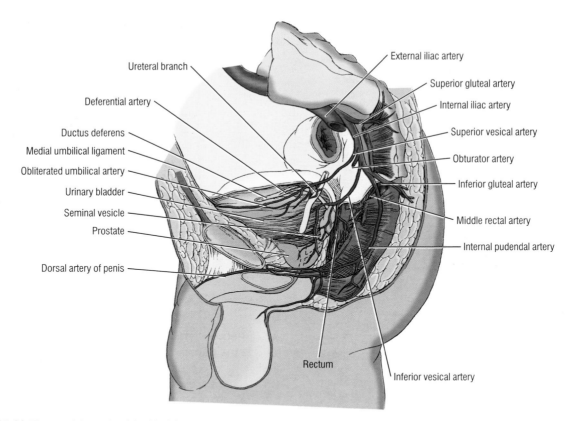

FIG. 24-11. The arterial supply of the bladder.

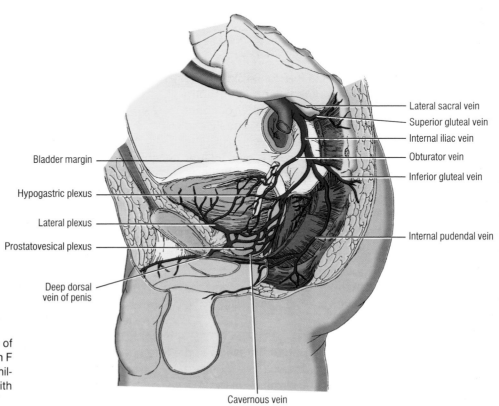

FIG. 24-12. The venous drainage of the bladder. (Modified from Hinman F Jr. Atlas of Urosurgical Anatomy. Philadelphia: WB Saunders, 1993; with permission.)

# Innervation

An excellent summary of the innervation of the urinary bladder was provided by de Groat[19]:

> *The central nervous regulation of the lower urinary tract is mediated by simple on-off switching circuits in the brain and spinal cord that are under voluntary control. Interruption of central inhibitory mechanisms can unmask primitive voiding reflexes that trigger bladder hyperactivity.*

The urinary bladder is innervated by neural fibers from the autonomic system (sympathetic system from T11 to L2, and parasympathetic system from S2 to S4) as well as from somatic nerves, from S2, S3 and S4 (pudendal nerve) and by several other routes not via the pudendal nerve.

## *Autonomic Nervous System*

### Sympathetic

Preganglionic sympathetics arise from the intermediolateral cell column at T11-L2 or at L1 and L2 forming white communicating rami which pass to the sympathetic trunk; from this the lumbar splanchnic nerves are formed. These nerves form several plexuses, such as the superior hypogastric plexus, which is the lower part of the aortic plexus (Fig. 24-13). The superior hypogastric plexus produces the right and left hypogastric nerves, which travel downward medial to the internal iliac artery and anterior to the sacral sympathetic chain. They enter the right and left inferior pelvic hypogastric plexuses close to the base of the bladder, and are responsible for the autonomic innervation of the superficial trigone musculature and the urethra.

### Parasympathetic

Preganglionic parasympathetic neurons arise in the intermediate gray of the spinal cord at S2, S3, and S4. These fibers leave the spinal cord and enter the ventral primary rami of the spinal nerves at those levels. The preganglionic neurons leave the ventral primary rami as the so-called pelvic splanchnic nerves (or nervi erigentes). The pelvic splanchnic nerves enter the right and left pelvic plexuses (Fig. 24-13) and the preganglionic fibers ultimately synapse in ganglia in the pelvic connective tissues or upon, or within, the walls of the pelvic organs, including the urinary bladder. Small islands of ganglionic cells and profuse nerve elements are distributed richly within the bladder. Postganglionic parasympathetic fibers provide motor stimulation for the detrusor musculature of the bladder.

Sensory fibers for vesical distension and other sensory modalities are carried to the sacral part of the spinal cord by way of the pelvic splanchnic nerves (Fig. 24-14). Sensory fibers for pain pass both by way of the pelvic splanchnic nerves, and by sympathetic pathways up through the pelvic, hypogastric, and preaortic plexuses to reach the sympathetic chains. Here they exit to gain access to the lower thoracic and upper lumbar segments of the cord. Because of the duality of the pathways for pain, presacral neurectomy does not materially reduce vesical pain; rather, bilateral anterolateral cordotomy may be required to attain relief.

Current thinking[20-22] regarding pain arising from pelvic viscera is that it follows the parasympathetic fibers back to the central nervous system (CNS) (S2-4) rather than following sympathetics, other than pain arising in the fundus of the uterus which is transmitted via sensory fibers which traverse the superior hypogastric plexus. (Thus the rationale for presacral neurectomy as treatment for dysmenorrhea.) Also, ovarian pain fibers accompany the arterial supply up to the origins of the gonadal arteries from the aorta; thus, such pain can be relieved by transecting the infundibulopelvic ligament containing ovarian nerves, arteries, veins, and lymphatics. Discussions of vesical pain in various references emphasize the parasympathetic pathways to the cord. In addition to the pelvic viscera, the pain fibers of the lower respiratory tract pass to the CNS by way of parasympathetic paths; pelvic splanchnic nerves carry pelvic pain and the vagi convey pain fibers of the lower respiratory tree.

## *Somatic Nerves*

Somatic neurofibers arise from the sacral cord at S2, S3, S4 (Figs. 24-13 and 24-14) and leave the ventral primary rami of those spinal nerves to form the pudendal nerve. This nerve is responsible for the innervation of the periurethral striated sphincteric apparatus that voluntarily stops urination, including the compressor urethrae muscle and the sphincter urethrae of the urogenital diaphragm and the bulbospongiosus muscle of the superficial perineal compartment. Unilateral sacrifice of sacral nerves results in little bladder or anorectal dysfunction.[23]

We quote from Fowler:[24]

> *To effect both storage and voiding, connections between the pons and the sacral spinal cord must be intact as well as the peripheral innervation which arises from the most caudal segments of the sacral cord. From there the peripheral innervation passes through the cauda equina to the sacral plexus and via the pelvic and pudendal nerves to innervate the bladder and sphincter. Thus, the innervation for physiological bladder control is extensive, requiring supra-*

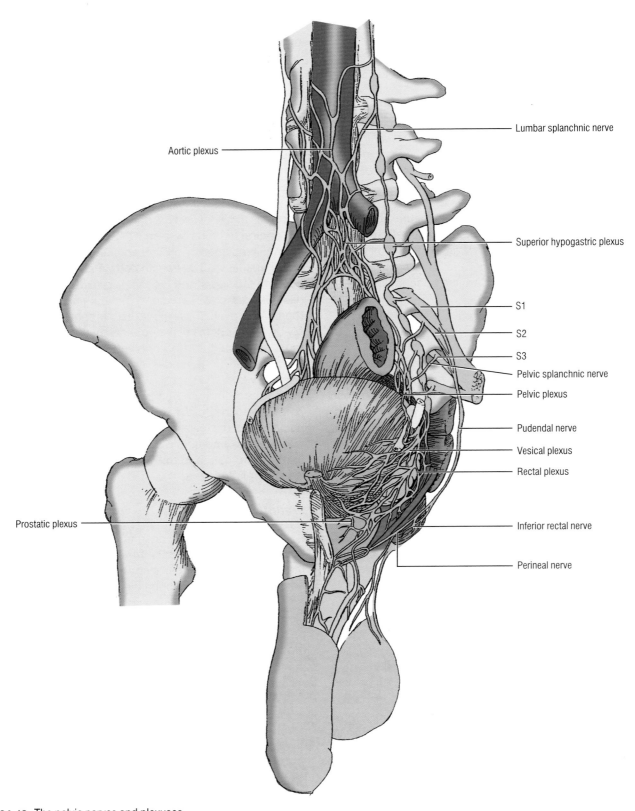

Lumbar splanchnic nerve

Aortic plexus

Superior hypogastric plexus

S1

S2

S3

Pelvic splanchnic nerve

Pelvic plexus

Pudendal nerve

Vesical plexus

Rectal plexus

Prostatic plexus

Inferior rectal nerve

Perineal nerve

FIG. 24-13. The pelvic nerves and plexuses.

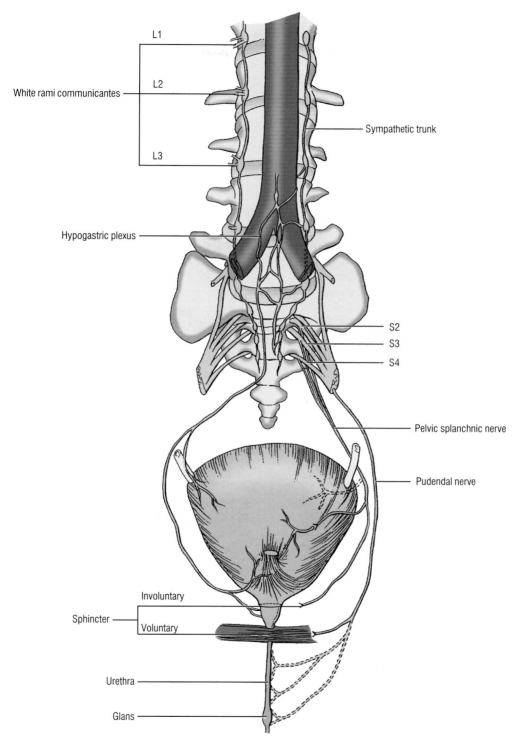

FIG. 24-14. The nerve supply of the bladder and urethra.

*pontine inputs, intact spinal spinal connections between the pons and the sacral cord, as well as intact peripheral nerves.*

REMEMBER:
- The neurophysiology of the lower urinary system is full of controversial and enigmatic speculations. It is not within the scope of this book to offer these controversial details. We present only the anatomy and surgical applications of this area, not the pathophysiology.
- The sympathetic nerves spring from the thoracolumbar portion of the spinal cord.
- The parasympathetic nerves spring from the sacral portion of the spinal cord at levels S2, S3, and S4.
- The male has two sphincteric networks. The proximal is at the bladder neck and is of smooth muscle origin. The distal is at the membranous urethra and consists of both smooth and striated muscle. The action of both networks produces the continence mechanism.
- In radical prostatectomy with removal of the bladder neck, the sphincteric apparatus of smooth muscle of the urethra may be able to control incontinence. Also, contraction of the pelvic floor probably constricts the membranous urethra.[25]
- The female has only one sphincteric network, at the bladder neck and proximal urethra, perhaps at the vesicourethral junction.
- The proximal half of the urethra is above the pelvic floor. Therefore, abdominal pressure compresses this part of the urethra. The pelvic floor relaxes voluntarily, producing a voluntary relaxation of the fibers of the external urethral sphincter.

## *Higher Level Representation*

According to Waxman,[26] micturation is mediated by the spinal cord, "but descending pathways from the brain modify, inhibit, or initiate the reflexes" (Fig. 24-15). Cortical representation of the urinary bladder is most likely present in the paracentral lobule, whose stimulation may evoke bladder contraction. Other higher levels may be present, but their identity and nature of participation are obscure. Whether this system initiates relaxation or contraction of the external sphincter in starting or stopping micturition is not known.

To initiate urination the person should be able to voluntarily relax the perineal muscles. The perineal muscles are:
- Levator ani
- Sphincter and compressor urethrae
- Bulbospongiosus (in the male)

The following muscles initiate voluntary contraction after urination:

- Ischiocavernosus
- Bulbospongiosus
- External sphincter

REMEMBER:
- The sympathetic trunk may bifurcate or trifurcate as it descends through the abdomen and pelvis. Branches may descend in the psoas-vertebral groove.
- Afferent fibers within the pudendal nerve convey sensation from the external sphincter and the posterior urethra.
- The internal sphincter is innervated by the autonomic nervous system. The external sphincter is supplied by the pudendal nerve, with skeletal motor fibers arising from the ventral horn of cord levels S2-S3-S4.

In the male, the rarely paralyzed internal sphincter is continuous with the smooth muscle of the trigone and the ureteric muscle. It is innervated by the sympathetic fibers from the hypogastric plexus. The external sphincter is innervated by the pudendal nerve (voluntary action) and is rarely affected by disease. If it is divided by surgery, incontinence results.

In the female, for all practical purposes the internal sphincter is continuous with the compressor urethra and urethrovaginal sphincter distally. These several muscular entities are inadequate to maintain urinary continence unless the bladder and urethra are supported. Without proper angulation of the urethra, incontinence results.

- Bladder dysfunction, failure of ejaculation, and impotence may result from injury to sympathetic and parasympathetic nerves during separation of the posterior wall of the rectum from the sacrum. The scissors and the palm of the dissecting hand must stay close to the wall of the rectum to avoid the nerves during mobilization of the anorectum.
- In males with retroperitoneal lymphadenopathy or undergoing bilateral sympathectomy, one should remove the sympathetic ganglionic segment at the L1 level only unilaterally. Clinically the left side is more important than the right side. Preserve the left if you can, and be more careful with it. This procedure will avoid failure of ejaculation and sterility, because the ductus deferens, ejaculatory duct, seminal vesical, and urethra are under sympathetic control. The second, third, and fourth lumbar ganglia can be removed bilaterally without disturbance of sexual function.
- Be sure to protect the genitofemoral nerve and the iliohypogastric nerves during lumbar sympathectomy.
- To maintain urinary continence, a synergistic action should take place between the sphincter of the bladder neck and the proximal urethral sphincter. The striated distal urethral

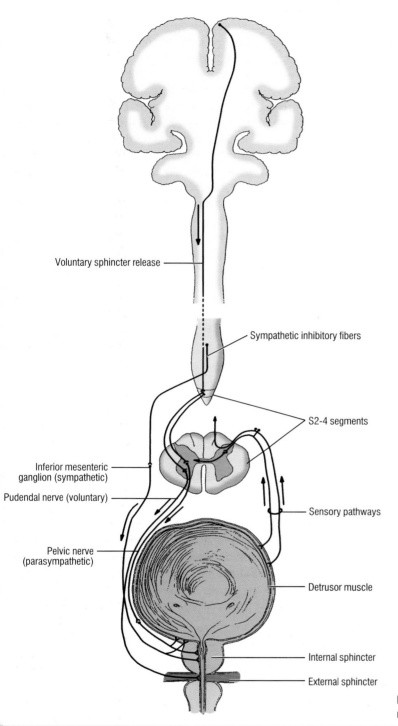

Voluntary sphincter release

Sympathetic inhibitory fibers

S2-4 segments

Inferior mesenteric ganglion (sympathetic)

Pudendal nerve (voluntary)

Sensory pathways

Pelvic nerve (parasympathetic)

Detrusor muscle

Internal sphincter

External sphincter

**FIG. 24-15.** Descending pathway and innervation of the urinary bladder.

sphincter (external), which is innervated by the pudendal nerve, prevents urination. Total, or stress incontinence will be produced by inactivation of these sphincters. In a large number of patients, the etiology of urge incontinence cannot be determined. They are classified as having idiopathic bladder disorder.

- Surgical treatment of intrinsic urethral dysfunction can be accomplished by use of injectable fat[27] or collagen or by sling procedures.[28] Pharmacologic treatment is based on the distribution of cholinergic receptors and

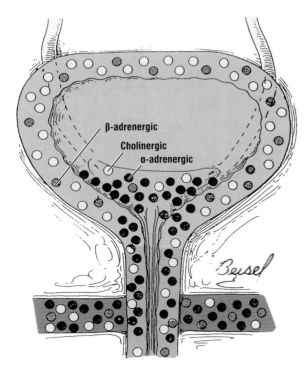

β-adrenergic
Cholinergic
α-adrenergic

Beisel

**FIG. 24-16.** Adrenergic and cholinergic receptor distribution in the bladder, urethra, and pelvic floor musculature. (Modified from Bellinger MF. Myelomeningocele and neuropathic bladder. In: Gillenwater JY, Grayhack JT, Howards SS, Duckett JW. Adult and Pediatric Urology (3rd ed). St. Louis: Mosby, 1996; with permission.)

α and β adrenergic receptors (Fig. 24-16).[29]
- The act of voiding has been difficult to study and early descriptions have blended a few known facts with an excess of imaginative conjecture. Recent studies have used elegant tracing techniques to examine the precise course of central nerve pathways and neural projections. These studies have helped to define the neuroanatomy of the central mechanisms that control bladder and urethral function in animals. Comparative anatomy and non-invasive imaging of human subjects have provided further evidence that would support a unifying concept for the anatomy of micturition.
- Bladder paragangliomas present with hypertensive attacks precipitated by micturition and hematuria. Demirkesen et al.[30] presented a case of bladder paraganglioma at pregnancy causing early preeclampsia.

## Neurogenic (Unstable) Bladder

As Abrams[31] stated, "The unstable bladder is well recognized, yet poorly understood." We quote from Freeman and Malvern:[32]

*The unstable bladder (or unstable detrusor) has been defined by the International Continence Society as one that has been shown objectively to contract (spontaneously or on provocation) during the filling phase while the patient is attempting to inhibit micturation. Unstable detrusor contractions may be asymptomatic or may be interpreted as a normal desire to void. The presence of these contractions does not necessarily imply a neurological disorder. Unstable contractions are usually phasic in type... A gradual increase in detrusor pressure without subsequent decrease is best regarded as a change of compliance.*

Neurogenic (neuropathic) bladder is found most commonly in children with meningomyelocele. The neural and bony abnormalities vary in meningomyelocele, and accordingly, the types of neurogenic bladder vary also. Most common is a lax sphincter with poorly contracting or non-contracting detrusor.

More ominous is the bladder in which there is a hyperactive detrusor and a sphincter that operates out of synch, often closing more tightly during detrusor contraction. This condition is called detrusor/sphincter dyssynergia. Elevated bladder pressure places the patient's upper tracts at great risk. Treating children for most neurogenic bladders involves using clean intermittent catheterization with or without anticholinergics/smooth muscle relaxants.

Although many classification systems for neuropathic bladder exist,[29] practically speaking there are two types. An *efferent bladder* is a hypertonic bladder with small capacity, presumably due to lack of inhibition from higher levels upon lower spinal cord segments. An *afferent bladder* is a hypotonic bladder of large capacity.

Some authors present "atonic" as a third type of neurogenic bladder. However, this is not a neurogenic bladder, but a condition secondary to long-standing obstruction.

### Efferent (Spastic) Neurogenic Bladder

The characteristics of efferent or spastic neurogenic bladder are:
- Tone is elevated
- Sensation is present
- Moderate distention produces pain
- Intravesical pressure is elevated

The patient reports the following symptoms regarding urination:
- Uncontrollable sense of need
- Frequency
- Urge incontinence
- Nocturia

Studies of patients with efferent (spastic) neurogenic bladder show that they may desire to void with the first or second filling (50 ml to 100 ml) of fluid[33] (Fig. 24-17). Moderate distention of the bladder causes severe pain. This type of bladder is commonly associated with disorders involving the pyramidal tracts. Lesions involving a single pyramidal tract have been alleged as causative factors in the production of hypertonic bladders. The internal sphincter slowly also becomes hypertonic, but not enough to withstand the effect of the hypertonic detrusor, which becomes more spastic. Dribbling and, perhaps, incontinence result.

Perhaps the production of spastic neurogenic bladder is responsible for the lack of inhibition from levels above to lower spinal cord levels. Treatment involves the use of anticholinergics or smooth muscle relaxants that act distal to the neuromuscular junction (e.g. oxybutynin).

## *Afferent (Flaccid) Neurogenic Bladder*

The filling capacity of afferent or flaccid neurogenic bladder is tremendous. Sensation is present but hyposensitivity produces a delay in stimulation to empty the bladder. It therefore empties by reflex, as in newborn infants. The pressure of the internal sphincter remains normal, but there is an inability to relax and the detrusor muscle is hypotonic due to some atrophy.

Patients with afferent (flaccid) neurogenic bladder can tolerate a volume of up to 2 liters of fluid, added in 50 ml quantities[33] (Fig. 24-18). Desire to void, distress, and pain are produced only when greater than usual amounts of fluid have been added. Hyposensitivity, or complete lack of sensitivity, can be associated with the problem, in which case the desire to void may not occur until after introduction of 500 ml. Distress and severe pain may be delayed until the bladder volume reaches 800 ml.

Internal sphincter pressure remains normal, irrespective of the presence of a hypotonic detrusor muscle. The voluntary abdominal muscles are therefore frequently required to facilitate micturition. This type of bladder is associated with disorders affecting the afferent pathway (end organs, posterior roots, or posterior spinal columns). Hyposensitivity of the bladder may lead to delayed awareness of the need to empty the bladder. Atrophy of the detrusor muscle, resulting from prolonged overdistention, plus inability of the internal sphincter to relax at the proper time may result.[33] Treatment for this problem may involve intermittent catheterization, Foley catheter, or a suprapubic tube. Urinary diversion with simple cystectomy will avoid later complications of a retained nonfunctioning bladder.[34]

Treatments for children with neurogenic bladder in-

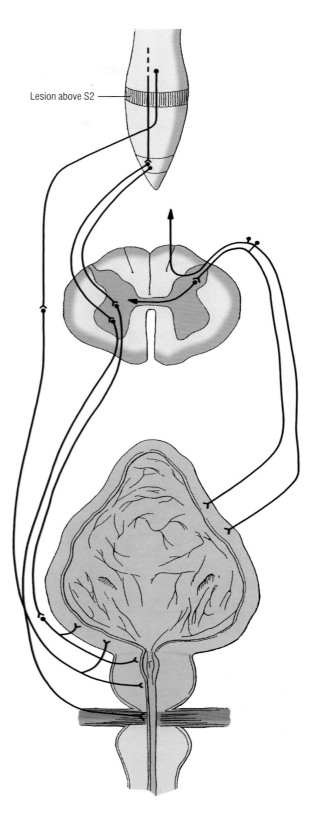

**FIG. 24-17.** Spastic neurogenic bladder, caused by a more or less complete transection of the spinal cord above S-2. Function may return with recovery from spinal shock.

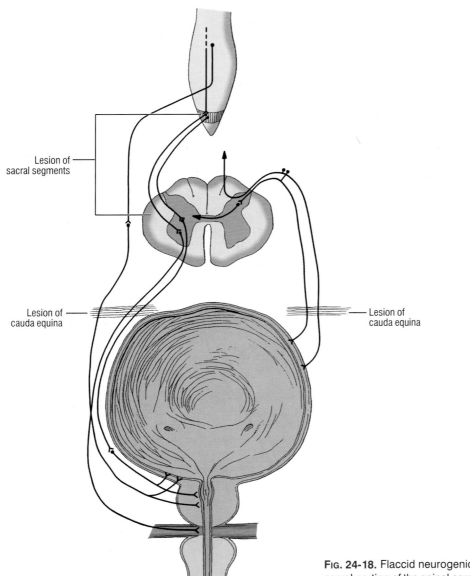

**Fig. 24-18.** Flaccid neurogenic bladder, caused by a lesion of either the sacral portion of the spinal cord or the cauda equina.

Lesion of
sacral segments

Lesion of
cauda equina

Lesion of
cauda equina

clude artificial urinary sphincter creation[35] and augmentation cystoplasty with clean intermittent self-catheterization.[36] However, Bertschy and colleagues[37] caution that complications associated with intestinal mucosa in the bladder occur with some frequency with enterocystoplasty for bladder augmentation.

## HISTOLOGY AND PHYSIOLOGY

Transitional epithelium lines the bladder. The color of the mucosa varies. When the bladder is empty, the color is red. When it is full, the color is pale.

We quote the excellent summary of Lewis[38] on the histology and physiology of the bladder epithelium:

*The mammalian urinary bladder epithelium (urothelium) performs the important function of storing urine for extended periods, while maintaining the urine composition similar to that delivered by the kidneys. The urothelium possesses four properties to perform this function. First, it offers a minimum epithelial surface area-to-urine volume; this reduces the surface area for passive movement of substance between lumen and blood. Second, the passive permeability of the apical membrane and tight junctions is very low to electrolytes and non-electrolytes. Third, the urothelium has a hormonally regulated sodium absorptive system; thus passive movement of sodium from blood to urine is countered by active sodium reabsorption. Last, the permeability properties of the apical membrane and tight junctions of the urothelium are not altered by most substances found in the urine or blood. The importance of the barrier function of the urothelium is illustrated by infectious cystitis. The loss of barrier function results in the movement of urinary constituents into the lamina propria and underlying muscle layers, resulting in suprapubic and lower back pain and frequent, urgent, and painful voiding.*

The nature of the vesical mucosa allows the bladder to expand. The mucosa becomes flattened when the bladder is full of urine. When the bladder is empty it becomes multilaminar, or wrinkled. However, the area at the trigone is always flat and smooth because it is fixed to the musculature below. The musculature of the trigone region is apparently continuous with the musculature of the ureters, and is thus predominantly under control of sympathetic neural innervation. The detrusor muscle is under parasympathetic control.

The mucosa of the urinary bladder is continuous superiorly with the mucosal lining of the ureters and is likewise continuous inferiorly with the mucosa of the urethra. It is believed that continence and urination are regulated by the musculature organized about the vesical neck, preprostatic muscular portion of the male urethra, and levator ani musculature. In addition the musculature includes vectors of urethral supporting tissues and the sphincteric musculature of the urogenital diaphragm. In other words, the pubococcygeus of the pelvic diaphragm which supports the vesical neck of the urinary bladder may, perhaps, be responsible for the relaxation of the neck since it moves the neck downward and relaxes the urethrae. Nonetheless, the histology and anatomy of the trigonal region and the precise mechanisms controlling both urinary continence and voluntary micturition are enigmatic, complex, and not yet fully understood.

Additional histologic information on the bladder was presented previously in this chapter under the heading "Bladder Wall."

The pathophysiology of the normal bladder is enigmatic and ill understood. The urinary bladder has a dual physiologic destiny:
- To act as a reservoir for urine — a very simple act. The bladder receives the urine from the ureters.
- To contract and expel the urine to the urethra — a complex procedure. This involves the innervation of the urinary bladder and the production of the micturition reflex. The detrusor muscle contracts and the urethral resistance falls.

From the physiologic standpoint, is the parasympathetic nervous system a fellow traveler of the somatic nervous system? Most likely yes.

## SURGERY OF THE URINARY BLADDER

## Indications

Many conditions and problems of the urinary bladder require surgery or other treatment. We present a few.

### Surgery for Bladder Exstrophy

Kasat and Borwankar[39] presented eleven important factors for successful primary closure in staged reconstruction of bladder exstrophy:
- Proper patient selection
- Staged approach
- Anterior approximation of pubic bones with placement of bladder and urethra in true pelvis
- Posterior bilateral iliac osteotomies in all indicated cases
- Double-layered closure of the bladder
- Two weeks of proper ureteric catheter drainage
- Prevention of infection
- Prolonged and proper postoperative immobilization
- Prompt treatment of bladder prolapse
- Prevention of postoperative abdominal distension
- Ruling out of bladder outlet obstruction before removal of bladder catheter

Females with exstrophy/epispadias demonstrate anterior displacement of the bladder, urethra, and vagina with lack of development of anterior pelvic floor musculature. Kropp and Cheng[40] recommend total urogenital complex mobilization to normal anatomical position.

### Bladder Injuries

Small retroperitoneal perforations of the bladder usually heal with only prolonged Foley catheter drainage. However, larger retroperitoneal injuries or perforations involving the dome of the bladder, which leak urine into the peritoneal cavity, require open surgical repair and extravesical drainage, in addition to prolonged Foley catheter drainage. Gravity cystogram should be performed prior to removal of the Foley catheter to exclude persistent urinary extravasation.

The absence of pelvic fluid on a trauma CT scan indicates that bladder rupture is unlikely, but Pao et al.[41] caution that a passively distended opacified bladder may be injured despite an absence of extravasated contrast material.

### Bladder Fistulas

Bladder fistulas are of the following types: enteric, colonic, vaginal, uteral, and cutaneous. All may be the result of inflammatory or neoplastic process, traumatic or iatrogenic.

Iatrogenic and traumatic bladder fistulas may be repaired immediately or delayed by 4 to 6 months to permit resolution of inflammation and edema. When repair is performed, the involved portion of the bladder and a small circumferential ring of normal tissue should be excised. The bladder should be closed in non-overlapping layers with absorbable suture. If possible, omentum or other vascularized tissue should be interposed between the fistula repair and the surrounding structures. Prolonged extravesical drainage and Foley catheter should be performed.

### Lithiasis

Bladder calculi can be treated by performing an open cystotomy and stone removal or by an endoscopic approach. If the latter is used, the surgeon may use a manual lithotrite to crush the stone into small fragments or an electrohydrolic, laser, or ultrasonic lithotriptor.

## Procedures

The three most important surgical procedures for the urinary bladder are cystoscopy, partial cystectomy, and total (radical) cystectomy. The last two are utilized for malignancy.

### Cystoscopy

Endoscopic evaluation of the bladder may be performed using a rigid or flexible cystoscope. Rigid cystoscopy has the advantage of a wide, clearer image. However, the flexible cystoscope is much more comfortable, especially in men, and permits better visualization of the dome and around an enlarged prostate. If performed in a gentle fashion, the majority of diagnostic cystoscopies can be done in the office.

Transurethral removal of noninvasive bladder cancer is performed for histologic study and curative resection of tumors that do not invade the detrusor muscle. Holzbeierlein and Smith[42] caution that there is a high rate of new tumor occurrence.

### Partial Cystectomy

Most bladder tumors are resected transurethrally using a resectoscope. Open partial cystectomy is indicated for superficial tumors that are too large to excise transurethrally or are in a bladder diverticulum. If partial cystectomy is being performed for an invasive tumor, it should be located in the dome so that a 1 cm margin of normal tissue can be circumferentially resected, and the remainder of the bladder should be free of other tumor. Typically, partial cystectomy can be performed using a retroperitoneal approach. The bladder should be entered at a site a few centimeters away from the tumor. The excised surgical specimen should be labeled and sent for frozen section histologic analysis to exclude positive margins. The bladder is closed in layers with absorbable suture. Prolonged extravesical drainage and Foley catheter are required.

Bladder augmentation ureterocystoplasty using the lower part of an extremely dilated megaureter was reported by Perovic et al.[43] Function of the ipsilateral kidney was preserved.

### Total (Radical) Cystectomy

Primary radical cystectomy is considered the standard for care of organ-confined muscle invasive bladder cancer.[44] Leissner and colleagues[45] recommend extensive lymphadenectomy as a potentially curative procedure for invasive bladder cancer, and state the need for a standardized lymph node resection.

In males, the procedure used is cystoprostatectomy in conjunction with urinary diversion. Complete removal of the prostate prevents residual disease in patients at higher risk for a second malignancy such as an unsuspected prostate cancer.[46] In females, the procedure is anterior exenteration (hysterectomy and bilateral removal of tubes and ovaries) along with urinary diversion.

Whittlestone and Persad[47] state that the ileal conduit is considered the "gold standard" following cystectomy. Tainio et al.[48] caution that a gastric segment should never be used as a conduit in the urinary tract.

### Laparoscopic Surgery

Denewer et al.[49] reported encouraging results using laparoscopic-assisted cystectomy and lymphadenectomy to treat 10 patients with carcinoma of the urinary bladder.

They emphasized, however, that the technique needs further modifications and refinements.

# Incisions

A midline incision or a Pfannenstiel incision is excellent for surgery of the urinary bladder (and, as a matter of fact, for any pelvic surgery). Redman[50] beautifully described the various incisions used.

Lower anterior abdominal wall incisions are of 3 types:
- Midline lower
- Lateral lower
- Transverse lower (Pfannenstiel)

The above incisions allow the surgeon several options.
- Entry and exploration of the peritoneal cavity
- After elevating the peritoneum, exploration of the retroperitoneal space, together with thin or thick vesicoumbilical connective tissue

The surgical anatomy for the incisions is covered in the chapter on the abdominal wall.

## Surgical Applications

This is not a book of technique; its emphasis is on surgical anatomy. In radical cystectomy for both males and females, the surgeon should have good knowledge of the anatomy of the following:
- Incision
- Pelvic lymphatics
- Iliac arteries and veins
- Peritoneal reflections
- Pelvic ureter
- Bladder and its ligamentous supports
- Rectum
- Deep dorsal vein of penis/clitoris
- Urethra

# ANATOMIC COMPLICATIONS OF RADICAL CYSTECTOMY

We present in detail the anatomic complications only of radical cystectomy. The excellent chapter of Lieber[51] in the book of Smith and Ehrlich and several other sources form the basis of this presentation.

In the majority of cases, urologic surgery is the surgery of older people. Lieber re-emphasizes the old axiom, "Elderly and poor-risk patients tolerate one major op-

eration very well, but they tolerate major complications and reoperation very poorly."[51]

We will discuss the following anatomic complications of radical cystectomy:
- Bleeding of arterial or venous origin
- Nerve injury
- Rectal injury
- Impotence
- Urinary incontinence
- Vaginal cuff complications
- Urinary diversion complications
- Wound dehiscence

## Bleeding of Arterial or Venous Origin

The common iliac artery, the external and internal iliacs, their branches, and their corresponding veins are responsible for bleeding in radical cystectomy. Clear delineation of the great vessels helps the ligation procedure of the small vessels toward the bladder. The internal iliacs can be temporarily occluded bilaterally or ligated permanently if the vascular supply to the gluteal region is protected (Fig. 24-19).

Bilateral ligation of the internal iliac arteries furnishes eight major pathways of collateral circulation. The very rich collateral circulation follows:
- Uterine artery with ovarian artery from the aorta
- Middle rectal artery with superior rectal artery from the inferior mesenteric
- Obturator artery with inferior epigastric from the external iliac
- Inferior gluteal with circumflex and perforating branches of the deep femoral
- Iliolumbar with lumbar branch from the aorta
- Lateral sacral with middle sacral from the aorta
- Anastomoses between vessels of the bladder wall and abdominal wall
- Anastomoses between the internal and external pudendal arteries

It is advisable to ligate the internal iliac artery distal to the origin of its posterior division, because it is the origin for the superior gluteal artery. This avoids postoperative gluteal pains secondary to ischemia (buttocks angina).

REMEMBER:
- In some cases the internal iliac artery has no distinct posterior division and one must search for the superior gluteal artery. It is also advisable for the surgeon to prepare, isolate, and ligate the arteries and veins that provide the blood supply of the urinary bladder.
- The three vesical arteries originate from the anterior division of the internal iliac artery. The vesical veins are

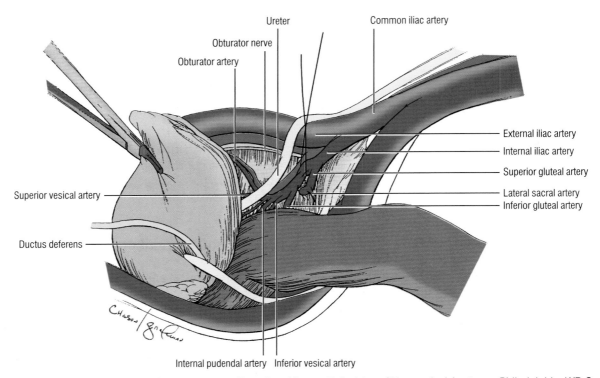

FIG. 24-19. Ligation of anterior pedicles for cystectomy. (Based on Hinman F Jr. Atlas of Urosurgical Anatomy. Philadelphia: WB Saunders, 1993.)

easily visible, because they are located in the same plane as the arteries. Lieber[51] advised the surgeon not to drift too far laterally in order to avoid the internal iliac vein.

- To avoid further bleeding, the ideal plane should be established between the bladder and the rectum. This plane is between the seminal vesicles and the rectum, ventral to the anterior lamina of the fascial septum of Denonvilliers. Therefore this blind procedure should be done slowly and carefully to avoid producing a false pathway between the seminal vesicles and the bladder.
- Another source of bleeding can be the deep dorsal vein of the penis and the plexus of Santorini.[52] Careful dissection of the vein as it passes over the bladder neck at the apex and ligation of its three branches are necessary. The venous plexuses can be exposed and ligated close to the incised endopelvic fascia near the pelvic side wall, and far away from the bladder and prostate.

## Nerve Injury

Because the surgeon normally avoids the lateral pelvic wall, the obturator is the only nerve open to injury; even

then it is only injured on very rare occasions. This nerve can be palpated by introducing the index finger into the retropubic space under the pubic ramus just lateral to the pubic symphysis. The surgeon will feel a cordlike formation containing the nerve and the obturator vessels (Figs. 24-20, 24-21). The obturator canal can be palpated with ease in many cases, helping one locate the obturator nerve and vessels.

Injury to the obturator nerve produces severe disability of the lower extremity by paralyzing the adductor muscles. Because we do not know the results of neurorrhaphy, use very careful dissection during pelvic lymphadenectomy.

## Rectal Injury

To avoid rectal injury, dissect away from the rectal wall. This may not be an option if the patient has had previous radiation because radiation often results in heavy fixation of the bladder and rectum. Therefore, preparation of the bowel with enemas and antibiotics is essential. If laceration is recognized in the operating room, closure in two or three layers with non-absorbable interrupted sutures will suffice. Occasionally, a sigmoid diverting colostomy will be necessary.

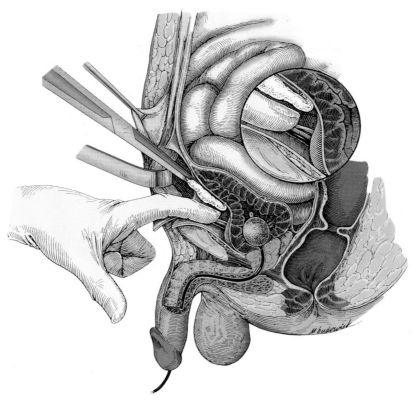

**FIG. 24-20.** A finger introduced into the retropubic space identifies the structures entering the obturator foramen. (Modified from Skandalakis LJ, Gadacz TR, Mansberger AR Jr, Mitchell WE Jr, Colborn GL, Skandalakis JE. Modern Hernia Repair: The Embryological and Anatomical Basis of Surgery. New York: Parthenon, 1996; with permission.)

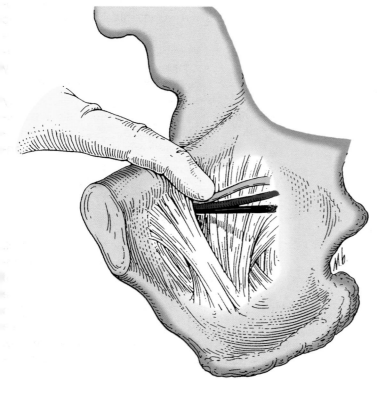

**FIG. 24-21.** Medial view of the right pelvis. The finger is inserted into the retropubic space under the pubic ramus just lateral to the pubic symphysis. A cordlike formation containing the obturator nerve, artery, and vein can be felt. The nerve appears as a shiny silver cord. (Modified from Skandalakis LJ, Gadacz TR, Mansberger AR Jr, Mitchell WE Jr, Colborn GL, Skandalakis JE. Modern Hernia Repair: The Embryological and Anatomical Basis of Surgery. New York: Parthenon, 1996; with permission.)

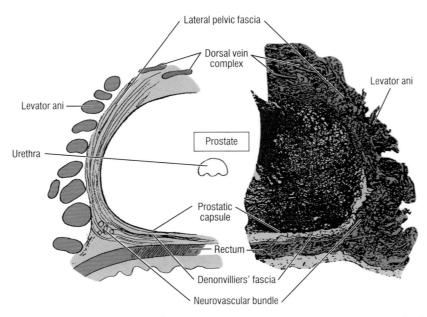

**FIG. 24-22.** Cross section through an adult prostate demonstrating the anatomic relations between the lateral pelvic fascia, Denonvilliers' fascia, and the neurovascular bundle. (Modified from Walsh PC, Lepor H, Eggleston JC. Radical prostatectomy with preservation of sexual function: anatomical and pathological considerations. Prostate 1983;4:473-485; with permission.)

## Impotence

To prevent impotence following radical cystectomy, the surgeon should preserve the autonomic plexus at the pelvic side walls by staying close to the seminal vesicles. Walsh et al.[53] developed this nerve-sparing technique. They were able to prevent injury to the nerves innervating the corpora by locating the neurovascular bundle between the lateral pelvic fascia and Denonvilliers' fascia (Figs. 24-22 to 24-25). For all practical purposes, the neural bundle is located within the envelope of endopelvic fascia adjacent to the posterolateral aspects of the prostate gland bilaterally.

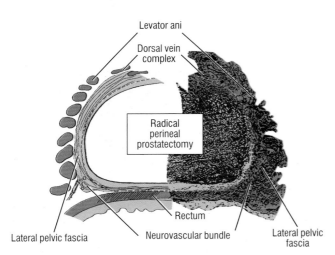

**FIG. 24-23.** The surgical plane employed in radical prostatectomy (dashed blue line indicates incision). (Modified from Walsh PC, Lepor H, Eggleston JC. Radical prostatectomy with preservation of sexual function: anatomical and pathological considerations. Prostate 1983;4:473-485; with permission.)

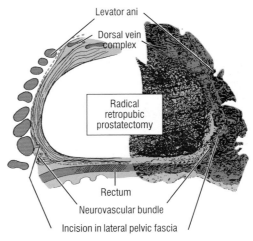

**FIG. 24-24.** The surgical plane employed in radical retropubic prostatectomy, indicating the site for incision (dashed blue line) in the lateral pelvic fascia which avoids injury to the neurovascular bundle. (Modified from Walsh PC, Lepor H, Eggleston JC. Radical prostatectomy with preservation of sexual function: anatomical and pathological considerations. Prostate 1983;4:473-485; with permission.)

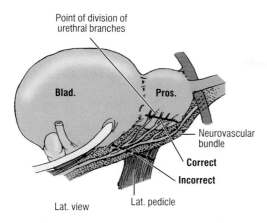

Point of division of
urethral branches

Blad.

Pros.

Neurovascular
bundle

**Correct**

**Incorrect**

Lat. pedicle

Lat. view

FIG. 24-25. The correct site for ligation of the lateral pedicle. (Modified from Walsh PC, Lepor H, Eggleston JC. Radical prostatectomy with preservation of sexual function: anatomical and pathological considerations. Prostate 1983;4:473-485; with permission.)

The student of radical cystoprostatectomy should study in detail the excellent work of Walsh and colleagues.[52-56] The apex of the prostate should be dissected very carefully, thereby avoiding injury to the neurovascular pedicle. Remember that the cavernous nerves have a posterolateral pathway in relation to the membranous urethra during their penetration of the urogenital diaphragm, where they pass laterally to reach the crura of the corpora cavernosa penis.

## Urinary Incontinence

In the male, the external sphincter circles the membranous urethra (Fig. 24-26). Avoid incontinence after radical prostatocystectomy by saving the sphincter when possible. In the female the external sphincter is located at the midurethral segment, where a horseshoe-shaped formation of striated muscle, the compressor urethra, is pre-

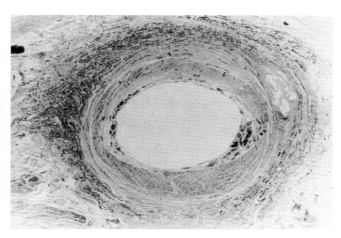

FIG. 24-26. Histologic section of the membranous urethra of a normal adult male shows the distribution of the smooth intrinsic musculature in the urethral wall, with circular fiber orientation. It is surrounded by an equally thick intrinsic coat of striated muscle fibers, essentially omega-shaped, with a defect in the midline posteriorly where it inserts in the perineal body. Note that the external sphincter constitutes an integral part of the musculature of the urethral wall at the level of the membranous urethra. (From Tanagho EA. Anatomy of the lower urinary tract. In: Walsh PC, Retik AB, Stamey TA, Vaughan ED Jr. (eds). Campbell's Urology (6th ed). Philadelphia: WB Saunders, 1992; with permission.)

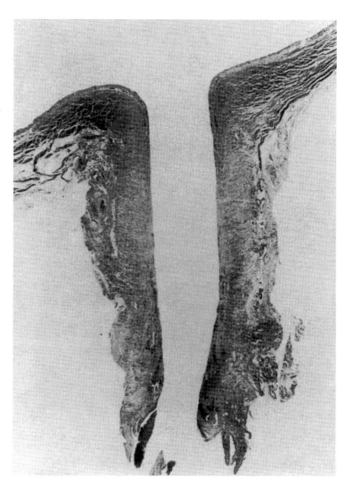

FIG. 24-27. Sagittal sections of the entire female urethra from the internal to the external meatus. Note the muscular nature of the entire urethral tube except at its most distal end, which is fibrous and opens to the outside at the level of the vaginal vestibule. The inner longitudinal fibers are embedded in dense collagen, whereas fibers constitute the bulk of the musculature of the urethral canal from the level of the internal meatus all the way down to the external meatus, as a direct continuation of the outer longitudinal fibers of the bladder wall. (From Tanagho EA, Smith DR. Mechanism of urinary continence. J Urol 1968;100:640-646; with permission.)

sent in continuity with the urethral musculature and the sphincter urethrovaginalis (Fig. 24-27).[17] Tanagho[8] stated that urodynamically this external female sphincter "shows its significance."

The complication of urinary incontinence resulting from radical cystectomy depends upon the proper management of the membranous urethra. Several techniques of neobladder construction exist. The surgeon should use the one with which he or she is familiar. The surgeon should also try to save as much of the urethra as possible if the urethra is not involved with a tumor.

## Vaginal Cuff Complications

When the bladder, urethra, and anterior vaginal wall are removed, a good closure of the defect will avoid leakage of the peritoneal contents or possible enteric contents secondary to small bowel fistula. The advice of Lieber[51] is to close the anterior vaginal wall distally or longitudinally, or perhaps to separate the posterior vaginal wall from the rectum, bringing it in an anteroposterior direction to close the defect. Absorbable suture should be used. The vaginal cuff can be closed with interrupted absorbable sutures to prevent the occurrence of hernias, but not closed watertight, so as to permit drainage of blood and urine. As for enteric fistulas, simple resection and closure after separation from the bladder is the procedure of choice. Colostomy or bowel resection is done in rare cases.

## Urinary Diversion Complications

A loop of small or large bowel can be used for neobladder formation. Therefore, the surgeon should be extremely careful to produce a good pouch with good blood supply and a perfect ureteroenteric anastomosis. Avoid kinking of ureters and twisting of the bowel which can produce intestinal obstruction or intestinal leakage.

## Wound Dehiscence

Good, intelligent, careful anatomic closure of the abdominal wall is the procedure of choice (see "Incisions" under "Surgery of the Urinary Bladder").

## REFERENCES

1. Hamilton, WJ, Mossman, HW. Hamilton, Boyd and Mossman's Human Embryology (4th ed). Baltimore: Williams & Wilkins, 1972.

2. Kelalis PP, King LR, Belman AB. Clinical Pediatric Urology. Philadelphia: WB Saunders, 1992.

3. Larsen WJ. Human Embryology (2nd ed). New York: Churchill Livingstone, 1997.

4. Moore KL, Persaud TVN. The Developing Human (5th ed). Philadelphia: WB Saunders, 1993.

5. Skandalakis JE, Gray SW. Embryology for Surgeons (2nd ed). Baltimore: Williams & Wilkins, 1994.

6. Gastol P, Baka-Jakubiak M, Skobejko-Wlodarska L, Szymkiewicz C. Complete duplication of the bladder, urethra, vagina, and uterus in girls. Urology 2000;55:578-581.

7. Basmajian JV, Slonecker CE. Grant's Method of Anatomy (11th ed). Baltimore: Williams & Wilkins, 1989.

8. Tanagho EA. Anatomy of the lower urinary tract. In: Walsh PC, Retik AB, Stamey TA, Vaughan ED Jr. (eds). Campbell's Urology (6th ed). Philadelphia: WB Saunders, 1992.

9. Elbadawi A. Pathology and pathophysiology of detrusor in incontinence. Urol Clin North Am 1995;22:499-512.

10. Malvern J. The anatomy and physiology of the unstable bladder. In: Freeman RM, Malvern J (eds). The Unstable Bladder. Boston: Wright, 1989, p. 5-9.

11. Bates CP, Whiteside G, Turner Warwick RT. Synchronous cine/pressure/flow cystourethrography with special reference to stress and urge incontinence. Br J Urol 1970;42:714.

12. Couillard DR, Webster GD. Detrusor instability. Urol Clin North Am 1995;22:593-612.

13. Rivas DA, Chancellor MB. Neurogenic vesical dysfunction. Urol Clin North Am 1995;22:579-591.

14. Tanagho EA, Pugh RCB. The anatomy and function of the uterovesical junction. Br J Urol 1963;35:154.

15. Nergardh A, Boreus LO. Autonomic receptor function in the lower urinary tract of man and cat. Scand J Urol Nephrol 1972; 6: 32-36.

16. Klück P. The autonomic innervation of the human urinary bladder, bladder neck and urethra: a histochemical study. Anat Rec 1980; 198:439-447.

17. Oelrich TM. The striated urogenital sphincter muscle in the female. Anat Rec 1983;205:223-232.

18. Geppert MK, Geppert JJ, Hirsch HA. Anatomy and tensile strength of the internal obturator muscle in the framework of a modified technic of the Marshall-Marchetti-Krantz operation. [German] Geburtshilfe Frauenheilkd 42(12):892-894, 1982.

19. de Groat WC. Anatomy of the central neural pathways controlling the lower urinary tract. Eur Urol 1998;34 (Suppl 1):2-5.

20. Dyson M (ed). Urinary system. In: Williams PL (ed). Gray's Anatomy (38th ed). New York: Churchill Livingstone, 1995, p. 1841.

21. Rosse C, Gaddum-Rosse P. Hollinshead's Textbook of Anatomy (5th ed). Philadelphia: Lippincott-Raven, 1997, p. 668.

22. Brodal P. The Central Nervous System, Structure and Function (2nd ed). New York: Oxford University Press, 1998, p. 522.

23. Nakai S, Yoshizawa H, Kobayashi S, Maeda K, Okamura Y. Anorectal and bladder function after sacrifice of the sacral nerves. Spine 2000;25:2234-2239.

24. Fowler CJ. Neurological disorders of micturition and their treatment. Brain 1999;122:1213-1231.

25. Hinman F Jr. Atlas of Urosurgical Anatomy. Philadelphia: WB Saunders, 1993, p. 377.

26. Waxman SG. Correlative Neuroanatomy (24th ed). New York: Lange Medical Books/McGraw-Hill, 2000.

27. Trockman BA, Leach GE. Surgical treatment of intrinsic urethral

dysfunction: injectables (fat). Urol Clin North Am 1995;22:665-672.

28. McGuire EJ, O'Connell HE. Surgical treatment of intrinsic urethral dysfunction: slings. Urol Clin North Am 1995;22:657-664.

29. Bellinger MF. Myelomeningocele and neuropathic bladder. In: Gillenwater JY, Grayhack JT, Howards SS, Duckett JW (eds.) Adult and Pediatric Urology (3rd ed). St. Louis: Mosby, 1996.

30. Demirkesen O, Cetinel B, Yaycioglu O, Uygun N, Solok V. Unusual cause of early preeclampsia: bladder paraganglioma. Urology (Online) 2000;56:154.

31. Abrams P. The unstable bladder. In: Fitzpatrick JM, Krane RJ. The Bladder. New York: Churchill Livingstone, 1995, p. 221.

32. Freeman RM, Malvern J (eds). The Unstable Bladder. Boston: Wright, 1989.

33. Chusid JG. Correlative Neuroanatomy & Functional Neurology (17th ed). Los Altos, CA: Lange Medical Publications, 1979, pp. 271-272.

34. Neulander EZ, Rivera I, Eisenbrown N, Wasjman Z. Simple cystectomy in patients requiring urinary diversion. J Urol 2000;164:1169-1172.

35. Kryger JV, Gonzalez R, Barthold JS. Surgical management of urinary incontinence in children with neurogenic sphincteric incompetence. J Urol 2000;163:256-263.

36. Arikan N, Turkolmez K, Budak M, Gogus O. Outcome of augmentation sigmoidocystoplasty in children with neurogenic bladder. Urol Int 2000;64:82-85.

37. Bertschy C, Bawab F, Liard A, Valioulis I, Mitrofanoff P. Enterocystoplasty complications in children. A study of 30 cases. Eur J Pediatr Surg 2000;10:30-34.

38. Lewis SA. Everything you wanted to know about the bladder epithelium but were afraid to ask. Am J Physiol Renal Physiol 2000;278:F867-F874.

39. Kasat LS, Borwankar SS. Factors responsible for successful primary closure in bladder exstrophy. Pediatr Surg Int 2000;16:194-198.

40. Kropp BP, Cheng EY. Total urogenital complex mobilization in female patients with exstrophy. J Urol 2000;164;1035-1039.

41. Pao DM, Ellis JH, Cohan RH, Korobkin M. Utility of routine trauma CT in the detection of bladder rupture. Acad Radiol 2000;7:309-310 and 317-324.

42. Holzbeierlein JM, Smith JA Jr. Surgical management of noninvasive bladder cancer (stages Ta/T1/CIS). Urol Clin North Am 2000;27:15-24.

43. Perovic SV, Vukadinovic VM, Djordjevic MLJ. Augmentation ureterocystoplasty could be performed more frequently. J Urol 2000;164:924-927.

44. Kim HL, Steinberg GD. The current status of bladder preservation in the treatment of muscle invasive bladder cancer. J Urol 2000; 164:627-632.

45. Leissner J, Hohenfellner R, Thüroff JW, Wolf HK. Lymphadenectomy in patients with transitional cell carcinoma of the urinary bladder; significance for staging and prognosis. BJU Int 2000;85:817-823.

46. Abbas F, Biyabani SR, Pervez S. Incidental prostate cancer: the importance of complete prostatic removal at cystoprostatectomy for bladder cancer. Urol Int 2000;64:52-54.

47. Whittlestone TH, Persad R. Radical cystectomy and bladder substitution. Hosp Med (London) 2000;61:336-340.

48. Tainio H, Kylmala T, Tammela TL. Ulcer perforation in gastric urinary conduit: never use a gastric segment in the urinary tract if there are other options available. Urol Int 2000;64:101-103.

49. Denewer A, Kotb S, Hussein O, El-Maadawy M. Laparoscopic assisted cystectomy and lymphadenectomy for bladder cancer: initial experience. World J Surg 23:608-611, 1999.

50. Redman JF. Anatomy of the genitourinary system. In: Gillenwater JY, Grayhack JT, Howards SS, Duckett JW (eds). Adult and Pediatric Urology (3rd ed). St. Louis: Mosby Yearbook, 1996.

51. Lieber MM. Complications of radical cystectomy. In: Smith RB, Erlich RM (eds). Complications of Urologic Surgery: Prevention and Management (2nd ed). Philadelphia: WB Saunders, 1990.

52. Reiner WG, Walsh PC. An anatomical approach to the surgical management of the dorsal vein and Santorini's plexus during radical retropubic surgery. J Urol 1979;121:198-200.

53. Walsh PC, Lepor H, Eggleston JC. Radical prostatectomy with preservation of sexual function: anatomical and pathological considerations. Prostate 1983;4:473-485.

54. Walsh PC, Donker PJ. Impotence following radical prostatectomy: insight into etiology and prevention. J Urol 1982;128:492-497.

55. Lepor H, Gregerman M, Crosby R, Mostofi FK, Walsh PC. Precise localization of the autonomic nerves from the pelvic plexus to the corpora cavernosa: a detailed anatomical study of the adult male pelvis. J Urol 1985;133:207-212.

56. Schlegel PN, Walsh PC. Neuroanatomical approach to radical cystoprostatectomy with preservation of sexual function. J Urol 1987;138:1402-1406.

# Chapter 25

# Male Genital System

JOHN E. SKANDALAKIS, GENE L. COLBORN, THOMAS A. WEIDMAN, ROBERT A. BADALAMENT, WILLIAM M. SCALJON, THOMAS S. PARROTT, NIALL T.M. GALLOWAY, PETROS MIRILAS

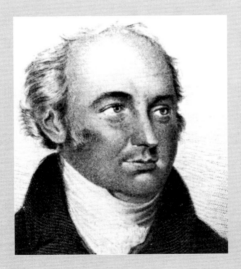

**Sir Astley Paston Cooper (1768-1841),** with his book *Treatise on Hernia,* became the founder of modern hernia repair.

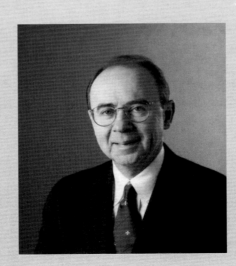

**Patrick C. Walsh (1938--)** is Professor and Director, Urology, Johns Hopkins School of Medicine and Johns Hopkins Hospital.

*At this time of life the testis is connected in a very particular manner with the parietes of the abdomen, at that place where in adult bodies the spermatic vessels pass out, and likewise to the scrotum. This connection is by means of substance which runs down from the lower end of the testis to the scrotum, and which at present I shall call the ligament or gubernaculum testis, it connects the testis with the scrotum, and directs its course in its descent.*

*John Hunter*[1]

The male genital system consists of the following genital organs:
- Testis
- Epididymis
- Ductus deferens (vas)
- Spermatic cord
- Scrotum
- Seminal vesicle
- Ejaculatory duct
- Prostate
- Bulbourethral gland
- Male urethra
- Penis

# *Testis, Epididymis, and Spermatic Cord*

## HISTORY

The anatomic and surgical history of the male genital system is shown in Table 25-1.

## EMBRYOGENESIS

### Normal Development

#### *Gonadal Genesis*

Although the gender of an individual is normally determined at conception by the sex chromosomes, the developing gonad shows no morphologic sex differentiation until the seventh to eighth week (indifferent stage). The gonads develop near the kidney in the retroperitoneal space at the lumbar area.

Formation of the gonad is dependent upon three primordia:
- Primordial germ cells
- Genital ridge. The genital ridge is formed by the mesenchyme of the ventromedial aspects of the mesonephros close to the root of the mesentery
- Coelomic epithelium overlying the mesenchyme

The arrival of primitive germ cells from the yolk sac is almost completed around the end of the sixth week. At the end of the seventh week or early in the eighth week, the differentiation stage takes place, perhaps with hormonal influence. During this period the testes are suspended by the mesorchium, a double peritoneal fold. The lower fold forms the hunterian gubernaculum. The upper fold transmits the spermatic vessels.

**TABLE 25-1. Anatomic and Surgical History of the Male Genital System**

| Testes, Epididymis, and Scrotum | | |
|---|---|---|
| Albert von Haller | 1749 | Stated that testes descend from abdominal cavity to scrotum through "vagina cylindrica" |
| K.F. Wolff | 1759 | Described mesonephric duct |
| John Hunter (1728-1793) | | Stated that during embryonal life, testes descend from retroperitoneal area to scrotum; cryptorchid gonads do not descend due to dysgenesis; first to use term "gubernaculum" |
| B.W. Seiler | 1817 | Interpreted action of gubernaculum as power for testicular descent |
| J. Müller | 1825 | Discovered paramesonephric duct |
| E.H. Weber | 1847 | Theorized that balloonlike swelling of gubernaculum is main force for testicular descent |
| C. Weil | 1884 | Rejected Weber's theory of involvement of gubernaculum in testicular descent, attributing descent to increased intraabdominal pressure |
| H. Klaatsch | 1890 | Proposed conus inguinalis as key factor in testicular descent |
| Neuhauser | 1900 | Argued that scrotum is sexual signal to female of capability to produce offspring |
| O. Frankl | 1900 | Studied testicular descent |
| C.R. Moore | 1924 | Observed degradation of intratubular epithelium in congenital and experimental cryptorchidism; thermoregulatory theory of testicular descent |
| E.R.A. Cooper | 1929 | Disputed Hunter's theory of cryptorchid dysgenesis; reported that cryptorchid testes in very young children were histologically normal |
| B. Schapiro | 1931 | Hormonal treatment for cryptorchidism |
| F. Rost | 1934 | Used water-soluble extracts of anterior pituitary hormone to induce testicular descent in rodents |
| A. Müller | 1938 | Stated that scrotum is an act of self-creativity in male body |
| A. Portman | 1938 | Supported Müller's theory; expression of male sex developed apart from any evolutionary or thermoregulatory factor |
| L. Moscowitch | 1938 | Hypothesized that posterior vesical ligament was responsible for failure of testicular descent |
| T. Martins | 1943 | Stated that administration of androgens (testosterone), not contractile forces, was cause of testicular descent |
| Busch & Sayegh | 1963 | Performed lymphography of testicle. Recognized and reported concept of primary and secondary nodes, and noted importance in surgical management of testicular carcinoma. |
| F. Hadžiselimović | 1980, 1983 | Described role of epididymis in testicular descent |
| M.K. Backhouse | 1981 | Experimental confirmation of Martins' theory; no histological evidence of paratesticular degeneration of gubernaculum |
| Chris F. Heyns, John M. Hutson | 1987 | Gubernaculum involvement in testicular descent |

*History table compiled by David A. McClusky III and John E. Skandalakis.*

**References for Testes, Epididymis, and Scrotum Table**
Busch FM, Sayegh ES. Roentgenographic visualization of human testicular lymphatics: a preliminary report. J Urol 1963;89:106-110.
Hæger K. The Illustrated History of Surgery. London: Harold Starke, 1989.
Hadžiselimović F. History and evolution of testicular descent. In: Hadžiselimović F (ed). Cryptorchidism: Management and Implications. New York: Springer-Verlag, 1983.
Heyns CF, Hutson J. Historical review of theories of testicular descent. J Urol 1995;153:754-767.
Garrison FH. History of Medicine, 4th ed. Philadelphia: WB Saunders, 1913; p. 452.
O'Rahilly R, Müller F. Human Embryology & Teratology, 2nd ed. New York: Wiley-Liss, 1996; p. 450.

## TABLE 25-1 *(cont'd)*. Anatomic and Surgical History of the Male Genital System

### Ductus Deferens (Vas)

| | | |
|---|---|---|
| Sir Astley Cooper | 1823 | First experimental work on vasectomy in dogs |
| H.C. Sharp | 1909 | Reported benefits of vasectomy in patients with "the habit of masturbation" |
| E. Steinach | 1927 | Advocated vasectomy as "rejuvenation operation" |
| L. Shun-Quiang | 1974 | Developed the no-scalpel vasectomy; introduced to West in late 1980s |

*History table compiled by David A. McClusky III and John E. Skandalakis.*

**References for Ductus Deferens Table**
Lipshultz LI, Benson GS. Vasectomy-1980. Urol Clin North Am 1980;7:89-105.
Sharp HC. Vasectomy as a means of preventing procreation in defectives. JAMA 1909;53:1897.
Shun-Quiang L. Vasal sterilisation techniques; teaching material for the National Standard Workshop. Chonguing, China: Scientific and Technical Literature Press, 1988:176.
Steinach E. Biological methods against the process of old age. Med J Rec 1927;125:77.

### Seminal Vesicles and Ejaculatory Ducts

| | | |
|---|---|---|
| Gabriele Falloppio (1523-1562) | | Proved the existence of the seminal vesicles |
| Zinner | 1914 | First report of congenital cysts of the seminal vesicle with associated renal dysgenesis |
| Aboul-Azin | 1979 | Studied and reported on the anatomy of the seminal vesicles and the ejaculatory ducts |
| Nguyen et al. | 1996 | Studied and reported on the anatomy of the ejaculatory duct |
| Okubo et al. | 1998 | First report of in vivo endoscopy of the seminal vesicle |

*History table compiled by David A. McClusky III and John E. Skandalakis.*

**References for Seminal Vesicles and Ejaculatory Ducts Table**
Aboul-Azin TE. Anatomy of the human seminal vesicles and ejaculatory ducts. Arch Androl 1979;3:287-292.
Mettler CC. History of Medicine. Blakiston: Philadelphia, 1947.
Nguyen HT, Etzell J, Turek PJ. Normal human ejaculatory duct anatomy: a study of cadaveric and surgical specimens. J Urol 1996;155:1639-1642.
Okubo K, Maekawa S, Aoki Y, Okada T, Maeda H, Arai Y. In vivo endoscopy of the seminal vesicle. J Urol 1998;159:2069-2070.
Zinner A. Ein Fall von intravesikaler Samenblasenzyste. Wien Med Wochenschr 1914;64:605.

### Prostate

| | | |
|---|---|---|
| Herophilus of Chalcedon | 300 BC | First to use term "prostate," because of organ's location "standing before" urinary bladder |
| Galen (AD 130-200) | | Reported findings of Herophilus |
| Nicolo Massa | 1536 | Anatomic studies (Padua) |
| Andreas Vesalius (1514-1564) | | Anatomic studies |
| Civillard | 1639 | Performed first perineal prostatic resection |
| Jean Zulema Amussat | 1832 | Removed part of prostate through suprapubic cystotomy |
| Louis August Mercier | 1837 | Penetrated prostate through perineum by "prostotome" |
| Max Nitze | 1877 | Produced cystoscope with lenses and electric lighting (Berlin) |
| A.F. McGill | 1889 | Reported 37 prostatectomies through bladder from above (Leeds) |
| Belfield | 1890 | Reported on 133 cases of partial prostatectomy by suprapubic or perineal approach; performed perineal, suprapubic prostatectomies with mortality rate of 14% in 80 cases (Chicago) |
| Goodfellow | 1891 | Performed first total perineal prostatectomy (removal of adenoma only) |
| Fuller | 1894 | Performed first total suprapubic prostatectomy |
| J.N. Langley and H.K. Anderson | 1894-1896 | Studied extrinsic innervation of prostate |

### TABLE 25-1 *(cont'd)*. Anatomic and Surgical History of the Male Genital System

| | | |
|---|---|---|
| H.H. Young | 1904<br>1909 | Performed first radical perineal prostatectomy<br>Introduced clod punch operation for prostatectomy |
| Van Stockum | 1909 | Performed first simple retropubic prostatectomy |
| O.S. Lowsley | 1912 | Detailed anatomic work on prostate which dominated anatomy and surgery for approximately 50 years |
| Jean Casimir Felix Guyton (1831-1920) | | Pioneered prostatic surgery; first to use Giviole cystoscope |
| Millin | 1945 | Popularized simple retropubic prostatectomy |
| Flocks | 1952 | Popularized interstitial colloidal gold treatment for prostate cancer |
| L.M. Franks | 1954 | Reported that benign prostatic hyperplasia arises in central zone, cancer in peripheral zone |
| Liebel, Bovie, Stern, Bumpus, R. Wappler, McCarthy, Foley, F. Wappler, Curtiss, Nesbit, Hirschowits, Peters | 1924-1957 | All made important advances in development of transurethral resection of prostate |
| Carlton | 1965 | Combined interstitial gold 198 and external beam irradiation |
| Charles Huggins | 1966 | Won Nobel Prize: antiandrogen therapy, castration or female estrogen |
| Whitmore | 1970 | Popularized retropubic iodine 125 brachytherapy |
| John E. McNeal | 1972 | Reported 4 prostatic zones; described pre-prostatic sphincter |
| S. Furuya et al. | 1982 | Suggested that almost 50% of prostatic obstruction is attributed to neural pathways on smooth muscle of bladder neck, and preprostatic and prostatic smooth muscle |
| Patrick C. Walsh | 1982 | Advocated identification and preservation of neurovascular bundle to avoid impotence after radical prostatectomy |
| Schuessler et al. | 1991 | Described laparoscopic pelvic lymphadenectomy |
| Onik & Cohen | 1993 | Popularized transperineal cryoablation for prostate cancer |

*History table compiled by David A. McClusky III and John E. Skandalakis.*

**References for Prostate Table**

Chapple CR. Anatomy and innervation of the prostate gland. In: Chapple CR (ed). Prostatic Obstruction: Pathogenesis and Treatment. New York: Springer-Verlag, 1994.

Hæger K. The Illustrated History of Surgery. London: Harold Starke, 1989.

Schuessler WW, Vancaillie TG, Reich H, Griffith DP. Transperitoneal endosurgical lymphadenectomy in patients with localized prostate cancer. J Urol 1991;145:988-991.

Walsh PC, Retik AB, Vaughn ED, Wein AJ (eds). Campbell's Urology, 7th Ed. Philadelphia: WB Saunders, 1998.

| **Bulbourethral Glands (of Cowper)** | | |
|---|---|---|
| William Cowper | 1699 | Described the bulbourethral glands. Usually referred to also as their discoverer. However, in spite of the fact that the glands are often called "Cowper's glands," they were really discovered by Jean Méry (1645-1722). Today their function is still obscure. |

*History table compiled by David A. McClusky III and John E. Skandalakis.*

**References for Bulbourethral Glands Table**

Persaud TVN. A History of Anatomy: The Post-Vesalian Era. Springfield, IL: Charles C. Thomas, 1997, p. 245.

**TABLE 25-1 *(cont'd)*. Anatomic and Surgical History of the Male Genital System**

| | | Male Urethra |
|---|---|---|
| Egyptians | 3000-2000 BC | Used sounds or similar devices to dilate strictures |
| Celsus | ca. 400 BC | Described urethrotomy for impacted urethral calculus |
| Heliodorus & Antyllus | ca. AD 150 | First to attempt hypospadias repair |
| Ferri | 1530 | Described first use of cutting sound |
| Bell | 1816 | Described external urethrotomy and placement of catheter to treat strictures. Also described excision of diseased segment, followed by catheter placement. |
| Civiale & Guillion | 1831 | Introduced blind urethrotomy with retractable blades |
| Dieffenbach | 1838 | Treated hypospadias by piercing glans to allow cannula to remain in position until channel became lined with epithelium |
| Mettauer | 1842 | Suggested multiple subcutaneous incisions to straighten chordee |
| Boisson | 1861 | Suggested transverse incision at point of greatest curvature of chordee. Also used scrotal tissue to reconstruct urethra during hypospadias repair. Performed first buttonhole flap. |
| Thiersch | 1869 | Used local tissue flaps to repair epispadias |
| Duplay | 1874 | Performed staged urethroplasty using central flap which is tubularized and covered by lateral penile skin flaps (later popularized by Browne in 1953, and Horton in 1973) |
| Otis | 1876 | Popularized internal urethrotomy with retractable blades |
| Rosenberger & Landerer | 1891 | Independently described burying penis in scrotum to obtain skin coverage for later hypospadias repair (later popularized by Cecil-Culp in 1951) |
| Hook | 1896 | Described vascularized preputial flap for urethroplasty (later popularized by Davis in 1950, and Broadbent in 1961) |
| Beck & Hacker | 1897 | Undermined and advanced urethra onto glans for subcoronal hypospadias repair (later popularized by Waterhouse in 1981) |
| Beck | 1897 | Used adjacent rotation flaps from scrotum for resurfacing after Duplay-type urethroplasty (later popularized by Turner-Warwick in 1979) |
| Nove-Josserand | 1897 | Used split-thickness skin grafts for hypospadias repair |
| Russell | 1900 | Described first one-stage hypospadias repair using urethral tube constructed from flap developed on ventrum of penis. Neourethra was passed through tunnel in glans and secured to tip of glans. |
| Edmunds | 1913 | First to transfer skin of prepuce to ventral surface of penis at time of chordee release (later popularized by Byars in 1955) |
| Bevan | 1917 | Used urethral meatus-based flap channeled through glans for distal hypospadias repair (later popularized by Mustarde in 1965) |
| Humby | 1941 | Described one-stage hypospadias repair using free full-thickness graft from groin or arm |
| Memmelaar | 1947 | Described one-stage urethroplasty using bladder mucosa as free graft |
| Berry | 1961 | First implant of acrylic prosthesis between bulbous urethra and bulbospongiosus muscle for treatment of incontinence |
| Hodgson | 1970-1972 | Described three procedures using vascularized preputial or penile skin grafts for one-stage hypospadias repair |
| Sachse | 1972 | Developed endoscopic internal urethrotomy using "cold knife" |
| Scott, Bradley & Timm | 1973 | Introduced artificial urinary sphincter |
| Duckett | 1980 | Described technique for transverse preputial island flap |
| Duckett | 1981 | Described meatal advancement and glanuloplasty incorporated procedure (MAGPI) |

*History table compiled by David A. McClusky III and John E. Skandalakis.*

**References for Male Urethra Table**
Walsh PC, Retik AB, Vaughn ED, Wein AJ (eds). Campbell's Urology, 7th Ed. Philadelphia: WB Saunders, 1998.

### TABLE 25-1 *(cont'd)*. Anatomic and Surgical History of the Male Genital System

| | | Penis |
|---|---|---|
| Egyptians, Amorites, Hittites | 3000-2000 BC | Described circumcision |
| Bible | ? | When Abraham made his covenant with God, he was told: "an uncircumcised male who does not circumcise the flesh of his foreskin shall be cut off from his kin." (Genesis 17:11) |
| Celsus | ca. 400 BC | Advocated surgical removal of presumed cancerous lesion of penis leaving margin of healthy tissue |
| Morgagni | 1761 | Mentioned procedure of partial penectomy, which was performed earlier by Valsalva |
| Thiersch | 1875 | First detailed description of penectomy for penile cancer |
| MacCormack | 1886 | Advocated total penile amputation with bilateral inguinal lymphadenectomy for penile cancer |
| Bogoras | 1936 | First surgically successful restoration of potency using rib cartilage implanted into a tube skin graft |
| Mohs | 1936 | Started use of micrographic surgery for penile cancer |
| Goodwin & Scott | 1952 | Used acrylic splints as penile implants for impotence |
| Beheri | 1966 | Reported over 700 successful penile implants for impotence |
| Small & Carrion | 1973 | Introduced first silicone semi-rigid prosthesis for impotence |
| Scott, Bradley & Timm | 1973 | Introduced first inflatable prosthesis for impotence |
| Cabanas | 1977 | Introduced concept of sentinel lymph node biopsy for penile cancer |

*History table compiled by David A. McClusky III and John E. Skandalakis.*

**References for Penis Table**
Walsh PC, Retik AB, Vaughn ED, Wein AJ (eds). Campbell's Urology, 7th Ed. Philadelphia: WB Saunders, 1998.

### Gubernaculum

The testicular gubernaculum is a gelatinous cylinder of mesenchymal origin. We agree with O'Rahilly and Müller[2] on several points concerning the gubernaculum.

- It does not pull the testis into the scrotum
- It does not possess the so-called "tails"
- Its increase in size prior to descent is an important factor in the passage of the testis through the inguinal canal

Perhaps Arey[3] was correct in stating that the destiny of the gubernaculum is to prepare the way and to provide the space for the testicular journey.

The proximal part of the gubernaculum is attached to the lower pole of the testicle. The organ reaches the scrotum but occasionally passes to the perineum, the pubopenile area, or the femoral area. These areas are the ectopic locations outside the line of physiologic descent. Cryptorchidism results when the descent of the testis is arrested along the normal course (abdominal, inguinal, or prepubic).

We quote Favorito et al.[4]:

> In fetuses without congenital malformations or epididymal alterations, such as tail disjunction or elongated epididymis, the proximal portion of the gubernaculum was attached to the testis and epididymis in all cases. In undescended testes there was an increased incidence of paratesticular structure malformations accompanied by gubernacular attachment anomalies compared to the testes in normal fetuses.

### Fascia

The coverings of the spermatic cord are formed by the evagination of the layers of the abdominal wall. The external spermatic fascia is formed by the fascia of the external oblique muscle, not the aponeurosis. The cremasteric fascia is formed by the internal oblique and transversus abdominis muscles. The internal spermatic fascia is formed by the transversalis fascia.

### Female Homologues

The proper ligament of the ovary and the round ligament of the uterus are the remnants of the gubernaculum in the female. To be more specific, the ovarian gubernaculum forms the ovarian ligament between the uterus and the ovary and the round ligament extending between the uterus and the labia majora. The round ligament of the uterus passes downward through the inguinal canal and into the labium majus. It is the homologue of the gubernaculum of the undescended testis, not of the spermatic cord of the descended testis. For all practical purposes, the gubernaculum disappears in the male.

## *Descent of the Gonads*

The testis that has not begun its descent is, together with the epididymis, attached to the posterior abdominal wall by a mesorchium that contains the blood vessels and the ductus deferens. It may lie at the level of the lower pole of the kidney, the iliac fossa, or in the pelvis (Fig. 25-1).

The downward journey commences at approximately the third month of gestation. The pathway is retroperitoneal.

During the seventh month the testes are found at the level of the anterior superior iliac spine. The epididymis is in a posterolateral location. The gubernaculum, whose circumference is as large as the testis and the epididymis, is approximately 1.8 cm long. The peritoneum dips into the inguinal canal ahead of the testes, but extends down the gubernaculum only part way. The testes and gubernaculum extend into the canal. The scrotum and the gubernaculum are not attached to each other. The "scrotal ligament" of Lockwood[5] fails to qualify as a ligament.

The testes begin to enter the internal ring as the gubernaculum emerges from the external ring. As the gubernaculum reaches the bottom of the scrotal sac, it begins to

shorten until its lower two-thirds has disappeared completely. At about the end of the seventh month, the testes pass through the inguinal canal. Although descent through the canal is accomplished in a few days, it takes four additional weeks for the testes to pass from the external ring to the bottom of the scrotum. The best description of testicular descent is that of Scorer.[6]

Descent may be complete early or may still be incomplete at birth. Among the premature births studied by Scorer,[6] the testes were undescended in 50% or more of the larger infants. After the testes emerge through the external ring, the ring contracts.

For a discussion of current theories of the role of androgen in testicular descent, the interested reader is referred to Barthold et al.[7]

### Processus Vaginalis

The proximal part of the processus vaginalis (from the peritoneal cavity to the testis) closes after descent is complete. Closure is complete by birth in 50% to 75% of infants. Scorer believed that this closure may be recognized by palpating the spermatic cord shortly after birth.[8]

Once the testes are in the scrotum, the distal part of

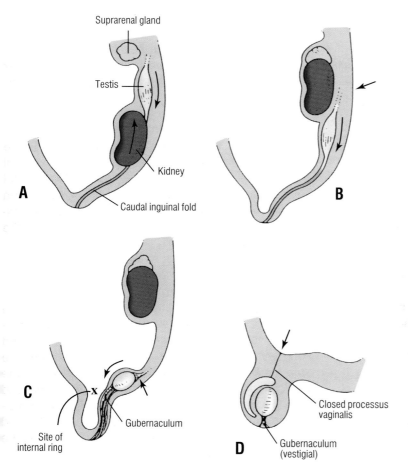

FIG. 25-1. Descent of testis. **A,** Fifth week. Testis begins its primary descent; kidney ascends. **B,** Eighth to ninth weeks. Kidney reaches adult position. **C,** Seventh month. Testis at internal inguinal ring; gubernaculum (in inguinal fold) thickens and shortens. **D,** Postnatal life. Testis in scrotum; processus vaginalis closed, and gubernaculum (vestigial). (Modified from Skandalakis JE, Gray SW, Rowe JS Jr. Anatomical Complications in General Surgery. New York: McGraw-Hill, 1983; with permission.)

the processus vaginalis forms the tunica vaginalis; the proximal part is usually obliterated. It is unknown, however, why the processus vaginalis closes. Further, it may persist throughout life. The two points of obliteration are the deep inguinal ring and just above the upper pole of the testis.

After the testicular descent, the lumen of the processus vaginalis becomes obliterated above the testis. In the adult, a fibrous band marks the upper (funicular) part of the processus, while the scrotal portion (tunica vaginalis) remains as an isolated peritoneal cavity. A homologous cavity in the female (canal of Nuck) is usually obliterated before birth.

How can we explain the descent of the testicles? Only the good Lord knows, we tell our students. We can mention, however, the influence of hormones and the gubernaculum upon the descent of the testicles. The gubernaculum is immature mesenchymal tissue, which most likely with the aid of the processus vaginalis helps the gonads travel downward by evagination of the lower abdominal wall.

### Hormonal Influence

Shapiro,[9] in 1930, demonstrated the role of hormones in the descent. Engle[10] later induced premature descent of the testes in the macaque with anterior pituitary hormone. Martins[11] controlled the descent of paraffin masses simulating the testes in rats and monkeys injected with testosterone. Wislocki[12] suggested that maternal chorionic gonadotropin stimulates androgen production in the adrenal cortex of the male fetus, which leads to normal descent. Although ordinary cryptorchidism often demonstrates normal, not low, androgen production, the high frequency of retained testes in various types of pseudohermaphrodites strongly suggests that androgen is an important factor in descent.

The prostate gland, the seminal vesicles, and the ductus deferens develop normally if the Y chromosome is present. If the fetal testicle secretes the müllerian inhibiting substance (MIS), then a regression of the female genital tract occurs. The Leydig cells produce testosterone, which is responsible for the differentiation of the wolffian system. Chorionic gonadotropin is used successfully for the treatment of bilateral undescended testes. However, surgery is the treatment of choice if that therapy is unsuccessful.

Hutson and Baker[13] hypothesize that in patients with persistent müllerian duct syndrome (PMDS), the gubernaculum fails to develop during the first phase of descent. They consider the possible role of MIS in initiating this first step, and await more experiments to evaluate its relevance. The etiology of PMDS implicates a role for müllerian inhibiting substance in gubernacular development.

### Gubernaculum and Descent

Hutson et al.[14] theorize that failure of masculinization of the development of the gubernaculum testes in persistent müllerian duct syndrome allows testicular herniation and perhaps plays a role in testicular descent. Androgens may direct gubernacular migration via release of a second messenger (a calcitonin gene-related peptide) from the genitofemoral nerve.

Although hormones probably regulate descent, the actual mechanics can only be conjectured. If a testis and a gubernaculum together form a cylindrical plug in the inguinal canal, this plug will be forced downward at each rise of pressure in the abdomen, such as from uterine pressure in prenatal life or from crying or straining in postnatal life. If the lower end of the gubernaculum is progressively destroyed, perhaps by hormonal action, the gubernaculum may serve to lower the testes slowly into the scrotum under the pressure of the abdomen. It thereby acts as a brake rather than as a positive traction force, as was originally proposed.

From their studies on the gubernaculum of the pig, Backhouse and Butler[15] believe that final descent results from invasion of the remaining gubernaculum by the growing epididymis. We concur with this conclusion.

In several recent publications, Hutson and co-workers[16-20] consider various concepts about testicular descent. We present verbatim their summary of these theories[21]:

> *The most plausible explanations for testicular descent in the human fetus are related to development of the gubernaculum, processus vaginalis, inguinal canal, spermatic vessels and scrotum since these structures differ substantially between male and female fetuses. The gubernaculum consists of primitive mesenchymal tissue around which the abdominal wall muscles differentiate, creating the inguinal canal. In the early fetus the gubernaculum serves to anchor the testis to the internal inguinal ring. Rapid growth of the gubernaculum before descent may dilate the inguinal canal and rings sufficiently to admit the testis.*
>
> *Growth of the processus vaginalis toward the tip of the gubernaculum provides a mechanism by which intra-abdominal pressure transmitted via the open processus can exert traction on the gubernaculum and, thereby, on the testis. However, this process of traction is not continuous since the length of the intra-abdominal gubernaculum increases significantly and the testis is freely mobile before inguinal descent, which is relatively rapid. It appears likely that growth of the gubernaculum and processus vaginalis must reach a critical stage before intra-abdominal pressure transmitted via the open processus can effect the rapid inguinal transit of the testis, which is possibly pre-*

*cipitated by fetal respiratory efforts or hiccuping.*

*Clearly, firm attachment of the gubernaculum to the testis, and adequate lengthening of the spermatic vessels and vas deferens as well as development of the scrotum are also indispensable for full descent. The absence of a firm scrotal attachment of the gubernaculum has discredited the traction theories but it is possible that intra-abdominal pressure exerted via the open processus vaginalis may stabilize the gubernacular tip, and so contraction of the gubernaculum can pull the testis down. The contractility demonstrated in the rodent gubernaculum should be investigated in large mammals since it remains unresolved whether the gubernaculum in these species may be capable of contraction, causing the rapid inguinal passage of the testis.*

*Although gonadotropins and androgens appear to have a role, their target structures and mechanisms of action remain undefined. It is generally accepted that the fetal spermatic vessels, vas deferens and scrotum are androgen target structures, but this hypothesis has not been biochemically proved in regard to the spermatic vessels. It appears unlikely that androgens are responsible for growth of the gubernaculum but regression of this structure may be androgen-dependent. The theory that androgens exert their effect on the gubernaculum via the spinal nucleus of the genitofemoral nerve and a "second messenger," such as calcitonin gene-related peptide, needs to be investigated in a nonrodent animal model. In addition, the possibility that growth of the gubernaculum is stimulated by a nonandrogenic fetal testicular hormone different from müllerian inhibiting substance should be further investigated. We hope that the controversy on the enigma of testicular descent will eventually be resolved as speculation gives way to scientifically proved fact.*

### Role of Temperature

The testicle is sensitive to the warm temperature of the abdominal cavity. Normal body temperature, abnormal for the undescended testicle, arrests spermatogenesis and enables only the Sertoli cells to survive. Spermatogenesis requires a cool climate, as provided in the scrotum. Moore[22] proved this when he insulated the scrotum of a ram with a tea cozy. After 80 days, no spermatozoa were found. The ram regained spermatogenesis when the insulating material was removed. Pituitary gonadotropin plays a significant role in these changes, as proven by its importance as a stimulus during puberty.

Much more work is needed to further our understanding of testicular descent. Though we do not understand the intricacies of testicular descent, we know it occurs so the organ can locate itself in a cooler environment. The testicle does not like the warmth of the retroperitoneal space; it is a warrior and does not want to have a fireplace chat with other retroperitoneal fellows. Instead, fighting, constantly alone, the testicle practically destroys the lower abdominal wall. It gloriously seeks out the bracing climate of the scrotum for its abode. This location helps prevent malignancies. It permits the testicle to fulfill its physiologic destiny of successfully producing spermatozoa.

Physicians must not forget the anxieties of young boys suspecting that they have an empty scrotum.

### Female Homologues

In females, ovarian descent normally ceases after the 12th week at the area of the pelvic brim. By definition, the canal of Nuck extends into the labium majus in the female; it corresponds to the processus vaginalis of the male. If the processus vaginalis is not obliterated by the 8th prenatal month, a hydrocele may be formed; perhaps an ectopic ovary may be found within the canal of Nuck, in the form of a congenital indirect inguinal hernia.

## Congenital Anomalies

Anomalies of the male reproductive tract may be appreciated in Table 25-2 and Fig. 25-2. Anomalies of the gonads are considered below.

### *Undescended Testis*

The proportion of undescended testes increases with prematurity of the neonate. Scorer[23] found undescended (cryptorchid) testes in 21 percent of premature neonates and in only 2.7 percent of full term neonates. By the end of the first year of life, testes were undescended in only 0.8 percent. Retraction of the testis by the cremaster muscle in young boys (cremasteric reflex) may produce a false diagnosis of undescended testis.[24]

An undescended testis may remain in the abdomen, or its descent may be arrested in any portion of the normal pathway from the abdomen to the scrotum (Fig. 25-3A). The most common site of arrest (62 percent) is the inguinal canal. Figure 25-3B shows the proportion of testes arrested at various locations.

Among premature infants, failure of descent is usually bilateral; among infants of normal birth weight, the right testis is much more often undescended than is the left. In adults, this proportion is reversed.

An undescended (cryptorchid) testis may or may not be normal. If it is brought down surgically before 2 years of age, a normal testis may become functional. If it is not

## TABLE 25-2. Anomalies of the Male Reproductive Tract

| Anomaly | Prenatal Age at Onset | First Appearance (or Other Diagnostic Clues) | Sex Chiefly Affected[a] | Relative Frequency | Remarks |
|---|---|---|---|---|---|
| Müllerian and mesonephric remnants in the male: | | | | | |
| Torsion of the appendix testis or appendix epididymis | | In adolescence | Male | Uncommon | Predisposing factors not known |
| Cysts of the prostate utricle | 12th week | In adulthood | Male | Uncommon (clinically significant) | |
| Absence of wolffian derivatives in the male: | | | | | |
| Complete absence | 4th week | At birth | Male | Rare | Associated with absence of kidneys and uterus: lethal if bilateral |
| Partial absence | After the 4th week | In adulthood | Male | Uncommon | Bilateral absence casues infertility; unilateral absence is asymptomatic |
| Duplications of the ductus deferens | Late 4th week | None | Male | Rare | |
| Absence of the seminal vesicle | 3rd month or earlier | Adulthood only if bilateral | Male | Unknown | Sterility if bilateral |
| Duplication of the seminal vesicle | 3rd month | Never | Male | Unknown | Asymptomatic |
| Anomalies of the prostate gland: | | | | | |
| Absence of the prostate | 12th week | In adulthood | Male | Rare | Associated with infantile genitalia and pituitary insufficiency |
| Other anomalies | ? | At any age | Male | Rare | May produce urethral obstruction |
| Agenesis of the penis | 4th week | At birth | Male | Very rare | |
| Agenesis of the glans penis | 4th month | At birth | Male | Very rare | |
| Defects of the corpus spongiosum and corpora cavernosa | 3rd month? | At birth | Male | Very rare | |
| Duplication of the penis | Various times | At birth | Male | Very rare | Similar duplication of the clitoris is even rarer |
| Transposition of the penis and scrotum | 9th week | At birth | Male | Very rare | |
| Duplications of the penile urethra | 10th to 14th weeks | At any age | Male | Uncommon | |
| Atresia and stenosis of the urethra | ? | In infancy | Male | Common | Present in females also |
| Hypospadias | 8th week or later | At birth | Male | Rare | Very rare in females; familial tendency suggested |

[a]These conditions may occur also in females with anomalous male organs.

*Source:* Skandalakis JE, Gray SW, eds. Embryology for Surgeons, 2nd Ed. Baltimore: Williams & Wilkins, 1994; with permission.

brought down until puberty, it will almost surely be nonfunctional. Remember that surgical correction of the undescended testis always involves repair of an indirect inguinal hernia.

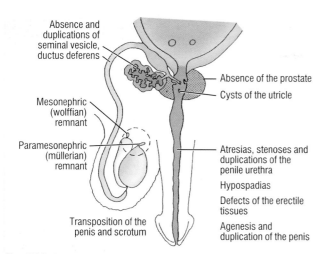

**FIG. 25-2.** Sites of developmental anomalies of male reproductive tract. (Modified from Skandalakis JE, Gray SW. Embryology for Surgeons (2nd ed). Baltimore: Williams & Wilkins, 1994; with permission.)

sents a 22-fold increase over the rate of 2.2 per 100,000 in adults who experienced the development of tumors in normally descended testes. In Martin's[29] earlier report, all patients with tumors had orchiopexy performed after 5 years of age. However, there currently are reports of tumors developing when surgery is performed earlier. Testicular seminoma which developed 14 years after orchiopexy for undescended testis in a patient with Noonan's syndrome was reported by Aggarwal et al.[31] Long-term follow-up of patients undergoing orchiopexy at any age seems advisable.

## Defects of Closure of the Processus Vaginalis

Defects of closure of the processus vaginalis are not unusual. They may be classified as diverticular defects and cystic defects.

A patent processus vaginalis may be unilateral or bilateral. Routine inguinal herniography to identify crypt-

### Histologic Changes

Even though at birth the volume of undescended testis is relatively normal, it decreases as time passes. Testicular histologic abnormalities accounting for this phenomenon can be summarized as a progressive deterioration of the number of germ cells. This change can be noted as early as the second year of life. It is common to find a total lack of germ cells in orchiectomy specimens of cryptorchid teenagers who have not been previously treated. Furthermore, more proximal testes (e.g., abdominal) are more severely affected.[25]

How histologic abnormalities relate to adult infertility in previously cryptorchid patients is not entirely clear. Several retrospective studies have not clearly defined a corelation between paternity and age at orchiopexy.[26,27] Despite a lack of good data, most surgeons prefer to offer correction before evidence of histologic abnormalities can be shown. Orchiopexy prior to age 2 is currently the accepted norm. It has been shown that early orchiopexy (age 1-2) correlates with improved fertility.[28]

### Malignancy

There is definitely an increased incidence of malignancy in cryptorchid testes. It appears that an undescended testis is thirty-five times more likely to be found in those with testicular tumors than in the general male population.[29] A calculation of the incidence of malignancy in cryptorchid patients, as contrasted with the increased presence of cryptorchid individuals in malignancy cases, is more difficult to ascertain and requires certain statistical assumptions.[30] It has been estimated to be 48.91 per 100,000. This repre-

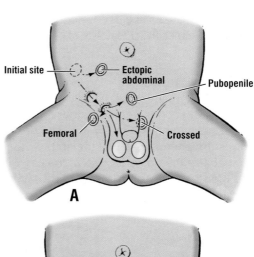

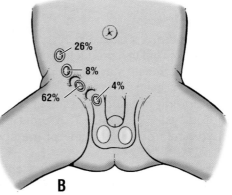

**FIG. 25-3. A,** Ectopic testes. Perineal ectopia not shown. **B,** Undescended testes. Percentages of testes arrested at different stages of normal descent. (Data from Campbell MF, Harrison JH. Urology (3rd ed). Philadelphia: Saunders, 1970. Modified from Skandalakis JE, Gray SW. Embryology for Surgeons (2nd ed). Baltimore: Williams & Wilkins, 1994; with permission.)

orchidism patients with a patent processus vaginalis, for whom nonsurgical treatment would be ineffective, was urged by Varela-Cives et al.[32] Owings and Georgeson[33] report that laparoscopic exploration of a symptomatic unilateral inguinal hernia to detect a contralateral patent processus vaginalis is safe and accurate.

### Diverticular Defects

There are three types of diverticular defects:
- Congenital indirect hernia
- Acquired indirect inguinal hernia
- Sliding indirect hernia

CONGENITAL INDIRECT HERNIA. A completely open processus vaginalis occurs in congenital indirect hernia (Fig. 25-4A). Herniation of intestine or omentum occurs at or shortly after birth.

ACQUIRED INDIRECT INGUINAL HERNIA. In this condition an unclosed cranial (funicular) portion of the processus opens into the peritoneal cavity (Fig. 25-4B). The lower portion of the processus is closed. Acquired indirect inguinal hernia increases the possibility of herniation later in life.

SLIDING INDIRECT HERNIA. A sliding indirect hernia forms when a "retroperitoneal" viscus, usually the cecum or the sigmoid colon, descends behind, rather than within, an open processus vaginalis (Fig. 25-4F). The descending viscus forms the posterior wall of the empty processus. Efforts to mobilize the posterior wall of the sac will jeopardize the blood supply to the viscus. The sac must be opened anteriorly, but is not to be dissected from the spermatic cord.

### Cystic Defects

When the processus is closed at the cranial end only, an accumulation of fluid can produce hydrocele (Fig. 25-4C). An infantile hydrocele may have a patent processus vaginalis (communicating hydrocele).

If the midportion of the processus is unclosed, it leaves a closed cyst (Fig. 25-4D). This forms a cystic or funicular hydrocele or a hydrocele of the spermatic cord.

Note: Collection of fluid in a normally developed tunica vaginalis produces adult hydrocele (Fig. 25-4E).

### Ectopic Testis

By definition, ectopic testes are outside the path of normal descent. If the testis is not in the scrotum or in the normal path of descent, it may be ectopic. When both testes migrate toward the same hemiscrotum, a symptomatic inguinal hernia may occur on the side of the migration.[34] Ectopic testes are baffling and, fortunately, very rare. Figure 25-3A shows some of the sites in which ectopic testes have been found.

The term cryptorchidism covers both undescended and ectopic (maldescended) testes. Both should be located and placed in the scrotum at an early age if at all possible. If surgery is performed on an adult, orchiectomy should be considered.

We quote Hutcheson et al.[35]:

*Similar pathological findings in ectopic and undescended testes as well as the association of ectopic testis with a contralateral undescended testis suggest that ectopic and undescended testes are variants of the same congenital anomaly. Thus, boys with ectopic testis may have an increased incidence of subfertility and testicular malignancy. This spectrum of abnormal testicular position, and its range of pathological conditions and complications may appropriately be called the undescended testis sequence.*

### Appendix Testis and Appendix Epididymis

The ductus epididymis arises from the mesonephric (wolffian) duct as does the ductus deferens. The ductuli efferentes drain the rete testes; as they leave the tunica albuginea on their way to open into the epididymis they beome highly convoluted so that each ductule forms a lobule at the head of the epididymis.

Superior aberrant ductules remain connected with the testis but not with the epididymis. They are reported to be the source of spermatoceles. Inferior aberrant ductules (aberrant vas of Haller) lose their connection with the testis but retain connections with the epididymis. They apparently are known to undergo torsion with varying levels of discomfort as the result.

The paradidymis (organ of Giraldes) comprises persistent remnants of mesonephric tubules which are connected to neither the epididymis nor the testis. No symptoms are attributed to this structure. The cranial part of the mesonephric duct becomes the appendix of the epididymis (hydatid of Morgagni).[36] It is a pedunculated structure which may undergo torsion. This produces aching that ranges in intensity from dull to marked and requires surgical intervention. Finally, the appendix of the testis is the remnant of the cranial end of the paramesonephric (müllerian) duct. It, too, may undergo torsion and cause severe discomfort to the patient.

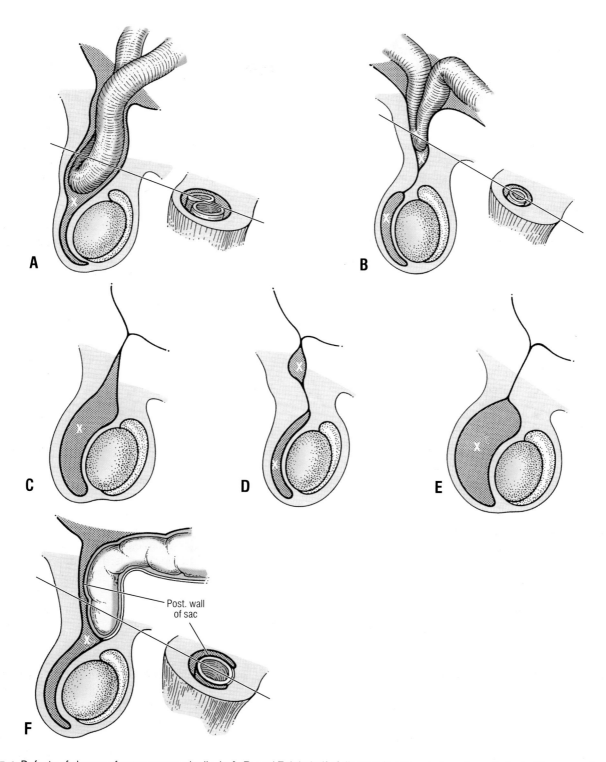

**Fig. 25-4.** Defects of closure of processus vaginalis. In **A, B,** and **F** right half of diagram is cross section of area indicated by connecting diagonal line. *X,* processus vaginalis. **A,** Completely unclosed processus. An intestinal loop or omentum may follow testis into scrotum (congenital indirect hernia). **B,** Cranial (funicular) portion of processus unclosed. Herniation may occur later in life (acquired indirect hernia). **C,** All but cranial portion unclosed. Serous fluid accumulates to form infantile hydrocele. **D,** Midportion of processus unclosed, forming cyst (cystic hydrocele). **E,** Normally closed processus. Fluid may accumulate in tunica vaginalis (adult hydrocele). **F,** Sliding indirect inguinal hernia. Descending viscus, usually colon, remains retroperitoneal. Sac (processus vaginalis) remains unclosed or becomes closed. (Modified from Skandalakis JE, Gray SW, Rowe JS Jr. Anatomical Complications in General Surgery. New York: McGraw-Hill, 1983; with permission.)

## SURGICAL ANATOMY

### Topography and Relations

#### *Testis*

The normally descended testis is ovoid and about 4 cm in length. The tunica vaginalis of peritoneum envelops the whole testis except its posterior border and its superior pole.

The testis itself is surrounded by a dense, irregular connective-tissue capsule, the tunica albuginea. Posteriorly, the tunica forms a median septum, the mediastinum testis, from which more delicate connective tissue divides the parenchyma into 200 to 300 compartments that contain the seminiferous tubules. These coiled tubules anastomose in the mediastinum of testis to form the rete testis, from which 6 to 12 ductuli efferentia pass to the head of the epididymis.

The testis has two free surfaces, the medial and the lateral, and two borders, the anterior and the posterior. The posterior border has a superior portion that is related to the head of the epididymis, and an inferior portion that is related to the body and tail of the epididymis.

The right testicle, in most cases, is at a higher level than the left. Occasionally, the right testicle is lower in total situs inversus, and, according to Chang et al.,[37] in left-handed men. For medicolegal reasons, this finding should be reported in the patient's chart.

#### *Epididymis*

The head of the epididymis is firmly fixed to the upper pole of the testis (Fig. 25-5). The body and the tail are less

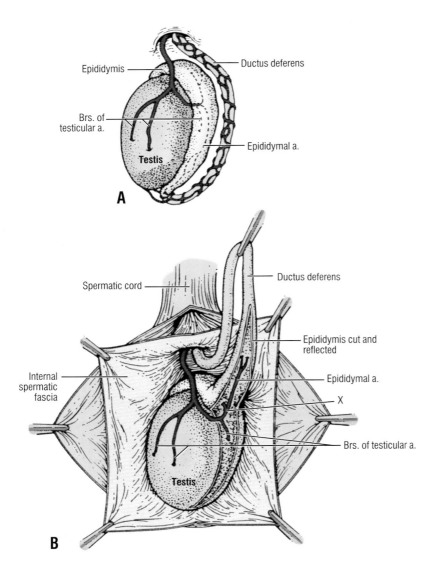

FIG. 25-5. Epididymectomy. **A,** An epididymal branch of testicular artery supplies epididymis. **B,** Epididymis dissected from below. Branch of testicular artery to testis must be preserved. Branch to epididymis (reflected upward) may be ligated at *X*. (Modified from Skandalakis JE, Gray SW, Rowe JS Jr. Anatomical Complications in General Surgery. New York: McGraw-Hill, 1983; with permission.)

firmly fixed to the posterior border of the testis. This posterior surface is not covered by the tunica vaginalis, but it is the site of the blood and nerve supply to both organs.

At the upper one-third of the posterior border, the testicular artery bifurcates into testicular and epididymal branches (Fig. 25-5). During epididymectomy, the surgeon should start from the lower pole and proceed upward about 2.5 cm. This will avoid injury to the testicular branch of the artery and testicular atrophy.

The surgeon should remember that the epididymis may not be in its normal position (Fig. 25-6A). It may be elongated (Fig. 25-6B) or dissociated from the testis (Fig. 25-6B through E). There may be a very small tunica vaginalis, or it may be wider than usual, forming a mesorchium (Fig. 25-6C).

Occasionally, the epididymis is descended and the testis is retained (Fig. 25-6E). Such separation of testis and epididymis usually results in blindly ending vasa efferentia dilated to form spermatoceles. The testis itself may or may not be normal. If the condition is bilateral, the patient will be sterile.[38]

## *Spermatic Cord*

The spermatic cord is a matrix of connective tissue con-

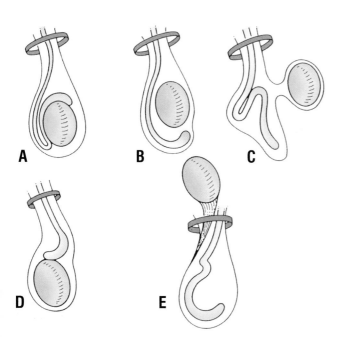

**Fig. 25-6.** Varieties of separation of testis and epididymis. **A,** Normal relations. **B, C, D, E,** One or both structures maldescended **E,** Epididymis normally descended: testis remains above internal ring. (Modified from Skandalakis JE, Gray SW, Rowe JS Jr. Anatomical Complications in General Surgery. New York: McGraw-Hill, 1983; with permission.)

tinuous proximally with the preperitoneal connective tissue. Concentrically invested by three layers of tissue, the cord contains the ductus deferens (vas), three arteries, three veins, the pampiniform plexus, and two nerves. One other nerve, the ilioinguinal, lies just lateral to the major layers of the cord.

The elements of the spermatic cord relate to each other as follows.
- Anterior: pampiniform plexus
- Posterior: ductus and remnant of processes vaginalis or hernial sac

These anatomic entities of the spermatic cord, as well as others, are covered by the spermatic fasciae. The spermatic cord on its way to the scrotum may be found deep under the fasciae of Scarpa and Colles.

The components of the spermatic cord are listed in Table 25-3. The key to remember is "three": three layers of fasciae, three arteries, three veins, three nerves, multiple lymphatics, and one ductus.

## *Fasciae*

The ductus deferens and the accompanying blood vessels of the spermatic cord are surrounded by three layers of fascia.
- *External spermatic fascia,* the outermost layer, is a continuation of the fascia of the external oblique muscle.
- *Cremasteric fascia* is primarily continuous with the musculature and fascia of the internal oblique and, in some

| TABLE 25-3. The Spermatic Cord and its Covering |
|---|
| Three fasciae: |
|     External spermatic (from external oblique fascia) |
|     Cremasteric (from internal oblique muscle and fascia) |
|     Internal spermatic (from transversalis fascia) |
| Three arteries: |
|     Testicular artery |
|     Cremasteric artery |
|     Deferential artery |
| Three veins: |
|     Pampiniform plexus and testicular vein |
|     Cremasteric vein |
|     Deferential vein |
| Three nerves: |
|     Genital branch of genitofemoral nerve |
|     Ilioinguinal nerve |
|     Sympathetic nerves (testicular plexus) |
| Lymphatics |

*Source:* Skandalakis JE, Colborn GL, Pemberton B, Skandalakis LJ, Gray SW. The surgical anatomy of the inguinal area. Part 2. Contemp Surg 38:28-38, 1991; with permission.

cases, the transversus abdominis muscle as well.

- *Internal spermatic fascia* is a continuation of the transversalis fascia.

Stoppa et al.[39] discuss the retroparietal spermatic sheath and present the posterior relations of the spermatic sheath of the spermatic cord to the external iliac vessels. They advise preservation of this part of the spermatic sheath when spermatic cord mobilization occurs during hernia repair. Preservation avoids perivascular sclerosis due to contact with a large prosthesis.

## Vascular Supply

### *Arteries*

The arteries of the testis and the epididymis are shown in Figures 25-7 and 25-8. The internal spermatic, or testicular, artery arises from the aorta. Shinohara et al.[40] reported a variation in which the left testicular artery originated from the aorta 1 cm above the origin of the left inferior phrenic artery. The testicular artery is the chief source of blood to the testis. The artery of the ductus deferens (deferential artery) emerges from the inferior vesicular artery. The external spermatic, or cremasteric, artery springs from the inferior epigastric artery.

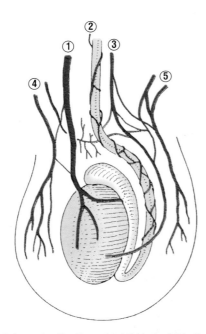

FIG. 25-7. Arterial supply of testis and epididymis. 1, Testicular artery. 2, Deferential artery. 3, Cremasteric artery. 4, Posterior scrotal artery. 5, Anterior scrotal artery. (Modified from Skandalakis JE, Gray SW, Rowe JS Jr. Anatomical Complications in General Surgery. New York: McGraw-Hill, 1983; with permission.)

Four other arteries anastomose with the testicular artery and each other to form a collateral circulation.[41] There are anastomoses between the testicular and deferential vessels (Fig. 25-7). A good anastomosis exists between the gonadal and the deferential arteries in all patients. There are also some anastomoses between these and the cremasteric arteries in approximately two-thirds of patients. Additional anastomoses appear to exist between the testicular, cremasteric, and scrotal vessels.

According to Neuhof and Mencher,[42] collateral circulation is sufficient to prevent gangrene upon division of the cord in 98% of their patients. Testicular atrophy occurred in 19 of the 24 patients. Among a larger group, Burdick and Higinbotham[43] found atrophy in 80% and gangrene in 2 percent.

If the cord is divided, it is advisable to keep the testicle in the scrotum and not bring it into the surgical field. Collateral circulation will probably be better served with this action.

Bifurcation of the testicular artery into the main testicular and epididymal branches occurs between the upper and middle one-third of the testicle. Dissection of the epididymis during epididymectomy should start at the lower pole of the testicle and proceed upward (approximately 2.5 cm). From there, the surgeon will find the bifurcation, and should ligate only the epididymal branch.

### *Veins*

According to Hinman,[44] the veins that drain the testis, epididymis, and spermatic cord connect with a deep and a superficial venous network. The deep network is the more common pathway and has three components:

- *Anterior:* Pampiniform plexus and testicular vein
- *Middle:* Deferential and funicular veins
- *Posterior:* Cremasteric veins

The pampiniform venous plexus is formed in the spermatic cord by 10 to 12 veins that segregate into anterior and posterior groups (Fig. 25-9). Each group is drained by three or four veins that join to form two veins proximal to the internal inguinal ring. These veins run in the extraperitoneal space on either side of the testicular artery. The vein on the right opens into the inferior vena cava; that on the left enters the left renal vein. The cremasteric venous network flows into the inferior epigastric veins. The deferential vein drains into the pelvic plexus.

The superficial venous network is described as follows by Hinman[44]:

> *The scrotal veins drain through the external pudendal veins into the internal saphenous vein or through the superficial perineal veins into the internal pudendal vein.*

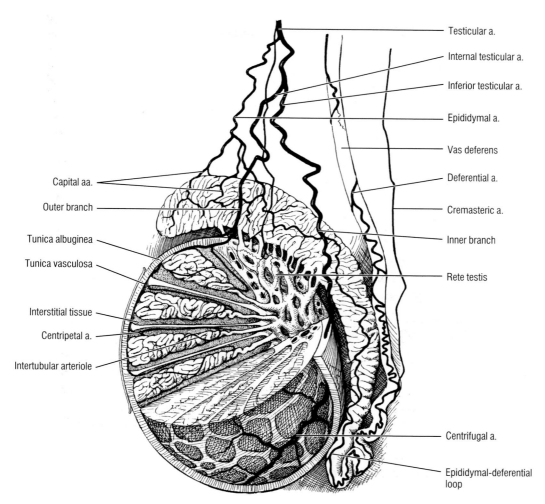

Testicular a.

Internal testicular a.

Inferior testicular a.

Epididymal a.

Vas deferens

Deferential a.

Cremasteric a.

Inner branch

Rete testis

Centrifugal a.

Epididymal-deferential loop

Capital aa.

Outer branch

Tunica albuginea

Tunica vasculosa

Interstitial tissue

Centripetal a.

Intertubular arteriole

**Fig. 25-8.** Internal arterial distribution of the testis and epididymis. (From Hinman F Jr. Atlas of Urosurgical Anatomy. Philadelphia: WB Saunders, 1993; with permission.)

*Within this system, the cremasteric vein joins the venous plexus of the spermatic cord and the inferior epigastric vein.*

Lechter and coworkers[45] dissected 100 cadavers (88 male, 12 female). They produced a beautiful and complete report on the anatomy of the gonadal vessels for both sexes, finding a 20% rate of variance from the typical pattern (Fig. 25-10, Fig. 25-11, Table 25-4, Table 25-5, Table 25-6).

## Lymphatics

A superficial plexus and a deep plexus of lymph vessels drain the testis and the epididymis upward through the spermatic cord to the lateral and preaortic lymph nodes.

## Innervation

The innervation of the testis is effected by sympathetic and general visceral sensory fibers associated with the collateral ganglia and plexuses of the aorta in the region of the superior mesenteric and renal arteries. These fibers course with the testicular arteries to the testes for sympathetic supply and sensory innervation (pain). The spinal cord levels involved in the pain pathway are those from which thoracic splanchnics arise, i.e., T5 to T12 (but chiefly from T10 and T11).

The genital branch of the genitofemoral nerve (L1, L2) enters the inguinal canal through the internal inguinal ring. This branch serves the cremasteric muscle. The ilioinguinal nerve (L1) emerges between the external and internal oblique muscles near the anterior superior iliac spine. It then enters the canal and subsequently exits from the

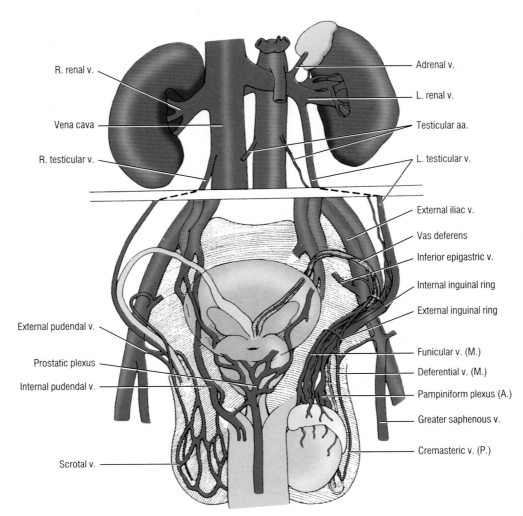

**Fig. 25-9.** Deep and superficial venous networks of testis, epididymis, and ductus deferens (vas). (A.), Anterior pathway. (M.), Middle pathway. (P.), Posterior pathway. (Modified from Hinman F Jr. Atlas of Urosurgical Anatomy. Philadelphia: WB Saunders, 1993; with permission.)

external inguinal ring. There, the ilioinguinal nerve supplies the skin of the penile root, the upper part of the scrotum, and the upper, medial thigh.[46-48]

The arteries of the cord and the ductus deferens receive their autonomic supply by sympathetic fibers originating from the prostatic portion of the pelvic plexus.

## HISTOLOGY

### Testis

The histology of the testis will be briefly described from outside to inside. The tunica vaginalis has two serous layers (parietal and visceral) which represent the out-

pocketing of the peritoneum. Under the visceral layer, the tunica albuginea is dense connective tissue enveloping the testicular parenchyma; its fibrous septa form approximately 300 pyramid-shaped lobules. The bases of the pyramids are related to the tunica albuginea; the apices are related to the posterior aspect of the tunica albuginea forming the mediastinum testis.

Each pyramidal lobule contains 2-4 convoluted seminiferous tubules which are responsible for the genesis of spermatozoa. Posteriorly, these convoluted tubules become straight and anastomose. They form the rete testis from which 10-12 efferent ducts are formed. The efferent ducts pierce the tunica albuginea and pass into the head of the epididymis.

The interstitial tissue lies between the tubules. It contains the Leydig cells which synthesize testosterone and other steroid hormones. The Sertoli cells lining the lumen

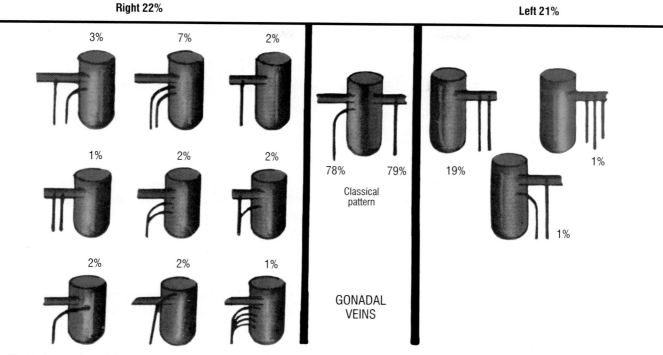

**Right 22%**

3%    7%    2%

1%    2%    2%

2%    2%    1%

78%    79%    Classical pattern

**Left 21%**

19%    1%

1%

GONADAL VEINS

**FIG. 25-10.** Anatomic variations of terminations. (Modified from Lechter A, Lopez G, Martinez C, Camacho J. Anatomy of the gonadal veins: A reappraisal. Surgery 1991;109:735; with permission.)

of the seminiferous tubules are epithelial cells and have some metabolic effect on the germinal cells.

Each testis contains approximately 500 seminiferous tubules, with a combined length of approximately 250 m.

## Epididymis

The epididymis is a long (4-6 m) and very tortuous tube. It is lined by pseudostratified columnar epithelium, which rests on a basement membrane with smooth muscle fibers. These fibers serve, perhaps, to propel the sperm to the ductus deferens.

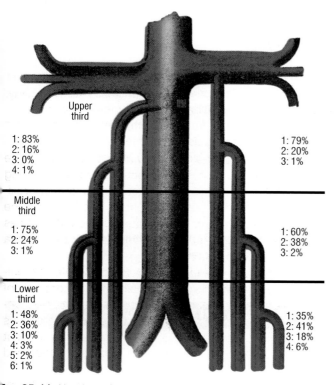

Upper third

1: 83%
2: 16%
3: 0%
4: 1%

1: 79%
2: 20%
3: 1%

Middle third

1: 75%
2: 24%
3: 1%

1: 60%
2: 38%
3: 2%

Lower third

1: 48%
2: 36%
3: 10%
4: 3%
5: 2%
6: 1%

1: 35%
2: 41%
3: 18%
4: 6%

**FIG. 25-11.** Number of venous trunks. (Modified from Lechter A, Lopez G, Martinez C, Camacho J. Anatomy of the gonadal veins: A reappraisal. Surgery 1991;109:735; with permission.)

**TABLE 25-4. Gonadal Veins: Age, Length, and Diameter Distribution**

|  | Minimum | Maximum | Mean | SD |
|---|---|---|---|---|
| Age (yr) | 16 | 76 | 34.6 | 14.9 |
| Length (cm) | 12 | 33 | 23.1 | 3.7 |
| Diameter (mm) | 0.1 | 0.8 | 0.31 | 0.11 |

*Source:* Lechter A, Lopez G, Martinez C, Camacho J. Anatomy of the gonadal veins: A reappraisal. Surgery 109:735-739, 1991; with permission.

**TABLE 25-5. Gonadal Veins: Location and Number of Valves**

| Level/Valved Veins | Right, 48% (%) | Left, 62% (%) |
|---|---|---|
| Ostial valve | 84 | 77 |
| Upper third | 12 | 13 |
| Middle third | 2 | 3 |
| Lower third | 2 | 7 |

The left gonadal vein is valvated more often than the right side (p = 0.001). Roughly 80% of valves are located at the ostium.

*Source:* Lechter A, Lopez G, Martinez C, Camacho J. Anatomy of the gonadal veins: A reappraisal. Surgery 109:735-739, 1991; with permission.

## Spermatic Cord

The histology of the spermatic cord is that of the anatomic entities it contains.

## PHYSIOLOGY

### Testis

The two testicular functions are spermatogenesis, which is the production of spermatozoa (gametes), and production of the steroid testosterone. After the sperm forms in the testis, it travels via the epididymis, the ductus deferens, and the urethra to be expelled by ejaculation.

Testosterone is responsible for the regulation, maintenance, well-being, and transport of the spermatozoa, as well as for the development of the reproductive glands and secondary sex characteristics.

Malignant testicular tumors are common (most are seminomas). Germ cell tumors are the most commonly diagnosed malignancies in male patients between the ages of 15 and 35.[49] Benign tumors are very rare. A palpable abdominal mass in childhood or early adulthood could be a metastasis from painless testicular tumors. Palpate both testes gently and very completely, and order a sonogram if the form of the testis is suspicious. For clinical stage I nonseminoma, retroperitoneal lymph node dissection is advised for staging, prognostic, and therapeutic purposes.[50] Nerve sparing retroperitoneal lymphadenectomy, with identification of the postganglionic nerves, results in the preservation of ejaculation in most patients with low-stage disease and in select patients with advanced disease.[51]

The following summarizes nodal infiltration in metastasis:

- Right testicle:
  - to the node or nodes located at the vicinity of the angle between the renal vein and the IVC
  - to the precaval nodes at the aortic bifurcation
- Left testicle:
  - to the paraaortic nodes
  - to the preaortic nodes (inferior mesenteric nodes)

NOTE: From either testicle, metastasis occasionally reaches into the pelvis and to the external iliac nodes.

## Epididymis

The epithelium of the epididymis contains nutrient fluid and hormones. The function of the epididymis is not well understood. Perhaps it helps with the motility of the sperm. With some assistance from the Sertoli cells, the epithelium of the epididymis may assist the maturation of the sperm and influence the sperm's ability to fertilize the ovum.

## Spermatic Cord

The physiology of the spermatic cord is that of the anatomic entities it contains.

**TABLE 25-6. Gonadal Veins: Collaterals**

| Level/Veins with Collaterals | Right, 49% % | G/R (%) | Left, 67% % | G/R (%) |
|---|---|---|---|---|
| Upper third | 26 | 61/39 | 42 | 88/12 |
| Middle third | 36 | 52/48 | 46 | 45/55 |
| Lower third | 10 | 0/100 | 12 | 0/100 |

G, Collaterals coming from Gerota's perirenal fat; R, collaterals coming from retroperitoneal tissues.
The right gonadal vein has fewer collaterals than the left gonadal vein (p = 0.001).

*Source:* Lechter A, Lopez G, Martinez C, Camacho J. Anatomy of the gonadal veins: A reappraisal. Surgery 109:735-739, 1991; with permission.

## SURGICAL APPLICATIONS

### Varicocelectomy

If the patient is symptomatic, the treatment of choice is ligation of the dilated veins. In adolescent boys with varicocele, some element of testicular growth arrest may be found, such that the testis ipsilateral to the varicocele is often significantly smaller. Current indications for correction in teenage boys are for repair of a large varicocele (particularly if symptomatic), and for a discrepancy in testicular size exceeding 10-20%. Surgical correction has been shown to restore testicular volume in a high percentage of cases. However, Grasso et al.[52] found that left spermatic vein ligation for low-grade varicocele in patients more than 30 years old did not improve sperm quality or rate of paternity when compared with an untreated control group.

Salerno et al.[53] studied vascular variants in anastomosis between the internal spermatic vein and visceral veins. They stressed the importance of accurate venography with a skilled interventional radiologist prior to sclerotherapy.

## Epididymectomy

In epididymectomy, the surgeon must free the epididymis from the testis. Dissect from below upward for about 2.5 cm (1 inch). Visualize the testis as three equal parts, i.e., the upper pole, the central segment, and the lower pole. The bifurcation of the testicular artery is found somewhere between the central segment and the upper pole. Small branches may be ignored, but the epididymal branch must be identified and ligated.

## Orchiopexy

An empty scrotal sac implies an undescended or maldescended testis. True agenesis of the testis is extremely rare. The retained testis should be brought down before the child is 2 years old. After the child reaches 10 years, the testis should be removed rather than brought down.

Early orchiopexy is recommended for the following reasons:

- Cosmetic considerations are important; children can be cruel to those who are "different."
- Preservation of function may be possible if the testis is relocated early enough. However, remember Hunter's[1] dictum that the testis failed to descend because it was defective and was not defective because it failed to descend.
- It reduces risk of trauma, especially to ectopic testis.
- It reduces risk of malignant changes in the retained testis.
- It repairs coexisting indirect inguinal hernia.

Hutcheson et al.[54] stated that good knowledge of the retroperitoneal fascial layers is the key to successful inguinal orchiopexy. We quote their anatomical description:

*The intermediate stratum of the retroperitoneum consists of the connective tissue between the transversalis fascia, also known as the endoabdominal fascia or outer stratum, and the connective tissue of the peritoneum or inner stratum. Proximally the ureter, spermatic vessels and vas are bound in an investing fascia comprising the intermediate stratum. As the vas joins the vessels, the fibers of the intermediate stratum attenuate and these structures are enveloped by the fascia of the inguinal canal, called the internal spermatic fascia, which is contiguous with the transversalis fascia. This investing fascia holds the hernial sac, vas, vessels and cremasteric fibers together. When the testis stops short of the scrotum in its course of descent, the vas and vessels may not be foreshortened. They may be folded in the retroperitoneum and held in place by this investing fascia, as though they were in a retroperitoneal felt.*

## Orchiectomy

Every effort should be made to save the testicle except in testicular necrosis due to spermatic torsion or malignancy. The most common testicular malignancy in children is a yolk sac tumor. Removal of the testicle may be approached through the scrotum in benign disease (e.g., hydrocele) or through an inguinal incision if malignancy is suspected (elevation of alpha-fetoprotein). The scrotal approach should be done through a transverse scrotal incision since the blood vessels run transversely.

With testicular malignacy, retroperitoneal lymphadenectomy may be necessary as well as high ligation and removal of the spermatic cord. Occasionally hemiscrotectomy must be done if there is a fixation of the testicle to the skin.

## ANATOMIC COMPLICATIONS

## Varicocelectomy

Persistence of varicosities is the most frequent complication. It results from failure to ligate all the varicosed veins. The ductus deferens and its artery, as well as the testicular artery, must be identified and protected. Best results with few complications have been obtained when the testicular artery and vein are ligated above their confluence with the ductus deferens and its accompanying deferential artery.[55]

## Epididymectomy

Every precaution must be taken to preserve the main trunk of the testicular artery (see Fig. 25-5). Injury to this artery will result in testicular atrophy at best and testicular necrosis at worst.

## Orchiopexy

The most common complication of orchiopexy is injury to the blood supply from ligation or excessive traction on a "short" spermatic cord. After careful lysis of all adhesions, if the cord is too short to place the testis in the scrotum, the internal ring should be opened. The spermatic vessels must not be sacrificed for an additional length of cord. Hunt et al.[56] described a method for increasing the available length of the spermatic cord. Caruso et al.[57] advocate a single high

scrotal incision for patients with a palpable undescended testicle below the external ring for dissection of the hernial sac and relocation of the testis.

Remember that the collateral blood supply to the normal descended testis is not available to the relocated testis.

## Orchiectomy

The primary complications of orchiectomy are bleeding and formation of hematoma (inguinal or scrotal). A vertical incision should never be used because the blood vessels of the scrotal wall run transversely.

Bleeding from the cut edge of the tunica vaginalis can be prevented by wrapping the scrotum with an elastic bandage for 24 hours. Pressure must be uniform and the bandage must be smooth to avoid local skin necrosis.

# Ductus Deferens (Vas)

## HISTORY

The anatomic and surgical history of the ductus deferens is shown in Table 25-1.

## EMBRYOGENESIS AND CONGENITAL ANOMALIES

The mesonephric ducts are stimulated by testosterone, which is produced by the Leydig cells. The ducts form the right and left ductus deferens.

Congenital anomalies are found in Table 25-2. They include the following malformations.

- Absence of ductus deferens (unilateral or bilateral)[58]
- Congenital atresia
- Duplication
- Ectopia
- Anomalous pathway
- Other possible associated anomalies

## SURGICAL ANATOMY

The ductus deferens starts where the epididymal duct (epididymal tail) ends, and terminates at the ejaculatory duct (Fig. 25-12). The ductus has a length of about 45 cm. Characteristically, its tortuous proximal part and almost straight distal part are dilated.

### Pathway

The pathway of the ductus is scrotal, inguinal, abdominal, and pelvic.

Within the scrotum, the ductus has an ascending course at the medial side of the epididymis and the posterosuperior area of the testicle.

Within the inguinal canal, the ductus is incorporated into the spermatic cord. It is located posteromedially in the cord, and is surrounded by the venous pampiniform plexus.

At the deep inguinal ring (abdominal), the ductus leaves the cord. It proceeds toward and into the pelvis after looping over the inferior epigastric artery and in front of the

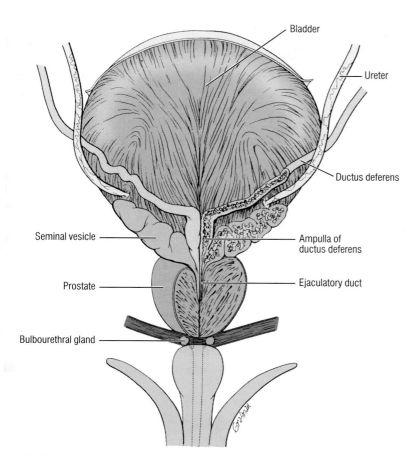

**FIG. 25-12.** Seminal vesicles and associated ducts. (Based on Hinman F Jr. Atlas of Urosurgical Anatomy. Philadelphia: WB Saunders, 1993.)

external iliac artery and vein. In the pelvis, the ductus descends from the pelvic sidewall with its deferential arterial supply, supported by a delicate mesentery.

## Relations

The ductus is related to the following anatomic entities during its backward pathway to the base of the bladder (Fig 25-13):
- lateral to the umbilical artery
- lateral to the obturator nerve and vessels
- lateral to the superior vesical vessels
- anteromedial side of the ureter
- posterior aspect of the bladder
- medial to the seminal vesicles where it becomes dilated as the ampulla

The ductus continues toward the base of the prostate, joining the duct of the seminal vesicle to form the ejaculatory duct. The ejaculatory duct passes anteroinferiorly through the prostate to reach the summit of the seminal colliculus, the expanded portion of the urethral ridge in the prostatic part of the urethra.

REMEMBER:
- The ductus can be palpated in the upper part of the scrotum as a firm cord.
- The ductus can also be palpated at the posterior aspect of the spermatic cord during open inguinal herniorrhaphy.
- The ductus deferens is located at the lateral side of the inferior epigastric artery, where the elements of the spermatic cord separate just inside and lateral to the internal abdominal ring. At the lower, inner part of the deep inguinal ring, from medial to lateral, are the cremasteric artery, the genital branch of the genitofemoral nerve, and the ductus.
- The topographic anatomy and relations of the ductus within the lower abdomen and pelvis should be kept in mind.

## HISTOLOGY AND PHYSIOLOGY

The ductus is a long tube with a very thick wall and a very narrow lumen. Its mucosa has the same epithelium as

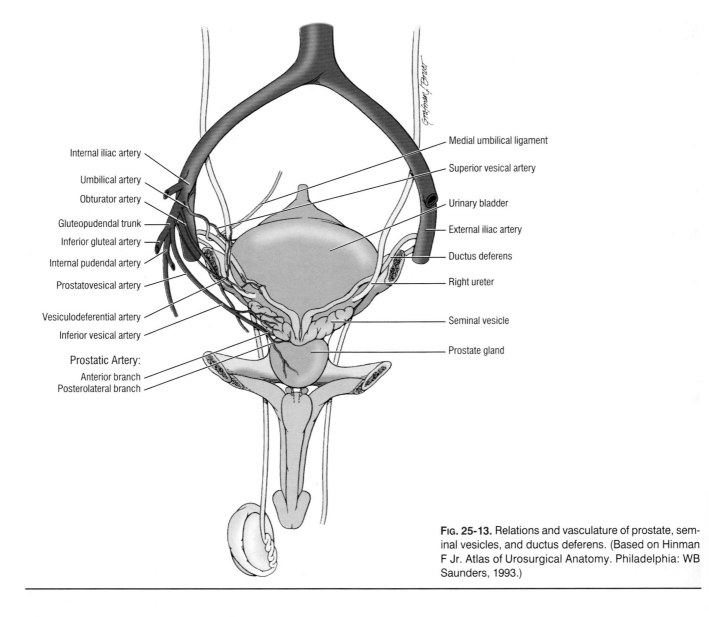

Internal iliac artery

Umbilical artery

Obturator artery

Gluteopudendal trunk

Inferior gluteal artery

Internal pudendal artery

Prostatovesical artery

Vesiculodeferential artery

Inferior vesical artery

Prostatic Artery:

Anterior branch
Posterolateral branch

Medial umbilical ligament

Superior vesical artery

Urinary bladder

External iliac artery

Ductus deferens

Right ureter

Seminal vesicle

Prostate gland

FIG. 25-13. Relations and vasculature of prostate, seminal vesicles, and ductus deferens. (Based on Hinman F Jr. Atlas of Urosurgical Anatomy. Philadelphia: WB Saunders, 1993.)

the epididymis, and its thick muscular wall is formed by smooth muscle cells.

A small portion of the sperm is stored in the epididymis, but the majority is stored in the ductus deferens.

## SURGICAL APPLICATIONS

The general surgeon encounters more and more patients requesting bilateral partial vasectomy as a contraceptive measure to provide elective sterility in men. The incision for vasectomy should be made high on the scrotum,

well away from the epididymis. The ductus deferens (vas) can be pulled out for 4 to 6 cm for ligation. Precautions must be taken in this procedure to avoid spontaneous recanalization of the ductus.

In vasectomy, simple ligation is not an adequate procedure. A segment of the ductus should be removed. Some surgeons cauterize both ends of the cut ductus,[59] or fold each end over and bury each in a different scrotal layer.[60] It has become commonplace, when a patient requests it, to perform vasectomy during laparoscopic or open herniorrhaphy.

Epididymectomy for treatment of scrotal pain following vasectomy was recommended by West et al.[61]

# ANATOMIC COMPLICATIONS

## Vascular Injury

During vasectomy, hemorrhage from the scrotal wall must be avoided. The blood vessels run transversely, so a vertical incision should never be used. Suture the subcutaneous layer with absorbable continuous or interrupted sutures when closing the incision. An elastic bandage will maintain gentle compression for 24 hours.

## Inadequate Procedure

Sperm granuloma is the result of leakage of sperm from the proximal cut end of the ductus. It can occur during the operation or later if the stump is inadequately occluded; rupture of an epididymal tubule is a rare but possible cause. The usual cause is from ligatures that cut through the wall of the ductus. The incidence can be as high as 60 percent.[62] Schmidt and Morris[63] considered sperm granuloma to be the most important complication of vasectomy.

The granuloma may be self-limiting and may respond to conservative treatment, but surgical excision is sometimes required. Pain, over a period of months, is suggestive of sperm granuloma.

Spontaneous restoration of the ductus deferens has been reported in as many as 6 percent of some series.[63] This is the result of inadequate ligation. Very rarely, duplication of the ductus is encountered. Usually, but not always, a supernumerary testis is also present.[65] A second ligation is required if sperm appear in the ejaculate.

# *Potential Spaces Above the Urogenital Diaphragm*

# SURGICAL ANATOMY

The fascial layers in the perineum are complicated and unpredictable to some degree. In brief, Camper's fascia of the anterior abdominal wall (Fig. 25-14) is continuous with the fatty layer in the perineum, thigh, and gluteal region. Scarpa's membranous layer extends into the perineum, but is referred to there as Colles' fascia. Further, Camper's fascia and Scarpa's fascia of the anterior abdominal wall blend, become thinner and coalesce with smooth muscle fibers to form the dartos tunic of the external genitalia.

The fascial layer on the external surface of the external oblique muscle and rectus sheath is called the fascia of Gallaudet (sometimes referred to as the innominate fascia). A similarly-named counterpart is to be found covering the muscles in the superficial compartment of the perineum. This deep fascial layer is called Buck's fascia on the penis, and forms the deep fascia of the penis.

The seeming simplicity of arrangement of fascial layers, as described above, is belied by variations in degree of lamination of fibrous tissue associated with Camper's fascia, and its intermingling with Scarpa's fascia in the lower part of the anterior abdominal wall and perineum. In addition, there may be some adipose tissue between Colles' fascia and the deep fascia of Gallaudet in the perineum. On the genitalia, the space between superficial fascia and Buck's fascia is easily determined.

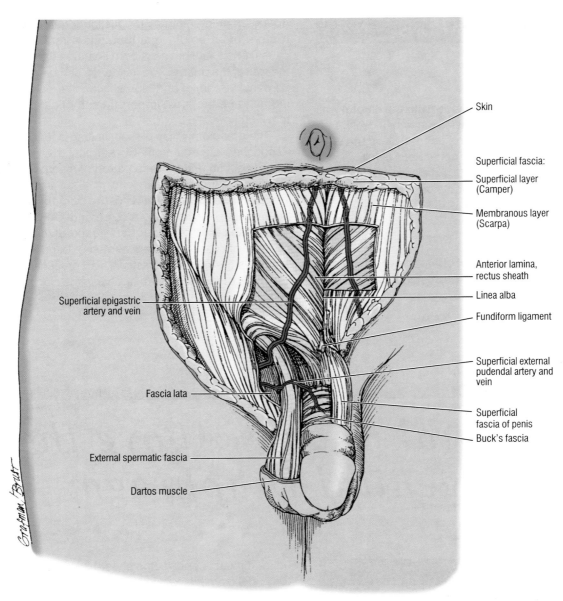

Skin

Superficial fascia:

Superficial layer
(Camper)

Membranous layer
(Scarpa)

Anterior lamina,
rectus sheath

Linea alba

Fundiform ligament

Superficial external
pudendal artery and
vein

Superficial
fascia of penis

Buck's fascia

Superficial epigastric
artery and vein

Fascia lata

External spermatic fascia

Dartos muscle

**Fig. 25-14.** Skin and fascia of inguinal area. (Based on Hinman F Jr. Atlas of Urosurgical Anatomy. Philadelphia: WB Saunders, 1993.)

# *Scrotum*

## HISTORY

The anatomic and surgical history of the scrotum is shown in Table 25-1 under the heading *Testes, Epididymis, and Scrotum.*

## EMBRYOGENESIS

### Normal Development

The formation of the scrotum is a result of the fusion of the right and left labioscrotal folds. A scrotal septum separates the scrotum into two halves. This separation is obvious externally by the raphe between the right and left scrotal halves.

### Congenital Anomalies

The congenital anomalies of the scrotum will be found in Table 25-2.

The cause of the venous dilation of varicocele is enigmatic. There is no solid embryologic or anatomic explanation for the condition. Varicocelectomy is the procedure of choice for testicular pain and infertility.

Accessory scrotum has been reported.[66]

## SURGICAL ANATOMY

### Layers of the Scrotum

The scrotum houses the testes and the epididymis. It is composed of eight layers that are derived and modified from the six layers of the abdominal wall (Fig. 25-15). Although the layers are continuous, their terminology changes as they pass from abdomen to scrotum (Table 25-7).

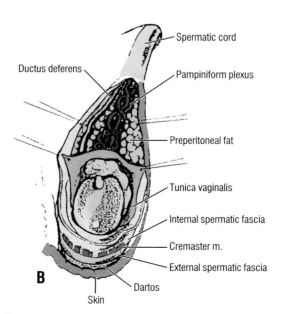

**FIG. 25-15.** Scrotal layers. **A,** Cross section of scrotum and testes; **B,** Anterior view of left testis (the parietal layer of the tunica vaginalis and spermatic cord has been opened). (Modified from Gray SW, Skandalakis JE, McClusky DA. Atlas of Surgical Anatomy for General Surgeons. Baltimore: Williams & Wilkins, 1985; with permission.)

**TABLE 25-7. The Corresponding Layers of the Abdominal Wall and Scrotum**

| Abdominal Wall | Scrotum |
|---|---|
| Skin | Skin |
| Superficial fascia (Camper's and Scarpa's) | Dartos and smooth muscle |
| External oblique (innominate) fascia | External spermatic fascia |
| Internal oblique muscle and aponeurosis | Cremasteric fascia and muscle |
| Transversus abdominis muscle and aponeurosis | Cremasteric fascia and muscle |
| Transversalis fascia | Internal spermatic fascia |
| Preperitoneal fat | Preperitoneal fat |
| Peritoneum | Tunica vaginalis |

*Source:* Modified from Skandalakis JE, Colborn GL, Pemberton B, Skandalakis LJ, Gray SW. The surgical anatomy of the inguinal area — Part 2. Contemp Surg 38:28-38, 1991; with permission.

## Scrotal Skin (Layer 1)

The first layer, the scrotal skin, is thin, pigmented, elastic, and corrugated. It is heavily fixed to the underlying superficial fascia. It contains many sebaceous glands that occasionally become cystic. In the midline is the raphe, the medial ridge, and the attachment of the septum.

## Dartos (Layer 2)

The second layer, the dartos muscle or tunic, is the superficial fascia of the scrotum. It is formed by the blending of Camper's fatty tissue, Scarpa's membranous fascia, and smooth muscle fibers. The dartos tunic is continuous over the penis, forming its superficial fascia. In the perineum the adipose layer of Camper and the membranous layer, now called Colles' fascia, again separate into more or less distinct layers. The first and second layers are scrotal in the strict sense.

The dartos tunic, composed of connective tissue and smooth muscle fibers, is fixed to the skin. Colles' fascia is attached posteriorly to the urogenital diaphragm and laterally to the periosteum of the ischiopubic rami. In the perineum, Colles' fascia lies superficial to the deep fascia which covers the superficial genital musculature.

A potential space, the superficial perineal cleft, is formed between Colles' fascia and the muscular fascia (of Gallaudet) that opens anteriorly and superiorly into the subcutaneous space of the lower abdomen, between the membranous fascia of Scarpa and the deep muscle fascia of Gallaudet. Extravasated urine may collect in this space.

The deep fascia of the perineum (the fascia of Gallaudet or external perineal fascia) is continuous with Buck's deep fascial layer of the penis.

## External Spermatic Fascia (Layer 3)

The external spermatic fascia is the third layer. This is the scrotal continuation of the external muscle fascia of the abdominal wall, referred to as the fascia of Gallaudet or innominate fascia. This fascial layer is continuous over the penis as the deep fascia, or Buck's fascia.

## Cremaster Muscle (Layers 4 and 5)

The cremaster muscle is derived primarily from the internal oblique muscle, but may also include the transversus abdominis muscle. Although the fibers are striated, they are not under voluntary control.

## Internal Spermatic Fascia (Layer 6)

The internal spermatic fascia is a prolongation of the transversalis fascia. Layers 3, 4, 5, and 6 form the coverings of the spermatic cord.

## Preperitoneal Fat (Layer 7)

A layer of preperitoneal fat may or may not be present.

## Tunica Vaginalis (Layer 8)

The tunica vaginalis is a serous membrane of peritoneum. Layers 7 and 8 are constituents of the cord.

Within these eight layers of the scrotum, the testes themselves move freely. Only the skin and the dartos are fixed. At the base of the scrotum, the scrotal ligament anchors the testis and deters torsion.

The subcutaneous superficial fascia in the scrotum contains little adipose tissue, this being replaced by smooth muscle that forms the tunica dartos scroti. The attachment of these muscle fibers to the skin forms the rugal folds of the scrotal skin.

# Vascular Supply

## Arteries

The scrotum is well supplied with blood. Branches of the superficial and deep external pudendal arteries (from the common femoral artery) supply the anterior part of the scrotum and anastomose with branches of the internal pudendal artery, which supply the posterior portion of the scrotum. The terminal branches in the scrotum lie transversely, so that exploration of the scrotum should be through a transverse incision to minimize bleeding. Good hemostasis is necessary to avoid hematomas. Good approximation of the dartos will help.

## Veins

The veins draining the anterior scrotum follow the external pudendal arteries to empty into the great saphenous vein. Veins from the posterior scrotum follow the internal pudendal artery to become tributaries to the internal iliac vein.

## Lymphatics

The skin of the scrotum, together with the perineal skin, is drained by lymph vessels that follow the external pudendal vessels to the superficial inguinal nodes.

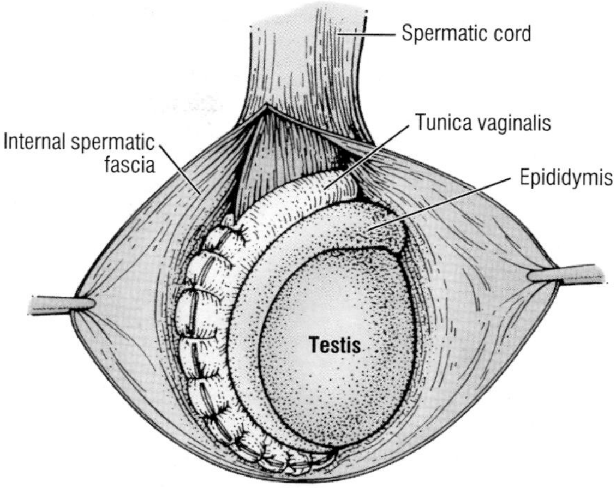

## Innervation

The skin of the anterior scrotum is innervated by anterior scrotal branches of the ilioinguinal nerve. There are some fibers from the external spermatic branch of the genitofemoral nerve that also supply the cremaster muscle. The posterior scrotum receives posterior scrotal nerves from the perineal branch of the pudendal nerve or the long scrotal branches of the posterior femoral cutaneous nerve.

## SURGICAL APPLICATIONS

For hydrocelectomy, two methods can be used. Ex-

FIG. 25-16. Hydrocelectomy: bottle neck procedure. (Modified from Skandalakis JE, Gray SW, Rowe JS Jr. Anatomical Complications in General Surgery. New York: McGraw-Hill, 1983; with permission.)

cision of the tunica vaginalis uses continuous, oversewn absorbable sutures to ensure hemostasis. The "bottle neck" procedure involves incision of the tunica, erection of the edges, and suturing posteriorly to the epididymis by interrupted or continuous absorbable sutures (Fig. 25-16).

## ANATOMIC COMPLICATIONS

Bleeding from the cut edge of the tunica vaginalis can be prevented by wrapping the scrotum with an elastic bandage for 24 hours. Pressure must be uniform and the bandage must be smooth to avoid local skin necrosis.

# Seminal Vesicles

## HISTORY

The anatomic and surgical history of the seminal vesicles is shown in Table 25-1.

## EMBRYOGENESIS AND CONGENITAL ANOMALIES

The seminal vesicles (seminal glands) are formed from

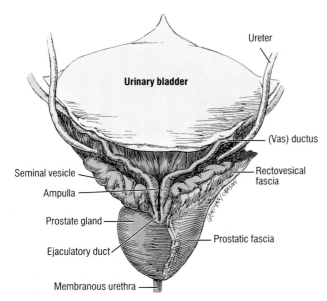

FIG. 25-17. Seminal vesicles and deferent ducts.

a lateral outgrowth of the caudal end of each mesonephric duct.

The congenital anomalies of the seminal vesicles are not well documented. They are associated with other malformations of the male reproductive system (see Table 25-2). These defects include unilateral or bilateral absence, duplications, and cysts.

## SURGICAL ANATOMY

The seminal vesicles are bilateral, saccular tubular glands (Figs. 25-17, 25-18). Each seminal vesicle measures approximately 5 cm x 1 cm; each is normally about 15 cm in length when uncoiled. The seminal vesicles are located at the posterior surface of the base of the bladder, lateral to the ductus deferens.

The topographic anatomy and relations of the seminal vesicles are as follows:

- Anterior and superior: urinary bladder, occasionally fixed
- Posterior and inferior: Denonvilliers' fascia (the rectovesical septum) and anorectum
- Above: peritoneum in the rectovesical fossa (may be occasionally reached by the tip of the seminal vesicles)
- Medial: ductus deferens
- Lateral: multiple vesicle vessels and levator ani
- Below: ejaculatory duct, where it unites with the ampulla of the ductus deferens

## Vascular Supply

### *Arteries*

The blood supply to the seminal vesicle (see Fig. 25-13) is presented very succinctly by Hinman.[44] We present his description:

> The blood supply to the seminal vesicle is from the vesiculodeferential artery. This artery arises from the superior vesical artery or, more frequently, from the site where the internal iliac artery takes off from the umbilical artery.[67] As it passes anterior to the ureter, it provides branches to that structure. At the seminal vesicle, it divides into three branches: (1) one to the bladder, (2) one to the vas, and (3) the largest to the anterior surface of the vesicle. This anterior vesicular artery divides on the surface of the vesicle to supply its anterior part. A second source of blood is the inferior vesicular artery, which may come either from the prostatovesical artery or directly from the gluteopudendal trunk. Its small branches supply the posterior portion of the vesicle and anastomose with branches of the anterior vesicular artery.

### *Veins*

The veins follow the arteries, draining into the prostatic venous plexus and then to the internal iliac vein.

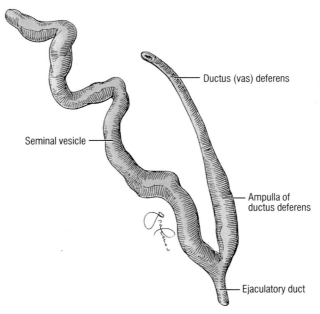

FIG. 25-18. Seminal vesicle unraveled. (Based on Basmajian JV, Slonecker CE. Grant's Method of Anatomy, 11th ed. Baltimore: Williams & Wilkins, 1989.)

## *Lymphatics*

The lymphatics drain into the external and internal iliac nodes together with the prostatic lymphatics. There are lymphatic interconnections with lymphatics from the ductus, the bladder, and the rectum.

## Innervation

According to Macwhinney,[68] the seminal vesicles are innervated by adrenergic fibers from the hypogastric nerve. If both sympathetic chain ganglia at the L1 spinal nerve level are removed by lumbar sympathectomy, sexual function may be affected.[69] Loss of ejaculatory ability occurs in 54% of these cases, and impotence in 63%, according to Whitelaw and Smithwick.[70]

Erection is primarily due to parasympathetic neural control. The ejaculatory response is principally under sympathetic control until ejaculate reaches the penile urethra within which somatic motor innervation comes into play.

## HISTOLOGY

The mucosal folds of the seminal vesicles consist of pseudostratified epithelium with columnar or cuboidal cells. Their mucosa is composed of columnar epithelium with some goblet cells. The lamina propria is formed by connective tissue and some smooth muscle.

## PHYSIOLOGY

The seminal vesicles do not store the spermatozoa, as

some have thought. Spermatozoa are stored in the epididymis until the first phase of sexual excitement, when they are held in the ampulla of the ductus. Tanagho[71] stated that the seminal vesicles have a considerable luminal storage capacity.

The seminal vesicles are secretory glands. The physiologic destiny of the seminal vesicles is to secrete a fluid which is responsible for the nutrition of the spermatozoa.

About 70% of the seminal fluid is formed in the seminal vesicle. Its complex secretion consists of water, mucoid fructose substances, potassium ions, prostaglandins, endorphins, fibronectin, and so on. When prostaglandin was first discovered it was so named because of the erroneous conclusion that it was secreted by the prostate. Soon it was discovered that, indeed, prostaglandin is secreted by the seminal vesicles, not the prostate. Fructose is produced nowhere else in the body, and provides a forensic determination of rape. The choline content, assayed as choline crystals, is the preferred test to determine the presence of semen (Florence test).

Emission of the ejaculate is effected by muscles that receive parasympathetic fibers and somatic nerve fibers from S2, 3, 4.

## SURGICAL APPLICATIONS

- Normal seminal vesicles cannot be felt by rectal examination in the majority of cases.
- Only seminal vesicles enlarged by disease (inflammatory process, etc) will be felt by rectal examination.
- The inferior vesicular artery should be clipped or controlled prior to removal of the seminal vesicle to avoid troublesome bleeding.
- Eastham et al.[72] presented a case of seminal vesicle abscess secondary to tuberculosis.

# Ejaculatory Ducts

## HISTORY

The anatomic and surgical history of the ejaculatory ducts is shown in Table 25-1.

## EMBRYOGENESIS AND CONGENITAL ANOMALIES

The ejaculatory ducts are formed from a portion of the mesonephric duct between the duct of the seminal vesicle and the urethra. Each ejaculatory duct is formed by the union of the ampulla of the ductus and the inferior part of the seminal vesicle.

Malformations of the ejaculatory ducts include agenesis, duplication, ectopia, congenital obstruction, and ureteric insertion into the duct.

## SURGICAL ANATOMY

The ejaculatory ducts pass distally through the prostate gland, with the posterior glandular part of the organ behind. The median lobe of the prostate is in front. The duct has a very thin wall, a length of approximately 2 cm, and a diameter of less than 1 mm. The ducts end as small openings on either side of the midline on the verumontanum of the urethral ridge (Figs. 25-19, 25-20).

Since a sphincter has not yet been found in this area, a fold of mucosa acting as a valve could be an obstacle, preventing retrograde passage of fluid up the ejaculatory duct. Perhaps the "curvy" pathway of the ducts is responsible for this action.[66] It is possible that the ducts are compressed by prostatic glandular tissue, except in orgasm when internal pressure caused by the ejaculation opens the duct.

It is not known if the smooth muscle of the ejaculatory duct walls is a sphincterlike anatomic entity. Its tissue paper consistency makes it very vulnerable. It is easily torn from the prostate.

## HISTOLOGY AND PHYSIOLOGY

Embryologically and anatomically, the ejaculatory duct is formed by the union of the seminal vesicle and the ampulla of the ductus deferens, so most likely their histology and physiology are the same.

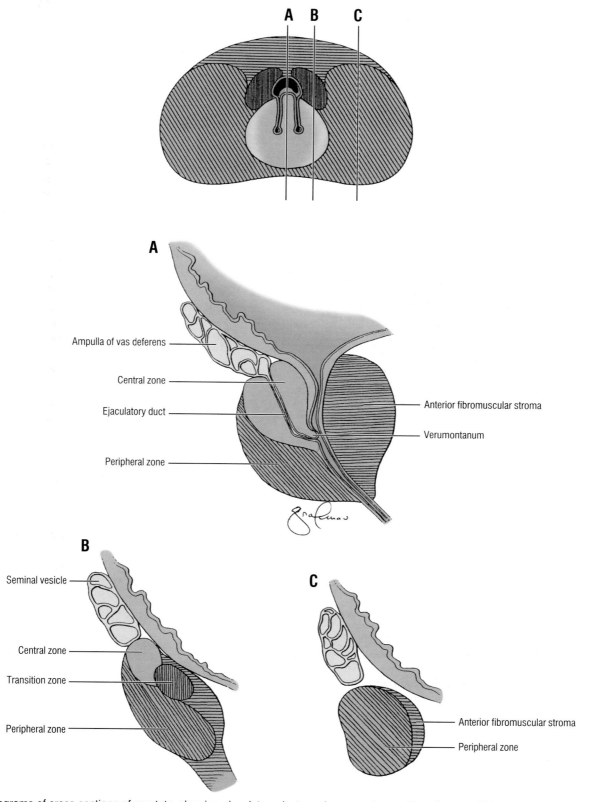

A B C

A

Ampulla of vas deferens

Central zone

Ejaculatory duct

Peripheral zone

Anterior fibromuscular stroma

Verumontanum

B

Seminal vesicle

Central zone

Transition zone

Peripheral zone

C

Anterior fibromuscular stroma

Peripheral zone

Fɪɢ. **25-19.** Diagrams of cross-sections of prostate, showing ejaculatory ducts and verumontanum. Top diagram: Oblique transverse section through the terminal portions of ejaculatory ducts. **A,** Near median section (peripheral zone, anterior fibromuscular stroma). **B,** Sagittal section, 1 cm from median plane (transitional, central, peripheral zones). **C,** Sagittal section, 2 cm from median plane (peripheral zone, anterior fibromuscular stroma.) (Based on Hinman F Jr. Atlas of Urosurgical Anatomy. Philadelphia: WB Saunders, 1993.)

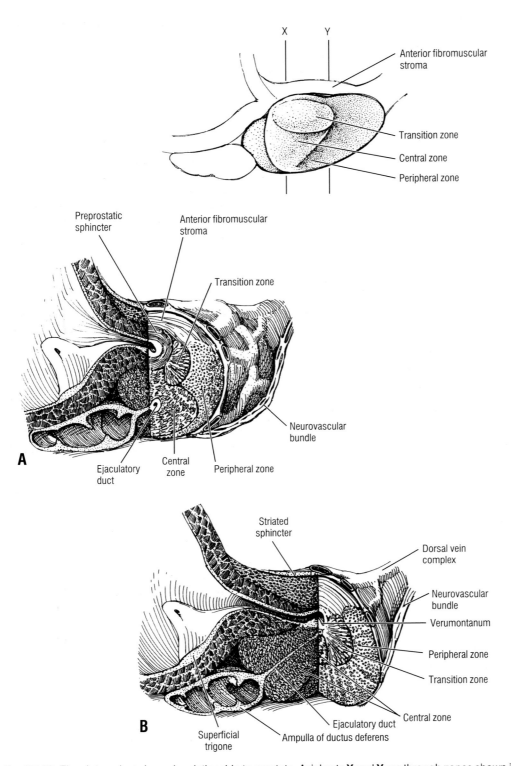

FIG. 25-20. Ejaculatory duct shown in relationship to prostate. Axial cuts **X** and **Y** are through zones shown in small diagram. **A,** Proximal cut on plane X. Sagittal section on left, axial section on right. **B,** Distal cut on plane Y. (From Hinman F Jr. Atlas of Urosurgical Anatomy. Philadelphia: WB Saunders, 1993; with permission.)

# *Prostate*

For the many men suffering from prostate cancer throughout the world, we must continue our efforts to improve
diagnosis, treatment, and basic understanding of this fatal
disease.

**Walsh and Brooks**[73]

The author of this chapter most senior in age (JES, 67 at
that time) had a complete physical examination by Dr. William
M. McClatchey in March, 1987, which was reported as negative. Because of pain in his left knee, he had another partial
examination in October, 1987.

WMcC:    I want to do a rectal.
JES:        But I had a rectal by you 6 months ago.
WMcC:    My professor told me that not one patient will
             leave my office without a recent rectal exami-
             nation.
JES:        (Unwillingly) O.K.

Rectal exam revealed a prostatic nodule. Prostate specific antigen (PSA) from the earlier exam had been 0.3
ng/ml; the current report was 0.4 ng/ml. Both were within
normal limits. But biopsy revealed adenocarcinoma.
Radical prostatectomy by Dr. Sam Ambrose 2 weeks later
revealed that the prostate (including its capsule) was full of
cancer. Five years later an LHRH (luteinizing hormone-re-
leasing hormone) agonist (Lupron) was started because
the PSA had risen to 5.3 ng/ml. At present, Dr. Skandalakis
is asymptomatic and the PSA is under 0.

## HISTORY

The anatomic and surgical history of the prostate is
shown in Table 25-1.

## EMBRYOGENESIS AND CONGENITAL ANOMALIES

The prostate gland is formed around the end of the third

month (first trimester) from the epithelium of the future prostatic urethra. The epithelium proliferates and penetrates
the surrounding mesenchyme, which is the future fibromuscular prostatic tissue.

Congenital anomalies of the prostate will be found in
Table 25-2. These include partial or complete agenesis,
persistence of the anterior lobe, enlargement of the prostatic utricle, and heterotopic prostate. All these anomalies
are rare.

## SURGICAL ANATOMY

### Topographic Anatomy and Relations

The classical description of the adult prostate is that it
has the size, shape, and consistency of a large chestnut.
The form of the prostate is that of a compressed inverted
cone: pyramidal, having a base and an apex. It is located
between the vesical neck of the bladder and the apex of
the urogenital diaphragm. According to Wilson et al.,[74] the
prostate apex is located above the ischial tuberosities in
99.3% of cases. This fact may help the radiologist-oncolo-
gist to deliver accurate external beam radiation.

The normal weight of the prostate in a young adult is
from 17 to 19 g. The numbers 4, 3, 2 are useful as a mnemonic for remembering the transverse, vertical, and sagittal dimensions in centimeters, respectively, of the gland.

The prostate is enveloped by extraperitoneal connective tissues that cover the thin anatomic capsule (true
capsule) of the organ, and it in turn envelops the proximal
male urethra.

### Fixation and Suspension

The following structures are responsible for the fixation
of the prostate in its bed:
- Puboprostatic ligaments
- Urogenital diaphragm
- Bladder
- Prostatic sheath
- Fascia of Denonvilliers

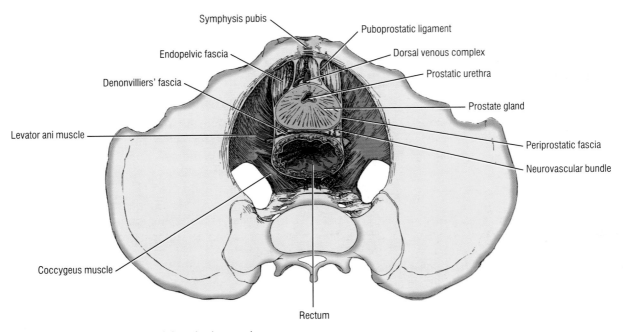

Symphysis pubis

Puboprostatic ligament

Endopelvic fascia

Dorsal venous complex

Denonvilliers' fascia

Prostatic urethra

Prostate gland

Levator ani muscle

Periprostatic fascia

Neurovascular bundle

Coccygeus muscle

Rectum

**FIG. 25-21.** Puboprostatic ligaments and dorsal vein complex.

Steiner[75] stated that the puboprostatic ligaments have a pyramidal shape that is part of a larger urethral suspensory mechanism which attaches the membranous urethra to the pubic bone (Fig 25-21).

Both males and females have a similar mechanism of suspension formed by 3 anatomic entities in continuity.

- A condensation of the endopelvic fascia between the prostate and the levator ani forms the "white line" (Fig. 25-22). This band attaches posteriorly to the ischial spine, where it is continuous with the transverse fascial septum formed by the fascia of Denonvilliers. Anteriorly, the arcus tendineus of the fascia pelvis attaches to the pubic bone approximately 1 cm from the lower edge of the pubis about a centimeter lateral to the symphysis. This band is intimately continuous with the puboprostatic and pubourethral ligaments on either side of the midline. The puboprostatic ligaments connect the pubic bone with the capsule of the gland.
- The fascial capsule (true capsule) of the prostate is continuous with the superior fascia of the urogenital diaphragm, the anterior thickened edge of which forms the transverse perineal ligament.
- The intermediate pubourethral ligament is formed by the pubic arcuate and the transverse perineal ligaments.

Steiner[75] stated that the attachment of the urethral suspensory mechanism is inserted bilaterally into the lateral urethral border, forming a sling from the pubic arch. A good anatomic understanding of the relationship of the urethral suspensory mechanism to the urethra and its striated muscle sphincter and dorsal vein may facilitate apical dissection during radical retropubic prostatectomy. Proper prostatic apical dissection will minimize bleeding, ensure positive surgical margins, and reduce the likelihood of urinary incontinence.

## Prostatic Urethra

The prostatic urethra (Fig. 25-23) begins at the urethral meatus at the apex of the trigone of the bladder. This opening is crescent-shaped, invaginated posteriorly by a protuberance caused by the underlying glandular tissue (median lobe of the prostate), thus forming the uvula vesicae. This is continuous with a posterior midline urethral ridge, or crest, in the urethra. The urethral ridge has a distinctly expanded portion called the verumontanum, or seminal colliculus. To better understand these structures, we can define some of the anatomic entities related to the prostate and the urethra (see also the discussion of the prostatic urethra in the male urethra section of this chapter).

The *urethral crest* is a ridge located on the floor of the posterior urethra between the bladder and the membranous urethra. It is wider at the vesical neck (the uvula) than on its pathway to the membranous urethra.

The *verumontanum (colliculus seminalis)* is a small elevated hillock at the middle area of the urethral crest.

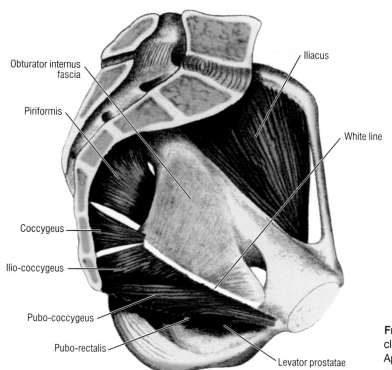

Obturator internus
fascia

Piriformis

Coccygeus

Ilio-coccygeus

Pubo-coccygeus

Pubo-rectalis

Iliacus

White line

Levator prostatae

**FIG. 25-22.** Levator ani muscle (left half), showing levator muscle of prostate. (Modified from Last RJ. Anatomy Regional and Applied (5th ed). Baltimore: Williams & Wilkins, 1972; with permission.)

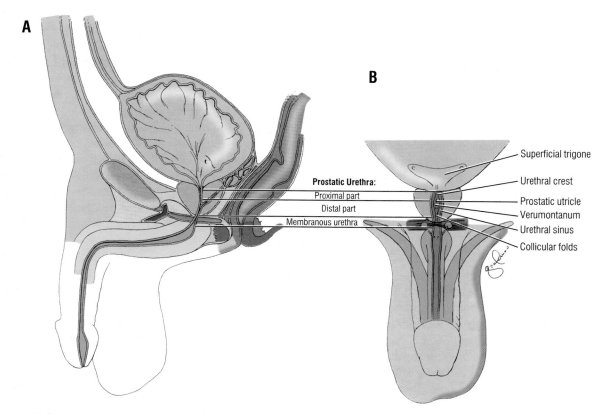

**A**

**B**

**Prostatic Urethra:**
Proximal part
Distal part
Membranous urethra

Superficial trigone

Urethral crest

Prostatic uticle

Verumontanum

Urethral sinus

Collicular folds

**FIG. 25-23.** Prostatic urethra. **A,** sagittal section. **B,** Oblique coronal view. (Based on Hinman F Jr. Atlas of Urosurgical Anatomy. Philadelphia: WB Saunders, 1993.)

The *prostatic utricle* or *uterus masculinus* is a crypt located in the middle portion of the verumontanum, approximately 6 mm deep. Garat et al.[76] and Varlet et al.[77] reported congenital dilatation of the utricle. Meisheri et al.[78] urge that patients with an enlarged prostatic utricle be carefully examined to ascertain whether this condition is associated with female internal organs.

The *orifices of the ejaculatory ducts* are located on the right and left sides of the verumontanum.

The *prostatic sinus* is a depression located on the right or left side of the urethral crest, home of the openings of the prostatic ductules and the urethral glands.

Ureteric ectopia occurs most commonly in the prostatic urethra, and in the seminal vesicle with less frequency. If an ectopic ureter is in the seminal vesicle, a normal ipsilateral kidney is uncommon.

## Prostatic Surfaces

There are four prostatic surfaces: one posterior, one anterior, and two inferolateral.

The *posterior surface* is flat transversely and convex vertically. It is separated from the rectal ampulla by the bilaminar fascia of Denonvilliers. This surface is characterized by a midline groove that is wider toward the base of the gland, and serves to partially separate the gland posteriorly into left and right lobes.

The posterior surface may be palpated by digital rectal examination. The vesicoprostatic junction is located at the upper border of the posterior surface.

The narrow and convex *anterior surface* is located between the apex and the base. Multiple large veins separate this surface from the symphysis pubis. According to Tanagho,[71] the distance between the pubic symphysis and the anterior surface is approximately 2 cm.

The avascular puboprostatic ligaments are fibrous cords, wide or narrow. They connect the upper limits of the anterior surface of the prostate to the pubic bone, at the right and left sides of the cartilaginous area.

The right and left *inferolateral surfaces* are embraced by the anterior part of the levator ani muscles. They are fixed to the levator by the arcus tendineus of the fascia pelvis ("white line"), sagittal connective tissue bands between the ischial spine, and the pubic bone (Fig. 25-22). Here there is a very rich venous network and fibrous tissue which contributes part of the lateral prostatic sheath.

The levator prostatae muscle is the most anterior and most medial part of the levator ani muscle. These muscle fibers pass about the prostate gland and insert into the perineal body beneath the prostate gland, related to the anterior parts of the levator ani muscle. Thus, the muscle en-

croaches upon the prostate behind by a U-shaped sling (Fig. 25-22). Last[79] astutely noted that "levator prostate" is not an apt term. We tend to agree; nonetheless, at orgasm, the pubococcygeus muscle contracts strongly and with this, the prostatic portion probably does, indeed, both lift and compress the prostate gland.

## Fascia of Denonvilliers

In early fetal peritoneal development, the peritoneum extends downward as a pouch reaching the muscular pelvic floor and perineal body. Later the pouch disappears as the growing organs lift the peritoneal covering, resulting in fusion of the more anterior and posterior parts of the peritoneal covering, producing a bilaminar transverse septum. This septum is continuous with the peritoneum above and the perineal body below, and is continuous between the ischial spines. Layers unite with each other, forming a potential space. The union of these two layers produces the fascia of Denonvilliers.

Van Ophoven and Roth[80] concluded: "Denonvilliers' fascia consists of a single layer arising from fusion of the 2 walls of the embryologic peritoneal cul-de-sac. Histologically, it has a double-layered quality. The fascia of Denonvilliers extends from the deepest point of the interprostatorectal peritoneal pouch to the pelvic floor. A so-called posterior layer is in reality the rectal fascia propria."

The potential space which was present embryologically between the two laminae discussed above may be retained as the space of Proust (Fig. 25-24). It has a strong anterior layer related to the prostate and a loose posterior layer related to the rectum. Jewett et al.[81] were not able to demonstrate the plane of cleavage of the potential space within the two layers of the Denonvilliers' fascia. It is more likely that the so-called posterior layer is in fact part of the lateral pillar of the rectum.

## Structure

Lowsley[82] reported that the prostate gland can be divided into six lobes: anterior, posterior, median, subcervical, right lateral, and left lateral (Fig. 25-25). His description is no longer accepted, however, because it was based on studies of fetal and newborn prostates, and is not an accurate description of the adult gland.

Avoiding use of the term "lobes" because of the confusion it engenders, McNeal[83-85] described four regions or zones in the prostate: peripheral, central, transition, and anterior fibromuscular stroma (Fig. 25-26). The urethra is the key anatomic entity defining these regions (Figs. 25-26

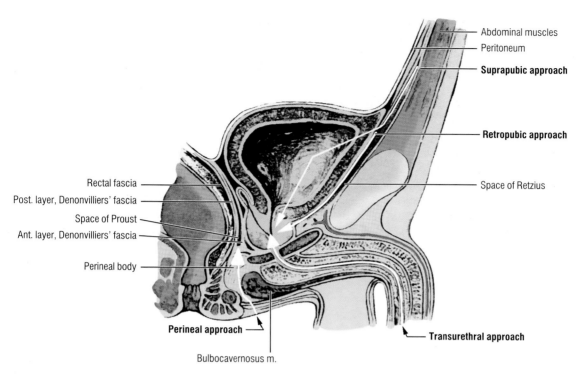

**FIG. 25-24.** Fascia of Denonvilliers and space of Proust. White lines and arrows show various approaches for prostatectomy. (Modified from Healey JE, Hodge J. Surgical Anatomy (2nd ed). Philadelphia: BC Decker, 1990; with permission.)

through 25-32). Posterior to the urethra is the glandular area. Anterior to the urethra is the fibromuscular area; that is, the ventral portion of the glandular prostatic tissue is covered by the fibromuscular stroma.

To describe the prostate, McNeal uses three reference planes (Fig. 25-27): sagittal, coronal, and oblique coronal.

- The *sagittal plane* bisects the prostate and incises the full length of the urethra, demonstrating its lumen. The urethra is thus the key anatomic entity related to all four of McNeal's zones.
- The *coronal section* shows both the distal urethra and the ejaculatory ducts in continuity with one another; that is, the ducts are parallel with the distal urethra.
- The *oblique coronal plane* passes along the long axis of the proximal urethral segment, which cannot be seen in the coronal plane. It has an upward pathway through the bladder neck, transecting the base of the verumontanum.

McNeal[84] wrote that marked histologic differences exist between the peripheral and central zones, suggesting important differences in biologic function. This information and some of the other findings from McNeal's brilliant embryologic, anatomic, histologic, and pathologic observations are summarized below.

## *The 4 Zones of McNeal from an Embryologic, Anatomic, Histologic, and Pathologic Viewpoint*

EMBRYOLOGY (SPECULATIVE)

| | |
|---|---|
| Peripheral | It is likely that the glands of this zone develop from the urogenital sinus and drain into the prostatic urethra. |
| Central | Ducts of this zone are probably of wolffian origin. |
| Transition | Glands in the transition zone are formed from the junction of the proximal and distal urethral segments. |
| Stroma | This region is formed by nonglandular tissue. |

ANATOMY

| | |
|---|---|
| Peripheral | Nearly 75% of the glandular prostate, the peripheral zone surrounds most of the central zone and much of the urethra; in other words, it surrounds the posterior and lateral areas of the prostate gland. Its glands drain into the prostatic urethra. |
| Central | The central zone, which is nearly 25% of the |

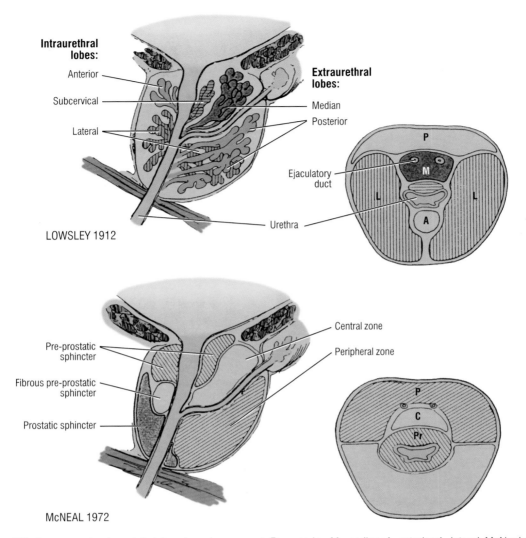

**FIG. 25-25.** Differing concepts of prostate lobes. Lowsley concept: P, posterior; M, median; A, anterior; L, lateral. McNeal concept: P, peripheral zone, C, central zone; Pr, prostatic sphincter. (Modified from Redman JF. Anatomy of the genitourinary system. In: Gillenwater JY, Grayhack JT, Howards SS, Duckett JW (eds). Adult and Pediatric Urology (2nd ed). St. Louis: Mosby Year Book, 1991, pp. 3-62; with permission.)

glandular prostatic parenchyma, envelops the ejaculatory ducts and extends toward the base of the urinary bladder.

Transition | This zone is less than 5% of the glandular prostate. The transition zone is composed of two minute glandular regions which are lateral to the preprostatic sphincter and directly related to the proximal urethral segment. The periurethral region is related to this zone and to the junction of the proximal and distal urethral segments. Periurethral ducts, which are responsible for the genesis of benign prostatic hyperplasia, are present.

Stroma | The anterior fibromuscular stroma is non-

glandular. It constitutes 1/3 of the prostatic tissue within the prostatic capsule but is in continuity with the detrusor muscle of the neck of the urinary bladder. It is heavily fixed with the anterior surfaces of the three glandular zones, and represents the periurethral gland region.

HISTOLOGY

Peripheral | This zone is formed by multiple tubulo-alveolar glands. The long, narrow ducts of this zone branch into small, round, regular acini with smooth, nonseptate walls. Epithelium is simple columnar; its pale cells have

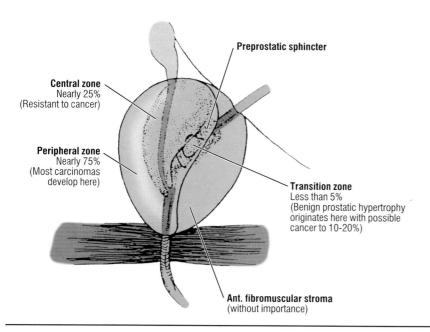

**Central zone**
Nearly 25%
(Resistant to cancer)

**Preprostatic sphincter**

**Peripheral zone**
Nearly 75%
(Most carcinomas
develop here)

**Transition zone**
Less than 5%
(Benign prostatic hypertrophy
originates here with possible
cancer to 10-20%)

**Ant. fibromuscular stroma**
(without importance)

FIG. 25-26. McNeal's 4 anatomic regions of the prostate from an anatomic and pathologic standpoint. Percentages represent the proportion of each region to the prostate as a whole. (Modified from Tanagho EA. Anatomy of the lower urinary tract. In: Walsh PC, Retik AB, Stamey TA, Vaughn ED Jr (eds). Campbell's Urology, 6th Ed. Philadelphia: WB Saunders, 1992; with permission.)

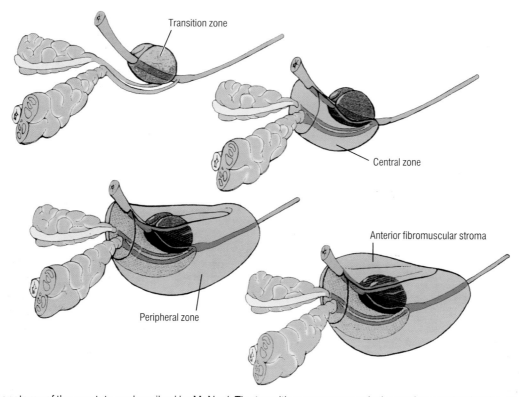

Transition zone

Central zone

Peripheral zone

Anterior fibromuscular stroma

FIG. 25-27. Zonal anatomy of the prostate as described by McNeal. The transition zone surrounds the urethra proximal to the ejaculatory ducts. The central zone surrounds the ejaculatory ducts and projects under the bladder base. The peripheral zone constitutes the bulk of the apical, posterior, and lateral aspects of the prostate. The anterior fibromuscular stroma extends from the bladder neck to the striated urethral sphincter. (Modified from Brooks JD. Anatomy of the lower urinary tract and male genitalia. In: Walsh PC, Retik AB, Vaughn ED Jr, Wein AJ (eds). Campbell's Urology, 7th Ed. Philadelphia: WB Saunders, 1998; with permission.)

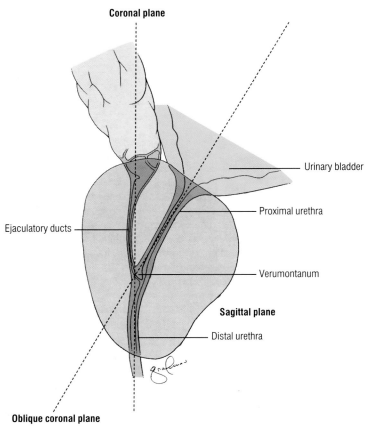

**FIG. 25-28.** Diagram of prostate, sagittal plane. Relationships to other planes of section, coronal and oblique coronal, are shown by dotted lines. Coronal plane follows ejaculatory ducts and distal urethra. Oblique coronal plane follows proximal urethra to bladder. (Based on McNeal JE. The zonal anatomy of the prostate. Prostate 1981;2:35-49.)

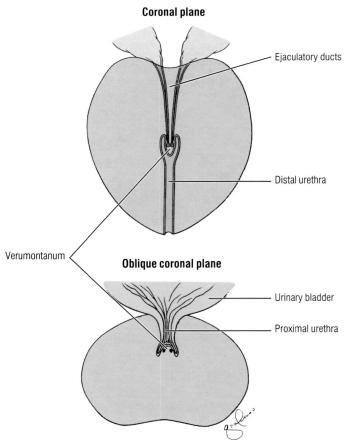

**FIG. 25-29.** Contour of prostate in coronal and oblique coronal planes. (Based on McNeal JE. The zonal anatomy of the prostate. Prostate 1981;2:35-49.)

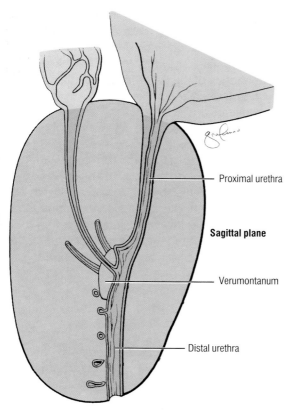

FIG. 25-30. Sagittal diagram of early embryo prostate shows area of stromal condensation. Laterally developing duct buds (circles) and proximally developing buds (in profile) shown in relationship to distal urethral segment and ejaculatory ducts, respectively. (Based on McNeal JE. The zonal anatomy of the prostate. Prostate 1981; 2:35-49.)

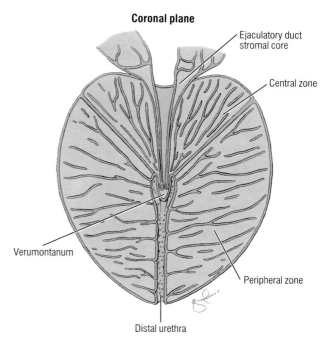

FIG. 25-31. Coronal plane diagram of central zone and peripheral zone. Boundary between them marked by heavy lines radiating from verumontanum. Relationships are shown to the distal urethral segment, verumontanum, and ejaculatory duct stromal core. (Based on McNeal JE. The zonal anatomy of the prostate. Prostate 1981;2:35-49.)

distinct borders and basally-placed small, dark nuclei.

Central   The central zone is continuous with the peripheral zone and, like the peripheral zone, is formed by several tubuloalveolar glands (mucosal, submucosal, main prostatic) which are located around the urethra. The acinar tissue consists of large, irregularly shaped spaces; the walls have intraluminal ridges or septa. The cells of the central zone differ significantly from those of the peripheral zone. They have more opaque, granular cytoplasm and less distinct cell membranes. Their cell length varies, they have an irregular luminal border, and they appear more crowded. Their nuclei, which are slightly larger than those of the peripheral zone and stain paler, are displaced to

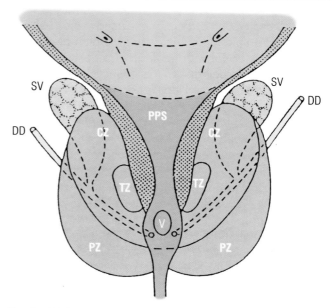

FIG. 25-32. Schematic diagram of adult prostate. Peripheral zone (PZ), central zone (CZ) and transitional zone (TZ) at apex of pre-prostatic sphincter (PPS). Seminal vesicles (SV) and ducti deferentes (DD) fuse to form ejaculatory ducts opening alongside verumontanum (V). (Modified from Chapple CR. Anatomy and innervation of prostate gland. In: Chapple CR (ed). Prostatic Obstruction: Pathogenesis and Treatment. New York: Springer-Verlag, 1994; with permission.)

variable levels from the basement membrane.

Transition    In this zone one observes a minimal number of glands.

Stroma    The fibromuscular stroma is composed of striated and smooth muscles, as well as elastin and collagen.

NOTE: The origin of the preprostatic sphincter described by McNeal is enigmatic; perhaps there is participation of wolffian and sinus tissue.

PATHOLOGY

Peripheral    Most carcinomas develop in the peripheral zone.

Central    Carcinoma seldom arises in the central zone.

Transition    The transition zone and other periurethral glands are the exclusive site of origin of benign prostatic hypertrophy. The area near or within the sphincter almost invariably produces the most numerous and largest nodules. Ten to twenty percent of carcinomas may develop in the transition zone.

Stroma    This area is without importance for prostatic function or pathology.

Wendell-Smith[86] has summarized the structural and functional description of the prostate used in the 1998 edition of the *Terminologia Anatomica*,[87] which blends the concepts of McNeal with findings of other workers on predilection for pathology and malignancy:

> The use of the term lobe *is confined to the right and left lobes and the variable middle lobe. The term* lobule *is used for the subdivisions, which are named from the anatomical position. Thus each side has a* supero-medial, *an* anteromedial, *an* inferoposterior, *and an* inferolateral lobule. *Also necessary to describe a site of predilection is a peri-urethral gland zone. In ultrasound diagnosis, the* trapezoid area *is important: its upper limit is the* rectoperinealis, *its anterior limit is the* intermediate part *of the urethra, its lower limit is the* anoperinealis, *and its posterior limit is the* anorectal junction. *Confusion at the bladder neck is resolved by recognizing that the position of the* internal urethral orifice *varies with functional state of the bladder: when it is filling the orifice lies above the base of the prostate; when voiding begins, the orifice descends to the base of the prostate; between the* filling internal orifice *and the* emptying internal orifice *is the* bladder neck part *of the urethra.*

We recommend Wendell-Smith's comprehensive article to the interested student.

Hricak et al.[88] studied the normal anatomy of the prostate by MRI. They reported that zones were seen very well. Cornud et al.[89] used endorectal MRI to study the zonal anatomy of the prostate. They reported clearly delineated anatomic boundaries of the transition zone, the prostatic capsule, the neurovascular bundles, and the caudal junction of the ejaculatory ducts.

Some workers believe that approximately 70-80% of prostatic cancers may develop in the peripheral zone. Cancer may develop in the central zone at a rate of only 5-10%. Remember: when a nodule forms, it can be palpated by rectal digital examination. Benign prostatic hyperplasia may appear lobar by digital examination, although the normal, non-hyperplastic prostate lacks lobar configuration.[90]

Reese et al.[91] suggested that the central zone of the prostate may be the selective site of origin of proteolytic enzymes in seminal fluids.

## Capsules of the Prostate

There are three capsules of the prostate; two (the true and false) are anatomic (Fig. 25-33), the third is pathologic (Fig. 25-34).

The *true capsule* is a very thin covering surrounding the gland in toto.

The *false capsule* (periprostatic fascia or prostatic sheath) is an extraperitoneal fascia (visceral layer of endopelvic fascia). This capsule is continuous with 4 fasciae:

- *Anterior:* fascia of the bladder, puboprostatic ligament
- *Lateral:* arcus tendineus of the fascia pelvis
- *Posterior:* fascia of Denonvilliers
- *Inferior:* superior fascia of the urogenital diaphragm

Between the true and false capsules is a venous plexus, the prostatic or pudendal venous plexus (Fig. 25-33).

Part of the normal aging process is progressive prostatic growth due to benign prostatic hyperplasia (BPH). The peripheral part of the prostate becomes compressed against the surrounding endopelvic connective tissue, forming a *surgical capsule (pathologic capsule)*. When enucleation of the prostate is performed, the plane between the compressed peripheral tissue and the adenomatous tissue permits removal of the adenoma, leaving behind the peripheral condensed prostatic tissue and the anatomic capsule.

The pathologic capsule is formed of essentially normal prostatic tissue peripheral to an adenoma, compressed against the false capsule (Fig. 25-34B). This remains after enucleation of the adenoma (Fig. 25-34C).

DiLollo et al.[92] studied the morphology of the prostatic capsule and its posterosuperior region. They advised the following:

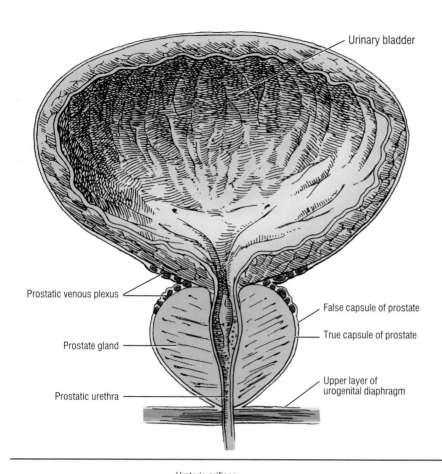

Urinary bladder

Prostatic venous plexus

False capsule of prostate

True capsule of prostate

Prostate gland

Upper layer of
urogenital diaphragm

Prostatic urethra

FIG. 25-33. Capsules of prostate.

Ureteric orifices

Prostate

Prostatic urethra

Membranous urethra

**A**

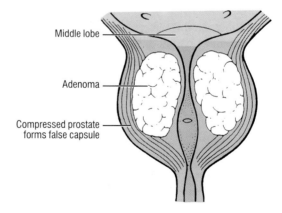

Middle lobe

Adenoma

Compressed prostate
forms false capsule

**B**

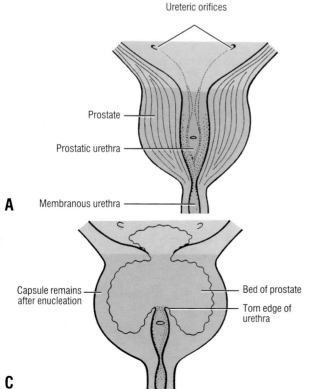

Capsule remains
after enucleation

Bed of prostate

Torn edge of
urethra

**C**

FIG. 25-34. Surgical anatomy of prostatectomy. **A,** Normal prostate (vertical section). **B,** Prostatic adenoma (benign hypertrophy) compresses normal prostatic tissue into false capsule. **C,** Prostatectomy removes adenoma but leaves capsule. (Modified from Ellis H. Clinical Anatomy (6th ed). Oxford UK: Blackwell Scientific, 1980; with permission.)

[I]n the prostatic zone limited by the ejaculatory ducts, the ventral surface of the seminal vesicles and the basal portion of the urinary bladder, there is no real connective tissue barrier around the prostate; on the contrary, a rich vascular network is present. Thus, a malignant tumor which begins in this zone should be considered from the very early stages potentially extracapsular. It is important to note that the present conclusions confirm the earlier observations of Denonvilliers.

## Vascular Supply

### Arteries

According to Clegg,[67] there are three arterial zones within the prostatic parenchyma: anterior or capsular, intermediate, and urethral.

Characteristically, the urethral vessels enter the prostatovesical junction at 7 to 11 o'clock and at 1 to 5 o'clock. The two sides have few anastomoses.

The blood supply of the prostate is derived primarily from the inferior vesical artery (Fig. 25-35). A branch of this artery enters the prostate laterally at the prostatovesical junction. This artery divides into two branches, the peripheral and the central. The peripheral branch serves the majority of the prostatic parenchyma; the central branch supplies the urethra and the periurethral tissues.

Other arteries contributing rami to the prostate are the internal pudendal and middle rectal arteries. Last[79] considered the middle rectal artery to be poorly named, since most of its blood goes to the prostate gland.

Remember that an accessory pudendal artery may arise in the pelvis and pass under the pubic arch with the deep dorsal vein to reach the penis. Such arteries usually arise from a branch of the anterior division of the internal iliac artery. Accessory pudendal arteries can arise unilaterally or bilaterally from the obturator artery, the internal pudendal artery prior to its exit from the pelvis, or directly from the internal iliac or the superior and inferior vesical arteries. The accessory pudendal artery leaves the pelvis by passing through the hiatus between the pubic arcuate ligament and the transverse perineal ligament.

An accessory pudendal artery may provide the dorsal artery of the penis, the deep artery to the corpus cavernosum, or both. Such branches are divided during radical prostatectomy. Their frequency of occurrence is only about 3% in females, but 10% in males.[93] This artery is always present in lower animals, and is called the urogenital artery, because it supplies the bladder.[94,95]

### Veins

There is a rich venous plexus (prostatic plexus) (Fig. 25-36) between the prostate gland and the prostatic sheath. It communicates with the internal iliac venous system and the presacral veins. The prostatic venous plexus receives the deep dorsal penile vein and the veins of the base of the bladder. The vesical and internal iliac veins receive most of the venous blood.

It has been said that the prostatic venous plexus does not have any valves. Part of the blood drains toward the extradural venous plexus of Batson;[96] this suggests an ex-

## Editorial Comment

The concept that the propensity for prostatic cancers to metastasize to the skull and the spine may be related to an absence of valves in the venous drainage of the prostate and the drainage of prostatic blood toward the extradural venous plexus of Batson[96] is time honored. It is a possible mechanism for cancer cells to reach these tissues, but cancer cells could also pass through the pulmonary circulation or the lymphatic circulation. For hematogenous metastases cells must first enter into the venous system (or pass through the lymphatic system into the venous system). Once the cancer cells arrive at a potential metastatic site the actual development of a metastasis is probably a rare event. Establishment of a metastasis is dependant upon a viable cell or cells attaching to the vascular endothelium, then traversing the endothelium, then being able to start to proliferate in the environment, and then eventually being able to provoke the host tissue into providing a tumor blood supply (angiogenesis). I believe that the propensity for hematogenous metastases to develop at a particular site is far more dependent on the interplay of the complex cell surface molecules and cellular messengers than on any vascular interconnections. (RSF Jr)

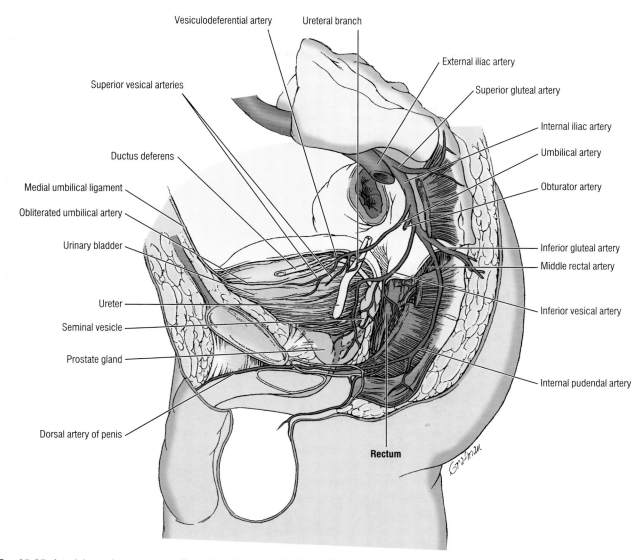

**FIG. 25-35.** Arterial supply to prostate. (Based on Hinman F Jr. Atlas of Urosurgical Anatomy. Philadelphia: WB Saunders, 1993.)

planation for the metastasis of cancer of the prostate to the spine and skull.

The deep dorsal vein of the penis reaches the prostatic venous plexus by passing through the cleft between the pubic arcuate ligament and the transverse perineal ligament of the urogenital diaphragm. According to Redman,[97] the vein trifurcates upon emerging through the opening, with a pathway toward the anterior lateral parts of the prostate, thereby forming Santorini's plexus. In the laboratory, we have seen low bifurcation. In cases of uncontrolled bleeding from the dorsal venous plexus during radical retropubic prostatectomy, the deep dorsal vein of the penis can be ligated.

## Lymphatics

From the prostatic acinus, large intraprostatic trunks are formed. These penetrate the prostatic capsule and form the periprostatic lymphatic plexus. This plexus yields lymphatic vessels which follow the vascular network of the prostatovesical arteries.

The lymph vessels that follow the prostatovesical arteries travel to the internal iliac lymph nodes (Fig. 25-37). The vessels also travel to the presacral lymph nodes and, occasionally, to the external iliac lymph nodes.

Hinman[66] emphasized that from a surgical standpoint, the primary sites of lymphatic drainage of the prostate are

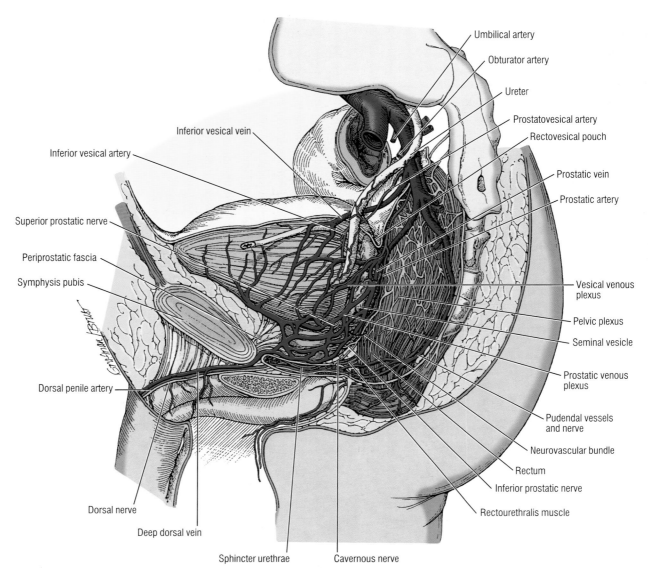

FIG. 25-36. Venous drainage of prostate. (Based on Hinman F Jr. Atlas of Urosurgical Anatomy. Philadelphia: WB Saunders, 1993.)

the obturator and external iliac nodes. He also stated that the presacral and presciatic nodes are less important as initial sites of prostatic lymphatic drainage. Hinman also mentioned the work of Whitmore and Mackenzie,[98] McLaughlin et al.,[99] and Wilson et al.[100]

The histologic studies of the glandular prostate by Fukuda et al.[101] demonstrated a high lymphatic density in the midbase region surrounding ejaculatory ducts. The authors concluded that the midbase region might be a route of lymphatic spread of prostate cancer.

Metastasis to other anatomic entities such as the penis[102] may occur.

## Innervation

The preganglionic sympathetic nerve supply to the smooth muscle of the seminal vesicles, ejaculatory ducts, and prostate gland arises in the intermediate gray area of spinal cord levels L1 and L2 (or L3). Postganglionic fibers arise in the preaortic or pelvic plexuses. The sympathetic fibers cause contraction of the smooth muscle and expulsion of seminal fluid.

Parasympathetic fibers from sacral cord levels S2, S3, and S4 synapse in pelvic ganglia and periprostatic ganglia. They act perhaps to dilate blood vessels and stimulate secretion from glands of the genital system, including the prostate.

The neurovascular bundles described by Walsh and Donker[103] are located on the dorsolateral surface of the prostate gland between the rectal wall and the prostate (Fig. 25-38). They are concealed within the periprostatic fascia. These nerve plexuses include branches of the preganglionic parasympathetic visceral efferent fibers (nervi erigentes or pelvic splanchnic nerves with cell bodies in the intermediolateral cell column of S2-S4), sensory fibers, and sympathetic fibers. Although these nerves are very small, their anatomic location can be estimated by looking for the capsular vessels. Preserve the neurovascular bundles during "nerve sparing" radical retropubic prostatectomy by avoiding tissues that are located posterolaterally. This *may* prevent impotence. Klotz[104] advocates intraoperative cavernous nerve stimulation

during radical prostatectomy to optimizing nerve sparing since these nerves are often difficult to visualize and may have a variable course.

Carlton[105] stated that visualization of the neurovascular bundle is better with perineal prostatectomy than with retropubic prostatectomy. The neurovascular bundle may be saved during prostate surgery by rotating the bladder and elevating the ureter, with close division of the tissues around the wall of the urinary bladder.

We quote Baskin et al.[106]:

*Perforating branches from the dorsal lateral neurovascular bundle do not exist based on serial step sectioning and microscopic examination of male genital specimens. Surgically it is possible to elevate the neurovascular bundle but the dissection needs to remain directly on top of the tunica albuginea to prevent neuronal injury. Small perforating branches into the*

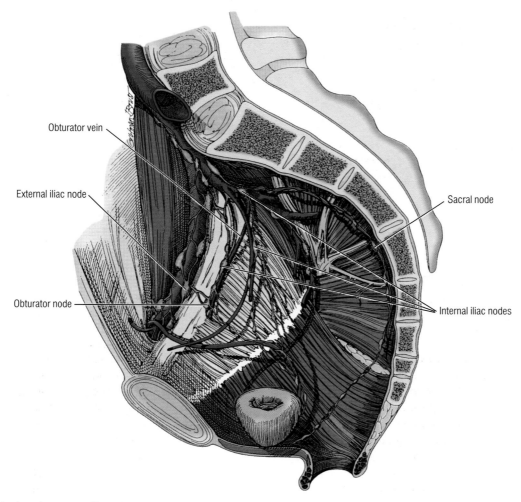

Obturator vein

External iliac node

Sacral node

Obturator node

Internal iliac nodes

**Fig. 25-37.** Lymphatics of prostate. (Based on Hinman F Jr. Atlas of Urosurgical Anatomy. Philadelphia: WB Saunders, 1993.)

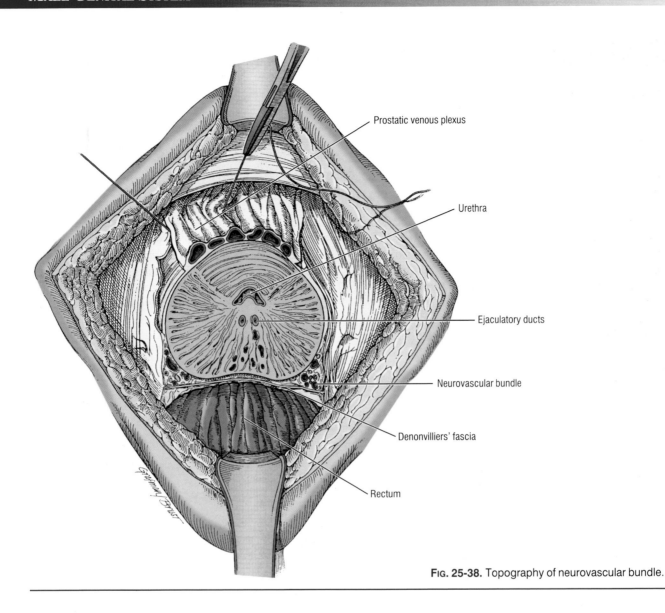

Prostatic venous plexus

Urethra

Ejaculatory ducts

Neurovascular bundle

Denonvilliers' fascia

Rectum

**FIG. 25-38.** Topography of neurovascular bundle.

*urethral spongiosum may be injured with unknown significance. We continue to advocate plication in the nerve-free zone at the 12 o'clock position for correction of penile curvature.*

It has become evident that four factors are involved in maintaining erectile function following radical prostatectomy: preservation of the neurovascular bundle, tumor category, age, and preservation of accessory pudendal arteries. Of these factors, preservation of the neurovascular bundle appears to be most important. Catalona and Basler[107] reported potency rates of 63% and 41% of patients undergoing bilateral and unilateral nerve-sparing radical prostatectomy, respectively. Investigators from Stanford University[108] report less favorable results: that the

ability to achieve unassisted intercourse with vaginal penetration occurred in 1.1% of men having non-nerve sparing radical prostatectomy, 13.3% with unilateral neurovascular bundle preservation, and 31.9% with bilateral neurovascular bundle preservation. Quinlan and associates[109] noted that advancing tumor categories and age result in lower potency rates. Polascik and Walsh[110] have discovered that when present, preservation of the accessory pudendal artery significantly increases potency rates among men undergoing radical prostatectomy.

For patients with clinically localized prostate cancer, Ghavamian and Zincke[111] advocate nerve dissection starting at the lateral aspect of the prostate with secondary urethral dissection to decrease dissection around the striated sphincter.

## HISTOLOGY

Seventy percent of the weight of the prostatic mass is glandular epithelium. Thirty percent is fibromuscular, mainly non-striated. The glandular part contains ducts and acini which are lined with columnar epithelium and drain in the posterior and lateral walls of the prostatic urethra.

According to McNeal,[84,85] the three glandular regions of the prostate differ histologically and biologically. In all regions, ducts and acini are lined with secretory epithelium, with a layer of basal cells and interspersed endocrine-paracrine cells beneath. The peripheral zone has small, rounded, uniform glands. The central and transitional zones have very large and irregular acini.

Perhaps autocrine, paracrine, endocrine (androgen-sensitive or androgen-insensitive), and other unknown factors play a role in the regulation and control of the growth of the prostate. Therefore, growth as well as metastasis of prostatic carcinomas may be controlled or altered by the above factors.

Enzyme-histologic studies of Zaviacic[112] support the belief that the prostate and the urethral and paraurethral glands in the female are homologous.

## PHYSIOLOGY

The prostate gland secretes a milklike alkaline fluid. This fluid is very important for the fertilization of the ovum, since sperm within both the ductus deferens and vaginal tissue produce fertilization-inhibiting acidity. Guyton[113] stated that prostatic fluid most likely neutralizes the acidity of the fluids of the ductus deferens and vagina after ejaculation, enhancing the motility and fertility of the sperm. The prostatic fluid also contains citric acid, calcium, phosphorus, and other substances.

We quote Hayward and Cunha[114]:

> The development of the prostate is controlled by steroid hormones that in turn induce and maintain a complex and little understood cross talk between the various cell types making up the gland. The result of this intracellular communication can be either new growth or growth quiescence, depending upon the differentiation state of the cell type being stimulated. Secretory function of the prostate is dependent upon direct stimulation of fully differentiated prostatic epithelial cells by androgens. The prostate thus seems to be regulated in a similar manner to other organs of the male and female genital tract with proliferative control mediated by cell-cell interactions, whereas differentiated function is determined by direct steroid action on the parenchymal cells.

## SURGICAL APPLICATIONS

- Remember Healey and Hodge's[115] axiom about the space of Proust: "It has been the lament of many that it is not always easy to find this passage between 'wind and water.'"
- The prostate will hypertrophy after middle age, causing partial or total obstruction of the prostatic urethra.
- The thick fibromuscular parenchyma anterior to the urethra forms the anterior third of the prostate. It may undergo fibromuscular hypertrophy, but not glandular hypertrophy.
- The transition zone lateral to the preprostatic sphincter is probably responsible for the origin of all prostatic hyperplasias, but almost never for malignancy.
- The peripheral zone is the site most commonly responsible for the formation of malignant nodules.
- The urogenital sinus is most likely responsible for the embryogenesis of the peripheral and transition zones, as well as of the periurethral glands.[71] The wolffian duct appears to be responsible for the genesis of the central zone, and thus may be a factor in the resistance of this zone to the formation of cancer.
- McNeal[116] stated:
  - Cancer originates from the peripheral and transition zones.
  - Benign nodular hyperplasia may also develop in these two zones.
  - Cancers with a volume of more than 5 cc and poor differentiation are the most likely to metastasize.
  - Morphologically favorable cancers have a volume of less than 4 cc; unfavorable cancers have a volume of more than 12 cc.
  - Metastasis to lymph nodes is strongly related to the size of the cancer and the percentage of high-grade tumor.
- With enucleation, the urologist's index finger is introduced between the benign prostatic mass and the pathologic capsule. This avoids the prostatic venous plexus, which is external to this plane.
- There are several approaches to the prostate gland:
  - Transurethral resection (TUR)
  - Transabdominal approach (through the urinary bladder)
  - Radical retropubic approach (through the space of Retzius)
  - Perineal approach

An excellent article by Carlin and Resnick[117] provides detailed descriptions of the anatomic entities related to radical perineal prostatectomy, from outside to deep, in order to "integrate this knowledge with the surgical approach to the radical perineal prostatectomy." The entities they describe are:

- Skin
- Subcutaneous tissues
- Colles' fascia
- Superficial transverse perineus muscle (Fig. 25-39)
- Deep transverse perineus muscle
- Central tendon (perineal body)
- Pelvic floor musculature
- Anorectum and external anal sphincter (Fig. 25-39)
- Rectourethralis muscle (Fig. 25-40)
- Denonvilliers' fascia (Figs. 25-41 through 25-44)
- Neurovascular bundle and neuroanatomy (Figs. 25-43, 25-45)
- Vascular supply (Fig. 25-46)

- In the perineal approach, with division of the central fibromuscular perineal body, the anterior and posterior layers of the potential space of Proust should be identified. This serves not only to protect the rectum, but also to avoid bleeding.
- Remember that the lower rectal wall is heavily fixed to the apical part of the prostate and, therefore, to the proximal urethra. The rectourethralis muscle might be responsible for this stout attachment. The proximity of the peritoneum in the rectovesical fossa must be borne in mind when using the perineal approach. This is the area where rectal perforation most commonly occurs during radical prostatectomy. When peritoneum in the rectovesical area is inadvertently opened, it is easy to think that the rectum has been perforated. Awareness of the anatomy will help in this situation.
- Koch[118] reminds us that knowledge of the prostatic dorsal venous anatomy facilitates dissection of the prostatic apex with little bleeding and with preservation of the

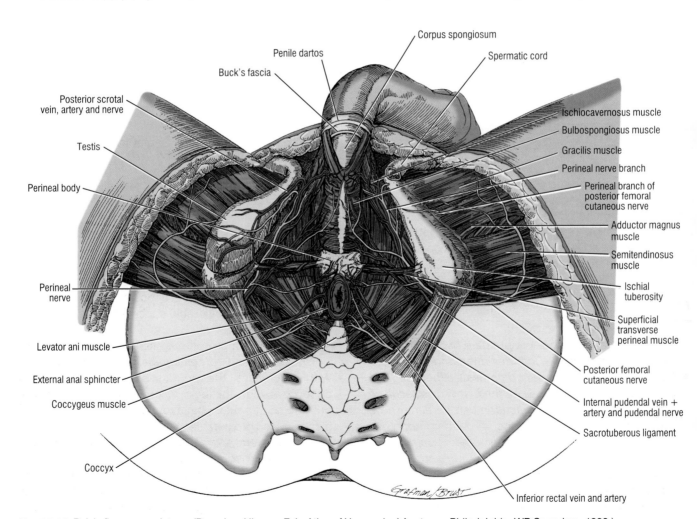

FIG. 25-39. Pelvic floor musculature. (Based on Hinman F Jr. Atlas of Urosurgical Anatomy. Philadelphia: WB Saunders, 1993.)

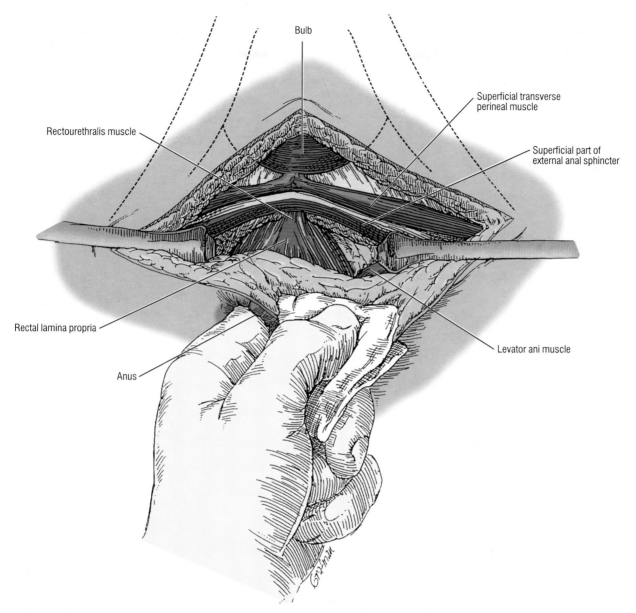

Bulb

Superficial transverse
perineal muscle

Rectourethralis muscle

Superficial part of
external anal sphincter

Rectal lamina propria

Levator ani muscle

Anus

FIG. 25-40. Rectourethralis muscle. (Based on Hinman F Jr. Atlas of Urosurgical Anatomy. Philadelphia: WB Saunders, 1993.)

rhabdosphincter, urethra, and neurovascular bundles.
- We are grateful to Dr. P.C. Walsh, who allowed us to reprint verbatim the anatomy of radical prostatectomy.[119]

*Radical perineal prostatectomy was first developed at The Johns Hopkins Hospital in 1904 by Hugh Hampton Young[120] and the retropubic approach was introduced in 1947 by Terrance Millin.[121] Although radical prostatectomy provided excellent cancer control, it never gained widespread popularity because of major side effects. Virtually all men who underwent radical prostatectomy were impotent, many had signif-*

*icant urinary incontinence, and when performed via the retropubic approach, excessive bleeding was common. With the introduction of external beam radiotherapy for the treatment of prostate cancer, by 1970 radical prostatectomies were rarely performed.*

*Recognizing that there was no better way to cure organ confined disease than to remove the primary organ, in 1974 I embarked on a series of anatomical studies in an attempt to understand the source for this morbidity with the hope that it might be avoided. In retrospect, it became clear that impotence was universal*

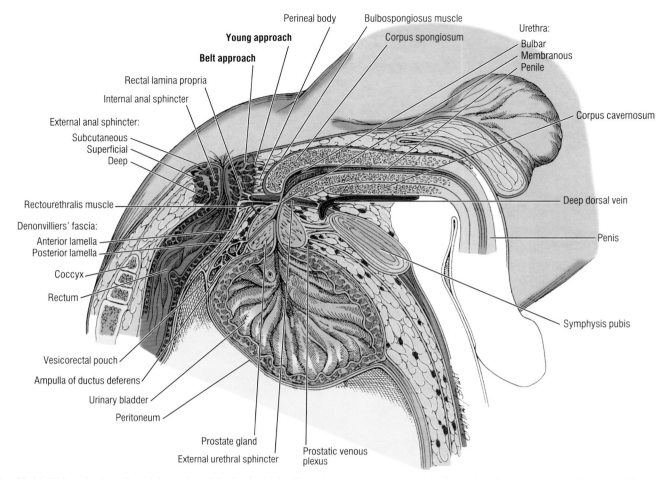

**FIG. 25-41.** Mid-sagittal section of the male pelvis. Dashed blue lines show various approaches for perineal prostatectomy. (Based on Hinman F Jr. Atlas of Urosurgical Anatomy. Philadelphia: WB Saunders, 1993.)

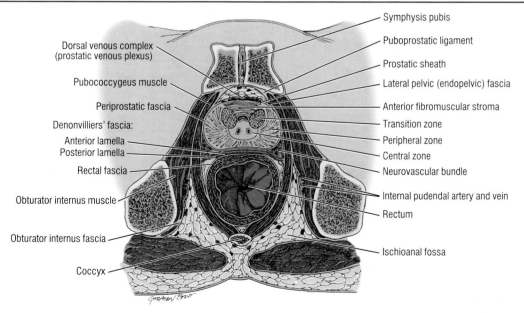

**FIG. 25-42.** Transverse section of male pelvis shows fascial layers surrounding prostate gland. (Based on Hinman F Jr. Atlas of Urosurgical Anatomy. Philadelphia: WB Saunders, 1993.)

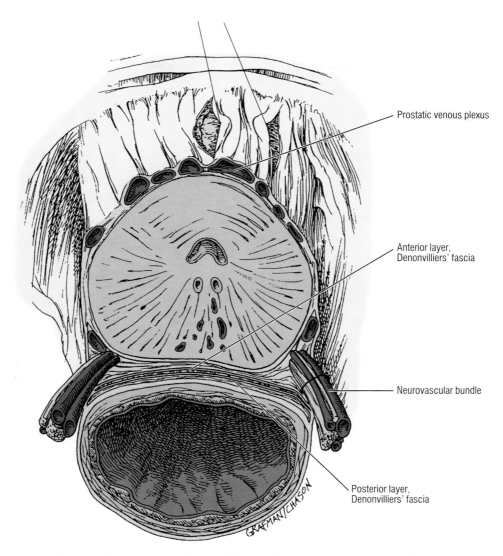

Prostatic venous plexus

Anterior layer,
Denonvilliers' fascia

Neurovascular bundle

Posterior layer,
Denonvilliers' fascia

**FIG. 25-43.** Transverse section of prostate gland shows anatomy of fascia of Denonvilliers and neurovascular bundles.

*because the location of the autonomic innervation to the pelvic organs and the corpora cavernosa was not known, incontinence was common because the anatomical understanding of the sphincteric complex was incorrect, and excessive bleeding occurred because the anatomy of the dorsal venous complex and Santorini's plexus was not charted. This deficit in the understanding of the peri-prostatic anatomy can be traced to the use of adult cadavers, which were not ideal for these investigations. The agents used for tissue fixation dissolve adipose tissue, thus obscuring normal tissue planes and the pelvic viscera compress the pelvic organs into a thick pancake of tissue, making anatomical dissection difficult... [T]hese problems were overcome by intra-operative anatomical dissections, and the use of infant cadavers for anatomical studies.*

*Anatomy of the Dorsal Venous Complex*

*During radical retropubic prostatectomy, excessive bleeding was common because the large venous complex that travels over the anterior surface of the urethra and prostate must be divided. This venous complex is covered by a thick sheath of dense fascia, which obscures the anatomical location of the venous tributaries. Anatomical studies showed that the deep dorsal vein leaves the penis under Buck's fascia between the corpora cavernosa and penetrates the urogenital diaphragm dividing into three major branches: the superficial branch and the right and left lateral venous plexus.[122] The superficial branch lies outside the pelvic fascia but the common trunk and lateral venous plexuses are covered and concealed by this fascia (Fig. 25-47). The lat-*

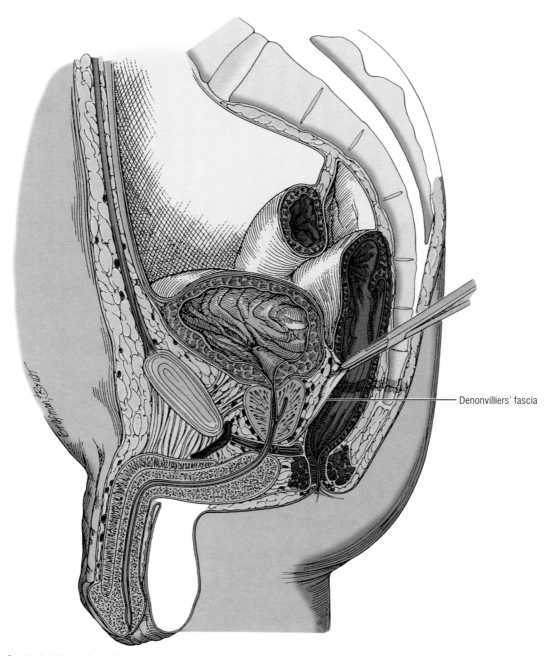

Denonvilliers' fascia

**Fig. 25-44.** Sagittal oblique view of male pelvis.

eral venous plexuses travel posterolaterally and communicate freely with the pudendal, obturator, and vesicle plexus. These anatomical observations made it possible to devise major alterations in the surgical technique that avoided excessive bleeding:

1. The endopelvic fascia was opened adjacent to the pelvic sidewall to avoid injury to the lateral venous plexus.
2. The puboprostatic ligaments were divided with care

not to injure the superficial branch of the dorsal vein nor to enter the anterior prostatic fascia covering Santorini's plexus and the dorsal venous complex.

3. The common trunk of the dorsal vein over the urethra was isolated with a right angle clamp, transected, and ligated, thus avoiding most of the major bleeding associated with this procedure. The development of this technique made the operation safer and provided a relatively bloodless field which made it

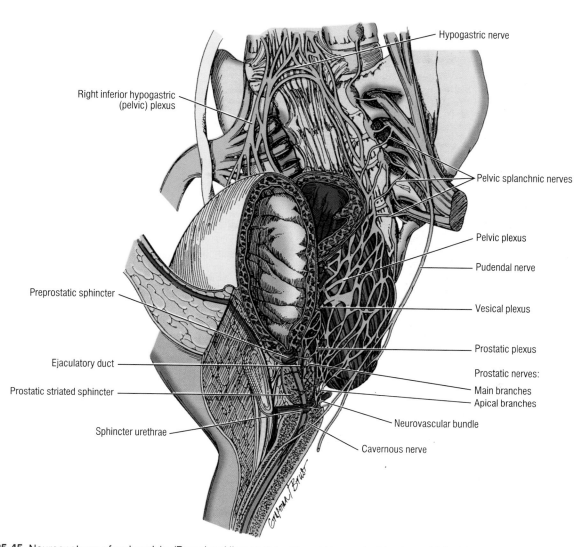

Hypogastric nerve

Right inferior hypogastric (pelvic) plexus

Pelvic splanchnic nerves

Pelvic plexus

Pudendal nerve

Vesical plexus

Preprostatic sphincter

Prostatic plexus

Prostatic nerves:
Main branches
Apical branches

Ejaculatory duct

Prostatic striated sphincter

Neurovascular bundle

Sphincter urethrae

Cavernous nerve

**FIG. 25-45.** Neuroanatomy of male pelvis. (Based on Hinman F Jr. Atlas of Urosurgical Anatomy. Philadelphia: WB Saunders, 1993.)

*possible to view the periprostatic anatomy in a way not possible previously. Shortly after this technique was developed, a patient reported that he was fully potent after surgery. This patient continues to do well 20 years postoperatively. Based on that experience, I questioned why any man was impotent after radical prostatectomy. At this time it was believed that impotence after radical prostatectomy was neurogenic in origin, and that it was caused by injury to the cavernous nerves that traveled through the prostate. For this reason, it was assumed that impotence was a necessary complication of a radical prostatectomy. From this one experience, I knew that was not true.*

*Autonomic Innervation of the Corpora Cavernosa*

*The autonomic innervation to the corpora cavernosa*

*is derived from the pudendal nerve and the pelvic plexus. The pudendal nerve provides both autonomic supply to the corpora cavernosa and sensory supply to the skin. Because the pudendal nerve is not close to the operative field, and because sensation is intact in impotent men after surgery, injury to the pudendal nerve could not be implicated. Rather, it was assumed that injury to the pelvic plexus or its branches must be responsible. The pelvic plexus provides autonomic innervation to all of the pelvic organs but, until the time of this work, the exact location of the pelvic plexus and the branches to the corpora cavernosa in man was not known.*

*In 1981 I had the opportunity to perform fetal dissections with Dr. Pieter Donker, Emeritus Professor of Urology at Leiden University, The Netherlands. Dr. Donker identified the fetus as an ideal model for these*

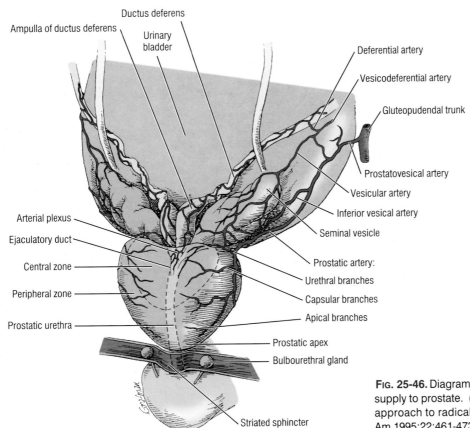

**FIG. 25-46.** Diagrammatic representation of posterior vascular supply to prostate. (Based on Carlin BI, Resnick MI. Anatomic approach to radical perineal prostatectomy. Urol Clin North Am 1995;22:461-473.)

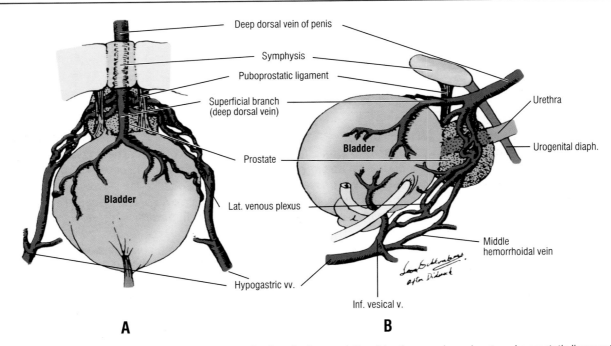

**A**                **B**

**FIG. 25-47.** Santorini's venous plexus. **A,** Trifurcation of dorsal vein of penis shows relationship of venous branches to puboprostatic ligaments (supine view). **B,** Anatomic relationship at trifurcation (lateral view, lateral pelvic fascia removed). (Modified from Reiner WB, Walsh PC. An anatomical approach to the surgical management of the dorsal vein and Santorini's plexus during radical retropubic surgery. J Urol 1979;121:198-200; with permission.)

studies because the fibrofatty tissue was less abundant, the pelvic structures were not disturbed by the pressure of the abdominal viscera, and the nerves were correspondingly larger in relationship to adjacent structures. At the time that I met Dr. Donker, he was performing dissections of the pelvic plexus to characterize the autonomic innervation to the bladder. After informing him that the branches of the pelvic plexus to the corpora cavernosa were also not known, we traced these pathways in stillborn male infants. The pelvic plexus, which provides autonomic innervation to all of the organs, rests on the lateral surface of the rectum. The branches that innervate the corpora cavernosa were seen clearly outside the capsule of the prostate and its surrounding tissue as they travel between the prostate and rectum before penetrating the urogenital diaphragm and innervating the corpora cavernosa[103]...This study showed clearly that the prostate could be removed completely with preservation of these nerves. This study provided the schematic anatomy of the pelvic plexus and cavernous nerves. Next, landmarks in the adult needed to be developed.

In the operating room, it became clear that the capsular arteries and veins of the prostate were located in the same region as the cavernous branches. This finding suggested that these vessels may serve as the scaffolding for these microscopic nerves and that the neurovascular bundle could be used as a visual landmark for their identification. To confirm this impression, an adult cadaver was perfused completely with Bouin's solution shortly after death. The pelvic organs were removed en bloc, 10,000 whole-mount step sections were prepared, and a 3-dimensional reconstruction performed.[123] This 3-dimensional reconstruction showed clearly that the cavernous nerves did travel in association with the capsular arteries and veins of the prostate outside the capsule and fascia of the prostate. Armed with these findings, we characterized the full neuroanatomy of the male pelvis using dissections performed in fresh cadavers.[124] This study showed that the pelvic plexus is located 5-11 cm from the anal verge traveling on the lateral surface of the rectum with its midpoint at the tip of the seminal vesicle. After providing branches to the bladder, lower ureter, and prostate, the branches from the pelvic plexus travel in association with the capsular arteries and veins of the prostate dorso-lateral to the prostate, where the nerves exit to innervate the corpora cavernosa.

*Anatomy of the Striated Sphincter Continence Mechanism*

For years it was widely believed that the urinary continence mechanism in man was composed of a group of horizontally oriented pelvic floor muscles contained in the levator ani complex. However, in 1980 Oelrich showed that the sphincteric complex responsible for passive urinary control was a vertically oriented tubular sheath.[125] In utero, this sphincter extends without interruption from the bladder to the perineal membrane. As the prostate develops from the urethra, it invades the sphincter muscle thinning the overlying parts and causing a reduction or atrophy of some of the muscle. In the adult, at the apex of the prostate the fibers are circular and form a tubular striated sphincter surrounding the membranous urethra (Fig. 25-48). Thus, as Myers and colleagues have shown, the prostate does not rest atop a flat transverse urogenital diaphragm like an apple on a shelf with no striated muscle proximal to the apex.[126] Rather, the external striated sphincter is more tubular and has broad attachments over the fascia of the prostate near the apex. This anatomy had important implications in transection of the dorsal vein complex (which is intimately associated with the striated sphincter), the apical dissection, and reconstruction of the urethra.[127]

*Pelvic Fascia*

The prostate is covered with two distinct and separate fascial layers: Denonvilliers' fascia, which covers the posterior surface of the prostate, and the lateral pelvic fascia, which covers the pelvic musculature. This fascia has also been called the prostatic fascia. All of these fascial layers are intimately associated with the dorsal vein complex, the neurovascular bundle, and the striated sphincter (Fig. 25-48). These intimate relationships must be well understood in order for the surgeon to completely remove localized prostate cancer.

## ANATOMIC COMPLICATIONS

### Transurethral Resection

Complications of transurethral resection include:
- Bleeding from the prostate parenchyma or bladder neck
- Injury of the bladder wall and prostatic capsule or intraperitoneal perforation into the space of Retzius
- Urethral strictures at the membranous urethra, penoscrotal junction, or fossa navicularis
- Incontinence

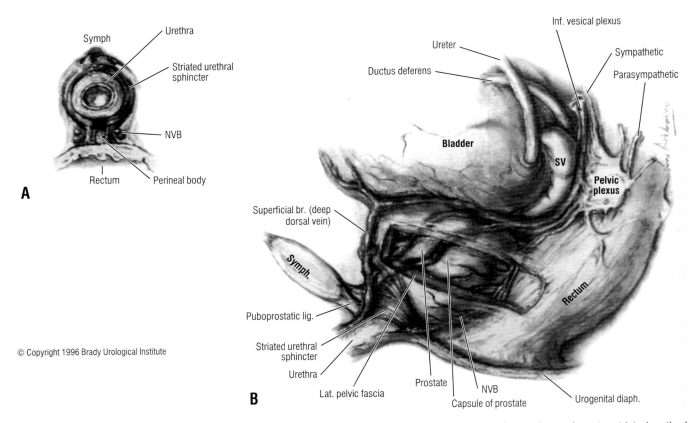

© Copyright 1996 Brady Urological Institute

Fɪɢ. 25-48. **A,** Cross-section of urethra just distal to apex of prostate demonstrating inner circular layer of smooth muscle, outer striated urethral sphincter, perineal body. **B,** Anatomic relationship of prostate to pelvic fascia, pelvic plexus, neurovascular bundle (NVB). Window of fascia removed to illustrate prostatic capsule. Note attachment of striated urethral sphincter to apex of prostate. SV, seminal vesicle. (Modified from Walsh PC. Anatomic radical prostatectomy: cancer control with preservation of quality of life. In: Fortner JG, Sharp PA (eds). Accomplishments in Cancer Research 1996. Philadelphia: Lippincott-Raven, 1997, pp. 41-53; with permission.)

Bleeding from the prostate parenchyma or bladder neck may occur with transurethral resection. Catheter traction will usually stop bleeding, if electrocautery is not successful. According to Smith,[128] the most common area for bleeding is the anterior bladder neck. The surgeon must visualize and inspect the prostatic fossa thoroughly. Occasionally, exploration, complete enucleation of the adenoma, direct fulguration/electrocautery and/or ligation may be necessary. The prostatic urethra as well as the prostatic fossa may be compressed with a balloon catheter to stop bleeding, if necessary.

Another complication is injury of the bladder wall and prostatic capsule, or intraperitoneal perforation into the space of Retzius. With intra- or extraperitoneal injury, laparotomy and repair should be performed. Small extraperitoneal perforations usually respond to prolonged Foley catheter drainage.

Urethral strictures may form at the membranous urethra, the penoscrotal junction, or the fossa navicularis. A soft and gentle technique is the only prophylactic measure against urethral strictures.

Incontinence may follow transurethral resection. There are two functional sphincters for urinary control. One, the internal sphincter, is at the bladder neck; this is the sphincter typically damaged during transurethral prostatectomy (TURP). Thus, after TURP, the patient is more reliant on the external sphincter. The best method to prevent incontinence is to avoid damage to the external sphincter caused by overzealous resection.

Anticholinergic treatment is used in dealing with incontinence resulting from sphincter damage; urologists try anticholinergics because their use is simple. Alpha-receptor stimulators, such as Ornade, are beneficial to some patients.

## Transabdominal Approach

Complications of the transabdominal approach (through the urinary bladder) include:
• Damage to the external sphincteric apparatus

- Injury to the posterior capsule with injury to the seminal vesicles
- Bleeding at the bladder neck

To avoid damage to the external sphincteric mechanism, the surgeon must cut apical attachments very carefully.

Inspect the prostatic fossa for bleeding or injury of the seminal vesicles. If injury to the seminal vesicles is discovered, repair the posterior capsule and anastomose it to the bladder neck.

Bleeding at the bladder neck can be controlled by ligating bleeding points using figure of eight at 5 and 7 o'-clock with 2-0 absorbable sutures. If bleeding continues, a purse-string suture around the bladder neck should be considered.

## Radical Retropubic Approach

Complications of radical retropubic prostatectomy (through the space of Retzius) include:
- Bleeding
- Rectal injury
- Ureteric injury
- Obturator nerve injury
- Impotence
- Bladder neck contracture
- Incontinence

Venous bleeding is the most common intraoperative complication during radical retropubic prostatectomy. The anatomic entities involved are the venous plexuses around the prostate and the deep dorsal vein of the penis; these are referred to collectively as the dorsal venous complex. During lymphadenectomy, any branch of the internal iliac vein can be involved.

To avoid venous bleeding
- Incise the endopelvic fascia carefully under direct vision. Large veins may lie directly behind the endopelvic fascia. These may be controlled with cautery or ligature.
- Carefully ligate the dorsal venous complex.
- Carefully divide the puboprostatic ligaments. Approach from lateral to medial. Blunt dissection between the puboprostatic ligaments will almost always cause bleeding. When transecting the puboprostatic ligaments, take care to avoid branches of the dorsal venous complex; these are located immediately behind the ligaments.

After successful control of the previous elements, follow with careful exposure of the prostatic apex. This cannot be accomplished unless the incision, ligation, and division described above have been followed.

Epidural anesthesia may result in a "regional" hypotension which can decrease blood loss.

Walsh[129] advises bulldog clamps to both hypogastric (internal iliac) arteries for reduction of blood flow to the prostate. Beware of the artery to the seminal vesicle at the very tip of the seminal vesicle; it can cause troublesome bleeding.

Rectal injury is very rare (1% according to Borland and Walsh[130]). It most commonly occurs during dissection of the apex of the prostate. This is where the prostatic fascia is most adherent to the rectal fascia. Upward retraction of the prostate will tent the rectum; this can increase the risk of iatrogenic injury to the rectum.

Close a rectal laceration in two layers. Interpose omentum between the rectum and the vesicourethral anastomosis through a small peritoneal opening. Administer antibiotics during and after surgery, along with copious irrigations. Rarely, it may be necessary to perform a diverting colostomy. However, if the bowel has not been prepared, the surgeon must weigh that risk when deciding whether the colostomy is appropriate.

Ureteric injury may occur after the lateral, anterior, and posterior surfaces of the prostate are free. Then the prostate is attached only to the bladder. Administer indigo carmine to assist in identifying the ureteric orifices. Incise the anterior bladder neck, and identify the orifices. Then, dissect the posterior bladder neck from the prostate, seminal vesicles, and ampullae of the ducti deferentes. Ureteric reimplantation is advised in instances of ureteric injury close to the trigone.

Division injury of the obturator nerve at the pelvic sidewall requires end-to-end re-anastomosis. Division of the obturator nerve will be followed by paralysis of the adductor muscle group, the gracilis, and the obturator externus. A sensory deficit will also be present along the medial part of the thigh.

Impotence is the result of excision of the neurovascular bundle (which was described previously with the innervation of the prostate). According to Walsh,[129] the father of nerve-sparing prostatectomy, "A number of factors may be responsible for postoperative impotence other than injury to the cavernous nerves."

Bladder neck contracture (vesicourethral anastomotic stricture) can be avoided by good mucosa-to-mucosa apposition of the bladder neck and the urethra. Use six interrupted 2-0 absorbable sutures at 2, 5, 7, and 10 o'clock.

Incontinence can be prevented by avoiding injury to the muscles of the pelvic floor and by leaving as much urethral length as possible. The surgeon should perform a good mucosa-to-mucosa vesicourethral anastomosis. Use of alpha-adrenergic agonists, anticholinergics, etc, is recommended.

Steiner[131] lists the anatomic components of the urethral sphincter complex whose preservation is necessary for continence:

- entire circumference of rhabdosphincter musculature
- periurethral fascial investments (pubourethral ligaments anterolaterally and median fibrous raphe posteriorly)

The innervation of the rhabdosphincter is preserved by way of the intrapelvic branch of the pudendal nerve (somatic). The innervation of the mucosal and smooth muscle components is preserved by way of the urethral branch of the inferior hypogastric plexus (autonomic).

## Perineal Prostatectomy

Complications of the perineal approach to the prostate include:

- Inability to identify the anterior rectal fascia and the pathway to the prostate and prostatic apex
- Bleeding
- Bladder neck injury and occlusion of ureteric orifices
- Urinary perineal leakage
- Stricture at the urethrovesical anastomosis
- Incontinence
- Impotence

The inability to find the pathway to the prostate by failure to identify the anterior rectal fascia is a true anatomic complication. Incise the central tendon very carefully. Avoid any injury to the bulbospongiosus muscle, the penile bulb, or the membranous urethra. Divide the variably distinct rectourethralis muscle without injury either to the rectal wall or the urethra.

Venous bleeding results from separation of the prostate from the bladder.

Avoid injury to the bladder neck by incising the posterior bladder neck transversely between 5 and 7 o'-clock, until the fascia enveloping the seminal vesicles can be identified. Care must be exercised during reconstruction of the bladder neck to avoid injury of the ureteric orifices.

Urinary perineal leakage is a very benign complication, and will heal rapidly. A Foley catheter should be positioned in the most dependent area of the urinary bladder.

In perineal prostatectomy, the complications of stricture at the urethrovesical anastomosis, incontinence, and impotence are similar to the conditions mentioned previously.

Ahearn et al.[132] reported two cases of transient lumbosacral polyradiculopathy after radical prostatectomy.

# *Bulbourethral Glands of William Cowper*

## HISTORY

Table 25-1 presents a historical note about the bulbourethral glands.

## EMBRYOGENESIS AND CONGENITAL ANOMALIES

The spongy urethra is responsible for the genesis of the urethral and bulbourethral glands.

Congenital anomalies of the bulbourethral glands include syringocele (retention cyst) and diverticulum of the anterior urethra. Syringocele may produce intraurethral urinary retention or incontinence.

## SURGICAL ANATOMY

The two round bulbourethral glands have an approximate diameter of 0.5-1.5 cm. They are located within the sphincter urethrae muscle, adjacent to the membranous part of the urethra; therefore, they are below the prostate (see Fig. 25-12). Each gland has a minute duct which penetrates the inferior fascia of the urogenital diaphragm. It enters and traverses the penile substance, ending in the lower aspect of the spongy urethra (bulbous) on either side at 3 and 9 o'clock.

## HISTOLOGY

Each bulbourethral gland is formed by several tubuloalveolar glands with columnar or cuboidal glandular epithelium.

Very rarely, the bulbourethral glands may develop an adenocarcinoma that invades the prostate. According to Hopkins and Grabstald,[133] it is possible in most cases to visualize the perineal mass and feel the prostate behind the tumor.

## PHYSIOLOGY

The bulbourethral and urethral glands secrete mucus consisting of sialoproteins and amino sugars. This mucus may aid in lubricating the urethra.

# *Potential Spaces Under the Urogenital Diaphragm*

## SURGICAL ANATOMY

Potential spaces under the urogenital diaphragm include the peripenile space, the periscrotal space, and the superficial perineal cleft.

It is well known that there is a potential space between the superficial fascia and the deep fascia on the anterior abdominal wall. This potential space is continuous superiorly with the retromammary space. It is also continuous inferiorly. Its continuation over the penis and the scrotum could be referred to as the peripenile and periscrotal spaces, respectively. In the perineal area, this potential space is named the superficial perineal cleft (see "Layers of the Scrotum" in this chapter).

The potential space is sealed off from the thighs laterally by the attachment of Colles' membranous fascia to the ischiopubic rami. It is closed off from the ischioanal fossae posteriorly by the fusion of Colles' fascia with the posterior edges of the superficial compartment (at the superficial transversus perineus muscle and the perineal body) and the urogenital diaphragm.

The superficial perineal cleft can always be found by blunt dissection, though the distinction between the fascial layers in the perineum may be difficult to visualize clearly. Begin in the perineum and probe upward. Or begin in the space between the superficial and the deep fascia on the anterior abdominal wall and probe inferiorly around the scrotum.

# *Male Urethra*

*Whereas the bladder is a muscular sac, the urethra is a muscular tube.*

*Emil A. Tanagho*[71]

## HISTORY

The anatomic and surgical history of the male urethra is shown in Table 25-1.

## EMBRYOGENESIS

### Normal Development

The pelvic part of the urogenital sinus in the male is responsible for the genesis of the prostatic and membranous parts of the urethra.

The endodermal and splanchnic mesoderm participate in the formation of the urethra, the former being responsible for the epithelium and the latter for the connective tissue and smooth muscle.

### Congenital Anomalies

Congenital anomalies of the male urethra can be found in Table 25- 2.

### *Atresia and Stenosis*

Atresia and stenosis may be caused by failure of the urethral plate to canalize. By definition, the urethral plate is "the endodermal layer of the attenuated distal portion of the urogenital sinus ... displayed on the caudal aspect of the phallus... [w]ith proliferation of mesenchyme within the genital folds, the urethral plate sinks into the body of the phallus forming a primary urethral groove," according to *Gray's Anatomy*.[134] Meatal stenosis is treated by meatomy. Urethral reconstruction or replacement are the procedures of choice for more extensive atresias.

### *Duplications of the Penile Urethra*

Duplication of the penile urethra is a rare anomaly. One can only speculate about the origin of this malformation. The existence of an extra endodermal canal or closing or splitting of the urethral plate are speculative etiologic factors.

Collateral duplications consist of complete duplication with diphallia and abortive duplication (one urethra is a blind sinus).

Treatment consists of excision of the more atretic accessory channel.

### *Dislocations of the Penile Urethra*

In *epispadias,* the opening of the urethra is located at the dorsum of the penis. This condition may be caused by a shift of the lateral anlage of the genital tubercle. Epispadias is treated surgically.

In *hypospadias,* the urethral opening may be on the underside of the penis, on the scrotum, or on the perineum. The urethral canal becomes a gutter secondary to partial or total failure of function of the urethral folds. Surgery is the preferred treatment. A study by Erol et al.[135] found that the urethral plate is well vascularized, and has a rich nerve supply and an extensive muscular and connective tissue backing. Based on the findings, they advocate preservation of the urethral plate and the onlay island flap for hypospadias reconstruction.

## SURGICAL ANATOMY

Fig. 25-49 will orient the reader to the relationships of the male urethra, which has a length of 8 inches (20 cm).

The urethra has 3 relatively narrow areas:
- at the membranous part of the urethra
- at the juncture of the glans penis with the corpus spongiosum
- at the external urethral meatus

### Topographic Anatomy

Tanagho[71] (Fig. 25-50) subdivides the urethra into pro-

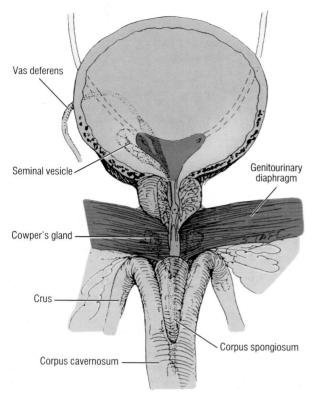

Vas deferens

Seminal vesicle

Cowper's gland

Crus

Corpus cavernosum

Genitourinary
diaphragm

Corpus spongiosum

**FIG. 25-49.** Anatomic relationship of bladder, prostate, prostatomembranous urethra, and root of penis. Prostate, situated just below bladder base, has its apex resting on genitourinary diaphragm, within which Cowper's glands, with ducts extending distally, open into bulbous part of the urethra, surrounded by corpus spongiosum. Two corpora cavernosa diverge at this point, each one gaining fixation to pubic arch. (From Tanagho EA. Anatomy of the lower urinary tract. In: Walsh PC, Retik AB, Stamey TA, Vaughan ED Jr (eds). Campbell's Urology (6th ed). Philadelphia: WB Saunders, 1992, pp. 40-69; with permission.)

static, membranous, bulbous, and penile areas.

Hinman,[66] however, considers the prostatic urethra an anatomic entity that belongs to the prostate. He defines the combined membranous-penile urethra to be composed of three segments (Fig. 25-51): bulbomembranous, bulbospongy, and penile. The bulbomembranous urethra is related to the urogenital diaphragm with the striated urethral sphincter and has a length of 2 cm. The bulbospongy urethra extends from within a few centimeters of the anatomic membranous urethra distally to the level of the suspensory ligament. The bulbourethral ducts (Cowper's) empty into this segment at 3 and 9 o'clock.

In our discussion below, we will use the following terminology: prostatic urethra (including the preprostatic part), membranous urethra, and spongy or penile urethra, as widely accepted.

### *Prostatic Urethra*

That part of the urethra from the vesical neck to the prostate is referred to as the preprostatic segment. It is 1-1.5 cm long, and has a stellate-shaped lumen. Smooth muscle of this segment of the urethra prevents retrograde ejaculation.

The segment of the prostatic urethra (Fig. 25-52) in the gland above the superior fascia of the urogenital diaphragm traverses the prostatic parenchyma, between the anterior and middle thirds of the gland. The prostatic urethra has a length of approximately 3 cm, and is the widest and most distensible of the segments. Its pathway is not straight, forming an acute angulation at the area of the verumontanum (Fig. 25-52, Fig. 25-53).

The student of urethral anatomy should remember the 3 elevations within the lumen of the prostatic urethra:
• crista urethralis
• verumontanum
• prostatic utricle

The *crista urethralis* (Fig. 25-52) is an elevation of the mucous membrane in the form of a median longitudinal ridge, located posteriorly on cross-section. For all practical

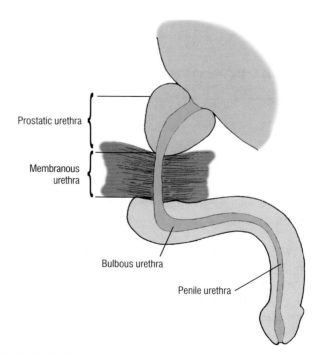

Prostatic urethra

Membranous
urethra

Bulbous urethra

Penile urethra

**FIG. 25-50.** Urethral lumen, prostatic urethra, membranous urethra, bulbous urethra, and penile urethra, which opens into external meatus after fusiform dilatation of navicular fossa. (Modified from Tanagho EA. Anatomy of the lower urinary tract. In: Walsh PC, Retik AB, Stamey TA, Vaughan ED Jr (eds). Campbell's Urology (6th ed). Philadelphia: WB Saunders, 1992, pp. 40-69; with permission.)

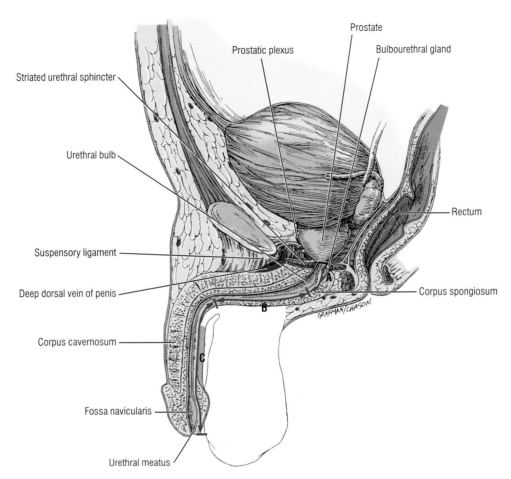

Prostate

Prostatic plexus

Bulbourethral gland

Striated urethral sphincter

Urethral bulb

Rectum

Suspensory ligament

Deep dorsal vein of penis

Corpus spongiosum

Corpus cavernosum

Fossa navicularis

Urethral meatus

A

B

C

GRAFMAN/CHASON

**FIG. 25-51.** Gross structure of urethra shows bulbomembranous urethra *(A)*, bulbospongy urethra *(B)*, and penile urethra *(C)*, as used by Hinman[66]. (Based on Hinman F Jr. Atlas of Urosurgical Anatomy. Philadelphia: WB Saunder, 1993.)

purposes, the crista urethralis is the downward continuation of the superficial trigone of the urinary bladder. It bifurcates into the bulbous urethra. The prostatic sinus is located on each side of the crista urethralis. The orifices of the prostatic ducts are found in the floor of the prostatic sinus.[71]

The *verumontanum* is an elevation at the middle area of the urethral crest.

The *prostatic utricle* (utriculus masculinus) and the orifices of the right and left ejaculatory ducts are located upon the summit of the verumontanum.

### Membranous Urethra

The membranous urethra is the urethral segment within the urogenital diaphragm. Tanagho[71] stated that it is the thickest segment. It is also the narrowest (except for the external urethral meatus), shortest (2-2.5 cm) and least di-

latable part of the urethra. The membranous urethra takes a curved pathway forward and downward through the urogenital diaphragm, becoming concave ventrally.

Smooth and striated muscle thickly invests this part of the urethra. The most important muscular component is the striated external coat, which is the voluntary urinary sphincter. The skeletal muscle is supplied by somatic motor fibers (from sacral levels S2-S4) carried by the perineal branch of the pudendal nerve. The muscle forms an incomplete ring at the posterior midline, resembling the Greek letter 'omega' (Ω). Therefore, its action is perhaps more compressive than truly sphincteric.

The bifurcation of the crista urethralis extends from the prostatic apex to the penile bulb.

Anteriorly, the deep dorsal vein of the penis enters the pelvis between the arcuate pubic ligament and the transverse perineal ligament.

The right and left bulbourethral glands (Fig. 25-52) are

located lateral to the membranous urethra. They drain into the proximal spongy urethra (bulbous). According to Tanagho,[71] the cavernous nerves also pass through the diaphragm (at 3 and 9 o'clock) before they penetrate the crura of the penis.

## Penile Urethra

The penile urethra is the distal part of the urethra. It extends from the inferior fascia of the urogenital diaphragm to the external meatus of the penis. The proximal segment is called the bulbar part, because it is enveloped by the penile bulb and the bulbospongiosus muscle. The distal part is called the pendulous part of the penile urethra. The penile (or spongy) urethra is located within the corpus spongiosum of the penis (Fig. 25-54). Its pathway is upward and downward as well as downward and forward when the penis is flaccid.

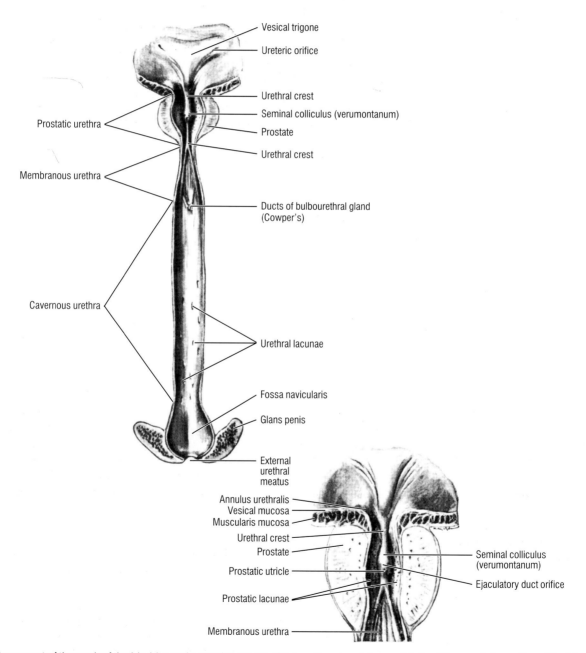

FIG. 25-52. Anterior aspect of the neck of the bladder and posterior aspect of the urethra. Inset shows details of the prostatic urethra. (Modified from McVay CB. Anson & McVay Surgical Anatomy, 6th Ed, Vol II. Philadelphia: WB Saunders, 1984; with permission.)

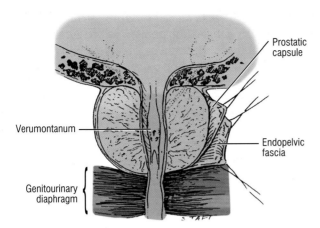

FIG. 25-53. Section of the prostate gland shows the prostatic urethra, verumontanum, and crista urethralis, in addition to the opening of the prostatic utricle and the two ejaculatory ducts in the midline. Note that the prostate is surrounded by the prostatic capsule, which is covered by another prostatic sheath derived from the endopelvic fascia. The prostate is resting on the genitourinary diaphragm. (Modified from Tanagho EA. Anatomy of the lower urinary tract. In: Walsh PC, Retik AB, Stamey TA, Vaughan ED Jr (eds). Campbell's Urology (6th ed). Philadelphia: WB Saunders, 1992, pp. 40-69; with permission.)

The lumen of the penile urethra is transversely slitlike until micturition, when it expands to about 6 mm. The adult spongy urethra has an approximate length of 15 cm. It is dilated at its intrabulbar part and distally at the navicular fossa, just internal to the meatus. The external meatus, which is also about 6 mm in length, is sagittal in orientation.

The termination of the urethra is characterized by the fossa navicularis (Fig. 25-52), a widening of the urethral lumen which corresponds to the entrance of the urethra to the glans penis. Its opening at the external meatus is the narrowest part of the entire urethra. A calculus can lodge at this point.

## Vascular Supply

### Arteries

The arterial supply of the prostatic, membranous, and penile urethra:

- Prostatic: inferior vesical artery, middle rectal artery
- Membranous: artery of bulb (from internal pudendal artery)
- Penile: urethral artery, bulbar artery, tiny branches from dorsal and deep arteries of penis

### Veins

The veins drain into the prostatic plexus by way of the deep dorsal vein and into the internal pudendal veins by way of the paired dorsal veins.

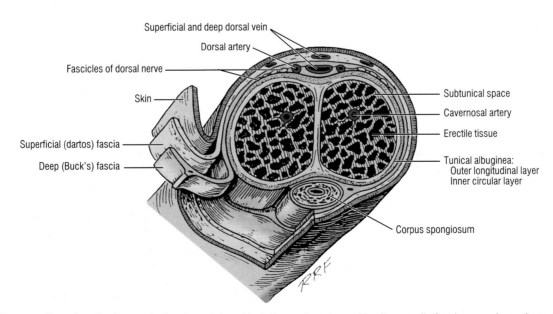

FIG. 25-54. Cross section of penis, demonstrating the relationship between the corporal bodies, penile fascia, vessels, and nerves. (Modified from Devine CJ Jr, Angermeier KW. The anatomy of stress incontinence. AUA Update Series, 1994; 13(2):10; with permission.)

## *Lymphatics*

The prostatic and membranous lymphatics drain into the internal and external iliac nodes. The spongy lymphatics drain into the deep inguinal lymph nodes, with a minority draining into the external iliac nodes.

## Innervation

The possible innervation of the prostatic urethra is by the prostatic plexus. The cavernous nerves from the prostatic plexus innervate the membranous urethra. The penile urethra is innervated by the pudendal nerve.

We quote Strasser and Bartsch[136] on the innervation of the rhabdosphincter:

> *The rhabdosphincter presents as a vertical structure extending from the bulb of the penis to the region of the bladder neck along the prostate and the membranous urethra. Inserting dorsally into the perineal body via a broad tendinous raphe, the striated muscle fibers form an omega-shaped loop around the anterior and lateral aspects of the membranous urethra. The existence of a "urogenital diaphragm" and a strong, circular, striated "external sphincter urethrae" completely encircling the urethra caudal to the apex of the prostate cannot be confirmed by anatomical and histological investigations. The rhabdosphincter is supplied by branches of the pudendal nerve after leaving the pudendal canal.*

## HISTOLOGY

The wall of the urethra is formed by 3 layers:
- muscular coat
- mucosal coat
- submucosal layer

The *muscular coat* of the prostatic and membranous urethra is the downward continuation of the detrusor muscle of the urinary bladder. Therefore, it is especially innervated by sympathetic nerve fibers. The sphincter urethra is formed by striated muscle which surrounds the membranous urethra.

After studying 50 male and 15 female cadavers, Rother et al.[137] stated that the volume of muscle cells and fibers in male and female urethral sphincter muscles decreases with age, beginning in early childhood.

The *mucosal coat* is composed proximally of transitional epithelium continuous with that of the bladder. This cell type terminates at the verumontanum, just distal to the openings of the ejaculatory ducts. Distally, a mixture of stratified columnar epithelium and pseudostratified epithelium with mucous glands can be found. The mucous membrane of the penile urethra is characterized by frequent recesses associated with the tubular mucous glands of Littre, particularly in the dorsal part of the urethra. Distally in the penile urethra, the mucosa becomes stratified squamous in character.

The *submucosal layer* has a rich vascular and erectile network.

## ANATOMIC COMPLICATIONS

If the male urethra is divided by traumatic injury or for clinical reasons, the pathway taken by extravasating urine and blood differs between the anterior (bulbous and pendulous) segments and the posterior (prostatic and membranous) segments, because of the anatomic arrangement of fascial layers and their connections.

If the deep fascial layer is torn from rupture of the anterior urethra, the extravasate can flow into the superficial perineal cleft (see preceding section "Potential Spaces Under the Urogenital Diaphragm" in this chapter). From this space, it can readily track superiorly into the periscrotal and peripenile spaces, and upward upon the abdominal wall, even reaching the level of the nipples. Rupture of the urethra is shown in Figs. 25-55 through 25-58. Hackler[138] stated that Colles' fascia resists the penetration of urine into the pelvis, the thigh, and the anal triangle.

Rupture of the anterior urethra at the junction of the penile bulb and the inferior fascial layer of the urogenital diaphragm (that is, the perineal membrane) results in extravasation of urine and blood. If there is no break in the continuous layer of deep fascia, which includes the perineal fascia of Gallaudet and the penile fascia of Buck, extravasation is limited to the penile shaft (Fig. 25-56).

Rupture of the posterior urethra at the junction of the prostatic apex and the urogenital diaphragm produces an extraperitoneal pelvic collection of urine and blood (Fig. 25-58). We believe that Denonvilliers' fascia posteriorly and the urogenital diaphragm inferiorly are the anatomic entities responsible for the limits of extravasation in the extraperitoneal area and into the space of Retzius.

According to Hackler,[138] pelvic fractures are responsible for 90% of the injuries of the posterior urethra (prostato-membranous), but the injury is significant in only 10% of male patients. Frick et al.[139] reported that approximately 13% will also have urinary bladder disruption.

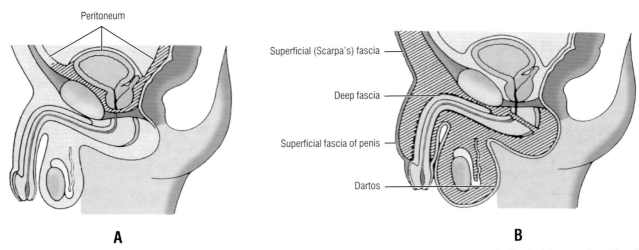

Peritoneum

Superficial (Scarpa's) fascia

Deep fascia

Superficial fascia of penis

Dartos

**A**

**B**

FIG. 25-55. **A,** Rupture of urethra above urogenital diaphragm. **B,** Rupture of bulbous urethra and muscle fascia (deep perineal fascia) of Gallaudet. Diagonal lines represent extravasation of urine. (Modified from Decker GAG, Du Plessis DJ. Lee McGregor's Synopsis of Surgical Anatomy (12th ed). Bristol UK: Wright, 1986; with permission.)

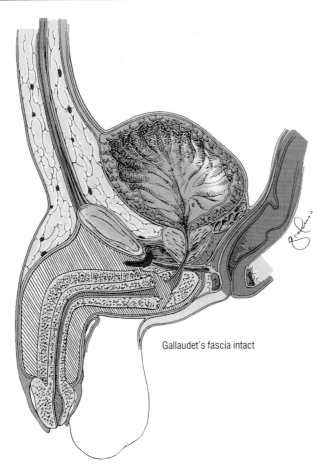

Gallaudet's fascia intact

FIG. 25-56. Anterior urethral rupture. Extravasation limited to penile shaft when Gallaudet's (Buck's) fascia remains intact. (Based on Hackler RH. Complications of urethral and penile trauma. In: Greenfield LJ (ed). Complications in Surgery and Trauma. Philadelphia: JB Lippincott, 1984, pp. 741-748.)

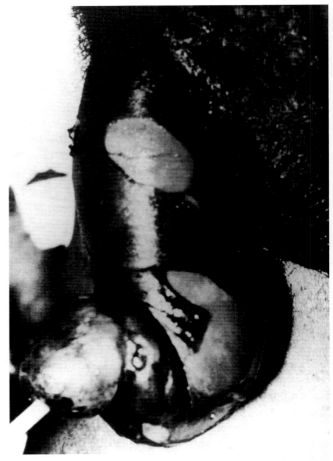

FIG. 25-57. Rupture of anterior urethra. Extravasation limited within Buck's fascia. (From Hackler RH. Complications of urethral and penile trauma. In: Greenfield LJ (ed). Complications in Surgery and Trauma (2nd ed). Philadelphia: JB Lippincott, 1990, pp.784-791; with permission.)

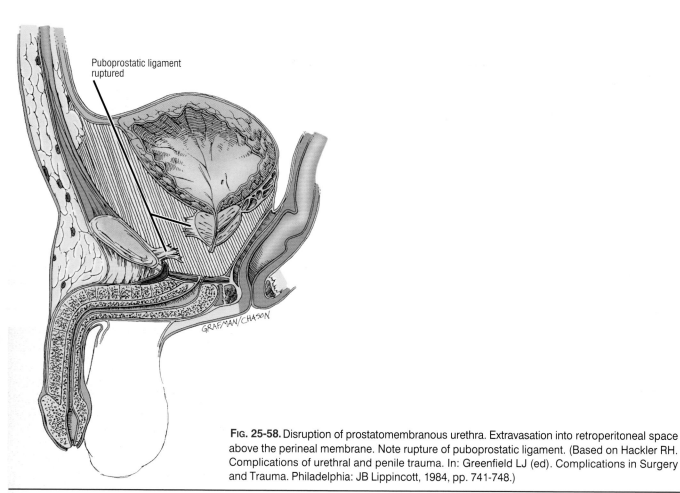

Puboprostatic ligament
ruptured

GRAFMAN/CHASON

**FIG. 25-58.** Disruption of prostatomembranous urethra. Extravasation into retroperitoneal space above the perineal membrane. Note rupture of puboprostatic ligament. (Based on Hackler RH. Complications of urethral and penile trauma. In: Greenfield LJ (ed). Complications in Surgery and Trauma. Philadelphia: JB Lippincott, 1984, pp. 741-748.)

The treatment of urethral injuries depends upon the severity of the injury. Observation, suprapubic cystostomy, or exploration with urethral realignment are the procedures of choice, according to the injury.

# *Penis*

## HISTORY

The anatomic and surgical history of the penis is shown in Table 25-1.

## EMBRYOGENESIS

### Normal Development

Under the influence of testosterone, the genital tuber-cle is responsible for the genesis of the penis.

### Congenital Anomalies

Congenital anomalies of the penis will be found in Table 25-2. These include agenesis of the glans penis, phimosis, duplication, transposition of the penis and scrotum, and defects of the corpus spongiosum and corpora cavernosa.

Agenesis of the penis may be associated with several other anomalies. The scrotum is normal and the testes may be descended or undescended. The embryogenesis of this malformation may be lack of formation of the genital tubercle, with no pars phallica to the urogenital sinus. Treatment includes reconstruction of the phallus and inflatable penile prosthesis.

Penoscrotal transposition is a rare anomaly with partial or complete positional exchange between the penis and scrotum. It may be associated with severe chordee and hypospadias.[140]

## SURGICAL ANATOMY

### Topographic Anatomy

#### Structure

The penis can be divided into three parts: the root, the body, and the glans. The root, or penile bulb, is located within the superficial perineal pouch. According to Tanagho,[71] it provides fixation and stability. The body is formed by the three spongy erectile anatomic entities: two corpora cavernosa and one corpus spongiosum. The glans is the distal end of the corpus spongiosum.

The paired *corpora cavernosa* are located on the dorsum of the pendulous part of the penis, partially separated by the penile septum. Proximally, each begins as a slender cylinder firmly attached to the ischiopubic ramus. From this origin to the pendulous part of the shaft, each of the two erectile bodies is referred to as a crus penis; the con-

tinuation is the corpus. The penile crus is surrounded by fibers of the ischiocavernosus muscle, stoutly attached to the ischiopubic ramus and the perineal membrane (Fig. 25-59).

The *corpus spongiosum,* or penile bulb, lies in the ventral midline area of the penis (Fig. 25-60). Its proximal part is covered by the bilateral bulbospongiosus muscles (Fig. 25-61). After taking origin from the perineal membrane and the perineal body, the muscle fibers pass anteromedially, inserting into the midline penile raphe. The corpus spongiosum surrounds the urethra, which is open at the end of the glans. The bulbospongiosus muscles and ischiocavernosus muscles are covered externally by a very distinct muscle fascia, the fascia of Gallaudet. This fascial layer is continuous from the crura to the bulb, and also attaches deeply to the perineal membrane.

#### Ligaments

The penis is supported by two ligaments, the fundiform and the suspensory. The fundiform ligament is a downward continuation of the superficial fasciae of Camper and Scarpa, which lose their individual identity as they merge to form the fundiform ligament (see "Potential Spaces Above the Urogenital Diaphragm" in this chapter). When approaching the penile dorsum, it splits, surrounds the body of the penis, and unites at the penile ventral area with the scrotal septum. The suspensory ligament under and deep to the fundiform ligament arises from the fascia of Gallaudet (deep fascia of the abdominal wall) and from the frontal aspect of the pubic bone and the symphysis, blend-

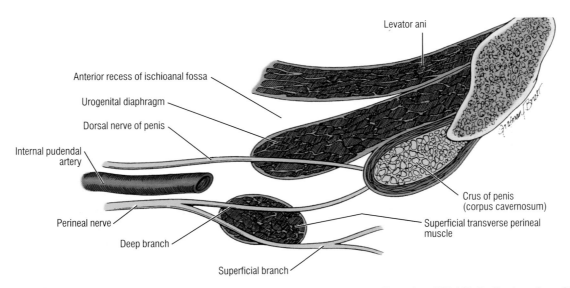

FIG. 25-59. Corpora cavernosa and crus penis. Parasagittal section of the perineum. (Based on O'Rahilly R. Gardner-Gray-O'Rahilly Anatomy (5th ed). Philadelphia: WB Saunders, 1986.)

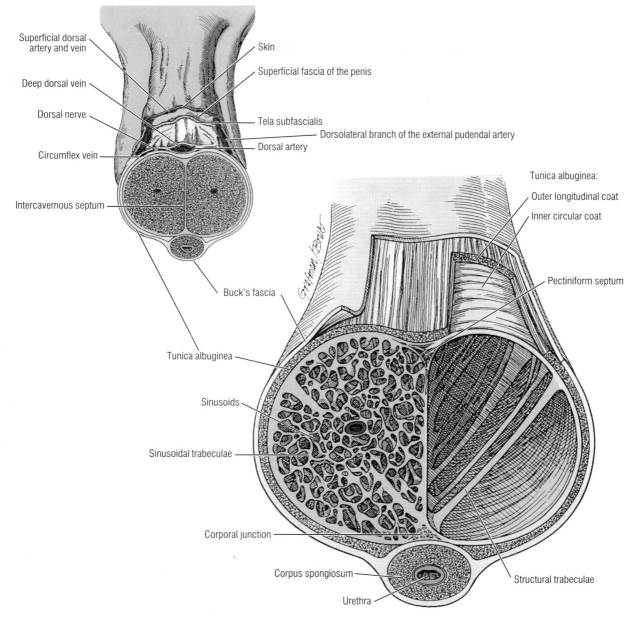

**FIG. 25-60.** Structural layers of penis. (Based on Hinman F Jr. Atlas of Urosurgical Anatomy. Philadelphia: WB Saunders, 1993.)

ing below with the deep penile fascia on each side.

Hoznek et al.[141] stated that the anatomy of the suspensory ligament of the penis consists of separate ligamentous structures, as follows:

> The suspensory apparatus consisted of separate ligamentous structures: the fundiform ligament, which is lateral, superficial and not adherent to the tunica albuginea of the corpora cavernosa; the suspensory ligament properly so-called, further back, stretching

between the pubis and the tunica albuginea of the corpora cavernosa and consisting of two lateral, circumferential, and one median bundles, which circumscribed the dorsal vein of the penis. These structures were identifiable in MRI and their supporting role was evidenced during tests of erection. The suspensory ligament seemed to maintain the base of the penis in front of the pubis and to behave as a major point of support for the mobile portion of the penis during erection.

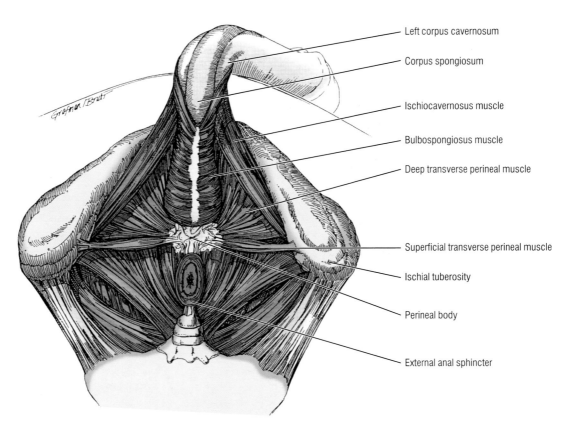

Left corpus cavernosum

Corpus spongiosum

Ischiocavernosus muscle

Bulbospongiosus muscle

Deep transverse perineal muscle

Superficial transverse perineal muscle

Ischial tuberosity

Perineal body

External anal sphincter

FIG. **25-61.** Bulbospongiosus and ischiocavernosus muscles cover corpora cavernosa and corpus spongiosum.

## *Penile Coverings*

From superficial to deep, the penile coverings are: the skin, the superficial fascia, the tela subfascialis, the deep fascia (Buck's), and the tunica albuginea (Fig. 25-60, Fig. 25-62). These structures cover the shaft of the penis and, therefore, the three erectile, cylindrical, tubelike entities (two corpora cavernosa and one corpus spongiosum).

The skin that covers the penis is thin, with a very thin areolar layer which covers, or is mixed with, the superficial penile fascia. The distal part of the skin forms two anatomic entities, the foreskin (prepuce) and the frenulum. The prepuce or foreskin is a fold of skin at the area of the penile neck. The frenulum is a narrow, midline ridge of redundant skin on the ventrum of the shaft which extends from the meatal groove to the coronal sulcus.

The *superficial penile fascia* is the downward continuation of the fasciae of Camper and Scarpa. It is without an adipose content, but with some smooth muscle fibers, like the dartos tunic of the scrotum.

Occasionally, the superficial fascia is called Colles' fascia in the literature. However, we like to reserve this eponym for the part of the fascia of Scarpa that continues immediately after the formation of the tunica dartos, and that terminates by fusing posteriorly with the urogenital diaphragm. Colles' fascia, therefore, participates in the formation of the superficial perineal cleft. Several authors also name the superficial pouch as the pouch of Colles.[142]

The *tela subfascialis* a very thin areolar tissue layer. It occupies the interval between the superficial dartos tunic and Buck's deep fascia over the extracorporal segments of the cavernous arteries, veins, and nerves.[66] Also in this interval are the bilateral dorsal arteries, dorsal veins, and dorsal nerves.

The *deep penile fascia* (fascia of Buck) covers the corpora cavernosa and the corpus spongiosum. Buck's fascia splits to invest the deep dorsal vein in the midline of the penile shaft.

The *tunica albuginea* is a thick white connective tissue matrix formed by two fibrous layers, the outer longitudinal and the inner circular, with little in the way of elastic tissue. It is strongly attached to the overlying fascia of Buck; or perhaps it is better to say that the fascia of Buck is firmly fixed to the tunica albuginea.

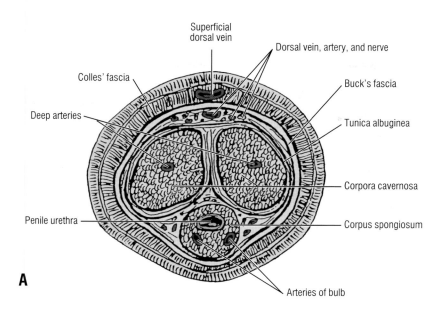

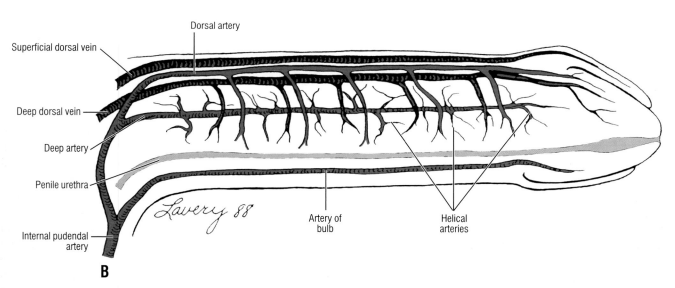

**FIG. 25-62. A,** Cross-section of penis. **B,** Arterial and venous supply. (Modified from Siegel SW. Anatomy and embryology. In: Novick AC (ed). Stewart's Operative Urology, 2nd ed. Baltimore: Williams & Wilkins, 1989, pp. 454-478; with permission.)

# Vascular Supply

## *Arteries*

The arterial blood supply of the penis is formed by a superficial and a deep system (Fig. 25-62B). The external pudendal artery is responsible for the formation of the

superficial system; the internal pudendal artery provides the deep system.

### Superficial System

The arterial blood supply of the skin of the penis is very good. It originates from the external pudendal artery (from the common femoral artery), which gives origin to a dorso-

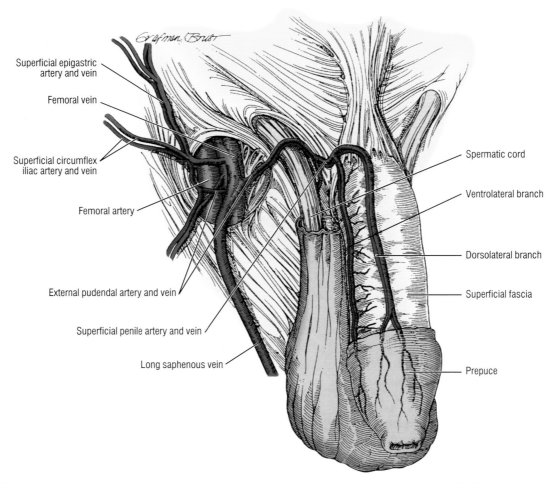

FIG. 25-63. Superficial arterial system. (Based on Hinman F Jr. Atlas of Urosurgical Anatomy. Philadelphia: WB Saunders, 1993.)

lateral and a ventrolateral branch (Fig. 25-63).

**Deep System**

The internal pudendal arteries, right and left, give origin to the penile artery. The penile artery gives three or four bilateral branches to the penis: the bulbourethral artery (the artery to the bulb and the urethral artery), the deep artery (central or cavernous), and the dorsal artery. Figure 25-64 summarizes both the superficial and deep systems.

The bulbourethral artery and the deep artery arise within the urogenital diaphragm. There are good anastomoses between the deep artery and the bulbourethral artery, but not between the deep and dorsal arteries.

The dorsal artery can be regarded as the terminal continuation of the internal pudendal artery (Fig. 25-65). The dorsal artery leaves the urogenital diaphragm by piercing the transverse perineal ligament (the fusion of the superior and inferior fasciae of the diaphragm) and by passing onto

the dorsum of the shaft beneath the superficial fascia.

The beneficiaries of the dorsal artery are the corpora cavernosa, the corpus spongiosum, the tunica albuginea, and the urethra which are pierced by branches of the dorsal artery. The dorsal artery also gives off laterally directed circumflex branches which pass to the corpus spongiosum, with similarly named tributaries to the deep dorsal vein. The fellow traveler with the dorsal artery is the more laterally situated dorsal nerve.

According to Gardner et al.,[143] the dorsal artery provides most of the blood supply to the glans. Remember that the dorsal arteries and nerves curve ventrally before entering the glans (Fig. 25-66). The dorsal artery terminates as the artery to the glans.

The bilateral deep artery of the penis (cavernous) enters each corpus cavernosum on the deep surface of the crus and continues its pathway toward the glans (Fig. 25-67). However, its branches terminate approximately at the

**ARTERIES OF THE PENIS**

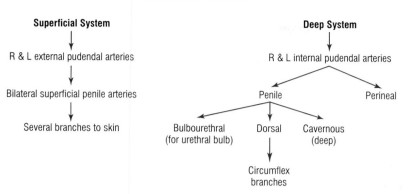

Fig. 25-64. Arteries of the penis.

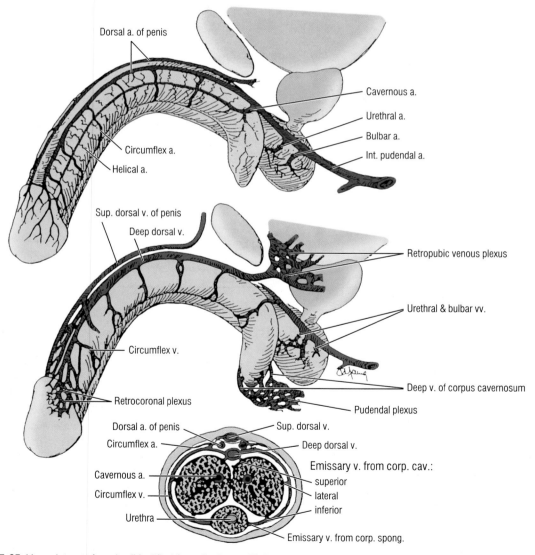

FIG. 25-65. Vasculature of penis. (Modified from Redman JF. Anatomy of the genitourinary system. In: Gillenwater JY, Grayhack JT, Howards SS, Duckett JW (eds). Adult and Pediatric Urology, 2nd ed. St. Louis: Mosby Year Book, 1991, pp. 3-62; with permission.)

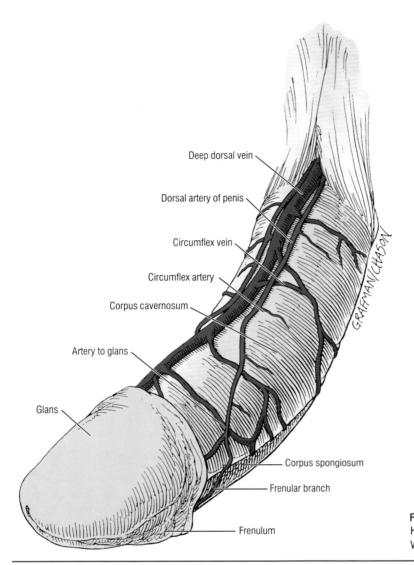

Deep dorsal vein

Dorsal artery of penis

Circumflex vein

Circumflex artery

Corpus cavernosum

Artery to glans

Glans

Corpus spongiosum

Frenular branch

Frenulum

**FIG. 25-66.** Blood supply to glans and frenulum. (Based on Hinman F Jr. Atlas of Urosurgical Anatomy. Philadelphia: WB Saunders, 1993.)

penile neck without anastomosing with the branches of the dorsal artery.

NOTE: The bulbourethral artery is presented in some anatomy books as the bulbar and urethral arteries (Fig 25-65), and in others as a a single artery (Fig. 25-67).

The bulbourethral artery is often short and wide. It enters the bulb of the penis after piercing the inferior fascia of the urogenital diaphragm. This artery supplies the bulb, the urethra, the corpus spongiosum and the glans. It may arise from the bulbar artery.

Droupy et al.[144] described three patterns of penile arterial supply based on dissection of twenty fresh cadavers.
- Type I arises from the internal pudendal arteries (3 of 20)
- Type II arises from both accessory and internal pudendal arteries (14 of 20)
- Type III arises from accessory pudendal arteries (3 of 20)

## Veins

The veins of the penis form a very peculiar and enigmatic system. The heterogeneity and complexity of this system approaches that of the human venous system as a whole. Moscovici et al.[145] studied the venous vasculature of 25 cadaveric penises and reported as follows:

*The superficial veins arising from the tegumentary layers drain into the superficial dorsal vein which in three-quarters of cases empties into the left great saphenous vein. The veins of the deep internal system, running below the deep fascia of the penis, emerge from the erective bodies and can be divided into two systems, one anterosuperior and the other postero-inferior. The anterosuperior system comprises the veins of the glans which will form the deep dorsal vein; the lat-*

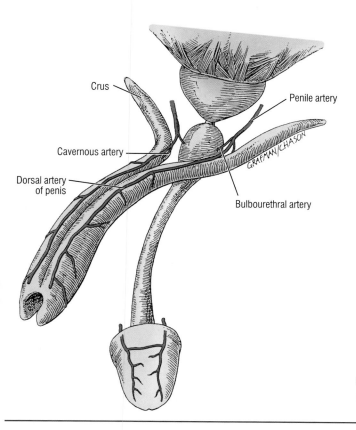

Crus

Penile artery

Cavernous artery

Dorsal artery
of penis

Bulbourethral artery

**FIG. 25-67.** Distal arterial distribution to penis. (Based on Hinman F Jr. Atlas of Urosurgical Anatomy. Philadelphia: WB Saunders, 1993.)

*ter receives blood from the medial portion of the the cor-pus spongiosum and from the free portion of the cor-pora cavernosum mainly via the circumflex veins. It ends in the pre-prostatic plexus. The posteroinferior system, issuing from the posterior portion of the erectile bodies, is composed of the bulbar, cavernous and crural veins which drain towards the pre-prostatic plexus and the in-ternal pudendal veins. Anastomoses link the two networks, superficial and deep. Study of the structure of the veins of the deep system reveals the presence of muscular cushions, which we have shown to have adrenergic innervation. (Fig. 25-68, Fig. 25-69, Fig. 25-70, Fig. 25-71)*

*...The blockage of the anterosuperior system during erection by the deep fascia of the penis and possibly by vasomotor changes involving polsters could play a role in maintaining erection. However, its main mecha-nism remains the compression of the sub-albugineal venous plexus inside the cavernous bodies. The posteroinferior system could be a preferential route for nutritive drainage of the penis.*

An excellent presentation of the penile veins is given by Hinman.[66] He divides the penile venous network into three systems: superficial, intermediate, and deep (Fig. 25-72).

**Superficial System**

The superficial dorsal vein is the major component of the superficial (subcuticular) venous penile network. The super-ficial dorsal vein, which is rarely double, is formed from sev-eral minute veins of the dorsolateral penile surface. The superficial venous system drains the penile skin.

**Intermediate System**

The intermediate system is formed by the following en-tities.
- Deep dorsal vein
- Circumflex vein
- Prostatic plexus
- Lateral venous plexus
- Retrocoronal plexus

These multiple veins are located under Buck's fascia. They drain the glans penis, corpus spongiosum, and distal two-thirds of the corpora cavernosa. The intermediate system drains into the deep dorsal vein or veins, which ter-minates into the internal iliac veins via the prostatic and vesical plexuses.

Topographicoanatomically the deep dorsal vein, in-vested by Buck's fascia, is disposed between the bilateral lymphatics, the dorsal artery, and the dorsal nerve. Small veins leave the deep dorsal vein before its passage into the

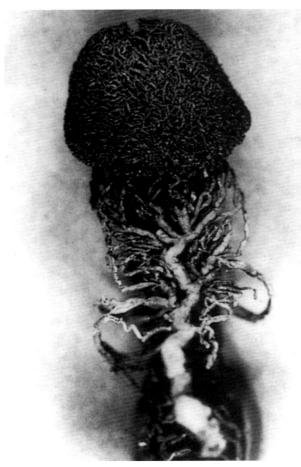

**FIG. 25-68.** Dorsal view of the penis after injection-corrosion showing the veins of the glans, the retrocoronal plexus and the deep dorsal vein. (From Moscovici J, Galinier P, Hammoudi S, Lefebvre D, Juricic M, Vaysse P. Contribution to the study of the venous vasculature of the penis. Surg Radiol Anat 1999;21:193-199; with permission.)

pelvis to drain into the internal pudendal vein. Passing through the perineum, the internal pudendal veins receive tributaries from the penile bulb and from the scrotum.

The deep dorsal vein is located between the two corpora cavernosa. It receives much of their venous drainage by way of deep perforating vessels. These vessels arise from minute tributaries of the corpus spongiosum, the adjacent corpora cavernosa, and the circumflex veins from the corpus spongiosum (Fig. 25-73). The perineal and penile veins are valveless.

### Deep System

The deep system drains into the deep dorsal vein which goes to the internal pudendal vein. It is formed by the following veins.

- Cavernous
- Bulbar
- Crural

We refer the student who wants to know more about the complicated relations of the deep system to the excellent book of Hinman.[66]

## *Lymphatics*

The lymphatic drainage of the penis is peculiar. The skin and prepuce drain into the superficial inguinal lymph nodes (Fig. 25-74). The lymphatics of the glans and penile

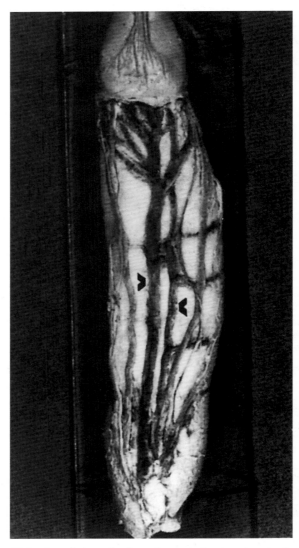

**FIG. 25-69.** Dorsal view of a dissection revealing two dorsal veins of unequal calibre. (From Moscovici J, Galinier P, Hammoudi S, Lefebvre D, Juricic M, Vaysse P. Contribution to the study of the venous vasculature of the penis. Surg Radiol Anat 1999;21:193-199; with permission.)

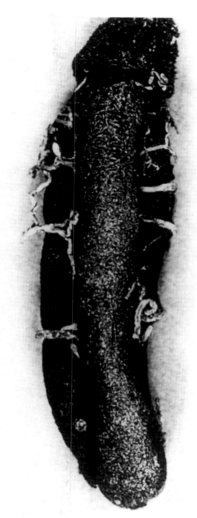

**FIG. 25-70.** Ventral view of the penis after injection-corrosion showing the inferior emissary veins and the origin of the circumflex veins. (From Moscovici J, Galinier P, Hammoudi S, Lefebvre D, Juricic M, Vaysse P. Contribution to the study of the venous vasculature of the penis. Surg Radiol Anat 1999;21:193-199; with permission.)

urethra drain into the deep inguinal and external iliac lymph nodes (Fig. 25-75).

# Innervation

## Somatic

The dorsal nerves originate from the pudendal nerve within Alcock's canal (Fig. 25-76). They enter the dorsum of the penis to innervate the skin and glans of the penis. The perineal nerves and their branches innervate the vessels of the erectile elements and the urethra. The sensory fibers

enter the dorsal gray of the cord at cord levels S2-S4. Likewise, the motor supply to the ischiocavernosus and bulbospongiosus muscles is supplied by motor fibers from the ventral gray area at the same cord levels. The ilioinguinal nerve innervates the skin of the root of the penis.

The dissection studies of Colombel et al.[146] showed evidence of communication between the cavernous nerves and the dorsal nerve of the penis.

## *Autonomic*

The sympathetic nerves arise from spinal cord levels L1 and L2, synapsing in the sympathetic chains at vertebral levels S2, S3, and S4. The postganglionic fibers join the sacral nerves and pass into the pudendal nerve. These nerve fibers are responsible for vasoconstriction. According to Andersson et al.,[147] they produce erection through a series of complex interactions. Stimulation of the sympathetic pathways also mediates detumescence and contributes to the maintenance of the penis in a non-erect state.

The parasympathetic nerves from S2, S3, and S4 (the nervi erigentes) produce vasodilation and resultant erection. The cavernous nerve originates from the prostatic plexus and supplies the corpus cavernosum (Fig. 25-77). Occasionally, it bifurcates. One branch is responsible for the erectile tissue of the corpus spongiosum and the penile urethra. The other branch is responsible for the erectile tissue of the corpora cavernosa.

REMEMBER:
- The terminology for the nerve plexuses in the lower abdomen and pelvis is inconsistent and confusing. In this regard, one hears of superior and inferior mesenteric

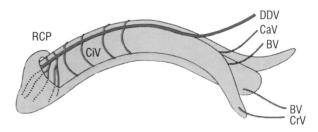

**FIG. 25-71.** The two drainage systems of the erectile bodies: the anterosuperior system comprising the veins of the glans, the retrocoronal plexus (RCP), the circumflex veins (CiV) and the deep dorsal vein (DDV); and the posteroinferior system comprising the bulbar (BV), cavernous (CaV), and crural (CrV) veins. (Modified from Moscovici J, Galinier P, Hammoudi S, Lefebvre D, Juricic M, Vaysse P. Contribution to the study of the venous vasculature of the penis. Surg Radiol Anat 1999;21:193-199; with permission.)

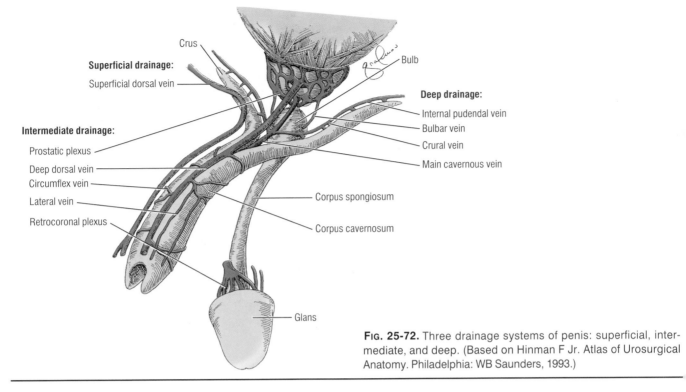

Crus

**Superficial drainage:**

Superficial dorsal vein

Bulb

**Deep drainage:**

Internal pudendal vein

Bulbar vein

Crural vein

Main cavernous vein

**Intermediate drainage:**

Prostatic plexus

Deep dorsal vein

Circumflex vein

Lateral vein

Retrocoronal plexus

Corpus spongiosum

Corpus cavernosum

Glans

**FIG. 25-72.** Three drainage systems of penis: superficial, intermediate, and deep. (Based on Hinman F Jr. Atlas of Urosurgical Anatomy. Philadelphia: WB Saunders, 1993.)

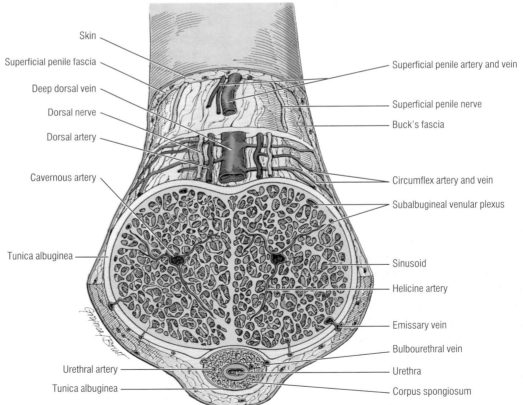

Skin

Superficial penile fascia

Deep dorsal vein

Dorsal nerve

Dorsal artery

Cavernous artery

Tunica albuginea

Urethral artery

Tunica albuginea

Superficial penile artery and vein

Superficial penile nerve

Buck's fascia

Circumflex artery and vein

Subalbugineal venular plexus

Sinusoid

Helicine artery

Emissary vein

Bulbourethral vein

Urethra

Corpus spongiosum

**FIG. 25-73.** Blood vessels and nerves of penile shaft (cross section). (Based on Hinman F Jr. Atlas of Urosurgical Anatomy. Philadelphia: WB Saunders, 1993.)

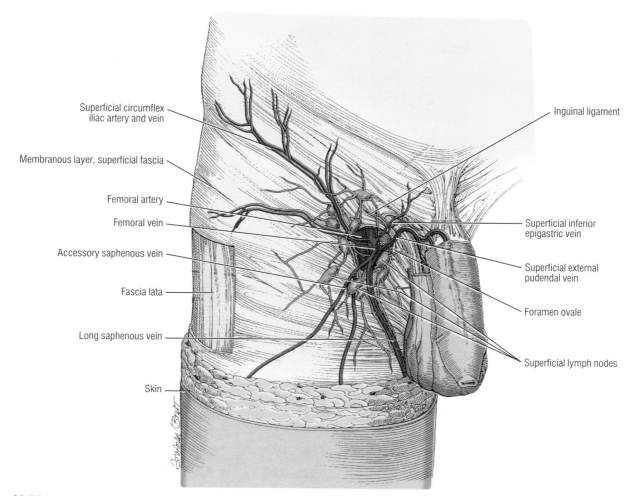

Superficial circumflex
iliac artery and vein

Membranous layer, superficial fascia

Femoral artery

Femoral vein

Accessory saphenous vein

Fascia lata

Long saphenous vein

Skin

Inguinal ligament

Superficial inferior
epigastric vein

Superficial external
pudendal vein

Foramen ovale

Superficial lymph nodes

FIG. 25-74. Superficial lymph drainage system. (Based on Hinman F Jr. Atlas of Urosurgical Anatomy. Philadelphia: WB Saunders, 1993.)

plexuses, preaortic plexuses, superior and inferior hypo-gastric plexuses, and so on. There is little doubt that many of the terms, such as "hypogastric," are outdated. It would perhaps be simpler to refer to a preaortic plexus that bifurcates into right and left pelvic plexuses. These, in turn, would give rise to more precisely named entities, such as the vesical plexus, the prostatic plexus, and so on. However, the prostatic plexus is formed by the inferior hypogastric plexus (autonomic) which is responsible for the genesis of the cavernous nerve (a forward continuation of the prostatic plexus).

- The inferior hypogastric plexus is synonymous with the pelvic plexus. It is located on the lateral pelvic wall (Fig. 25-78). It is formed by:
  - postganglionic sympathetic nerves that have descended through the hypogastric plexus from ganglia in the lumbar part of the sympathetic chains
  - preganglionic parasympathetic fibers that arise directly

from the ventral rami of S2-S4 as pelvic splanchnic nerves
  - sensory fibers for pain and other modalities from the pelvic organs
- The nervi erigentes from S2-S4 are responsible for general sensations from the left colon and the pelvic organs. Parasympathetic functions include the sense of distention and reflex behavior for emptying of the urinary bladder and rectum. Pain from the epididymis is also carried by these nerves.
- Pain fibers from visceral structures are usually carried by nerves which are principally associated with the sympathetic nervous system; this is obviously a primary protective feature of the "fight or flight" function of that system. Pain from the urinary bladder passes upward through the hypogastric plexus. Passing into the sympathetic chains by way of the sacral and lumbar splanchnic nerves, these pain fibers then ascend in the chains to

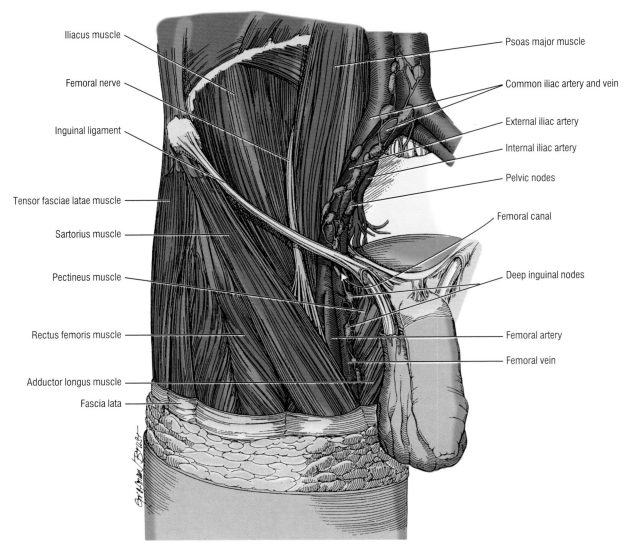

FIG. **25-75.** Deep inguinal drainage system. (Based on Hinman F Jr. Atlas of Urosurgical Anatomy. Philadelphia: WB Saunders, 1993.)

spinal cord levels T10-L2, where they gain access to the spinal cord. It is for this reason that lumbar sympathectomy can alleviate pain from the uterus and certain other pelvic tissues. However, the innervation of the pelvic organs does not enjoy complete unanimity among those who study the neurophysiology in this area.

- Initially, the penile neurovascular bundle is located posterolateral to the prostate and anterior to Denonvilliers' fascia, together with branches of the prostatovesicular artery and veins. To be more specific concerning penile surgery, the neurovascular bundle is located between Buck's fascia above and the tunica albuginea below. It can be uncovered by an incision lateral to the midline.
- Below we reprint a very interesting exchange between in-

vestigators of penile innervation. The subject under consideration is the anatomy of the lateral rectal ligaments, anatomic entities related to the pelvirectal spaces above the levator ani which divide the spaces into anterior and posterior compartments. Rutegård et al.[148] stated:

*The contents of the so-called lateral rectal ligaments are defined differently in surgical and anatomical texts. In surgical texts the middle rectal arteries are referred to as the main structures within them.[149-151] In contrast, the meticulous anatomical work by Sato and Sato[152] has shown that arteries are found in only about 20 per cent of cadaver dissections, whereas nerve branches from the pelvic plexuses, also called the neurovascular bundles, are uniformly constant structures within the liga-*

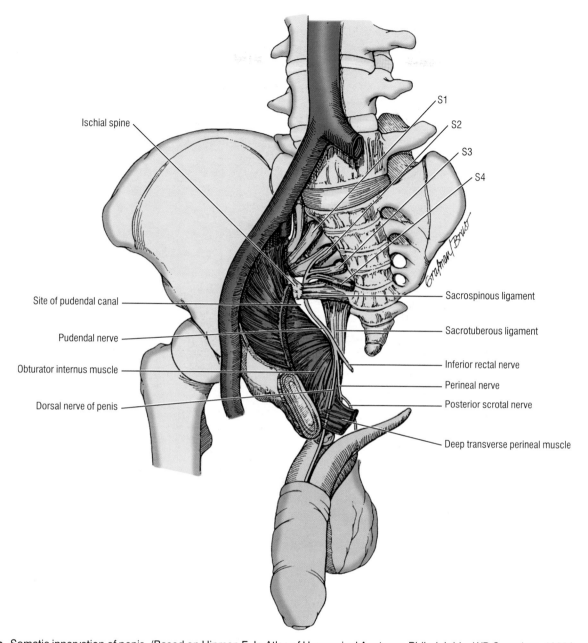

FIG. 25-76. Somatic innervation of penis. (Based on Hinman F Jr. Atlas of Urosurgical Anatomy. Philadelphia: WB Saunders, 1993.)

*ments. This view of the lateral ligaments as important nerve-containing structures is supported by clinico-physiological results after sphincter-saving surgery reported in the Japanese literature.*[153,154]

*The autonomic nerve supply of the lower rectum has been postulated to arise from the pelvic side wall plexuses.*[152,155] *The close relationship of the ligaments to the pelvic plexuses, which contain merging sympathetic and parasympathetic nerve fibres, makes the dissection of the ligaments crucial in maintaining*

*genitourinary function.*[156,157]

*However, Enker et al.*[158] *recently considered the ligaments to be structures that are surgically developed by medial traction during operation. This view has been further established by the same group after cadaveric studies.*[159]

In disagreement with the hypothesis of Enker et al.,[158] Rutegård et al.[148] continued:

*In fact, the lateral ligaments encountered in rectal*

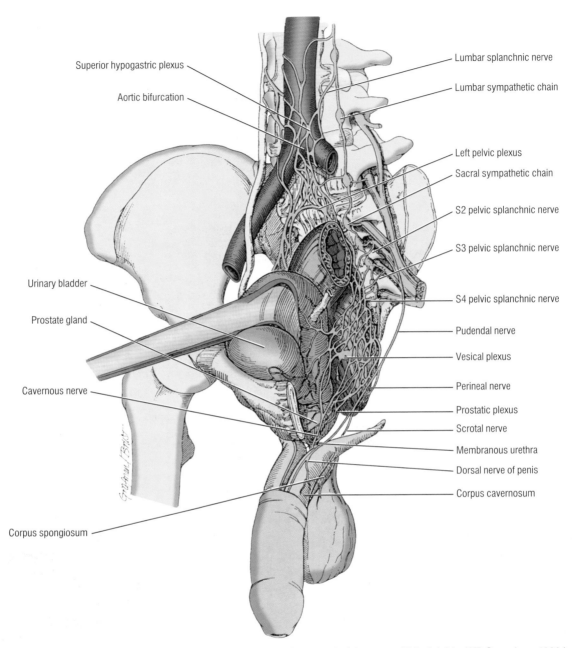

Superior hypogastric plexus

Aortic bifurcation

Lumbar splanchnic nerve

Lumbar sympathetic chain

Left pelvic plexus

Sacral sympathetic chain

S2 pelvic splanchnic nerve

S3 pelvic splanchnic nerve

Urinary bladder

S4 pelvic splanchnic nerve

Prostate gland

Pudendal nerve

Vesical plexus

Perineal nerve

Cavernous nerve

Prostatic plexus

Scrotal nerve

Membranous urethra

Dorsal nerve of penis

Corpus cavernosum

Corpus spongiosum

**FIG. 25-77.** Autonomic innervation of penis. (Based on Hinman F Jr. Atlas of Urosurgical Anatomy. Philadelphia: WB Saunders, 1993.)

*surgery correspond well to the medial portion of the lateral ligaments of the rectum as described by Sato and Sato.[152] Accordingly, the authors consider the ligaments to be real anatomical findings and not merely surgically developed structures, as recently described.[158,159]*

Rutegård et al.[148] show the right lateral rectal ligament in a highly diagrammatic fashion in Fig. 25-79.

Liang et al.[160] responded to the findings of Rutegård

et al.[148] as follows:

*We endorse the presence of the lateral ligament demonstrated by Rutegård et al. (Br J Surg 1997;84: 1544-5). The lateral ligaments are closely interrelated to the pelvic plexus which is a fenestrated rectangular plate of sympathetic and parasympathetic fibres. This provides innervation to the bladder, ureter, prostate, seminal vesicles, membranous urethra and corpora cavernosa via anterolateral branches, and to the distal*

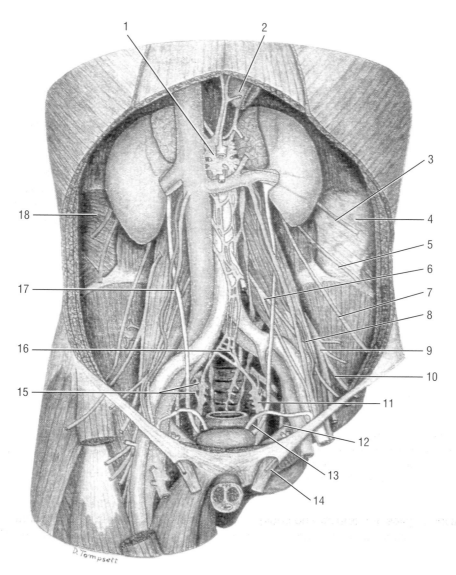

**FIG. 25-78.** Nerves of posterior abdominal wall. 1, Celiac ganglia. 2, Cardia of stomach. 3, Subcostal nerve. 4, Transversus abdominis. 5, Iliohypogastric nerve. 6, Genitofemoral nerve. 7, Ilioinguinal nerve. 8, Testicular artery (unusual origin from renal artery). 9, Femoral nerve. 10, Lateral cutaneous nerve of thigh. 11, Inferior hypogastric (pelvic) plexus. 12, Obturator nerve. 13, Ductus deferens. 14, Ilioinguinal nerve. 15, Nervi erigentes. 16, Superior hypogastric plexus. 17, Testicular vessels. 18, Internal oblique muscle. (From Last RJ. Anatomy Regional and Applied (5th ed). Baltimore: Williams & Wilkins, 1972; with permission.)

rectum via medial branches.[161] Conceivably, the nerve fibres elegantly illustrated by the authors by immuno-histochemistry were the rectal branches of the pelvic plexus. It is only the medial segment of the lateral ligament that is included in the resection during rectal cancer surgery.[152] Before sharp dissection of the lateral ligament we routinely find the location of the plexus by tracing the exposed hypogastric nerve or direct palpation. The pelvic plexus is, therefore, rarely injured during the division of the lateral ligament. Partial injury of the pelvic plexus results in temporary loss of genitourinary function.

The periprostatic plexus represents a further challenge for the colorectal surgeons endeavouring to perform autonomic nerve-preserving lower rectal cancer surgery. The periprostate plexus, running between the anterolateral rectal wall and the prostate, is vulnerable to inadvertent dissection which results in sexual dysfunction.[162]

Whether the middle rectal artery is included in the

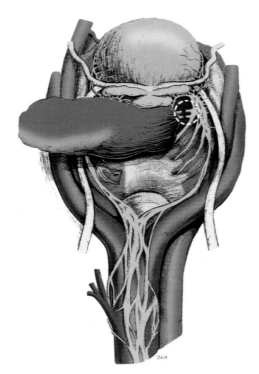

**FIG. 25-79.** Diagram of the autonomic nerve supply in the pelvis. Surgeon's view from the head end of the patient. Within the dashed circle, notice that two nerve fibers in the right lateral rectal ligament are divided as they bridge over from the pelvic plexus to the rectum. (Modified from Rutegård J, Sandzén B, Stenling R, Wiig J, Heald RJ. Lateral rectal ligaments contain important nerves. Br J Surg 84:1544-1545, 1997; with permission.)

*lateral ligament or not is of little clinical significance because its small size allows easy control by cautery.*

In the same journal, Rutegård's reply was as follows:
*We appreciate the comments from Liang et al. and agree with their description of the nerve anatomy. Their illustration [Editors' note: We have not reproduced the illustration in this chapter] has the advantage of clearly showing the sympathetic trunk which can often be visualized even in the presacral area but may give rise to the misunderstanding that the hypogastric nerves and the pelvic plexuses lie close to the rectal wall; in fact they can usually be found on the pelvic side wall.*

- Finally, we quote the cadaveric studies of penile innervation and vascularization by Benoit et al.[163]:
*The pelvic nerve plexus had both parasympathetic and sympathetic roots. It was distributed to the external urethral sphincter giving rise to cavernous nerves which anastomosed in 70% of the cases with the pudendal nerve in the penile root. Accessory pudendal*

*arteries were present in the pelvis in 70% of the cases, anastomosing in 70% of the cases with the cavernous arteries that originated from the pudendal arteries. Transalbugineal anastomoses were always seen between the cavernous artery and the spongiosal arterial network. There were 2 venous pathways, 1 in the pelvis and 1 in the perineum with a common origin from the deep dorsal penile vein. It is concluded that there are two neurovascular pathways destined for the penis that are topographically distinct. One is located in the pelvis and the other in the perineum. We were unable to determine the functional balance between these two anastomosing pathways but experimental data have shown that they are both involved in penile erection. These 2 neurovascular pathways, above and below the levator ani, together with their anastomoses, form a neurovascular loop around the levator ani.*

## HISTOLOGY

Both dorsally located corpora cavernosa are covered partially by tunica albuginea; also, the tunica albuginea completely envelops the ventrally located corpus spongiosum of the urethra. All three cylindrical masses are composed of dilated blood vessels lined by epithelium.

## PHYSIOLOGY

The anatomy and physiology of erection is beautifully presented in Table 25-8, which describes the blood circulation during tumescence and detumescence. In brief, in response to psychic and tactile stimuli, parasympathetic fibers act to cause vasodilation of the arterial branches supplying the spongy tissues of the corpora cavernosa and the corpus spongiosum, resulting in profuse inflow of blood to them. The relatively inelastic tunica albuginea impedes venous return as the erectile tissue becomes engorged with blood. Contraction of the overlying skeletal musculature is also a part of these processes.

Erection of the penis occurs as the cavernous bodies become rigid. The tunica of the corpus spongiosum is not as dense or inelastic as the corpora cavernosa. The tunica of the corpus spongiosum and the terminal glans do not become so turgid as to impede the ejaculate. Following ejaculation, an act principally under sympathetic control, sympathetic domination causes vasoconstriction and detumescence.

### TABLE 25-8. Blood Circulation During Erection and Detumescence

| Arterial Supply | Venous Drainage |
|---|---|
| Tumescence | Detumescence |
| **Corpora Cavernosa** | |
| Principal cavernous arteries (accessory cavernous arteries) *to* (dorsal arteries) *to* helicine arteries *to* sinusoids | 1. Emissary veins *to* circumflex veins *to* deep dorsal vein *to* periprostatic plexus |
| | 2. Cavernous vein *to* internal pudendal vein |
| | 3. Crural vein *to* internal pudendal vein |
| **Corpus Spongiosum** | |
| Bulbourethral arteries *to* urethral arteries *to* circumflex branches of dorsal arteries | Vein of the bulb *to* periprostatic plexus *to* internal pudendal vein |
| **Glans** | |
| Dorsal artery *to* urethral artery | Retrocoronal venous plexus *to* deep dorsal vein *to* periprostatic plexus |

*Source:* Hinman F Jr. Atlas of Urosurgical Anatomy. Philadelphia: WB Saunders, 1993; with permission.

## SURGICAL APPLICATIONS

The following are the most common surgical procedures of the penis:

- Dorsal slit
- Circumcision
- Release of chordee
- Hypospadias repair
- Epispadias repair
- Partial penectomy
- Total penectomy
- Insertion of penile prosthesis
- Correction of penile curvature
- Excision and incision of Peyronie's disease
- Surgical procedures for priapism
- Surgery for penile trauma
- Penile replantation
- Penile reconstruction

## ANATOMIC COMPLICATIONS

Complications of penile surgery can be avoided by good anatomic knowledge. The most important anatomic compli-

cations are injury of the urethra, which was described previously in the section on the male urethra, and bleeding.

Bleeding is avoided by good ligation of the vascular network (superficial dorsal veins, deep dorsal vein, two dorsal arteries). Be sure to ligate the frenulum above its division. This will ligate the frenular branch of the artery to the glans, which originates from the dorsal artery of the penis.

Also presented here are anatomic complications of circumcision in adults and of the amputated penis.

Circumcision in adults consists of partial removal of the excess foreskin of the penis. Bleeding, with hematoma formation, is the most frequent complication of this simple operation. A number of iatrogenic complications have been reported:

- Removal of too much or too little skin
- Amputation of the glans
- Skin pathology, such as adhesions, epidermal inclusion cysts, and trapped deposits of smegma. The latter is the result of a bad suture line that does not approximate the mucosal and cutaneous edges.

Laumann et al.[164] reported the following:

*[C]ircumcision provides no discernible prophylactic benefit and may in fact increase the likelihood of STD [sexually transmitted disease] contraction ...circumcised men have a slightly lessened risk of experiencing sexual dysfunction, especially among older men ...circumcised men displayed greater rates of experience of various sexual practices. While evidence regarding STD experience contributes to ongoing debates, our results concerning sexual dysfunction and practice represent largely unprecedented effects. These findings suggest the need for continued research that should further aid parents in weighing the benefits and risks of circumcising their sons.*

For the survival of an amputated penis, microsurgery must be performed. Hackler[138] recommended anastomosis of at least one of the dorsal arteries, the deep dorsal vein, and the superficial dorsal vein. Necrosis of the penile

### Editorial Comment

*A study of the risk of heterosexual transmission to male partners of the immunodeficiency virus (HIV-1) found that transmission was much higher in uncircumcised men than in circumcised men.*[165] *(RSF Jr)*

skin should be treated by total distal excision to 0.5 cm from the glans penis, and graft of split-thickness skin from the defect to the coronal sulcus. According to Peters and Sagalowsky,[166] this will avoid the production of lymphedema.

# REFERENCES

1. Hunter J. Works of John Hunter (1786). vol 4. Palmer JF (ed). London: Longman, 1839.

2. O'Rahilly R, Müller F. Human Embryology & Teratology, 2nd ed. New York: Wiley-Liss, 1996, p. 308.

3. Arey LB. Developmental Anatomy, 7th ed. Philadelphia: WB Saunders, 1965.

4. Favorito LA, Samapaio FJB, Javaroni V, Cardoso LE, Macedo C, Waldemar S. Proximal insertion of gubernaculum testis in normal human fetuses and in boys with cryptorchidism. J Urol 2000;164:792-794.

5. Lockwood CB. The development and transition of the testicles: Normal and abnormal. Br Med J 1:444, 1887.

6. Scorer CG. The anatomy of testicular descent: Normal and incomplete. Br J Surg 49:357, 1962.

7. Barthold JS, Kumasi-Rivers K, Upadhyay J, Shekarriz B, Imperato-McGinley J. Testicular position in the androgen insensitivity syndrome: implications for the role of androgens in testicular descent. J Urol 2000;164:497-501.

8. Scorer CG. The incidence of incomplete descent of the testicle at birth. Arch Dis Child 1956;31:198.

9. Shapiro B. Kann man mit Hypophysenvorderlappen den unterentwickelten mannlichen Genitalapparat bein Menschen zum Wachstum Anregen? Dtsch Med Wochenschr 1930;56:1605.

10. Engle ET. Experimentally induced descent of the testis in the macaque monkey by hormone from the anterior pituitary and pregnancy urine. Endocrinology 16:513, 1932.

11. Martins T. Mechanism of descent of testicle under action of sex hormones. In: Essays in Biology in Honor of Herbert M. Evans. Berkeley: University of California Press, 1943, pp 387-397.

12. Wislocki GB. Observations on descent of testes in macaque and in chimpanzee. Anat Rec 57:133, 1933.

13. Hutson JM, Baker ML. A hypothesis to explain abnormal gonadal descent in persistent müllerian duct syndrome. Pediatr Surg Int 1994;9:542-543.

14. Hutson JM, Davidson PM, Reece LA, Baker ML, Zhou BY. Failure of gubernacular development in the persistent müllerian duct syndrome allows herniation of the testes. Pediatr Surg Int 1994;9:544-546.

15. Backhouse KM, Butler H. The gubernaculum testis of the pig (sus scropha). J Anat 1960;94:107.

16. Hutson JM, Hasthorpe S, Heyns CF. Anatomical and functional aspects of testicular descent and cryptorchidism. Endocr Rev 1997;18:259-280.

17. Clarnette TD, Hutson JM. Is the ascending testis actually "stationary"? Normal elongation of the spermatic cord is prevented by a fibrous remnant of the processus vaginalis. Pediatr Surg Int 1997;12:155-157.

18. Hutson JM, Terada M, Zhou B, Williams MP. Normal testicular descent and the aetiology of cryptorchidism [Review]. Adv Anat

Embryol Cell Biol 1996;132:1-56.

19. Clarnette TD, Hutson JM. The genitofemoral nerve may link testicular inguinoscrotal descent with congenital inguinal hernia. Aust NZ J Surg 1996;66:612-617.

20. Hutson JM. Testicular descent: the first step towards fertility. Int J Androl 1994;17:281-288.

21. Heyns CF, Hutson JM. Historical review of theories on testicular descent. J Urol 1995;153:754-767.

22. Moore CR, Oslund R. Experiments on sheep testes, cryptorchidism, vasectomy and scrotal insulation. Am J Physiol 1924;67:595.

23. Scorer CG. The descent of the testis. Arch Dis Child 1964;39:605.

24. Scorer CG. Undescended testicle. Br Med J 1960;1:1359.

25. Hadžiselimović F, Duckett JW Jr, Snyder HM III, Schnaufer L, Huff D. Omphalocele, cryptorchidism, and brain malformations. J Pediatr Surg 1987;22:654-656.

26. Cendron M, Keating MA, Huff DS, Koop CE, Snyder HM III, Duckett JW. Cryptorchidism, orchiopexy and infertility: A critical long-term retrospective analysis. J Urol 1990;142:559-562.

27. Puri P, O'Donnell B. Semen analysis of patients who had orchiopexy at or after seven years of age. Lancet 1988;8614(vol II): 1051.

28. Ludwig G, Potempa J. Der optimale Zeitpunkt der Behandlung des Kryptorchismus. Dtsch Med Wochenschr 1975;100:680.

29. Martin DC. Germinal cell tumors of the testis after orchidopexy. J Urol 1979;121:422.

30. Kogan S. Cryptorchidism. In: Kelalis PP, King LR, Belman AB (eds). Clinical Pediatric Urology (3rd ed). Philadelphia: WB Saunders, 1992.

31. Aggarwal A, Krishnan J, Kwart A, Perry D. Noonan's syndrome and seminoma of undescended testicle. South Med J 2001;94:432-434.

32. Varela-Cives R, Bautista-Casanovas A, Gude F, Cimadevila-Garcia A, Tojo R, Pombo M. The predictive value of inguinal herniography for the diagnosis and treatment of cryptorchidism. J Urol 2000;163:964.

33. Owings EP, Georgeson KE. A new technique for laparoscopic exploration to find contralateral patent processus vaginalis. Surg Endosc 2000;14:114-116.

34. Chen KC, Chu CC, Chou TY. Transverse testicular ectopia: preoperative diagnosis by ultrasonography. Pediatr Surg Int 2000;16:77-79.

35. Hutcheson JC, Snyder HM III, Zuñiga ZV, Zderic SA, Schultz DJ, Canning DA, Huff DS. Ectopic and undescended testes: 2 variants of a single congenital anomaly? J Urol 2000;163:961.

36. Ambrose SS, Skandalakis JE. Torsion of the appendix epididymis and testis: report of six episodes. J Urol 1957;77:51-58.

37. Chang KS, Hsu FK, Chan ST, Chan YB. Scrotal asymmetry and handedness. J Anat 1960;94:543.

38. Hanley HG, Hodges RD. The epididymis in male sterility: a preliminary report of microdissection studies. J Urol 1959;82:508.

39. Stoppa R, Diarra B, Mertl P. The retroparietal spermatic sheath –an anatomical structure of surgical interest. Hernia 1997;1:55-59.

40. Shinohara H., Nakatani T., Fukuo Y., Morisawa S., Matsuda T. Case with a high-positioned origin of the testicular artery. Anat Rec 1990;226(2):264-266.

41. Hanley HG, Harrison RG. Nature and surgical treatment of varicocele. Br J Surg 1962;50:64.

42. Neuhof H, Mencher WH. The viability of the testis following complete severance of the spermatic cord. Surg Gynecol Obstet 1960;8:672.

43. Burdick CG, Higinbotham NL. Division of the spermatic cord as

an aid in operating on selected types of inguinal hernia. Ann Surg 1935;102:863.

44. Hinman F Jr. Atlas of Urosurgical Anatomy. Philadelphia: WB Saunders, 1993.

45. Lechter A, Lopez G, Martinez C, Camacho J. Anatomy of the gonadal veins: A reappraisal. Surgery 1991;109:735.

46. Skandalakis JE, Skandalakis LJ, Colborn GL. Testicular atrophy and neuropathy in herniorrhaphy. Am Surg 62(9):775-782, 1996.

47. Skandalakis JE, Colborn GL, Gray SW, Skandalakis LJ, Pemberton LB. The surgical anatomy of the inguinal area — Part 1. Contemp Surg 38:20-34, 1991.

48. Skandalakis JE, Colborn GL, Pemberton LB, Skandalakis LJ, Gray SW. The surgical anatomy of the inguinal area — Part 2. Contemp Surg 38:28-38, 1991.

49. Nahleh Z, Gallardo J, Tabbara IA. Advanced germ cell tumors in male patients. South Med J 2001;93:1054-1066.

50. Foster RS, Donohue JP. Retroperitoneal lymph node dissection for the management of clinical stage I nonseminoma. J Urol 2000;163:1788-1792.

51. Klein EA. Open technique for nerve sparing retroperitoneal lymphadenectomy. Urology 2000;55:132-135.

52. Grasso M, Lania C, Castelli M, Galli L, Franzoso F, Rigatti P. Low-grade left varicocele in patients over 30 years old: the effect of spermatic vein ligation on fertility. BJU Int 2000;85:305-307.

53. Salerno S, Cannizzaro F, Lo Castro A, Romano P, Bentivegna E, Lagalla R. [Anastomosis between the left internal spermatic and splanchnic veins. Retrospective analysis of 305 patients]. Radiol Med 2000;99:347-351.

54. Hutcheson JC, Cooper CS, Snyder HM III. The anatomical approach to inguinal orchiopexy. J Urol 2000;164:1702-1704.

55. Parrott TS, Hewatt L. Ligation of the testicular artery and vein in adolescent varicocele. J Urol 1994;152:791.

56. Hunt JB, Witherington R, Smith AM. The midline preperitoneal approach to orchiopexy. Am Surg 1981;47:184.

57. Caruso AP, Walsh RA, Wolach JW, Koyle MA. Single scrotal incision orchiopexy for the palpable undescended testicle. J Urol 2000;164:156-159.

58. Weiske WH, Salzler N, Schroeder-Printzen I, Weidner W. Clinical findings in congenital absence of the vasa deferentia. Andrologia 2000;32:13-18.

59. Sender MB, Koyle MA, Rajfer J. Complications of scrotal surgery. In: Smith RB, Ehrlich RM. Complications of Urologic Surgery (2nd ed). Philadelphia: WB Saunders, 1990, pp. 526-533.

60. Dale GA. Complications of scrotal surgery. In: Smith RB, Skinner DG (eds). Complications of Urologic Surgery. Philadelphia: WB Saunders, 1976, pp. 395-407.

61. West AF, Leung HY, Powell PH. Epididymectomy is an effective treatment for scrotal pain after vasectomy. BJU Int 2000;85:1097-1099.

62. McDonald SW. Vasectomy review: sequelae in the human epididymis and ductus deferens. Clin Anat 1996;9:337-342.

63. Schmidt SS, Morris RR. Spermatic granuloma: The complication of vasectomy. Fertil Steril 1973;24:941.

64. Hackett RE, Waterhouse K. Vasectomy - reviewed. Am J Obstet Gynecol 1973;116:438.

65. Skandalakis JE, Gray SW. Embryology for Surgeons (2nd ed). Baltimore: Williams & Wilkins, 1994.

66. Budhiraja S, Pandit SK. Accessory scrotum. Urol Int 2000;63:210-211.

67. Clegg EJ. The arterial supply of the human prostate and seminal vesicles. J Anat 89:209, 1955.

68. Macwhinney MG. Male accessory sex organs and androgen action. In: Lipshultz LI, Howards SS (eds). Infertility of the Male. New York: Churchill Livingstone, 1983, pp. 135-163.

69. Hardy JD. Complications in Surgery and Their Management (4th ed). Philadelphia: WB Saunders, 1981.

70. Whitelaw GP, Smithwick RH. Some secondary effects of sympathectomy with particular reference to disturbance of sexual function. N Engl J Med 1951;245:221.

71. Tanagho EA. Anatomy of the lower urinary tract. In: Walsh PC, Retik AB, Stamey TA, Vaughn ED Jr (eds). Campbell's Urology (6th ed). Philadelphia:WB Saunders, 1992, pp. 40-69.

72. Eastham JA, Spires KS, Abreo F, Johnson JB, Venable DD. Seminal vesicle abscess due to tuberculosis: role of tissue culture in making the diagnosis. South Med J 92(3):328-329, 1999.

73. Walsh PC, Brooks JD. The Swedish prostate cancer paradox [editorial]. JAMA 1997;277:497-498.

74. Wilson LD, Ennis R, Percarpio B, Peschel RE. Location of the prostatic apex and its relationship to the ischial tuberosities. Int J Radiat Oncol Biol Phys 1994;29:1133.

75. Steiner MS. The puboprostatic ligament and the male urethral suspensory mechanism: an anatomic study. Urology 1994;44:530.

76. Garat JM, Viladoms JM, Gosalbez R Jr. Megautricles: embryogenic hypothesis. Urology 1992;40:265.

77. Varlet F, Coupris L, Laumonier F, Duverne C. Congenital dilatation of the prostatic utricle. Ann Urol (Paris) 1992;26:39.

78. Meisheri IV, Motiwale SS, Sawant VV. Surgical management of enlarged prostatic utricle. Pediatr Surg Int 2000;16:199-203.

79. Last RJ. Anatomy Regional and Applied (5th ed). Baltimore: Williams & Wilkins, 1972.

80. van Ophoven A, Roth S. The anatomy and embryological origins of the fascia of Denonvilliers: A medico-historical debate. J Urol 157:3-9, 1997.

81. Jewett HJ, Eggleston JC, Yawn DH. Radical prostatectomy in the management of carcinoma of the prostate: probable causes of some therapeutic failures. J Urol 1972;107:1034.

82. Lowsley OS. The development of the human prostate gland with reference to the development of other structures at the neck of the urinary bladder. Am J Anat 1912;13:299.

83. McNeal JE. The prostate and prostatic urethra: a morphologic synthesis. J Urol 1972;107:1008-1016.

84. McNeal JE. Normal histology of the prostate. Am J Surg Pathol 1988;12:619.

85. McNeal JE. The zonal anatomy of the prostate. Prostate 1981; 2:35.

86. Wendell-Smith C. Terminology of the prostate and related structures. Clin Anat 2000;13:207-213.

87. Federative Committee on Anatomical Terminology (FCAT). Terminologia Anatomica: International Anatomical Terminology. Stuttgart: Thieme, 1998.

88. Hricak H, Dooms GC, McNeal JE, Mark AS, Marotti M, Avallone A, Pelzer M, Proctor EC, Tanagho EA. MR imaging of the prostate gland: normal anatomy. AJR 1987;148:51.

89. Cornud F, Belin X, Melki P, Helenon O, Cretien Y, Dufour B, Moreau JF. Zonal anatomy of the prostate using endorectal MRI. J Radiol 1995;76:11.

90. Myers RP. Structure of the adult prostate from a clinician's standpoint. Clin Anat 2000;13:214-215.

91. Reese JH, McNeal JE, Redwine EA, Stamey TA, Freiha FS. Tissue type plasminogen activator as a marker for functional zones within the human prostate gland. Prostate 1988;12:47.

92. Di Lollo S, Menchi I, Brizzi E, Pacini P, Papucci A, Sgambati E, Carini M, Gulisano M. The morphology of the prostatic capsule with particular regard to the posterosuperior region: an anatomical and clinical problem. Surg Radiol Anat 1997;19:143-147.

93. Tramier D, Argeme M, Huguet JF, Juhan C. Radiological anatomy of the internal pudendal artery (a. pudenda interna) in the male. Anat Clin 1981;3:195-200.

94. Hafferl A. Das Arteriensystem. In: Bolk L, Goppert E, Kallius E, Lubosch W (eds). Handbuch der vergleichenden Anatomie der Wirbeltiere (Bd VI). Amsterdam: Asher, 1967.

95. Lippert H, Pabst R. Arterial Variations in Man. Classification and Frequency. Munich: J.F. Bergmann Verlag, 1985, p. 59.

96. Batson OV. The function of the vertebral veins and their role in the spread of metastases. Ann Surg 1940;112:138.

97. Redman JF. Anatomy of the genitourinary system. In: Gillenwater JY, Grayhack JT, Howards SS, Duckett JW (eds). Adult and Pediatric Urology (2nd ed). St. Louis: Mosby Year Book, 1991, pp. 3-62.

98. Whitmore WF Jr, Mackenzie: Experiences with various operative procedures for the total excision of prostatic cancer. Cancer 1959; 12:396.

99. McLaughlin AP, Saltzstein SL, McCullough DL, Gittes RF. Prostatic carcinoma: Indications and location of unsuspected metastases. J Urol 1976;115:89.

100. Wilson CS, Dahl DS, Middleton RG. Pelvic lymphadenectomy for the staging of apparently located prostatic cancer. J Urol 1977;117:197.

101. Fukuda H, Yamada T, Kamata S, Saitoh H. Anatomic distribution of intraprostatic lymphatics: implications for the lymphatic spread of prostate cancer - a preliminary study. Prostate 2000;44:322-327.

102. Celebi MM, Venable DD, Nopajaroonsri C, Eastham JA. Prostatic cancer metastatic only to the penis. South Med J 1997; 90:959-961.

103. Walsh PC, Donker PJ. Impotence following radical prostatectomy: Insight into etiology and prevention. J Urol 128:492-497, 1982.

104. Klotz L. Intraoperative cavernous nerve stimulation during nerve sparing radical prostatectomy: how and when? Curr Opinion Urol 2000;10:239-243.

105. Carlton CE Jr. Commentary. Prostate excision: perineal prostatectomy. In: Hinman F Jr. Atlas of Urologic Surgery (2nd ed). Philadelphia: WB Saunders, 1998.

106. Baskin LS, Erol A, Li YW, Liu WH. Anatomy of the neurovascular bundle: is safe mobilization possible? J Urol 2000;164:977-980.

107. Catalona WJ, Basler JW. Return of erections and urinary continence following nerve sparing radical retropubic prostatectomy. J Urol 150:905, 1993.

108. Geary ES, Dendinger TE, Freiha FS, Stamey TA. Nerve sparing radical prostatectomy: a different view. J Urol 154:145-149, 1995.

109. Quinlan DM, Epstein JI, Carter BS, Walsh PC. Sexual function following radical prostatectomy: influence of preservation of neurovascular bundles. J Urol 145:998, 1991.

110. Polascik TJ, Walsh PC. Radical retropubic prostatectomy: the influence of accessory pudendal arteries on the recovery of sexual function. J Urol 153:150-152, 1995.

111. Ghavamian R, Zincke H. Technique for nerve dissection. Semin Urol Oncol 2000;18:43-45.

112. Zaviacic M. The adult human female prostate homologue and the male prostate gland: a comparative enzyme-histochemical study. Acta Histochem 1985;77:19.

113. Guyton AC. Textbook of Medical Physiology (7th ed). Philadelphia: WB Saunders, 1986, p. 957.

114. Hayward SW, Cunha GR. The prostate: development and physiology. Radiol Clin North Am 2000;38:1-14.

115. Healey JE, Hodge J. Surgical Anatomy (2nd ed). Philadelphia: BC Decker, 1990.

116. McNeal JE. Cancer volume and site of origin of adenocarcinoma in the prostate: relationship to local and distant spread. Hum Path 1992;23:258-266.

117. Carlin BI, Resnick MI. Anatomic approach to radical perineal prostatectomy. Urol Clin North Am 1995;22:461.

118. Koch MO. Management of the dorsal vein complex during radical retropubic prostatectomy. Semin Urol Oncol 2000;18:33-37.

119. Walsh PC. Anatomic radical prostatectomy: cancer control with preservation of quality of life. In: Fortner JG, Sharp PA (eds). Accomplishments in Cancer Research 1996. Philadelphia: Lippincott-Raven, 1997, pp. 41-53.

120. Young HH. The early diagnosis and radical cure of carcinoma of the prostate: being a study of 40 cases and presentation of a radical operation which was carried out in 4 cases. Johns Hopkins Hosp Bull 1905;16:315-321.

121. Millin T. Retropubic Urinary Surgery. London: Livingstone, 1947.

122. Reiner WB, Walch PC. An anatomical approach to the surgical management of the dorsal vein and Santorini's plexus during radical retropubic surgery. J Urol 1979;121:198-200.

123. Lepor H, Gregerman M, Crosby R, Mostofi FK, Walsh PC. Precise localization of the autonomic nerves from the pelvic plexus to the corpora cavernosa: a detailed anatomical study of the adult male pelvis. J Urol 1985;133:207-212.

124. Schlegel PN, Walsh PC. Neuroanatomical approach to radical cystoprostatectomy with preservation of sexual function. J Urol 1987;138:1402-1406.

125. Oelrich TM. The urethral sphincter muscle in the male. Am J Anat 1980;158:229-246.

126. Myers RP, Goellner JR, Cahill DR. Prostate shape, external striated urethral sphincter and radical prostatectomy: the apical dissection. J Urol 1987;138:543-550.

127. Walsh PC, Quinlan DM, Morton RA. Radical retropubic prostatectomy-improved anastomosis and urinary continence. Urol Clin North Am 1990;17:679-684.

128. Smith RB. Complications of transurethral surgery. In: Smith RB, Ehrlich RM (eds). Complications in Urologic Surgery (2nd ed). Philadelphia: WB Saunders, 1990, pp. 355-376.

129. Walsh PC. Radical retropubic prostatectomy. In: Walsh PC, Retik AB, Stamey TA, Vaughn ED Jr (eds). Campbell's Urology (6th ed). Philadelphia:WB Saunders, 1992, pp. 2865-2886.

130. Borland RN, Walsh PC. The management of rectal injury during radical retropubic prostatectomy. J Urol 1992;147:905.

131. Steiner MS. Anatomic basis for the continence-preserving radical retropubic prostatectomy. Semin Urol Oncol 2000;18:9-18.

132. Ahearn GS, Bedlack RS, Price DT, Robertson CN, Morgenlander JC. Transient lumbosacral polyradiculopathy after prostatectomy: Association with spinal stenosis. South Med J 1999;92: 809-811.

133. Hopkins SC, Grabstald H. Benign and malignant tumors of the

male and female urethra. In: Walsh PC, Gittes RE, Perlmutter AD, Stamey TA (eds). Campbell's Urology (5th ed). Philadelphia: WB Saunders, 1986, pp. 1441-1458.

134. Williams PL (ed). Gray's Anatomy (38th ed). New York: Churchill Livingstone, 1995.

135. Erol A, Baskin LS, Li YW, Liu WH. Anatomical studies of the urethral plate: why preservation of the urethral plate is important in hypospadias repair. BJU Int 2000;85:728-734.

136. Strasser H, Bartsch G. Anatomy and innervation of the rhabdosphincter of the male urethra. Semin Urol Oncol 2000;18:2-8.

137. Rother P, Löffler S, Dorschner W, Reibiger I, Bengs T. Anatomic basis of micturition and urinary continence: Muscle systems in urinary bladder neck during ageing. Surg Radiol Anat 18: 173-177, 1996.

138. Hackler RH. Complications of urethral and penile trauma. In: Greenfield LJ (ed). Complications in Surgery and Trauma (2nd ed). Philadelphia: JB Lippincott, 1990, pp. 784-791.

139. Frick J, Schulman CL, Marberger H. Traumatic lesion of the urethra: Immediate and delayed treatment. Eur Urol 1975;1:3.

140. Kolligian ME, Franco I, Reda EF. Correction of penoscrotal transposition: a novel approach. J Urol 2000;164:994-997.

141. Hoznek A., Rahmouni A., Abbou C., Delmas V., Colombel M. The suspensory ligament of the penis: an anatomic and radiologic description. Surg Radiol Anat 1998;20:413-417.

142. Grant JCB, Basmajian JV. Grant's Method of Anatomy (7th ed). Baltimore: Williams & Wilkins, 1965.

143. Gardner E, Gray DJ, O'Rahilly R. Anatomy (4th ed). Philadelphia: WB Saunders, 1975.

144. Droupy S, Benoît G, Giuliano F, Jardin A. Penile arteries in humans. Surg Radiol Anat 1997;19:161-167.

145. Moscovici J, Galinier P, Hammoudi S, Lefebvre D, Juricic M, Vaysse P. Contribution to the study of the venous vasculature of the penis. Surg Radiol Anat 1999;21:193-199.

146. Colombel M, Droupy S, Paradis V, Lassau JP, Benoît G. Cavernopudendal nervous communicating branches of the penile hilum. Surg Radiol Anat 1999;21:273-276.

147. Andersson KE, Hedlund P, Alm P. Sympathetic pathways and adrenergic innervation of the penis. Int J Impotence Res 2000;12 (Suppl 1):S5-12.

148. Rutegård J, Sandzén B, Stenling R, Wiig J, Heald RJ. Lateral rectal ligaments contain important nerves. Br J Surg 84:1544-1545, 1997.

149. Goligher JC. Surgery of the Anus, Rectum and Colon, 4th ed. London: Baillière Tindall, 1980.

150. Corman ML. Carcinoma of the rectum. In: Corman ML (ed). Colon and Rectal Surgery, 3rd ed. Philadelphia: JB Lippincott,

1993, pp. 596-720.

151. Enker WE. Potency, cure, and local control in the operative treatment of rectal cancer. Arch Surg 127: 1396-1402, 1992.

152. Sato K, Sato T. The vascular and neuronal composition of the lateral ligament of the rectum and the rectosacral fascia. Surg Radiol Anat 13:17-22, 1991.

153. Shoji Y, Kusunoki M, Fujita S, Yamamura T, Utsunomiya J. Functional role of the preserved rectal cuff in ileoanal anastomosis. Surgery 111:266-273, 1992.

154. Ikeuchi H, Kusnoki M, Shoji Y, Yamamura T, Utsunomiya J. Clinico-physiological results after sphincter-saving resection for rectal carcinoma. Int J Colorectal Dis 11:172-176, 1996.

155. Gordon PH. Anatomy and physiology of the anorectum. In: Fazio VW, ed. Current Therapy in Colon and Rectal Surgery. Philadelphia: BC Decker, 1990, pp. 1-9.

156. Heald RJ. The 'Holy Plane' of rectal surgery. J R Soc Med 81: 503-508, 1988.

157. Havenga K, Enker WE, McDermott K, Cohen AM, Minsky BD, Guillem J. Male and female sexual and urinary function after total mesorectal excision with autonomic nerve preservation for carcinoma of the rectum. J Am Coll Surg 182:495-502, 1996.

158. Enker WE, Thaler HT, Cranor ML, Polyak T. Total mesorectal excision in the operative treatment of carcinoma of the rectum. J Am Coll Surg 181:335-346, 1995.

159. Havenga K, DeRuiter MC, Enker WE, Welvaart K. Anatomical basis of nerve-preserving total mesorectal excision for rectal cancer. Br J Surg 83:384-388, 1996.

160. Liang JT, Chang KJ, Wang SM. Lateral rectal ligaments contain important nerves (Letter to Editor). Br J Surg 85:1157-1164, 1998.

161. Nivatvongs S, Gordon PH. Surgical anatomy. In: Gordon PH, Nivatvongs S, eds. Principles and Practice of Surgery for the Colon, Rectum and Anus. St Louis, MO: Quality Medical Publishing, 1992: 31-36.

162. Weinstein M, Roberts M. Sexual potency following surgery for rectal carcinoma. Ann Surg 1977; 185:295-300.

163. Benoît G, Droupy S, Quillard J, Paradis V, Guiliano F. Supra and infralevator neurovascular pathways to the penile corpora cavernosa. J Anat 1999;195:605-615.

164. Laumann EO, Masi CM, Zuckerman EW. Circumcision in the United States. JAMA 1997;277:1052-1057.

165. Quinn TC, Wawer MJ, Sewankambo N, et al. Viral load and heterosexual transmission of human immunodeficiency virus type 1. N Engl J Med 2000;342:921-929.

166. Peters PC, Sagalowsky AF. Genitourinary trauma. In: Walsh PC, Gittes RF, Perlmutter AD (eds). Campbell's Urology (5th ed). Philadelphia: WB Saunders, 1986, pp. 1217-1226.

# Chapter 26

# Female Genital System

ROBERT M. ROGERS JR., GENE L. COLBORN, THOMAS A. WEIDMAN,
JOHN E. SKANDALAKIS, PETROS MIRILAS, NIALL T.M. GALLOWAY

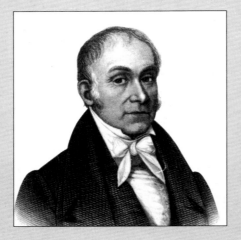

**Ephraim McDowell (1771-1830),** one of the pioneers in the United States of removal of huge ovarian cysts without anesthesia.

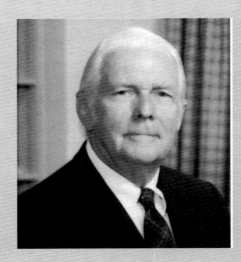

**John Ridley (1914--),** contemporary surgeon and author of the beautiful book, *Gynecologic Surgery: Errors, Safeguards, Salvage.*

*A knowledge of anatomy and physiology is just as essential to the gynecologist as a familiarity with the general principles of surgery; indeed, the very foundation stones of successful work are laid in envisaging the relations of the parts to be dealt with so clearly that the operator divides layer from layer almost as if the coverings of the body were transparent. Without this accurate knowledge of the component parts of the pelvis and abdomen and their mutual relations, to be gained only by actual dissections, surgery is not an art, but at best a haphazard procedure guided by luck; without a knowledge of physiology an operator will often ruthlessly sacrifice organs or parts of organs whose functional activity is essential to the happiness and well-being of the patient.*

*Howard A. Kelly (1898)[1]*

# INTRODUCTION

The female reproductive system consists of the ovaries, uterine tubes, uterine body and cervix, and the vaginal canal leading to the external genitalia of the vulva. These female viscera are in close proximity to the urethra and bladder anteriorly, and the rectum and anal canal posteriorly.

An overview of the embryogenesis of the female reproductive system must include the anatomic entities produced from the wolffian and müllerian primordia (Table 26-1). Specifics about the possible development of each entity will be found in the corresponding sections throughout the chapter.

All the organs of the female reproductive system are concerned with storage and evacuation, functions that can be sustained only if normal anatomic relationships are maintained. In the normal, standing nulliparous female patient, the following anatomic relationships are found:

- The lower one-third of the vagina is almost vertical in orientation, while the upper two-thirds of the vagina is almost horizontal.
- The cervix is found approximately at the level of the ischial spines, but suspended anterior to a line drawn between the spines.
- The urethra is almost vertical in orientation, whereas the bladder lies on top of the almost horizontal anterior wall of the vagina.
- The anal canal is almost vertical in orientation, whereas

the rectum lies on top of the almost horizontal levator plate (Fig. 26-1).

The goal of successful reparative gynecological surgery, whether via the abdominal or vaginal approach, is to restore these natural anatomic relations.

How can these pelvic organs maintain their central anatomic positions while fulfilling their unique roles of distension and storage? The answer is found in a detailed examination of the endopelvic fascia. This connective tissue network is located in the retroperitoneal areas of the pelvis between the parietal peritoneum and parietal fascia of the muscles of the pelvic wall and floor.[2] This three-dimensional meshwork of perivascular and visceral fascial sheaths is ultimately anchored to the parietal fascia lining the pelvic basin. The visceral endopelvic fascia will be further discussed later in this chapter, as well as in the chapter on the pelvis and perineum.

It is not within the scope of this chapter to provide detailed physiology of the female genital system, or of the major hormones associated with it, namely luteinizing hormone, follicle stimulating hormone, estrogen, and progesterone.

# HISTORY

The history of the anatomy and surgery of the female genital system is shown in Table 26-2.

## TABLE 26-1. Derivation of Reproductive Tract Structures from Wolffian and Müllerian Primordia

| Male | Female |
| --- | --- |
| Genital ridges | |
|   Testis | Ovary |
|     Seminiferous tubules (medulla) | Pfluger's tubules[a] |
|     Rete testis | Rete ovarii[a] |
|     Gubernaculum testis | Round ligament of uterus and ovary |
|     Ligament of testis | Ligament of ovary |
|     Mesorchium | Mesoovarium |
| Wolffian derivatives | |
|   Mesonephric tubules | |
|     Ductuli efferentes | Epoophoron[a] |
|       Ductuli abberantes[a] | Ductuli aberrantes (Haller)[a] |
|       Paradidymis (tubules)[a] | Paroophoron[a] |
|     Paradidymis collecting duct | ? |
|   Mesonephric duct | |
|     Ureter, pelvis, and collecting tubules of kidney | Ureter, pelvis, and collecting tubules of kidney |
|     Trigone of bladder | Trigone of bladder |
|     Proximal ductus epididymis | Duct of the epoophoron[a] |
|     Distal ductus epididymis | ? |
|     Proximal ductus deferens | ? |
|     Ductus deferens | Gartner's duct[a] |
|     Ejaculatory duct | ? |
|     Seminal vesicle | ? |
|     Appendix epididymis[a] | Appendix vesiculosa epoophoron[a] |
| Müllerian derivatives | |
|   Appendix testis[a] | Uterine tube distal (fimbria) Hydatid of Morgagni?[a] |
|   ? | Oviduct |
|   ? | Uterus |
|   ? | Cervix and upper vagina |
|   Prostatic utricle[a] | Lower vagina |
|   Colliculus seminalis | Hymen? |
| Urogenital sinus derivatives | |
|   Bladder | Bladder |
|   Prostatic urethra above colliculus seminalis | Urethra |
|   Urethra below colliculus seminalis | Lower vagina and vestibule |
|   Membranous urethra | Lower vagina and vestibule |
|   Cavernous urethra | Lower vagina and vestibule |
|   Corpus cavernosum urethra | Vestibule of bulb |
|   Corpus cavernosum penis | Corpus cavernosum clitori |
|   Bulbourethral glands (Cowper's) | Vestibular glands (Bartholin's) |
|   Urethral glands (Littré) | Minor vestibular glands |
|   Prostate gland | Paraurethral glands of Skene? |
|   Urethral crest & colliculus seminalis | Hymen |
| External genitalia | |
|   Glans penis | Glans clitoris |
|   Floor of penile urethra | Labia minora |
|   Scrotum | Labia majora |
|   Processus vaginalis testis | Canal of Nuck |

[a]Vestigial structures.

*Source:* Skandalakis JE, Gray SW (eds). Embryology for Surgeons, 2nd Ed. Baltimore: Williams & Wilkins, 1994; with permission.

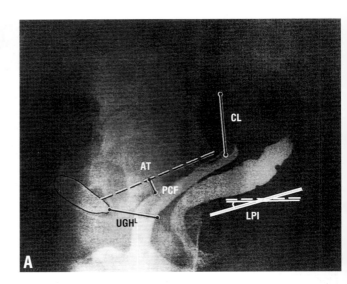

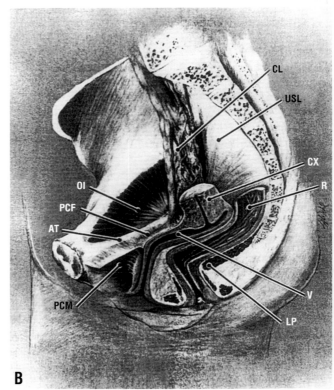

FIG. 26-1. **A,** Lateral radiograph of the opacified vagina and rectum. **B,** Support structures: lateral view. Bladder, urethra, and uterine corpus have been removed from this diagrammatic sagittal section to reveal attachments of the vagina. A line with a dot at each end indicates the distance spanned by the indicated structure; a line ending in a single dot points to the structure. CL, Cardinal ligament; AT, Arcus tendineus fasciae pelvis; PCF, Pubocervical fasciae; LPI, Levator plate inclination; UGH^L, Urogenital hiatus length; USL, Uterosacral ligament; CX, Cervix; R, Rectum; OI, Obturator internus muscle; V, Vagina; LP, Levator plate; PCM, Pubococcygeus muscle. (DeLancey JOL. Vaginographic examination of the pelvic floor. Int Urogynecol J 1994;5:19-24; with permission.)

## TABLE 26-2. Anatomic and Surgical History of the Female Genital System

| | | |
|---|---|---|
| Soranus of Ephesus (fl. 117) | | Wrote an often-translated chapter on the anatomy of the female genitalia |
| Galen (130-ca. 200) | | Wrote tracts on dissection of the uterus (probably infraprimate) for midwives. Assumed the human uterus to be bicornuate. |
| Hendrik van Deveter (1651-1724) | | Wrote an authoritative and well-illustrated obstetrics text |
| William Hunter | 1774 | Wrote *Anatomy of the Human Gravid Uterus* |
| McDowell | 1809 | Removed a giant pseudomucinous cystadenoma |
| Roux | 1832 | Performed the first suture of a ruptured female perineum |
| Sims | 1852 | Invented the speculum |
| Keith | 1878 | Removed large ovarian cysts |
| Tait | 1879 | Devised a method of flap splitting for plastic repair of the perineum |
| Emmet | 1882 | Repaired childbirth injury anatomically. Great master and teacher of plastic surgery of the perineum, vagina, cervix, uterus, and bladder. |
| Kelly | 1897 | Advocated individual ligation of uterine and ovarian vessels prior to hysterectomy or oophorectomy |
| | 1914 | Developed anterior vaginal repair and Kelly plication for stress urinary incontinence |
| Brunschwig Parsons | 1948 1954 | Proposed radical hysterectomy with exenteration procedures |
| Marshall, Marchette, and Krantz | 1949 | Developed retropubic cystourethropexy |
| Bricker | 1952 | Devised ileal bladder |
| Mulligan | 1953 | Inserted plastic tubes into stenosed uterine fallopian tubes to treat infertility |
| Meigs | 1954 | Popularized total hysterectomy |
| Pereyra | 1959 | Developed needle suspension of the bladder |
| Burch | 1961 | Performed retropubic colposuspension |
| Stamey | 1973 | To needle suspension of the bladder, introduced several concepts including cystoscopic control of needle placement, visualization of bladder neck closure with elevation of sutures, and the use of bolsters to support the bladder neck |
| Raz | 1981-1985 | Introduced an inverted U-shaped incision for needle suspension of the bladder |
| Gittes and Loughlin | 1987 | Developed the no-incision modification of the Pereyra technique |
| Nezhat et al. | 1992 | Described laparoscopic radical hysterectomy with laparoscopic paraaortic lymphadenectomy |
| Querleu | 1993 | Described complete laparoscopic surgical staging procedure for ovarian carcinoma |

*History table compiled by David A. McClusky III and John E. Skandalakis.*

**References**

Garrison FH. An Introduction to the History of Medicine (4th ed). Philadelphia: WB Saunders, 1960.

Nezhat CR, Burrell MO, Nezhat FR, Benigno BB, Welander CE. Laparoscopic radical hysterectomy with paraaortic and pelvic node dissection. Am J Obstet Gynecol 1992;166:864-865.

Querleu D. Laparoscopic paraaortic node sampling in gynecologic oncology: a preliminary experience. Gynecol Oncol 1993;49:24-29.

# *Ovaries*

## EMBRYOGENESIS

### Normal Development

The bilateral mesonephric ducts and genital ridges develop from the intermediate mesoderm at approximately the fifth week of gestation. Primordial germ cells from the yolk sac endoderm migrate to the genital ridge to develop as gonads.

Around the seventh week, sex can be determined by XX or XY genotype. Gross identification of the ovary is possible at 10 weeks. Two X chromosomes (several genes) are required for complete development of the ovary. Female sexual differentiation does not depend on hormones.

At approximately the 12th week, the ovary is located at the inferior part of the pelvic brim. The gubernaculum of the ovary produces the ovarian and round ligaments of the uterus. The persistence of a portion of the processus vaginalis forms the canal of Nuck.

Primordial ovarian follicles are present at approximately the 16th week. Each one forms one oogonium. At birth, each ovary contains 200,000-250,000 follicles.

### Congenital Anomalies

The ovarian anomalies (Table 26-3 and Table 26-4) are very closely related to the anomalies of the urinary system. When nephric structures are absent on one side, the ovarian agenesis is primary and the germ cells have migrated to the normal side. In some cases, the solitary ovary is larger than normal. With bilateral (müllerian) agenesis, hormonal treatment is needed. In a patient with müllerian agenesis, Vaughn and Jones[3] separated ovaries within bilateral inguinal hernias. Two cases of a rare supernumerary ovary located in the omentum of a neonate were reported by Kuga et al.[4]

We quote from Vendeland and Shehadeh,[5] who reported the seventh case of accessory ovary in the literature:

> *Supernumerary and accessory ovaries are rare anomalies. The reported incidence of these conditions is 1:29,000-700,000 gynecologic admissions. Since 1864 there have been only six cases of accessory ovary reported in the literature. Additionally, there have been 26 reported cases of supernumerary ovaries...In 36% of reported cases [of accessory ovary], associated congenital anomalies have been identified. Defects have included accessory fallopian tube, bifid fallopian tubes, accessory tubal ostium, bicornuate and unicornuate uteri, septate uterus, agenesis of kidney or ureter, bladder diverticulum, accessory adrenal gland and lobulated liver...Since accessory ovaries are likely to be asymptomatic, they may be underreported. This condition is associated with a high risk of pelvic and renal anomalies and should lead to further evaluation to allow physicians to provide advice about future reproductive function and management of congenital anomalies.*

| TABLE 26-3. Absence of the Ovaries | | | | |
|---|---|---|---|---|
| | **Sex Chromosomes** | **Germ Cells** | **Nephrogenic Ridge** | **Ovary** |
| Phenotypic females | | | | |
|   Normal | XX | Present | Present | Present |
|   Anovarism  { | XX | *Absent* on affected side | *Absent* | *Absent* (agenesis)[a]; unilateral, rare |
| | XX | *Absent* | Present | *Absent* (secondary dysgenesis); bilateral or unilateral, very rare |
|   Turner's syndrome | XO | *Absent* | Present | *Absent* (primary dysgenesis); bilateral, uncommon |

[a]Associated with absence of the kidney, ureter, uterine tube and hemiuterus on the affected side.

*Source:* Skandalakis JE, Gray SW (eds). Embryology for Surgeons, 2nd Ed. Baltimore: Williams & Wilkins, 1994; with permission.

**TABLE 26-4. Anomalies of the Ovaries**

| Anomaly | Prenatal Age at Onset | First Appearance (or other diagnostic clues) | Relative Frequency | Remarks |
| --- | --- | --- | --- | --- |
| Congenital absence of one or both ovaries (excluding Turner's syndrome) | Atrophy after 4th week | At menarche, if bilateral; otherwise discovery is accidental | Very rare | |
| Congenital absence of one ovary and homolateral kidney and ureter | 4th week | In childhood | Rare | Uterine and tubal anomalies |
| Inguinal herniation and ectopia of ovary | Around birth | In childhood or later | Rare | Some cases are acquired, not congenital |

Adapted from Skandalakis JE, Gray SW (eds). Embryology for Surgeons, 2nd Ed. Baltimore: Williams & Wilkins, 1994, Table 20.6; with permission.

# SURGICAL ANATOMY

## Topography

The ovaries, right and left, are traditionally described as "almond-shaped," measuring 1 cm × 2 cm × 3 cm, and weigh approximately 3 to 4 grams each. They are white in color. The ovaries are asymmetrical, the right larger than the left. The roughened appearance of the surface of each ovary after puberty is due to degenerating corpora lutea. In addition to producing a woman's ova, the ovaries are important endocrine organs.

Each ovary is located in the ovarian fossa on the lateral pelvic sidewall, and is attached to the posterior and superior aspect of the broad ligament by a double peritoneal fold, called the mesovarium. The mesovarium does not cover the ovaries; it only "attaches" to their anterior borders. The mesovarium is a reduplication of the posterior lamina of the broad ligament. It is cuboidal epithelium (formerly referred to as "germinal epithelium," a misnomer) that covers the ovaries.

The utero-ovarian ligament (proper ovarian ligament, commonly referred to as the ovarian ligament [Fig. 26-2]), which is derived from the embryonic ovarian gubernaculum, attaches the ovary to the body of the uterus. The continuations of the embryonic gubernacula form the round ligaments of the uterus (Fig. 26-2) and pass through the deep inguinal rings to enter the inguinal canals, then attach to the labia majora. The infundibulopelvic ligament (suspensory ligament of the ovary) (Fig. 26-3) is simply the peritoneal covering over the ovarian vessels and accompanying

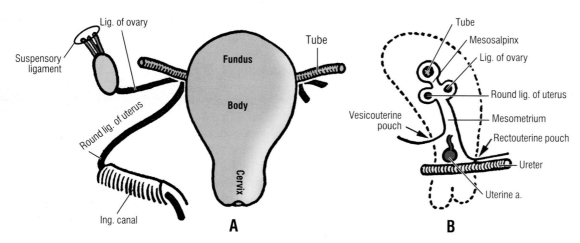

FIG. 26-2. **A,** Derivatives of the gubernaculum ovarii: ligament of ovary and round ligament of uterus. **B,** Sagittal section through broad ligament of uterus. (Modified from Basmajian JV, Slonecker CE. Grant's Method of Anatomy (11th ed). Baltimore: Williams & Wilkins, 1989; with permission.)

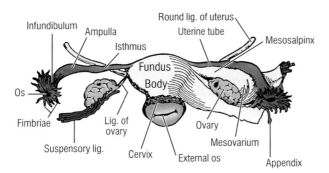

FIG. 26-3. Uterus and appendages (from behind). (Modified from Basmajian JV, Slonecker CE. Grant's Method of Anatomy (11th ed). Baltimore: Williams & Wilkins, 1989; with permission.)

lymph channels and nodes and visceral nerves, as they pass just over and just lateral to the ureter at the pelvic brim.

The position of the ovaries is variable. Normally each is located on the lateral pelvic sidewall on either side of the uterus, below and posterior to each uterine tube, resting within the ovarian fossa. Bazot et al.[6] stated that the suspensory ligament is a good anatomic landmark for localization of the ovaries and lymph nodes related to ovarian tumors. The ovaries of multiparous women may have a lower position. Hill and Breckle[7] stated that the position of the uterus and ovaries can be affected by the degree to which the bladder is filled.

The ovary may be in an abnormal position
- Within the posterior wall of the broad ligament (therefore, the mesovarium is absent)
- Within the rectouterine pouch (cul-de-sac of Douglas)
- Within the sac of a femoral hernia

The ovarian fossa is a very shallow depression of the peritoneum on the lateral pelvic sidewall, bounded as follows:
- Superior: External iliac vessels, obturator nerve
- Anterior: Attachment of the broad ligament to the pelvic sidewall
- Posteroinferior: Ureter

## Relations

For descriptive purposes, the ovary has two borders — anterior and posterior; two poles — upper and lower; and two surfaces — medial and lateral.

### *Borders*

- The anterior ovarian border is related to the mesovarium,

which contains the vessels and nerves for the hilum.
- The posterior ovarian border is free.

### *Poles*

- The upper pole (tubal extremity) has a special relationship with the uterine tube. The proximity of the tubal extremity and the uterine tube allows the fimbriae to touch the surface of the ovary. The tubal extremity of the upper pole is also related to the peritoneum by the infundibulopelvic ligament (suspensory ligament of the ovary).
- The lower pole is connected to the lateral wall of the uterus by the utero-ovarian ligament (proper ligament of the ovary).

### *Surfaces*

- The medial surface is related to the uterine tube. A small uncovered area relates to loops of small and large bowel. The medial surface is closely related to the fimbriated end of the uterine tube which practically covers this surface.
- The lateral surface is related to the ovarian fossa.

## Ligaments

### *Utero-Ovarian Ligament*

The utero-ovarian ligament (proper ligament of the ovary) (Fig. 26-2) is a cordlike structure invested with the posterior layer of the broad ligament. It consists of smooth muscle and connective tissue. The ovarian ligament extends from the lower ovarian pole to the lateral uterine wall. It is located between the mesosalpinx and the mesovarium.

### *Infundibulopelvic Ligament*

The infundibulopelvic ligament (suspensory ligament of the ovary) (Fig. 26-3) is a fan-shaped band of fibromuscular visceral connective tissue containing arteries, veins, lymphatics, and visceral nerves extending from the upper ovarian pole to the lateral pelvic wall. This ligament passes from the abdominal cavity into the pelvic cavity at the level of the pelvic brim, superficial to the bifurcation of the common iliac artery, just lateral to where the ureter passes over the bifurcation of the common iliac vessels. This relationship is not evident unless the operator retracts the infundibulopelvic ligament anteriorly at the level of the pelvic brim.

## *Mesovarium*

The mesovarium (Fig. 26-3) is a short peritoneal fold from the posterior surface of the broad ligament to the anterior ovarian wall. It facilitates the passage of ovarian vessels and nerves into the ovarian portae (hila). The mesovarium, the infundibulopelvic ligament, and the utero-ovarian ligament together support the ovary in its position along the pelvic sidewall.

# Vascular Supply

## *Arteries*

The blood supply to the ovaries originates from the aorta as the ovarian arteries, below the renal arteries on the anterolateral surface of the aorta. The ovarian arteries (Fig. 26-4, Fig. 26-5, Fig. 26-6) supply the uterine tubes and the upper portion of the body and fundus of the uterus, and anastomose on the lateral aspects of the uterus with the uterine arteries.

The ovarian arteries travel obliquely downward in the retroperitoneum; they, together with accompanying veins, nerves, lymphatics, and overlying peritoneum, form the in-fundibulopelvic ligament (suspensory ligament) at the level of the pelvic brim. These vessels are medial to the ureter in the abdominal cavity, and then cross at the pelvic brim to travel laterally and anteriorly (very occasionally, posteriorly) to the ureter in the pelvis.

REMEMBER:
* The ovarian artery and the ovarian branch of the uterine artery are responsible for the blood supply of the ovary.
* The tubal branch of the uterine artery supplies the tube. The uterine artery also supplies the uterus and the upper vagina.

A detailed anatomic description is necessary for the surgeon to understand the arterial blood supply of the ovaries and the uterine tubes, especially when dealing with microsurgery. The details of the vascular anatomy are illustrated in Figures 26-6 and 26-7.

## *Veins*

The multiple ovarian veins form a plexus that is located in the area of the mesovarium and the infundibulopelvic ligament. The plexus coalesces to form two veins that are ad-

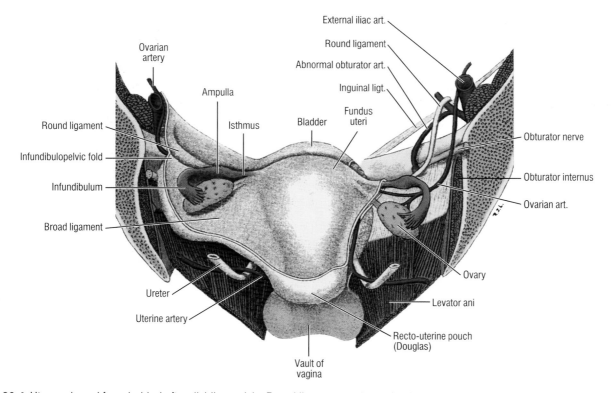

**FIG. 26-4.** Uterus viewed from behind after dividing pelvis. Broad ligament and a parietal peritoneum have been removed from right side. Drawn from a dissection. (Modified from Last RJ. Anatomy Regional and Applied (5th ed). Baltimore: Williams & Wilkins, 1972, p. 514; with permission.)

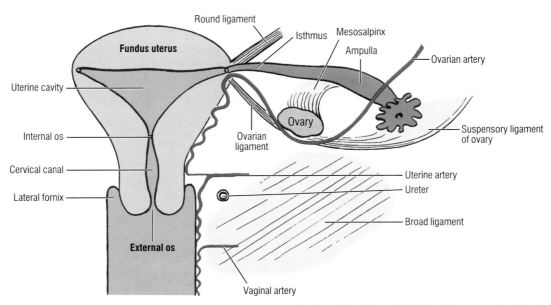

**FIG. 26-5.** Pathway of ovarian artery, uterine artery, and vaginal artery. (Modified from Brantigan OC. Clinical Anatomy. New York: McGraw-Hill, 1963; with permission.)

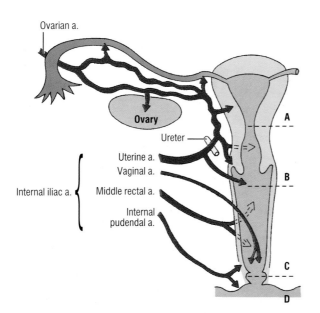

**FIG. 26-6.** The blood supply to the female reproductive system. Extensive anastomoses occur between the ovarian and uterine arteries. Cervical branches of the uterine arteries anastomose across the median plane. The four-tiered concept of the reproductive system (A, B, C, D) is based on anatomic, physiologic, and pathologic data and may perhaps have embryologic implications. (Modified from Gardner E, Gray DJ, O'Rahilly R. Anatomy (5th ed). Philadelphia: WB Saunders, 1986; with permission.)

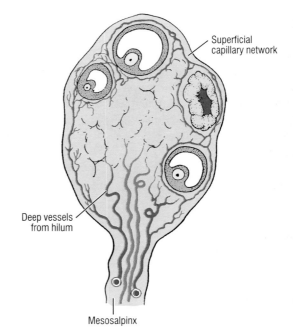

**FIG. 26-7.** Vascular anatomy of ovary pertinent to ovarian resection and reconstruction. (Modified from Cohen BM. Surgery of the ovary, including anatomic derangements of the fimbrial-gonadal ovum-capture mechanism. In: Hunt RB (ed). Atlas of Female Infertility Surgery (2nd ed). St. Louis: Mosby Year Book, 1992, pp. 389-403; with permission.)

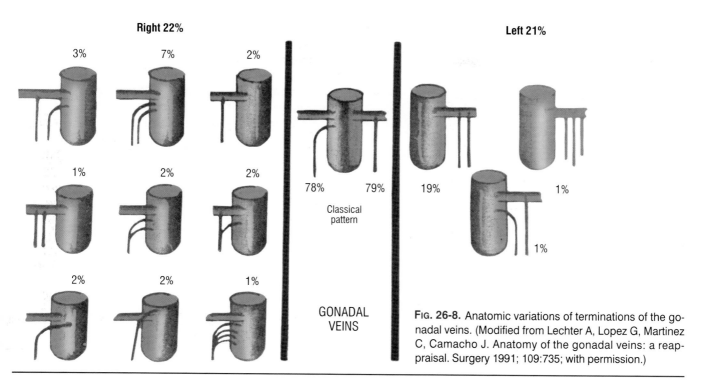

GONADAL
VEINS

**FIG. 26-8.** Anatomic variations of terminations of the gonadal veins. (Modified from Lechter A, Lopez G, Martinez C, Camacho J. Anatomy of the gonadal veins: a reappraisal. Surgery 1991; 109:735; with permission.)

jacent to the ovarian artery. The two veins then unite to form a single vein. The single vein on the right empties into the inferior vena cava; the single vein on the left empties into the left renal vein.

In an interesting study of both male and female gonadal vein anatomy, Lechter et al. reported several variations in the patterns of vessels emptying into the main gonadal veins[8] (Fig. 26-8, 26-9). In this study 88 cadavers were male and 12 were female. To determine whether there are any gender-based differences in gonadal vein formation patterns it may be useful to conduct a study of only female cadavers.

## Lymphatics

The ovarian lymphatics drain to the upper paraaortic nodes, which are located close to the origin of the right and left ovarian arteries, just below the renal vessels.

## Innervation

The ovary receives its visceral sympathetic innervation from the aorticorenal plexus. However, as each ovarian plexus travels with the ovarian vessels to each infundibulopelvic ligament, other sympathetic input may originate from the superior and inferior hypogastric plexuses. The preganglionic sympathetic fibers responsible for ovarian

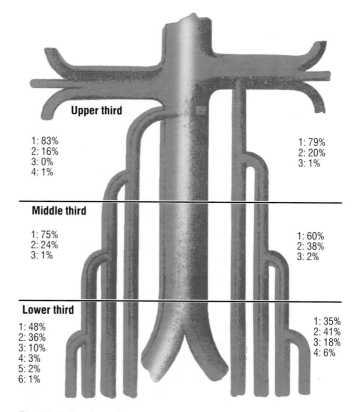

**FIG. 26-9.** Number of venous trunks of the gonadal veins. (Modified from Lechter A, Lopez G, Martinez C, Camacho J. Anatomy of the gonadal veins: a reappraisal. Surgery 1991;109:735; with permission.)

supply are believed to originate in the intermediolateral cell column of the spinal cord at T10 and T11 and travel into the abdomen in the thoracic splanchnic nerves; these fibers synapse in ganglia near the superior mesenteric artery. According to Williams et al.,[9] the parasympathetic fibers are provided by the inferior hypogastric plexus, arising, therefore in the pelvic splanchnic nerves at S2, S3, and S4. This innervation is probably vasodilatory in effect.

Visceral sensory fibers from the ovary are carried by way of the thoracic splanchnic nerves to reach spinal nerve levels T10, T11 of the spinal cord. With referral of pain sensations, ovarian pain may therefore be experienced in the periumbilical region, like appendicitis. Unremitting ovarian pain may be treated by division of the infundibulopelvic ligament and the nerves within it.

Ovarian pain may occasionally be distributed by the pathway of the obturator nerve to the triangle of Scarpa at the inner surface of the thigh and down to the knee (Howship-Romberg sign). This could be due to supply of pain fibers to the peritoneum by the obturator nerve. A more likely explanation is the proximity of the obturator nerve to the ovarian fossa in the lateral wall of the pelvis. This allows it to be, at times, readily affected by the troubles of the adjacent ovary, with sensory fibers of the obturator nerve referring the pain of the ovary to the lower limb. Such a sign may also manifest itself with an obturator hernia.

## HISTOLOGY

Each ovary is covered with germinal cuboidal epithelium. Characteristically, the cuboidal cells become continuous with the mesothelial cells of the mesovarium at the ovarian porta. This superficial ovarian stroma is not peritoneum.

The ovarian parenchyma under the stroma of the cuboidal cells is formed by two parts: a superficial cortex and a deep medulla. The cortex is dense. It contains reticular fibers and fusiform cells that secrete estrogens. With age, the cortex is changed into a smooth tunica albuginea.

The medulla is more vascular than the cortex, according to Bannister and Dyson.[10] It is formed by thin connective tissue, many elastic fibers, and nonstriated myocytes.

## PHYSIOLOGY

The preovulatory follicle and the subsequent corpus luteum establish the cycle of ovarian hormones, primarily estrogen and progesterone, that orchestrates the release of a properly matured ovum with a properly coordinated endometrial development in order to receive a fertilized ovum. This ovarian cycle modulates the hypothalamic-pituitary-ovarian axis through both negative and positive feedback on GnRH (gonadotropin releasing hormone), FSH (follicle stimulating hormone), and LH (luteinizing hormone). A significant amount of ovarian tissue may be surgically excised without loss of ovarian function. Luciano et al.[11] concluded that surgical trauma is well tolerated by the ovaries without impairing ovarian function.

We quote from Slowey[12] on polycystic ovary syndrome:

*Polycystic ovary syndrome is the most common endocrinopathy in women of reproductive age...resulting from insulin resistance and the compensatory hyperinsulinemia. This results in adverse effects on multiple organ systems and may result in alteration in serum lipids, anovulation, abnormal uterine bleeding, and infertility.*

Ovaries growing large cysts and/or tumors predispose the ovary to torsion which twists the ovarian vessels in the infundibulopelvic ligament. This leads to ischemia of the ovary. Modern observations show that the ovary may be untorsed. If this maneuver allows the ovary to regain a healthy color, there is no need to do an oophorectomy. Entrapment of the ovary within scar tissue or various hernial sacs within the pelvis may also predispose to acute and/or chronic pain syndromes.

We quote from Kokoska et al.[13] on acute pediatric ovarian torsion:

*Ultrasonography with color doppler is helpful for differentiating acute ovarian torsion from appendicitis. Although the twisted ovary can rarely be salvaged, the etiology is usually benign. Preoperative serum markers and contralateral ovary biopsy may be unnecessary.*

## SURGICAL APPLICATIONS

- The ovaries are most commonly evaluated by vaginal/rectal palpation and vaginal probe ultrasound study. The ovaries may be palpated at the time of vaginal examination. However, because the ovaries lie posterior to the broad ligament, within reach of a finger in the rectum, a rectovaginal examination is encouraged in order to better assess the condition and size of each ovary. Many practitioners also perform in their offices vaginal probe ultrasound scans with the bladder empty to assess follicular activity of the ovaries, and to determine the presence of cystic or solid tumors.

- The infundibulopelvic ligament with accompanying ovarian vessels travels just lateral to, and on top of, the ureter at the level of the pelvic brim. In order to avoid injuring the ureter during ligation or coagulation of the infundibulopelvic ligament, the operator needs to retract this ligament away from the ureter and positively identify the ureter before any procedures are performed on the infundibulopelvic ligament.

- The vessels that arise at the hilum and travel into the ovarian parenchyma are difficult to see. Electrocoagulation with compression by absorbable sutures may be used in this area. Oelsner et al.[14] reported that through-and-through sutures for ovarian reconstruction have a "detrimental" effect on the ovarian parenchyma.

- After removing a paratubal cyst, be certain that the uterine tube itself has not been damaged and remember to close the mesosalpinx.

- The cortical ovarian zone has a vascular network under the epithelial covering. Hemostasis is important whenever working with the ovary. This is especially important when excising benign ovarian cysts or tumors.

- Treatment of ovarian cysts in the newborn is controversial. Hengster and Menardi[15] concluded that "cystectomy is the treatment of choice for larger asymptomatic cysts because of their potential malignancy and serious potential complications." However, in an editorial von Schweinitz[16] advised against operation because a study he coauthored found that ovarian cysts in the newborn demonstrated continuous regression leading to the cyst vanishing in most cases. He advised regular ultrasound of uncomplicated ovarian cysts, and determination of serum levels of α-fetoprotein and β-human chorionic gonadotropin to rule out a malignant germ-cell tumor.

- Benign tumors include:
  – Ovarian cysts (polycystic ovary syndrome)
  – Solid tumors

- The incidence of malignant tumors by histologic type[17] is:
  – 60% serous cystadenocarcinoma
  – 15% pseudomucinous carcinoma
  – 10% solid undifferentiated adenocarcinoma
  – 6% granulosa cell carcinoma
  – 2% dysgerminoma
  – 7% other types

- Infantile primary ovarian lymphoma has been reported.[18]

- Montero et al.[19] studied transcoelomic, lymphatic, and hematogenous spread of ovarian tumors to the peritoneum, pelvic and paraaortic lymph nodes, lung, and pleura.

## Partial Oophorectomy, Total Unilateral Oophorectomy, Bilateral Oophorectomy

In the presence of persistent benign ovarian cysts or benign ovarian tumors, a partial oophorectomy can easily be accomplished either at the time of laparoscopy or at the time of laparotomy. Experience has shown that much of the ovary can be excised without compromising ovarian function as regards hormonal and ovum production. Hemostasis can be achieved with sutures, electrocoagulation, or laser energy. Various substances and materials have been used in the past to help avoid subsequent scarring at the operative site.

If the benign process encompasses most of the ovary, a total unilateral oophorectomy may be performed by isolating the ovarian vessels in the supplying infundibulopelvic ligament, appropriately ligating or coagulating them, and then transecting these vessels and removing the entire ovary. In the case of malignant ovarian tumors and cysts, both ovaries need to be surgically removed, and appropriate lymph node sampling within the pelvis and periaortic areas is mandated. In very select cases of chronic pelvic pain, endometriosis, pelvic inflammatory disease and scarring, removal of one or both ovaries may alleviate some or all of the chronic pelvic pain. However, even in light of "obvious" pathology that may cause chronic pelvic pain, not all patients who have bilateral oophorectomy will have relief of their pain. In the case of prior oophorectomy and persistence of pelvic pain, one may have to open and explore the lateral pelvic wall, and ligate the ovarian vessels in the infundibulopelvic ligament in search of an ovarian remnant.

## ANATOMIC COMPLICATIONS OF OVARIAN SURGERY

Ovarian surgery, as mentioned above, consists of partial unilateral oophorectomy, partial bilateral oophorectomy, total unilateral oophorectomy, and total bilateral oophorectomy. During surgery, the primary complication is bleeding.

Postoperative complications include intraperitoneal bleeding and occasional small bowel obstruction.

# *Uterine Tubes*

*...it is indisputable that the surgeon's knowledge of current facts regarding the anatomy and physiology of the oviduct and a conscientious attempt to respect and preserve these facts have helped considerably in achieving the desired clinical results.*

**Jerome J. Hoffman**[20]

## EMBRYOGENESIS

### Normal Development

The genital ducts are of two types: mesonephric or wolffian in the male, and paramesonephric or müllerian in the female (see Table 26-1). The paramesonephric ducts form the uterine tubes.

### Congenital Anomalies

Just as anomalies of the ovary may be related to anomalies of the urinary system, anomalies of the uterine tubes may be associated with anomalies of other anatomic entities (Table 26-5). Duplication of the uterine tubes is an extremely rare condition formed by splitting of the müllerian system. It may be unilateral or bilateral, and may be associated with double ovaries and uterus, but not double vagina.

## SURGICAL ANATOMY

### Topography and Relations

The uterine tubes are variously known as the fallopian tubes or oviducts, tubes, or salpinges, from the Greek "salpinx" which means trumpet. Each uterine tube is a cylindrical, convoluted canal with a variable length from 7 to 14 cm. This does not include the intramural portion within the uterine cornu, which has a length of approximately 1.5 cm.

The uterine tube is enclosed within the upper margin of the broad ligament.

Three of the four parts of the uterine tube are shown in Fig. 26-10:

- Infundibulum, with its abdominal, or pelvic, orifice (external tubal ostium) which is related to the ovary via its fimbria
- Ampulla
- Isthmus
- The fourth, or uterine part, with its uterine orifice (internal ostium), is not shown. This portion is also known as the intramural segment of the tube.

### *Infundibulum*

The infundibulum is the funnel-shaped part of the ampulla, related to the ovary. It is characterized by a peritoneal opening 2 mm in diameter at its proximal end, surrounded by fimbria. The infundibulum belongs to the ampulla. One particularly long fimbria, the fimbria ovarica, is attached to the ovary and assists in ovum pick-up.

The topographic anatomy of the fimbriated end of the salpinx in relation to the ovarian surface is very important for ovum pick-up. According to Cohen,[21] the salpingo-ovarian relation may be violated by several occurrences:

- Uterine retroversion may produce proptosis of the fimbriae away from the ovary (Fig. 26-11A)
- Uterine anteversion may produce the same phenomenon due to traction of the infundibulopelvic ligament and upward displacement (Fig. 26-11B) of the ovary
- Fimbriae related to a small surface of a large ovary (Fig. 26-12B)
- Stenosis of the peritoneal opening, secondary to pelvic inflammatory disease, endometriosis, or other adhesive processes (Fig. 26-13)
- Occasionally, the fimbria ovarica may have a length of more than 4 cm (Fig. 26-14), and therefore have less contact with the ovarian surface, decreasing its efficiency in picking up the released ovum from the ovary
- Other pathologic anatomic entities creating obstacles between the ovary and ostium (Fig. 26-15)
- Multiple (accessory) fimbriae (Fig. 26-16)

Donnez and Casanas-Roux[22] stated that the pregnancy rate after fimbrial surgery is related to ampullary dilatation,

**TABLE 26-5. Anomalies of the Female Reproductive Tract**

| Anomaly | Prenatal Age at Onset | First Appearance (or Other Diagnostic Clues) | Sex Chiefly Affected[a] | Relative Frequency | Remarks |
|---|---|---|---|---|---|
| Aplasia and atresia of the uterus and vagina | | | | | |
|   Complete absence of uterus and vagina | 8th week | At birth | Female | Rare | Familial tendency suggested |
|   Absence of vagina | 9th week | At birth | Female | Uncommon | Familial tendency suggested |
|   Rudimentary, solid uterus, and vagina | 17th week | At birth | Female | Rare | |
|   Imperforate hymen | 5th month | In infancy or childhood | Female | Common | |
| Duplication of the uterine tubes | 6th to 7th weeks | Found only with ectopic pregnancy | Female | Very rare | Small asymptomatic duplications may be more frequent |
| Incomplete fusion of the müllerian ducts: | | | | | |
|   Separate hemiuteri | 3rd week? | At birth | Female | Very rare | Two separate vaginae |
|   Uterus didelphys | 9th week | | | Uncommon | May have septate vagina |
|   Uterus unicornis | 9th week | | | Rare | |
|   Uterus duplex | 9th week | Asymptomatic until pregnancy occurs | Female | Common | May have single or double cervix and septate vagina |
|   Uterus septus | 12th week | | | Uncommon | |
|   Uterus arcuatus | 7th month | | | Common? | |
| Fusion of the labia | ? | Infancy | Female | Rare | May not be congenital |

[a]Although these conditions may occur in males with anomalous or vestigial female structures, these anomalies all occur chiefly in females.

*Source:* Skandalakis JE, Gray SW (eds). Embryology for Surgeons, 2nd Ed. Baltimore: Williams & Wilkins, 1994; with permission.

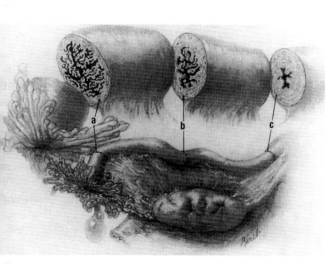

FIG. 26-10. Uterine tube of an adult woman with cross section illustrations of the gross structure of the epithelium in several portions. a, Infundibulum; b, Ampulla; c, Isthmus. (Cunningham FG, MacDonald PC, Gant NF, Leveno KJ, Gilstrap LC III. Williams Obstetrics (19th ed). Stamford CT: Appleton & Lange, 1993; with permission.)

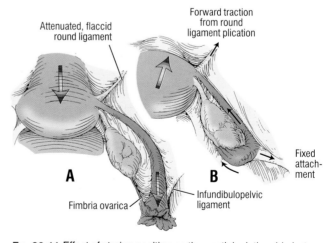

FIG. 26-11. Effect of uterine position on the spatial relationship between the ovary and the uterine tube fimbriae. **A,** Uterine retroversion, ligaments lax, proptosis of the fimbriae. **B,** Uterine anteversion, ligaments taut, fimbriae brush against the ovary. (Modified from Cohen BM. Surgery of the ovary, including anatomic derangements of the fimbrial-gonadal ovum-capture mechanism. In: Hunt RB (ed). Atlas of Female Infertility Surgery (2nd ed). St. Louis: Mosby Year Book, 1992, pp. 389-403; with permission.)

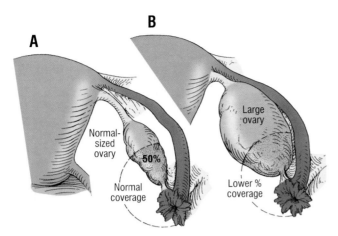

FIG. 26-12. Relationship between tubal ostium and ovarian surface affected by gonadal enlargement. **A,** Normal-sized ovary. **B,** Large ovary. (Modified from Cohen BM. Surgery of the ovary, including anatomic derangements of the fimbrial-gonadal ovum-capture mechanism. In: Hunt RB (ed). Atlas of Female Infertility Surgery (2nd ed). St. Louis: Mosby Year Book, 1992, pp. 389-403; with permission.)

the percentage of ciliated cells, and thickness of the tubal wall.

## Ampulla

The ampulla constitutes the remaining two-thirds of the uterine tube. Anatomically it extends from the distal part of the isthmus to the fimbriated vestibule. It is the widest segment of the tube, being 1 cm in diameter.

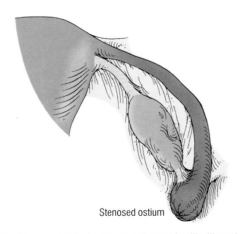

FIG. 26-13. Stenosed tubal ostium reduces the likelihood of ovum pickup. (Modified from Cohen BM. Surgery of the ovary, including anatomic derangements of the fimbrial-gonadal ovum-capture mechanism. In: Hunt RB (ed). Atlas of Female Infertility Surgery (2nd ed). St. Louis: Mosby Year Book, 1992, pp. 389-403; with permission.)

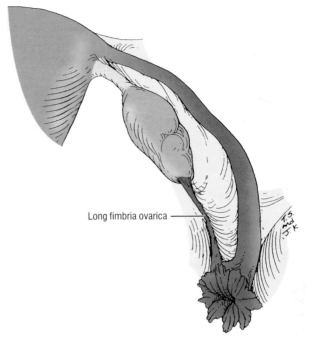

FIG. 26-14. Effect of elongation of fimbria ovarica. (Modified from Cohen BM. Surgery of the ovary, including anatomic derangements of the fimbrial-gonadal ovum-capture mechanism. In: Hunt RB (ed). Atlas of Female Infertility Surgery (2nd ed). St. Louis: Mosby Year Book, 1992, pp. 389-403; with permission.)

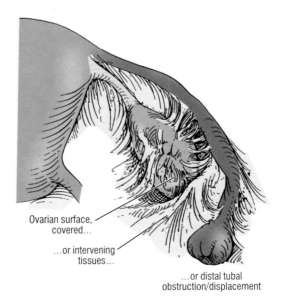

FIG. 26-15. Major causes of damage to fimbrial ovum pickup mechanism. (Modified from Cohen BM. Surgery of the ovary, including anatomic derangements of the fimbrial-gonadal ovum-capture mechanism. In: Hunt RB (ed). Atlas of Female Infertility Surgery (2nd ed). St. Louis: Mosby Year Book, 1992, pp. 389-403; with permission.)

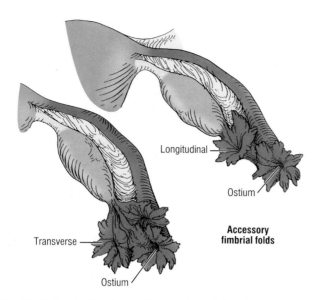

**FIG. 26-16.** Surgical anatomy of accessory fimbriae. Note transverse and longitudinal accessory folds. (Modified from Cohen BM. Surgery of the ovary, including anatomic derangements of the fimbrial-gonadal ovum-capture mechanism. In: Hunt RB (ed). Atlas of Female Infertility Surgery (2nd ed). St. Louis: Mosby Year Book, 1992, pp. 389-403; with permission.)

## Isthmus

The isthmus extends from the tubocornual junction to the most proximal part of the ampulla. It has a diameter of approximately 2 mm. It represents the medial one-third of the tube. Ectopic pregnancy may occur in this segment. DeCherney and Boyers[23] reported that segmental resection with anastomosis is preferable to salpingostomy. Hoffman[20] stated that the ciliated cells in this segment constitute approximately 54% of the cellular makeup.

## Intramural Segment

The uterine segment (intramural) has a length of approximately 1 cm. It is the narrowest portion of the tube, with a diameter of approximately 1 mm. It is the part between the end of the isthmus and the uterine cornu, located within the uterine wall.

## Vascular Supply

### Arteries

Two arteries participate in supplying the uterine tubes:
- The uterine artery supplies a fundal-cornual branch and

a true tubal branch.
- The ovarian artery contributes a true tubal branch from its end.

As may be seen in Fig. 26-17, there is rich anastomosis along the mesenteric area of the tube.

Manuaba[24] reemphasized the possibility of damage to ovarian blood vessels during tubal occlusion for voluntary sterilization.

### Veins

The veins draining the uterine tube parallel the arteries.

### Lymphatics

The tubal lymphatics have practically the same pathway as the lymphatics of the uterine fundus. These lymphatics follow the uterine and ovarian vessels to the pre-aortic and aortic lymph nodes.

## Innervation

The tubes are innervated by the sympathetic and parasympathetic systems, through the ovarian and inferior hypogastric plexuses. Pain sensation from the oviduct is transmitted back to the T11, T12, L1, and L2 levels of the spinal cord and corresponding dermatomes.

## HISTOLOGY

Each uterine tube has an external layer (serosal), an intermediate layer (muscular), and the innermost layer (mucosal). The serosa is the peritoneum that covers the extrauterine portion of the tube entirely except for its lower part, which is related to the mesosalpinx. The intermediate portion, the muscular layer, consists of two strata: outer longitudinal and inner circular. However, there is an extra stratum located between the circular layer and the mucosa at the uterotubal junction. Hoffman[20] presents these strata as inner circular, middle oblique, and outer longitudinal. The rich vascularity in this area has an enigmatic physiologic function.

According to Hoffman,[20] the mucosa lining the lumen of the uterine tube is composed of four types of cells: peg, indifferent, secretory, and ciliated. According to the same author, only the secretory and ciliated cells appear to play a role in ovum transport.

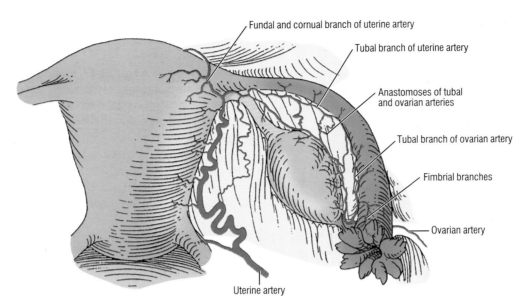

**FIG. 26-17.** Arterial blood supply of the uterine tube. (Modified from Hoffman JJ. Anatomy and physiology of the uterine tube. In: Hunt RB (ed). Atlas of Female Infertility Surgery (2nd ed). St. Louis: Mosby Year Book, 1992, pp. 3-11; with permission.)

## PHYSIOLOGY

The physiology of the uterine tube is not well known; the anatomy is much better appreciated. But Hoffman[20] was correct when he emphasized that both disciplines should be respected. Diverse attempts at substituting other structures for the uterine tubes (including artificial tubes, veins or arteries, and the appendix), have not been successful. The tube largely maintains its many physiologic secrets.

How is sperm transport aided? How do the sperm reach the ampulla in an hour and a half? How does the tube transport ova, sperm, zygote, the preimplantation morula, and finally the blastocyst? Are the ciliated mucosal cells responsible for the transmittal of the ovum to the ampulla? More studies are needed to better understand the unknown potentialities of these anatomic entities.

## SURGICAL APPLICATIONS

- Salpingectomy (removal of the uterine tube) is a very common operative procedure on the tube. It is performed in situations where there is irreversible and severe damage to the tube, such as for a tubal hydrosalpinx or pyosalpinx with pelvic inflammatory disease. It

is also performed in conditions of the tube that may be life-threatening to the patient, such as in ectopic pregnancy (Fig. 26-18) with or without tubal rupture, and neoplastic tubal tumor.

We quote from Piura and Rabinovich[25]:

*Fallopian tube carcinoma is rarely suspected preoperatively. The symptom complex of "hydrops tubae profluence," said to be pathognomonic for this tumor, is rarely encountered. The treatment approach is similar to that used for ovarian carcinoma and includes primary surgery comprised of total abdominal hysterectomy, bilateral salpingo-oophorectomy and staging*

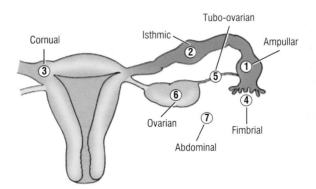

**FIG. 26-18.** Ectopic pregnancy. Diagram shows the various implantation sites, numbered in order of decreasing frequency of occurrence. (Modified from Sabiston DC, Jr. Textbook of Surgery, 15th. ed. Philadelphia: WB Saunders, p. 1518; with permission.)

*followed by chemotherapy. The prognosis for patients with primary fallopian tube carcinoma is similar to that of patients with primary ovarian carcinoma.*

- Surgically, great care must be taken in separating the tube away from the ovary in order not to damage the ovarian blood supply. In addition, when removing the tube, whenever possible the operator should leave a 1 cm segment of the tube attached to the cornual region of the uterus in order to decrease the chances of a utero-peritoneal fistula into the pelvic cavity, which can lead to a cornual pregnancy.

- A cornual pregnancy is a potentially life-threatening condition. Pressure from a growing cornual pregnancy can cause catastrophic sudden rupture of the uterine cornua which leads to immediate and massive intraperitoneal hemorrhage.

- When performing a salpingectomy, the operator should try to preserve as much of the ovary as possible. However, even a partial oophorectomy can be accomplished, yet still allow full hormonal function of the remaining ovarian tissue.

- Mild cases of pelvic inflammatory disease, endometriosis externa, prior pelvic and abdominal surgeries, and other adhesion-producing processes can cause occlusion of a tube, thus leading to infertility due to the inability of the released ovum to pass through the tube to become fertilized by the upswimming sperm. Occlusion of the tube can occur at any point along the tube, from the cornual region out to the infundibulum.

- In many cases the tube is simply kinked by adhesive disease. The actual lumen, when straightened out, is truly patent.

- Gentle microsurgical techniques, both at open laparotomy and through the laparoscope, have been developed in order to lyse adhesions and straighten out the tubal lumen. In cases of actual tubal occlusion due to scar tissue or prior tubal sterilization, microsurgical techniques have been developed to actually excise the scarred portion of the tube that contains the tubal occlusion and then reanastomose the healthy, presumably functioning, portions of the tube. These techniques have evolved since the early 1970s. Textbooks have been written on the details and specific indications for microsurgery for the many different conditions of peritubal adhesive disease and tubal occlusive disease.

Microsurgery pertaining to tubal functioning and fertility is an art and science unto itself. Its techniques and surgical procedures are well addressed in postgraduate gynecological fellowships dealing with reproductive medicine.

- The key to microsurgical techniques is the gentle pinpoint handling of the tissues, in order to limit any damage to the tubal lumen and the delicate blood supply to the tube. In addition, observation has shown that as much healthy tube must be preserved as possible.

- A healthy tube that is too short will not allow for proper ovum pickup and proper fertilization of any egg that may be picked up by the tube. In addition to the restoration of a damaged tube to as normal a state as possible, microsurgical techniques also concentrate on the restoration of normal fimbriae. This includes proper length of the fimbria ovarica and the relation of the fimbriae to the ovary, which also needs to be freed of any adhesive disease.

- The implantation of a fertilized egg into a uterine tube is an ectopic pregnancy which may cause rupture and subsequent hemorrhage. The tube is also a very rare source of pelvic cancer.

- Ectopic gestational remnants in the fallopian tube and broad ligament with characteristics of proliferation of intermediate trophoblast were reported by Kouvidou et al.[26] The placental site nodule was asymptomatic and benign.

- Torsion of the tube is a rare event but can occur in both benign and malignant situations. A rare leiomyoma of the fallopian tube with torsion at the ampullary-isthmic junction of the oviduct was reported by Misao et al.[27] Ovarian torsion is usually accompanied by tubal torsion.

## ANATOMIC COMPLICATIONS OF UTERINE TUBE SURGERY

The anatomic complications of surgery of the uterine tubes are closely related to the surgery of hysterectomy or other gynecological procedures involving one or both uterine tubes.

- Tubal ligation, if inadequately performed, can fail to provide sterilization.

- Tuboplasty, if inadequately performed, may not promote conception.

- Prolapse of the tube after abdominal or vaginal hysterectomy has been reported. The situation usually presents as a painful vaginal cuff with a friable edematous mass at the vaginal apex. It appears to be granulation but persists after application of silver nitrate. Manipulation of this area is very painful for the patient.

# *Uterus*

## EMBRYOGENESIS

### Normal Development

The paramesonephric or müllerian ducts, which are formed in the mesonephros by invaginations of the coelomic epithelium, are responsible for the genesis of the uterus and the upper vagina (Table 26-1).

Uterine epithelium is formed from the urogenital sinus. The uterine walls are formed by the splanchnic mesenchyme. The cervix may be of paramesonephric origin.

### Congenital Anomalies

Despite the fact that uterine anomalies, as well as anomalies of some other entities of the female genital tract, are secondary to an incomplete partial or total fusion of the paramesonephric ducts, the question remains whether these anomalies are developmental arrests. Perhaps they are due to genetic factors.

The uterus may be aplastic or hypoplastic. Uterine duplications may be total (uterus didelphys) or partial (uterus arcuatus or uterus bicornis, which is most common). Double uterus may be associated with obstructed hemivagina and renal agenesis[28].

We quote from Homer et al.[29] on the septate uterus:

> *A bicornuate uterus results from failure of fusion of the mullerian ducts, whereas a septate uterus results from failure of resorption of the intervening septum. The fibromuscular septum so formed may project minimally from the uterine fundus or may extend to the cervical os, almost completely dividing the uterine cavity in two. Septa also may be segmental, resulting in partial communication between the two sides.*

Giraldo et al.[30] advise gynecologists to be aware of the possibility of cervical duplication associated with longitudinal vaginal septum and septate uterus. The anomalies can be ameliorated surgically by resection of the uterine and vaginal septum.

Several variations are shown in Fig. 26-19. Further information about congenital anomalies will be found in Table 26-5.

## SURGICAL ANATOMY

### Topography

The adult uterus is a thick, flattened, pear-shaped muscular organ. It is located between the bladder anteriorly and the rectum posteriorly; laterally it is enveloped by the right and left broad ligaments. The uterus can be subdivided into the fundus, body, and cervix (see Fig. 26-2A).

The shape and the size of the uterus are variable, depending upon the age and parity of that patient. The uterus weighs approximately 40 to 60 grams in the nulliparous patient and approximately 60 to 80 grams in the multiparous patient. The uterus is typically 8 cm in length from the external os of the cervix to the top of the fundus, and is approximately 5 cm in width at the level of the uterine ostia, which defines the widest part of the uterus.

The endometrial cavity (Fig. 26-20) is a flattened potential space which is triangular in shape, with the apex pointing inferiorly toward the cervix. The walls of the uterus are approximately 2 cm in thickness, principally due to the muscular portion known as the myometrium.

The numbers 1, 2, 3 serve as a useful mnemonic for the length of the uterus:
- 1 inch (2.5 cm) equals the length of the cervix (supravaginal and vaginal)
- 2 inches (5.0 cm) equals the body, including the isthmus
- 3 inches (7.5 cm) equals the total length of the organ

The widest portion of the uterus at the cornua measures 2 inches.

The uterus is normally anteflexed, with the body bending forward at the isthmus, indenting the bladder. The typical uterus is also anteverted, with the endocervical canal oriented at a 90° angle to the lumen of the vagina (Fig. 26-21).

In retroversion (Fig. 26-21A, Fig. 26-22), the uterus is inclined posteriorly toward the rectum. The cervix faces anteriorly.

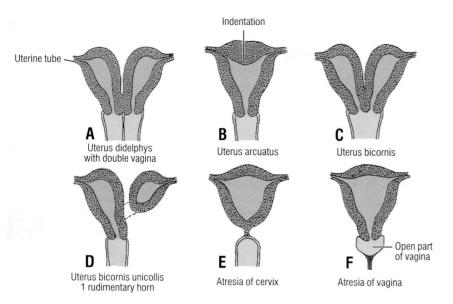

Indentation

Uterine tube

**A** Uterus didelphys with double vagina

**B** Uterus arcuatus

**C** Uterus bicornis

**D** Uterus bicornis unicollis 1 rudimentary horn

**E** Atresia of cervix

**F** Atresia of vagina — Open part of vagina

**FIG. 26-19.** Schematic representation of the main abnormalities of the uterus and vagina, caused by persistence of the uterine septum or obliteration of the lumen of the uterine canal. (Modified from Sadler TW. Langman's Medical Embryology, 8th ed. Philadelphia: Lippincott Williams & Wilkins, 2000; with permission.)

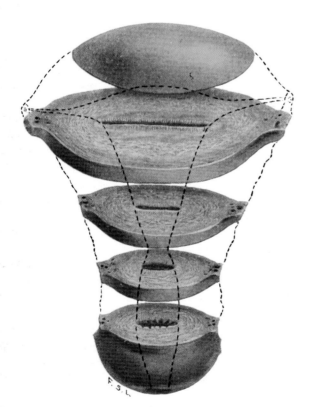

**FIG. 26-20.** Reconstruction of uterus, showing shape of its cavity and cervical canal. (Modified from Eastman NJ. Williams Obstetrics (10th ed). New York: Appleton-Century-Crofts, 1950; with permission.)

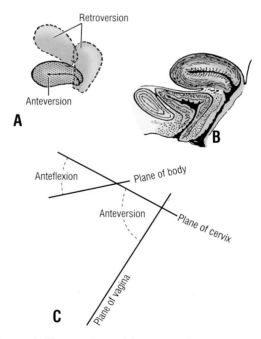

Retroversion

Anteversion

**A**

**B**

Anteflexion — Plane of body

Anteversion — Plane of cervix

Plane of vagina

**C**

**FIG. 26-21. A,** Three outlines of the uterus, showing a more normal position (anteversion) and a moderate and a more extreme degree of retroversion. The last is most often brought about by filling of the bladder. **B,** The normal adult uterus is anteverted (i.e., at an angle with respect to the vagina) and anteflexed (i.e., flexed somewhat on it-self). **C,** The solid lines indicate the planes and the angles of antever-sion and anteflexion. These are not fixed positions. (Modified from Gardner E, Gray DJ, O'Rahilly R. Anatomy (4th ed). Philadelphia: WB Saunders, 1975; with permission.)

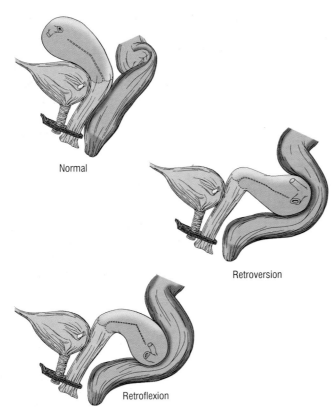

Normal

Retroversion

Retroflexion

FIG. 26-22. Uterine positions. Note that the diagram of retroversion represents an extreme position. The malpositions of the uterus vary in degree according to several factors.

In retroflexion (Fig. 26-22), the body of the uterus is curved posteriorly at the isthmus of the uterus. The cervix is in its normal position.

Various combinations of retroversion and retroflexion can occur. These positions are not pathological but simply normal variations on the position of the uterus (Fig. 26-22). It is not uncommon to find a uterus retroflexed and/ or retroverted toward the rectum posteriorly.

Fullness of bladder and rectum also plays a great role in the position of the uterus.

## Relations

### *Fundus*

The thick, convex fundus is that portion of the uterus at and above the level where the uterine tubes enter the uterus; it is covered with peritoneum. The fundus essentially forms the roof for the uterine cavity.

### *Body*

The body of the uterus lies within the pelvic cavity. The uterine cavity lies almost totally within the uterine body. Its right and left lateral aspects are related to the broad ligament.

### *Isthmus*

The narrowed, waistlike, isthmic portion of the uterus leads into the more inferior cervix. The isthmus is known obstetrically as the lower uterine segment. The isthmus was described by Aschoff,[31] who stated that the lowest part of the uterine cavity becomes very narrow, forming a canal.

### *Cervix*

The cervix is approximately 3 to 4 cm in length and consists of a vaginal portion, which is easily seen during speculum examination of the vagina, and a supravaginal portion, which is very important to the endopelvic fascial support system of the cervix and upper vagina. The anterior area of the supravaginal part is related closely to the base of the urinary bladder and is not covered by peritoneum. Its posterior area is covered by peritoneum which forms the rectouterine pouch of Douglas above and the posterior vaginal fornix below. The pouch of Douglas separates the uterus from the rectum.

The cervix enters the vagina by coursing perpendicularly to the anterior vaginal wall, thus explaining the shorter length of the anterior vaginal wall (7 cm) when compared with the posterior vaginal wall (9-10 cm).

The cervix normally has a very dense consistency like a "nose." During pregnancy, however, this consistency softens significantly, so that the cervix may very well have the consistency of "lips." The protrusion of the vaginal portion of the cervix into the vagina allows segregation of the proximal portion of the vagina into anterior, posterior, and lateral fornices. Each ureter passes within 1.5 cm of the supravaginal portion of the cervix as the ureter makes it knee-bend underneath the uterine artery to pass medially and anteriorly across the anterolateral fornix to enter the bladder.

Surrounding the supravaginal portion of the cervix is a dense ring of endopelvic fascia into which is anchored the pubocervical fascia, as well as the uterosacral and cardinal ligaments. This endopelvic fascial ring is known as the pericervical fascial ring. This pericervical ring of visceral connective tissue is a key link in the important mechanical continuity of the endopelvic fascia associated with the vagina and cervix, consisting of contributions both from the suspensory ligaments (cardinal and uterosacral ligaments) and the pubocervical fascia.

REMEMBER: The ureter is very close (approximately 1-1.5 cm) to the lateral wall of the supravaginal part of the cervix.

### *Anterior, Posterior, and Lateral Relations of the Uterus*

- Anterior (Fig. 26-23)
  - Vesicouterine pouch
  - Some loops of small bowel
  - Supravaginal and intravaginal cervix
  - Anterior fornix of vagina
- Posterior (Fig. 26-23)
  - Rectouterine pouch of Douglas with small bowel loops
- Lateral (Fig. 26-23)
  - Broad ligament with the anatomic entities enveloped
  - Ureter with uterine vessels and nerves
  - Vesical vessels and nerves

## Uterine Cavity

The cavity of the body has a triangular shape (Fig. 26-24), which changes with pregnancy. The cavity is wide at the fundus and becomes narrower and narrower approaching the isthmus (internal os). For all practical purposes, the anterior and posterior walls are in apposition. The isthmic cavity is very narrow but has the ability to dilate. Last[32] stated that this part is the "lower uterine segment," as referred to by the obstetrician.

There is some confusion in the literature about the internal os and its relation to the isthmus. Is the isthmus the upper one-third of the cervix? Or does it belong to the lowest part of the body, forming the "lower uterine segment"? Regardless, the most important fact is that during pregnancy the isthmus expands, and practically becomes a segment of the body cavity in which the fetus rests.

The endocervical canal is narrow proximally and distally. Its peculiar anatomy includes the formation of one vertical fold anteriorly and one posteriorly. The canal is closed not by apposition but by palmate folds originating from the anterior and posterior vertical folds, which fit against each other.

## Pelvic Peritoneum and Its Uterine Relations

The peritoneal relations to the endopelvic female genital organs are illustrated in Fig. 26-25 and Fig. 26-26. The peritoneum travels downward to the pelvic cavity after cov-

ering anterior and posterior uterine surfaces. Two spaces are formed: the deep rectouterine space of Douglas and the shallow vesicouterine space.

In covering the posterior uterine area, the peritoneum covers the posterior area of the cervix completely. However, anteriorly it covers fundus, body, and the supravaginal (isthmic) part of the cervix. The reader will find more details as well as surgical applications in the chapter about the peritoneum.

## Endopelvic Fasciae

The suspensory mechanism of greatest direct support for the pelvic organs is supplied by the cardinal ligament/ uterosacral ligament complex. These structures are part of a continuous network called the endopelvic fascia (Fig. 26-

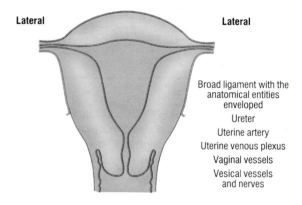

Lateral                                   Lateral

Broad ligament with the anatomical entities enveloped
Ureter
Uterine artery
Uterine venous plexus
Vaginal vessels
Vesical vessels and nerves

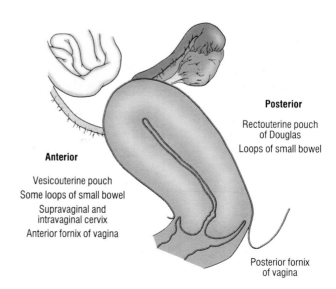

**Posterior**

Rectouterine pouch of Douglas
Loops of small bowel

**Anterior**

Vesicouterine pouch
Some loops of small bowel
Supravaginal and intravaginal cervix
Anterior fornix of vagina

Posterior fornix of vagina

FIG. 26-23. Relational anatomy of the uterus.

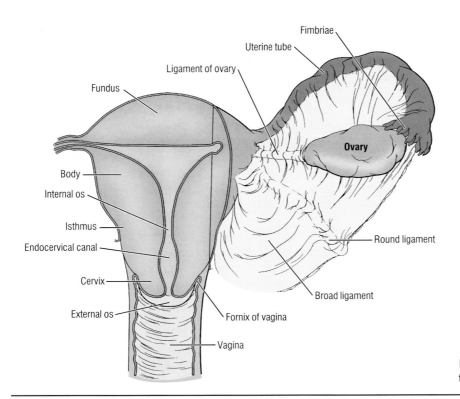

FIG. 26-24. Female reproductive organs, posterior view.

27A) between the peritoneum and the parietal fascia over the muscular pelvic basin. Microscopically, endopelvic fascia is a three-dimensional meshwork of collagen, elastin, and smooth muscle. This meshwork surrounds and supports the viscera in both the abdominal and pelvic cavities. Anatomists and surgeons have artificially described this whole network in a piecemeal fashion, assigning various names to isolated segments.

On visual inspection at the time of detailed anatomic dissections, the endopelvic fascia is actually an interconnected system of sheaths, continuous and interdependent.

The endopelvic fascia serves two important purposes. First, it serves to provide mechanical conduits and supports for the visceral arteries and veins, visceral nerves, and lymph nodes and channels that course in the sub-

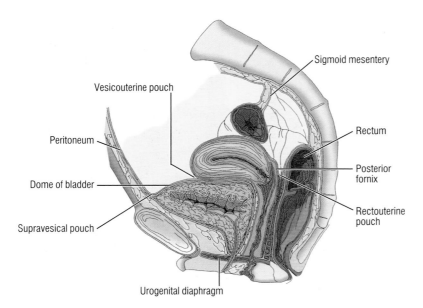

FIG. 26-25. The peritoneum of the female pelvis in paramedian section.

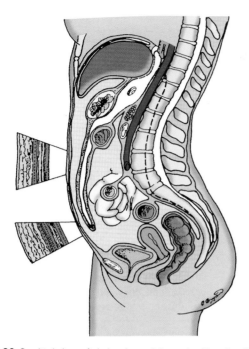

**FIG. 26-26.** Sagittal view of abdominopelvic cavity. Details of layering of abdominal wall are shown in insets to left. Dotted line indicates extension of peritoneal space lateral and dorsal to spine. (Modified from DeLancey JOL, Richardson AC. Anatomy of genital support. In: Hurt WG (ed). Urogynecologic Surgery. Gaithersburg MD: Aspen, 1992, pp. 19-33; with permission.)

peritoneal areas of the pelvis. Secondly, the endopelvic fascia surrounds the organs within the pelvis and serves to anchor them to the parietal fascia of the muscular pelvic basin, thus positioning these organs within the pelvis in their normal anatomic positions.

The vesicovaginal fascia is a fusion of two fasciae, one from the urinary bladder and one from the vagina. Both of these fasciae are derived from the intermediate stratum (the fascia enclosing the adrenals, kidney, ureters, urinary bladder, uterus, and the supplying vessels). If one kidney is absent, the intermediate stratum (i.e., the renal fascia) does not develop in that area.

## Levator Plate

The uterus and cervix, as well as the upper two-thirds of the vagina, are suspended over the levator plate.[2] This constitutes the most important source of indirect mechanical support for these organs. The levator plate (Fig. 26-28) is formed by the midline fusion of the levator ani muscles between the rectoanal junction and the coccyx.

When a woman is standing upright, the healthy levator plate is almost horizontal in orientation (see Fig. 26-1). When the patient performs a Valsalva maneuver, such as in coughing or laughing, the downwardly directed intra-abdominal and intrapelvic forces push the upper two-thirds

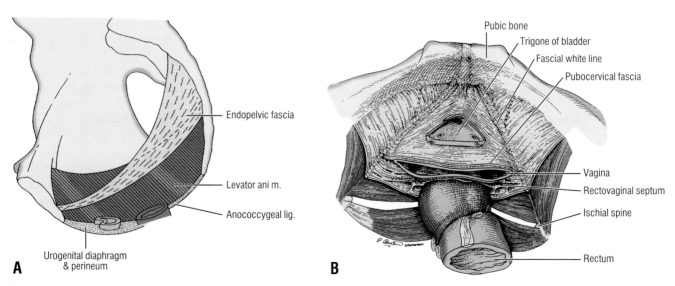

**FIG. 26-27. A,** Endopelvic fascia. **B,** The pubocervical fascia (ligament) supports the urethra (only the trigone is shown) and is attached laterally to the fascial white lines. The rectovaginal septum is a thin layer of fascia between the vagina and rectum. (**A,** Modified from Skandalakis LJ, Gadacz TR, Mansberger AR Jr, Mitchell WE Jr, Colborn GL, Skandalakis JE. Modern Hernia Repair: The Embryological and Anatomical Basis of Surgery. New York: Parthenon, 1996; **B,** Courtesy of Dr. Cullen Richardson. Modified from Brubaker LT, Saclarides TJ (eds). The Female Pelvic Floor: Disorders of Function and Support. Philadelphia: FA Davis, 1996; with permission.)

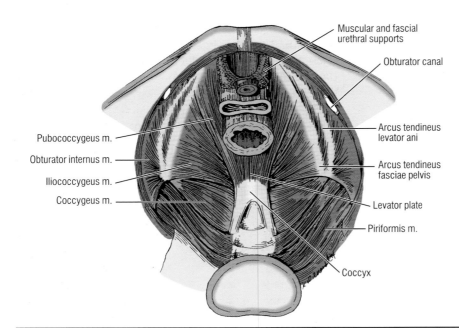

Pubococcygeus m.

Obturator internus m.

Iliococcygeus m.

Coccygeus m.

Muscular and fascial
urethral supports

Obturator canal

Arcus tendineus
levator ani

Arcus tendineus
fasciae pelvis

Levator plate

Piriformis m.

Coccyx

**FIG. 26-28.** Superior view of pelvic floor. (Modified from Retzky SS, Rogers RM, Richardson AC. Anatomy of female pelvic support. In: Brubaker LT, Saclarides TJ (eds). The Female Pelvic Floor: Disorders of Function and Support. Philadelphia: FA Davis, 1996; with permission.)

of the vagina and cervix against the tensed levator plate in a flap-valve action. By this mechanism, these pelvic viscera are impinged within the pelvic cavity and prevented from prolapsing through the levator hiatus toward the vaginal introitus. In addition, the tensing of the levator plate is also accompanied by contraction of the pubococcygeus muscles surrounding the levator hiatus, which further blocks any movement of the vagina and cervix downward. This flap-valve mechanism is dependent upon the suspension of the upper two-thirds of the vagina and cervix over the levator plate.

## Ligaments of the Uterus and Cervix

We refer the interested student to the excellent work of DeLancey and Richardson[33] on the anatomy of the support of the female pelvic organs. The ligaments that attach to the uterus are:
- Broad ligament
- Round ligament
- Cardinal ligament
- Uterosacral (sacrocervical) ligament
- Anterior uterine (uterovesical) ligament
- Posterior uterine (rectovaginal) ligament
- Pubocervical fascia
- Utero-ovarian ligament
- Rectouterine ligament

The utero-ovarian ligament will not be considered here because it has been discussed in the preceding sections

on topography, poles, ligaments, and mesovarium of the ovaries.

There is confusion in the literature about the name, origin, and "anatomy" per se of several of these ligaments. For example, the sacrocervical ligament is occasionally referred to as the uterosacral. Are both the same? Another example is the pubocervical ligament which is perhaps nothing but the pubocervical fascia (Fig. 26-27B). Is the anatomic term "ligament" correct or is it just a fascia?

### *Broad Ligament*

After covering the uterus anteriorly and posteriorly, the pelvic visceral peritoneum extends from each side of the uterus to both lateral pelvic walls, forming the two layered right and left portions of the broad ligament (Fig. 26-29, Fig. 26-30). The broad ligaments have an almost triangular shape. Together with the uterus, they divide the pelvic cavity into an anterior, or vesicouterine, fossa and a posterior, or rectouterine fossa - also known as the cul-de-sac of Douglas (see Figs. 26-2, 26-4). This peritoneal reflection also invests the round ligaments (ligamentum teres uteri), which travel laterally and anteriorly to leave the pelvis via the internal inguinal rings. The broad and round ligaments offer no useful mechanical support to the uterus, cervix, or vagina, in contrast to the cardinal ligaments and uterosacral ligaments, which offer significant suspensory support to the lower uterine segment, cervix, and upper portion of the vagina.

The broad ligament is the mesentery of the uterus, tubes,

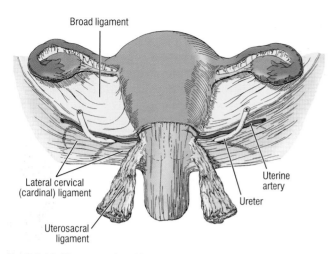

**FIG. 26-29.** Uterosacral and lateral cervical (cardinal) ligaments from above and behind.

and ovaries. Each double-folded broad ligament has four borders — medial, lateral, superior, and inferior. Each of these borders relates with several anatomic entities. The medial border is related to the lateral edge of the uterus and encloses the uterine vessels and the uterus. The lateral border is related to the lateral pelvic wall. The superior border is free and directed anteriorly. It envelops the uterine tube, its vessels, and the ovarian ligament from above downward. It also contains the ovarian vessels and the round ligament. The inferior border forms an extension over the floor of the true pelvis.

Anatomy, embryology, nomenclature, and convenience fight each other for recognition when the broad ligament is being described. The mesosalpinx (Fig. 26-31) is that part of the broad ligament located just beneath the uterine tube. It contains the epoophoron (the parovarium or organ of Rosenmüller), Gartner's duct, and other vestigial structures from the mesonephric wolffian duct. The mesovarium, an extension of the broad ligament originating from its posterior surface, suspends the ovary. The mesometrium is the area of the broad ligament below the mesovarium. The parametrium consists of the connective tissue elements within the broad ligament just lateral to the body and lower uterine segment of the uterus.

The inferior border or base of the broad ligament is wide as well as thick. This area contains the portion of the cardinal ligament that invests the uterine vessels and the lower portion of the ureter. The cardinal ligament then continues to follow the uterine artery into the cervix, lower uterine segment, and upper one-third of the vagina.

REMEMBER: from the front of the broad ligament, the round ligament stands out; from the back of the broad ligament, the uteroovarian ligament stands out.

The distal portion of the ureter penetrates the cardinal ligament, which forms a ureteric tunnel around the ureter. At this point, the ureter passes underneath the obliquely coursing uterine artery ("water under the bridge"). The uterine venous plexus surrounds the ureter and uterine artery within the base of the cardinal ligament, which is in the base of the broad ligament.

Remember the 4 U's related to the broad ligament:
- **U**terine artery (Fig. 26-29)
- **U**reter (Fig. 26-29)
- **U**terovesical pouch
- **U**terorectal pouch

Remember the four M's from above downward associated with the posterior surface of the broad ligament:

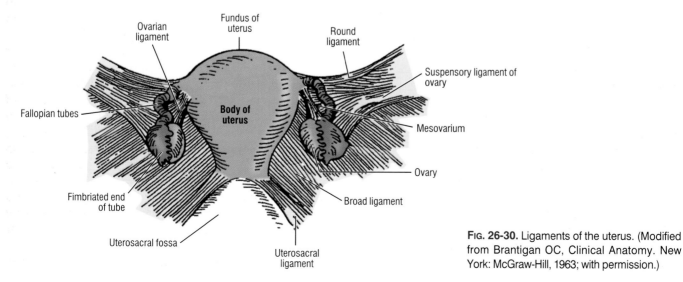

**FIG. 26-30.** Ligaments of the uterus. (Modified from Brantigan OC, Clinical Anatomy. New York: McGraw-Hill, 1963; with permission.)

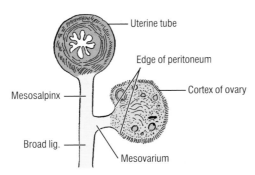

**FIG. 26-31.** Diagram of the peritoneal relations of the ovary in a section through the upper part of the broad ligament. At the peritoneal edge about the hilum of the ovary the mesothelium of the peritoneum is continuous with the epithelium of the ovarian cortex. (Modified from Hollinshead WH. Anatomy for Surgeons, vol. 2. New York: Hoeber-Harper, 1961; with permission.)

- Mesosalpinx
- Mesovarium (Fig. 26-30)
- Mesometrium
- Mackenrodt ligament (cardinal, transverse cervical) (Fig. 26-29).

### Round Ligament

The round ligaments (Fig. 26-32, Fig. 26-33, Fig. 26-34A) are two flat, narrow cords some 10-12 cm long. They arise from the lateral aspects of the upper part of the body of the uterus. Each travels laterally and anteriorly through the mesometrium and leaves the pelvic cavity through the internal inguinal ring to pass through the inguinal canal (see Fig. 26-2). Near the uterus the round ligament contains much smooth muscle (the continuation of the smooth muscular uterine wall) and connective tissue. More distally, the ligament consists principally of fibrous tissue in its termination near the mons pubis. Together with the ovarian ligament, it represents the embryologic homologue of the male gubernaculum.

The round ligament has a diameter of approximately 3 to 5 mm. It is attached to the anterior and lateral aspects of the uterus just below the insertion of the ovarian ligament and the tubes. The round ligament travels within the broad ligament just beneath its anterior leaflet running upward and outward.

The pathway of the round ligament is as follows: lateral aspect of the uterus to the broad ligament, across the umbilical and obturator vessels to the superior pubic ramus, crossing the external iliac vessels, entering the inguinal canal at the deep inguinal ring, passing through the inguinal canal and usually inserting into the fibrofatty tissue of the mons pubis, and into the proximal part of the labium majus, the homologue of the scrotum. Attah and Hutson[34]

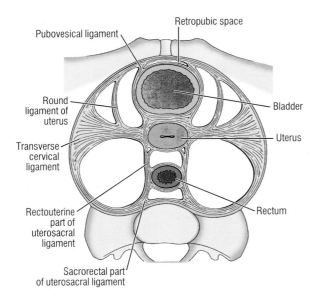

**FIG. 26-32.** Superior view of ligaments of the uterus. (Modified from Slaby FJ, McCune SK, Summers RW. Gross Anatomy in the Practice of Medicine. Philadelphia: Lea & Febiger, 1994; with permission.)

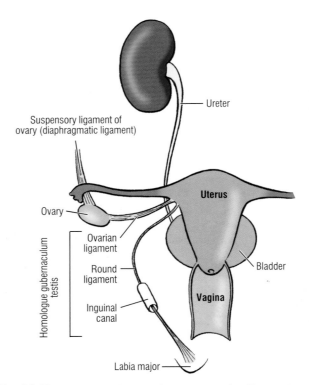

**FIG. 26-33.** Pathways of round ligament, ovarian ligament, and suspensory ligament. (Modified from Brantigan OC. Clinical Anatomy. New York: McGraw-Hill, 1963; with permission.)

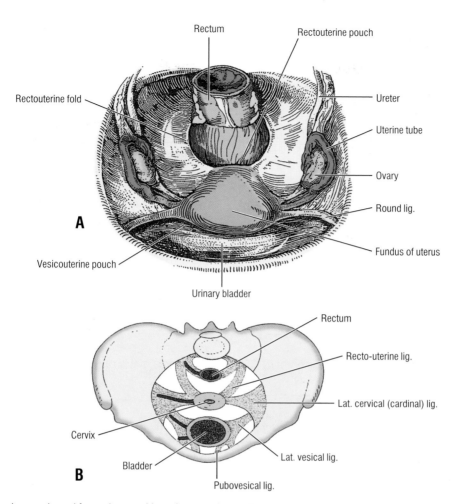

**FIG. 26-34. A,** The pelvic viscera viewed from above, with peritoneum intact. **B,** Horizontal section of the pelvic viscera, showing the ligaments of the uterus. The arteries shown are, from posterior to anterior, the middle rectal, uterine, and inferior and superior vesical. (Modified from Gardner E, Gray DJ, O'Rahilly R. Anatomy: A Regional Study of Human Structure (5th ed). Philadelphia: WB Saunders, 1986; with permission.)

stated that the round ligament does not reach the labium majus.

Within the inguinal canal, the round ligament is accompanied by an arterial branch (the counterpart of the cremasteric artery) of the inferior epigastric artery and the genital branch of the genitofemoral nerve. These two structures are located just behind the shelving edge of the inguinal ligament and in front of the pectineal line. A branch of the uterine artery passes outward along the round ligament. This vessel, referred to as "Sampson's artery," anastomoses with the cremasteric branch of the inferior epigastric artery.

## Cardinal Ligament

The cardinal ligament has many names:

- Ligament of Mackenrodt
- Ligament of Kocks
- Uterine retinaculum of Martin
- Lateral ligament
- Transverse cervical ligament (transverse ligament of cervix)

Sheathlike investments of pelvic structures are provided by the endopelvic fascia. In the example of the cardinal ligament/uterosacral ligament complex (Fig. 26-29, Fig. 26-32, Fig. 26-34, Fig. 26-35, Fig. 26-36), a sheath consisting of collagen bundles, elastic fibers, and smooth muscle surrounds the internal iliac artery and vein and follows the branching of the uterine artery to the endopelvic fascial capsule surrounding the lower uterine segment, cervix, and upper one-third of the vagina.

Range and Woodburne[35] observed that the cardinal lig-

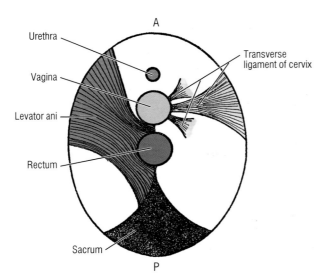

**FIG. 26-35.** Important anatomic features of female pelvic floor. On the viewer's left the arrangement of levator ani is shown. On the viewer's right the transverse ligament of the cervix (visceral pelvic fascia) is shown. Note the multiple points of origination of the transverse (cardinal) ligament. A, Anterior; P, Posterior. (Modified from McGregor AL, Du Plessis DJ. A Synopsis of Surgical Anatomy (10th ed). Baltimore: Williams & Wilkins, 1969; with permission.)

ament is connective tissue enveloping the uterine vessels. They found that although the ligament is composed of much delicate tissue, the collective strength of these fibers is great in affording support to the uterus.

The cardinal ligament follows the pathway of the uterine artery and uterine veins into the base of the broad liga-

ment. Approximately 1.5 cm lateral to the edge of the cervix, the ureter passes underneath the uterine vessels and enters the ureteric tunnel, as mentioned above.

The cardinal ligament is anchored posteriorly to the parietal fascia over the piriformis muscle, the obturator internus muscle, and along the anterior bony border of the greater sciatic foramen. Remember that the piriformis muscle together with its fascia, large nerves, and vessels passes through and fills the greater sciatic foramen. Thus the cardinal ligament may be considered a "vascular leash" that suspends the cervix and upper two-thirds of the vagina over the levator plate. Remember, the levator plate is a dynamic muscular platform that allows entrapment of the upper third of the vagina within the pelvis during stress in order to prevent prolapse of the uterocervix and upper third of the vagina.

Posteriorly continuous with the uterosacral ligament, the cardinal ligament is anteriorly continuous with the arcus tendineus fasciae pelvis. This is the stout connective tissue band that provides a line of fusion between the pubocervical fascia on the anterior wall of the vagina and the superior fascia of the pelvic diaphragm.

### Uterosacral Ligament

The uterosacral (or sacrocervical) ligament (Fig. 26-29, Fig. 26-30, Fig. 26-32, Fig. 26-36) is a complex band of connective tissue and smooth muscle. It receives contributions from the tough, presacral fascia of Waldeyer over the 2nd, 3rd, and 4th sacral vertebrae and the piriformis muscle fascia. Within this fascia and invested by it are the pelvic

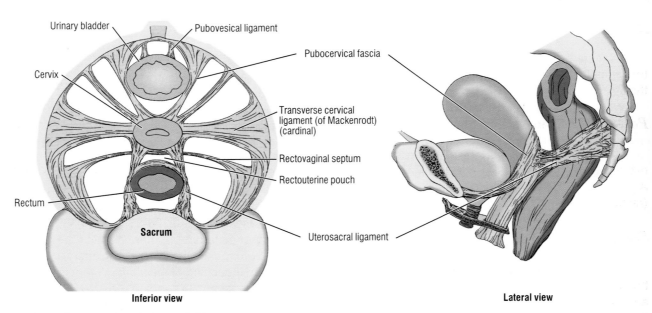

**FIG. 26-36.** Uterine ligaments from below and side.

splanchnic nerves and the more inferior portions of the pelvic nerve plexus. Thus the uterosacral ligament may be considered a "neural leash" or "sacral leash," while, as previously indicated, the cardinal ligament may be thought of as a "vascular leash" in providing direct organ support. Along with the cardinal ligament, the uterosacral ligament helps suspend the upper third of the vagina and cervix over the levator plate.

The uterosacral ligaments are the lateral boundaries of the uterorectal space of Douglas. Campbell[36] stated that they are composed of smooth muscle, fibrous tissue, and nerves.

This band of tissue passes lateral to the rectum on a horizontal plane in the standing patient and attaches to the posterior and lateral aspects of the pericervical ring of endopelvic fascia. Just before reaching the pericervical ring, the uterosacral ligament contributes to the formation of the rectovaginal septum, thereby providing a connective tissue hammock for the upper part of the vagina, a stratum of tissue attached above to the peritoneum of the pouch of Douglas, attached below to the perineal body, and suspended laterally between the right and left ischial spines. As noted previously, the uterosacral ligament is continuous anteriorly with the cardinal ligament complex.

The uterosacral ligaments are substantial cords of endopelvic fascia that have a distinct appearance at the time of laparotomy or laparoscopy. They are readily appreciated by palpation during pelvic examination and at the time of surgery. Remember, the uterosacral ligaments are the lateral borders of the uterorectal space or pouch of Douglas, also known as the cul-de-sac of Douglas.

## *Anterior Uterine Ligament*

The anterior uterine ligament (Fig. 26-37) is the peritoneal fold extending from the anterior uterine surface to the urinary bladder. It is the floor of the uterovesical fossa.

## *Posterior Uterine Ligament*

The posterior uterine ligament is a peritoneal fold extending from the posterior uterine surface to the rectum. Again, it is simply the floor of the cul-de-sac of Douglas (rectouterine pouch) (Fig. 26-2, Fig. 26-38).

## *Pubocervical Fascia*

The pubocervical fascia (ligament?) (Fig. 26-36) follows the anterior uterine aspect and upper vagina. It passes around the urethra to the posterior surface of the pubic bones.

## *Rectouterine Ligament*

The rectouterine ligament is that portion of the network of pelvic visceral fascia that travels from the pericervical ring and upper vagina, around the rectum, to attach to the presacral fascia over the lower sacrum.

## Vascular Supply

### *Arteries*

The uterine artery (see Fig. 26-6) is the medial off-shoot from the internal iliac artery, as the internal iliac artery terminates to become the umbilical artery, the source of the superior vesical artery just proximal to the beginning of the obliterated segment of the umbilical artery. The uterine artery is the chief blood supply to the uterus.

From its origin the uterine artery descends along the pelvic sidewall and then proceeds medially, surrounded by the fibers of the cardinal ligament. The uterine artery then passes over the ureter and ascends tortuously along the lateral aspect of the uterus within the broad ligament (see Figs. 26-4 and 26-5). At the junction of the uterine tubes with the uterus, the uterine artery turns laterally toward the ovarian hilum (see Fig. 26-17, Fig. 26-37).

The uterine artery gives the following branches along its course:
- Vaginal artery (Fig. 26-39)
- Cervical artery
- Anterior and posterior uterine branches
- A tubal branch and an ovarian branch that anastomose

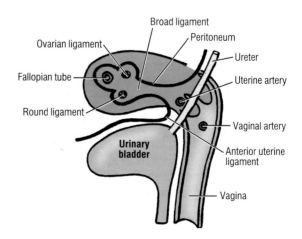

**FIG. 26-37.** Relations of the ureter, the uterine and vaginal arteries, and ligaments. (Modified from Brantigan OC. Clinical Anatomy. New York: McGraw-Hill, 1963; with permission.)

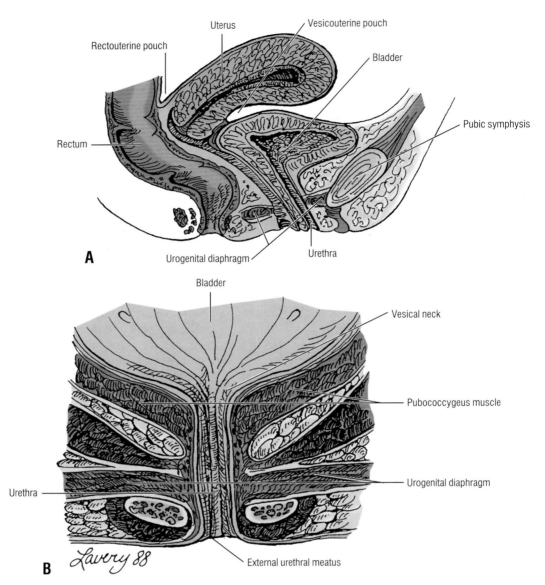

FIG. 26-38. **A,** The floor of the rectouterine pouch or cul-de-sac of Douglas is the posterior uterine ligament. The female urethra is about 4 cm long, beginning at the vesical neck and ending at the external meatus. It lies beneath the pubic symphysis with the vesical neck in a high retropubic position. **B,** The female urethra has a strong muscular wall, composed of smooth and striated muscle. The urethral lining is composed of transitional epithelium, with portions of pseudostratified epithelium. (Modified from Siegel SW. Anatomy and embryology. In: Novick AC (ed). Stewart's Operative Urology (2nd ed). Baltimore: Williams & Wilkins, 1989, pp. 454-478; with permission.)

with the similar branches from the ovarian artery (see Fig. 26-17)

The ovarian artery (see Fig. 26-6) also contributes significantly to the blood supply of the uterus. The ovarian arteries originate from the abdominal aorta approximately 1-2 cm below the origin of the renal arteries. On their way downward, they pass over the ureters. These arteries assist vascularization of the ureter by their ureteric branches. They cross the common iliac vessels superficial to the ureter and enter the infundibulopelvic ligament at the pelvic brim just

superficial to the bifurcation of the common iliac artery into the external and internal iliac arteries. The ovarian arteries participate in the blood supply of the uterine tubes as well as portions of the broad ligament and upper portion of the uterus.

The branches of the uterine and ovarian arteries invade the uterine wall obliquely. At approximately the middle of the muscular stroma, they form the arcuate arteries. The arcuate arteries produce radial branches, which are destined to take care of the endometrium by their own

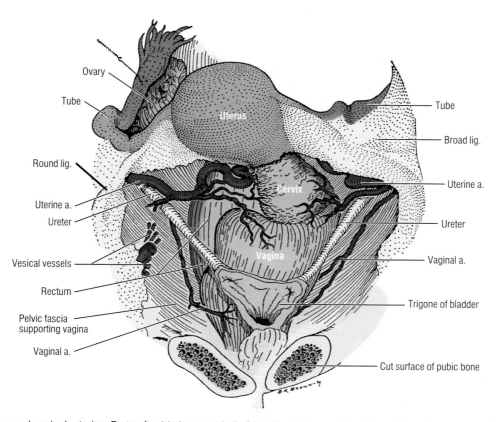

**FIG. 26-39.** Uterine and vaginal arteries. Parts of pubic bone and all of the bladder (except for trigone) have been removed. The uterus is asymmetrically placed; hence, one ureter is close to the cervix and the other is far removed from it. (Modified from Basmajian JV, Slonecker CE. Grant's Method of Anatomy (11th ed). Baltimore: Williams & Wilkins, 1989; with permission.)

spiral and basal branches.

The distribution of the uterine artery is as follows:

- The vaginal artery arises just before the uterine artery passes over the ureter. There may be two, or even three, vaginal arteries. It (or they) passes underneath the ureter to continue inferiorly toward the vaginal wall. There the vaginal artery forms anterior and posterior branches which, by rich anastomoses between vaginal and uterine arterial branches, form anterior and posterior "azygos arteries" of the vagina. The vaginal artery supplies the vaginal mucosa, the base of the bladder, the vestibular bulb, and provides additional supply to the rectum.
- The cervical branch arises from the uterine artery at the area of the isthmus or lower uterine segment. It bifurcates into an anterior and posterior branch.
- These branches anastomose with the anterior and posterior branches of the opposite side, thus forming the so-called coronary artery of the cervix. Anterior and posterior uterine branches also arise from the uterine artery. These take care of the anterior and posterior parts of the uterus.

- Tubal and ovarian branches are produced by the bifurcation of the uterine artery close to the fundus of the uterus. Both branches pass laterally. The tubal branch goes to the mesoappendix of the uterine tube, and the ovarian branch passes toward the mesovarium of the ovary. The tubal artery anastomoses with the tubal branch of the ovarium. The ovarian branch anastomoses with the main ovarian artery (see Figs. 26-6, 26-17).

According to Clark as cited in Eastman,[37] the two uterine sides communicate very well, since fluid injected into one side escapes from the opposite side.

### *Veins*

The venous network of the uterus is very rich. These veins form the uterovaginal venous plexus that accompanies the uterine artery. It communicates posteriorly with the rectal or hemorrhoidal plexus and anteriorly with the vesical plexus. The uterovaginal plexus can be divided into two parts: the upper part drains to the uterine veins; the lower part drains to the internal iliac vein via the internal pudendal vein.

A portosystemic anastomosis is located below the rectouterine pouch, or pouch of Douglas, connecting the uterovaginal plexus with the superior rectal vein. The arcuate veins form the right and left uterine veins, which empty into the internal iliac vein. Ovarian and upper broad ligament venous blood is collected in the pampiniform plexus via small veins, and drains into the ovarian vein. The right ovarian vein drains directly into the inferior vena cava, whereas the left ovarian vein drains into the left renal vein.

Pelvic varices may be found in the infundibulopelvic and broad ligaments, with lateral extensions to the cervix and vagina and below the peritoneum of the vesicouterine and rectouterine pouch. The ovarian vein crosses the ureter close to the infundibulopelvic ligament at the pelvic brim.

## Lymphatics

A rich lymphatic network is present under the peritoneum, especially at the posterior uterine wall; the lymphatic vessels form a peculiar and complicated network (Fig. 26-40). The lymphatics of the uterotubal area drain to the superficial inguinal lymph nodes, following the pathway of the round ligament. The round ligament leaves the pelvis via the internal inguinal ring and inguinal canal to enter the external inguinal ring and area of the mons pubis. The upper part of the uterus (the fundus and part of the upper body) drains into the paraaortic lymph nodes. The lower part of the body of the uterus drains into the external iliac nodes. The cervical lymph nodes drain into the internal and external iliac as well as sacral nodes.

Scheidler et al.[38] stated that lymphangiography (LAG), computed tomography (CT), and magnetic resonance (MR) imaging perform similarly in the detection of lymph node metastasis from cervical cancer. As CT and MR imaging are less invasive than LAG and also assess local tumor extent, they should be considered the preferred adjuncts to clinical evaluation of invasive cervical cancer.

## Innervation

Much is yet unknown regarding the innervation of the uterus, with respect to both the anatomic and physiologic aspects of the nerve supply. The uterus has no somatic innervation, only visceral innervation from sympathetic and parasympathetic sources (Fig. 26-41). The parasympathetic efferent (motor) fibers and afferent (sensory) (Fig. 26-42) fibers travel within the nervi erigentes, which pass into the pelvic plexus after leaving the anterior rami of the second, third, and fourth sacral spinal nerve branches. The sympathetic efferent supply (Fig. 26-42, Fig. 26-43) de-

scends through the hypogastric and pelvic plexuses.

The parasympathetic efferent nerve supply originates from the intermediolateral cell column from the second, third, and fourth sacral segments of the spinal cord. The afferent or sensory nerve fibers carry nociceptive as well as sexual sensations to the dorsal root ganglia and posterior horn of the same spinal cord segments.[39]

The postganglionic sympathetic visceral nerves to the uterus originate from several sources, although the preganglionic fibers arise principally from the intermediolateral cell column of the spinal cord at levels T12 and L1. A considerable portion of the uterine tubes, upper portion of the broad ligament, and perhaps a portion of the uterus are supplied by the sympathetic nerves of the ovarian plexus (Fig. 26-44) that travel with the ovarian vessels in the infundibulopelvic ligament.

A second sympathetic source originates from the inferior hypogastric plexus. This is a 3 cm × 5 cm plexus of visceral nerves surrounding the ureter and internal iliac artery and branches in the lateral pelvic sidewall, lateral to the uterosacral ligament at the base of the broad ligament. The inferior hypogastric plexus and nerves have sympathetic input from the sacral splanchnic nerves of the sympathetic

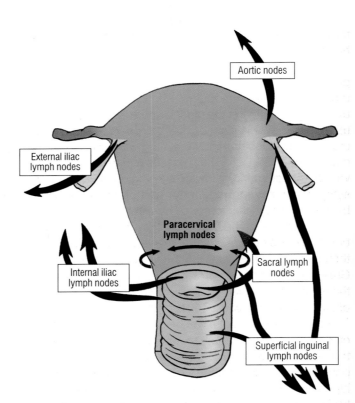

**FIG. 26-40.** Lymphatic drainage of the uterus and vagina. (Based on Ellis H. Clinical Anatomy: A Revision and Applied Anatomy for Clinical Students, 4th Ed. Philadelphia: FA Davis, 1969.)

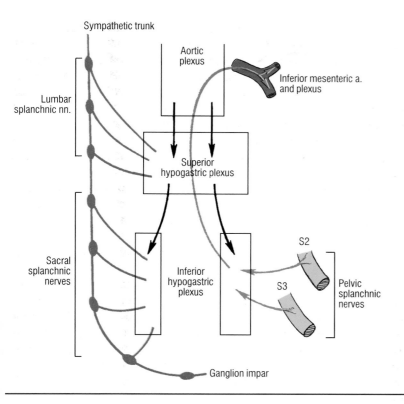

Sympathetic trunk

Aortic plexus

Inferior mesenteric a. and plexus

Lumbar splanchnic nn.

Superior hypogastric plexus

S2

Sacral splanchnic nerves

Inferior hypogastric plexus

S3

Pelvic splanchnic nerves

Ganglion impar

**FIG. 26-41.** Autonomic plexuses in pelvis. (Modified from Hall-Craggs ECB. Anatomy as a Basis for Clinical Medicine (3rd ed). Baltimore: Williams & Wilkins, 1995; with permission.)

trunk as well as from the superior hypogastric plexus via the hypogastric nerves (see Fig. 26-41).

The inferior hypogastric plexus divides into further plexuses in order to service the bladder, rectum, and the uterovaginal area. The uterine nerves originate from the uterovaginal plexus (of Frankenhäuser) and enter the upper part of the vagina, cervix, and lower portion of the uterus via the uterine vessels. An aggregation of ganglion cells is found typically near the cervix. Contraction and vasoconstriction of the uterine vessels are produced by sympathetic action, whereas vasodilatation is produced by parasympathetic stimulation.

Many of the pain fibers from the uterine fundus and body pass upward through the hypogastric plexus and then into the lumbar segments of the sympathetic chains. Grasping the cervix will produce severe pain. Division of the hypogastric nerves will produce anesthesia at the area of the fundus but not in the cervix.

Pain fibers from the vagina, cervix, and isthmic regions of the uterus pass to the central nervous system by way of the pelvic splanchnic nerves, accompanying the pelvic parasympathetic nerve supply. Because of the relatively high failure rate of uterosacral ligament transection in relieving chronic pelvic pain, it is believed that most visceral nerve fibers enter into, and travel from, the uterus along the uterine vessels and not necessarily through the uterosacral

ligaments. Perhaps the accepted view is that noxious stimuli from the uterine fundus are referred to dermatomes T11, T12, L1, and L2.

Gardner et al.[40] stated that doubt surrounds the role of these nerves in uterine function. Perhaps the sympathetic is not only a vasoconstrictor but also is a producer of some motor action. The pathway of S2-S3 (nervi erigentes) is responsible for cervical pain. The lower thoracic and hypogastric nerves are the pathway of pain from the body of the uterus, as during labor.

The above summary of sympathetic and parasympathetic innervation appears relatively simple but, in addition, hormones play a role in uterine function. Presumably there are synergistic and antagonistic actions between the two systems.

The pathway of afferent uterine nerve fibers is as follows:

- Uterine body: hypogastric nerves → T11-T12 → spinal cord
- Cervix: lumbar sympathetics → first two lumbar ganglia → dorsal root ganglia of L1 and L2 → spinal cord, *or:* pelvic splanchnic nerves → dorsal root ganglia of S2-S4 → spinal cord

In summary, we know very little about uterine innervation. Much of our current thought is speculation based upon studies of rats and cats and a few human studies. Is the uterine body innervated only by the sympathetics?

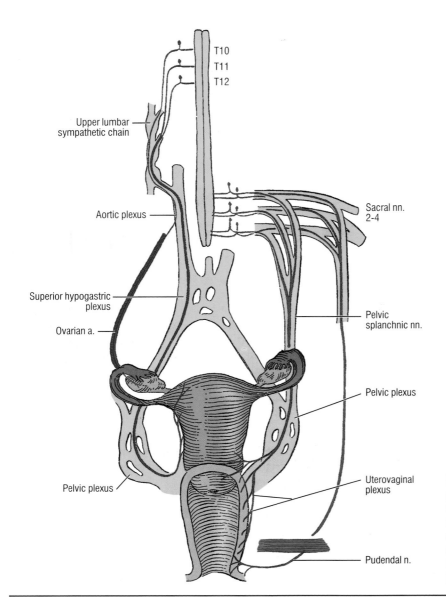

T10
T11
T12

Upper lumbar
sympathetic chain

Aortic plexus

Sacral nn.
2-4

Superior hypogastric
plexus

Ovarian a.

Pelvic
splanchnic nn.

Pelvic plexus

Pelvic plexus

Uterovaginal
plexus

Pudendal n.

**Fɪɢ. 26-42.** Probable afferent innervation of female genital tract. Fibers entering the spinal cord through sacral nerves are shown on viewer's right (blue lines). Fibers associated with sympathetic system and entering spinal cord through thoracic nerves are shown on viewer's left (red lines). (Modified from Hollinshead WH. Anatomy for Surgeons. New York: Hoeber-Harper, 1961; with permission.)

Perhaps. Are cholinergic and adrenergic fibers present only in the cervical musculature[10] and the submucosal layers? Perhaps.

## HISTOLOGY

The uterus is composed of 3 layers:
● Serosa
● Muscular coat
● Mucosa

The serosa is the pelvic peritoneum (perimetrium). It covers the fundus and the body of the uterus (Fig. 26-45).

The muscular coat (myometrium) is formed by an abundance of smooth muscle fibers which contain a rich neurovascular network (Fig. 26-46, Fig. 26-47). The myometrium is continuous laterally with the muscular coat of the uterine tube. The fundus and body of the uterus contain more muscular tissue, whereas the cervix contains more fibrous tissue.

The mucosa of the uterus, or the endometrium, lines the inner surface of the uterine cavity. It is composed of many tortuous glands. The endometrium significantly changes in thickness and cellular character with the cyclical hormonal variation, the menstrual cycle. The endometrium does not have a submucosa. The endometrium is

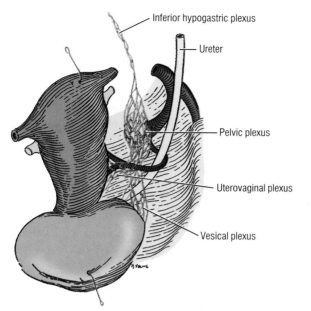

**FIG. 26-43.** Uterovaginal plexus. (Modified from Hollinshead WH. Anatomy for Surgeons. New York: Hoeber-Harper, 1961; with permission.)

directly fixed to the muscular coat and has tremendous regenerating potential. The endometrium of the nonpregnant uterus presents in three basic phases: menstruation, proliferation (Fig. 26-48A), and secretory (Fig. 26-48B) activity. After a cervical dilatation and curettage, the endometrium is able to regenerate because the mucosa dips deep within the muscular stroma. These intramuscular mucosal glands are not mechanically violated during the procedure. It is not within the scope of this chapter to give detailed histologic descriptions.

## PHYSIOLOGY OF UTERUS

The uterus is a very thick-walled, muscular organ with three layers. The thin external layer is simply the visceral peritoneum. The thick middle muscular layer, or myometrium, consists of interlacing, circular, longitudinal, and oblique spiral bundles of smooth muscle and large venous

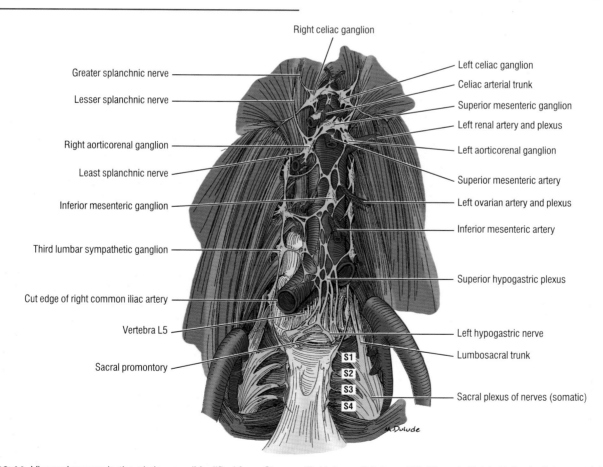

**FIG. 26-44.** Visceral nerves in the abdomen. (Modified from Steege JF, Metzger DA, Levy BS. Chronic Pelvic Pain: An Integrated Approach. Philadelphia: WB Saunders, 1998; with permission.)

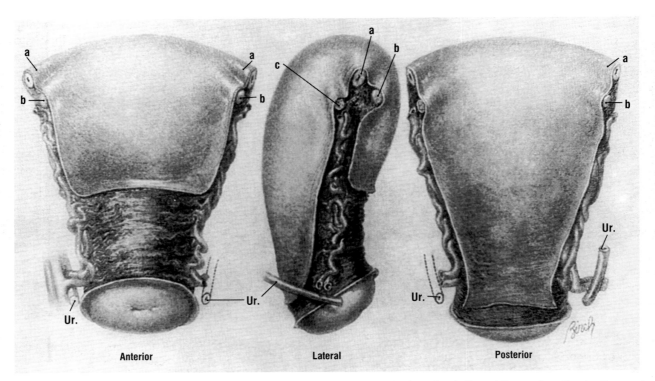

**FIG. 26-45.** Anterior, right lateral, and posterior views of uterus of adult woman. a, Uterine tube; b, Round ligament; c, Ovarian ligament; ur, Ureter. (Cunningham FG, MacDonald PC, Gant NF, Leveno KJ, Gilstrap LC III. Williams Obstetrics (19th ed). Stamford CT: Appleton & Lange, 1993; with permission.)

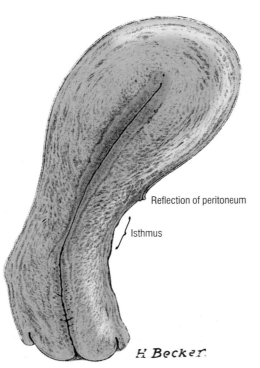

**FIG. 26-46.** Myometrium: sagittal section of normal adult uterus. (Modified from Eastman NJ. Williams Obstetrics (10th ed). New York: Appleton-Century-Crofts, 1950; with permission.)

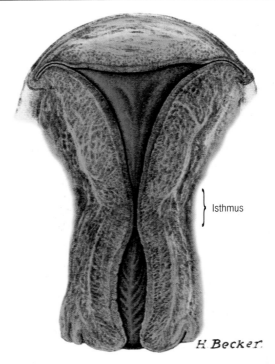

**FIG. 26-47.** Frontal section of normal adult uterus, showing myometrium and shape of cavity and isthmus. (Modified from Eastman NJ. Williams Obstetrics (10th ed). New York: Appleton-Century-Crofts, 1950; with permission.)

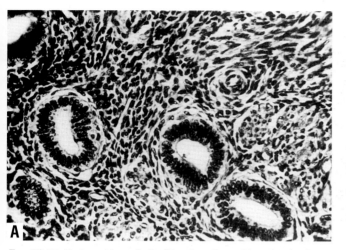 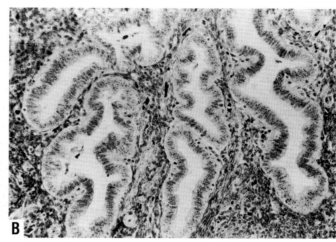

**FIG. 26-48.** Endometrium. **A,** Proliferative phase. The gland cells are usually organized in a simple array. **B,** Secretory phase (21st day of the menstrual cycle). Uterine glands are tortuous, with lumens dilated by accumulation of secretory material. (Junqueiro LC, Carneiro J, Contopoulos AN. Basic Histology, 2nd ed. Los Altos, CA: Lange Medical Publications, 1971; with permission.)

plexuses. The myometrium is sensitive to estrogen and progesterone hormones. The endometrium is a mucous membrane from 1 to 6 mm in thickness, depending upon hormonal stimulation. The endometrium develops day by day in specific histologic changes when stimulated by estrogen and/or progesterone according to the ovarian cycle (see Fig. 26-48). The visceral vasculature to the uterus, as well as in the myometrium and endometrium, is likewise very sensitive to the ovarian hormones.

Dysmenorrhea is uterine pain associated with menses. Current theories suggest that the rapid release of synthesized prostaglandins act directly on the myometrium causing intense smooth muscle contractions with resulting constriction of small endometrial blood vessels, tissue ischemia, and subsequent pain. Prostaglandin synthetase inhibitor medication has been shown to be very effective in inhibiting prostaglandin synthesis and in significantly decreasing pain in primary dysmenorrhea. Wilson and colleagues[41] found insufficient evidence in controlled trials to recommend the use of uterine nerve ablation to treat primary or secondary dysmenorrhea.

Endometrial tissue may be found associated with anatomic entities close to the uterus such as the uterine tubes and ovaries, and more remote locations in the gastrointestinal tract (e.g., abdominal wall). This ectopic mucosa menstruates in the pelvic cavity or with the organ where it is located. La Greca et al.[42] advised that endometriosis of the ileum may produce symptoms mimicking inflammatory bowel disease.

After menopause, with the removal of estrogen and progesterone stimulation, both the myometrium and endometrium atrophy.

## SURGICAL APPLICATIONS

*[In abdominal hysterectomy, the] dissection is always anatomic, bleeding is always under prompt control, and modifications because of pelvic disease are easily undertaken.*

*Tiffany J. Williams*[43]

### Abdominal Hysterectomy

If at all possible, perform a total abdominal hysterectomy in preference to a supracervical hysterectomy. Leaving the cervix in situ may eventually lead to cervical dysplasia and/or cervical cancer. It should be noted, however, that some gynecologic surgeons prefer a supracervical hysterectomy for two reasons: first, to preserve an intact pericervical ring of endopelvic fascia for support; second, to preserve sexual pleasure at the level of the cervix.

### Vaginal Hysterectomy

During vaginal hysterectomy, the round and ovarian ligaments, as well as the uterine tubes, are brought down into the vagina as a result of the downward pull on the uterus. Postoperative enterocele or cul-de-sac hernia is prevented in many surgical cases by plicating the uterosacral ligaments in the midline and attaching the vaginal cuff to them. During any pelvic surgery, the operator must always know the whereabouts of the ureters, as well as the bladder and rectosigmoid.

During surgical procedures, division of the round ligament allows for ready, safe access to the retroperitoneal areas of the vesical space-obturator space, and to the pelvic sidewall adjacent to the space of Retzius, the region between the bladder and the pubic bone and rectus muscles. This area is well above the course of the ureter as it travels through the base of the broad ligament and cardinal ligament.

## Coagulation and Embolization of Uterine Vessels

Embolization of the pelvic vasculature is used to treat postpartum and postsurgical bleeding. Dover et al.[44] reported success in treating symptomatic fibroids by uterine artery embolization. Laparoscopic bipolar occlusion of uterine vessels was employed by Liu[45] to reduce the size of symptomatic leiomyomas.

REMEMBER:
- The cardinal ligament, uterosacral ligament, and the levator plate are of special significance in supporting the uterus.
- The distal ureter is related to the supravaginal cervix within the broad ligament, below the uterine vessels, and above the level of the lateral fornix, approximately 1.3 cm (approximately ½ inch) or less lateral to the cervix. It can be injured, divided, and ligated during total hysterectomy. Accidental division during surgery produces a very serious anatomic complication.
- The ureter runs from the pelvic wall toward the urinary bladder through the base of the cardinal ligament, or it may have a close relation to the pubovesicocervical fascia. These facts should be remembered during abdominal hysterectomy.
- During vaginal hysterectomy, the round and ovarian ligaments as well as the uterine tubes are exposed as the uterus is drawn downward.
- In vaginal hysterectomy, the uterosacral and cardinal ligaments can be divided and ligated. This represents lower ligation of the broad ligament. Ligation of tubes, ovaries, and round ligaments is upper ligation.
- Because their biopsy studies showed a greater density of autonomic nerves and ganglia in the uterosacral ligaments than in the cardinal ligaments at the level of a radical hysterectomy (RH), and because RH disrupts more

nerve tissue than does simple hysterectomy, the study of Butler-Manuel et al.[46] supports the neurogenic etiology of pelvic morbidity after RH.
- The round ligament becomes hypertrophied in pregnancy and may be palpated.
- The uterosacral ligament is exposed by cutting the posterior leaflet of the broad ligament. Stay close to the uterine wall to avoid injury to the ureters.
- When sutured together, the uterosacral ligaments practically close the posterior pelvis.
- Be sure to recognize the urinary bladder, the ureter, and the rectosigmoid.
- Both leaflets of the broad ligament should be incised and separated carefully to free the urinary bladder.
- Be sure to free the bladder during abdominal hysterectomy. Proceed from the anterior surface of the uterus by a peritoneal incision that is not close to the anterior uterine wall. If necessary, leave myometrium on the bladder rather than the bladder on the uterus.[43]
- When bleeding occurs during hysterectomy, internal iliac (hypogastric) ligation is occasionally required, and may be done with impunity.
- To avoid ureteric injuries, the best surgical dissection involves the upper $1/3$ of the uterine side; in other words, the best area is close to the fundus.
- Remember the relationship between the pubovesicocervical fascia and the ureter. The fascia covers the area between the cardinal ligament and the cervical surface. The ureter is within this fascia, but at the base of the cardinal ligament. Therefore, dissect within the fascial plane above the base of the cardinal ligament.
- The cardinal ligaments and uterosacral ligaments are different parts of the same endopelvic fascial complex that suspends the upper third of the vagina and cervix over the levator plate. This suspensory action allows forces from above in the standing female patient to entrap the upper third of the vagina and cervix against the levator plate in order to prevent vaginal and cervical prolapse. This is known as a flap-valve mechanism. The cardinal and uterosacral ligaments and the pubovesicocervical fascia are the main supporters of the female contents after abdominal hysterectomy. They should be sutured to the vaginal angles.
- The infundibulopelvic and round ligaments provide minimal support for the vaginal vault. However, their approximation to the vault will help to cover the sutured vaginal wall with peritoneum.
- Smith-Bindman et al.[47] strongly recommended endovaginal ultrasound for postmenopausal women with vaginal bleeding to diagnose or rule out endometrial cancer and other endometrial disease.

# ANATOMIC COMPLICATIONS OF HYSTERECTOMY

## Anatomic Complications of Abdominal Hysterectomy

The following are possible anatomic complications of abdominal hysterectomy:

- Intrinsic sphincter deficiency[48]
- Injury to the bladder
- Injury to one or both ureters
- Somatic nerve injury
- Intestinal injury
- Hemorrhage

During the performance of a "routine" hysterectomy, whether abdominal or vaginal, injuries to the bladder, ureters, rectosigmoid, and blood vessels have been reported. Injuries to somatic nerves are very unlikely, but have been reported in relation to patient positioning for a particular surgery, particularly in the dorsolithotomy position for a vaginal hysterectomy.

### *Injury to the Bladder*

Always keep in mind the relationship between the bladder and anterior abdominal wall and between the bladder and the cervix. If injury to the bladder is not recognized in the operating room, results may be catastrophic for both the patient and the surgeon.

The urinary bladder can be injured:

- During the abdominal incision. It is important to open the peritoneal cavity by incising the peritoneum very high.
- During dissection within the vesicouterine and vesicovaginal space. This dissection is best performed sharply trying to find the white shiny surface of the pubocervical fascia.

If the bladder is opened inadvertently, the surgeon must determine whether the ureters are involved also. If the ureters are not involved, then the defect should be closed in two layers, trying to avoid the bladder mucosa. Absorbable 2-0 or 3-0 sutures with an atraumatic continuous or interrupted suture are acceptable. The first layer should be inverted by a continuous or interrupted absorbable suture. A transurethral catheter should drain the bladder for several days to a week, depending upon the size and location of the injury.

### *Unilateral or Bilateral Ureteric Injury*

*In spite of the greatest care and knowledge of the anatomic relations, the ureter may occasionally be unexpectedly injured. In fact, this may occur more frequently than is usually recognized.*

**Michael Newton & John R. Lurain**[49]

*The only gynecologist who has not injured a ureter or bladder is one who has done little surgery.*

**Lawrence R. Wharton, Jr.**[50]

The distal ureter travels within the base of the broad ligament through the base of the cardinal ligament as the uterine vessels travel toward the cervix. The crossing of the ureter below the uterine vessels (Fig. 26-49 and see Fig. 26-37) is in relation to the lateral vaginal fornix and is approximately 1.5-2 cm from the side of the cervix. The ureter can be injured during clamping, ligation, and cutting in this area during a total hysterectomy.

Accidental occlusion of the ureter at this point may eventually lead to hydroureter, hydronephrosis, and eventual renal failure of that side. After passing through the ureteric tunnel in the base of the cardinal ligament, the ureter makes a "knee-bend" and travels anteriorly and medially across the anterolateral fornix of the vagina for several centimeters before it enters the bladder.

Injury to the ureter can occur:

- When clamping uterine vessels or the uterosacral ligament

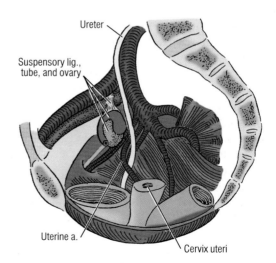

FIG. 26-49. Some relations of the ureter in the female pelvis. (Modified from Hollinshead WH. Anatomy for Surgeons, Vol. 2. New York: Hoeber-Harper, 1961; with permission.)

**1515**

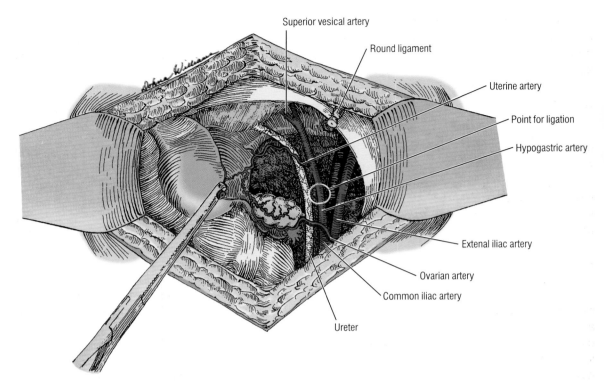

**Fig. 26-50.** Retroperitoneal anatomy, showing relative positions and courses of uterine, ovarian, and iliac vessels as well as ureter and bladder. (Modified from Williams TJ. Abdominal hysterectomy, myomectomy, and presacral neurectomy: with management of bladder injury and attention to thromboembolic disease. In: Ridley JH (ed). Gynecologic Surgery: Errors, Safeguards, and Salvage (2nd ed). Baltimore: Williams & Wilkins, 1981; with permission.)

- When clamping the infundibulopelvic ligament at the pelvic brim
- When clamping at the lateral wall of the proximal vagina
- During pelvic retroperitonealization

The most common sites of ureteric injury are:
- At the lateral pelvic sidewall where the uterine vessels pass over the ureter
- At the ureterovesical junction, particularly during the performance of anterior colporrhaphy
- At the infundibulopelvic ligament

The damaged ureter should be recognized and repaired immediately. Such repair may include a ureteroureteric anastomosis or a ureterovesical anastomosis.

During any gynecologic surgery, it is recommended that one visualize and/or palpate the ureter as much as possible. The description by Williams[43] may be helpful in identifying the ureter: "Peristalsis and the characteristic wavy blood vessels on the ureteral surface are not duplicated by any other structure" (Fig. 26-50).

### Nerve Injury

Nerve injury is an extremely rare phenomenon during abdominal hysterectomy. Nerves of the anterior abdominal wall such as the iliohypogastric or ilioinguinal nerve can be injured during the performance or closure of an anterior abdominal incision. Injury to the sacral plexus and nerves is unusual but may occur when performing deep aggressive clamping and ligation of vessels deep in the pelvis near the ischial spine or over the sacrum.

The femoral nerve is located in the iliopsoas groove, well above and well lateral to any operative field for hysterectomy. However, the deep lateral blade of a self-retaining retractor may rest upon the psoas muscle and impinge the femoral nerve against the iliacus muscle which is against the bony backstop of the iliac fossa. Therefore, when placing lateral retractors during the performance of a hysterectomy in a low transverse skin incision, the operator must be sure that the lateral blades of the retractors are not impinging upon the psoas muscle.

During radical hysterectomies and the performance of obturator space lymph node dissections, the obturator nerve may be inadvertently cut. An intraoperative neurosurgical consult is a necessity if this occurs.

## *Intestinal Injury*

Intestinal injury in the operating room is a serious matter. Intra-operative recognition of the problem is essential. A lacerated viscus, whether small or large bowel, should be closed with interrupted nonabsorbable suture. If the injury is extensive and the laceration is long, in some cases a segmental resection and end-to-end anastomosis may be necessary.

## *Hemorrhage*

Bleeding within the pelvis as a result of a hysterectomy may result from injury to the ovarian vessels, uterine vessels, and/or their tributaries. The surgeon can avoid bleeding by careful localization of the site of bleeding, followed by careful ligation of the bleeding vessel. The course of the ureter must always be known. Never use blind clamping. Open the broad ligament and ligate the vessel that is bleeding. If necessary, an internal iliac (hypogastric) artery ligation may be needed to decrease pulse pressure within the pelvis, and thus promote hemostasis.

# Anatomic Complications of Vaginal Hysterectomy and Repair

*The technical difficulties in the vaginal hysterectomy are principally raised by the spatial conceptualization of the normal anatomy in the craniocaudal direction and the topographical modifications from the surgical manipulations.*

*P. Kamina*[51]

Anatomic complications of vaginal hysterectomy include:
- Bleeding (very common)
- Ureteric injury
- Nerve injury
- Intestinal injury
- Bladder injury
- Shortening of the vagina
- Stenosis of the introitus

## *Bleeding*

Bleeding may result from incomplete ligation of the in-

fundibulopelvic ligament around the ovary, or more commonly, from incomplete hemostasis at the level of the vaginal cuff, with a resultant vaginal cuff hematoma.

## *Ureteric Injury*

Ureteric injury is less common in vaginal hysterectomy than in total abdominal hysterectomy, because release of the bladder pillars at the beginning of vaginal hysterectomy allows the ureters to retract superiorly and laterally away from the uterine vessels that will soon be clamped.

Kamina[51] stated that during vaginal hysterectomy, caudal continuous traction of the cervix is imperative to avoid ureteric injury. Caudal and continuous traction makes dissection easier by:
- Breaking the uterus away from its visceral connections
- Individualizing the various ligaments
- Restoring the peritoneum and fornices

## *Nerve Injury*

Nerve injury during the actual performance of vaginal hysterectomy is rare. The few cases of injury to somatic nerves reported during vaginal hysterectomy are due to patient positioning in the dorsolithotomy position.

## *Intestinal Injury*

A lacerated viscus, whether small or large bowel, should be closed with interrupted nonabsorbable suture. If the injury is extensive and the laceration is long, in some cases a segmental resection and end-to-end anastomosis may be necessary. Intestinal injury from adhesion of the rectosigmoid or small bowel to the fundus of the uterus is unusual and very rare.

## *Bladder Injury*

Bladder injury most commonly occurs during attempts to enter the vesicouterine fold in order to enter the anterior cul-de-sac and retract the bladder anteriorly away from the lower uterine segment. In many instances bladder injury is due to prior scarring in this area from a previous cesarean delivery.

## *Shortening of the Vagina*

Shortening of the vagina occurs very rarely but may be due to excessive excision of vaginal cuff epithelium, thus shortening the vagina to below the level of the ischial spines.

We quote from Yamamoto et al.[52]:

*Preservation of the ovaries appeared to be important in preventing vaginal shortening, and post-operative hormone replacement therapy was not as effective as the preservation of the ovaries. The effect of external irradiation on vaginal shortening was not conspicuous in the case[s in which] the ovaries were preserved.*

### Stenosis of the Introitus

Stenosis of the vaginal vault as well as the vaginal introitus is, again, due to excessive excision of vaginal epithelium during the performance of an anterior colporrhaphy or posterior colpoperineorrhaphy. After these procedures, a "three-finger" vaginal introitus is preferred, with the vaginal cuff located just above the level of the ischial spines.

# Vagina

## EMBRYOGENESIS

### Normal Development

The embryogenesis of the vagina is enigmatic. Its genesis may be said to be dual: the upper part of the vagina is of mesodermal origin; the lower part (urogenital sinus) is of endodermal origin.

### Congenital Anomalies

Congenital anomalies of the vagina are associated, in most cases, with uterine and vulvar anomalies. The anomalies of the vagina include embryologic agenesis, imperforate hymen, formation of various septa within the vagina itself, and cysts such as a Gartner's duct cyst or Skene's duct cyst. Primary vaginal adenocarcinoma arising from a metanephric duct remnant has been reported.[53] Asymptomatic cysts do not have to be removed. For further information see Fig. 26-19 and Table 26-5.

## SURGICAL ANATOMY

### Topography and Relations

The vagina is a musculomembranous tube between the bladder anteriorly and the rectum posteriorly (Fig. 26-51). The vagina starts at the vestibule of the vulva and extends posteriorly to the cervix and uterus. The vagina has a configuration of an "H" cleft with the anterior and posterior walls in apposition. Each anterolateral sulcus of the vagina is attached to the fascial white line (arcus tendineus fasciae pelvis) from the sidewall of the pelvis. The vagina is very distensible, obviously, to accommodate the erect male penis during sexual intercourse and to allow for the birth of an infant.

The cervix projects through the upper anterior wall of the vagina. Therefore, the length of the anterior wall of the vagina, from introitus to cervix is approximately 7 cm anteriorly; the length of the posterior wall to the posterior fornix is approximately 9-10 cm.

### Orientation of the Vagina

The following description is presented for the purposes of anatomic orientation. In the normal nulliparous standing female, the bladder, the upper two-thirds of the vagina, and the rectum lie along an almost horizontal axis. The levator plate of the levator ani muscles forms a parallel, horizontal muscular hammock or dynamic back-stop for these viscera. When the upper portion of the vagina is in its normal position, the cervix is found at the level of the ischial spines. The posterior vaginal fornix extends more posteriorly to lie over the coccyx and lower sacrum medially and the sacrospinous ligaments laterally.

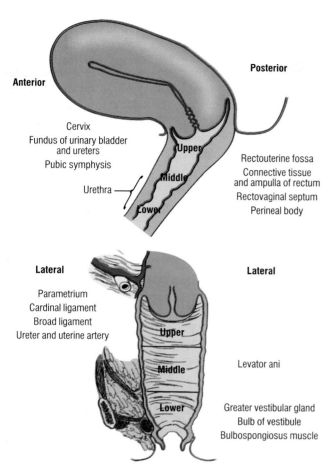

**Fig. 26-51.** Highly diagrammatic representation of the relations of the vagina to several anatomic entities (anteriorly, posteriorly, and laterally).

## Vaginal Support

The supports of the vagina include the:
- Arcus tendineus fasciae pelvis
- Cardinal ligament/uterosacral ligament complex
- Levator ani
- Perineal body
- Pubocervical fascia

### Arcus Tendineus Fasciae Pelvis

The epithelial lining of the vagina is intimately surrounded by a fibromuscular coat, which is thickened anteriorly by the external layer of connective tissue (clinically or surgically named the pubocervical fascia). An oblique band of endopelvic fascia connects each anterolateral sulcus of the vagina to the musculature of the pelvic floor. The arcus tendineus fasciae pelvis, or fascial white line, is a thickening of the parietal fascia over the levator ani mus-

cles which extends from the pubic arch in a straight line to the ischial spine.

Remember, portions of the levator ani, that is, the iliococcygeus muscle and part of the pubococcygeus anteriorly, originate from the arcus tendineus levator ani or muscle white line, which is a thickening of the parietal fascia overlying the obturator internus muscle. This line extends from the lateral posterior aspect of the pubic bone in a curvilinear fashion toward the ischial spine. The muscle white line and the fascial white line usually merge into one white line as they pass posteriorly toward the ischial spine.

### Cardinal Ligament/Uterosacral Ligament Complex

The supports of the vagina include the cardinal ligament/uterosacral ligament complex, which was described with the uterus. These ligaments suspend the upper third of the vagina over the levator plate in order to allow the flap-valve mechanism to come into full effect and thus prevent vaginal prolapse.

### Levator Ani Muscle

In contrast to the horizontal orientation of the bladder, upper vagina, and rectum, the urethra, the distal one-third of the vagina and the anal canal are almost vertical in orientation. These lower structures are supported by the pubococcygeus muscles of the levator hiatus and the structures of the perineum — the perineal body and the anatomic structures of the urogenital and anal triangles. When these normal anatomic relationships are disrupted, physiologic dysfunctions such as urinary and fecal incontinence, and prolapse of the pelvic organs and vagina can ensue.

### Perineal Body

The opening of the vagina is supported by the perineal body. The perineal body is a pyramidal-shaped fibromuscular structure, with the base of the pyramid found between the anus and introitus of the vagina and parallel with the floor in the standing female patient. The apex of the pyramid is located between the lower third and the middle third of the vagina, at the point where the vagina turns from its vertical orientation into its almost horizontal orientation. Supporting structures that stabilize the perineal body include the pubococcygeus muscles, the transverse perinei muscles, and the perineal membrane.

### Pubocervical Fascia

"Pubocervical fascia" is simply a clinical/surgical term for the thickened anterior portion of the fibromuscular coat that surrounds the vaginal epithelium. The pubocervical fascia extends from underneath the urethra, laterally to the fascial white lines, and posteriorly to the pericervical ring of endopelvic fascia around the cervix. The cardinal ligament/uterosacral ligament complex from each side inserts into the same pericervical fascia. The pubocervical fascia is a horizontal hammock upon which the bladder rests.

The purpose of the intact pubocervical fascia is to prevent cystocele. Dr. A. Cullen Richardson of Atlanta (personal communication, 1989) has observed that approximately 85% of cystoceles result from a tearing away of the pubocervical fascia from one or both fascial white lines. This constitutes the "paravaginal defect."

Zacharin[54] stated that the levator ani complex and pelvic cellular tissues must be restored in patients with pulsion enterocele.

## Vascular Supply

### Arteries

The internal iliac artery and its several branches are responsible for the rich blood supply of the vagina.

The upper part of the vagina is supplied by branches from the uterine artery (see Fig. 26-6).

The middle part of the vagina is supplied by multiple branches from the vaginal artery, with some anastomoses with branches from the middle rectal arteries. These anastomoses form two longitudinal vessels anterior and posterior — the azygos arteries of the vagina.

The lower part of the vagina is fed by branches of the vaginal artery and from the artery of the bulb of the vestibule, a branch from the perineal artery from the pudendal artery.

### Veins

The vaginal venous blood returns to the vaginal venous plexus and then to the uterine, as well as to the vesical, plexuses. All this venous blood eventually drains into the internal iliac (hypogastric) veins.

### Lymphatics

The upper part of the vagina contains lymphatic vessels that follow the uterine artery and drain into the external and internal iliac lymph nodes (see Fig. 26-40). The middle portion of the vagina contains lymphatic vessels that follow the vaginal artery and drain into the internal iliac nodes.

The lymph from the lower part of the vagina drains to the sacral and common iliac nodes. The introitus of the vagina or hymenal area drains to the superficial inguinal nodes.

## Innervation

The uterovaginal plexus is responsible for the innervation of the vagina (see Fig. 26-42). The uterovaginal plexus, which is derived from the inferior hypogastric plexus, contains autonomic fibers for the muscular coat of smooth muscle of the vagina. Some vasomotor fibers exist here also; however, there is no vaginal sensation except in the most distal part, which is innervated by pudendal nerve branches.

## HISTOLOGY

The vaginal wall is formed by three layers:
- Innermost (epithelium — often inaccurately called mucosa)
- Intermediate (connective tissue and smooth muscle fibers)
- External (superficial muscular coat)

## Epithelial Layer (Vaginal Mucosa)

The innermost layer is covered by stratified squamous epithelium. Its appearance is dominated by hormonal influences, responding with cyclic changes. Both anterior and posterior vaginal mucosa possess longitudinal ridges (columns of vagina) and several transverse ridges.

## Intermediate Layer

The intermediate tissue between the mucosal and muscular layers consists of connective tissue investing a rich venous network as well as smooth muscle fibers originating from the muscular layer.

## External Muscular Coat

The muscular layer is of smooth muscle origin. It consists of two layers, one external longitudinal and the other circular. At its distal, most narrow end, the vagina is surrounded by the striated bulbospongiosus muscles.

The vagina may be envisioned most simply as a hollow fibromuscular tube that is lined on the inside by stratified squamous epithelium. There are no mucosal glands in this epithelium. Lubrication of the vagina during sexual excitement occurs as a result of transudation of serosanguinous fluid from the surrounding venous engorgement. The vaginal epithelium is hormonally manipulated, having cyclic changes. Both the anterior and posterior vaginal epithelium demonstrate longitudinal ridges. These ridges are formed of elastin found in the fibromuscular coat surrounding the epithelium. Loss of these longitudinal ridges is an indication of breaks within the pubocervical fascia (fibromuscular coat around the vagina).

## PHYSIOLOGY

The physiological destiny of the vagina is threefold:
- Organ of copulation
- Birth canal
- Tube for the excretions of uterus, menstrual period, etc.

Details of the vasocongestive and orgasmic reflex are not within the scope of this chapter.

## ANATOMY OF THE VAGINAL EXAMINATION

The vaginal examination is accomplished by inspection and by bimanual examination. Inspection includes visualization of the vulva and surrounding cutaneous areas for pathologic processes such as condylomata, infection of the Bartholin's glands, imperforate hymen, prolapse of urethral mucosa, or dermatitis.

With the insertion of the speculum into the vagina, the vaginal epithelium can be evaluated for discharges, leukoplakia, cystoceles, prolapse, or rectoceles. Visualization of the cervix and subsequent Pap smear allows cytological examination of the cervix.

A bimanual gynecologic examination allows the physician to evaluate the vaginal introitus, to determine the character or texture of the vaginal epithelium, to detect support defects in and surrounding the vagina, and to palpate the uterus, tubes, ovaries, and any other pelvic mass. The urethra, urinary bladder, and pubic symphysis can be felt anteriorly. Apically, evaluation of cervical and uterine support and the presence of vaginal prolapse and/or cul-de-sac hernia can be determined. Posteriorly, support to the rectum can be evaluated, particularly with a rectovaginal examination.

A rectal examination at this time will also allow the examiner to obtain a small sample of stool which can then be tested for the presence of occult blood. Bimanual examination also allows the practitioner to feel the midplane and outlet of the bony pelvis to evaluate the size of the pelvis in relation to childbearing.

Inspection of the vaginal introitus may include a measurement of the vaginal outlet, which is normally 4 to 6 cm in length in multiparous women. A gaping vaginal introitus points to the disruption of the superficial perineal muscles and detachment of the lower one-third of the vagina from the perineal body. The perineal body itself should not demonstrate an excursion of more than 1 cm upon palpation. A relaxed vaginal outlet with a disrupted perineal body indicates a damaged pelvic floor.

After disassembling a Graves bivalve speculum and placing the lower half in the vagina, the examiner may then assess the anterior, apical, and posterior vaginal walls for defects (Fig. 26-52A). The posterior vaginal wall may be depressed in order to inspect the anterior vaginal wall. Loss of anterior wall support indicates the development of a cystocele (Fig. 26-52B, Fig. 26-53). Lateral tears or paravaginal defects can be diagnosed by both inspection and palpation of the vagina.

A ring forceps can be placed gently along the lateral vaginal sulci from the vaginal introitus to the level of the ischial spines. This maneuver reapproximates the pubocervical fascia to the fascial white lines. If the cystocele is due to a lateral or paravaginal defect, the cystocele will disappear. If the bulging cystocele does not disappear with this maneuver, then a midline, or perhaps a transverse, cervical break in the pubocervical fascia is diagnosed. During vaginal palpation, the ischial spine and fascial white line can be felt laterally on each side.

With the lower half of the Graves speculum rotated 180° to support the anterior vaginal wall, the examiner can assess weakness in the posterior vaginal wall or the presence of a rectocele. A rectocele results from a break in the rectovaginal septum, usually being torn from the perineal body. The rectovaginal septum is a separate sheet of endopelvic fascia between the vagina anteriorly and the rectum posteriorly. An intact rectovaginal septum is of great importance in the prevention of rectocele and enterocele formation. A rectovaginal examination in many cases allows the examiner to palpate the rectovaginal septum. This allows for identification of the site of an endopelvic fascial break allowing the formation of the rectocele.

The rectovaginal exam also allows the examiner to assess the integrity of the perineal body. At this time, there is no universally used system for defining and describing the severity of pelvic floor defects such as cystocele, enterocele, and rectocele, though a formal system has been recommended.[55]

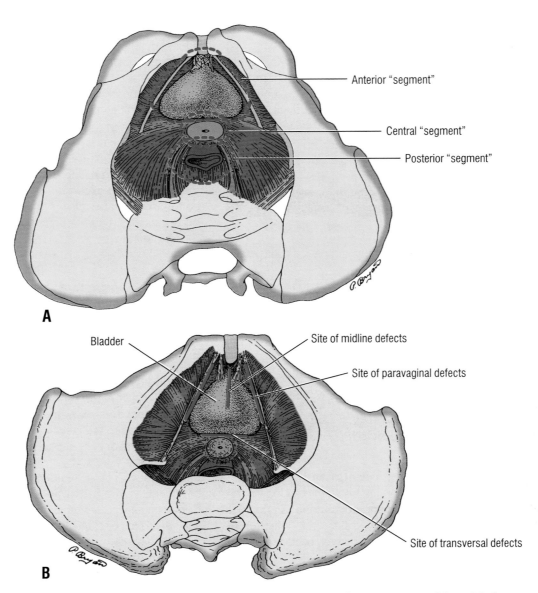

FIG. 26-52. Sites of pelvic support defects. **A,** Defects in the pelvic supports may occur in three different segments of the pelvic floor: anterior, central, and posterior. **B,** A cystocele can result from any break in the continuity of the pubocervical fascial, hammocklike supports of the bladder. The three sites of possible defects are indicated. The paravaginal break is the most common, accounting for about 85 percent of all cystoceles and urethroceles. (Modified from Skandalakis LJ, Gadacz TR, Mansberger AR Jr, Mitchell WE, Jr., Colborn GL, Skandalakis JE. Modern Hernia Repair: The Embryological and Anatomical Basis of Surgery, revised 2nd ed. New York: Parthenon, 1996. Plate 2-27; with permission.)

Palpation of the vagina should be performed with the patient both at rest and during straining. An enterocele is manifested as a bulging of the apical portion of the vagina during straining. This usually indicates a break in the attachment of the rectovaginal septum with the uterosacral ligaments.[56]

Cervical support should also be evaluated during the vaginal examination. The cervix is suspended over the levator plate by the two cardinal-uterosacral ligament complexes. If these structures are intact, the cervix has very little lateral movement. Though pelvic examinations are traditionally done in the dorsolithotomy position in the United States, occasionally pelvic floor defects are not readily apparent until the patient is examined in the standing position.[57]

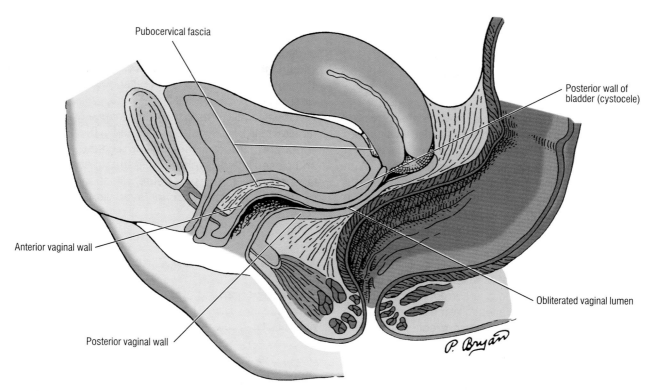

**FIG. 26-53.** Diagrammatic sketch showing the pubocervical fascia separated from its attachment into the pericervical ring. Note that the bladder is covered only by vaginal mucosa over the cystocele. (Modified from Skandalakis LJ, Gadacz TR, Mansberger AR Jr, Mitchell WE Jr, Colborn GL, Skandalakis JE. Modern Hernia Repair: The Embryological and Anatomical Basis of Surgery, revised 2nd ed. New York: Parthenon, 1996. Plate 2-30; with permission.)

## SURGICAL APPLICATIONS

- A patient voiding normally but also experiencing constant urinary leakage should be evaluated for ureterovaginal or vesicovaginal fistula.
- Ridley[58] advised repair of vesicovaginal fistula by closure of the bladder in two layers, with closure of the vaginal mucosa as a third layer.

## ANATOMIC COMPLICATIONS OF ANTERIOR AND POSTERIOR COLPORRHAPHY

Possible complications involved with the performance of anterior and posterior colporrhaphies to repair cystoceles and rectoceles of the vagina include:
- Bleeding

- Urethral injury
- Bladder injury
- Ureteric injury
- Intestinal injury
- Vaginal strictures
- Dyspareunia

### Bleeding

The vaginal wall has an extremely rich blood supply, particularly laterally. Avascular surgical planes such as in the vesicovaginal space and the rectovaginal space are very important to identify and use surgically.

### Urethral Injury

Urethral injury may take place during dissection in performing anterior colporrhaphy. Because the vaginal wall envelops the distal urethra, too vigorous a dissection may produce injury or scarring to the urethra. Overmobilization of the urethra will disrupt its nerve and blood supply. Resulting fibrosis and urethral dysfunction may ensue.

## Bladder Injury

Aggressive dissection in the vesicovaginal space may result in an inadvertent entry into the bladder. It is important that this be recognized as soon as possible so that ureteric function can be assessed via cystoscopy. With knowledge that the ureters are not involved in the bladder injury, the injury site may then be closed with a running 2-0 absorbable suture and then imbricated with interrupted 2-0 absorbable suture, exercising care to avoid damage to the ureters in the process.

The bladder should be drained with a Foley catheter for approximately a week postoperatively. Hurt and Dunn[59] stated: "[I]t is important not to overcorrect the cystocele." The good surgeon should always remember that "the enemy of good is better." Moderate correction, not overcorrection, of a cystocele is important. Preservation of the posterior ureterovesical angle is important in avoiding postoperative anatomic genuine stress urinary incontinence.

## Ureteric Injury

Ureteric injury can occur during aggressive lateral dissection during anterior colporrhaphy or performance of a vaginal paravaginal defect repair. In some techniques of anterior colporrhaphy, ureteric occlusion can also occur during wide plication of the bladder to correct a midline cystocele.

## Intestinal Injury

During the performance of a posterior colporrhaphy to repair a rectocele, the operator may lacerate or perforate the anterior rectal wall, or even damage the sphincteric apparatus of the surgical anal canal. Again, such lacerations should be repaired in two layers with absorbable sutures. The sphincters of the anal canal should also be repaired when seen.

Occasionally during the performance of an enterocele repair, small bowel may be lacerated in the cul-de-sac. It is important that such lacerations be recognized immediately and closed with 2 layers of 2-0 permanent suture: the first layer of bowel (mucosa) closure with absorbable (chromic or Vicryl), and the second layer with nonabsorbable sutures.

## Vaginal Strictures

When performing reparative vaginal surgery, the surgeon must be careful not to excise too much of the vaginal epithelium. Vigorous excision of "excess" vaginal epithelium may very well lead to a short vagina with narrow diameter. It is recommended that the patient leave the operating room with her vagina three fingers in diameter (approximately 4 cm), with a length approximately at or superior to the level of the ischial spines.

## Dyspareunia

A narrow, shortened vagina may certainly lead to dyspareunia. According to Hurt and Dunn,[59] "The construction of a high perineum is of no advantage to the patient and is often the cause of dyspareunia."

While Weber et al.[60] found that the combination of Burch colposuspension and posterior colporrhaphy was especially likely to result in dyspareunia, they reported that sexual function and satisfaction improved or did not change in most women following surgery for prolapse and/or urinary incontinence.

# Female Urethra

## EMBRYOGENESIS

### Normal Development

The endoderm is responsible for the epithelium of the urethra. The splanchnic mesoderm is responsible for the surrounding smooth muscles and connective tissue.

### Congenital Anomalies

Absence of the urethra may be congenital. This deformity occurs secondary to complete hypospadias.

## SURGICAL ANATOMY

The female urethra (Fig. 26-38, Fig. 26-54) will be considered in this chapter for surgical purposes only.

### Topography and Relations

The length of the female urethra is approximately 4 cm, but is extremely variable. Its diameter is about 6 mm, and it can be dilated up to 1 cm with ease. It extends from the neck of the bladder to the external urethral orifice, which is located between the labia minora, anterior to the vaginal opening, and approximately 2.5 cm below the glans clitoris.

The female urethra is oriented almost vertically in the standing patient. It is fused with the anterior vaginal wall and also with the symphysis pubis by the perineal membrane.

O'Connell et al.[61] performed detailed dissection on 2 fresh and 8 fixed human female cadavers ranging in age from 22 to 88. They wrote:

> The female urethra, distal vaginal wall and erectile tissue are packed into the perineum caudal (superficial) to the pubic arch, which is bounded laterally by the ischiopubic rami, and superficially by the labia minora and majora. This complex is not flat against the rami as is commonly depicted but projects from the bony landmarks for 3 to 6 cm. The perineal urethra is embedded in the anterior vaginal wall and is surrounded by erectile tissue in all directions except posteriorly where it relates to the vaginal wall. The bulbs of the vestibule are inappropriately named as they directly relate to the other clitoral components and the urethra. Their association with the vestibule is inconsistent and, thus, we recommend that these structures be renamed the bulbs of the clitoris.

O'Connell et al.[61] concluded that the dissections "suggest that current anatomical descriptions of female human urethral and genital anatomy are inaccurate."

### Female Continence Mechanism

Tanagho[62] wisely stated that the female urethra represents the entire sphincteric mechanism of the urinary bladder in the female. Its two muscular layers (inner longitudinal and outer semicircular) form the sphincteric urethral apparatus in continuation with the detrusor muscle of the urinary bladder. This sphincteric apparatus is more obvious at the middle one-third, according to Tanagho,[62] because of the formation of an incomplete ring posteriorly where the arms of the ring travel laterally and fuse to the urethrovaginal septum.

Siracusano et al.[63] reported that the following elements contribute to the maintenance of continence:
- Maximum urethral closure pressure
- Anatomic and functional length of urethra
- Ability of perineum to increase the urethral pressure simultaneously with the Valsalva maneuver
- Appropriate location of the sphincteric unit

We are grateful to Drs. Sandra S. Retzky and Robert M. Rogers Jr. for permission to quote the following material on urinary incontinence in women:[57]

> The continence mechanism in women centers on the proximal urethra and urethrovesical (U-V) junction. Continence is maintained by multiple structural and physiologic mechanisms that regulate closure of

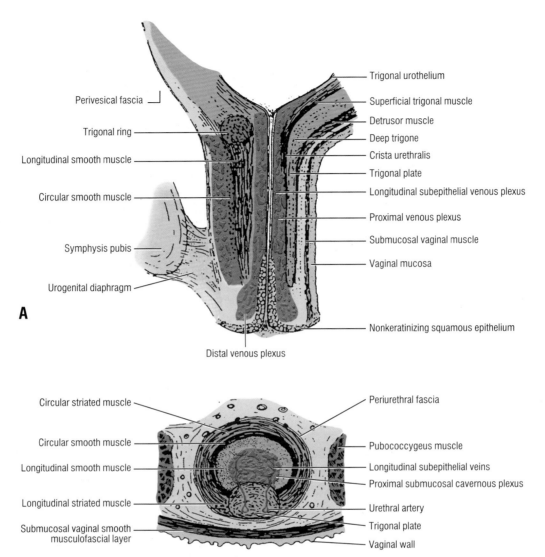

**FIG. 26-54.** Anatomy of the urethra. **A,** Sagittal section. **B,** Cross section. (Modified from Lentz GM. Urogynecology. London: Arnold [a member of Hodder Headline Group. Co-published by Oxford University Press Inc, New York], 2000; with permission.)

*the urethra and support of the bladder and urethrovesical junction. Actual closure of the urethra is produced by three different systems: the involuntary internal sphincter at the vesical neck, the voluntary external sphincter muscles of the urethra, and mucosal coaptation produced by the urethral submucosal vascular plexus. Anatomic support for these structures primarily comes from a fascial layer, the pubocervical fascia, which is attached to the levator ani muscles of the pelvic floor.*

### Internal Sphincter

Located at the urethrovesical junction, the internal

sphincter (Fig. 26-55) is formed by a ring of involuntary smooth muscle from the bladder trigone and two U-shaped loops of smooth muscle derived from the detrusor (bladder) muscle. The trigone, located at the bladder base, is composed of specialized smooth muscle that is histologically distinct from the rest of the bladder. The trigonal musculature (ring) encircles the urethral lumen at the urethrovesical junction. Below the trigonal ring, the detrusor loops open in opposite directions. The more prominent loop (loop of Heiss) passes in front of the internal urethral meatus and opens posteriorly. The second, smaller loop passes under the trigone and opens anteriorly. The proximal urethra passes between these two loops.

The muscles of the internal sphincter are innervated by

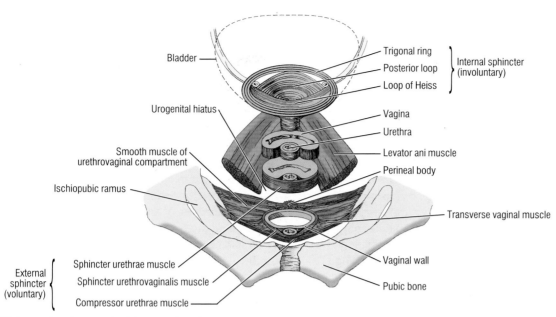

Bladder

Urogenital hiatus

Smooth muscle of
urethrovaginal compartment

Ischiopubic ramus

Trigonal ring
Posterior loop          } Internal sphincter
Loop of Heiss           } (involuntary)

Vagina
Urethra
Levator ani muscle
Perineal body

Transverse vaginal muscle

External
sphincter {
(voluntary) {

Sphincter urethrae muscle
Sphincter urethrovaginalis muscle
Compressor urethrae muscle

Vaginal wall
Pubic bone

**FIG. 26-55.** Internal and external sphincters of the female urethra.

autonomic fibers. Continuous contraction of the trigonal ring and detrusor loop mechanism is important for maintaining continence at rest. Conditions that affect pudendal nerve function (childbirth injury, prior antiincontinence procedures, myelodysplasia) can damage the internal sphincter and lead to urinary incontinence even when support for this area is normal.

### *External Sphincter*

The second system of urethral closure comprises three small skeletal muscles that envelop the urethra below the level of the internal sphincter. The most proximal and largest of these muscles is the urethral sphincter muscle (sphincter urethrae) (Fig. 26-55, Fig. 26-56). It almost com-

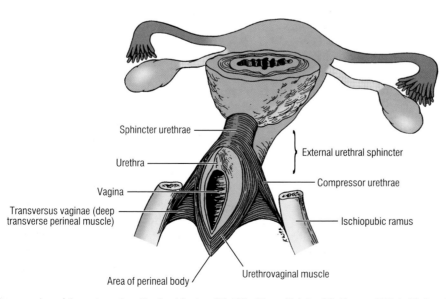

Sphincter urethrae

Urethra

Vagina

Transversus vaginae (deep
transverse perineal muscle)

Area of perineal body

External urethral sphincter
}

Compressor urethrae

Ischiopubic ramus

Urethrovaginal muscle

**FIG. 26-56.** The muscles of the external urethral sphincter. (Modified from Retzky SS, Rogers RM Jr, Richardson AC. Anatomy of Female Pelvic Support. In: Brubaker LT, Saclarides TJ (eds). The Female Pelvic Floor: Disorders of Function and Support. Philadelphia: FA Davis, 1996; with permission.)

pletely encircles the upper portion of the urethra, except posteriorly where the inferior extension of the trigone fills the gap. The compressor urethrae and urethrovaginal muscles form the distal portion of the external urethral sphincter. The urethrovaginal muscle wraps around the distal portion of the urethra and vagina, inserting into the perineal body. The compressor urethrae muscles originate from the medial surfaces of the ischiopubic rami, overlap the urethrovaginal muscle, and course over the anterior surface of the urethra. Both of these muscles act as sphincters of the vagina as well as of the urethra. They are located just above the perineal membrane in the deep compartment of the urogenital triangle in the perineum.

The delicate muscles of the external sphincter act as a unit. They contract voluntarily and prevent incontinence if urine gets past a marginally functioning internal sphincter. The resting tone of the external sphincter muscles also contributes to the pressure inside the urethral lumen. An intraurethral pressure higher than bladder pressure helps maintain continence. Like the internal sphincter, the external sphincter is innervated by fibers from the pudendal nerve and is subject to damage from childbirth injuries and surgery.

## Mucosal Coaptation

In addition to the internal and external sphincters, the submucosal vasculature of the urethra is considered to be a part of the continence mechanism. This arteriovenous complex is located between the smooth muscle coat of the urethra and its epithelial lining. Filling of this vasculature with blood improves mucosal coaptation by causing the urethral walls to seal, thus increasing urethral resting pressure and preventing involuntary urine loss. The submucosal plexus and epithelium of the urethra are estrogen-sensitive; during menopause, hormone replacement therapy can improve blood flow to this area.

## Endopelvic Fascia

The following material on the endopelvic fascia and muscles of the pelvic floor is based on a chapter written by Retzky, Rogers, and Richardson.[2] We recommend the chapter to the reader.

In the normal, nulliparous standing woman, the bladder, proximal two-thirds of the vagina, and rectum lie in an almost horizontal axis. In contrast, the urethra, distal one-third of the vagina, and anal canal are oriented almost vertically. Support for the vesical neck, proximal urethra, and vagina is absolutely critical for female continence. The pelvic element most responsible for maintaining normal relationships between the structures of the lower urinary

tract is the endopelvic fascia.

Microscopically, endopelvic fascia is a three-dimensional meshwork of collagen, elastin, and smooth muscle. This matrix surrounds and supports the viscera in both the abdominal and pelvic cavities and extends from the pelvic floor to the respiratory diaphragm. Endopelvic fascia is histologically and functionally different from parietal fascia, which covers the skeletal musculature of the pelvic floor. Endopelvic fascia is a latticework of tissue that encapsulates, suspends, and anchors these organs in a central position. Normal function of the pelvic organs is, to a great extent, position-dependent.

The specific area of endopelvic fascia important for urethrovesical junction support is the pubocervical fascia, or paravaginal tissue. Pubocervical fascia, a sheet of thick fibrous tissue, is located on the vagina underneath the bladder. Pubocervical fascia is anterior vaginal fascia that fuses with vaginal skin, providing a hammock (or sling) for the urethra and bladder. Proximally, the pubocervical fascia attaches to the cervix; distally, it travels beneath the urethra and fuses with the perineal membrane of the urogenital triangle; and laterally, it is connected to the pelvic wall at the fascial white line (arcus tendineus fasciae pelvis). The fascial white line is a linear thickening of the parietal fascia of the levator ani muscles. The fascial white line extends from the ischial spine to the posterior aspect of the pubic bone and forms the lateral support for the bladder, vagina, and rectum.

The pubocervical fascia forms the horizontal platform that supports the bladder, and its anterior portion supports the urethra. The proximal urethra and urethrovesical junction are almost vertical and held in close proximity to the posterior aspect of the pubic symphysis. With increased abdominal pressure, the lower urinary tract is forced inferiorly and compressed against the pubocervical fascia. This urethrovesical junction "trapping" promotes continence.

## Muscles of the Pelvic Floor

The levator ani muscles assist in maintaining the proper position of the urethrovesical junction and urethra within the pelvis. They do so through their attachments to the pubocervical fascia at the fascial white lines. The levator ani muscles include the pubococcygeus and iliococcygeus muscles and are part of the pelvic floor. The levator muscles are dually innervated by motor efferents from S2-S4 on their pelvic surface and by branches of the pudendal nerve on their perineal surface.

The terms "pelvic floor" or "pelvic diaphragm" refer to all the muscular components that close the pelvic cavity and their respective parietal fascial coverings. Unlike striated muscles in other areas of the body, the muscles of the pelvic floor, including the coccygeus muscles, are in a constant state of contraction, which allows for the efficient positioning of the urethrovesical junction.

Remember: Multiple structures and physiologic mechanisms ensure continence in women. The primary mechanism of continence is produced by loops of specialized detrusor muscle at the internal urethral sphincter. The urethra, resting on a hammock of connective tissue called the pubocervical fascia, is held in a position that prevents rotational descent into the vagina. Therefore, increases in intraabdominal pressure compress the anterior urethral wall against the posterior urethral wall, which is fixed against the pubocervical fascial backstop. This action adds additional closing pressure to that generated by the internal sphincter mechanism. To further secure urinary continence, the external sphincter mechanism closes the middle portion of the urethra. The submucosal plexus plays a role in the prevention of leakage by sustaining urethral pressure. Usually, incontinence becomes clinically apparent only when multiple failures of these systems take place.

Interesting material on the urethra, urogenital sphincter, and continence can be found in the writings of Oelrich[64] and DeLancey.[65,66]

## Vascular Supply

### Arteries

The inferior vesical artery is responsible for the blood supply of the proximal urethra. The uterine artery and inferior vesical artery supply the middle part of the urethra. The distal portion is supplied by the internal pudendal artery.

### Veins

Venous blood returns into the vesical plexus and also the internal pudendal vein.

### Lymphatics

The urethral lymphatics follow the pathway of the internal pudendal artery. The majority drain into the internal iliac nodes, with some draining into the external iliac nodes.

## Innervation

Somatic and autonomic nerve fibers innervate the female urethra: the somatic by the pudendal nerve for stri-

ated muscle, and the autonomic by parasympathetic fibers.[62]

## HISTOLOGY

The wall of the female urethra is formed by 3 principal layers with a rich vascular submucosa: the muscular layer described above, a transitional mucosal layer proximally, and a stratified squamous layer distally.

According to Stothers et al.,[67] the three walls of the female urethra can be well demonstrated with MRI.

After studying 50 male and 15 female cadavers, Rother et al.[68] stated that the volume of muscle cells and fibers in male and female urethral sphincter muscles decreases with age, beginning in early childhood.

## PHYSIOLOGY

Four mechanisms affect female urinary continence at the level of the urethra: 1) the involuntary smooth muscle of the internal sphincter at the urethrovesical junction; 2) the voluntary skeletal muscle that comprises the external urethral sphincter; 3) the rich vascular network forming the submucosal seal surrounding the urothelium; and 4) the "flap-valve" mechanism of the "hammock hypothesis" of DeLancey.[66]

The internal sphincter is primarily under the control of the sympathetic nervous system and alpha-adrenergic receptors, with norepinephrine being the chief neurotransmitter. The external urethral sphincter has innervation from both the pudendal nerve and pelvic plexus of nerves. Aggressive surgical dissection around the urethra can denervate the urethra and weaken its ability to hold back urine. The submucosal vascular seal generates approximately one-third of the total urethral closing pressure. This mucosal seal has a high concentration of estrogen receptors and is definitely affected by estrogen. The attachment of the "hammock" of pubocervical fascia underneath the urethrovesical junction from its lateral attachment to one or both "fascial white lines" allows intrapelvic pressure to compress the urethra against the backstop of pubocervical fascia. The purpose of a retropubic urethropexy or sling procedure is to reestablish this backstop in order to allow the "flap-valve" mechanism to come into full play.

## SURGICAL APPLICATIONS

- Each surgical approach to the female urethra should be tailored to the local pathology and the final diagnosis.
- Repositioning of the vesical neck and proximal urethra is the goal of surgery to relieve urinary stress incontinence.
- A cystocele or enterocele must be corrected if present.
- Ridley[58] advocated the following approaches for treating urinary stress incontinence:
  - Plication of the paraurethral and bladder neck tissues
  - Sling procedures with application of various materials beneath the posterior urethra and bladder neck
  - Repositioning of the bladder next to the urethra in the retropubic area
  - Combining the above procedures

## ANATOMIC COMPLICATIONS OF FEMALE URETHRAL SURGERY

Bredael et al.[69] stated that injury of the female urethra is rare with pelvic fractures.

Ridley[58] listed the following anatomic complications of female urethral surgery:

- Overcorrection or partial obstruction of the urethra by plication
- Overcorrection or formation of a posterior urethrovesical angle by the sling or retropubic fixation
- Undercorrection of the urethra and bladder weakness by insufficiency of plication, tension on the sling, or retropubic fixation
- Injury to the bladder neck during placement of the sling.
  Remember to avoid sling tension, but do not place the sling loosely.
- Absence of the urethra from surgical or obstetrical errors.[70]

If bleeding or urethral or bladder injury occurs, the wound should be drained suprapubicly.

# *Vulva*

## EMBRYOGENESIS

### Normal development

The urogenital folds form the labia minora. They do not fuse except at the caudal ends, which form the frenulum of the labia minora.

The labial folds fuse anteriorly to form the mons pubis and the anterior labial commissure; they fuse posteriorly to form the posterior labial commissure. The unfused portions of the labial folds form the labia majora.

In the female, the phallus becomes the clitoris.

### Congenital Anomalies

The anomalies of the vulva are the anomalies of the anatomic entities forming this region (see Table 26-5).

## SURGICAL ANATOMY

### Topography and Relations

The term "vulva" is essentially equivalent to the urogenital region of the perineum. The following anatomic entities collectively form the vulva (Fig. 26-57):

- Mons pubis (mons veneris)
- Labia majora
- Labia minora
- Clitoris
- Vestibule and its related entities

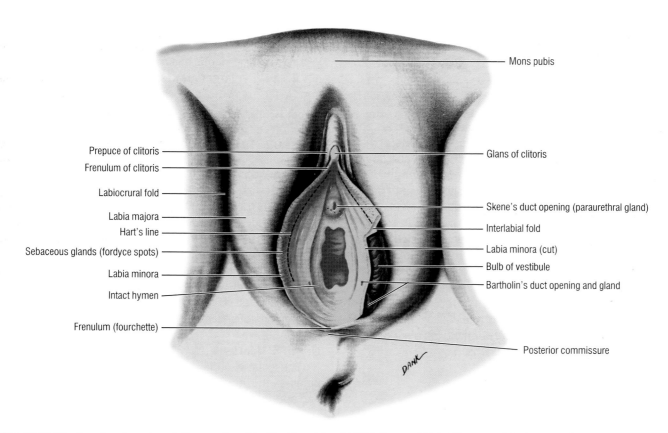

Mons pubis

Prepuce of clitoris

Frenulum of clitoris

Labiocrural fold

Labia majora

Hart's line

Sebaceous glands (fordyce spots)

Labia minora

Intact hymen

Frenulum (fourchette)

Glans of clitoris

Skene's duct opening (paraurethral gland)

Interlabial fold

Labia minora (cut)

Bulb of vestibule

Bartholin's duct opening and gland

Posterior commissure

**FIG. 26-57.** The female external genitalia, or vulva. (Modified from Tovell HMM, Young AW Jr. Diseases of the Vulva in Clinical Practice. New York: Elsevier Science Publishing Co., 1991; with permission.)

## *Mons Pubis (Mons Veneris)*

In Latin, *mons* means "a hill;" *veneris* originates from the name Venus, the Roman goddess of love. The ancient Greeks called this anatomic area the Hill of Aphrodite (the Greek goddess of love). It consists of fibrofatty tissue (mostly fat) and forms a cushion, resting upon the anterior surface of the symphysis pubis like a dome.

After puberty this area is covered by coarse hair which is said to be different in females and males. It is said that the upper end of the hair pattern in the female is limited in a horizontal fashion, whereas the pubic hair of the male extends upward toward the navel, although this upward extension of the hair is more similar to that elsewhere on the body, not possessing the character of pubic hair. The student occasionally will see the term "escutcheon" applied to this trigonic hairy area. *Escutcheon,* a word which means shield, comes from the old French or Latin scutum.

## *Labia Majora*

The labia majora, the analogues of the scrotum, are prominent folds on each side of the mons veneris. They form the boundaries of the pudendal cleft, into which the urethra and vagina open. In front, the right and left labia majora unite and form the so-called anterior commissure. The labia majora gradually terminate near the center of the perineum, but occasionally their posterior ends unite to form the posterior commissure, just posterior to the fourchette.

Each labium majus is formed by fibrofatty tissue that is covered by pigmented skin, with typically stiff pubic hair and possessing sebaceous follicles. The internal surface of the labia majora is smooth and without hair. The round ligaments of the uterus may often be traced from the external ring of the inguinal canal to the more proximal, or superior, part of each labium.

The so-called posterior commissure is not usually a union of the labia, but a projection of the perineal body into the pudendal cleft. In extremely rare cases, a foldlike union takes place just behind the fourchette.

The contents of the labia majora are:
- Round ligament (partial)
- Fibrofatty tissue
- Multiple blood vessels
- Smooth muscle fibers similar to the dartos muscle of the male

- Cutaneous nerves
- Lymphatics

## *Labia Minora*

The labia minora are the analogues of the corpus spongiosum of the male. The labium minus is a bilateral, hairless, pinkish fold, thin and flat, of variable size and shape. The labia minora are approximately 4 cm in length. They are covered by stratified squamous epithelium and have a very rich network of nerves. Sebaceous follicles are numerous on the apposing surfaces.

At their posterior ends, the labia minora may unite with the labia majora or the two minora may be joined by a transverse fold, the fourchette or frenulum, seen more commonly in virgins. The labia minora bifurcate anteriorly. The lateral parts unite and form the prepuce; the medial parts unite and form the frenulum of clitoris. Gottlicher[71] found a third labium located between the labia majora and labia minora in 5.3% of 1180 patients.

## *Clitoris*

The clitoris is the analogue of the male penis without the urethra. The clitoris consists of two crura, the corpus, and the glans. The two crura arise from the bony pelvis; specifically, from the internal surface of the ischiopubic rami, anterior to the ischial tuberosities. Both fuse together approximately at the middle of the pubic arch to form the body, which bends acutely downward and backward. It is fixed to the symphysis pubis by the suspensory ligament of clitoris.

The shaft of the clitoris is formed almost entirely by the junction and fusion of the bilateral corpora cavernosa, which arise from the ischiopubic rami as crura. The crura are covered by the ischiocavernosus muscles, which contract in clitoral erection.

The two corpora are encased in tough fibrous connective tissue and separated by a midline connective tissue septum. The corpus spongiosum of the pendulous part of the male penis does not exist as a counterpart in the female. However, in its place, there are two slender, cord-like structures of erectile tissue which are extensions of the vestibular bulbs into the shaft of the clitoris, wherein they fuse at a commissure, thereafter terminating at the glans clitoris.

The lower, spongy end of the clitoris is slightly enlarged to form the glans clitoris. It is innervated profusely by the terminal branches of the dorsal clitoral nerves, the terminal branches of the pudendal nerves, and is exquisitely sensi-

tive. It, and the lower part of the clitoral shaft, are normally covered by the prepuce provided by the labia minora. When erect, the clitoris has a length of 1-2.5 cm; occasionally it is very enlarged. Barrett and Gonzales[72] and Ansell and Rajfer[73] reported successful reduction clitoroplasties.

## *Vestibule And Its Related Entities*

According to Woodruff and Friedrich,[74] the vestibule is "a 'collision zone' formed at the junction of different germ layers." It is an opening between the right and left labia minora, extending from the clitoris to the fourchette. Between the vaginal orifice and the fourchette is the vestibular fossa.

The vestibule is perforated by several openings:
- Opening of the urethra
- Opening of the vagina
- Right and left ducts of the glands of Bartholin
- Openings of several other ducts (Skene's, etc)[75]

### Urethral Meatus
The external urethral meatus, or opening (Fig. 26-38), is between the labia minora, anterior to the vaginal opening, and approximately 2.5 cm below the glans clitoris.

### Opening of the Vagina
The opening of the vagina is a posterior midline cleft with variable appearance due to the variable morphology of the hymen.

### Major Vestibular Glands
The major vestibular glands, homologous to the male bulbourethral glands of Cowper, are the glands of Bartholin. They are round or ovoid, the size of a pea or small bean. They are located on either side of the vaginal opening beneath the bulb of the vestibule. The opening of each duct is located between the hymen and the labia minora at the sides of the vestibule, opening at about the 5 o'clock and 7 o'clock positions of the vestibule. During coitus they secrete a small amount of mucus to lubricate the distal vagina.

Sarrel et al.[76] reported 4 patients with pain during intercourse due to Bartholin gland pathology. They performed removal of the gland in 3 cases and marsupialization in 1 case with good results.

### Minor Vestibular Glands
There are also several other mucous glands. The glands of Skene have ducts opening at the upper portion of the vestibule, lateral to the urethral orifice,[75] and into the urethra. These glands may be divided into upper and lower parts as they are related to the urethra. The lower ones

open into the vestibule and are identified as paraurethral glands. The upper ones open into the urethra and are known as periurethral glands.

The periurethral glands are considered by some to be the homologues of the prostate. Others, however, disagree. Tepper et al.,[77] for instance, reported that the female paraurethral Skene's glands are homologues of the prostate. These authors stated that 83% were positive for prostate-specific antigen and 67% for prostate-specific acid phosphatase.

Major and minor vestibular glands may suffer infection and become abscessed. Treatment starts with incision and drainage; later, the recurrent cyst may be marsupialized or excised completely.

## *Vestibular Bulbs*

The vestibular bulbs, erectile tissue homologues of the penile bulb, consist of erectile tissue on each side of the opening of the vagina, and are covered by the bulbospongiosus muscles. Approximately 3 cm in length, the bulbs unite in front, forming a thin strand of tissue passing along the inferior surface of the body of the clitoris to reach the glans. The posterior ends of the vestibular bulbs cover the pea-sized vestibular glands of Bartholin.

## *Hymen*

The hymen is a peculiar anatomic entity without any known function, but is responsible for several medicolegal problems. The hymen is a folded mucous membrane inside the vaginal orifice with an opening of variable shape (semilunar, concave, cribriform, fringed, etc). Occasionally, the hymen does not exist.

Rarely, there is no opening (imperforate hymen), responsible for a condition named hematocolpos (accumulation of menstrual blood and other secretions). The treatment of hematocolpos is simple incision and drainage.

Mor et al.[78] reported a high incidence of hymenal tags (5.75%) and bands (2.7%) in an examination of 974 female neonates.

Berenson[79] studied the appearance of the hymen at birth and 1 year of age in 62 female babies, and reported the following observations: in 8% the inferior half of the hymen was obscured secondary to labial agglutination at 1 year of age; 58% of the remainder had a marked decrease in the amount of their hymenal tissue between birth and 1 year.

# Vascular Supply

## *Blood Supply*

In brief, the blood supply for the region of the vulva is derived by way of the superficial and deep external pudendal branches of the femoral vessels and the posterior labial vessels, derived from the perineal branches of the internal pudendal arteries and veins. Anastomoses of the vulvar vasculature are profuse. Because of the rich blood supply — both arterial and venous — hemorrhage from vulvar injuries or during surgical procedures in the region can be grave. The blood supply is described in greater detail in chapters on the surgical anatomy of the inguinal region and the perineum.

## *Lymphatics*

The pattern of lymphatic drainage of the region of the vulva is described in the chapter on the perineum. Lymphedema of the external genitalia was reported by Huang and colleagues,[80-82] who performed successful microsurgery.

Bartholdson et al.[83] reported that lymph of the labia majora drains to bilateral inguinal nodes and pelvic lymph nodes. These authors advised that carcinoma of the vulva should be treated accordingly. Eicher et al.[84] reported that unblocked vulvar lymphatics drain over or under the mons bilaterally into the pelvis through the obturator foramen or the space of Retzius. When the lymphatics are blocked by pressure, they drain to the perianal or the deep external pudendal areas. They travel laterally to the thigh and then to deep femoral nodes. Spread is bilateral.

# Innervation

The anterior cutaneous nerve supply of the vulva is derived from the ilioinguinal nerve and genital branch of the genitofemoral nerve. Posterior labial cutaneous supply arises from the perineal branch of the pudendal nerve and the perineal branch of the posterior femoral cutaneous nerve of the thigh. The anterior sensory supply is gained principally from the first lumbar spinal nerve. The posterior supply originates primarily from the third sacral spinal nerve.

To gain adequate anesthesia of the anterior region, therefore, the differing levels of supply must be given serious and thoughtful consideration. For further details regarding the nerve supply of the region and its surgical applications, please consult the chapters on the abdominal wall, the inguinal region, and the perineum.

## HISTOLOGY

The vulva is the obvious external appearance of the female genitalia. This structure is contained within the urogenital triangle and consists of the mons pubis, the labia majora, the labia minora, the clitoris, the urethral meatus, the vestibule, and the hymen. The mons pubis is the lower border of the lower abdominal wall and is a mound of fibrofatty tissue overlying the pubic crest area. The skin is keratinized squamous epithelium containing eccrine glands and hair follicles. The subcutaneous tissue is very fibrous in order to suspend this structure from the aponeuroses and linea alba of the lower abdominal wall. The round ligament passes through the lateral aspect of the mons pubis from the external inguinal ring on its journey to insert into subcutaneous tissue of the ipsilateral labium majus.

The labia majora, or the larger lateral folds of the vulvar skin, course inferiorly and posteriorly to surround the labia minora. The lateral aspects of the labia majora have the same histology as the mons veneris, while the more medial aspects are thinner without hair follicles but with a higher concentration of sebaceous glands. The subcutaneous tissue is very vascularized, areolar, and continuous with Camper's fascia.

The labia minora are covered by thin, keratinized squamous epithelium overlying dense connective tissue containing erectile tissues that are abundantly vascularized. Its epithelium contains no hair follicles or eccrine glands.

The clitoris is located anteriorly near the meeting of the two labia majora in the midline. The clitoris consists of two crura, a shaft, and a glans. The two crura attach to the inferior pubic rami and are composed of elastic and vascular erectile tissue (corpora cavernosa). Each crus courses anteriorly to unite with its counterpart in the midline to form the shaft of the clitoris. The shaft is suspended from the pubic symphysis by a suspensory ligament. The shaft leads into the glans, which is composed of erectile tissues surrounded by a prepuce anteriorly and a frenulum posteriorly. These structures are covered with a thin keratinized squamous epithelium without glands or hair follicles. The glans is densely innervated by branches from the deep dorsal nerve from the pudendal nerve.

## PHYSIOLOGY

Vulvar tissues act to keep foreign material from entering up into the vagina and assist in directing the urinary stream during voiding. During sexual intercourse, the vulva enhance sexual pleasure through sensory and erectile functions.

In little girls, labial tissues can be fused (synechiae) requiring the use of topical estrogens to dissolve the synechiae and allow separation of the labia. The density of glands and hair follicles in the moist vulvar environment frequently predisposes to acute and chronic folliculitis and attendant itching and burning. Dermal infections are very common in this region of the body. Non-specific irritation of the vestibular glands may lead to vulvar vestibulitis and entry dyspareunia.

## SURGICAL APPLICATIONS AND ANATOMIC COMPLICATIONS

The most common vulvar procedures are:
• Incision and drainage of infected Bartholin's gland
• Removal of Bartholin's gland
• Vulvectomy (simple and radical)

Any lesion found on the vulva should be biopsied because benign and malignant tumors cannot always be readily differentiated by sight. Frequent biopsy of vulvar lesions is advised. Many lesions may easily be biopsied with local anesthesia, a Keyes skin punch, and Monsel's solution.

REMEMBER:
• To prevent breakdown at the "3-point skin union" over the symphysis pubis, produce a "tongue-shaped" mid-incisional flap (Fig. 26-58).
• If the tip of the "tongue-shaped" flap does not have good blood supply, remove more skin until bleeding occurs, avoiding necrosis.
• Removal after dissection of the ganglion of Cloquet (lymphoganglion of Rosenmüller) should be performed carefully. Avoid entrance into the peritoneal cavity. If femoral hernia is present, it should be repaired at the same time. Use the "below the inguinal ligament technique" by suturing the inguinal ligament to the pectineal fascia or to the Cooper's ligament.
• Avoid bleeding in the operating room by isolating and ligating the following vessels:
  – Superficial circumflex iliac artery

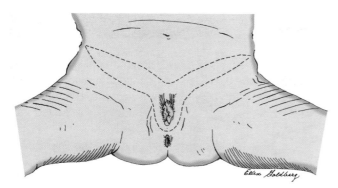

**FIG. 26-58.** Outline of the incision used for one-step radical vulvectomy and groin dissection. (Modified from Woodruff JD, Julian CJ. Surgery of the vulva; vulvectomy. In: Ridley JH (ed). Gynecologic Surgery: Errors, Safeguards, and Salvage (2nd ed). Baltimore: Williams & Wilkins, 1981; with permission.)

– Superficial epigastric artery
– Great saphenous vein
– Dorsal artery and vein of the clitoris
– Posterior labial branches of the internal pudendal vessels (Fig. 26-59)

- Ligate the lymphatic tissue at the apex of the femoral triangle in the femoral canal to avoid lymphorrhea or lymphocyst.
- Use the sartorius muscle (Fig. 26-60) to cover the femoral artery and vein, thus avoiding exposure and secondary bleeding.
- With a "fall astraddle," the vessels most likely to be injured and produce hematoma are:
  – Perineal branches of the internal pudendal vessels and their branches
  – Branches from superficial and deep external pudendal vessels
  – Clitoral vessels
  – Rectal vessels
- The branches from the superficial and deep external pudendal vessels are in the vicinity of the round ligament.
- The internal pudendal vessels are occasionally responsible for the formation of varices in the area of buttocks.
- Part of the skin, but most of the fibrofatty tissue of the mons veneris, is removed during vulvectomy for cancer. The justification is to try to contain superficial lymphatics with malignant cells.
- During bartholinectomy, bleeding may take place be-

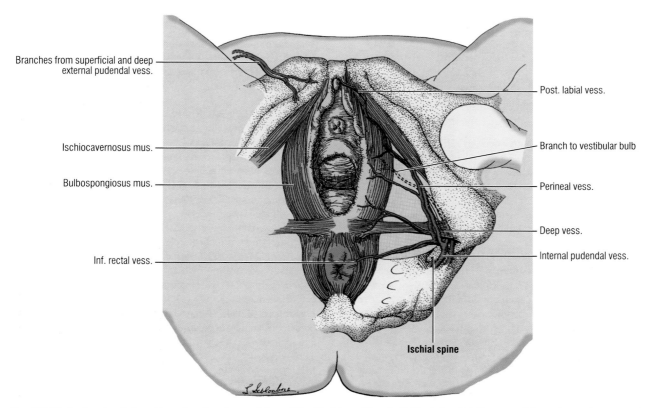

Branches from superficial and deep external pudendal vess.

Ischiocavernosus mus.

Bulbospongiosus mus.

Inf. rectal vess.

Post. labial vess.

Branch to vestibular bulb

Perineal vess.

Deep vess.

Internal pudendal vess.

**Ischial spine**

**FIG. 26-59.** Anatomic relationships of perineal vasculature. (Modified from Woodruff JD, Julian CJ. Surgery of the vulva; vulvectomy. In: Ridley JH (ed). Gynecologic Surgery: Errors, Safeguards, and Salvage. Baltimore: Williams & Wilkins, 1974; with permission.)

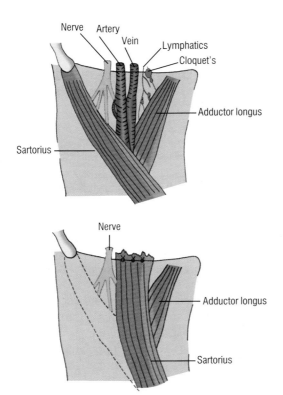

**FIG. 26-60.** Transplantation of sartorius muscle over femoral vessels. (Modified from Woodruff JD, Julian CJ. Surgery of the vulva; vulvectomy. In: Ridley JH (ed). Gynecologic Surgery: Errors, Safeguards, and Salvage (2nd ed). Baltimore: Williams & Wilkins, 1981; with permission.)

cause of the close relation of the Bartholin glands to the highly vascular bulb. Make the incision lateral to the groove but close to the labia minora.

# REFERENCES

1. Kelly HA. Operative Gynecology. New York: D. Appleton, 1898.
2. Retzky SS, Rogers RM, Richardson AC. Anatomy of female pelvic support. In: Brubaker LT, Saclarides TJ (eds). The Female Pelvic Floor: Disorders of Function and Support. Philadelphia: FA Davis, 1996.
3. Vaughn TC, Jones HL. Laparoscopic repair of bilateral inguinal hernias in a patient with mullerian agenesis. Fertil Steril 2000;73:1238-1240.
4. Kuga T, Esato K, Takeda K, Sase M, Hoshii Y. A supernumerary ovary of the omentum with cystic change: report of two cases and review of the literature. Pathol Int 49(6):566-570, 1999.
5. Vendeland LL, Shehadeh L. Incidental finding of an accessory ovary in a 16-year-old at laparoscopy: a case report. J Reprod Med 2000;45:435-438.
6. Bazot M, Deligne L, Boudghène F, Buy JN, Lassau JP, Bigot JM. Correlation between computed tomography and gross anatomy of the suspensory ligament of the ovary. Surg Radiol Anat 1999;21:341-346.
7. Hill LM, Breckle R. Value of a postvoid scan during adnexal sonography. Am J Obstet Gynecol 1985;152:23-25.
8. Lechter A, Lopez G, Martinez C, Camacho J. Anatomy of the go-
nadal veins: a reappraisal. Surgery 1991;109:735-739.
9. Berry M, Bannister LH, Standring SM (eds). Nervous system. In: Williams PL (ed). Gray's Anatomy (38th ed). New York: Churchill Livingstone, 1995, p. 1307.
10. Bannister LH, Dyson M. Reproductive system. In: Williams PL. Gray's Anatomy (38th ed). New York: Churchill Livingstone, 1995, pp. 1847-1880.
11. Luciano AA, Marana R, Kratka S, Peluso JJ. Ovarian function after incision of the ovary by scalpel, $CO_2$ laser, and microelectrode. Fertil Steril 1991;56:349.
12. Slowey MJ. Polycystic ovary syndrome: new perspective on an old problem. South Med J 2001;94:190-196.
13. Kokoska ER, Keller MS, Weber TR. Acute ovarian torsion in children. Am J Surg 2001;180:462-465.
14. Oelsner G, Graebe RA, Boyers SP, Pan SB, Barnea ER, DeCherney AH. A comparison of three techniques for ovarian reconstruction. Am J Obstet Gynecol 1986;145:569.
15. Hengster P, Menardi G. Ovarian cysts in the newborn. Pediatr Surg Int 71:372-375, 1992.
16. von Schweinitz D. Ovarian cysts in the newborn [Letters to the Editor]. Pediatr Surg Int 9:463-464, 1994.
17. Hammond CB. Gynecology: The female reproductive organs. In: Sabiston DC. Textbook of Surgery, 15th ed. Philadelphia: WB Saunders, 1997, p. 1516.
18. Turken A, Ciftci AO, Akcoren Z, Koseoglu V, Akata D, Senocak ME. Primary ovarian lymphoma in an infant: report of a case. Surg Today 2000;30:305-307.
19. Montero CA, Gimferrer JM, Baldo X, Ramirez J. Mediastinal metastasis of ovarian carcinoma. Eur J Obstet Gynecol Reprod Biol 2000;91:199-200.

20. Hoffman JJ. Anatomy and physiology of the fallopian tube. In: Hunt RB. Atlas of Female Infertility Surgery. 2nd ed. St. Louis: Mosby Year Book, 1992, pp. 3-11.

21. Cohen BM. Surgery of the ovary, including anatomic derangements of the fimbrial-gonadal ovum-capture mechanism. In: Hunt RB. Atlas of Female Infertility Surgery (2nd ed). St. Louis: Mosby Year Book, 1992, pp. 389-403.

22. Donnez J, Casanas-Roux F. Prognostic factors of fimbrial microsurgery. Fertil Steril 1986;46:200.

23. DeCherney AH, Boyers SP. Isthmic ectopic pregnancy: segmental resection as the treatment of choice. Fertil Steril 1985;44:307.

24. Manuaba IB. Nontraumatic tubal occlusion as a new technique for female voluntary sterilization. Adv Contracept 1993;9:303.

25. Piura B, Rabinovich A. Primary cancer of the fallopian tube: study of 11 cases. Eur J Obstet Gynecol Reprod Biol 2000;91;169-175.

26. Kouvidou C, Karayianni M, Liapi-Avgeri G, Toufexi H, Karaiossifidi H. Old ectopic pregnancy remnants with morphological features of placental site nodule occurring in the fallopian tube and broad ligament. Pathol Res Pract 2000;196:329-332.

27. Misao R, Niwa K, Iwagaki S, Shimokawa K, Tamaya T. Leiomyoma of the fallopian tube. Gynecol Obstet Invest 2000;49:279-280.

28. Phupong V, Pruksananonda K, Taneepanichskul S, Tresukosol D, Virutamasen P. Double uterus with unilaterally obstructed hemivagina and ipsilateral renal agenesis: a variety presentation and a 10-year review of the literature. J Med Assoc Thai 2000;83:569-574.

29. Homer HA, Li TC, Cooke ID. Septate uterus: a review of management and reproductive outcome. Fertil Steril 2000; 73:1-14.

30. Giraldo JL, Habana A, Duleba AJ, Dokras A. Septate uterus associated with cervical duplication and vaginal septum. J Am Assoc Gynecol Laparosc 2000;7:277-279.

31. Aschoff L. Zur Cervixfrage. Monatschr f Geburtsh u Gynäk 1905; 22:611.

32. Last RJ. Anatomy Regional and Applied (5th ed). Baltimore: Williams & Wilkins, 1972, p. 515.

33. DeLancey JOL, Richardson AC. Anatomy of genital support. In: Hurt WG (ed). Urogynecologic Surgery. Gaithersburg MD: Aspen, 1992, pp. 19-33.

34. Attah AA, Hutson JM. The anatomy of the female gubernaculum is different from the male. Aust N Z J Surg 1991;61:380.

35. Range RL, Woodburne RT. The gross and microscopic anatomy of the transverse cervical ligaments. Am J Obstet Gynecol 1964;90:460.

36. Campbell RM. The anatomy and histology of the sacrouterine ligaments. Am J Obstet Gynecol 1950;59:1.

37. Eastman NJ. Williams Obstetrics (10th ed). New York: Appleton-Century-Crofts, 1950, p. 46.

38. Scheidler J, Hricak H, Yu KK, Subak L, Segal MR. Radiological evaluation of lymph node metastases in patients with cervical cancer: a meta-analysis. JAMA 278(13):1096-1101, 1997.

39. Rogers RM. Basic pelvic neuroanatomy. In: Steege JF, Metzger DA, Levy B (eds). Chronic Pelvic Pain: An Integrated Approach. Philadelphia: WB Saunders, 1998.

40. Gardner E, Gray DJ, O'Rahilly R. Anatomy (4th ed). Philadelphia: WB Saunders, 1975.

41. Wilson ML, Farquhar CM, Sinclair OJ, Johnson NP. Surgical interruption of pelvic nerve pathways for primary and secondary dysmenorrhea. Cochrane Database System Rev 2000;2:CD001896.

42. La Greca G, Catanuto G, Pontillo T, Sichel I, Di Carlo I, Russello D, Latteri F. [Ileal endometriosis. A clinical case and a review of the literature]. Giornale Chir 2000;21:12-16.

43. Williams TJ. Abdominal hysterectomy, myomectomy, and presacral neurectomy: with management of bladder injury and attention to thromboembolic disease. In: Ridley JH (ed). Gynecologic Surgery: Errors, Safeguards, and Salvage. Baltimore: Williams & Wilkins, 1944, pp. 1-43.

44. Dover RW, Torode HW, Briggs GM. Uterine artery embolisation for symptomatic fibroids. Med J Aust 2000;172:233-236.

45. Liu WM. Laparoscopic bipolar coagulation of uterine vessels to treat symptomatic leiomyomas. J Am Assoc Gynecol Laparosc 2000;71:125-129.

46. Butler-Manuel SA, Buttery LD, A'Hearn RP, Polak JM, Barton DP. Pelvic nerve plexus trauma at radical hysterectomy and simple hysterectomy: the nerve content of the uterine supporting ligaments. Cancer 2000;89:834-841.

47. Smith-Bindman R, Kerlikowske K, Feldstein VA, Subak L, Scheidler J, Segal M, Brand R, Grady D. Endovaginal ultrasound to exclude endometrial cancer and other endometrial abnormalities. JAMA 280(17):1510-1517, 1998.

48. Morgan JL, O'Connell HE, McGuire EJ. Is intrinsic sphincter deficiency a complication of simple hysterectomy? J Urol 2000;164: 767-769.

49. Newton M, Lurain JR. Complications of gynecologic surgery. In: Hardy JR. Complications in Surgery and Their Management (4th ed). Philadelphia: WB Saunders, 1981, pp. 860-898.

50. Wharton LR Jr. Vaginal hysterectomy: anterior and posterior colporrhaphy; repair of enterocele; and prolapse of vaginal vault. In: Ridley JH (ed). Gynecologic Surgery: Errors, Safeguards, and Salvage. Baltimore: Williams & Wilkins, 1974, pp. 44-77.

51. Kamina P. De l'anatomie à la technique de l'hystérectomie vaginale. Rev Fr Gynecol Obstet 1990;85:435.

52. Yamamoto R, Okamoto K, Ebina Y, Shirato H, Sakuragi N, Fujimoto S. Prevention of vaginal shortening following radical hysterectomy. Br J Obstet Gynaecol 2000;107:841-845.

53. Shimao Y, Nabeshima K, Inoue T, Higo T, Wada T, Ikenoue T, Koono M. Primary vaginal adenocarcinoma arising from the metanephric duct remnant. Virchows Archiv 2000;436;622-627.

54. Zacharin RF. Pulsion enterocele: review of functional anatomy of the pelvic floor. Obstet Gynecol 1980;55:135.

55. Bump RC, Mattiasson A, Bo K. The standardization of terminology of female pelvic organ prolapse and pelvic floor dysfunction. Am J Obstet Gynecol 1996:175:10-17.

56. Richardson AC. The anatomic defects in rectocele and enterocele. J Pelvic Surg 1995;1:214-221.

57. Retzky SS, Rogers RM. Urinary incontinence in women. Ciba Clin Symp 1995;47:2-32.

58. Ridley JH. Stress urinary incontinence. In: Ridley RH (ed). Gynecologic Surgery: Errors, Safeguards, and Salvage. Baltimore: Williams & Wilkins, 1944, pp. 114-154.

59. Hurt WG, Dunn LJ. Complications of gynecologic surgery and trauma. In: Greenfield LJ (ed). Complications in Surgery and Trauma (2nd ed). Philadelphia: JB Lippincott, 1990, pp. 833-842.

60. Weber AM, Walters MD, Piedmonte MR. Sexual function and vaginal anatomy in women before and after surgery for pelvic organ prolapse and urinary incontinence. Am J Obstet Gynecol 2000;182: 1610-1615.

61. O'Connell HE, Hutson JM, Anderson CR, Plenter RJ. Anatomical relationship between urethra and clitoris. J Urol 159(6): 1892-1897, 1998.

62. Tanagho EA. Anatomy of the lower urinary tract. In: Walsh PC, Retik AB, Stamey TA, Vaughn ED Jr (eds). Campbell's Urology (6th ed). Philadelphia: WB Saunders, 1992, pp. 40-69.

63. Siracusano S, Mandras R, Belgrano E. [Physiopathology of the pelvic elements of support in stress urinary incontinence in women]. (Italian) Arch Ital Urol Androl 66(4 Suppl):151-153, 1994.

64. Oelrich TM. The striated urogenital sphincter muscle in the female. Anat Rec 1983;205:223-232.

65. DeLancey JO. Structural aspects of the extrinsic continence mechanism. Obstet Gynecol 1988;72:296-301.

66. DeLancey JO. Structural support of the urethra as it relates to stress urinary incontinence: the hammock hypothesis. Am J Obstet Gynecol 1994;170:1713-1723.

67. Stothers L, Chopra A, Raz S. Vaginal reconstructive surgery for female incontinence and anterior vaginal-wall prolapse. Urol Clin North Am 1995;22:641-655.

68. Rother P, Löffler S, Dorschner W, Reibiger I, Bengs T. Anatomic basis of micturition and urinary continence: Muscle systems in urinary bladder neck during ageing. Surg Radiol Anat 18:173-177, 1996.

69. Bredael JJ, Kramer SA, Cleeve LK, Webster GA. Traumatic rupture of the female urethra. J Urol 122:560, 1979.

70. Ridley JH. Surgery for vaginal fistulae. In: Ridley RH (ed). Gynecologic Surgery: Errors, Safeguards, and Salvage. Baltimore: Williams & Wilkins, 1944, pp. 155-201.

71. Gottlicher S. Uber das Labium tertium pudendi feminae. Zentralbl Gynakol 1994;116:419.

72. Barrett TM, Gonzales ET Jr. Reconstruction of the female external genitalia. Urol Clin North Am 1980;7:455.

73. Ansell JS, Rajfer J. A new and simplified method for concealing the hypertrophied clitoris. J Pediatr Surg 1981;16:681.

74. Woodruff JD, Friedrich EG Jr. The vestibule. Clin Obstet Gynecol 1985;28:134.

75. Chretien FC, Berthou J. Les glandes vestibulaires majeures de Bartholin et leur secretion: anatomie, proprietes physiques et roles physiologiques. Contracept Fertil Sex (Paris) 1994;22:720.

76. Sarrel PM, Steege JF, Maltzer M, Bolinsky D. Pain during sex response due to occlusion of the Bartholin gland duct. Obstet Gynecol 1983;62:261.

77. Tepper SL, Jagirdar J, Heath D, Geller SA. Homology between the female paraurethral (Skene's) glands and the prostate. Immunohistochemical demonstration. Arch Pathol Lab Med 1984;108: 423.

78. Mor N, Merlob P, Reisner SH. Tags and bands of the female external genitalia in the newborn infant. Clin Pediatr (Phila) 1983; 22:122.

79. Berenson AB. Appearance of the hymen at birth and one year of age: a longitudinal study. Pediatrics 1993;91:820.

80. Huang GK, Hu RQ, Shen YL, Pan GP. Microlymphaticovenous anastomosis for lymphedema of external genitalia in females. Surg Gynecol Obstet 1986;162:429.

81. Huang GK. Results of microsurgical lymphovenous anastomoses in lymphedema: report of 110 cases. Langenbecks Arch Chir 1989; 374:194.

82. Huang GK. Microsurgical therapy of lymphedema of the external female genitalia. Geburtshilfe Frauenheilkd 1989;49:876.

83. Bartholdson L, Hultborn A, Hulten L, Roos B, Rosencrantz M, Ahren C. Lymph drainage from the vulva and the foot as demonstrated by 198Au. Acta Radiol Ther Phys Biol 1977;16:209.

84. Eicher E, Danese C, Katz G. Vulvar lymphatics as demonstrated by vital dyes and lymphangiography. Int Surg 1983;68:175.

# Chapter 27

# Adrenal (Suprarenal) Glands

John E. Skandalakis, Gene L. Colborn,
Thomas A. Weidman, Robert A. Badalament,
Thomas S. Parrott, Petros Mirilas,
William M. Scaljon, Lee J. Skandalakis

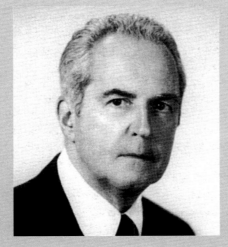

**H. William Scott, Jr. (1916-1998),** who knew everything about the adrenals.

*The various glands distributed throughout the entire body must be divided into two great classes: those which extract from the blood certain particular principles which impart to each secretion its individual characteristics; and those which, on the contrary, appear to secrete into the blood itself, if I may use the expression, or those which are intended to enrich the circulating blood with products manufactured in the interior of their own tissues. Such are the haematopoietic glands, among which are included the spleen, the thymus, the suprarenal capsules and other glands rich in blood-vessels, and which do not possess excretory ducts.*

*Claude Bernard*[1]

## HISTORY

The anatomic and surgical history of the adrenal glands is shown in Table 27-1.

## EMBRYOGENESIS

### Normal Development

The adrenal glands form from two separate primordia: the neuroectodermal component develops into the adrenal medulla, and the mesodermal component becomes the adrenal cortex. The cells of the future medulla are identified by the 21st to the 22nd day, and are among the wide variety of cells that migrate out of the neural crest (neuroectoderm) in the sixth and seventh weeks[2] (Fig. 27-1). These cells travel along the nerves of the 6th to 12th segments into the developing cortical primordia.

Within the cortical tissue, the migrating cells proliferate and differentiate into chromaffin cells at around the third month of gestation. This process is not complete until 12 to 18 months after birth. Some cells do not reach the adrenal organs, but differentiate into chromaffin cells along the aorta. They form nodules of extraadrenal medullary tissue.

The mesodermal component of the cortex is visible as

*Note to readers:* We have used the term "adrenal" rather than "suprarenal" in this text because in spoken language such lengthy terms as "suprarenalectomy" are so cumbersome they are not used.

early as the fourth week. The first indication of the cortex is increased division among the peritoneal epithelial cells of the posterior abdominal wall in the groove between the mesentery and the cranial end of the mesonephric ridge (Fig. 27-2). From this epithelium, cords of cells invade the mesenchyme, while surface cells form a cap over the region (Fig. 27-3A). This epithelial cap represents the future zona glomerulosa of the permanent cortex (Fig. 27-3B). Other derivatives of the neural crest cells such as chromaffin cells of the adrenal medulla and the aortic bodies are shown in Fig. 27-4 and Table 27-2.

Differentiation of cortical zones begins in the eighth week. The outer layer will become the adult zona glomerulosa. Beneath this is the proportionally large "fetal cortex" (Fig. 27-5A), which will decrease in relative size and form the zona fasciculata and the zona reticularis of the adult. These zones may be distinguished at birth (Fig. 27-5B), although they do not appear in the final adult form until the fourth year of postnatal life (Fig. 27-5C).

In the words of Sucheston and Cannon,[3] the adult zones appear to be established by "proliferation of the permanent cortex, maturation of the fetal cortex and growth of the medulla," and are finally completed by 11 to 15 years of age. However, some writers disagree with that view, and believe that shortly after birth, the fetal cortex degenerates and is replaced or reorganized,[4] or that the fetal zone cells remodel and reduce in size.[5]

Due to the large size of the fetal cortex, the volume of the adrenal glands of the human fetus is 20 times larger than that of the adult gland in relation to the weight of the body. The adrenal medulla, however, is small, and enlarges slightly after birth.

At birth, the volume of the adrenals is about 40 ml. Two months after birth, the volume has decreased to about 10 ml, owing to regression and replacement of the fetal cortex

## TABLE 27-1. The History of Anatomy and Surgery of the Adrenal Glands

| | | |
|---|---|---|
| Eustachius | 1522 | Discovered the adrenals. Reported his findings in 1563. |
| Spigelius | 1627 | Described the adrenals as "capsulae renales" |
| Riolan | 1629 | Described the adrenals as supra-renal capsules |
| Valsalva (1666-1732) | | Argued that the adrenal arteries were ducts running from the "glandula renalis" to the epididymis |
| Bartholinus (Bartolin) | 1656 | Described the adrenals as "capsulae atrabilariae" because he observed that they were filled with black fluid. This was later misconstrued to mean they were filled with black bile. |
| Diemerbroek | 1694 | Called the adrenals "deputy kidneys" |
| Winslow | 1732 | Provided a detailed and accurate description of the adrenals |
| Bordeau | 1775 | Reported his belief that the adrenals distribute substances into the blood |
| Schmidt | 1785 | Stated that the adrenals secreted substances that helped the action of the heart |
| J.F. Meckel ("The Younger Meckel") | 1805 | Reported on the form, color, and weight of the adrenals in 30 species of animals |
| Cuvier | 1805 | Studied the adrenals of the human fetus, claiming that they were large during embryological growth |
| Henle | 1843 | Stated that the adrenals could be extirpated with impunity "without sensation or motion suffering in the least" |
| Ecker | 1846 | Provided a detailed description of the microscopic anatomy of the adrenal glands |
| Remak | 1847 | Postulated that the adrenal medulla originates from sympathetic ganglia |
| Addison | 1849 & 1855 | Described the effects of diseases of the adrenals, including primary adrenocortical insufficiency (Addison's disease) |
| Vulpian | 1856 | Reported that the adrenal medulla developed a green color when in contact with ferric chloride |
| Brown-Séquard | 1856 | Established that the adrenals were essential for life |
| Gerlach and Welcher | 1857 | First to stain the adrenals |
| Harley | 1858 | Used carmine stain to provide a histological description of the adrenals. Stated that the removal of the adrenals prolonged life in some species. |
| Henle | 1865 | Used chromium salts to develop a brown-yellow color in the medulla (thus the term pheochrome, or "dark color") |
| Arnold | 1866 | Presented a classification of the adrenal cortex based on three zonae (glomerulosa, fasciculata, and reticularis) |
| Leydig | 1866 | Claimed that the adrenal gland is part of the nervous system rather than a blood gland, with the medulla functioning like a nervous ganglion |
| Frey | 1875 | Noted the presence of a rich blood supply in the adrenals |
| Gottschau | 1883 | Grouped the zona reticularis and the medulla together as the zona consuptiva. Stated that the cells of the cortex grew inward toward the medulla. |
| Frankel | 1886 | Described what is now known as pheochromocytoma |
| Tizzoni | 1889 | Showed that removing the adrenals caused changes in the brain and in the nervous system |
| Thorton | 1889 | Removed a tumor that "reminded the observer of the structure of an adrenal" when studied microscopically |
| Stilling | 1890 | Noted that accessory cortical bodies caused differing results after bilateral adrenalectomy |
| Oliver and Schafer | 1894-1895 | Found that a rise in blood pressure occurred after administration of an extract from the medulla, which they called adrenalin |
| Osler | 1896 | Administered an adrenal extract to temporarily treat Addison's disease |
| Abel | 1897 | Referred to Oliver and Schafer's extract called "adrenalin" (see above) as "epinephrine" |
| Takamine and Aldrich | 1901 | Working independently, they both isolated epinephrine/adrenalin |
| Blum | 1901 | Found that adrenal extracts caused glycosuria |
| Kohn | 1902 | Demonstrated that the cells of the adrenal medulla, the carotid body, the abdominal paraganglia, and the organ of Zuckerkandl contained cells positive to chromaffin; described the "chromaffin system" |
| Stolz | 1904 | Synthesized epinephrine and norepinephrine |
| Pick | 1912 | First used the term pheochromocytoma |
| Cushing | 1912-1932 | Described the syndrome of pituitary basophilism (Cushing's syndrome) and connected it with pituitary-adrenal hyperactivity |

## TABLE 27-1 *(cont'd)*. The History of Anatomy and Surgery of the Adrenal Glands

| | | |
|---|---|---|
| Elliot | 1913 | Described the association of the adrenal medulla with the sympathetic nervous system |
| Sargent | 1914 | Removed a 1,025-gram adrenal tumor |
| Rogoff and Stewart | 1921 | Wrote a series of reports on the removal of the adrenal glands |
| Vaquez and Donzelot | 1926 | Made the first clinical diagnosis of pheochromocytoma |
| Roux (Switzerland) Mayo (U.S.) | 1926 | Independently extirpated pheochromocytomas |
| Hartman, Dean and McArthur | 1928 | Purified adrenocortical extracts and published a paper about this new isolate which prolonged life in adrenalectomized animals |
| Pincoffs | 1929 | First to preoperatively diagnose pheochromocytoma |
| Rabin | 1929-1930 | Identified an epinephrine-type substance in a pheochromocytoma |
| Crile | 1932 | Surgically denervated an adrenal gland |
| Broster | 1933 | Used a transthoracic approach during surgery of the adrenals |
| Walters | 1934 | Used a lateral lumbar approach during surgery of the adrenals |
| Kendall | 1934 | Isolated cortisone |
| Young | 1936 | Noted the importance of direct observation of both adrenals. Recommended bilateral subtotal adrenalectomy to treat bilateral hyperplasia. |
| Holtz, Credner and Kronenberg | 1945 | Rediscovered norepinephrine |
| Roth and Kwale | 1945 | Introduced the histamine provocative test |
| Huggins and Scott | 1945 | Attempted to treat advanced prostatic cancer with a bilateral total adrenalectomy |
| Von Euler | 1946 | Reported that norepinephrine can be found in sympathetic nerve endings |
| Holtz | 1947 | Found norepinephrine in the adrenal medulla |
| Langino | 1949 | Introduced the Regitine (phentolamine) test |
| Thorn and Forsham | 1949 | Used cortisone acetate to treat Addison's disease |
| Wendlet | 1950 | Synthesized cortisol |
| Priestley | 1951 | With his colleagues at the Mayo Clinic, reported 29 patients who underwent subtotal adrenalectomy to treat Cushing's disease, noting that perioperative cortisol treatment greatly decreased postoperative complications |
| Pati o | 1951 | Successful transplantation of human fetal adrenal cortical tissue in patient with Addison's disease |
| Grundy and Reichstein | 1952 | Isolated aldosterone |
| Conn | 1955 | Described primary aldosteronism (Conn's syndrome) |
| Liddle | 1961 | Labeled hydrocortisone as the most important hormone in the adrenal cortex, noting its secretion after ACTH stimulation |
| Bartter | 1962 | Reported sodium-wasting condition (Bartter's syndrome) |
| Pearce | 1968-1978 | Described APUD (amine precursor uptake decarboxylation) system, including cells that produced peptide hormones of neural crest or neuroectodermal origin |
| Vingerhoeds et al. | 1976 | Described primary cortisol and glucocorticoid resistance |
| Viveros et al. | 1979 | Discovered enkephalins in the chromaffin vesicle |
| Forest et al. | 1982 | Studied (and discounted) relationship between adrenarche and gonadarche |
| Hricak & Williams | 1984 | Studied normal and pathologic adrenal anatomy with MRI |
| Madrazo et al. | 1987 | Autologous transplation of medullary tissue to treat Parkinson's disease |
| Counts et al. | 1987 | Studied (and discounted) relationship between adrenarche and gonadarche |

*History table compiled by David A. McClusky III and John E. Skandalakis*

**Recommended Reading (History):**

Bourne GH. The Mammalian Adrenal Gland. Oxford: Clarendon Press, 1949, pp. 1-28.

DeGroot LJ (ed). Endocrinology (3rd ed) Vol. II Part VI. Adrenal Cortex. Philadelphia: WB Saunders, 1995, pp. 1627-1880.

Hughes S, Lynn J. Surgical anatomy and surgery of the adrenal glands. In: Lynn J, Bloom SR (eds). Surgical Endocrinology. London: Butterworth Heinemann, 1993, pp. 458-467.

Scott HW. Surgery of the Adrenal Glands. Philadelphia: J.B. Lippincott Company, 1990, pp. 1-16.

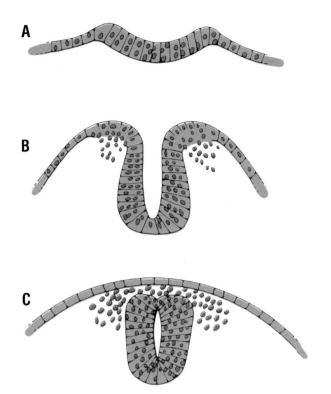

**FIG. 27-1.** Formation of neural tube and origin of cells of neural crest from neuroectoderm. (Modified from Skandalakis JE, Gray SW, Rowe JS Jr. Anatomical Complications in General Surgery. New York: McGraw-Hill, 1983; with permission.)

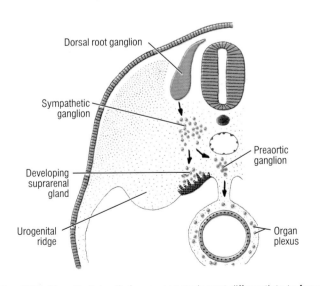

**FIG. 27-2.** Mesothelial cells from mesenteric root differentiate to form cortex. (Modified from Sadler TW. Langman's Medical Embryology (8th ed). Baltimore: Lippincott, Williams & Wilkins, 2000; with permission.)

(by whatever means). Growth begins again in the second year of postnatal life and accelerates after puberty. Final adult size (40 ml) is reached by age 17.[6]

Bocian-Sobkowska[7] studied the adrenal gland in the first postnatal year:

*The postnatal decrease in adrenal volume was caused mainly by a rapid fall of fetal zone volume (from 70% to 3% of total adrenal volume) that can be divided into two phases: rapid phase (from birth to the end of the second week) and a slow phase from the 3rd week on. Involution was accompanied by increase of zona glomerulosa (from 10% to 25% of total adrenal volume), zona fasciculata (from 10% to 38%) and zona reticularis volume (from 1% to 23%). During the whole investigated period the volume of medulla remained constant. The volume fraction of stroma (connective tissue and blood vessels) was highest at the beginning of the first postnatal week and then decreased rapidly at the end of the 2nd week, with the most pronounced changes in the fetal zone and medulla.*

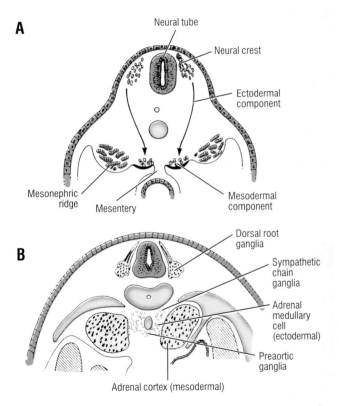

**FIG. 27-3.** Migration of neural crest cells into mesodermal components of adrenal gland during the sixth week **(A)** and seventh week **(B)**. (Modified from Skandalakis JE, Gray SW, Rowe JS Jr. Anatomical Complications in General Surgery. New York: McGraw-Hill, 1983; with permission.)

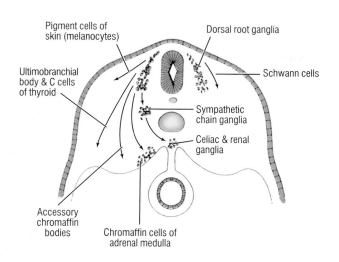

**FIG. 27-4.** Derivatives of neural crest. (Modified from Skandalakis JE, Gray SW, Rowe JS Jr. Anatomical Complications in General Surgery. New York: McGraw-Hill, 1983; with permission.)

The adrenal glands maintain their position in the abdomen, neither ascending with the kidney, nor descending with the testis. Their arterial supply is from segmental mesonephric arteries, greatly altered in their arrangement.

## Congenital Anomalies

Congenital anomalies of the adrenal glands are shown in Table 27-3 and Figure 27-6.

### *Agenesis of the Adrenal Glands*

Unilateral adrenal agenesis is almost always as-

---

**TABLE 27-2. Derivatives of the Neural Crest Cells**

- Dorsal root ganglion cells
- Sympathetic trunk ganglia
- Parasympathetic ganglia
- Schwann cells
- Ultimobranchial bodies
- Epidermal pigment cells
- Glial cells of peripheral ganglia (the satellite or capsule cells)
- Leptomeninx
- Parts of all the cranial nerve ganglia (except olfactory), connective tissue surrounding the eye and the ciliary muscle
- All derivatives of the pharyngeal arches (except skeletal muscles), dermis, and hypodermis of the face and neck, and trunco-conal septum (heart outflow tracts)

---

sociated with renal agenesis on the same side, but in 90 percent of patients with unilateral renal agenesis, the adrenal gland is present. Absence of the kidney is usually the result of defective ureteric bud development, which does not affect the adrenal gland. Only a failure of formation of the entire nephrogenic ridge results in the absence of both the kidney and the adrenal gland.

### *Fusion of the Adrenal Glands*

Fusion of the adrenal glands behind the aorta may accompany fusion of the kidneys (horseshoe kidney).[8]

### *Hypoplasia of the Adrenal Glands*

Adrenal hypoplasia is represented by two types: anencephalic and the type in which the marginal fetal cortex does not exist. According to Kerenyi,[9] Winquist,[10] and others all patients survived no longer than a few months.

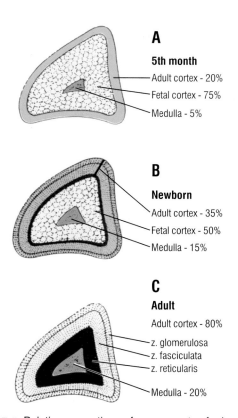

**A**

**5th month**
- Adult cortex - 20%
- Fetal cortex - 75%
- Medulla - 5%

**B**

**Newborn**
- Adult cortex - 35%
- Fetal cortex - 50%
- Medulla - 15%

**C**

**Adult**
Adult cortex - 80%
- z. glomerulosa
- z. fasciculata
- z. reticularis
- Medulla - 20%

**FIG. 27-5.** Relative proportions of components of adrenal gland: **A**, fifth month of gestation; **B**, at birth; **C**, adult. (Modified from Skandalakis JE, Gray SW, Rowe JS Jr. Anatomical Complications in General Surgery. New York: McGraw Hill, 1983; with permission. Data from Sucheston ME, Cannon MS. Development of zonular patterns in the human adrenal gland. J Morphol 1968;126:477.)

**TABLE 27-3. Anomalies of the Adrenal Glands**

| Anomaly | Prenatal Age at Onset | First Appearance (or Other Diagnostic Clues) | Sex Chiefly Affected | Relative Frequency | Remarks |
|---|---|---|---|---|---|
| Agenesis of the adrenals | 4th week | None, when unilateral | ? | Uncommon | Associated with absence of kidney on the same side |
| Fusion of the adrenals | 6th week | None | Male | Rare | Associated with fused kidneys |
| Hypoplasia of the adrenals | Probably late in gestation | At birth | Male | Very rare, except in anencephalic infants | Usually lethal in infancy |
| Heterotopia of the adrenals | 8th week | None | ? | Uncommon | Usually found within the capsule of the liver or the kidney |
| Accessory adrenal glands | 4th-6th weeks | None | Probably equal | Common | Rarely contain medullary tissue |
| Adrenal gland hemorrhage | At birth | Hypovolemic shock or corticosteroid deficiency at birth | ? | Rare; second most common source of hemoperitoneum in newborn | |
| Neuroblastoma | Approximately 4-5 weeks (?) (Originates in neural crest) | 2-5 years of age | Males slightly more than females | In up to 1:7000 children; most frequent solid tumor in children | It has been noted to occur with other congenital syndromes |

Modified from Skandalakis JE, Gray SW. Embryology for Surgeons (2nd ed). Baltimore: Williams & Wilkins, 1994, p. 726. Used with permission.

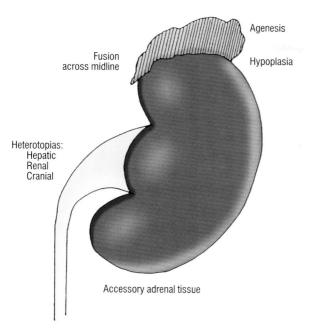

**FIG. 27-6.** Chief congenital anomalies of adrenal glands. (Modified from Skandalakis JE, Gray SW. Embryology for Surgeons (2nd ed). Baltimore: Williams & Wilkins, 1994; with permission.)

## Adrenal Heterotopia

Occasionally, the adrenal gland is in its normal location but is also beneath the capsule of the kidney (adrenorenal heterotopia) or that of the liver (adrenohepatic heterotopia) (Fig. 27-7A). Renal tubules or bile ducts may be intermingled with adrenal cells in the area of fusion of the organs. Such fusion renders adrenalectomy more difficult.

## Accessory Adrenal Tissue

Small nodules of adrenal tissue may be found throughout the abdomen (Figs. 27-8 - 27-9). The largest may contain both cortical and medullary tissue.[11] These are true accessory adrenal glands. They are usually found near the aorta, between the origin of the celiac axis and that of the superior mesenteric artery.

Accessory cortical tissue alone is not rare. Most such cortical nodules are under the renal capsule, in the broad ligament in the female or in the spermatic cord of the male.[12,13] These sites have surgical significance when the suspected lesion is not found within the substance of the normally situated adrenal glands. All these cortical structures are as susceptible to adenomas as is the normal adrenal gland (Fig. 27-7A).

Chromaffin tissue distributed around the aorta near the origin of the inferior mesenteric artery, in the lumbar sympathetic chain, and in and about the celiac plexus is normal (Fig. 27-7B). Such tissue represents chromaffin cells from the neural crest that were not incorporated into the adrenal medulla. The largest of these are the paraaortic bodies (organs of Zuckerkandl); they regress in size with age.[14]

These structures may be sites of pheochromocytomas in childhood. They may also be sites of "nonfunctioning" paragangliomas with no clinical evidence of hormonal activity.[15] Medullary (chromaffin) tissue outside the normal adrenal gland is much more frequently found than is cortical tissue, and is more frequently associated with hyperfunction than is cortical tissue. O'Riordain et al.[16] studied extraadrenal functional paragangliomas and their locations (Fig. 27-10).

## Pheochromocytoma

Pheochromocytoma is a benign or malignant medullary

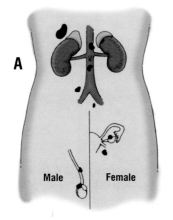
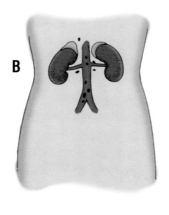

**FIG. 27-7.** Sites of heterotopic adrenal glands and nodules of cortical tissue (**A**), and chromaffin tissue (**B**). Masses (colored black) on and near aorta are retroperitoneal extraadrenal paraganglia. (Modified from Skandalakis JE, Gray SW, Rowe JS Jr. Anatomical Complications in General Surgery. New York: McGraw-Hill, 1983; with permission.)

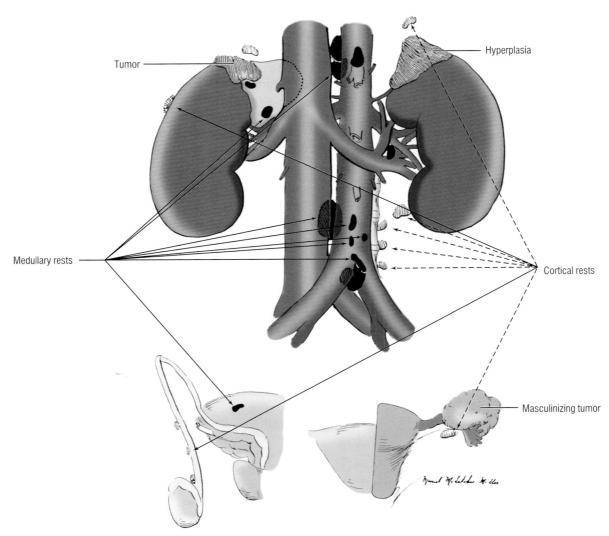

Tumor

Hyperplasia

Medullary rests

Cortical rests

Masculinizing tumor

**FIG. 27-8.** Reported locations of adrenocortical and medullary tissue. (Modified from Fonkalsrud EW. The adrenal glands. In: O'Neill JA, Rowe MI, Grosfeld JL, Fonkalsrud EW, Coran AG (eds). Pediatric Surgery, 5th ed. St. Louis: Mosby, 1998, pp. 1155-1574; with permission.)

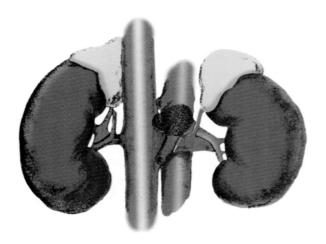

**FIG. 27-9.** Most frequent location of accessory gland (shaded area) on aorta between celiac and superior mesenteric arteries. (Modified from Graham LS. Celiac accessory suprarenal glands. Cancer 1953;6:149-152.)

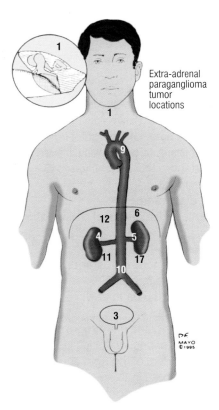

Extra-adrenal
paraganglioma
tumor
locations

**FIG. 27-10.** Anatomic location of extraadrenal tumors. Numbers indicate number of patients with tumors in particular location. (Note: patients with multiple tumors are counted more than once if they had tumors at different locations.) (Modified from O'Riordain DS, Young WF Jr, Grant CS, Carney JA, van Heerden JA. Clinical spectrum and outcome of functional extraadrenal paraganglioma. World J Surg 1996;20:916-922.)

tumor. "Functioning" tumors produce catecholamines, either epinephrine, norepinephrine, or both. Hypertension, tachycardia, sudoresis, and anxiety reaction result from the hormonal excess.[17]

Lo et al.[18] stated that "[a]drenal pheochromocytoma is potentially lethal if undetected and is associated with long-term morbidity." They cited the results of studies in which pheochromocytoma was diagnosed in 4 of 8486 autopsies (0.05%); in 3 of these cases, it was the immediate cause of death.

Ito et al.[19] stated that parenchymal degeneration of pheochromocytomas produces paroxysmal hypertension in most cases. Pheochromocytoma is a rare tumor that is found in only 0.1% of patients with diastolic hypertension, according to Favia et al.[20] They presented 55 patients with pheochromocytoma as a rare cause of hypertension.

### *Adrenal Gland Hemorrhage*

Adrenal gland hemorrhage is the second most common

source of hemoperitoneum in newborns. The right side is involved in 70% of cases, the left in 25%; the condition is bilateral in 5%.[21] This phenomenon has several etiologic factors. The large size of the neonatal adrenal gland makes it vulnerable to traumatic injury. Involution of the inner fetal cortical zone leaves central vessels unsupported.

### *Neuroblastoma*

Neuroblastoma is the second most common tumor of infancy, and the most common abdominal tumor of infancy. Fifty percent of the tumors originate in the adrenal gland; the remainder originate in the sympathetic chain. Genetic basis, autosomal dominance, autosomal recessive inheritance patterns, and chromosomal abnormalities are probably all responsible for the genesis of neuroblastoma.

We quote Alexander[22]:

> *Neuroblastoma is a malignant tumor of neural crest origin that may arise anywhere along the sympathetic ganglia or within the adrenal medulla. The median age of diagnosis is 2 years; however occurrence is skewed toward younger children, with nearly 35% of cases occurring under 1 year of age and the remainder under 10 years of age. Seventy-five percent of neuroblastomas originate within the abdomen or pelvis, and half of these occur within the adrenal medulla, whereas 20% originate within the posterior mediastinum and 5% within the neck.*

### *Adrenal Cyst*

Dermoid cyst of the adrenal gland has been reported.[23]

## SURGICAL ANATOMY

## Topography and Morphology

The adult adrenal gland weighs 4 to 8 g and measures ~4 × 3 × 1 cm. It is larger in women than in men. The adrenal glands are composed of two distinct parts, with differing functions and embryonic origins (see "Embryogenesis of the Adrenal Glands"). The volume of the larger portion, the cortex, is 8 to 20 times that of the medulla.[6]

The adrenal glands lie on the anteromedial surface of the kidneys near the superior poles; both the glands and the kidneys are retroperitoneal. The two glands differ in shape. The left is more flattened and has more extensive contact with the kidney. It is crescentic or semilunar in form, and may extend on the medial surface of the kidney almost to the hilum. The right gland is more triangular or pyramidal and lies higher on the kidney. This positioning is the reverse of that of the kidneys, in that the left kidney is higher. Each gland is capsulelike, covered by a thin connective tissue stroma.

Each adrenal gland, together with the associated kidney, is enclosed in the renal fascia (of Gerota) and is surrounded by fat, although the adrenal gland is separated from the kidney by a partition of connective tissue. The perirenal fat is more yellow and of a firmer consistency than fat elsewhere in the abdomen.

The adrenal glands are firmly attached to the fascia, which is in turn firmly attached to the abdominal wall and to the diaphragm. The inferior phrenic arteries pass superior to the adrenals to reach the diaphragm. The inferior phrenic arteries give off a series of branches, the superior adrenal arteries, like teeth of a comb. These, their associated connective tissue, and other adrenal arteries and veins assist in holding the adrenal glands *in situ*.

A layer of loose connective tissue separates the capsule of the adrenal gland from that of the kidney. Because the kidney and the adrenal gland are thus separated, the kidney can be ectopic or ptotic without a corresponding displacement of the gland. Fusion of the kidneys, however, is often accompanied by fusion of the adrenal glands.[8]

Occasionally, the adrenal gland is fused with the kidney so that separation is almost impossible. Davie[24] found six such cases in 1,500 autopsies. A partial or total nephrectomy in such individuals would require a coincidental adrenalectomy.

Normal adrenal glands can be visualized with computed tomography. They appear as triangular shadows, 2 cm in width, with their bases over the upper poles of the kidneys.[25] Linos and Stylopoulos[26] reported that computed tomography underestimates the actual size of adrenal tumors; even when corrected, the size of the tumor cannot predict its clinical behavior.

Anand et al.[27] reported that "[t]he commonest shape of the [adrenal] glands on the left side was semilunar but on the right side it was highly variable: triangular, tetrahedral, inverted Y or V shaped. On comparison of the gross measurements with available ultrasound and CT scan data it was found that both the length and thickness in the population studied were greater than reported in the literature. A knowledge of these variations is very important in diagnosis of abnormalities of the [adrenal] gland, of which tumoral enlargement is rather common."

## Relations

Each adrenal gland has only an anterior and posterior surface. Their relationships to other structures are as follows: (Figs. 27-11 - 27-12)

- Right adrenal gland:
  - Anterior surface:
    Superior: "bare area" of the liver
    Medial: inferior vena cava
    Lateral: "bare area" of the right lobe of the liver
    Inferior: peritoneum (very rarely, if ever) and first part of the duodenum (occasionally)
  - Posterior surface:
    Superior: diaphragm
    Inferior: anteromedial aspect of the right kidney
- Left adrenal gland:
  - Anterior surface:
    Superior: peritoneum (posterior wall of the omental bursa) and the stomach
    Inferior: body of the pancreas
  - Posterior surface:
    Medial: left crus of the diaphragm
    Lateral: medial aspect of the left kidney

The medial borders of the right and left adrenal glands are about 4.5 cm apart. In this space, from right to left, are the inferior vena cava, the right crus of the diaphragm, part of the celiac ganglion, the celiac trunk, the superior mesenteric artery, the other part of the celiac ganglion, and the left crus of the diaphragm.

REMEMBER:
- The right adrenal gland is located posterior to the duo-

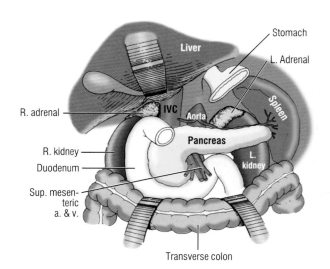

FIG. **27-11**. Relations of adrenal glands from anterior approach. (Modified from Skandalakis JE, Gray SW, Rowe JS Jr. Anatomical Complications in General Surgery. New York: McGraw-Hill, 1983; with permission.)

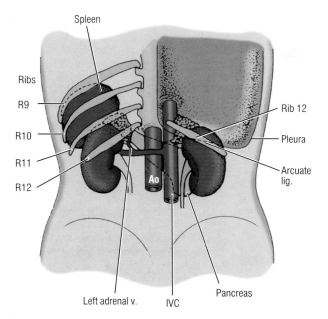

**FIG. 27-12.** Anatomy of adrenal glands. Ao, Aorta (Modified from Hughes S, Lynn J. Surgical anatomy and surgery of the suprarenal glands. In: Lynn J, Bloom SR (eds). Surgical Endocrinology. Oxford: Butterworth Heinemann, 1993, pp. 458-467; with permission.)

denum and the right lobe of the liver.
- In many cases, the medial part of the right adrenal gland is related to the inferior vena cava.
- The right adrenal gland may be closely related to the right hepatic vein as it passes to drain into the inferior vena cava.
- The right adrenal vein is short, and is difficult to ligate.
- The right adrenal gland is anterior to the diaphragmatic and pleural reflections.
- The left adrenal gland is located posterior to the stomach and pancreas and medial to the splenic porta.
- The left adrenal gland is located in front of the reflections of the diaphragm and the pleura.
- The left adrenal gland is related to the medial aspect of the upper pole of the left kidney, occasionally extending to the left renal porta.

## *Adrenal Zones*

The outer portion of the adrenal gland, the adrenal cortex, is composed of three zonae: glomerulosa, fasciculata, and reticularis. The innermost region of the adrenal gland is the medulla. Figs. 27-4 and 27-7 demonstrate chromaffin cells of the adrenal medulla and of heterotopic adrenal glands.

To help the student remember the layers of the adrenal

gland, every year in our clinical and surgical anatomy classes we repeat the mnemonic "**G**ood **F**or **R**eason **M**other" (Fig. 27-13). Another mnemonic device which is currently popular with medical students relates the architecture of the cortical region of the adrenal gland and its regulatory functions: **G**reat **f**at **r**ats: salt, sugar, sex.

## **Vascular Supply**

### *Arterial Supply*

The adrenal glands and the thyroid gland are the viscera having the greatest blood supply per gram of tissue. As many as 60 arterial twigs may enter the adrenal gland. The arterial supply of the adrenal glands arises, in most cases, from three sources (Fig. 27-14):
- The superior adrenal arteries. A group of six to eight arteries arises separately from the inferior phrenic arteries. One artery may be larger than the others, or all may be of similar size.
- The middle adrenal artery arises from the aorta just proximal to the origin of the renal artery. It can be single, multiple, or absent. It supplies the perirenal fat only.
- One or more inferior adrenal arteries arise from the renal artery, an accessory renal artery, or a superior polar artery. Small twigs may arise from the upper ureteric artery.

All these arteries branch freely before entering the adrenal gland, so 50-60 arteries penetrate the capsule over the entire surface.[28] It is possible that this branching of arteries before entering the adult adrenal gland indicates the outline of the surface of the much larger gland of the embryonic period, when the fetal cortex was present.

The sources of arterial supply to the adrenal gland are subject to variation.[29-31] In 61 percent of individuals, the supply by middle or inferior adrenal arteries may be lacking; the superior adrenals are absent in only about 2 percent of cases. In about 5 percent of individuals, the arterial supply is derived wholly from one source — a singular vessel supplying the superior, middle, and inferior branches.

### *Venous Drainage*

The adrenal venous drainage does not accompany the arterial supply, and is much simpler (Fig. 27-14). A single vein drains the adrenal gland, emerging at the hilum. The left vein passes downward over the anterior surface of the gland. This vein is joined by the left inferior phrenic vein before entering the left renal vein.

The right vein is typically very short; it may be 0.5 cm

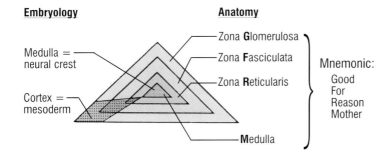

**Embryology**

Medulla =
neural crest

Cortex =
mesoderm

**Anatomy**

Zona **G**lomerulosa
Zona **F**asciculata
Zona **R**eticularis
**M**edulla

Mnemonic:
Good
For
Reason
Mother

**Physiology**

Zona Glomerulosa =
aldosterone (mineralocorticoid)

Zona Fasciculata and Reticularis =
cortisol (glucocorticoids), androgens

Medulla = catecholamines (epinephrine,
norepinephrine, dopamine)

**Pathology**

Pheochromocytoma and related tumors

Syndromes of corticosteroid excess

Neuroblastomas

Feminizing and masculinizing syndromes

**FIG. 27-13.** Summary of embryology, anatomy, physiology, and pathology of adrenal glands. (Modified from Skandalakis JE, Gray SW. Embryology for Surgeons (2nd ed). Baltimore: Williams & Wilkins, 1994.)

long, or even less. The right adrenal vein passes obliquely to open into the posterior side of the inferior vena cava. The right adrenal vein does not usually have any tributaries other than from the adrenal gland. If the adrenal gland must be mobilized or removed, it is wise to ligate the right adrenal vein first, then divide and ligate the arteries later, because the right vein is so easily torn from the inferior vena cava.

The right adrenal vein may drain into the right hepatic vein, close to the junction of the hepatic vein with the infe-

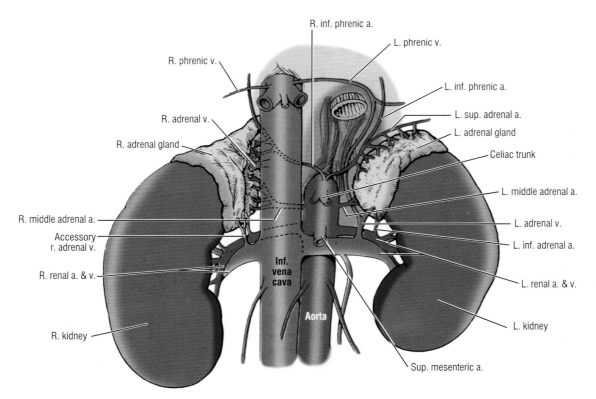

**FIG. 27-14.** Arterial supply and venous drainage of adrenal glands. (Modified from Skandalakis JE, Gray SW, Rowe JS Jr. Anatomical Complications in General Surgery. New York: McGraw-Hill, 1983; with permission.)

rior vena cava.[32] Occasionally there are two veins: one having a normal course, and an accessory vein entering the inferior phrenic vein.[33] In his 40 years in the dissecting room, the senior author of this chapter (JES) has encountered accessory veins several times. Some variations of the venous drainage are shown in Fig. 27-15.

When using the posterior approach to the adrenal gland, the left adrenal vein is found on the anterior sur-face of the gland. The right adrenal vein is found between the inferior vena cava and the gland. Careful mobilization of the gland is necessary for good ligation of the vein.

In the early studies of Dobbie and Symington,[34] it was observed that the adrenal gland appeared to be divisible into three regions: the head, the body, and the tail. The head region, in which the medullary tissue was most prominent,

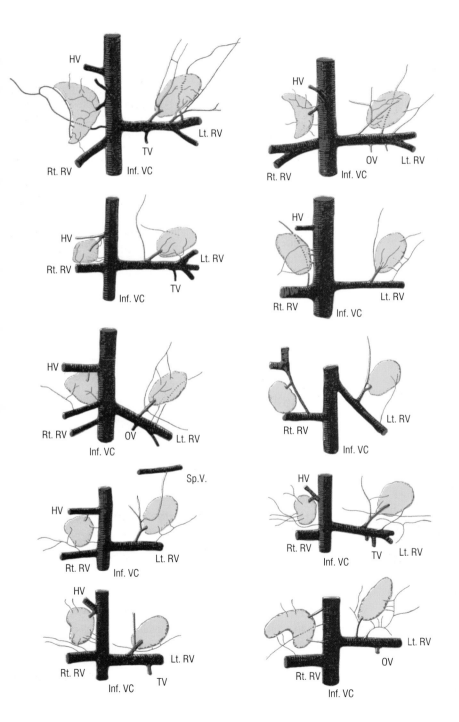

FIG. 27-15. Venous drainage of adrenals. HV, hepatic vein; Rt. RV, right renal vein; Inf. VC, inferior vena cava; TV, testicular vein; Lt. RV, left renal vein; OV, ovarian vein; Sp. V, suprarenal vein. (Modified from Johnstone FRC. The surgical anatomy of the suprarenal glands with particular reference to the suprarenal vein. Surg Clin North Am 1964;44: 1315-1385; with permission.)

was that part closest to the emergence of the adrenal vein from the gland. The tail, where medulla was almost absent, was the most lateral part. The ventral surface of the gland was characterized by an anterior groove. The dorsal surface possessed a ridgelike elevation, the crest, which increased in prominence near the lateral tip of the gland. The crest is flanked by two alar parts.

The central adrenal vein carries with it a cuff of cortical tissue into the substance of the gland. The vein is characterized by unique longitudinal muscle fibers, especially thick on its dorsal surface, which may be related to effective closure of its tributaries upon contraction. Shortly after entering the adrenal gland, the central vein receives a large muscular branch which curves backwards and drains the head of the gland. Several other main tributaries enter the main vein from the body and tail region.

In the studies of Monkhouse and Khalique,[35] in almost all cases venous interconnections were found between the adrenal venous system and the azygos, hemiazygos, and lumbar veins, in addition to accessory connections with the renal veins. The study was initiated by the finding (in a patient with a left-sided pheochromocytoma) of high levels of catecholamines in the superior vena cava and right atrium, rather than in the inferior vena cava, as one would normally expect.

### Lymphatic Drainage

The lymphatics of the adrenal gland are usually said to consist of a profuse subcapsular plexus that drains with the arteries and a medullary plexus that drains with the adrenal veins. Merklin[36] could find no evidence of lymphatic vessels within the parenchyma of the adrenal glands.

Drainage is to renal hilar nodes, lateral aortic nodes, and to nodes of the posterior mediastinum above the diaphragm by way of the diaphragmatic orifices for the splanchnic nerves (Fig. 27-16). Rouvière[37] stated that lymphatics from the upper pole of the right adrenal gland may enter the liver. The majority of capsular lymphatic vessels pass directly to the thoracic duct without the intervention of lymph nodes.[36]

## Innervation

The adrenal cortex appears to have only vasomotor innervation. Most of the fibers reaching the gland from the splanchnic nerves, the lumbar sympathetic chain, the celiac ganglion, and the celiac plexus enter the medulla (Fig. 27-17). These fibers are preganglionic[38] and end on the medullary chromaffin cells. This arrangement is not as anomalous as it might appear; chromaffin cells arise from the same embryonic source as do the postganglionic neurons elsewhere. Most of these preganglionic fibers in humans are nonmyelinated.[39]

## HISTOLOGY

### Adrenal Cortex

The vascularity of the adrenal cortex is among the greatest in the entire body. The adrenal cortex is composed of three zones: the zona glomerulosa, the zona fasciculata, and the zona reticularis. In all three zones, all cells produce steroids.

In the zona glomerulosa (the outermost layer), small cells are arranged in roughly spherical groups. This zone secretes the mineralocorticoid aldosterone.

In the zona fasciculata, larger cells are arranged in columns which are oriented radially. The carbohydrate-active steroid, cortisol, and the adrenal sex steroids are produced here. Vitamin C is abundant in these cells.

In the third layer, the zona reticularis, small cells are arranged in strands forming an irregular network. These cells secrete cortisol, androgens, and estrogens. Cholesterol is present as a precursor to the genesis of the steroids.

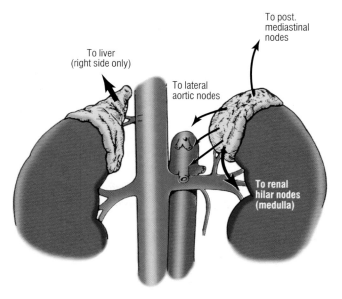

**FIG. 27-16.** Lymphatics of adrenal glands. (Modified from Skandalakis JE, Gray SW, Rowe JS Jr. Anatomical Complications in General Surgery. New York: McGraw-Hill, 1983; with permission.)

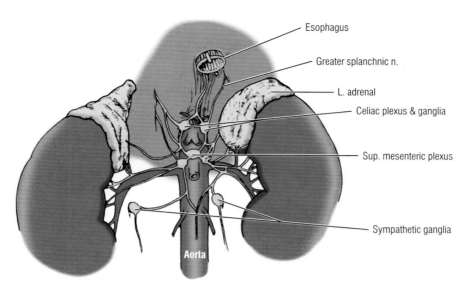

FIG. 27-17. Nerve supply to adrenal glands. (Modified from Skandalakis JE, Gray SW, Rowe JS Jr. Anatomical Complications in General Surgery. New York: McGraw-Hill, 1983; with permission.)

## Adrenal Medulla

The cells in the adrenal medulla are large and pale. They secrete epinephrine and have a chromaffin reaction. These cells are called chromaffin cells, or pheochromocytes. Distributed throughout the medulla, but few in number, are postganglionic sympathetic neurons.

Most medullary cells secrete epinephrine, but some secrete norepinephrine instead.

An abundance of round or oval secretory granules is located within the cellular cytoplasm of the adrenal medulla.

## PHYSIOLOGY

As mentioned above, the following corticosteroid hormones are secreted by the adrenal cortex:[40]
- aldosterone (in the zona glomerulosa)
- cortisol
- carbohydrate-active cortisol and androgens (in the zonae fasciculata and reticularis)

Secretion of aldosterone is controlled by angiotensin II, serum potassium, and the adrenocorticotropic hormone (ACTH) (Fig. 27-18).

Cortisol secretion is controlled by ACTH from the anterior pituitary gland (Fig. 27-19).

An excess of androgenic sex steroids almost always arises from carcinoma. Enzymatic defects (Fig. 27-20) are responsible for congenital adrenal hyperplasia with sexual ambiguity.[41] By blocking the adrenal production of cortisol, the defects result in the loss of negative feedback to the hypothalamus. There is continued stimulation and excess production of androgens and possibly mineralocorticoids. The result is congenital adrenal hyperplasia syndrome. The most common enzymatic deficiencies are 21-hydroxylase, 11-β-hydroxylase and 3-β-hydroxysteroid dehydrogenase.

In the adrenal medulla, sympathetic stimulation is responsible for the secretion of epinephrine and norepinephrine.

An excellent paper by Hiatt and Hiatt[42] presents the triumphal conquest of Addison's disease. It includes the discovery of the glands, identification of their hormonal products, use of the hormones for therapy, and biosynthesis for pharmacologic applications. We recommend it to all our readers.

Ito et al.[43] reported that the assay for urine metanephrine and normetanephrine is an effective test for the diagnosis of pheochromocytoma and management of incidentaloma.

We present Del Rio[44] verbatim:

*The sympathoadrenal system (SAS) represents a major contributor to body homeostasis, regulating blood pressure, heart rate, energy balance and intermediary metabolism. Thus, it is not unexpected that in the last decades a consistent literature has been focused on the possible role of the sympathoadrenal*

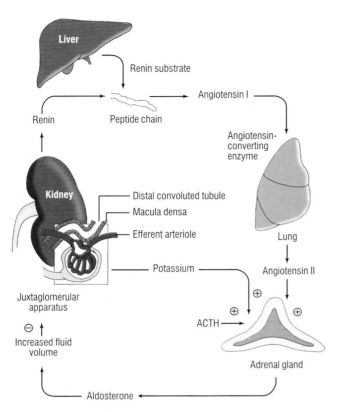

FIG. 27-18. Relations of renin, angiotensin I, angiotensin II, and their anatomic sites of production and enzymatic conversion. ACTH, adrenocorticotropic hormone. (Modified from Newsome HH. Suprarenal glands. In: Greenfield LJ (ed). Surgery: Scientific Principles and Practice. Philadelphia: JB Lippincott, 1993, pp. 1209-1223; with permission.)

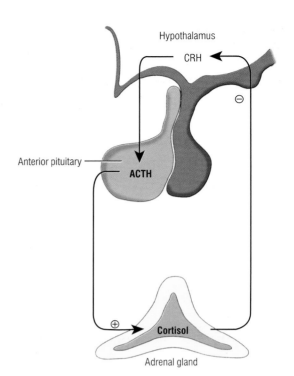

FIG. 27-19. Feedback relations between adrenal gland, hypothalamus, and anterior pituitary. CRH, corticotropin-releasing hormone; ACTH, adrenocorticotropic hormone. (Modified from Newsome HH. Suprarenal glands. In: Greenfield LJ (ed). Surgery: Scientific Principles and Practice. Philadelphia: JB Lippincott, 1993, pp. 1209-1223; with permission.)

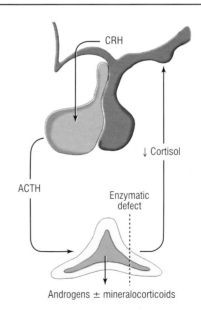

FIG. 27-20. Adrenal production of cortisol blocked by heritable enzymatic defects. CRH, corticotropin-releasing hormone; ACTH, adrenocorticotropic hormone. (Modified from Newsome HH. Suprarenal glands. In: Greenfield LJ (ed). Surgery: Scientific Principles and Practice. Philadelphia: JB Lippincott, 1993, pp. 1209-1223; with permission.)

*system in the pathogenesis of human obesity. There are, however, many factors confounding a comparison of sympathoadrenal system activity between lean and obese subjects. Among these, one should be aware that SAS should be functionally separated into sympathetic nervous system (SNS) and adrenal medulla (AM), and that each of these two systems can be activated independently from the other by distinct physiological stimuli; this phenomenon in fact underlies the discordant pattern of findings for adrenomedullary and sympathetic activity in human obesity. While, in fact, obese subjects often display an increased basal SNS activity, there are numerous reports of blunted AM function in the obese. Recent evidence suggests that this reduced adrenaline secretion is an acquired feature of human obesity, a finding that fits in well with the hypothesis that the hormonal milieu, particularly sex steroids and cortisol, plays a role in the determination of blunted AM activity. Catecholamines have been recently demonstrated to play a role also in the regulation of the whole energy balance. Adrenaline in fact acutely reduces both leptin mRNA as well as circulating leptin in human obese subjects, suggesting that catecholamines may influence the cross-talk between energy stores and the centrally mediated modulation of food intake.*

# SURGICAL APPLICATIONS

*...it should be recognized that the surgical approach and exposure to the suprarenal gland will be tailored to the underlying disease process...*

**Richard Bihrie and John P. Donahue**[45]

Surgery is the treatment of choice for all benign functioning or malignant adrenal tumors. Stratakis and Chrousos[46] summarized several studies of adrenal cancer, which showed these neoplasias accounting for 0.05-0.2% of all cancers and occurring at every age:

*A bimodal age distribution has been reported, with the first peak occurring before the age of 5 years and the second in the fourth to fifth decade. In all published series, females predominate, accounting for 65% to 90% of the reported cases. Several studies have shown a left-sided prevalence in adrenal cancer, whereas others have reported a right-sided preponderance. In approximately 2% to 10% of patients, adrenal cancer is found bilaterally.*

Khorram-Manesh et al.[47] reported the rarity of adrenocortical carcinoma and the need for better treatment alternatives. Though surgery is the treatment of choice, its role in advanced disease has been questioned.

Cook and Christie[48] reminded us that a unilateral adrenal mass may be secondary to *Mycobacterium kansasii* in patients with AIDS. The only conservative treatment applies to congenital adrenal hyperplasia with adrenal hyperfunction syndromes.

The adrenal glands may be approached by three open methods. These are: anterior, posterior, and lateral (transthoracic).

Harrison et al.[49] reported that the prognosis of adrenocortical carcinomas after curative resection depends on tumor size, hemorrhage, and mitotic count.

Paul et al.[50] advocated adrenalectomy for isolated adrenal metastases for selected patients presenting with long disease-free intervals and favorable tumor biology. Tsui et al.[51] provided a thoughtful analysis of the role of adrenalectomy in radical nephrectomy:

*With a low incidence of 0.6%, adrenal involvement is not likely in patients with localized, early stage renal cancer cell carcinoma and adrenalectomy is unnecessary, particularly when CT is negative. In contrast, the 8.1% incidence of adrenal involvement with advanced renal cell carcinoma supports the need for adrenalectomy. Careful review of preoperative imaging is required to determine the need for adrenalectomy in patients at increased risk with high stage lesions, renal vein thrombus and upper pole or multifocal intrarenal tumors. With a negative predictive value of 99.4%, negative CT should decrease the need for adrenalectomy. In contrast, positive findings are less reliable...[and] may not necessarily indicate adrenalectomy....*

## Anterior Approach for Left Adrenalectomy

The anterior approach is preferred when
- Adrenal disease is bilateral (10 percent of patients)[52]
- Tumor is over 10 cm in size
- Adrenal tumor has invaded surrounding structures

The anterior approach has the advantage of enabling the surgeon to inspect, palpate, and biopsy both glands. The incision chosen for an anterior approach may be vertical, midline or paramedian, transverse, or chevron. The chevron transabdominal incision provides bilateral exposure (Fig. 27-21).

### *Exposure and Mobilization of Left Adrenal Gland*

Exposure of the left adrenal gland begins with the incision of the posterior parietal peritoneum lateral to the left colon. The incision is carried upward, dividing the splenorenal ligament (Fig. 27-22). Care must be taken to avoid injury to the spleen, the splenic capsule, or the splenic vessels and the tail of the pancreas. The latter are enveloped by the splenorenal ligament.

Another approach to the left adrenal gland is by opening the lesser sac through the gastrocolic omentum, which may be incised longitudinally outside the gastroepiploic arcade (Fig. 27-23). In this approach, care must be taken to avoid traction on the spleen or the splenocolic ligament. The ligament may contain tortuous or aberrant inferior polar renal vessels or a left gastroepiploic artery.

Following either approach, the peritoneum under the lower border of the pancreas should be incised halfway along the tail; the incision should be extended laterally for about 10 cm. The pancreas can be gently retracted up-

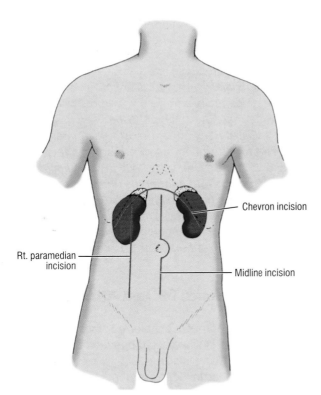

**FIG. 27-21.** Incisions for anterior exposure of adrenal glands. (Modified from Skandalakis JE, Gray SW, Rowe JS Jr. Anatomical Complications in General Surgery. New York: McGraw-Hill, 1983; with permission.)

ward, avoiding injury. This maneuver will expose the left adrenal gland on the superior pole of the left kidney; both the gland and the kidney are covered with renal fascia (of Gerota). The adrenal gland will be lateral to the aorta, about 2 cm cranial to the left renal vein. Incision of the renal fascia exposes the adrenal gland completely, and permits access to the adrenal vein. If the operation is for pheochromocytoma, the adrenal vein should be ligated at once to prevent the release of catecholamines into the circulation during subsequent manipulation of the gland.

A retractor must be placed gently to avoid tearing the inferior mesenteric vein from the splenic vein. Although the inferior mesenteric vein may be ligated without sequelae, it is prudent to refrain from the use of retractors in this area if possible.

A third approach, useful in patients whose left adrenal lesion is anterior, is exposure of the gland by an oblique incision of the left mesocolon (Fig. 27-24). The arcuate vessels can be divided and the marginal artery can be sectioned, but the major branches of the middle and left colic arteries must be preserved. Care to avoid excessive retraction will prevent injury to the wall of the left colon.

In some lesions, such as primary aldosteronism, the adrenal gland is hypervascular and friable; meticulous attention to hemostasis is essential. Adenoma can be disguised or mimicked by hematomas from operative trauma.[53] The surgeon can use a part of the adjacent periadrenal fascia to handle the gland. Manipulation should be with fine forceps only. Hemostasis from the numerous arteries can be maintained by clips, ligatures, or by electrocoagulation.

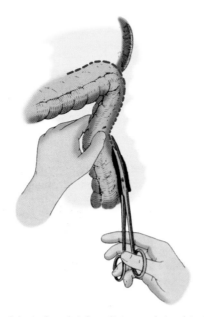

**FIG. 27-22.** Incision of parietal peritoneum lateral to left colon. Incision divides splenorenal ligament. (Modified from Skandalakis JE, Gray SW, Rowe JS Jr. Anatomical Complications in General Surgery. New York: McGraw-Hill, 1983; with permission.)

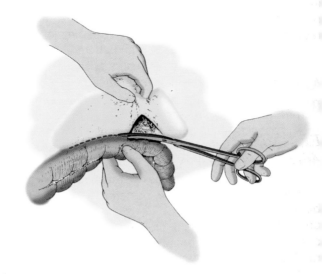

**FIG. 27-23.** Approach to the left adrenal through the gastrocolic omentum by opening the lesser sac. (Modified from Skandalakis JE, Gray SW, Rowe JS Jr. Anatomical Complications in General Surgery. New York: McGraw-Hill, 1983; with permission.)

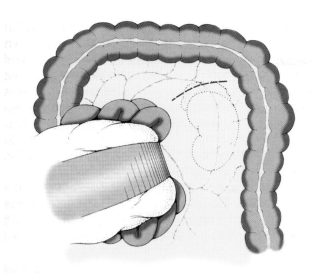

FIG. 27-24. Approach to the adrenal by incision of the left mesocolon near the splenic flexure. (Modified from Skandalakis JE, Gray SW, Rowe JS Jr. Anatomical Complications in General Surgery. New York: McGraw-Hill, 1983; with permission.)

Dissection should start at the inferolateral aspect of the left adrenal gland and should proceed superiorly (Fig. 27-25). The surgeon should keep in mind the possible presence of a superior renal polar artery. The gland can be retracted superiorly. Remember that the left adrenal gland extends downward, close to the left renal artery and vein.

After removal of the adrenal gland, its bed should be inspected for bleeding points. Surrounding organs, especially the spleen, should be inspected for injury. Splenic injury can be repaired with sutures over a piece of retroperitoneal fat, Gelfoam, or Avitene. More severe injury may require partial or even total splenectomy.

## Anterior Approach for Right Adrenalectomy

### Exposure and Mobilization of Right Adrenal Gland

On the right, the anterior approach to the adrenal gland begins with the mobilization of the hepatic flexure of the colon. Sharp dissection is necessary to divide posterior adhesions of the liver to the peritoneum. Remember that medial attachments can contain hepatic veins.

Mobilization of the colon will expose the duodenum. The second portion of the duodenum is freed by incision of its lateral avascular peritoneal reflection. It can now be separated from retroperitoneal structures and reflected forward

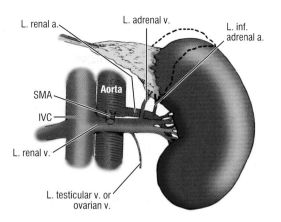

FIG. 27-25. The left adrenal gland exposed by an upward dissection. Note position of left adrenal vein. (Modified from Skandalakis JE, Gray SW, Rowe JS Jr. Anatomical Complications in General Surgery. New York: McGraw-Hill, 1983; with permission.)

and to the left (Kocher maneuver). This maneuver will expose the vena cava, the right adrenal gland, and the upper pole of the right kidney (Fig. 27-26). The surgeon must remember that the common bile duct and the gastroduodenal artery are in this area.

Unlike the left adrenal gland, the right gland rarely extends downward to the renal pedicle. The right adrenal vein usually leaves the gland on its anterior surface close to the cranial margin, and enters the vena cava on its posterior surface (Fig. 27-26). To prevent the release of catecholamines and to avoid stretching the vein, hemostatic clips should be placed as soon as both borders of

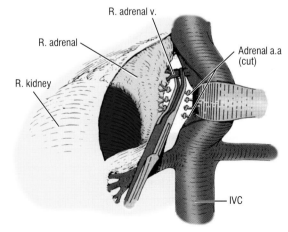

FIG. 27-26. Right adrenal gland and upper pole of right kidney are exposed following Kocher maneuver. Note position of right adrenal vein. (Modified from Skandalakis JE, Gray SW, Rowe JS Jr. Anatomical Complications in General Surgery. New York: McGraw-Hill, 1983; with permission.)

the vein are visible. Stretching the vein invites hemorrhage from the vena cava.

Tominaga et al.[54] advised resection of pheochromocytoma by completely isolating the IVC and using extracorporeal charcoal hemoperfusion, thereby preventing systemic distribution of catecholamines during manipulation of the tumor.

## Posterior Approach for Adrenalectomy

### *Exposure and Mobilization*

In spite of the advantage of being able to inspect, palpate, or biopsy both glands by using the anterior approach, improvements in preoperative diagnosis (such as computed tomography and selective adrenal angiography) have increased the use of the posterior approach.[55] The posterior approach can be used for any adrenalectomy except that in which a large or ectopic tumor is a strong possibility.

Nagesser et al.[56] have different parameters for surgery: "Although laparoscopic adrenalectomy is the treatment of choice for small and benign adrenal lesions, larger lesions and/or adrenal malignancy require open adrenalectomy. In these cases the retroperitoneal approach is the preferred route."

With the patient prone, a curvilinear incision is made through the latissimus dorsi muscle to the posterior lamella of the thoracolumbar fascia (Fig. 27-27). This will expose the erector spinae muscle. Lumbar cutaneous vessels must be ligated or cauterized. The surgeon must be sure to be over the 12th, not the 11th, rib. Dissection of the pleural fold at the 11th rib can result in pneumothorax. Remove the 12th rib on the left, and the 11th rib on the right.[57]

The erector spinae muscle attachments to the dorsal aspect of the 12th rib should be detached, exposing the rib. The rib must be removed subperiosteally to avoid damaging the underlying pleura. Periosteum should be stripped on the superior surface from medial to lateral and on the inferior surface from lateral to medial. Avoid injury to the 12th intercostal nerve bundle at the inferior angle of the rib. The nerve is separate from, but parallel with, the blood vessels. The vessels can be ligated if necessary.

The pleura must be separated from the upper surface of the diaphragm, and the diaphragm should be incised from lateral to medial. The fascia can be opened, and the upper pole of the kidney identified. Inferior retraction of the kidney will usually bring the adrenal gland into the field. Care must be taken to avoid tearing the renal capsule or stretching a possible superior polar artery.

Dissection of the left adrenal gland should begin on the medial aspect, with clips for the arteries encountered. Remember that the pancreas lies just beneath the gland; it is easily injured. In this approach, the last step is to identify the left adrenal vein, which usually emerges from the medial aspect of the gland and courses obliquely downward to enter the left renal vein. Undue traction on the gland can tear the renal vein.

The right adrenal gland is approached by retracting the superior pole of the right kidney inferiorly; the posterior surface of the adrenal gland can then be dissected free from fatty tissue. The liver must be retracted upward as the apex of the gland is reached. The lateral borders are freed up, leaving only the medial margins attached.

The right adrenal gland should be retracted laterally. Branches from the inferior phrenic artery, aorta, and right renal artery to the gland should be ligated. The right adrenal vein, also, should be ligated (Fig. 27-26). We recommend freeing the vena cava far enough to ensure room for an angle clamp should hemorrhage from the vena cava

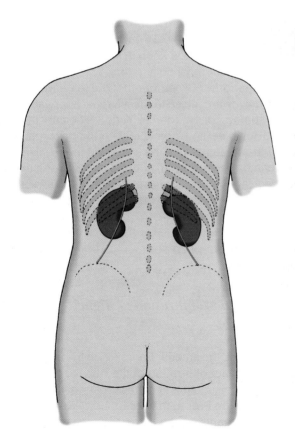

**FIG. 27-27.** Incisions for posterior approach to adrenal glands. (Modified from Skandalakis JE, Gray SW, Rowe JS Jr. Anatomical Complications in General Surgery. New York: McGraw-Hill, 1983; with permission.)

or the adrenal vein require it. After removing the gland, carefully inspect for air leaks and bleeding before closing the incision.

## Thoracoabdominal Approach for Adrenalectomy

### Exposure and Mobilization

The thoracoabdominal approach provides a better exposure for large tumors of a single adrenal gland.[58] It will permit removal of the spleen and the distal pancreas, should they be involved with the adrenal tumor.[59]

The incision starts at the angle of the 8th to the 10th rib. It extends across the midline to the midpoint of the contralateral rectus muscle just above the umbilicus (Fig. 27-28). The 10th rib is removed, the pleura is opened, and the diaphragm is incised from above. The remainder of the procedure is the same as for the anterior approach.

## LAPAROSCOPIC ADRENALECTOMY

Laparoscopic adrenalectomy may be performed by a lateral transabdominal or a posterior retroperitoneal approach. Duh et al.[60] reported that both methods are safe. They used the posterior approach for bilateral tumors; for tumors of more than 6 cm, the lateral approach was preferable. Walz et al.[61] supported the posterior retroperitoneoscopic approach for adrenalectomy.

Imai et al.[62] stated that laparoscopic transperitoneal lateral adrenalectomy is the technique of choice for removing functioning adenomas and adrenal masses less than 6 cm in diameter. They reported that patients undergoing the laparoscopic procedure experience greater comfort, less blood loss, and shorter hospital stays with no increase in cost.

Thompson et al.[63] found transabdominal laparoscopic adrenalectomy preferable to open posterior adrenalectomy, despite its greater expense. They reported improved patient comfort and satisfaction, and "dramatically" fewer complications. Rutherford et al.[64] presented 67 successful adrenalectomies employing the unilateral transabdominal approach; postoperative bleeding occurred in 1.5% of cases, as did port site herniation.

Basso et al.[65] advised that laparoscopic supragastric approach for left adrenalectomy gives a good visualization of the left adrenal, avoiding anatomic complications during mobilization of the spleen, pancreatic tail, and splenic flexure of the colon. Good visualization of

the left adrenal vein is also accomplished.

Horgan et al.[66] found laparoscopic adrenalectomy safe and effective for benign adrenal tumors. Jossart et al.[67] stated "Laparoscopic adrenalectomy can now be considered the standard of care for most adrenal neoplasms." Using data on pheochromocytoma surgery, Fern ndez-Cruz et al.[68] reached the same conclusion. Walther et al.[69] reported the following: "Laparoscopic partial adrenalectomy is technically feasible in patients with a hereditary form of pheochromocytoma, and may preserve adrenocortical function. Laparoscopic ultrasound was necessary to identify 2 of the seven pheochromocytomas removed."

Shen et al.[70] advised laparoscopic adrenalectomy for patients with primary hyperaldosteronism. The authors report that this laparoscopic procedure yields similar results with respect to blood pressure and hypokalemia and is accompanied by lower morbidity than the open procedure. Patients with less severe hypertension and hypokalemia are now undergoing this procedure.

A seven-year study of laparoscopic adrenalectomies by Brunt et al.[71] concluded the following:

*Laparoscopic adrenalectomy is a safe and effective procedure and has several advantages over open adrenalectomy. Laparoscopic adrenalectomy should become the preferred operative approach for the treatment of patients with small, benign adrenal neoplasms.*

In commentary on the Washington University findings, Prinz[72] wisely stated that adrenal glands should be removed in toto with their capsule intact. Prinz agreed with Brunt and colleagues that increased tumor size greatly decreased the advisability of laparoscopy. Siperstein et al.[73]

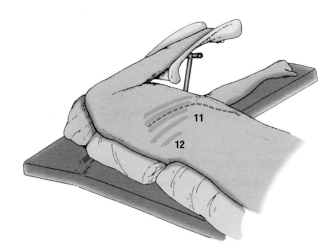

FIG. 27-28. Incision for thoracoabdominal approach to adrenal gland. (Modified from Skandalakis JE, Gray SW, Rowe JS Jr. Anatomical Complications in General Surgery. New York: McGraw-Hill, 1983; with permission.)

stated that laparoscopic posterior adrenalectomy should be considered in patients with tumors less than 6 cm. Staren and Prinz[74] concluded that more than 60 percent of surgically treatable adrenal disease may be approached laparoscopically.

Walz et al.[75] stated that in selected cases subtotal adrenalectomy via posterior approach retroperitoneoscopically is a safe procedure.

Kollmorgen et al.[76] compared acute-phase response and wound healing in laparoscopic and open posterior adrenalectomy in 40 pigs. They concluded that laparoscopic adrenalectomy compared favorably enough that study of its use should continue. Ting et al.[77] stated that laparoscopic adrenalectomy is replacing posterior adrenalectomy.

Barry et al.[78] stated that for small incidentalomas considered benign or nonfunctioning the appropriate treatment is conservative management, rather than laparoscopic removal.

Barresi and Prinz[79] stated the following:

*Conventional surgical approaches, particularly the transabdominal and thoracoabdominal approaches, will undoubtedly be required to treat certain lesions of the adrenal gland. This is especially true when dealing with larger tumors, and those suspicious for malignancy. Surgeons with an interest in treating patients with adrenal disorders must become proficient in the technique of laparoscopic adrenalectomy. This will allow them to offer their patients the most appropriate means of operative therapy suitable for their individual problems.*

Gill et al.[80] provided cautious support for outpatient adrenalectomy, "Ambulatory adrenalectomy is feasible and safe, and results in high patient satisfaction. However, ambulatory adrenalectomy should be restricted to highly select patients and performed by minimally invasive surgeons who have considerable experience with laparoscopic surgery."

Smith et al.[81] have written that "laparoscopic adrenalectomy has become the gold standard for adrenalectomy."

## ANATOMIC COMPLICATIONS

## Anterior Approach for Left Adrenalectomy

### *Vascular Injury*

#### Inferior Mesenteric Vein

The inferior mesenteric vein can be avulsed by excessive traction at its junction with the splenic vein. Bleeding is difficult to control, and the vessel may have to be ligated.

#### Middle and Left Colic Arteries

The middle and left colic arteries, or their larger branches, can be severed by sharp dissection through the left mesocolon. A segmental colectomy may be necessary if the blood supply is compromised. Excessive traction on the colon may lead to a tear of the spleen's capsule due to splenocolic attachment to the inferior pole of the spleen.

#### Superior Renal Polar Arteries

Superior renal polar arteries are present in about 15 percent of subjects.[30] Their position, superior to the renal arteries, renders them vulnerable. They can be ligated if necessary.

#### Renal Artery and Vein

The left adrenal gland extends down the medial surface of the left kidney almost to the hilum; thus, it is possible to injure the renal vessels while mobilizing the gland. Careful repair is required. If repair is not possible, nephrectomy may be necessary.

Remember, however, that the left kidney can be saved if the left renal vein is ligated proximal to its junction with the adrenal and gonadal veins; this is particularly true when operating on a right kidney tumor with an inferior vena caval thrombus. If ligation must be distal to these tributaries, venous infarction will occur; repair of the vein or nephrectomy is mandatory.

If nephrectomy is performed, ligate the renal and gonadal veins separately. Carlton and Guerriero[82] stated that major divisions of the renal vein at the hilum can be ligated with impunity. They believed that intrarenal collateral circulation will compensate for the segmental venous ligation.

### *Organ Injury*

#### Splenic Capsule and Spleen

Excessive traction on the spleen with tearing of the capsule is the greatest single operative risk in anterior left adrenalectomy. Nash and Robbins[83] reported splenic injury requiring splenectomy in up to 20 percent of adrenalectomy patients. We believe that partial splenectomy should be performed whenever possible.

#### Pancreas

The pancreatic parenchyma can be injured during upward reflection of the organ; this may result in clinical pancreatitis with the formation of a pseudocyst in some cases. Injury to the tail of the pancreas requires resection and drainage. If injury to the inferior border is minor, drain; if major, repair and drain, or resect the entire distal pancreas and drain.

### Renal Capsule

Sharp dissection of the inferior medial margin of the left adrenal gland can injure the capsule of the left kidney. Such injury should be repaired.

### Left Colon

Incision of the left mesocolon or excessive retraction of the colon could injure the colon wall, or even perforate it. The colon should be prepared with enemas and antibiotics before surgery, in case inadvertent perforation occurs and repair is necessary.

## Anterior Approach for Right Adrenalectomy

### *Vascular Injury*

### Hepatic Veins

Remember that the medial posterior attachments of the liver contain the hepatic veins. Retract with care. A right hepatic vein can be ligated.[84] Hepatic resection after major hepatic vein ligation is necessary in some animals, but not in humans.

### Inferior Vena Cava

Avoid aggressive lateral retraction of the adrenal gland. Traction on the right adrenal vein may rupture the vena cava; hemorrhage here is difficult to control, and immediate repair is necessary.

### Superior Renal Polar Artery

As on the left, the occasional polar artery lies close to the operative field and can be injured. If injured, it can be ligated.

### Gastroduodenal Artery

The gastroduodenal artery should be identified and avoided during the Kocher maneuver. If it is injured, ligation is necessary.

### *Organ Injury*

### Liver

Injury to the liver can result from excessive retraction. Pressure, cautery, Gelfoam, or Avitene can be used in repair.

### Duodenum

Mobilization and reflection can injure the duodenum and may result in a catastrophic postoperative duodenal fistula. Avoid sharp dissection, and be prepared to repair the defect.

## Posterior Approach for Adrenalectomy

### *Vascular Injury*

### Superior Renal Polar Arteries

As in other approaches, the superior renal polar arteries, which are inconstant, are vulnerable to inadvertent injury. They can be ligated if necessary.

### Left Adrenal Vein

Before mobilizing and clamping the left adrenal vein, the inferior vena cava should be freed up sufficiently to place a clamp on it in case ligation of either vessel should become necessary.

### Right Hepatic Vein

The right hepatic vein lies just cephalad to the right adrenal vein. It can be torn by excessive traction. It can be ligated.

### Inferior Vena Cava

In a right adrenalectomy, the vena cava can be injured by retraction or sharp dissection. Such injury must be repaired. Remember in retracting the liver that the veins from the caudate lobe often drain directly into the anterior surface of the inferior vena cava. Such veins, like the right adrenal vein, are often very short.

### *Organ Injury*

### Pleura

The pleura at the 12th rib must be identified and pushed out of the way. Flint and Bartels[58] found 4 cases of perforated pleura among 29 exposures of the adrenal glands.

If perforation occurs, it is necessary to evacuate air from the pleural cavity by catheter, with pulmonary inflation. Repair the pleural defect if possible.

### Twelfth Subcostal Nerve

The 12th subcostal nerve should be protected. Its injury will result in hyperesthesia or dysesthesia in the groin.

### Renal Capsule

Excessive retraction can tear the renal capsule. Repair

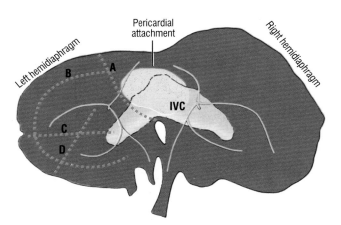

FIG. 27-29. Schematization showing chief branches of phrenic nerves on cranial surface of diaphragm. *Dashed lines* indicate location of incisions that will avoid phrenic nerves. *A,* The diaphragmatic component of a combined abdominothoracic incision extending down into the esophageal hiatus. *B,* Circumferential incision. *C, D,* Incisions extending from lateral (midaxillary) and posterior costal areas into the central tendon (from above). (Modified from Merendino KA. The intradiaphragmatic distribution of the phrenic nerve. Surg Clin North Am 1964;44:1217; with permission.)

it if necessary. The adrenal gland, in some cases, receives inferior adrenal arterial supply from capsular branches of the renal arteries.

**Pancreas**

Remember that in the posterior approach, the pancreas lies just beneath the left adrenal gland. See details in the "Anterior Approach for Left Adrenalectomy" section.

## Thoracoabdominal Approach for Adrenalectomy

### *Vascular Injury*

These injuries are the same as in anterior approaches.

### *Organ Injury*

In the thoracoabdominal approach, the lung and phrenic nerve are at risk in addition to the organs that are subject to injury in an anterior approach to the adrenal glands (splenic capsule and spleen, pancreas, left renal capsule, left colon, liver, duodenum).

If the pleura is entered, there is a possibility of injury to the lung; such injury must be repaired.

Incision of the diaphragm must be planned to avoid sectioning major branches of the phrenic nerve. Fig. 27-29 shows permissible incisions of the diaphragm from above.[85]

In a select group of patients with Cushing's syndrome, bilateral adrenalectomy is necessary and effective. However, this surgery is associated with occasional morbidity and mortality. According to O'Riordain et al.,[86] long-term sequelae are not well known.

NOTE: For further reading about the adrenal glands, the authors highly recommend *Surgery of the Suprarenal Glands,* edited by H. William Scott, Jr.[87]

## REFERENCES

1. Quoted in: Bourne GH. The Mammalian Adrenal Gland. Oxford: Clarendon Press, 1949, p. 17.

**Editorial Comment**

*This chapter provides an excellent summary of the embryology, surgical anatomy, and the more common surgical approaches for adrenalectomy. In addition to the approaches described in this chapter, I have found a transthoracic-transdiaphragmatic approach useful for occasional large high-lying tumors. The thoracoabdominal approach is necessary much less frequently than in the past because of the availability of retractors fixed to the table that can provide strong elevation of the cephalad portion of the abdominal incision.*

*The availability of sensitive biochemical tests and of highly specific preoperative localizing procedures permits the surgeon to select from a variety of operative approaches to the adrenal glands. Selection of the approach depends in part on whether the lesion is benign or malignant. Many surgeons have developed the skill to remove the smaller adrenal tumors laparoscopically. (RSF Jr)*

2. Crowder RE. The development of the adrenal gland in man, with special reference to origin and ultimate location of cell types and evidence in favor of the "cell migration" theory. Contrib Embryol Carnegie Inst Wash 1957;36:193.

3. Sucheston ME, Cannon MS. Development of zonular patterns in the human adrenal gland. J Morphol 1968;126:477.

4. Yeasting RA. Selected morphological aspects of human suprarenal glands. In: Mulrow PJ (ed). The Adrenal Gland. New York: Elsevier, 1986, pp. 45-63.

5. Winter JSD. Fetal and neonatal adrenocortical development: embryogenesis and morphology. In: James VHT (ed). The Adrenal Gland (2nd ed). New York: Raven Press, 1992. pp. 88-89.

6. Swinyard CA. Volume and corticomedullary ratio of the adult human suprarenal gland. Anat Rec 1940:76:69.

7. Bocian-Sobkowska J. Morphometric study of the human suprarenal gland in the first postnatal year. Folia Morphol (Warszawa) 2000;58: 275-284.

8. Potter EL. Pathology of the Fetus and the Newborn. Chicago: Year Book Medical Publishers, 1952.

9. Kerenyi N. Congenital adrenal hypoplasia: report of a case with extreme adrenal hypoplasia and neurohypophyseal aplasia, drawing attention to certain aspects of etiology and classification. Arch Pathol 71:336-343, 1961.

10. Winquist PG. Adrenal hypoplasia. Arch Pathol 71:324-329, 1961.

11. Graham LS. Celiac accessory adrenal glands. Cancer 1953;6:149.

12. Falls JL. Accessory adrenal cortex in broad ligament: incidence and functional significance. Cancer 1955;8:143.

13. Dahl EV. Aberrant adrenal cortical tissue near the testis in human infants. USAF Sch Aerospace Med 1961;61:1.

14. Weinberger MA. Pheochromocytoma. Arch Intern Med 1963;112:677.

15. Skandalakis JE, Vincenzi ER, Rand EO, Poer DH. Extraadrenal retroperitoneal "nonfunctioning" paraganglioma: report of a case and review of the literature. South Med J 1959;52:1368.

16. O'Riordain DS, Young WF Jr, Grant CS, Carney JA, van Heerden JA. Clinical spectrum and outcome of functional extraadrenal paraganglioma. World J Surg 1996;20:916-922.

17. Newsome HH Jr. Adrenal glands. In: Greenfield LJ, Mulholland MW, Oldham KT, Zelenock GB, Lillemoe KD (eds). Surgery: Scientific Principles and Practice (2nd ed). Philadelphia: Lippincott-Raven, 1997, pp. 1331-1347.

18. Lo CY, Lam KY, Wat MS, Lam KS. Adrenal pheochromocytoma remains a frequently overlooked diagnosis. Am J Surg 2000;179: 212-215.

19. Ito Y, Obara T, Yamashita T, Kanbe M, Iihara M. Pheochromocytomas: tendency to degenerate and cause paroxysmal hypertension. World J Surg 1996;20:923-927.

20. Favia G, Lumachi F, Polistina F, D'Amico DF. Pheochromocytoma, a rare cause of hypertension: long-term follow-up of 55 surgically treated patients. World J Surg 22:689-694, 1998.

21. Cywes S. Hemoperitoneum in the newborn. S Afr Med J 1967;41:1063-1073.

22. Alexander F. Neuroblastoma. Urol Clin North Am 2000;27:383-392.

23. Kaneko N, Kubota Y, Nakada T, Sasagawa I, Yaguchi H, Suzuki H. Dermoid cyst in the adrenal gland. Urol Int 2000;64:104-107.

24. Davie TB. Renal-adrenal adherence. Br J Surg 1935;22:428.

25. Hamilton WJ, Simon G, Hamilton SGI. Surface and Radiological Anatomy (5th ed). Baltimore: Williams and Wilkins, 1971, p. 240.

26. Linos DA, Stylopoulos N. How accurate is computed tomography in predicting the real size of adrenal tumors? Arch Surg 132:740-743, 1997.

27. Anand MK, Anand C, Choudhry R, Sabharwal A. Morphology of human suprarenal glands: a parameter for comparison. Surg Radiol Anat 1998;20:345-349.

28. Anson BJ, Cauldwell EW, Pick JW, Beaton LE. The blood supply of the kidney, suprarenal gland, and associated structures. Surg Gynecol Obstet 1947;84:313.

29. Edsman G. Angionephrography and suprarenal angiography. Acta Radiol 1957;155(suppl):5-141.

30. Merklin RJ, Michels NA. The variant renal and suprarenal blood supply with data on the inferior phrenic, ureteral and gonadal arteries. J Int Coll Surg 1958;29:41-46.

31. Merklin RJ. Arterial supply of the suprarenal gland. Anat Rec 1962;144:359-371.

32. Johnstone FRC. The surgical anatomy of the adrenal glands with particular reference to the suprarenal vein. Surg Clin North Am 1964;44:1315-1325.

33. Cade S. Adrenalectomy for hormone dependent cancers: breast and prostate. Ann R Coll Surg Engl 1954;15:71.

34. Dobbie JW, Symington T. The human adrenal gland with special reference to the vasculature. J Endocrin 1966;34:479-489.

35. Monkhouse WS, Khalique A. The adrenal and renal veins and their connections with the azygos and lumbar veins. J Anat 1986;146:105-115.

36. Merklin RJ. Suprarenal gland lymphatic drainage. Am J Anat 1966;119:359-374.

37. Rouvière H. Anatomy of the Human Lymphatic System. Tobias MJ (trans). Ann Arbor MI: Edwards Brothers, 1938.

38. MacFarland WE, Davenport HA. Adrenal innervation. J Comp Neurol 1941;75:219.

39. Coupland RE. Electron microscopic observations on the structure of rat adrenal medulla. I: The ultrastructure and organization of chromaffin cells in the normal adrenal medulla. J Anat 1965; 99:231.

40. Greenfield LJ, Mulholland MW, Oldham KT, Zelenock GB (eds). Surgery: Scientific Principles and Practice. Philadelphia: JB Lippincott, 1993.

41. Guyton AC. Textbook of Medical Physiology (8th ed). Philadelphia: WB Saunders, 1991.

42. Hiatt JR, Hiatt N. The conquest of Addison's disease. Am J Surg 174:280-283, 1997.

43. Ito Y, Obara T, Okamoto T, Kanbe M, Tanaka R, Iihara M, Okamoto J, Yamazaki K, Jibiki K. Efficacy of single-voided urine metanephrine and normetanephrine assay for diagnosing pheochromocytoma. World J Surg 22, 684-688, 1998.

44. Del Rio G. Adrenomedullary function and its regulation in obesity. Int J Obes Related Metab Disord 2000; 24 Suppl 2:S89-91.

45. Bihrie R, Donahue JP. Complications in adrenal surgery. In: Smith RB, Ehrlich RM (eds). Complications of Urologic Surgery (2nd ed). Philadelphia: Saunders, 1990.

46. Stratakis CA, Chrousos GP. Adrenal cancer. Endocrinol Metab Clin North Am 2000;29:15-25.

47. Khorram-Manesh A, Ahlman H, Jansson S, Wängberg B, Nilsson O, Jakobsson CE, Eliasson B, Lindstedt S, Tisell LE. Adrenocortical carcinoma: surgery and mitotane for treatment and steroid profiles for follow-up. World J Surg 1998;22:605-612.

48. Cook PP, Christie J. Unilateral adrenal mass due to *Mycobacterium*

*kansasii* in an AIDS patient. South Med J 91(10):981-982, 1998.

49. Harrison LE, Gaudin PB, Brenman MF. Pathologic features of prognostic significance for adrenocortical carcinoma after curative resection. Arch Surg 1999;134:181-185.

50. Paul CA, Virgo KS, Wade TP, Audisio RA, Johnson FE. Adrenalectomy for isolated adrenal metastases from non-adrenal cancer. Int J Oncol 2000;17:181-187.

51. Tsui KH, Shvarts O, Barbaric Z, Figlin R, deKernion JB, Belldegrun A. Is adrenalectomy a necessary component of radical nephrectomy? UCLA experience with 511 radical nephrectomies. J Urol 2000;163:437-441.

52. Graham JB. Pheochromocytoma and hypertension: an analysis of 207 cases. Int Abst Surg 1951;92:105.

53. Hunt TK, Schambelan M, Biglieri EG. Selection of patients and operative approach in primary aldosteronism. Ann Surg 1975;182: 353.

54. Tominaga M, Ku Y, Iwasaki T, Muramatsu S, Kuroda Y, Shima Y, Takao Y, Obara H. Resection of pheochromocytoma under inferior vena caval isolation and extracorporeal charcoal hemoperfusion. Arch Surg 1998;133:1016-1018.

55. Auda SP, Brennan MF, Gill JR Jr. Evolution of the surgical management of primary aldosteronism. Ann Surg 1980;191:1.

56. Nagesser SK, Kievit J, Hermans J, Krans HM, van de Velde CJ. The surgical approach to the adrenal gland: a comparison of the retroperitoneal and the transabdominal routes in 326 operations on 284 patients. Jpn J Clin Oncol 2000;30:68-74.

57. Bergland RM, Harrison TS. Pituitary and adrenal. In: Schwartz SI (ed). Principles of Surgery (4th ed). New York: McGraw-Hill, 1984.

58. Flint LD, Bartels CC. Ten years experience with 15 operated cases of pheochromocytoma. Surg Clin North Am 1962;47:721.

59. Chute R, Soutter L. Thoracoabdominal nephrectomy for large kidney tumors. J Urol 1949;61:688.

60. Duh QY, Siperstein AE, Clark OH, Schecter WP, Horn JK, Harrison MR, Hunt TK, Way LW. Laparoscopic adrenalectomy. Arch Surg 1996;131:870-876.

61. Walz MK, Peitgen K, Hoermann R, Giebler RM, Mann K, Eigler FW. Posterior retroperitoneoscopy as a new minimally invasive approach for adrenalectomy: results of 30 adrenalectomies in 27 patients. World J Surg 1996;20:769-774.

62. Imai T, Kikumori T, Ohiwa M, Mase T, Funahashi H. A case-controlled study of laparoscopic compared with open lateral adrenalectomy. Am J Surg 1999;178:50-54.

63. Thompson GB, Grant CS, van Heerden JA, Schlinkert RT, Young WF Jr, Farley DR, Ilstrup DM. Laparoscopic versus open posterior adrenalectomy: a case-control study of 100 patients. Surgery 1997;122:1132-1136.

64. Rutherford JC, Stowasser M, Tunny TJ, Klemm SA, Gordon RD. Laparoscopic adrenalectomy. World J Surg 1996;20:758-761.

65. Basso N, DeLeo A, Fantini A, Genco A, Rosato P, Spaziani E. Laparoscopic direct supragastric left adrenalectomy. Am J Surg 178:308-310, 1999.

66. Horgan S, Sinanan M, Helton WS, Pellegrini CA. Use of laparoscopic techniques improves outcome from adrenalectomy. Am J Surg 1997;173:371-374.

67. Jossart GH, Burpee SE, Gagner M. Surgery of the adrenal glands.

Endocrinol Metab Clin North Am 2000;29:57-68.

68. Fern ndez-Cruz L, Taur P, S enz A, Benarroch G, Sabater L. Laparoscopic approach to pheochromocytoma: hemodynamic changes and catecholamine secretion. World J Surg 1996;20:762-768.

69. Walther MM, Herring J, Choyke PL, Linehan WM. Laparoscopic partial adrenalectomy in patients with hereditary forms of pheochromocytoma. J Urol 2000;164:14-17.

70. Shen WT, Lim RC, Siperstein AE, Clark OH, Schecter WP, Hunt TK, Horn JK, Duh Q-Y. Laparoscopic vs open adrenalectomy for the treatment of primary hyperaldosteronism. Arch Surg 1999;134:628-32.

71. Brunt LM, Doherty GM, Norton JA, Soper NJ, Quasebarth MA, Moley JF. Laparoscopic adrenalectomy compared to open adrenalectomy for benign adrenal neoplasms. J Am Coll Surg 1996;183:1-10.

72. Prinz RA. Laparoscopic adrenalectomy. (Editorial). J Am Coll Surg 1996;183:71-73.

73. Siperstein AE, Berber E, Engle KL, Duh QY, Clark OH. Laparoscopic posterior adrenalectomy: technical considerations. Arch Surg 2000;135:967-971.

74. Staren ED, Prinz RA. Adrenalectomy in the era of laparoscopic surgery. Surgery 1996;120:706-711.

75. Walz MK, Peitgen K, Saller B, Giebler RM, Lederbogen S, Nimtz K, Mann K, Eigler FW. Subtotal adrenalectomy by the posterior retroperitoneoscopic approach. World J Surg 22: 621-627, 1998.

76. Kollmorgen CF, Thompson GB, Grant CS, van Heerden JA, Byrne J, Davies ET, Donohue JH, Ilstrup DM, Young WF. Laparoscopic versus open posterior adrenalectomy: comparison of acute-phase response and wound healing in the cushingoid porcine model. World J Surg 22:613-620, 1998.

77. Ting ACW, Lo C-Y, Lo C-M. Posterior or laparoscopic approach for adrenalectomy. Am J Surg 175:488-490, 1998.

78. Barry MK, van Heerden JA, Farley DR, Grant CS, Thompson GB, Ilstrup DM. Can adrenal incidentalomas be safely observed? World J Surg 22, 599-604, 1998.

79. Barresi RV, Prinz RA. Laparoscopic adrenalectomy. Arch Surg 1999;134:212-217.

80. Gill IS, Hobart MG, Schweizer D, Bravo EL. Outpatient adrenalectomy. J Urol 2000;163:717-720.

81. Smith CD, Weber CJ, Amerson JR. Laparoscopic adrenalectomy: New gold standard. World J Surg 1999;23:386-396.

82. Carlton CE, Guerriero WG. Complications in the management of renal trauma. In: Smith RB, Skinner DG (eds). Complications of Urologic Surgery. Philadelphia: Saunders, 1976.

83. Nash AG, Robbins GF. The operative approach to the left adrenal gland. Surg Gynecol Obstet 1973;137:670.

84. Mays ET, Conti S, Fallahzadeh H, Rosenblatt M. Hepatic artery ligation. Surgery 1979;86:536.

85. Merendino KA. The intradiaphragmatic distribution of the phrenic nerve. Surg Clin North Am 1964;44:1217.

86. O'Riordain DS, Farley DR, Young WF Jr, Grant CS, van Heerden JA. Long-term outcome of bilateral adrenalectomy in patients with Cushing's syndrome. Surgery 1994;116:1088.

87. Scott HW Jr (ed). Surgery of the Adrenal Glands. Philadelphia: JB Lippincott, 1990.

# Chapter *28*

# *Pelvis and Perineum*

GENE L. COLBORN, ROBERT M. ROGERS JR.,
JOHN E. SKANDALAKIS, ROBERT A. BADALAMENT,
THOMAS S. PARROTT, THOMAS A. WEIDMAN

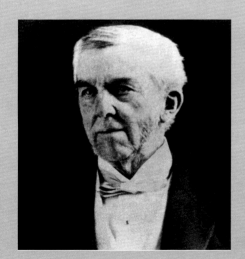

**Oliver Wendell Holmes (1809-1894),** who was famous for his wit, served as Dean of Harvard Medical School, as well as professor of anatomy and physiology, and wrote *Medical Essays,* a beautiful book of medical history.

*Indeed, the fitting together of these bones is so marvelous that it is not easy to explain.*

*Galen*[1]

*When lecturing to his students about the female pelvis... Oliver Wendell Holmes is said to have stated, "Gentlemen, this is the triumphal arch under which every candidate for immortality has to pass."*[2]

## HISTORY

The history of surgery of the pelvic sidewall, pelvic floor, and perineum is the history of the organs within. Therefore, this history is not addressed here, but is presented in the chapters that pertain to each individual organ.

# *Pelvic Sidewall*

## EMBRYOGENESIS

The anterior and posterior compartments of the limb bud mesoderm are responsible for the genesis of the pelvic bones. Specifically, the pubis and ischium are of anterior origin, and the ilium is of posterior origin. The scope of this chapter does not include embryologic details of the several anatomic entities forming the pelvic wall or their congenital anomalies.

## SURGICAL ANATOMY

### Introduction

During lower abdominal surgery, the pelvic wall is the source of most of the surgical problems, anatomic complications, and technical difficulties. General surgeons, urologists, and gynecologists must be very familiar with the topographic anatomy of the pelvic wall. Oncologic surgeons depend on this information to perform their radical operations for the cure of cancer.

Fragmented knowledge of pelvic anatomy has resulted, perhaps predictably, from the development of specialties related to specific organ systems. Thus, specialists in the treatment of colorectal, urologic, and gynecologic problems, for example, may operate in adjacent regions and yet possess very restricted knowledge of the clinical anatomy of nearby structures. Whorwell et al.[3] have pointed out, for instance, the tenfold increase in instability of the bladder detrusor muscle in patients who exhibit irritable bowel syndrome. It is important for the pelvic organ specialist to become familiar with the disorders of neighboring pelvic structures and the techniques for evaluating them.[4]

## "True" and "False" Pelvis

The concept of "true" and "false" pelvis is useful for the urologist, gynecologist, and urogynecologist, but for many surgeons operating in the lower areas of the abdomino-peritoneal cavity, this distinction is of little practical value.

It is difficult to pinpoint the organs that reside only in the true or the false pelvis. In this chapter, we include descriptions of anatomic entities that extend, or can extend, above the pelvic brim. We hope this does not confuse our reader.

### True (Lesser or Minor) Pelvis

The true pelvis is the area between the pelvic brim and the floor of the pelvic cavity, bounded by the linea terminalis above and the pelvic and urogenital diaphragms below.

The pelvis contains portions of the urinary, genital, and digestive tracts. The distal portions of the ureters, urinary bladder, female genitalia, prostate gland, rectosigmoid, proximal rectum, and small bowel are discussed in other chapters of this book.

The promontory of the sacrum and the iliopectineal line form the pelvic brim. The pelvic diaphragm below, with participation of the urogenital diaphragm, forms the floor of the pelvis. The sacrum, hip bones, and the two paired muscles (piriformis and obturator internus) and associated fasciae form the pelvic wall. The greater sciatic foramen transmits the piriformis muscle, sciatic nerve (Fig. 28-1) and other vessels and nerves of the gluteal and perineal regions.

The linea terminalis separates the false pelvis above from the true pelvis below. It is formed by the bilateral pubic crests and superior extent of the symphysis pubis, pectineal lines, arcuate lines, and midline sacral promontory. Inferior to the linea terminalis one typically finds the rectum, empty urinary bladder, non-pregnant uterus and its adnexa, vagina, terminal parts of the male reproductive system, sacral plexus, and pelvic neurovascular structures. Other elements, such as the greater omentum, transverse colon, sigmoid colon, and loops of small bowel (particularly ileum) provide unpredictable quantities of "temporary residents."

### False Pelvis

The intraperitoneal anatomy of the false pelvis is the downward continuation of the greater sac of the general abdominoperitoneal cavity. Its osseous boundaries are provided by the wings of the ilia (the flaring parts of the iliac bones of the pelvic girdle), the superior rami of the pubic bones, and the fourth and fifth lumbar vertebrae.

## Bony Wall, Its Ligaments, and Its Internal Coverings

The relatively unyielding framework of the pelvis consists of several bones together with their associated ligaments. This includes the two os coxae or hipbones, the sacrum, and the coccyx. The piriformis and obturator internus muscles arise from the bony surfaces of the true pelvis. With their fascial coverings, these constitute the primary sections of the pelvic sidewall.

In addition, the bony foramina and their contents provide secondary limitations on the dimensions of the cavity of the true pelvis.

Structures occupying the foramina include distinctly occlusive entities, such as the obturator membranes. Also occupying the foramina are soft, yielding elements. Soft structures entering or leaving the pelvic cavity include the sciatic nerve and its branches, the obturator nerves and vessels, the gluteal neurovascular elements, and the internal pudendal arteries and veins.

### Bones

The pelvis is bounded by the sacrum and coccyx posteriorly, and by the os coxae or hip bones anteriorly and laterally. The pelvic inlet (upper opening) is formed by the body and superior rami of the pubic bones and their pectineal lines, the arcuate lines of the ilia, and the sacral promontory. The pelvic outlet (lower opening) is formed anteriorly and laterally by the inferior rami of the pubis, the pubic symphysis and pubic arcuate ligament, and the rami and tuberosities of the ischia. Ligaments, sacrum, and coccyx are located posterolaterally and posteriorly.

### Ligaments

The sacrotuberous and sacrospinous ligaments participate in the formation of the pelvic walls. They also serve to convert the greater and lesser sciatic notches into the greater and lesser sciatic foramina by their attachments to the sacrum and coccyx medially and the ischial tuberosity and ischial spine laterally.

#### Sacrotuberous Ligament
The sacrotuberous ligament (Fig. 28-1) originates at the posterior superior iliac spine and the lateral border of the sacrum and coccyx. It inserts upon the ischial tuberosity.

#### Sacrospinous Ligament
The origin of the sacrospinous ligament (Fig. 28-1) is

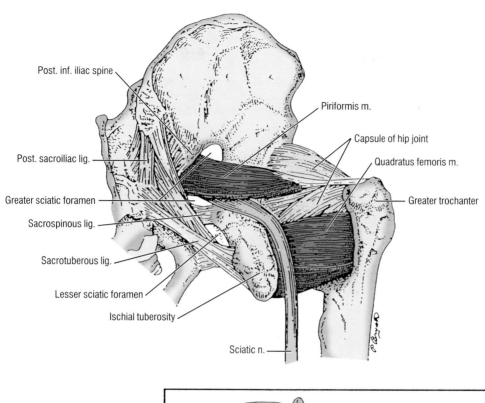

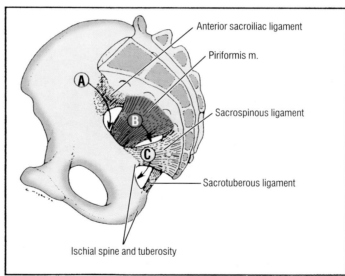

**Fig 28-1.** *Top:* Right posterior view of pelvis. *Inset:* Right lateral internal view showing sites of potential hernias through sciatic foramina. **A,** Suprapiriformic sciatic hernia. **B,** Infrapiriformic sciatic hernia. **C,** Subspinous sciatic hernia through lesser sciatic foramen. (Modified from Skandalakis LJ, Gadacz TR, Mansberger AR Jr, Mitchell WE Jr, Colborn GL, Skandalakis JE. Modern Hernia Repair: The Embryological and Anatomical Basis of Surgery. New York: Parthenon, 1996, Plate 2-1C; with permission. *Inset* modified from Skandalakis JE, Gray SW, Akin JT Jr. Surgical anatomy of hernial rings. Surg Clin North Am 1974;54:1227-1246; with permission.)

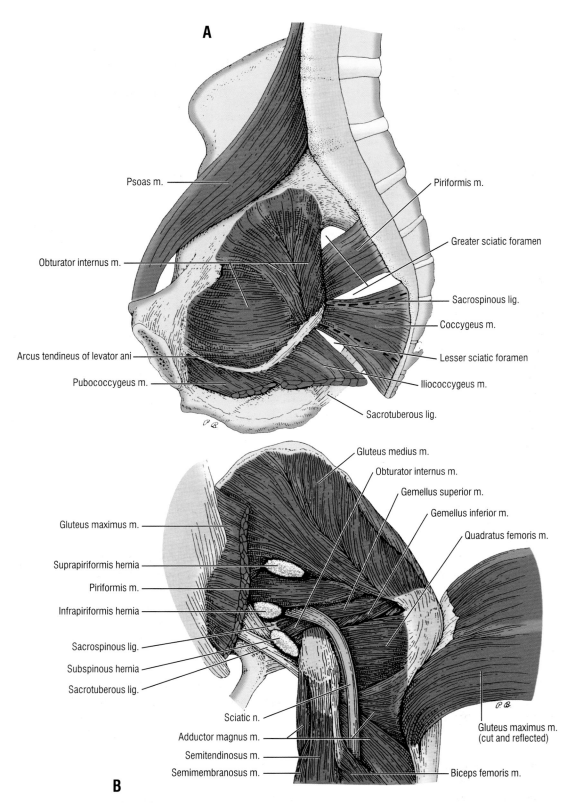

**A**

Psoas m.

Obturator internus m.

Arcus tendineus of levator ani

Pubococcygeus m.

Piriformis m.

Greater sciatic foramen

Sacrospinous lig.

Coccygeus m.

Lesser sciatic foramen

Iliococcygeus m.

Sacrotuberous lig.

Gluteus medius m.

Obturator internus m.

Gemellus superior m.

Gemellus inferior m.

Quadratus femoris m.

Gluteus maximus m.

Suprapiriformis hernia

Piriformis m.

Infrapiriformis hernia

Sacrospinous lig.

Subspinous hernia

Sacrotuberous lig.

Sciatic n.

Adductor magnus m.

Semitendinosus m.

Semimembranosus m.

Gluteus maximus m.
(cut and reflected)

Biceps femoris m.

**B**

FIG 28-2. **A,** Right pelvic wall with deep muscles and sciatic foramina. **B,** Right gluteal region with sites of sciatic hernias. Gluteus maximus transected and reflected. (Modified from Skandalakis LJ, Gadacz TR, Mansberger AR Jr, Mitchell WE Jr, Colborn GL, Skandalakis JE. Modern Hernia Repair. Pearl River NY: Parthenon, 1996; with permission.)

the lateral border of the sacrum and coccyx. Insertion is upon the ischial spine.

## *Foramina*

### Greater Sciatic Foramen

The greater sciatic foramen is five times larger than the lesser. It is formed by conversion of the greater sciatic notch into a foramen by the sacrospinous ligament.

The following anatomic entities leave the pelvis through the greater sciatic foramen (Fig. 28-2).
* Piriformis muscle
* Superior gluteal vessels and nerve (located superior to the piriformis)
* Inferior gluteal vessels and nerve (located inferior to the piriformis)
* Internal pudendal vessels and nerve (located inferior to the piriformis)
* Sciatic nerve
* Posterior femoral cutaneous nerve
* Nerves of the quadratus femoris, obturator internus, and gemelli muscles (all leave the pelvis inferior to the piriformis)

### Lesser Sciatic Foramen

The lesser sciatic foramen is formed by conversion of the lesser sciatic notch into a foramen by the sacrotuberous and sacrospinous ligaments (Fig. 28-2).

Several structures leave and enter from the lesser sciatic foramen. Leaving are the obturator internus and gemelli muscles, which arise from the edges of the foramen. The pudendal nerve, internal pudendal vessels, and the nerve to the obturator internus gain access to the perineum by passing through the lesser sciatic foramen.

REMEMBER: The supra- and infrapiriformis foramina and the lesser sciatic foramen are potential sites of herniation (Fig. 28-1, Fig. 28-2).

## *Soft Tissues of the Pelvic Sidewall*

The soft tissues of the pelvic sidewall consist of several layers. Their sequence from inside to outside is as follows.
* Peritoneum
* Endopelvic fasciae
* Internal iliac vessels, their branches, and associated smooth muscle and connective tissues
* Parietal layer of pelvic fascia
* Pelvic nerves
* Paired obturator internus muscles
* Piriformis muscles

## Anatomic Layers

We present here, as a series of three anatomic layers, the various elements of the pelvic sidewall in the order in which they are seen when dissecting one layer of tissue at a time from the peritoneum to the bone of the pelvic sidewall (Fig. 28-3).

### *First Anatomic Layer*

The first anatomic layer includes the peritoneum and ureter. The ureter is held to the peritoneum by connective tissue elements, which, in some respects, resemble a mesentery.

### *Second Anatomic Layer*

The second anatomic layer consists of the visceral branches of the internal iliac artery and vein, the endopelvic fascia, and the visceral nerves. Included in this layer are the vessels and nerves of the bladder, the internal reproductive organs, and the pelvic colon, together with the "pillars" of these organs. In the female, this layer also includes the specialized tissues of organ support, such as the cardinal and uterosacral ligament complexes and the pubovesicocervical fascia.

### *Third Anatomic Layer*

The third anatomic layer includes the parietal fascia, obturator nerves and vessels, other neurovascular elements of the pelvic sidewall, and the obturator internus and piriformis muscles and their various fasciae.

## Surgicoanatomic Layers

We acknowledge that the preceding order, although useful for anatomic clarity, does not fully reflect the layering of the pelvic elements as they are encountered in most pelvic surgical procedures. To the gynecologic or urologic surgeon especially, the following organization into five *surgicoanatomic* layers is more appropriate from a pragmatic point of view.

Now we present the anatomic entities of the pelvis both from a more technical, "surgicoanatomic" point of view, and also from a strictly "surgical," practical viewpoint. We trust that the details of the anatomy and its application in

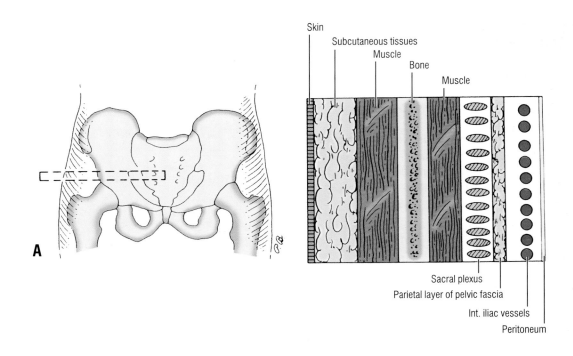

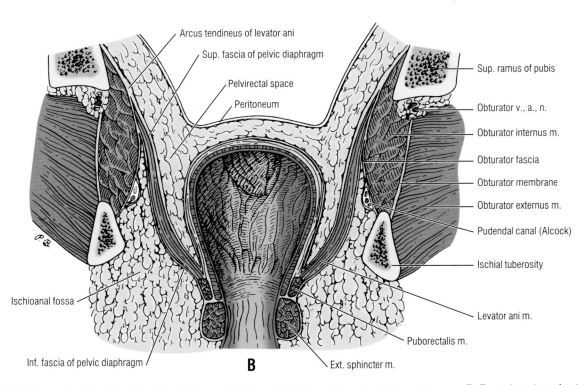

FIG. 28-3. Anatomy of pelvic wall and pelvic diaphragm. **A,** Elements of the pelvic wall: skin to peritoneum. **B,** Frontal section of pelvis showing fasciae of pelvic diaphragm, obturator fascia, and pudendal (Alcock's) canal. (Modified from Skandalakis LJ, Gadacz TR, Mansberger AR Jr, Mitchell WE Jr, Colborn GL, Skandalakis JE. Modern Hernia Repair. Pearl River NY: Parthenon, 1996; with permission.)

## TABLE 28-1. Ligaments of the Bladder

| Ligament | Location |
| --- | --- |
| *True Ligaments* | |
| Median umbilical ligament (urachus) (unpaired) | Dome of bladder to umbilicus |
| Lateral true ligament | Lateral wall of bladder to tendinous arch of pelvic fascia |
| Medial umbilical ligament (obliterated umbilical arteries) | Inguinal ligament |
| Medial puboprostatic ligament (male) | Pelvic wall to prostate gland |
| Lateral puboprostatic ligament | Pelvic wall to prostate gland |
| *False Ligaments* | |
| Superior false ligament (unpaired) | Covers the urachus |
| Lateral false ligament | Bladder to wall of pelvis |
| Lateral superior ligament | Covers the medial umbilical ligament |
| Posterior ligament (sacrogenital fold) | Side of bladder, around rectum to anterior aspect of sacrum |

*Source:* Skandalakis LJ, Gadacz TR, Mansberger AR Jr, Mitchell WE Jr, Colborn GL, Skandalakis JE. Modern Hernia Repair: The Embryological and Anatomical Basis of Surgery. New York: Parthenon, 1996; with permission.

these two differing approaches will converge in the mind of the reader. By employing these two schema, we hope to present the data as completely as we can without creating confusion.

### *First Surgicoanatomic Layer: Pelvic Peritoneum and Its Specializations*

The pelvic peritoneum is described in the chapter on the peritoneum. Here we emphasize only the most important entities from a surgical standpoint.

REMEMBER:
- The peritoneum does not reach the floor of the true pelvis in the adult.
- Several organs of the digestive, urinary, and genital tracts are not completely covered by the peritoneum.
- The pelvic peritoneum is associated medially with the urinary bladder, uterus, and rectosigmoid.
- The pelvic peritoneum is associated laterally with the uterine adnexa, ureter, and the ductus deferens.
- The ureter is fused intimately to the lateral surface of the peritoneum. If the peritoneum is incised and reflected medially, the ureter will be carried with it. The ureter can be re-

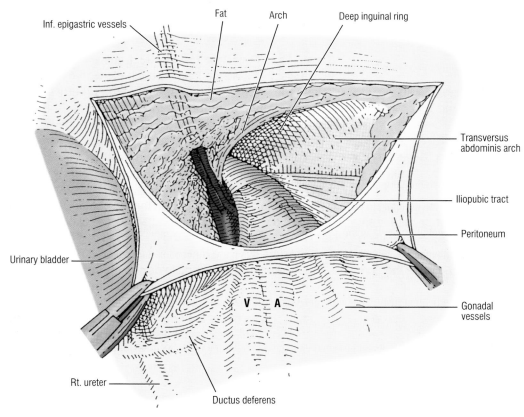

Fat    Arch    Deep inguinal ring

Inf. epigastric vessels

Transversus abdominis arch

Iliopubic tract

Peritoneum

Urinary bladder

V    A

Gonadal vessels

Rt. ureter

Ductus deferens

**FIG 28-4.** Path of inferior epigastric vessels. V, Vein; A, Artery. (Modified from Skandalakis LJ, Gadacz TR, Mansberger AR Jr, Mitchell WE Jr, Colborn GL, Skandalakis JE. Modern Hernia Repair. Pearl River NY: Parthenon, 1996; with permission.)

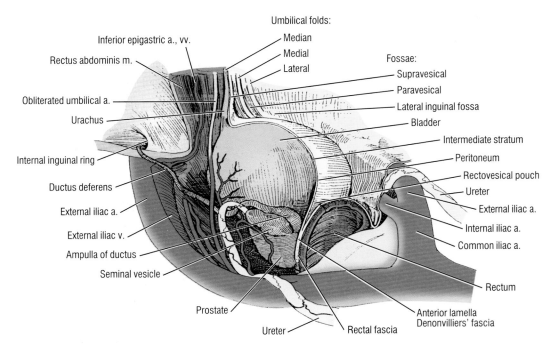

FIG. 28-5. Peritoneal relationships in the male. (Modified from Hinman F Jr. Atlas of Urosurgical Anatomy. Philadelphia: WB Saunders, 1993; with permission.)

leased from the peritoneum only by sharp dissection, which carries the risk of producing localized ureteric ischemia.

- The peritoneum of the pelvic wall is complicated by folds and fossae as it drapes over the midline organs of the urinary, genital, and digestive tracts.

### Urinary Tract Reflections and Spaces

Several folds of peritoneum are associated with the urinary bladder. When these folds or ligaments seem to have some support function, they are called true ligaments; when they seem less supportive, they are called false ligaments. This distinction is arbitrary and unconvincing. The most important of these peritoneal ligaments are listed in Table 28-1.

LATERAL UMBILICAL LIGAMENT. The bilateral, lateral umbilical ligament (peritoneum over the inferior epigastric artery and vein) (Fig. 28-4) is a helpful landmark for finding the ductus deferens when performing laparoscopic pelvic lymph node dissection and also for locating other inguinal entities in laparoscopic herniorrhaphies.

MEDIAL UMBILICAL LIGAMENT. The bilateral, medial umbilical ligament (peritoneum over the obliterated portions of the umbilical artery) can be seen passing upward and medially toward the umbilicus (Fig. 28-5). Above the urinary bladder, at its apex, are the supravesical fossae. The supravesical fossae are separated by the median umbilical ligament (peritoneum over the urachus of the bladder). Lateral

to the bladder are the paravesical fossae. The paravesical fossae are separated from the supravesical fossae by the transverse vesical fold, a horizontal fold of peritoneum which is most distinct when the bladder is empty.

### Genital and Digestive Tract Reflections and Spaces

FEMALE. The vesicouterine pouch of the female lies between the upper posterior aspect of the urinary bladder and the body and fundus of the uterus (Fig. 28-6). The broad ligaments extend laterally to the pelvic sidewall. The uterosacral ligaments in the female extend backward from the cervix, embracing the rectum in their course. The uterosacral ligaments form the rectouterine folds with overlying peritoneum.

The rectouterine folds bound the rectouterine pouch (of Douglas) on each side. The rectouterine fossa or pouch separates the urinary bladder, or the uterus and posterior vaginal fornix in front, from the rectum and rectal ampulla behind.

Between the uterosacral folds and the lateral wall of the rectal ampulla are the pararectal fossae, which communicate with the rectouterine pouch.

MALE. In the male, the counterparts of the uterosacral ligaments are the sacrogenital ligaments.

The rectovesical fossa, the male counterpart of the pouch of Douglas, separates the rectum from the urinary bladder and seminal vesicles in front. More superiorly in the pelvis on the left is the intersigmoid fossa (Fig. 28-7).

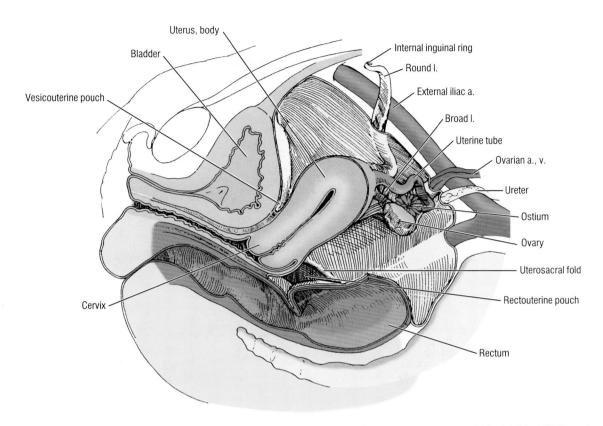

**FIG 28-6.** Peritoneal relationships in the female. (Modified from Hinman F Jr. Atlas of Urosurgical Anatomy. Philadelphia: WB Saunders, 1993; with permission.)

### Relations of the Intersigmoid Fossa

The peritoneum is anterior to the intersigmoid fossa. Posterior to the fossa are the bifurcation of the left common iliac artery and the passage of the left ureter into the true pelvis. The sigmoid mesocolon and its contained vessels, such as the sigmoid artery, are above and to the right of the fossa.

REMEMBER: The apex of the intersigmoid fossa is a landmark for finding the left ureter. With a finger in the fossa, the left ureter can be rolled on the underlying left common iliac artery.

## *Second Surgicoanatomic Layer: Blood Vessels of the Pelvis*

### General Topography of the Vessels

Between the peritoneum and the parietal pelvic fascia are the arteries and veins for the pelvic wall and viscera. The two main vessels are the bilateral internal iliac artery (Fig. 28-8) and internal iliac vein (hypogastric artery and vein) (Fig. 28-9). In the upright anatomic position, the artery

and vein pass in the vertical plane along the pelvic sidewall. Their branches generally pass medially and inferiorly to reach the pelvic viscera. They carry with them the heavy connective tissue mantle called the hypogastric sheath that assists the vessels in providing direct support to the

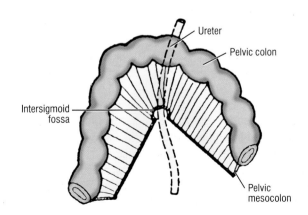

**FIG 28-7.** Intersigmoid fossa. (Modified from Decker GAG, du Plessis DJ. Lee McGregor's Synopsis of Surgical Anatomy (12th ed). Bristol: Wright, 1986; with permission.)

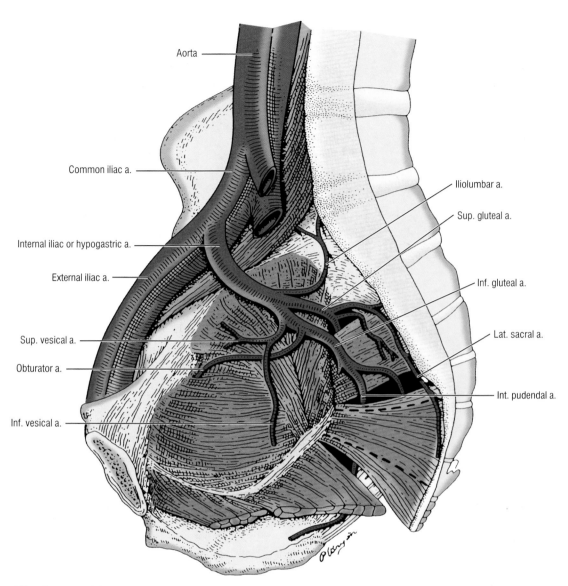

Aorta

Common iliac a.

Internal iliac or hypogastric a.

External iliac a.

Sup. vesical a.

Obturator a.

Inf. vesical a.

Iliolumbar a.

Sup. gluteal a.

Inf. gluteal a.

Lat. sacral a.

Int. pudendal a.

FIG 28-8. Internal iliac (hypogastric) artery branches into anterior and posterior division. Superior gluteal artery passes through superior portion of greater sciatic foramen. Inferior gluteal artery enters foramen below piriformis muscle. Inferior gluteal artery gives off superior and inferior vesical arteries and obturator artery before entering foramen. [Two unpaired arteries in the pelvis, the median sacral and superior rectal, are not shown.] All these arteries enter the pelvis extraperitoneally and may be ligated with impunity. (Modified from Skandalakis LJ, Gadacz TR, Mansberger AR Jr, Mitchell WE Jr, Colborn GL, Skandalakis JE. Modern Hernia Repair. Pearl River NY: Parthenon, 1996; with permission.)

organs. The reader should consult the classic and beautiful work of Uhlenhuth et al.[5] for a detailed description of the hypogastric sheath and its derivatives.

The visceral branches of the internal iliac artery and vein, together with visceral nerves, endopelvic connective tissues, and smooth muscle form the "second surgical layer" for the surgeon operating on the pelvic organs. When attempting to arrest hemorrhage arising from visceral blood vessels, it is within this layer that one attempts

to clamp, ligate, or clip the injured vessel or its ultimate source.

Other arteries are the unpaired median (middle) sacral, the distal portion of the inferior mesenteric artery with sigmoid branches and superior rectal branch. All enter the pelvis retroperitoneally and all can be safely ligated.

The rectal venous plexus (Fig. 28-9) is formed by the superior and middle rectal veins. The rectal venous plexus drains the rectosigmoid. From this plexus, drainage is to

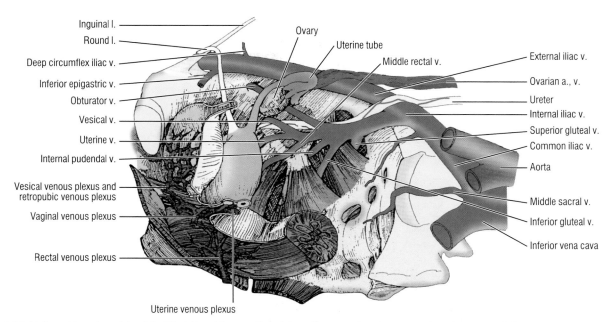

**FIG. 28-9.** Veins of female pelvis. (Modified from Hinman F Jr. Atlas of Urosurgical Anatomy. Philadelphia: WB Saunders, 1993; with permission.)

the inferior mesenteric vein (portal) and internal iliac vein (systemic). The uterine venous plexus drains to the internal iliac vein (systemic).

### Topography of the Branches

The surgeon should remember the topography of the bifurcations of the arterial and venous systems.

**ABDOMINAL AORTA.** The abdominal aorta (Fig. 28-8) bifurcates into the two common iliac arteries approximately at L4, 1 cm to 2 cm below and to the left of the umbilicus. When a thin, supine individual elevates the pelvis to displace the intestine, the pulse can be palpated at the bifurcation and the external iliac arteries can be felt at the pelvic brim.

**SACRAL ARTERIES.** The median sacral artery (which springs from the posterior aortic wall) is often forgotten by the surgeon. Despite its small size, it can produce bleeding when lacerated in the operating room. In some individuals, branches of this artery and the lateral sacral arteries ascend through the ventral sacral foramina to supply sacral and lumbar nerve roots and even contribute to the arterial supply of the caudal part of the spinal cord.

**INFERIOR VENA CAVA.** The inferior vena cava is formed from the two common iliac veins about 2 cm to 3 cm inferior to the umbilicus (Fig. 28-9, Fig. 28-10).

REMEMBER: The right common iliac artery crosses in

front of the left common iliac vein. This relationship is thought to be associated with the greater frequency of deep venous thromboses of the left common iliac vein and veins of the left lower limb. Inferior vena cava reflux associated with tricuspid regurgitation has been implicated in pelvic congestion syndrome.[6]

Wohlgemuth et al.[7] recommend percutaneous transluminal angioplasty, stenting, or both to treat pelvic vein stenosis following surgical thrombectomy.

**COMMON ILIAC ARTERY.** The bifurcation of the common iliac artery into internal and external iliacs is located at the level of the pelvic brim, opposite the sacroiliac joint (Fig. 28-8). Less commonly, however, this bifurcation may be just above or below the joint. This is especially true in individuals with more tortuous vessels, in some cases associated with vascular disease.

**INTERNAL ILIAC BIFURCATION.** The bifurcation of the internal iliac into anterior and posterior divisions is usually very close or slightly distal to its origin at the common iliac. After this last bifurcation the key number to remember is three. The posterior division has three parietal branches. The anterior division has three parietal branches and three visceral branches.

These patterns are quite variable. Branches of the internal iliac can arise as a "spray" of vessels with no distinct formation of anterior and posterior divisions.

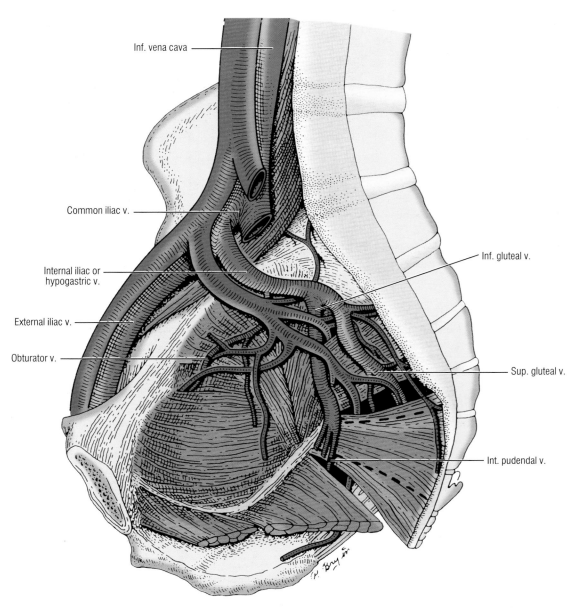

Inf. vena cava

Common iliac v.

Internal iliac or
hypogastric v.

External iliac v.

Obturator v.

Inf. gluteal v.

Sup. gluteal v.

Int. pudendal v.

FIG. 28-10. Venous pathways. (Modified from Skandalakis LJ, Gadacz TR, Mansberger AR Jr, Mitchell WE Jr, Colborn GL, Skandalakis JE. Modern Hernia Repair. Pearl River NY: Parthenon, 1996; with permission.)

*Terminal Branches of Posterior Division of Internal Iliac Artery.* Three parietal arterial branches typically originate from the posterior division of the internal iliac. These are the iliolumbar, superior gluteal, and lateral sacral arteries (Fig. 28-8), discussed below.

ILIOLUMBAR ARTERY. The iliolumbar artery is located behind the obturator nerve. It passes deep and laterally under the psoas muscle to supply the iliacus muscle and other tissues in the iliac fossa.

SUPERIOR GLUTEAL ARTERY. The superior gluteal artery is related to the sacral plexus. It most commonly passes be-

tween the lumbosacral trunk (formed by the junction of descending branches from L4 and L5) and the ventral ramus of S1 at the upper border of the piriformis muscle. As they pass through the greater sciatic foramen, the superior gluteal artery and the superior gluteal nerve (from L4, L5, S1) lie against the rather sharp edge of the upper bony margin of the foramen. Here the artery is quite vulnerable to laceration or avulsion.

The superficial branch of the superior gluteal supplies the upper half of the gluteus maximus. The deep branch courses transversely anteriorly between the gluteus medius and minimus, supplying them. Both the superficial and deep branches have extensive anastomoses with other regional vessels, including the inferior gluteal, medial circumflex, lateral femoral circumflex, and perhaps others.

LATERAL SACRAL AND INFERIOR GLUTEAL ARTERIES. The lateral sacral arteries are in front of the sacral plexus. There are one to three lateral sacral arteries. These pass through the ventral sacral foramina, providing branches to supply vertebrae and spinal nerve roots. They may contribute to the blood supply of the spinal cord by long, ascending branches. The inferior gluteal artery, usually a terminal branch of the anterior division of the internal iliac, may leave the pelvis by passing between S1 and S2. In a significant number of individuals the inferior gluteal and obturator arteries arise from the posterior division.

*Terminal Branches of Anterior Division of Internal Iliac Artery.*

VISCERAL BRANCHES. The anterior division gives origin to the following three or four visceral branches. All these branches remain within the pelvic cavity.
- Umbilical, whose patent segment is the source of the superior vesical arteries
- Uterine
- Inferior vesical
- Middle rectal artery, in some cases

NOTE: The visceral branches of the anterior division of the internal iliac will be described in greater detail in other chapters on the organs to which the branches are related.

To the urogynecologist in particular, the visceral branching pattern can be of use in locating the uterine artery. After observing the obliterated portion of the umbilical artery, one can trace it proximally toward its origin from the anterior division of the internal iliac. The surgeon can then identify the superior vesical branch of the artery passing medially toward the bladder. Proceeding further proximally, one can then identify the uterine artery passing medially toward the vicinity of the isthmus of the uterus, and then note the passage of the uterine artery over the ureter (Fig. 28-11).

PARIETAL BRANCHES. The anterior division also provides three parietal branches: the obturator, the internal pudendal, and the inferior gluteal. These arteries and their related structures (accessory pudendal, middle rectal, uterine and vaginal arteries) are discussed below.

Obturator Artery. The obturator artery is located below the obturator nerve at the sidewall of the pelvis. It passes through and exits the obturator foramen. In about 20 percent of individuals, the obturator artery arises from the superior gluteal artery. In 33 percent[8] (or even more commonly), an aberrant or accessory obturator artery is present, arising from the inferior epigastric artery.

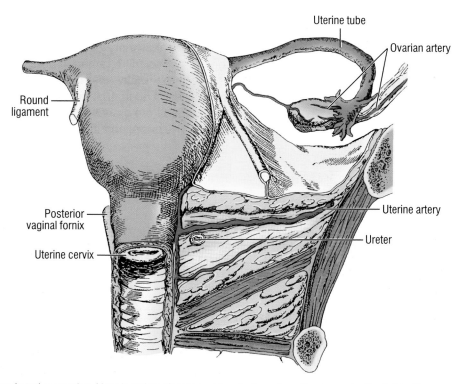

FIG. 28-11. Ovarian and uterine arteries. Note location of ureter under uterine artery ("water under the bridge").

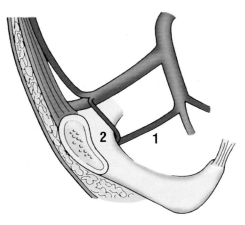

FIG. 28-12. Schematic view of the right side of the pelvis showing normal (1) and variant (2) positions of obturator vessels. (Modified from Gilroy AM, Hermey DC, DiBenedetto LM, Marks SC Jr, Page DW, Lei QF. Variability of the obturator vessels. Clin Anat 1997; 10:328-332; with permission.)

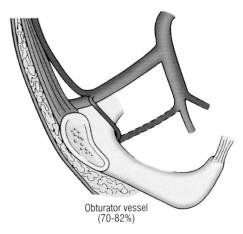

Obturator vessel
(70-82%)

FIG. 28-14. Summary schematic of the likelihood of encountering a variant obturator vessel on an individual pelvic side. (Modified from Gilroy AM, Hermey DC, DiBenedetto LM, Marks SC Jr, Page DW, Lei QF. Variability of the obturator vessels. Clin Anat 1997;10:328-332; with permission.)

Gilroy et al.[9] (Fig. 28-12, Fig. 28-13, Fig. 28-14) reported that 70-82% of pelvic halves and 83-90% of whole pelves had an artery, vein, or both in the variant position. Arteries were found predominantly in the normal position only, but normal and anomalous veins were most frequently found together. These data show that it is far more common than not to find a vessel coursing over the pelvic brim at this site; the implications for both pelvic surgeons and anatomists are obvious.

Aberrant Obturator. When it originates from the inferior epigastric artery, the aberrant obturator is closely related to the ligament of Gimbernat. The aberrant obturator crosses medial to, lateral to, or directly over the femoral ring and over

Cooper's ligament. Infrequently, both an aberrant obturator artery and a normal obturator artery are present, with rich anastomoses at the obturator canal. Such a vascular arrangement is called the "circle of death"[10] because of the profuse bleeding that can occur when either vessel is severed.

Internal Pudendal Artery and Vein. The internal pudendal artery is the more anterior of the two terminal branches of the anterior division of the internal iliac (Fig. 28-8). The internal pudendal artery leaves the pelvis by passing through the greater sciatic foramen. It crosses the sacrospinous ligament externally, just medial to the tip of the ischial spine. Here it accompanies the pudendal nerve (Fig. 28-15), formed from branches from S2, S3, and S4 at this location. The artery and its companion vein (Fig. 28-10) lie

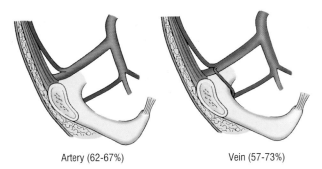

Artery (62-67%)        Vein (57-73%)

FIG. 28-13. Schematic summarizing the most common pattern for obturator arteries and veins with the range of percentages from the United States and China in parentheses. (Modified from Gilroy AM, Hermey DC, DiBenedetto LM, Marks SC Jr, Page DW, Lei QF. Variability of the obturator vessels. Clin Anat 1997;10:328-332; with permission.)

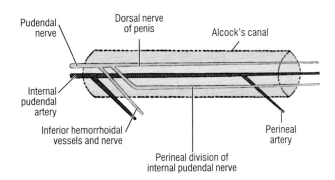

Pudendal nerve — Dorsal nerve of penis — Alcock's canal — Internal pudendal artery — Inferior hemorrhoidal vessels and nerve — Perineal division of internal pudendal nerve — Perineal artery

FIG. 28-15. Alcock's canal (dotted) and its contents. (Modified from McGregor AL, DuPlessis DJ. A Synopsis of Surgical Anatomy (10th ed). Baltimore: Williams & Wilkins, 1969; with permission.)

lateral to the nerve as they exit the pelvis inferior to the piriformis muscle. After crossing the external surface of the sacrospinous ligament and under the shelter of the more externally placed sacrotuberous ligament, the internal pudendal artery and its nerve enter Alcock's canal to supply the tissues of the ischioanal (ischiorectal) fossa and the urogenital structures. Their distribution is described later in this chapter and in the chapters on the genital systems.

Accessory Pudendal Artery. Rather frequently, an accessory pudendal artery arises from the internal pudendal artery just prior to the departure of the internal pudendal through the greater sciatic foramen. This relatively unknown artery leaves the pelvis beneath the pubic arcuate ligament. It is related unilaterally or bilaterally to the midline deep dorsal vein of the penis or clitoris. The accessory pudendal artery occurs in about 10 percent of males, including its origins from the internal pudendal, obturator artery, and other, less common sources.[11]

Inferior Gluteal Artery. The inferior gluteal artery (Fig. 28-8) passes through the greater sciatic foramen with its companion inferior gluteal nerve (L5, S1, S2), medial to the sciatic nerve. This artery supplies approximately the lower half of the gluteus maximus and anastomoses richly with other arteries deep to that muscle.

Middle Rectal Artery. The middle rectal artery arises most commonly from or with the vesical, internal pudendal, or inferior gluteal arteries. It can arise directly from the anterior division of the internal iliac, as well as from the uterine artery.

The middle rectal artery has 3 characteristic features which caused Last[8] to state that it is inappropriately named.
- It is often reduced in size and sometimes absent, especially in the female.
- Very little of the blood it transports goes to the rectum.
- Most of its blood goes to the prostate.

Uterine Artery. The uterine artery crosses the floor of the pelvis in the parametrial tissue of the broad ligament. It arises most commonly from the same vascular stem that provides origin for the umbilical artery.

To find the uterine artery, identify the obliterated portion of the umbilical artery where it passes the urinary bladder. Here one can observe the origin of the superior vesical branch(es) to the bladder. Proceed proximally toward the origin of the umbilical artery, where one can then identify the uterine artery as it arises from the same vascular stem. From its origin, the uterine artery passes medially toward the uterine isthmus, accompanied by its veins and abundant connective tissue, soon crossing over the ureter ("water under the bridge") (Fig. 28-11). This occurs approximately 1.5 cm (variably, 1 cm to 4 cm) from the uterine cervix. At the cervix, the uterine artery turns upward on the lateral wall of the body of the uterus in the broad ligament.

At the entrance of the uterine tube into the uterus, the uterine artery anastomoses end on with the tubal branch of the ovarian artery.[8] The uterine artery is the principal source of arterial supply to the uterine tube in about 60 percent of cases.

NOTE: The uterine artery is the direct anterior visceral branch from the internal iliac artery. In many cases it arises as a branch of the patent portion of the umbilical artery. In the male, the homologue of the uterine artery is the deferential branch of the inferior vesical artery.

Vaginal Artery. The vaginal artery is often a separate branch of the internal iliac artery. In many cases the vaginal artery comes from the uterine artery. There may be more than one vaginal artery; multiple vaginal arteries may arise from the internal iliac or from the internal iliac and uterine artery. The vaginal artery supplies the highly vascular walls of the upper part of the vagina.[8]

According to Killackey,[12] the rich anastomotic blood supply to the uterus from the ovarian, uterine, and vaginal vessels makes it difficult to cause devascularization injury when the uterus is removed during colorectal surgery, even with the most radical resection.

#### SUMMARY OF THE PELVIC ARTERIES
- Three parietal arterial branches leave the pelvis via the greater sciatic foramen:
  - Superior gluteal
  - Inferior gluteal
  - Internal pudendal
- The obturator artery leaves the pelvis via the obturator foramen.

NOTE: Any of these arteries leaving the pelvis can be ligated with relative impunity, taking care not to injure their fellow travelers, the nerves. If the internal iliac artery is occluded at its origin, however, or both gluteal arteries are ligated, gluteal ischemia can result.

All arteries of the pelvis enter it extraperitoneally. They are:
- Unpaired median sacral artery (runs from L4 to the coccyx and behind the left common iliac vein, superior hypogastric plexus, and rectum)
- Unpaired superior rectal artery
- Paired internal iliac arteries

### Collateral Circulation in the Pelvis
ARTERIAL CIRCULATION IN THE PELVIS. The eight potentially major pathways of collateral circulation after bilateral internal iliac ligation are:
- Uterine artery with ovarian artery from aorta
- Middle rectal artery with superior rectal artery from inferior mesenteric artery
- Obturator artery with inferior epigastric artery from external iliac artery

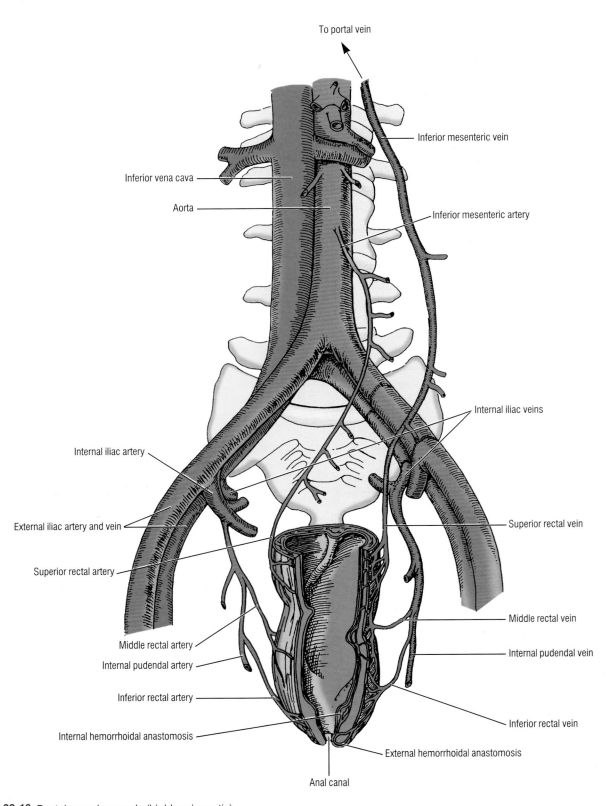

To portal vein

Inferior mesenteric vein

Inferior vena cava

Aorta

Inferior mesenteric artery

Internal iliac artery

Internal iliac veins

External iliac artery and vein

Superior rectal vein

Superior rectal artery

Middle rectal vein

Middle rectal artery

Internal pudendal artery

Internal pudendal vein

Inferior rectal artery

Inferior rectal vein

Internal hemorrhoidal anastomosis

External hemorrhoidal anastomosis

Anal canal

FIG. 28-16. Rectal vascular supply (highly schematic).

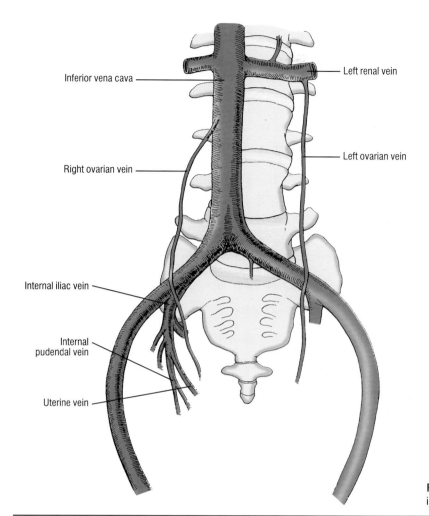

FIG. 28-17. Right and left ovarian veins and branches of internal iliac vein.

- Inferior gluteal artery with circumflex artery and perforating branches of the deep femoral artery
- Iliolumbar artery with lumbar artery from aorta
- Lateral sacral artery with median sacral artery from aorta
- Anastomoses between vessels of bladder wall and abdominal wall
- Anastomoses between internal and external pudendal arteries

The anastomosis of the middle rectal artery with the superior rectal artery and that of their corresponding veins can be extensive and significant (Fig. 28-16). The superior rectal artery is the terminal extension and downward continuation of the inferior mesenteric artery. It touches, but does not cross, the medial side of the left ureter, crosses the bifurcation of the left common iliac vessels, and descends into the base of the inferior limb of the sigmoid mesocolon to the rectum. The common iliac artery bifurcates at the pelvic brim opposite the sacroiliac joint.

**VENOUS CIRCULATION IN THE PELVIS.** Multiple small veins (Figs. 28-10, 28-16, 28-17) from the rectal plexus coalesce to form the superior rectal vein, draining by way of the infe-

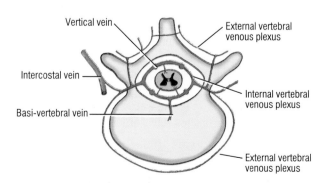

FIG. 28-18. Vertebral system of veins. (Modified from Decker GAG, du Plessis DJ. Lee McGregor's Synopsis of Surgical Anatomy (12th ed). Bristol: Wright, 1986; with permission.)

## Editorial Comment

*Retrograde venous reflux of prostatic cancer cells via Batson's plexus is a time-honored concept to explain the predilection for prostatic cancer to metastasize to the vertebrae and the skull. It would be difficult to prove that tumor cells do not reach these bone tissues via this mechanism rather than passing through the lungs and then into the systemic arterial system, but even if they do, there need to be many other mechanisms at play. Many cancer cells enter the systemic circulation, but the development of metastases is very inefficient. The growth of circulating tumor cells to form a metastasis depends on a relatively unique interaction between the tumor cell(s) and the host tissue. Ultimately there must be a molecular recognition system by which tumor cells interact with host endothelial cells in specific tissues and migrate through the capillary vessels to establish residence, to grow, and to eventually evoke a neovascular response from the host tissue. The mechanism for the rarity of metastatic disease in the distal extremities is yet to be explained, but it would seem unlikely that it has a simple anatomic explanation related to the circulation. The predilection for tumors such as prostate cancer and breast cancer to metastasize to the skull, vertebrae, and pelvis while sparing the bones of the distal extremities suggests that there may be biologic mechanisms that could potentially be modulated for therapeutic benefit. (RSF Jr)*

rior mesenteric vein to the portal system of the liver. Other rectal veins combine to form the middle rectal vein.

Superior and inferior gluteal veins emerge through the suprapiriformic and infrapiriformic apertures of the greater sciatic foramen and form the internal iliac (hypogastric) vein. Veins from the uterine, vesical, or prostatic venous plexus unite with the middle rectal vein to contribute to the internal iliac vein. The internal pudendal vein emerges through the lesser sciatic foramen to join the inferior gluteal or internal iliac vein. There are many variations of venous drainage.

The internal vertebral venous plexus (Batson's veins) (Fig. 28-18) is located within the extradural fat of the spinal canal. It communicates with the lateral sacral veins (a valveless system), then drains into the internal iliac vein.

NOTE: A sudden increase in pelvic pressure, such as from coughing, may produce venous reflux into the internal vertebral plexus. This can cause emboli because the blood courses through the posterior intercostal veins and into the superior vena cava via the azygos system. This route also provides an explanation for metastasis of cancer to the vertebrae and the skull. The brain and pelvic viscera are brought into association by this system.

**LYMPHATIC DRAINAGE IN THE PELVIS.** Lymphatic drainage of the pelvic organs is shown in Table 28-2.

### *Third Surgicoanatomic Layer: Pelvic Fasciae*

#### Parietal Fascia

According to Last,[13] the fascia of the pelvic wall is a strong, membranous layer covering the obturator internus and piriformis muscles that form the wall. The fascia is firmly attached to the periosteum at the muscles' margins.

From our observations, the parietal fascia should also include that fascia which covers the pelvic surface of the pelvic diaphragm, that is, the levator ani and coccygeus muscles. This is consistent with the concept that the endo-abdominal fascial lining is a continuum and called the fascia transversalis. This term refers to the apparent continuity of muscle fascia lining the abdominal muscles, including the inferior surface of the respiratory diaphragm above. Following this line of thought, we can view the muscle fascia lining the pelvic basin, both its sidewalls, and the floor as a continuing entity.

The parietal fascia of the pelvic basin is continuous with the parietal fascia of the false pelvis above. The parietal fascia also covers the "cracks" in the wall that are formed by the foramina. The superior and inferior gluteal blood vessels pierce this fascia to go to the buttocks, and the obturator nerve and vessels penetrate it to pass through the obturator canal.

#### Visceral Fascia

The visceral fascia (Fig. 28-19) is essentially the connective tissue that encapsulates the individual organs within the pelvis. This fascia can be named according to the organ it covers, such as vesical, rectal, or prostatic. The fascial encapsulation varies greatly in thickness over the organs of the pelvis. Where the organ passes through the pelvic floor, the visceral fascial capsule fuses with the adjacent parietal fascia of the floor.

**TABLE 28-2. Lymphatic Drainage of Pelvic Organs**

| Organs | Groups of Nodes Receiving Vessels Draining Pelvic Organs |
|---|---|
| Ovary (along ovarian a.) | Lumbar |
| Uterine tube (except part near uterus) (along ovarian a.) | Lumbar |
| Uterus | |
|   Upper part of body | Lumbar |
|   Lower part of body | External iliac |
|   Cervix | External iliac, internal iliac, and sacral |
|   Regional near uterine tube (along round ligament) | Superficial inguinal |
| Vagina | |
|   Upper part (along uterine a.) | External and internal iliac |
|   Middle part (along vaginal a.) | Internal iliac |
|   Lower part | Sacral and common iliac |
|   Part below hymen (with those from vulva and skin of perineum) | Superficial inguinal |
| Testis and epididymis (along testicular a.) | Lumbar |
| Seminal vesicle | External and internal iliac |
| Ductus deferens (pelvic portion) | External iliac |
| Prostate | Internal iliac mainly; sacral and external iliac |
| Scrotum | Superficial inguinal |
| Penis (clitoris) | |
|   Skin and prepuce | Superficial inguinal |
|   Glans | Deep inguinal and external iliac |
| Ureter (lower part) | External or internal iliac |
| Bladder | |
|   Superior and inferolateral aspects | External iliac |
|   Base | External iliac mainly; internal iliac |
|   Neck | Sacral and common iliac |
| Urethra | |
|   Female (along internal pudendal a.) | Internal mainly; external iliac |
|   Male | |
|     Prostatic and membranous parts (along internal pudendal a.) | Internal iliac mainly; external iliac |
|     Spongy part | Deep inguinal mainly; external iliac |
| Rectum | |
|   Upper part | Inferior mesenteric |
|   Lower part | Sacral, internal iliac, and common iliac |
| Anal canal | |
|   Above pectinate line (along inferior rectal and internal pudendal aa.) | Internal iliac |
|   Below pectinate line | Superficial inguinal |

*Source:* O'Rahilly R. Gardner-Gray-O'Rahilly Anatomy: A Regional Study of Human Structure, 5th Ed. Philadelphia: WB Saunders, 1986; with permission.

In certain areas, adjacent structures display a nearly common fascia, and it is practical to apply a more inclusive name. For instance, beginning anteriorly at the pubic bones, there is a continuing mantle of feltlike connective tissue and smooth muscle fibers known as the pubocervical, pubovesical, or pubovesicocervical fascia. It covers the anterior wall of the vagina and joins the superior fascia of the pelvic diaphragm lateral to the vagina (or prostate gland). Here it forms a bilateral band extending from about 1 cm above the lower border of the pubic bone to the ischial spine, the arcus tendineus fascia pelvis, or "white line of the pelvis." This connective tissue mantle is continuous also with the visceral fascia encapsulating the individual organs.

The relative density of the visceral fascia conforms with the distensibility of the organ. For example, the fascia covering the bladder and rectum is loose, while the fascia over the prostate is dense. The fascia that invests the organs contains the collecting channels of the lymphatic drainage from the organs. As noted by Uhlenhuth et al.,[5] surgeons are well aware that after a malignant growth in an organ invades the connective tissue capsule, metastatic spread is likely.

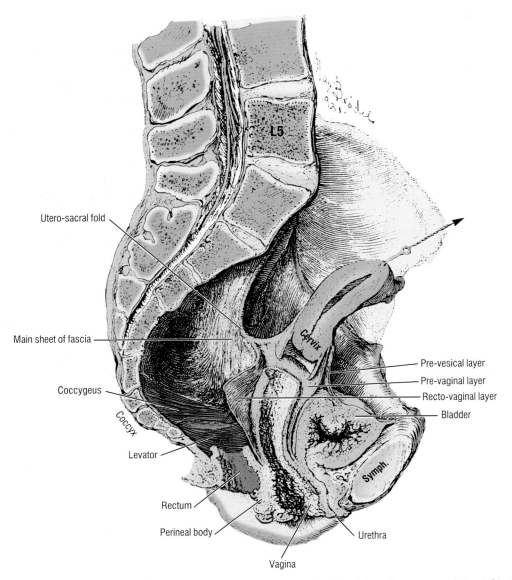

FIG. 28-19. Visceral fascia. (Modified from Sears NT. The fascia surrounding the vagina, its origin and arrangement. Am J Obstet Gynecol 1933; 25:484-492; with permission.)

### Specializations of Endopelvic Fasciae

The connective tissues separating the peritoneum, visceral capsules, and parietal fascia of the pelvis and lower anterior abdominal wall are organized distinctively and predictably into several forms. Their variations in density and quantity of tissue are attributable factors of age, sex, state of health, obesity, and so on.

Numerous past and current studies of these structures show a lack of unanimity regarding both the nomenclature and details of the organization and significance of these bands, sheaths, and visceral ligaments. Sidestepping some of the more obvious areas of controversy, we suggest

summarizing some of the fascial condensations as follows:
- Neurovascular connective tissue sheaths and "pillars"
- Derivatives of parietal fascia
- Condensations of extraperitoneal connective tissue laminae
- Peritoneal derivatives
- "Bands" supporting organs from the fusion of visceral and parietal fascia
- "Filling" tissue

Condensations of connective tissues and smooth muscle fibers accompany the vessels and nerves supplying the pelvic organs.

One such major "band" of tissue extends from and incorporates the branches of the internal iliac vessels to the midline pelvic organs. We compare this to a "vascular leash" to the viscera. This structure, with its derivatives, appears to be comparable with Uhlenhuth's "hypogastric wings."[5] We find the cardinal ligament (also called the lateral cervical ligament, transverse cervical ligament, retinacula uteri or ligament of Mackenrodt) to be part of this complex, accompanying the uterine artery. Anteriorly, the so-called lateral pillar of the urinary bladder is also derived from this tissue. It continues superiorly toward the navel with the obliterated part of the umbilical artery.

Another condensation of connective tissue and smooth muscle is formed largely by presacral connective tissue with contributions from the piriformis muscle fascia. It appears to incorporate splanchnic nerve branches from the sacral plexus and elements of the pelvic plexus (inferior hypogastric plexus). We liken it to a "neural leash" for the viscera. Several important derivatives appear from this "confederacy" of connective tissue, smooth muscle, and neural elements arising as laminae passing into successive horizontal planes.

Muntean[14] discussed the rectum and its fasciae and pelvic relations, observing the continuity of the presacral fascia with the lateral pillars of the rectum and with the arcus tendineus fascia pelvis, thereby forming a hammocklike support for the rectum. Further, the presacral fascia initially invests the pelvic splanchnic nerves and thereafter the right and left pelvic plexuses. We have observed that these nerve elements, plus connective tissue, smooth muscle, and overlying peritoneum, form the uterosacral ligaments. The left pelvic rectal stalk is usually thicker than that on the right side, because of the great number of ascending parasympathetic fibers destined to supply the descending and sigmoid colon.

We believe the forward extension of presacral fascia (fascia of Waldeyer) is continuous with the lateral pillar of the rectum. It receives the contributions of the superior and middle rectal vessels and their associated fasciae.

Just beneath the peritoneum of the wall of the pararectal fossa, this band is evident as the uterosacral ligament.

Anterior to the cul de sac of Douglas, the presacral band splits. Part of it continues as the uterosacral ligament and part diverges to continue with the rectovaginal septum (fascia of Denonvilliers).

At the level of the ischial spine, the neural and vascular leashes appear to be convergent with one another and with the arcus tendineus fascia pelvis.

The vesicoumbilical fascia is a triangular condensation of extraperitoneal connective tissue. It extends upward from the urinary bladder toward the umbilicus at the apex of the triangle. The urachus is in the triangle's middle and the obliterated umbilical arteries arise laterally. A variable quantity of adipose tissue is incorporated between the anterior and posterior laminae of this fascia. This interesting, well-localized condensation of extraperitoneal connective tissue lies between the peritoneum and the transversalis fascia.

The bilaminar rectovaginal septum of the female separates the rectum from the posterior vaginal wall. Similarly, the bilaminar rectogenital septum of the male separates the rectum from the prostate gland anteriorly. The septum extends from one ischial spine to the other and is attached inferiorly to the perineal body (perineal center) and floor of the pelvis. The potential space (of Proust) lies between the two laminae of the rectogenital septum, and has been referred to, facetiously, as the "space between wind and water."

The septum (fascia of Denonvilliers) is derived from the original attachment of the peritoneum to the pelvic floor. The septum is then lifted by the growth of the pelvic organs as a bilaminar layer of tissue that fuses at the floor of the rectogenital fossa. It varies in thickness by individual and is often bilaminar. The septum is of great value both in limiting the spread of disease and in providing a plane of access for surgical procedures.

The visceral capsules, vascular and neural sheaths, and the extraperitoneal spaces are occupied by widely varying quantities of adipose and areolar tissues and smooth muscle fibers. The vesicoumbilical specialization of the extraperitoneal connective tissue also varies greatly in the quantity of fat between the upper margin of the bladder and the umbilicus.

In the upright position, the bladder, uterus (anteflexed and anteverted), the majority of the vagina, and the rectal ampulla lie in horizontal planes, essentially parallel with the floor beneath the feet. These organs are suspended by hammocklike arrangements of connective tissue that extend from one side of the pelvis to the other. Following is a description of the hammock configuration.

- The *urinary bladder and urethra* rest upon a hammock provided by the pubovesicocervical fascia that extends posteriorly from the pubis to the posterior fornix. This hammock is secured to the levator ani muscle laterally by way of the arcus tendineus fascia pelvis. The hypogastric sheath suspends the hammock from above.

- The *vagina* reclines in a hammock formed by the rectovaginal septum which is attached below to the perineal body and laterally to the ischial spines (Fig. 28-20). This lateral attachment adds to reinforcement and suspension by the convergence of the cardinal and uterosacral ligaments at the pericervical ring and the adjacent region of posterior fornix.

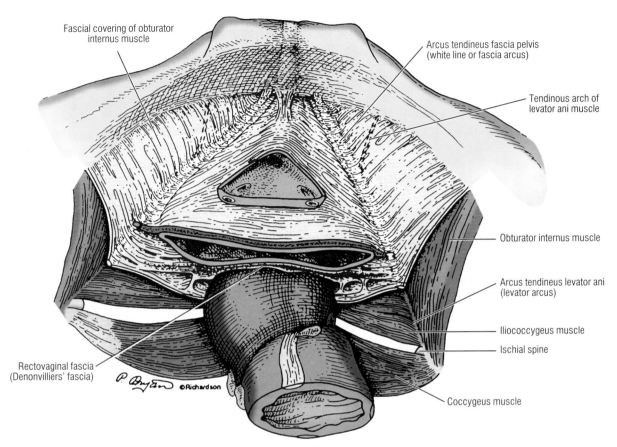

Fascial covering of obturator internus muscle

Arcus tendineus fascia pelvis (white line or fascia arcus)

Tendinous arch of levator ani muscle

Obturator internus muscle

Arcus tendineus levator ani (levator arcus)

Iliococcygeus muscle

Ischial spine

Coccygeus muscle

Rectovaginal fascia (Denonvilliers' fascia)

**FIG. 28-20.** Cross section of the pelvis through the vagina. Note the difference between the tendinous arch of the pelvic fascia (white line) and the tendinous arch of levator ani muscle. (Modified from Skandalakis LJ, Gadacz TR, Mansberger AR Jr, Mitchell WE Jr, Colborn GL, Skandalakis JE. Modern Hernia Repair. Pearl River NY: Parthenon, 1996; with permission.)

- The *rectum* is supported by the presacral fascia and the diverging connective tissues of the lateral rectal pillars.

REMEMBER:
- In the female, the visceral fascia envelops the bladder, urethra, vagina, and rectum, and extends downward and anterior to the vagina and between the rectum and vagina. Here further specialization occurs posterior to the vagina in the fascia of Denonvilliers.
- The cardinal ligament (lateral cervical ligament, transverse cervical ligament, retinacula uteri, or ligament of Mackenrodt) is a condensation of the endopelvic fascia. It is a thickening around the uterine vessels from the sidewall of the pelvis laterally to the cervix. It is considered by many to be formed merely of condensations of the blood vessel connective tissue sheaths, although it is recognized by others that the collagenous and elastic fibers are supplemented by smooth muscle fibers. The cylindrical shape of the uterine cervix is testimony to the

fact that it lies within a ring of connective tissue investment, lacking the direct connective tissue attachments that act to flatten the vagina and bladder in the coronal plane.
- The endopelvic fascia is a downward continuation of the endoabdominal fascia. As Davies[15] noted, it is multilaminar with an outer membranous component and an inner layer characterized by adipose elements. These fascial layers lie between the peritoneum and the transversalis, lumbar, iliacus, or diaphragmatic fascia throughout the abdominopelvic cavity.
- Urologists and gynecologists consider the pelvic floor to be formed by endopelvic fascia, the pelvic diaphragm and its fascial layers, undergirded by the urogenital diaphragm.
- The pelvic parietal fascia covers the superior surface of the levator ani muscle (pelvic diaphragm). Both its superior and inferior fascial layers are continuous with the superior fascia of the urogenital diaphragm at the margin

of the urogenital hiatus. The pelvic parietal fascia, a continuation of the transversalis fascia, covers two muscles (internal obturator and piriformis) and the pelvic diaphragm (levator ani and coccygeus).

- The presacral fascia is part of the parietal layer of pelvic fascia. It is located posterior to the retrorectal space. Thick and strong, it covers the concave surface of the sacrum. Multiple veins, several arteries, and nerves reside beneath this fascia.

- Some authors believe the urogenital diaphragm is covered with fascia superiorly and inferiorly and that both fasciae are continuous with the internal, or superior, parietal fascia of the pelvic diaphragm. McGregor and Du Plessis[16] stated: "The inferior layer of the urogenital diaphragm has nothing to do with the pelvic fascia. At one time during evolution the pelvis had no gap beneath the symphysis. This was filled by a mass of bone. With the advent of mammals there was insufficient room at the pelvic outlet for the passage of the fetal head: the bony mass became replaced by fascia – the inferior fascia of the urogenital diaphragm. This is therefore the morphological representative of this one-time bony layer."

- More accurate evaluation of female pelvic abnormalities is becoming possible with advancements in newer high resolution CT scanners combined with mechanical intravenous contrast medium injection and thinner sections. Foshager and Walsh[17] state that in order to reap maximum benefit from these improved technologies, medical professionals should be familiar with the CT appearance of the normal female pelvic anatomy and its variations.

- Pozzi and Shariat[18] have found that, even though the pelvic fascia and ligaments are very thin, they are well demonstrated (thanks to the natural contrast of pelvic fat) by high quality images of the latest CT scanners. The same authors report[19] that the normally thin fasciae and ligaments tend to appear thicker in abnormal conditions, as in the presence of pelvic neoplasms. These thickenings are easily demonstrated on axial scans. They emphasize, though, that there are many possible reasons for thickening other than neoplastic disease.

- Fritsch and Hötzinger,[20] using CT scan and MRI, report that pelvic connective tissue consists of three compartments: presacral, perirectal, and paravisceral. Readers wanting to know more about these compartments should consult the work of Fritsch and Hötzinger.

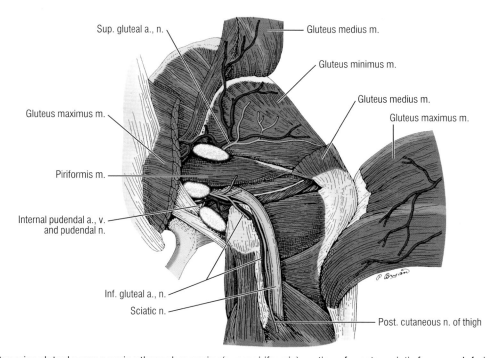

**FIG. 28-21.** Superior gluteal nerve passing through superior (suprapiriformic) portion of greater sciatic foramen. Inferior gluteal nerve and posterior cutaneous nerve of thigh passing, with sciatic nerve, through inferior (infrapiriformic) portion of greater foramen. Lesser sciatic foramen traversed by pudendal nerve, nerve to obturator internus muscle, and internal pudendal artery and vein. (Modified from Skandalakis LJ, Gadacz TR, Mansberger AR Jr, Mitchell WE Jr, Colborn GL, Skandalakis JE. Modern Hernia Repair. Pearl River NY: Parthenon, 1996; with permission.)

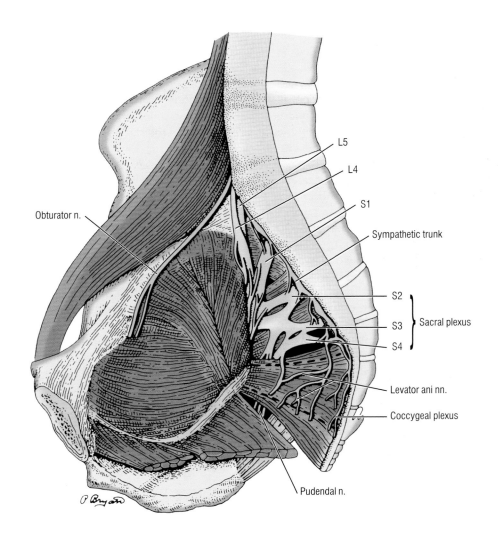

Obturator n.

L5

L4

S1

Sympathetic trunk

S2

S3 } Sacral plexus

S4

Levator ani nn.

Coccygeal plexus

Pudendal n.

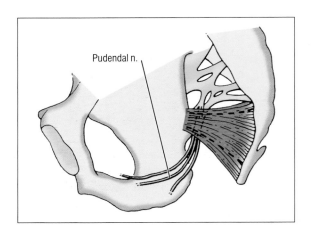

Pudendal n.

FIG. 28-22. Right pelvic wall and nerve supply. Sacral and coccygeal plexus. *Inset:* Course of pudendal nerve. (Modified from Skandalakis LJ, Gadacz TR, Mansberger AR Jr, Mitchell WE Jr, Colborn GL, Skandalakis JE. Modern Hernia Repair. Pearl River NY: Parthenon, 1996; with permission.)

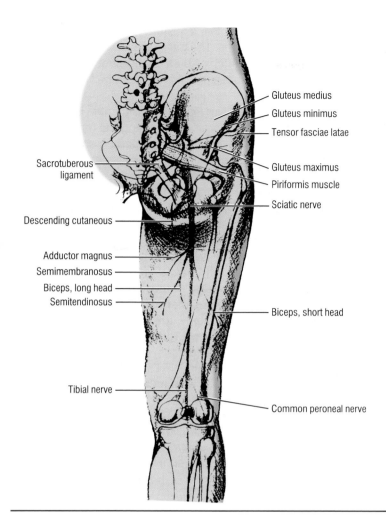

Gluteus medius

Gluteus minimus

Tensor fasciae latae

Gluteus maximus

Piriformis muscle

Sciatic nerve

Sacrotuberous
ligament

Descending cutaneous

Adductor magnus

Semimembranosus

Biceps, long head

Semitendinosus

Biceps, short head

Tibial nerve

Common peroneal nerve

**FIG. 28-23.** Diagrammatic representation of the course of the sciatic nerve and the common peroneal and tibial nerves, and the nerve to the hamstring muscles. (Modified from Nakano KK. Sciatic nerve entrapment: the piriformis syndrome. J Musculoskel Med 1987;4:33-37; with permission.)

## *Fourth Surgicoanatomic Layer: Nerves of the Pelvis*

Some pelvic surgeons include the visceral nerves (Fig. 28-21, Fig. 28-22, Fig. 28-23) within the second surgico-anatomic layer, together with the vascular supply of the pelvic viscera. The parietal nerves then reside in the third surgical layer of the pelvis. For all practical purposes, from this philosophically pragmatic approach, the third layer includes the obturator nerve and vessels, external iliac vessels, and genital branch of the genitofemoral nerve (all residing on the medial pelvic surface of the psoas muscle) and the obturator internus and piriformis muscles and their muscle fasciae.

Havenga et al.[21] define the autonomic nerves of the pelvis to include the paired sympathetic hypogastric nerve, sacral splanchnic nerves, and the pelvic autonomic nerve plexus. We quote from their excellent article:

*The anatomy of the pelvic autonomic nerves is* *closely related to the anatomy and the fascial planes which form the retrorectal space. The rectum is surrounded by a layer of fatty tissue which contains the blood vessels, draining lymph vessels, and the lymph nodes of the rectum itself. This layer is referred to as the mesorectum. ... Bladder and sexual dysfunction after rectal cancer surgery can be avoided in the majority of cases by identifying and preserving the pelvic autonomic nerves ... [and] by teaching surgeons the anatomy of the pelvic autonomic nerves and the pelvic fascial planes ...*

Anatomically, several plexuses and nerves are related to anatomic entities within the pelvis. They are as follows.

- Most superficial: anterior aspect of pelvic plexus for the rectum
- Superficial: urogenital fibers for the urinary bladder, prostate, upper urethra, root of penis
- Intermediate to deep: posterior aspect of pelvic plexus

within the endopelvic fascia, passing forward in the endopelvic fascia just above the levator ani for the urinary bladder and prostate

- Deepest: pudendal and sacral nerves anterior to the Waldeyer's fascia (described previously in this chapter). The nerve to the levator ani (from S4 or S5) courses upon the pelvic surface of the coccygeus, iliococcygeus, and pubococcygeus and provides branches that pierce the superior fascia of the pelvic diaphragm to innervate the muscles.

The nerves of the pelvis include branches of the lumbar and sacral plexuses, the abdominal sympathetics, and sensory fibers. The pelvic nerves include the following bilateral neural elements:

- Obturator nerves
- Pelvic, sacral, and coccygeal plexuses and their derivatives
- Pelvic splanchnic nerves
- Sacral part of the sympathetic nervous system

### Visceral Nerves of the Pelvis

The visceral nerve elements present within the pelvis include the nerves and plexuses supplying the pelvic organs with autonomic and visceral afferent supply.

The innervation of visceral peritoneum is poorly localized. Innervation is carried by nerves whose principal function is sympathetic ("fight or flight"). Pain is usually referred to the levels of the body wall associated with the cord levels at which the pain fibers enter. T11 - L2 serves the majority of lower abdomen and pelvis.

PELVIC PLEXUSES. The pelvic plexuses are seen especially well in the endopelvic tissues of the pelvic sidewall.

These plexuses contain a mixture of parasympathetic and sympathetic ganglia. The pelvic plexuses are a mixture of sensory and autonomic fibers on the sidewall of the pelvis lateral to the rectum and within the endopelvic and visceral fasciae.

*Inferior Hypogastric Plexus.* Considerable lack of agreement exists in the literature regarding the terminology for the nerve plexuses in the lower abdomen and pelvis. The term "inferior hypogastric plexus" seems as unacceptable a name for a pelvic plexus of nerves as "hypogastric artery" for the internal iliac artery. Nonetheless, the name "hypogastric" is fixed securely in clinical parlance.

Anatomically, the inferior hypogastric nerves are located at the lateral pelvic wall, 1 cm to 2 cm medial to and paralleling the ureter. The nerves create a bridge between the superior hypogastric plexus and the pelvic plexus. According to Church et al.,[22] the hypogastric nerves originate posterior to the superior rectal artery and move distally to 2 cm to 4 cm below the peritoneum (Fig. 28-24). Here, they continue downward with the pelvic parasympathetic nerves (nervi erigentes) which arise from S2 to S4 and form the pelvic plexus.[23,24] The pelvic plexus is located at the lateral pelvic wall and at the level of the distal one-third of the rectum.

NOTE: The hypogastric nerves originate in the superior hypogastric plexus, located at the aortic bifurcation. When ligating the inferior mesenteric artery, be extremely careful not to violate the plexus and the left hypogastric nerves. We advise careful isolation of the artery.

*Superior Hypogastric Plexus.* The superior hypogastric plexus is located at the aortic bifurcation and has no named ganglia. It can be considered as the continuation of the preaortic plexus beyond the inferior mesenteric part of

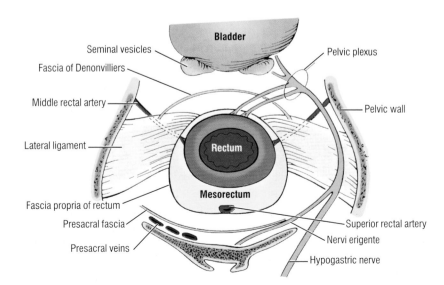

FIG. **28-24.** Relationship of rectum to surrounding fasciae, blood vessels, and nerves at various depths in male pelvis (schematic transverse section). Most of pelvic nerve plexus is laterally embedded in endopelvic fascia on pelvic wall. Middle rectal artery is separated from lateral ligaments. (Modified from Church JM, Raudkivi PJ, Hill GL. The surgical anatomy of the rectum: A review with particular relevance to the hazards of rectal mobilization. Int J Colorect Dis 1987;2:158-166; with permission.)

the plexus. The superior hypogastric (or, more simply, hypogastric) plexus divides into the right and left pelvic (inferior hypogastric) plexus.

**SYMPATHETIC FIBERS.** The sympathetic fibers of the pelvic plexus are vasomotor, motor to sphincters, inhibitory to peristalsis, and sensory for painful sensations for most of the pelvic viscera. The smooth muscle of the vesical trigone and the internal sphincter of the urethra are innervated through the hypogastric (presacral) sympathetic nerves. As far as we know, the testes and ovaries have good sympathetic supply but no definable or demonstrable parasympathetic supply.

The sympathetic contribution to the pelvic plexus derives in large part from the hypogastric plexus (mixture of pre- and postganglionic fibers) in front of the body of L5, forming the so-called "hypogastric nerve." In addition, several branches arise as sacral splanchnic nerves from the sacral portions of the sympathetic chains and join the plexus.

NOTE: "Sacral splanchnic" nerves should not be confused with the "pelvic splanchnic" nerves, which are parasympathetic in function.

The sacral sympathetic trunks cross the pelvic brim just behind the common iliac artery and vein. They travel downward close to the concavity of the sacrum – in most cases medial to the anterior sacral foramina. The foramina are useful landmarks for the topography of the trunks.

The final destinations of the sacral sympathetic trunks is the conjunction of the two sympathetic chains, anterior to the coccyx. Here the right and left chains unite to form a ganglion, the so-called ganglion impar. All the sacral ventral primary rami receive gray communicating rami (postganglionic sympathetic fibers) from the sympathetic trunks.

Sir William Turner, when asked by a student where the sympathetic nervous system begins, roared in his deep voice, "the sympathetic begins nowhere."[8] Many advances have been made in our knowledge since those days, but much still remains to be learned about the autonomic system.

These statements characterize pelvic sympathetics:
- Sympathetic fibers provide motor supply for the ducts and glands for ejaculation, including the urethra.
- The sympathetic system seems to have little effect upon the colon and rectum.
- Presacral neurectomy (resection of the superior hypogastric plexus) can be carried out with impunity only in females. Menstruation, pregnancy, and parturition can occur normally in the absence of sympathetic fibers to the pelvis. In the male, however, section of the presacral nerve results in sterility in 50 to 60 percent of patients.

- Chen[25] states that laparoscopic presacral neurectomy is an effective treatment for chronic pelvic pain and dysmenorrhea.

**PARASYMPATHETIC FIBERS.** The parasympathetic part of the pelvic plexus is derived from branches of S2-S4. These are the pelvic splanchnic nerves (nervi erigentes). The nervi erigentes are motor and secretomotor to the gut from the splenic flexure to the rectum. The muscle of the bladder (detrusor muscle) and rectum are also innervated by the nervi erigentes, as are the smooth muscles of the internal sphincter of the anal canal. The erectile tissues of the penis and clitoris also receive their functional fibers for erection from the pelvic splanchnic nerves.

### Parietal Nerves of the Pelvis

The parietal neural structures present within the pelvis include the paired obturator nerves, lumbosacral plexus, coccygeal plexus, and derivatives of these.

**OBTURATOR NERVE.** The obturator nerve (anterior divisions of L2-L4) (Figs. 28-22, 28-25) is the chief nerve supply for the adductor compartment of the thigh. It contains skeletal motor fibers for the following muscles: obturator externus, adductor longus, adductor brevis, adductor magnus (anterior part), and gracilis. It provides sensory fibers for the intermediate part of the medial surface of the thigh and some sensory fibers for the knee joint.

The obturator nerve traverses the pelvis only through extraperitoneal fatty tissue. The path of the obturator nerve follows.
- Appears from beneath the psoas muscle
- Crosses the pelvic brim medial to the sacroiliac joint to

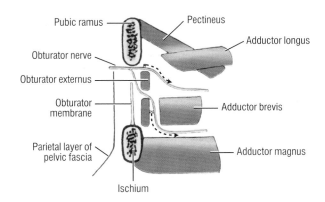

**FIG. 28-25.** Sagittal section of thigh showing the course of obturator hernia (dashed arrows) along obturator nerve and its branches. (Modified from McGregor AL, DuPlessis DJ. A Synopsis of Surgical Anatomy (10th ed). Baltimore: Williams & Wilkins, 1969; with permission.)

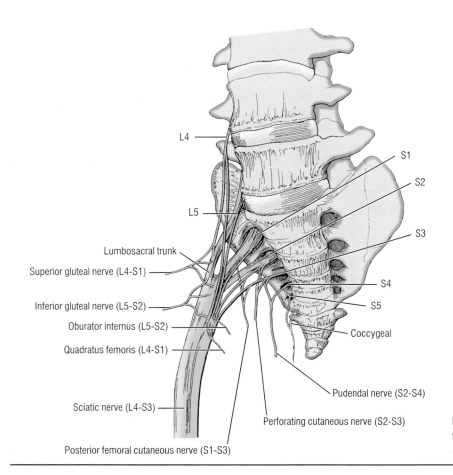

L4

S1

S2

L5

S3

Lumbosacral trunk

Superior gluteal nerve (L4-S1)

Inferior gluteal nerve (L5-S2)

S4

Oburator internus (L5-S2)

S5

Quadratus femoris (L4-S1)

Coccygeal

Pudendal nerve (S2-S4)

Sciatic nerve (L4-S3)

Perforating cutaneous nerve (S2-S3)

Posterior femoral cutaneous nerve (S1-S3)

**FIG. 28-26.** Formation of lumbosacral trunk and further formation of sciatic and pudendal nerves (highly diagrammatic).

the angle between the external and internal iliac vessels, very close to the ovary. (Ovarian pain can be referred to the medial side of the thigh).

- Passes vertically downward to the obturator foramen
- Traverses the muscle fibers of the obturator externus at the obturator foramen
- Divides into anterior and posterior divisions at the obturator foramen or somewhat more distally

The anterior division supplies the adductor longus and gracilis. The posterior division provides innervation for the adductor brevis and magnus.

Pellegrino and Johnson[26] report bilateral obturator nerve injury secondary to prolonged urologic surgery. The nerve injury was believed to have resulted from stretching at the bony obturator foramen.

Ali[27] reports a case of left tubal ectopic pregnancy presenting with left obturator nerve pain. More likely, however, tubal and ovarian pain is simply referred to dermatomes of intermediate lumbar spinal nerve levels, especially L2. This dermatome is supplied by the obturator nerve, in part.

The accessory obturator nerve, when present, passes

over the superior pubic ramus and behind the femoral sheath. It supplies the pectineus muscle.

**LUMBOSACRAL PLEXUS.** The lumbosacral plexus (L4-S5) (Fig. 28-26) is formed in the posterior wall of the pelvis by the lumbosacral trunk and the anterior primary rami of spinal nerves L4-S5.

NOTE: L4 is shared both by the lumbar and sacral plexuses. A branch from L4 (the so-called furcal nerve) joins L5 to form the lumbosacral trunk. This trunk carries the L4 and L5 contributions to join the nerves of the sacral plexus.

The sacral nerves emerge from the anterior sacral foramina. They unite in front of the piriformis where they are joined by the lumbosacral trunk. Several of the branches from this plexus provide origin for nerves supplying the pelvic viscera (pelvic splanchnic nerves). Other branches provide innervation for the muscles of the pelvic floor and sidewalls. The motor branches of the sacral plexus lie deep to the endopelvic fascia and exit via the greater sciatic foramen (except for the nerve to the levator ani).

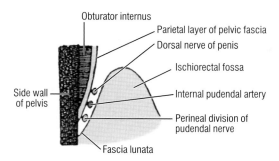

**FIG. 28-27.** Alcock's canal (formed by pelvic fascia and fascia lunata). (Modified from McGregor AL, DuPlessis DJ. A Synopsis of Surgical Anatomy (10th ed). Baltimore: Williams & Wilkins, 1969; with permission.)

Branches of the lumbosacral plexus exiting the greater sciatic foramen include the pudendal nerve, nerves to the gluteal region, and the sciatic nerve. These nerves provide motor and sensory supply to the perineum, gluteal area, posterior thigh, leg, and foot.

**PUDENDAL NERVE.** The pudendal nerve (S2-S4) is the nerve of the pelvic floor and perineum (see Fig. 28-21, Fig. 28-22, Fig. 28-26). It emerges through the greater sciatic foramen in company with and medial to the internal pudendal vessels. The nerve passes over the sacrospinous ligament, then through the lesser sciatic foramen to gain access to the perineum. Laterally, in the ischioanal fossa of the perineum, the pudendal nerve traverses the pudendal canal of Alcock (Fig. 28-27), providing motor and sensory branches to the perineal skin, the external anal sphincters, and the muscles of the urogenital region.

REMEMBER: A single nerve, the pudendal, and a single artery, the internal pudendal, are responsible for most of the innervation and blood supply of the perineum.

The pudendal nerve (from S2, S3, S4) has three divisions and covers five territories. The divisions of the pudendal nerve are rectal, perineal, and dorsal genital nerve of the penis or clitoris.

*Rectal Nerve.* The inferior rectal (inferior hemorrhoidal) supplies the external sphincter ani, assists in supplying the levator ani, and provides cutaneous innervation for the skin around the anus and the mucosal lining of the anal canal below the pecten.

*Perineal Nerve.* The perineal branch divides into posterior scrotal or labial cutaneous branches and deep muscular branches. The latter supply the muscles of the superficial perineal pouch and deep perineal pouch (the urogenital diaphragm).

*Dorsal Genital Nerve of the Penis or Clitoris.* The dorsal nerve of the penis supplies the glans, the prepuce, and the

skin of the penis/spongy urethra in the male and the clitoris in the female.

The territories the pudendal nerve supplies are pelvic, pudendal, deep perineal pouch, dorsum of penis or clitoris, and gluteal. The gluteal territory, however, is disputed by several anatomists, since the nerve only passes through the area.

**CUTANEOUS NERVES OF UROGENITAL TRIANGLE.** The cutaneous nerves of the urogenital triangle (Fig. 28-28 A&B) supply the following areas:
* Ilioinguinal nerve (L1): anterior 1/3 of the labia majora/ scrotum
* Dorsal nerve: skin of the clitoris/penis
* Perineal branch of posterior cutaneous nerve of thigh: lateral, posterior 2/3 of labia majora/scrotum. It may replace the pudendal nerve in much of the cutaneous supply.
* Labial/scrotal branches of perineal branch of pudendal nerve: medial, posterior 2/3 of labia majora/scrotum
* L1: dorsal aspect of root of penis
* S2-S3: areas distal to axial line, penile skin, and adjoining scrotum

**SCIATIC NERVE.** The sciatic nerve (L4-S3) is the largest nerve of the body. The pudendal and sciatic nerves are the terminal branches of the sacral plexus.

The path of the sciatic nerve (Fig. 28-1, Fig. 28-21, Fig. 28-23) is described below.
* It emerges from the greater sciatic foramen beneath the lower border of the piriformis muscle and under the gluteus maximus
* It crosses the posterior surface of the ischium and descends on the adductor magnus, deep to the long head of the biceps femoris
* Near the ischial tuberosity, it provides motor branches for the long head of the biceps femoris, the semitendinosus, the semimembranosus, and the distal part of the adductor magnus muscles
* At midthigh (variably), it divides into the tibial (L4-S3) and common fibular (peroneal) nerves (L4-S2)
* The tibial division of the sciatic nerve supplies the three longer components of the hamstring muscles (long head of biceps, semimembranosus, semitendinosus) and also the adductor magnus (the superior part of which is innervated by the obturator nerve)
* The common peroneal division innervates only the short head of the biceps in its course in the thigh, but supplies all of the musculature and most of the cutaneous supply to the leg and foot

**SEGMENTAL CUTANEOUS SUPPLY OF THE LOWER LIMB**
* L1-L3 supplies the anterior thigh from above down, in-

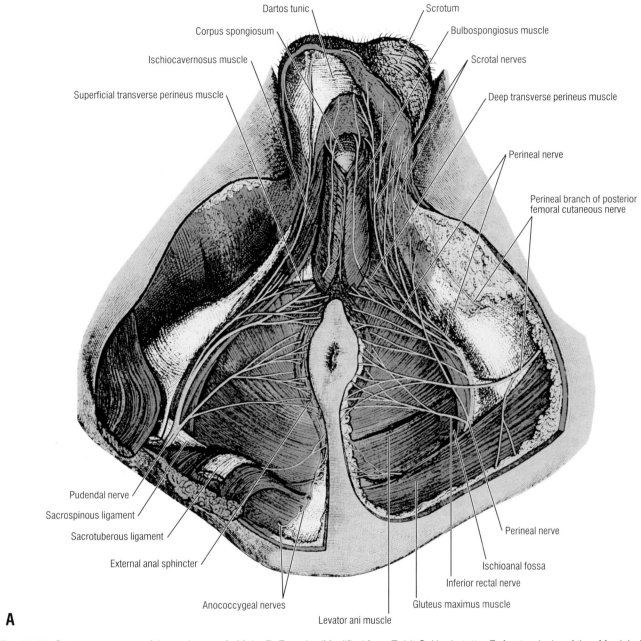

Dartos tunic

Corpus spongiosum

Ischiocavernosus muscle

Superficial transverse perineus muscle

Scrotum

Bulbospongiosus muscle

Scrotal nerves

Deep transverse perineus muscle

Perineal nerve

Perineal branch of posterior
femoral cutaneous nerve

Pudendal nerve

Sacrospinous ligament

Sacrotuberous ligament

External anal sphincter

Anococcygeal nerves

Levator ani muscle

Gluteus maximus muscle

Inferior rectal nerve

Ischioanal fossa

Perineal nerve

**A**

**FIG. 28-28.** Cutaneous nerves of the perineum. **A,** Male; **B,** Female. (Modified from Toldt C, Hochstetter F. Anatomischer Atlas. Munich: Urban & Schwarzenberg, 1976; with permission.)

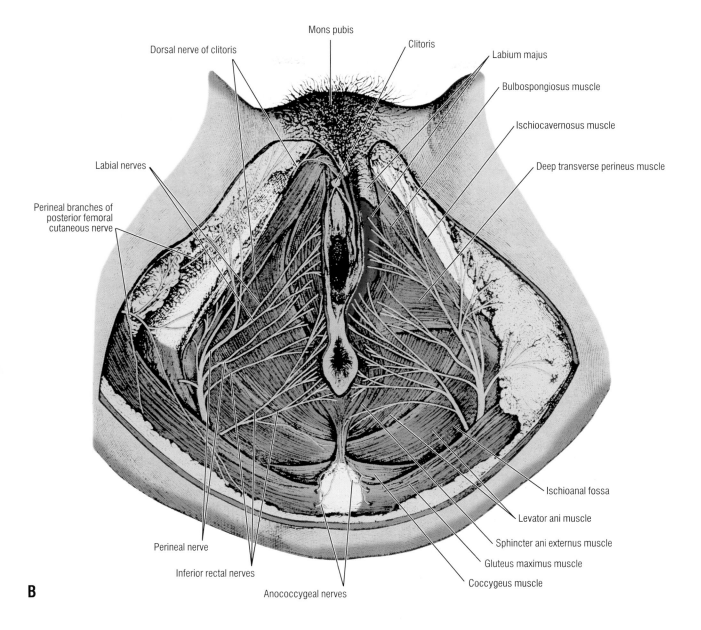

Mons pubis

Dorsal nerve of clitoris

Clitoris

Labium majus

Bulbospongiosus muscle

Ischiocavernosus muscle

Deep transverse perineus muscle

Labial nerves

Perineal branches of posterior femoral cutaneous nerve

Ischioanal fossa

Levator ani muscle

Perineal nerve

Sphincter ani externus muscle

Inferior rectal nerves

Gluteus maximus muscle

Coccygeus muscle

Anococcygeal nerves

B

cluding the anterior scrotum (vulva)
- L4 supplies the leg and foot medially
- L5 supplies:
  – Leg anterolaterally
  – Dorsum and sole of the foot
- S1 supplies:
  – Band of skin on the posterior thigh surface (by the posterior femoral cutaneous nerve)
  – Posterior side of the calf (medial and lateral sural cutaneous nerves)
  – Lateral side of the foot (sural nerve and lateral cutaneous nerve of the foot)
- S2 contributes sensory fibers to the posterior surface of the thigh and leg
- S3 and S4 supply the skin of the buttocks and lateral aspects of the perineum (including the posterior scrotum or vulva) by the perineal branch of the posterior femoral cutaneous nerve

REMEMBER: L1 supplies the anterior scrotum or vulva. S3 supplies the posterior scrotum or vulva.

NOTE: In some individuals, most of the sensory fibers to the perineum are derived from the posterior femoral cutaneous nerve. In such cases, pudendal nerve block may not be totally successful in achieving anesthesia.

A little aid for memory follows:
- 5 supplies 1, and 1 supplies 5 (meaning that L5 supplies the 1st toe and S1 supplies the 5th toe)

**MYOTOMES OF THE LOWER LIMB.** In general, the motor supply to the lower limb can be summarized as follows. Remember that the large muscles of the lower limb are, in almost every case, supplied by two or more spinal nerve levels.
- L1, L2, hip flexion (iliopsoas)
- L2, L3 [anterior divisions], adductor musculature
- L2, L3 [posterior divisions], quadriceps femoris muscles, sartorius (L4 carries the sensory limb of the patellar reflex)
- L4, foot inversion (tibialis anterior and posterior)
- L4, L5, foot dorsiflexion (extensores hallucis and digitorum)
- L5, foot dorsiflexion and inversion; great toe extension (extensor hallucis longus); hip abduction (gluteus medius, minimus); knee flexion (long hamstrings)
- S1, foot eversion (peroneal musculature); hip extension (gluteus maximus); knee flexion (short head of biceps femoris); plantar flexion of the foot (gastrocnemius, soleus)
- S2, toe pushoff (flexor hallucis and digitorum longus)
- S2, S3, intrinsic muscles of the sole of the foot

The following statements are usually true regarding pelvic sensation.
- Pain from upper pelvic viscera (ovaries, uterine fundus and body, most of the bladder) is carried by sympathetic routes. Pain from lower visceral elements (cervix, upper vagina, vesical trigone) is carried by the pelvic splanchnic nerves. Clinical data indicate that there can be considerable variation in the pain pathways between individual patients.
- Sensations of bladder distention are carried by pelvic splanchnic nerves (nervi erigentes). Bladder pain, especially from its lower segment, is transmitted by the sacral parasympathetics and not through the hypogastric plexus.
- Sensations of rectal distention are carried by pelvic splanchnic nerves (nervi erigentes). Rectal pain is carried by sacral nerves.
- Pain of the body of the uterus is carried by the hypogastric nerve, lumbar splanchnic nerves, and sympathetic chains. The cell bodies are found in the dorsal root ganglia of T11-L2 spinal nerves.
- Pain fibers from the cervix travel in the pelvic splanchnic nerves and have their cell bodies in the dorsal root ganglia of S2, S3 and S4.
- Pain from inflamed viscera is due to excessive dilation or swelling, muscle spasm, tension of the mesenteric folds, or involvement of the parietal peritoneum.
- Intensity of pain perception indicates the nerve carrying the pain. Visceral nerve branches carry a dull perceived pain from above the anal pecten. Somatic nerve branches of the pudendal nerve carry sharp, precisely located pain from the pecten outward. Robert et al.[28] report on the role of the pudendal nerve in perineal pain. They propose treatment by infiltrations at the level of the ischial spine or at the pudendal canal, and by surgery by a transgluteal route.
- Presacral resection for pain is disappointing and unpredictable in results.

## *Fifth Surgicoanatomic Layer: Muscles*

The pelvic muscles (Fig. 28-2) can be divided into lateral pelvic muscles (piriformis and obturator internus) and the muscles of the pelvic diaphragm. First we consider the muscles of the lateral pelvic wall. Muscles of the pelvic diaphragm are considered in the following section on the pelvic floor.

The following paragraphs consider place of origin, insertion, nerve supply, and action of the lateral pelvic muscles (piriformis and obturator internus).

### Piriformis
The piriformis muscle:

- Is a part of the lateral pelvic wall
- Originates from the anterior sacrum, greater sciatic notch, and sacrotuberous ligament
- Inserts at the upper border of the greater trochanter
- Is supplied by the L5-S2 nerves
- Rotates the extended thigh laterally and abducts the flexed thigh

REMEMBER: Within the pelvis, the piriformis is related to the rectum, sacral plexus, branches of the internal iliac vessels and, inferiorly, the coccygeus muscle. Outside the pelvis, the piriformis is related to the posterior surface of the ischium, the capsule of the hip joint, and the gluteus maximus (Figs. 28-1 and 28-8).

## Obturator Internus and Obturator Hernia

The obturator internus:

- Lies partly within the pelvis and partly posterior to the hip joint
- Originates on the internal surface of the ilium, pubic bone and ischium, ischiopubic rami, and inner surface of the obturator membrane
- Inserts at the medial surface of the greater trochanter
- Is supplied by the L5-S1 nerves
- Rotates the extended thigh laterally and abducts the flexed thigh

REMEMBER: The pelvic surface of the obturator internus forms the lateral boundary of the ischioanal fossa of the perineum. This boundary consists of fat-filled, pyramid-shapes on either side of the anus (Fig. 28-2B). Outside the pelvis, the obturator internus muscle is first joined by the superior and inferior gemelli, following their origin from the margin of the lesser sciatic foramen; thereafter, it is covered by the gluteus maximus and crossed by the sciatic nerve (Fig. 28-2).

The tendinous arch of the levator ani muscle, a specialization of the internal fascia of the obturator muscle, follows a line from the ischial spine to the posterior aspect of the body of the pubic bone. This fascial thickening gives origin to the lateral part of the pubococcygeus muscle and the entire iliococcygeus muscle. Along its path, the arcus tendineus of the levator ani is very closely related anteriorly to the proximal urethra and the neck of the urinary bladder. Klutke and Siegel[29] correctly identify the arcus tendineus as a fascial ring at the pelvic outlet that laterally secures the pelvic floor and several ligaments (Fig. 28-29).

NOTE: Part of the lateral wall of the false pelvis is formed by the iliacus muscle, which completely fills the iliac fossa. We do not consider the psoas major and minor muscles as musculature belonging to the lateral pelvic wall. Their presence on the bony rim of the pelvic sidewall does effectively deepen the true pelvic cavity, as can be appreciated in sectional imaging. We believe that, for all practical purposes,

these muscles belong to the posterior abdominal wall and lower limb. The only relationship between the psoas and iliacus muscles is that the tendon of the psoas major unites with the tendon of the iliac close to and above the inguinal ligament. The tendon of the combined iliopsoas then passes underneath the ligament and inserts into the lesser trochanter of the femur.

An obturator hernia is an abnormal protrusion of preperitoneal fat or an intestinal loop through the obturator canal. It characteristically affects the right side of middle-aged women. Its relation to groin hernia is seen in Fig. 28-30A.

The obturator *region* is bounded superiorly by the superior ramus of the pubic bone, laterally by the hip joint and the shaft of the femur, medially by the pubic arch, the perineum, and the gracilis muscle, and inferiorly by the insertion of the adductor magnus on the adductor tubercle of the femur.

The obturator *foramen* is the largest bony foramen in the body and is formed by the rami of the ischium and pubis. It lies inferior to the acetabulum on the anterolateral wall of the pelvis. Except for a small area, the obturator canal, the foramen is closed by the obturator membrane. Fibers of the membrane are continuous with the periosteum of the surrounding bones and with the tendons of the internal and external obturator muscles. Embryologically, the foramen and its membrane represent an area of potential bone formation that never proceeds to completion. In this sense the obturator foramen is a la-

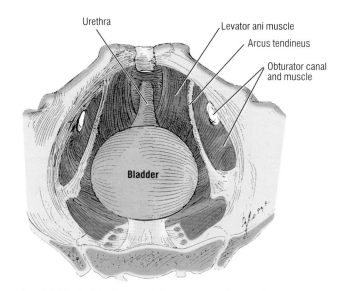

Urethra          Levator ani muscle
                 Arcus tendineus
                 Obturator canal
                 and muscle

Bladder

FIG. 28-29. Pelvic floor with levator muscle attached laterally to arcus tendineus (abdominal view). (Modified from the American Urological Association, Inc. The Anatomy of Stress Incontinence. AUA Update Series, Lesson 39, Volume IX, 1990, p. 306; with permission.)

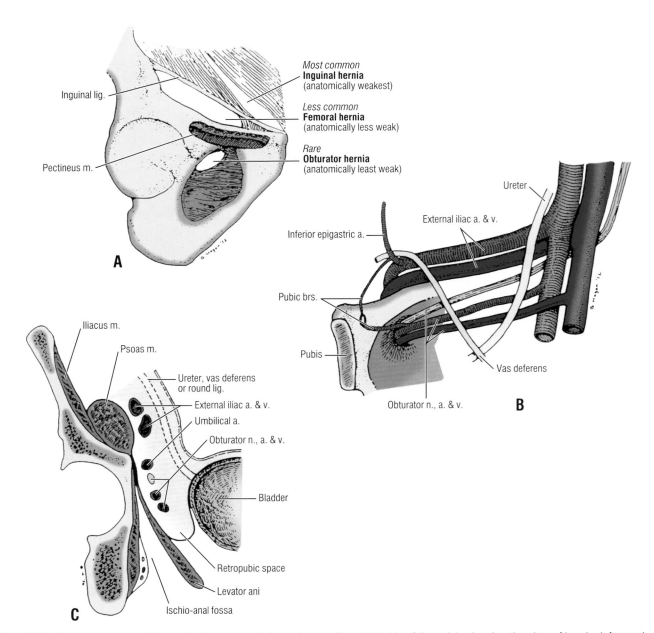

FIG. 28-30. Surgical anatomy of the obturator region. **A,** Lateral view of the right side of the pelvis showing the sites of inguinal, femoral, and obturator hernias. **B,** View of the medial wall of the male pelvis showing the obturator canal and structures passing through it. **C,** Diagrammatic coronal section of the lateral wall of the male pelvis showing the relation of obturator nerve, artery, and vein to other pelvic structures. **D,** The course and distribution of the right obturator nerve. **E,** Diagram of long section of the upper thigh through the obturator foramen showing the potential paths of obturator hernia. The hernia may follow the anterior or posterior division of the nerve. **F,** As it emerges through the obturator canal, the obturator artery divides to form an arterial ring around the obturator foramen. (**A, D, F** from Skandalakis JE, Gray SW. Obturator hernia. In Nyhus LM, Condon RE (eds). Hernia (4th ed). Philadelphia: Lippincott, 1995; with permission. **B, C, E** from Gray SW, Skandalakis JE, Soria RE, Rowe JS Jr. Strangulated obturator hernia. Surgery 1974;75:20-27; with permission.)

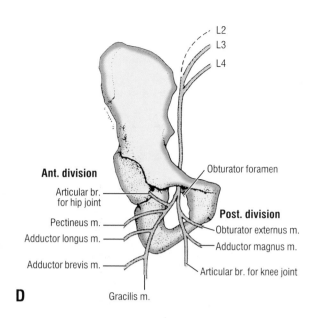

Ant. division

Articular br.
for hip joint

Pectineus m.

Adductor longus m.

Adductor brevis m.

Gracilis m.

L2
L3
L4

Obturator foramen

Post. division

Obturator externus m.

Adductor magnus m.

Articular br. for knee joint

**D**

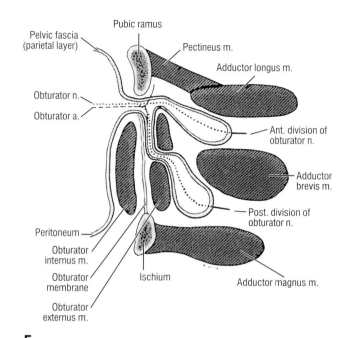

Pelvic fascia
(parietal layer)

Pubic ramus

Pectineus m.

Adductor longus m.

Obturator n.

Obturator a.

Ant. division of
obturator n.

Adductor
brevis m.

Post. division of
obturator n.

Peritoneum

Obturator
internus m.

Obturator
membrane

Ischium

Adductor magnus m.

Obturator
externus m.

**E**

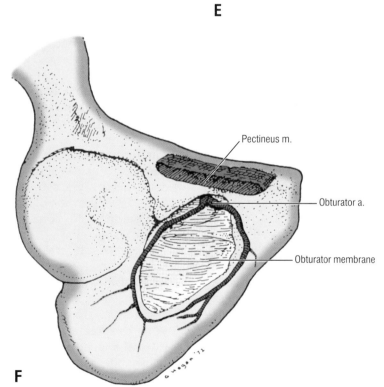

Pectineus m.

Obturator a.

Obturator membrane

**F**

cuna and the obturator canal is the true foramen.

The obturator *canal* is a tunnel 2 to 3 cm long beginning in the pelvis at the defect in the obturator membrane. It passes obliquely downward to end outside the pelvis in the obturator region of the thigh. The canal is bounded above and laterally by the obturator groove of the pubis and inferiorly by the free edge of the obturator membrane and the internal and external obturator muscles. Through this canal pass the obturator artery, vein, and nerve (Fig. 28-30A&B), and the hernial sac, if an obturator hernia is present.

The obturator nerve is usually superior to the artery and vein (Fig. 28-30C). The nerve separates into anterior and posterior divisions as it leaves the canal (Fig. 28-30D). The hernial sac may follow either division of the nerve (Fig. 28-30E). The obturator artery divides to form an arterial ring around the foramen (Fig. 28-30F). In the majority of cases, this artery provides the artery to the head of the femur.

The approach for the repair of an obturator hernia may be abdominal, retropubic, obturator, inguinal, laparoscopic, or a combination. Decision as to the approach depends upon whether there is a certain diagnosis. With certain diagnosis, we advise a lower suprapubic transverse incision. Without certain diagnosis, we advise lower midine incision.

## SURGICAL CONSIDERATIONS

- The retropubic space of Retzius communicates with the space occupied by areolar tissue in front of and to the sides of the bladder but not behind it. The retropubic space is also indirectly continuous with an inferior abdominal wall area, the space of Bogros.
- We quote from Killackey[12] on female colorectal cancer surgery:

   *The most important principle of curative surgical therapy is total resection of the mesorectum with careful, deliberate, hemostatic dissection along parietal pelvic fascia. .... To completely mobilize the rectum and treat most midrectal cancers, the rectovaginal septum must be dissected creating a rectovaginal space down to the pelvic floor. ... The boundaries of the rectovaginal space are: the pouch of Douglas (base of the cul de sac) cranially; perineal body caudally; and the pararectal spaces laterally.*

- The neck of the bladder or upper part of the prostate is attached to the distal part of the symphysis pubis by a cordlike ligament, a specialized thickening of the endopelvic fascia. This forms the puboprostatic or pubovesical ligaments.

- The pelvic splanchnic nerves are contained within a fine areolar fold, located at each side of the retrorectal space. It is essential in pelvic surgery to avoid injuring these nerves. An injury can cause bladder and rectal physiological impairment, and in the male, problems with erection.
- The presacral venous plexus can produce bleeding during pelvic surgery, especially with mobilization of the posterior rectal wall. The bleeding can be controlled with a tack or by using muscular plugs.
- Qinyao et al.[30] stated that large ventral neural foramina, 2 mm to 5 mm in diameter, were located in the 3rd, 4th, and 5th segments of the sacral body in 16 percent of their cases. The walls of the presacral veins are fixed to the sacral periosteum and the presacral fascia. In an effort to perform a better cancer operation, the surgeon removes the presacral fascia and sometimes the sacral periosteum. This can produce copious venous bleeding that is difficult to control because of the retraction of the veins within the foramina.
- The presacral fascia is part of the parietal fascia. Because of its paucity of lymphatics, it is not necessary to remove it. Invasion of the fascia by cancer is not curable.
- The obturator test is used to diagnose appendicitis. If the acute appendix is located over the pelvic brim, and if stretching the obturator internus muscle by flexing and rotating the thigh inward results in pain, the diagnosis is confirmed. The pain is due to inflamed fascia and peritoneum.
- Damage to the sciatic nerve creates paralysis of the hamstring muscles and all the muscles of the leg and foot. In gynecologic surgery, footdrop deformity can occur as a complication of injury to the fibers of the common peroneal division of the sciatic nerve within the true pelvis.
- Other nerves subject to injury by direct manipulation, retraction, or inadvertent clamping or laceration are:
   – Genitofemoral (lumboinguinal)
   – Ilioinguinal
   – Lateral cutaneous of thigh
   – Intermediate cutaneous of thigh
   – Medial cutaneous of thigh
   – Iliohypogastric
   – Obturator
   – Femoral
- Compression neuropathies must be considered in the differential diagnosis of sciatic pain. In the most common anatomic arrangement, the entire sciatic nerve passes inferior to the piriformis muscle. In somewhat less than 10 percent of individuals, the common fibular (common peroneal) division of the sciatic nerve passes through the piriformis muscle. In rarer cases, the whole

sciatic nerve passes through the piriformis. Either variation can result in "piriformis entrapment," causing gluteal pain and/or sciatica, described below. Even less frequently, the peroneal division leaves the pelvis superior to the piriformis, and the tibial division of the sciatic nerve pierces the muscle.

- Recognized more often in recent years as a cause of sciatic pain, piriformis syndrome can occur when the peroneal division of the sciatic nerve is compressed by contractions of the piriformis muscle. Piriformis syndrome (entrapment of the sciatic nerve on the sharp lower edge of the greater sciatic notch) may cause symptoms along the course and distribution of its component parts. Patients with piriformis syndrome complain of pain and/or paresthesia in the distribution of the sciatic nerve. These complaints can seem almost identical to those experienced with compression of the S1 nerve root by vertebral disk herniation at the level of the fifth lumbar vertebra. The symptomatology can be considerably greater than this, depending upon the nature of the entrapment and its severity. Complete nerve palsy is rare.

- Electromyography and nerve conduction studies are needed to confirm the diagnosis of piriformis entrapment. Look for normal activity in the gluteus maximus, gluteus medius, gluteus minimus, and tensor fasciae latae muscles, and abnormalities in innervation below this. Prescribe conservative measures (physical therapy, bed rest, antiinflammatory analgesics, and muscle relaxants) initially. If these fail, and if the diagnosis of piriformis syndrome has been substantiated, try division of one of the heads of origin of the piriformis muscle and operative neurolysis.[31]

- The fascia propria of the rectum is an enigmatic anatomic entity (Fig. 28-31). It envelops the rectum and its vessels, lymphatics, and nerves, but does not invest the rectal wall. It is located anterior to the retrorectal space. The so-called rectal mesentery (or mesorectum or fatty tissue) at the posterior part of the rectum is enclosed by the fascia propria.

- Many elements of the pelvic plexus are located below the uterine vessels in the cardinal ligament. Numerous visceral nerve fibers from the hypogastric plexus do, however, surround the ureter and the uterine vessels. If the nerves to the uterus are severed, it is usually in association with removal of the uterus, so that the nerve loss is of no consequence. Therefore, significant injury to the plexus during hysterectomy (not radical) is an uncommon sequela.

- Most rectoceles are caused by obstetrical trauma. If Denonvilliers' fascia is torn from the perineal body, a low

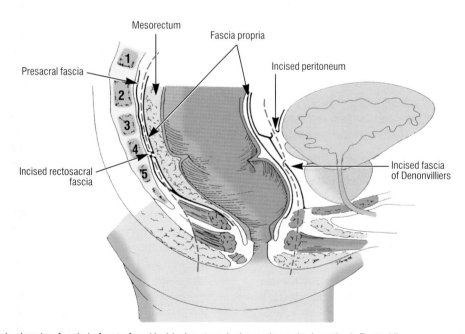

**FIG. 28-31.** Male pelvis showing fascia in front of and behind rectum (schematic sagittal section). Dotted lines represent paths of incisions in abdominoperineal resection for cancer. Note the incision of anterior peritoneum in front of fascia of Denonvilliers. Fascia of Denonvilliers is incised lower down, opposite seminal vesicles. Rectosacral fascia is incised posteriorly, disconnecting rectum from hollow of sacrum. (Modified from Church JM, Raudkivi PJ, Hill GL. The surgical anatomy of the rectum: A review with particular relevance to the hazards of rectal mobilization. Int J Colorect Dis 1987;2:158-166; with permission.)

## Editorial Comment

*After surgical resection alone for carcinoma of the rectum, high rates of pelvic recurrence have been commonly reported. Such high recurrence rates have led to a general recommendation that adjuvant radiation therapy be used for patients with Stage II (local recurrence rates of 30% to 35% reduced to 5%) and Stage III rectal cancer (local recurrence rates of 45% to 65% reduced to 10%). These high pelvic recurrence rates are probably re-*

*lated to less than complete resection of the lateral rectal tissue, as surgeons[23,24] who routinely employ surgical techniques that carefully excise the lateral rectal ligaments and their surrounding lymphatic tissues (total mesorectal excision) are able to report much lower rates of pelvic cancer recurrence along with good preservation of function. (RSF Jr)*

rectocele can form. If the fascia is torn at higher levels, midvaginal or high vaginal rectoceles or enteroceles can result, especially if the rectovaginal septum separates from its central attachments to the uterosacral ligaments. An enterocele usually consists of herniating peritoneum from the cul-de-sac, with small intestine within the peritoneal sac. Treatment must include restoration of the integrity of the rectovaginal septum.

- Operative trauma is a rare cause of rectovaginal fistula. According to Killackey,[12] with procedures that manipulate the rectovaginal space, such as vaginal hysterectomy, rectocele and vaginal vault prolapse repair, low anterior resection, ileal pouch-anal anastomosis and anorectal surgery, there is a 1%-2% possibility of rectovaginal fistula.

- Brunschwig and Walsh[32] found it possible to remove large segments of both the internal iliac vein and the common iliac vein in individuals with laterally extended malignant neoplasms.

- Batson[33] emphasized that blood-borne infections or malignant cells from pelvic organs reach the spinal column and brain without passing through the lungs (as we noted earlier in the chapter).

- When treating cancer involving the anterior rectal wall, the fascia propria and the proximal part of Denonvilliers' fascia should be removed.

- When treating cancer involving the posterior rectal wall, all the fatty tissue should be removed, including the fas-

cia propria. Do not remove the presacral fascia. Also, the posterior part of the pelvic plexus and the pelvic parasympathetics are close to the anterolateral part of the distal colon. Thus, if the cancer is located at the posterior rectal wall, the dissection should be close to the anterolateral aspect of the rectum. The nerves, however, should be sacrificed for a good cancer operation.

## ANATOMIC COMPLICATIONS

The anatomic complications of the pelvic wall are the complications of surgery of the several anatomic entities related to the lateral pelvic wall.

We appreciate the concise wisdom of Wagner and Russo[36]:

*Iatrogenic injury has become the most common etiology of genitourinary trauma. Careful attention to detail during the pre-operative and intra-operative periods is critical in avoiding these vexing complications. Unfortunately, the proximity of the pelvic organs along with disease processes will continue to result in some untoward urologic complications. The complexity of these complications mandates a multidisciplinary approach with the pelvic surgeon and urologist leading the team.*

# *Pelvic Floor*

## SURGICAL ANATOMY

### Form, Function, and Development

The floor of the pelvis is composed of musculature, erectile tissues, and connective tissues (including the perineal membrane) of the perineum below and the pelvic diaphragm and its superior and inferior fasciae above.

Almost by convention, the floor of the pelvis is usually described with the organs that occupy the cavity of the true pelvis. The perineum is presented separately, as though it is a totally separate entity. This, we believe, adds to the confusion experienced by the student, the practitioner, and the anatomist in attempting to understand the anatomy and many of the clinical problems of the pelvis.

In reality, the musculofascial pelvic floor and the entities of the perineum are very closely related embryologically, structurally, and functionally. The various elements that support the pelvic viscera and participate in their functions are presented here together, artificially separable, but interdependent by development and design.

The integrity of the floor of the pelvic basin is dependent upon the proper architectural form and vitality of both the levator ani and urogenital structures. This becomes exceedingly clear when one comes to understand the significance of the true and proper orientation of the bony pelvis in humans in the standing position.

When one stands upright, the anterior superior iliac spines and the pubic tubercles lie in the same vertical plane (Fig. 28-32). Although the truth of this is acknowledged in most modern anatomy textbooks, illustrations of the bony pelvis in many of the same reference texts exhibit an error of almost 60° in its orientation, often labeling the true anterior view as one from a superior point of view (Fig. 28-33).[2]

Because of the relatively vertical orientation of the pelvic inlet, with the pubic symphysis and much of the ventral surface of the sacrum oriented essentially downward, the long axis of the symphysis slopes downward at an approximate angle of 30° to the horizontal from anterior to posterior in the female, slightly more than this in the male (Fig. 28-34). The ischiopubic ramus essentially parallels the ground. Thus, much of the pressure and the weight of organs within

the abdominopelvic cavity is directed toward the region of the urogenital triangle, the interval between the inferior rami of the pubic bones. Because of the pelvic orientation in humans, the urogenital muscular and fascial elements interconnecting the ischiopubic rami undergird the musculofascial floor of the pelvis, the pelvic diaphragm, providing essential assistance to its role in support and its multiple roles in pelvic visceral functions.

The integrity of the support of the pelvic organs is dependent upon the following complex of structural features:
- Extraperitoneal smooth muscle and associated visceral ligaments passing from the pelvic sidewalls to the viscera
- Musculature, aponeurotic tissues, and fasciae of the pelvic diaphragm
- Muscles, cavernous tissues, and fasciae of the urogenital triangle, including the perineal membrane

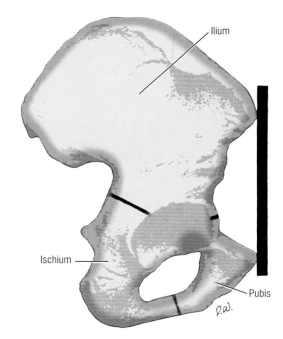

**FIG. 28-32.** Properly oriented hip bone (os coxae) (side view). Top part contacts black vertical bar at anterior superior iliac spine; bottom part contacts at pubic tubercle. Smaller black bars mark approximate boundaries between bones of os coxae. (Modified from Stromberg MW, Williams DJ. The misrepresentation of the human pelvis. J Biocommun 1993;20:14-28; with permission.)

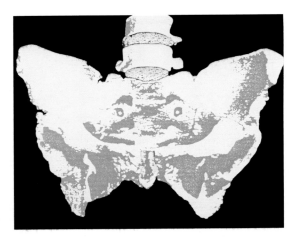

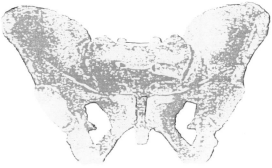

FIG. 28-33. *Upper,* Commonly presented, but incorrect, "front view" of bony pelvis, rotated about 60° to 75° from proper position. *Lower,* Similar incorrect view of bony pelvis, originally published in 1801. (Modified from Stromberg MW, Williams DJ. The misrepresentation of the human pelvis. J Biocommun 1993; 20:14-28; with permission.)

The first of these structural support systems is well described by Power,[37] and is elucidated elsewhere in this text in the chapter on the female genital system. The third of these structures, the urogenital triangle, will be considered later in this chapter under the section on the perineum. The pelvic diaphragm is reviewed in the following paragraphs.

## Pelvic Diaphragm

The pelvic diaphragm (Fig. 28-35, Fig. 28-36, Fig. 28-37) provides a musculofascial floor for the true pelvis. This floor is complete except for the midline openings between the two halves of the diaphragm. These openings are the urogenital hiatus and the rectal hiatus.

The rectum, urethra, and vagina pass together with fascia of the levator ani through the pelvic diaphragm. The diaphragm is composed of two paired muscles, the levator ani and coccygeus.

Anteriorly, between the inferior pubic rami, where the stress upon the pelvic floor is greatest in the upright posture, the floor is reinforced by the underlying urethrogenital complex of structures, including the so-called urogenital diaphragm.

The muscles of the pelvic diaphragm originate in the spine of the ischium, the white line (arcus tendineus) of the obturator fascia, and the body of the pubis. These muscles insert into the coccyx, the anococcygeal raphe, the perineal body, and the midline viscera (Fig. 28-38). The musculature of the pelvic diaphragm produces a gutterlike formation that slopes forward and downward.

### *Levator Ani*

The levator ani can be considered to be made up of three contributing muscular entities: iliococcygeus, pubococcygeus, and puborectalis (Fig. 28-38). This last component is essential to maintaining rectal continence. Shafik[38] considers the puborectalis to be part of the external sphincter and not a part of the levator ani.

**Iliococcygeus**
The posterior edge of the pubococcygeus is in some

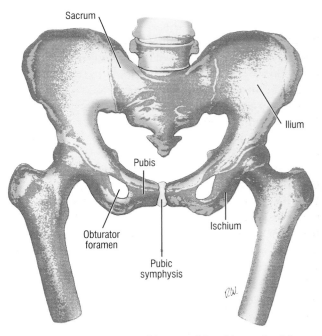

FIG. 28-34. Properly oriented bony pelvis with proximal femora attached (front view). Note that most of sacrum recedes from observer. Compare to Fig 28-33. (Modified from Stromberg MW, Williams DJ. The misrepresentation of the human pelvis. J Biocommun 1993;20:14-28; with permission.)

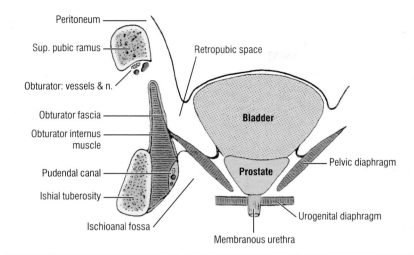

**FIG. 28-35.** Coronal section of male pelvis illustrating main part of funnel-shaped pelvic diaphragm formed mainly by two levator ani muscles. Pelvic diaphragm forms floor of abdominal and pelvic cavities and consists of paired levator ani and coccygeus muscles with their superior and inferior fasciae. Rectum is anchored to pelvic diaphragm in middle (see Fig. 28-41). Only pelvic diaphragm (levator ani portion) intervenes between ischioanal fossa and retropubic space. (Modified from Moore KL. Clinically Oriented Anatomy (2nd ed). Baltimore: Williams & Wilkins, 1985; with permission.)

cases separated by a narrow aponeurosis from the thinner and more aponeurotic iliococcygeus. In other cases they are continuous.

The iliococcygeus arises from the arcus tendineus levator ani, the more or less apparent specialization of the fascia of the internal obturator and fascia of the levator ani. The iliococcygeus inserts in the midline raphe (Fig. 28-38) and upon the coccyx.

### Pubococcygeus

The lateral borders of the urogenital hiatus of the pelvic diaphragm are formed by the medial borders of the pubococcygeus; the puborectalis takes a more lateral course from its origin.

In a study of histologic sections and grossly dissected specimens, Delancey and Starr[39] note that smooth muscle, collagen, and elastic fibers of the vaginal wall and paraurethral tissues interdigitate directly with the most medial muscle fibers of the levator ani. This occurs in the vicinity of the proximal part of the urethra. This strong attachment extends from the level of the entrance of the ureters into the bladder inferiorly to the urogenital diaphragm. They conclude that the inseparable nature of the vagina and lower urethra and the lateral attachments to the levator ani make it possible for the medial levator ani muscle to play a role in controlling the position of the vesical neck, and thus perhaps in voiding and continence. Mostwin[40] observes that disruption of the attachments of the pubococcygeus to the vaginal wall can result in herniation, with accompanying secondary posterior bladder descent.

In our dissections, we observed the strong intermingling of the most anterior and medial part of the pubococcygeus with the superolateral aspect of the vagina and the paraurethral musculature in the female and the prostatic

capsule in the male. In both male and female, some fibers pass deeply around these structures to insert into the perineal body. External to this lamina of fibers from the pubococcygeus, another fleshy muscular band arises partially from the pubic bone and partially from the fascia of the obturator internus. It passes behind the rectum to become continuous with fibers from the opposite side. As noted by Oelrich[41] in studies of the gorilla and humans, the pubococcygeus has no attachment to the coccyx.

**LEVATOR PLATE.** The striated musculature between the coccyx and the rectum, including the iliococcygeus and the posterior part of the pubococcygeus, forms the "levator plate." The strength of the levator plate and its degree of angulation with the horizontal plane from the coccyx to the rectum are both of importance in maintaining fecal continence.

The levator plate is also responsible for prevention of prolapse of the upper vagina, the uterus, and the rectum. With coughing, laughing, or straining, the vertical pressures exerted by the Valsalva maneuver bear directly upon these organs. The normal levator plate ascends to meet the organs, impinging upon them and preventing their prolapse.

### Puborectalis

The puborectalis arises from the lower posterior surface of the pubic bone. It is lateral and external to the pubovaginalis (levator prostatae) and pubococcygeus. Also, some of its deeper fibers take origin from fibrous tissue intervening between it and the sphincter urethrae muscle.[42] This gives further credence to the possible influence of contraction of the levator ani muscle upon urethral function and continence. Fibers from the left and right puborectalis

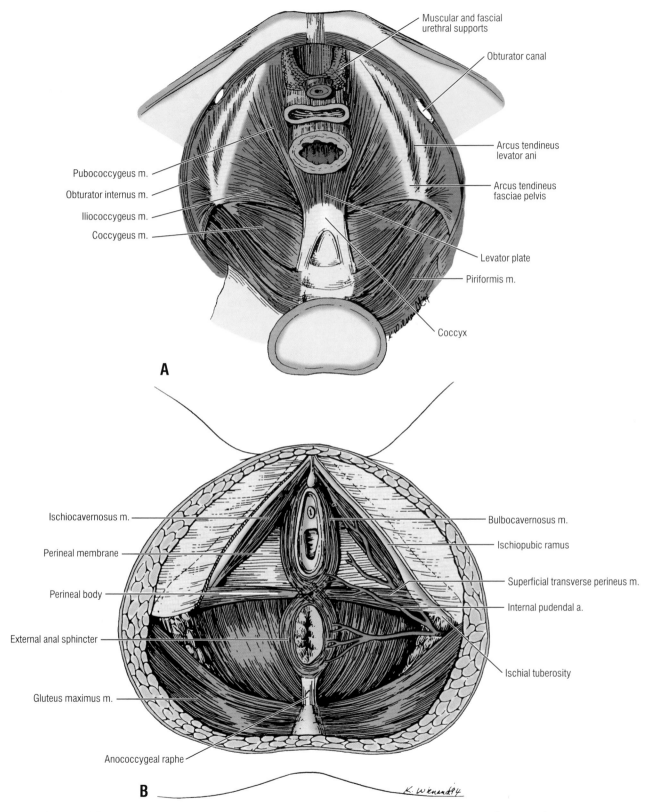

Muscular and fascial urethral supports

Obturator canal

Arcus tendineus levator ani

Arcus tendineus fasciae pelvis

Pubococcygeus m.

Obturator internus m.

Iliococcygeus m.

Coccygeus m.

Levator plate

Piriformis m.

Coccyx

**A**

Ischiocavernosus m.

Perineal membrane

Perineal body

External anal sphincter

Gluteus maximus m.

Anococcygeal raphe

Bulbocavernosus m.

Ischiopubic ramus

Superficial transverse perineus m.

Internal pudendal a.

Ischial tuberosity

**B**

FIG. 28-36. Muscles of female pelvic diaphragm. **A,** Seen from above. **B,** Seen from below. (Modified from Gray SW, Skandalakis JE. Atlas of Surgical Anatomy for General Surgeons. Baltimore: Williams & Wilkins, 1985; with permission.)

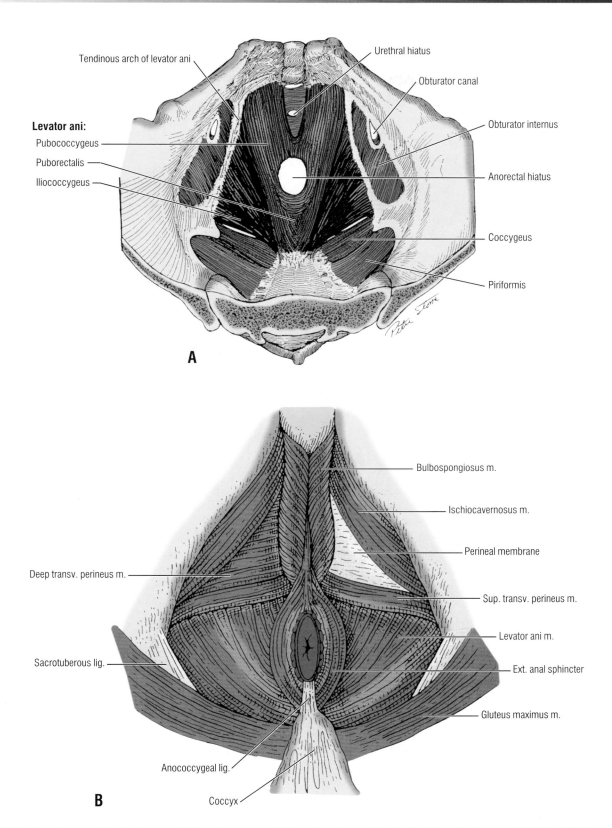

**FIG. 28-37.** Muscles of male pelvic diaphragm. **A,** Seen from above. **B,** Seen from below. (**A,** Modified from Christensen JB, Telford IR. Synopsis of Gross Anatomy (5th ed). Philadelphia: JB Lippincott, 1988; with permission. **B,** Modified from Skandalakis LJ, Gadacz TR, Mansberger AR Jr, Mitchell WE Jr, Colborn GL, Skandalakis JE. Modern Hernia Repair. Pearl River NY: Parthenon, 1996; with permission.)

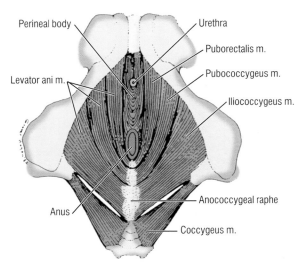

FIG. 28-38. Pelvic diaphragm from below. Levator ani composed of three muscles: puborectalis, pubococcygeus, and iliococcygeus. (Modified from Skandalakis JE, Gray SW, Rowe JS Jr. Anatomical Complications in General Surgery. New York: McGraw-Hill, 1983; with permission.)

muscles pass posteriorly. They then join posterior to the rectum, forming a well-defined sling (Fig. 28-39). Here, they blend with and pass external to the more cranial part of the deep external sphincter.

The puborectalis forms the so-called anorectal ring with the superficial and deep parts of the external sphincter and the proximal part of the internal sphincter. This ring can be palpated. Because cutting through it will produce anal incontinence, it must be identified and protected during surgical procedures. Further details of the external sphincter will be discussed with the morphology of the anal canal.

### *Coccygeus*

Another contributor to the pelvic diaphragm musculature is the coccygeus (Fig. 28-39). It arises from the spine of the ischium and the pelvic surface of the sacrospinous ligament, overlapping it somewhat. The coccygeus inserts upon the lateral aspects of the lower two sacral vertebrae and upon the upper two coccygeal vertebrae.

The funnel shape of the pelvic floor and anal canal is uniquely developed to provide discriminatory continence of gas, liquid, and solid. Many of the physiologic factors involved in this discrimination and control are poorly understood.[43] It has become conventional to speak of two diaphragms associated with the pelvic outlet, the pelvic diaphragm and the urogenital diaphragm. In fact, these structures are more closely related anatomically and func-

tionally than most sources recognize.

In embryologic development, the sphincter urethrae muscle and the other muscles of the perineum, including the external anal sphincter, arise from the cloacal sphincter and form an accessory pelvic diaphragm.[44] The levator ani arises from the caudal musculature. In lower animals, the caudal musculature is responsible for movements of the tail. It is modified in its human form to provide support functions.[45] Levi et al.[46] emphasize that the puborectalis is, indeed, a part of the levator ani, citing its common embryologic origin with the pubococcygeus and iliococcygeus muscles. On the other hand, Cherry and Rothenberger[43] state that the puborectalis is anatomically, neurologically, and functionally merged with the deep portion of the external sphincter ani muscle.

## Innervation of the Pelvic Diaphragm

The pelvic diaphragm receives nerve supply on its

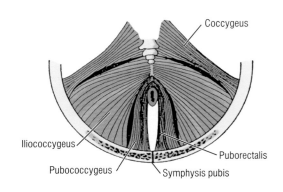

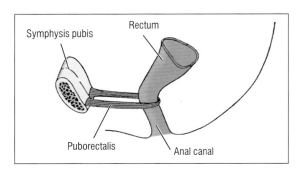

FIG. 28-39. Floor of pelvis seen from above showing levatores ani. *Inset:* How the anorectal junction is angulated by the sling formed by the puborectalis muscles. (Modified from McGregor AL, DuPlessis DJ. A Synopsis of Surgical Anatomy (10th ed). Baltimore: Williams & Wilkins, 1969; with permission.)

pelvic surface by the nerve to the levator ani, which arises from the ventral primary ramus of S4 or S5. A perineal branch arising either from this nerve or directly from the ventral primary ramus of S4 may pierce the coccygeus muscle, supply it, and then further supply the external sphincter ani. Additionally, the nerve to the levator ani may provide origin for a branch that joins the pudendal nerve at the entrance to the pudendal canal.

## Observations Regarding the Pelvic Floor

- The pelvic diaphragm prevents evisceration and never prolapses. Together with the anal sphincters, the ano-coccygeal ligament, and the perineal body, it supports the rectum and anal canal (Fig. 28-40).
- Several slings form and support the pelvic floor. In the

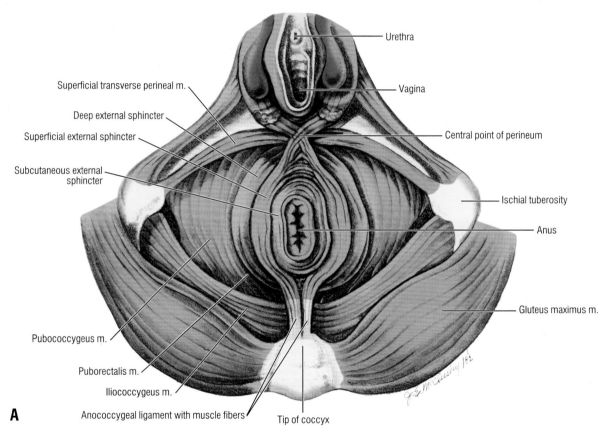

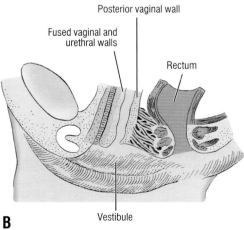

FIG. 28-40. Female pelvic diaphragm. **A,** Its formation by several muscles, from below. **B,** The perineal body (light gray) in sagittal section. It is larger, and contains more muscle, in the female than in the male. (**A,** Modified from Gray SW, Skandalakis JE. Atlas of Surgical Anatomy for General Surgeons. Baltimore: Williams & Wilkins, 1985; **B,** Modified from Hollinshead WH. Anatomy for Surgeons, Vol 2. New York: Hoeber-Harper, 1956; with permission.)

male, a sling forms around the prostate (levator prostatae or prostate levator) and passes behind it in a U-like formation. Both limbs insert into the perineal body. In the female, a sling at the internal sphincter of the vagina (pubovaginalis) passes behind the vagina in a U-like formation to insert into the perineal body. This "sphincter" of the pelvic floor should not be confused with the sphincter of the introitus (sphincter urethrovaginalis and bulbospongiosus muscles). In both male and female, the puborectalis (see Fig. 28-39 inset) is the most important sling.

- The puborectalis forms a sling that is responsible for the closing of the anorectal canal.
- The pelvic floor slopes downward and forward to receive the lowest part of the fetus (Fig. 28-41).
- The passive stretching and active contraction of the iliococcygeus participates in the mechanisms of defecation, micturition, and parturition.
- The levator ani, arcus tendineus fascia pelvis, and visceral fascia collaborate to create the integrity of the pelvic floor.

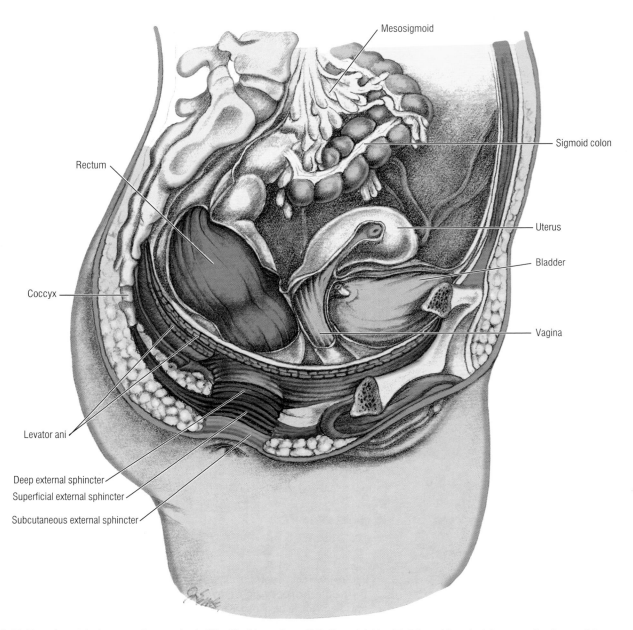

**FIG. 28-41.** Female pelvis (paramedian section). (Modified from Gray SW, Skandalakis JE. Atlas of Surgical Anatomy for General Surgeons. Baltimore: Williams & Wilkins, 1985; with permission.)

- The obturator nerve supplies the adductor muscles of the thigh. It is the most important nerve to protect in the superolateral wall of the true pelvis (see Fig. 28-30D).
- It is not known what nerve(s) innervates the visceral peritoneum.
- The pudendal nerve and internal pudendal artery and vein provide neural and vascular supply for the perineum and, in part, for the pelvic floor.
- The internal iliac vessels, the hypogastric nerve, and the pelvic splanchnic nerves provide the blood supply and innervation to the rectum and urinary bladder.
- The pelvic diaphragm musculature, its aponeurotic tissues, and its fascial coverings provide the fibromuscular pelvic floor and include the levator ani and coccygeus muscles. The endopelvic fascial lining of the muscles (pelvic surface) is essentially continuous with the transversalis fascial layer of the abdominal cavity.

## Structures of the Fasciae of the Pelvic Floor

The fasciae of the pelvis were described earlier in this chapter in discussing the pelvic sidewalls. We now relate some of the points discussed there to the structures of the pelvic floor.

The three different forms of fasciae associated with the pelvic floor are the parietal, visceral, and diaphragmatic fasciae. They are discussed below.

### *Parietal Fascia*

The parietal portion of the pelvic fascia is in large measure the fascia of the obturator internus, piriformis, and pelvic diaphragm muscles because it covers these muscles during its journey to reach and attach to the bones and ligaments of the pelvic outlet. The fascia of the obturator internus is seemingly interrupted within the pelvis by the narrow band of origin of the levator ani. This fascia, however, continues below that origin, thereby forming the lateral boundaries of the perineum below the floor of the pelvis. To be more specific, this fascia is responsible for the formation of Alcock's canal (Fig. 28-3) at the lateral wall of the ischioanal fossa where it covers the obturator internus muscle.

### *Visceral Fascia*

The visceral portion of the pelvic fascia is in continuity with the endopelvic connective tissues that intervene between the peritoneum and the parietal fascia of the pelvic sidewall and floor. The visceral fascia invests almost all of the pelvic surfaces of the organs within the pelvis. The possible exception to this may be parts of the fundus of the uterus and bladder. The visceral fascia is also continuous with the endopelvic connective tissue that provides connective tissue sheaths for the nerves and vessels supplying the organs. In addition, the coverings of the organs, nerves, and vessels are particularly reinforced by the following supporting structures:

- "Pillars" of the rectum and bladder
- Uterosacral and lateral cervical (Mackenrodt) ligaments of the uterus
- Rectovaginal (rectoprostatic) septum
- Arcus tendineus fascia pelvis
- Pubovesical fascial covering joining the bladder, vagina, and cervix
- Extrinsic prostatic capsule

### *Diaphragmatic Fascia*

The diaphragmatic fascia covers the superior surface (supraanal fascia) and the inferior surface (infraanal fascia) of the pelvic diaphragm. The diaphragmatic fascia is commonly accepted to be related to the superior fascia of the urogenital diaphragm. But this point should be understood in the context of the following section on the perineum.

The superior layer of the urogenital diaphragm is continuous (at least at its peripheral edges) with the pelvic parietal fascia that clothes the superior surface of the pelvic diaphragm. The inferior fascia (perineal membrane) is perhaps a different embryologic entity. However, it is reasonable that the envelope of the urogenital diaphragm could be of endopelvic origin. From a surgical standpoint this embryologic problem, if there is one, does not affect the functioning of the urogenital diaphragm in health and disease.

## Perineal Body (Center) and Perineal Hernia

The perineal body (center) (see Fig. 28-19, Fig. 28-38 and Fig. 28-40A&B) in the male represents the central tendinous point, a bolus of tissue between the anus and bulb. In the female it is the "perineum" of the gynecologist, a fibromuscular mass of tissue between the anus and vagina.

The perineal body, located under the pelvic floor, is formed by the attachments of several muscles. These include the following:

- Superficial transverse perineus
- Bulbospongiosus
- Sphincter urethrae in the male

- Sphincter urethrovaginalis and deep transverse perineus muscles in the female
- Superficial part of the external anal sphincter
- Levator prostatae and pubovaginalis of the levator ani

The perineal body is a midline landmark between the anterior and posterior triangles of the perineum. It gives some support to the levator ani muscle and thus to the pelvic organs.

A perineal hernia (Fig. 28-42) is the protrusion of a viscus through the floor of the pelvis (pelvic diaphragm) into the perineum. A hernial sac is present. The hernia may be primary, or it may be secondary to pelvic surgery. Only primary hernias are of concern here.

Perineal hernia is among the rarest of human hernias. Unlike inguinal hernia, which appears to be related to the erect posture of humans, perineal hernia is more common

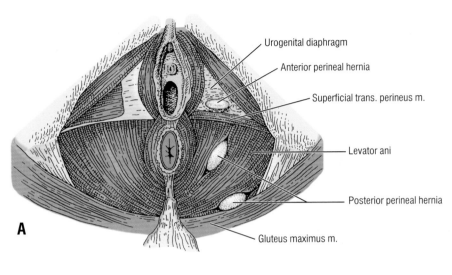

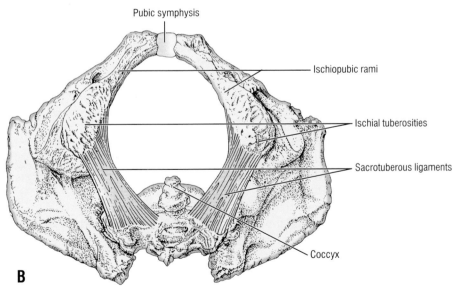

**Fig 28-42.** The female perineum. **A,** The female perineum seen from below showing possible sites of perineal hernias. A primary perineal hernia may occur anterior or posterior to the superficial transverse perineus muscle. An anterior hernia protrudes through the urogenital diaphragm into the triangle formed by the bulbospongiosus muscle medially, the ischiocavernosus muscle laterally, and the superficial transverse perineus muscle inferiorly. Anterior hernias occur only in females. A posterior perineal hernia may emerge between component muscle bundles of levator ani muscle or between that muscle and coccygeus muscle midway between the rectum and the ischial tuberosity. **B,** Boundaries of the perineum seen from above. This diamond-shaped area can be divided by a line connecting the ischial tuberosities into an anterior or urogenital triangle and a posterior or anal triangle. (Modified from Skandalakis LJ, Gadacz TR, Mansberger AR Jr, Mitchell WE Jr, Colborn GL, Skandalakis JE. Modern Hernia Repair. Pearl River NY: Parthenon, 1996; with permission.)

in quadrupeds than in humans.

By definition the pelvic diaphragm is the floor of the pelvic basin and the roof of the perineum. The hernial sac passing through any abnormal opening of the pelvic diaphragm will eventually appear in the perineal area. It may be anterior or posterior to the superficial transverse perineus muscle.

A primary perineal hernia may occur anterior or posterior to the superficial transverse perineus muscle (Fig. 28-42).

An anterior perineal hernia passes through the pelvic and urogenital diaphragms, lateral to the urinary bladder and vagina, and anterior to the urethra. It has been variously called pudendal, labial, lateral, or vaginal-labial. It is found only in women; it is hard to see how this kind of perineal hernia could occur in males.

A posterior perineal hernia passes between components of the pelvic diaphragm or through the hiatus of Schwalbe, when present, lateral to the urethra, vagina, and rectum. The hiatus is formed by the nonunion of the obturator internus and levator ani muscles. There are two possible locations: (1) an upper posterior hernia between the pubococcygeus and iliococcygeus muscles; and (2) a lower posterior hernia between iliococcygeus and coccygeus muscles, below the lower margin of the gluteus maximus muscle.

In males the perineal hernia enters the ischioanal fossa. In females it may enter the fossa or the labium majus, or it may lie close to the vaginal wall or below the lower margin of the gluteus maximus muscle.

A perineal hernia may be approached for repair through the perineum or through the abdomen.

## SURGICAL CONSIDERATIONS

• If the membranous urethra is injured proximal to (above) the urogenital diaphragm, extravasating urine and blood will pass into the space of Retzius in an extraperitoneal position. If the membranous urethra is injured distal to (below, or inferior to) the urogenital diaphragm, extravasating urine and blood will pass into the superficial perineal cleft. Extension upward to the anterior abdominal wall between the membranous superficial fascia of Scarpa and the deep muscular fascia (Gallaudet) is also possible. Details about repairing rupture of the urethra and urinary extravasations can be found in the chapter on the urethra.

• The lower posterior wall of the vagina is supported by the central perineal tendon. Damage to the tendon during delivery is the cause of vaginal prolapse.

• Infection of the nonpalpable Bartholin glands may present as unilateral or bilateral painful cystic swellings. Incision and drainage, with total excision of the cyst and marsupialization of the edges, is the treatment of choice.

• There are several approaches to reconstructive surgery of the pelvis and perineum. Jurado et al.[47] recommend a rectus abdominis flap for primary vaginal and pelvic floor reconstruction.

• For pelvic floor reconstruction after surgery for locally advanced rectal carcinoma, Small et al.[48] stress the role of muscle and myocutaneous flaps as biologic spacers to help prevent radiation injury, post-radiation fistulas, small bowel obstruction, and pelvic sidewall adherence.

NOTE: The numerous surgical considerations in this area will be discussed individually with each pertinent organ in other chapters.

## ANATOMIC COMPLICATIONS

The anatomic complications of the pelvic floor are the complications of surgery of the several anatomic entities that are related to the pelvic floor.

# *Perineum*

*In the female uterus, in the male perineum.*

**Rufus of Ephesus (115 AD)**[49]

The chapter in this book on the anorectum covers much of the same subject matter as that presented here, but if we discussed the pelvis without some accompanying discussion of the perineum, it would be incomplete. Therefore a very brief discussion of the perineum follows.

## EMBRYOGENESIS

The hindgut of the gastrointestinal tract, with its endodermal lining, ends blindly in the cloaca. At its ventral aspect, the cloaca characteristically has a diverticulumlike formation (the allantois), which is the urachus in the adult.

The urorectal septum, of mesodermal origin, divides the cloaca into anterior and posterior parts. The anterior (urogenital) portion contains several perineal muscles. The posterior segment (terminal hindgut) encompasses the external sphincter of the anus.

One tubular structure, the mesonephric duct (ductus in the male), enters the anterior part of the cloaca. The duct (or vas) produces another tubular structure (the ureter) that travels upward to meet the metanephros. The common channel of ductus and ureter is located close to the posterior wall of the urinary bladder and is absorbed later. Each of these tubes has different openings and, therefore, different embryologic and anatomic destinies.

The reader will find more details on the perineum in the chapters on the anal and genital areas.

## SURGICAL ANATOMY

### Introduction

#### *Definition of Perineum*

In the anatomic (upright or erect) position, the perineum is a narrow area of soft parts located between the mus-

culature of the gluteal and thigh areas (Fig. 28-43). With abduction of the thighs, the perineum has a diamond-shaped configuration (Fig. 28-44). The diamond is bordered by the ischiopubic rami and pubic symphysis in its anterior half, the urogenital triangle. In its posterior half, or anal triangle, boundaries are provided by the inferior border of the gluteus maximus muscle, the ischial tuberosities, the sacrotuberous ligaments, and the coccyx.

To some gynecologists, "perineum" refers to the midline, fibromuscular structure between the urethra and anus. Others apply the term "perineal body" to this central fixation body into which the levator ani, external sphincter ani, bulbospongiosus, and transverse perineus muscles insert or originate in part. As per Rufus[49] in this section's introduction, the ancients used the word "perineum" to refer to the male genitalia and the word "uterus" to indicate its female counterparts. It is apparent that the term has been broadened considerably in its applications.

### *Orientation and Relations of the Perineum*

The perineum as presently defined is located below the pelvic diaphragm, the musculofascial floor of the pelvis. The fascia of the pelvic diaphragm in the region of the urogenital hiatus is fused with the inferior fascia (perineal membrane) of the "urogenital diaphragm."[50,51] It provides a plane of connective tissue that serves as the meeting point of the pelvic floor and the superior extension of the perineum-based entities, chiefly the sphincter urethrae musculature. The terminal portions of the digestive tract and the male and female urogenital tracts pass through the midline hiatuses of the pelvic diaphragm and emerge in the perineum. For all practical purposes, the bony, muscular, and fascial elements of the pelvic diaphragm and perineum support the viscera and aid the function or limit the outlets of pelvic organs.

When learning or reviewing relations of perineal structures, remember that the term "superficial" implies a relationship closer to the skin. "Superficial" is synonymous with "inferior." The terms "deep" and "superior" mean that a structure is farther away from the skin or genitalia of the per-

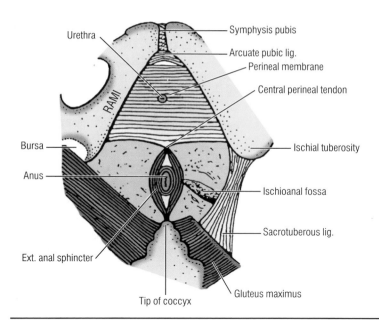

Urethra
Symphysis pubis
Arcuate pubic lig.
Perineal membrane
Central perineal tendon
RAMI
Ischial tuberosity
Bursa
Anus
Ischioanal fossa
Ext. anal sphincter
Sacrotuberous lig.
Tip of coccyx
Gluteus maximus

**FIG. 28-43.** Boundaries and subdivisions of perineum (diamond-shaped region) (see Fig. 28-42). Perineal membrane is pierced by urethra. Female vagina also pierces this perineal membrane. (Modified from Moore KL. Clinically Oriented Anatomy (2nd ed). Baltimore: Williams & Wilkins, 1985; with permission.)

ineum. For example, the bulbospongiosus muscles are relatively superficial in the perineum. The sphincter urethrae muscle is relatively deep.

## General Topography

### *Boundaries of the Perineum*

The perineum is a diamond-shaped region. The arcuate pubic ligament, the tip of the coccyx, and the ischial tuberosities form its angles (Fig. 28-43, Fig. 28-44).
Following are the boundaries of the perineum:
• Anterior: pubic symphysis
• Anterolateral: ischiopubic rami
• Inferolateral: ischial tuberosities
• Posterolateral: sacrotuberous ligaments and gluteus maximus
• Posterior: coccyx

### *Subdivisions of the Perineum*

An imaginary line between the two ischial tuberosities divides the perineal diamond into two triangles: a ventral or anterior urogenital triangle and a dorsal or posterior anal triangle (Fig. 28-44).
In some books the posterior triangle is called the anorectal triangle. This is not correct terminology because the rectum ends at the puborectal sling. The puborectal sling is where the puborectalis muscle causes the critical angulation affecting fecal continence between the anteriorly

directed rectum and the posteroinferiorly aligned anal canal.

### *Perineum Complex* (Fig. 28-45)

The list that follows is of anatomic entities and spaces

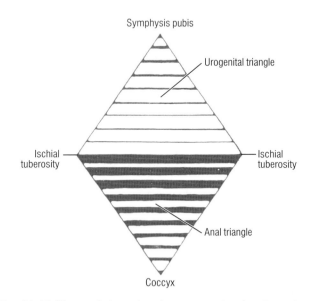

Symphysis pubis

Urogenital triangle

Ischial tuberosity

Ischial tuberosity

Anal triangle

Coccyx

**FIG. 28-44.** Diamond-shaped perineum or perineal region extends from symphysis pubis to coccyx. Transverse line between right and left ischial tuberosities divides perineum into two triangular areas: urogenital region or triangle, anteriorly, and anal region or triangle, posteriorly. (Modified from Moore KL. Clinically Oriented Anatomy. Baltimore: Williams & Wilkins, 1980; with permission.)

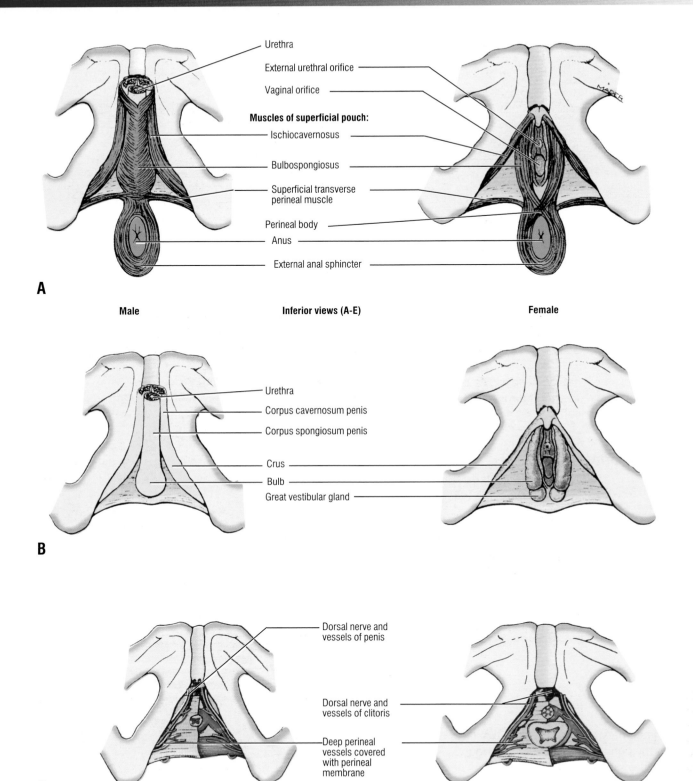

Urethra

External urethral orifice

Vaginal orifice

**Muscles of superficial pouch:**

Ischiocavernosus

Bulbospongiosus

Superficial transverse perineal muscle

Perineal body

Anus

External anal sphincter

**A**

**Male**

**Inferior views (A-E)**

**Female**

Urethra

Corpus cavernosum penis

Corpus spongiosum penis

Crus

Bulb

Great vestibular gland

**B**

Dorsal nerve and vessels of penis

Dorsal nerve and vessels of clitoris

Deep perineal vessels covered with perineal membrane

**C**

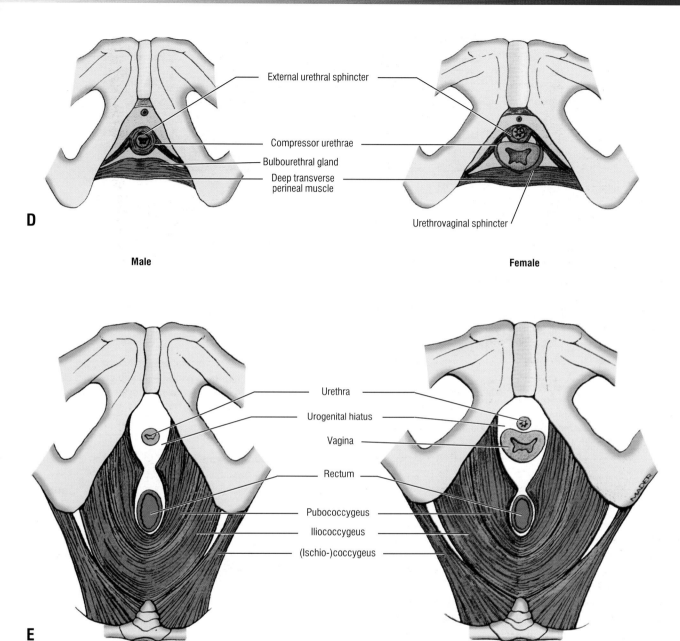

**FIG. 28-45.** Layers of perineum from superficial to deep. Male, left; female, right. Below the perineal membrane, the superficial perineal pouch or space contains the muscles **(A)** associated with the erectile bodies. In **B,** the erectile bodies themselves are shown. The urogenital hiatus, which is sealed inferiorly by the perineal membrane that extends between the ischiopubic rami **(C)**, contains the external urethral sphincter and deep transverse perineal muscles **(D)**. In **E,** the pelvic outlet is almost filled by the pelvic diaphragm (levator ani and coccygeus muscles), which forms the roof of the perineal compartment. The urethra (and vagina in females) passes through the urogenital hiatus anteriorly and the rectum posteriorly. (Modified from Moore KL, Dalley AF. Clinically Oriented Anatomy, 4th ed. Philadelphia: Lippincott, Williams & Wilkins, 1999; with permission.)

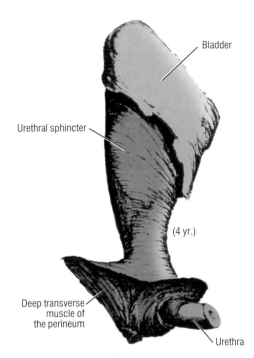

FIG. 28-46. Perineal view of bladder and urethral sphincter showing sphincter relations to urethra and deep transverse muscle of perineum (4-year-old male). (Modified from Oelrich TM. The urethral sphincter muscle in the male. Am J Anat 1980;158:229-246; with permission.)

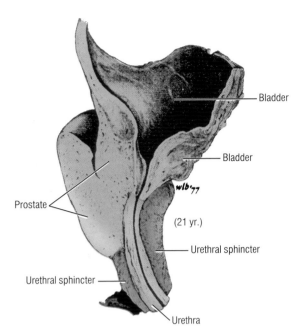

FIG. 28-47. Median section of bladder, urethra, prostate, and urethral sphincter showing extent of contact between urethra and urethral sphincter muscle (21-year-old male). (Modified from Oelrich TM. The urethral sphincter muscle in the male. Am J Anat 1980;158:229-246; with permission.)

related to the perineum and pelvic floor. Some of these entities and spaces have been discussed previously in this chapter or elsewhere in this book. We mention them in the context of the perineum and pelvic floor to better explain a complex area of the human body.

- Membranous fascial layer of Colles and superficial perineal cleft below (see "Superficial Fascia" under "Inguinofemoral Area" in chapter on abdominal wall and hernias)
- Superficial perineal pouch (superficial compartment)
- Deep perineal pouch (urogenital diaphragm)
- Ischioanal (formerly ischiorectal) fossae (see "Ischioanal Fossa" under "Rectum and Anal Canal" in chapter on large intestine and anorectum)
- Various fasciae of the perineum
- Perineal center (perineal body)
- Pelvic diaphragm

Figure 28-45 illustrates the perineal layers in a highly diagrammatic way to aid orientation. The deeper structures appear more realistically in Figures 28-46 through 28-49.

## Layers of the Urogenital Triangle

Progressing from superficial to deep (or inferior to superior), the urogenital triangle contains the following layers (Fig. 28-45):

- Skin and adipose layer (Camper's fascia, continuous

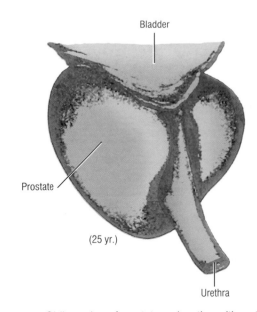

FIG. 28-48. Oblique view of prostate and urethra with urethral sphincter muscle removed (25-year-old male). (Modified from Oelrich TM. The urethral sphincter muscle in the male. Am J Anat 1980;158:229-246; with permission.)

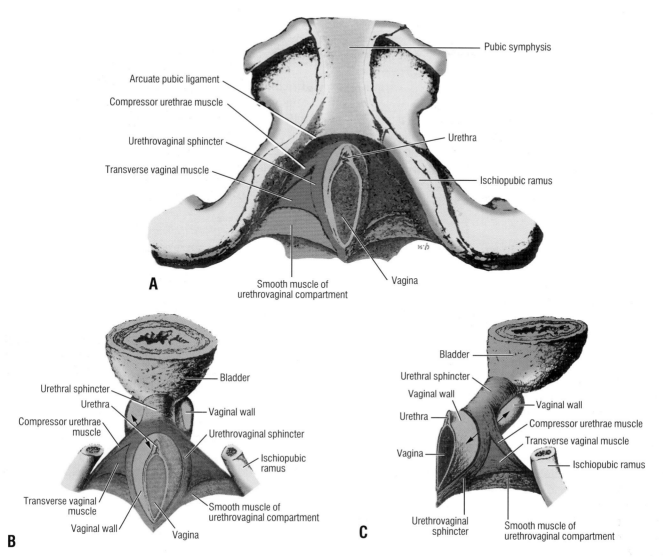

**FIG. 28-49.** Urogenital views of 27-year-old woman. **A,** Perineal view of urogenital sphincter musculature with perineal membrane removed. **B,** Complete urogenital sphincter musculature, bladder, and vagina with pubic symphysis removed and ischial rami spread. **C,** Oblique view of complete urogenital sphincter muscles, bladder, and vagina. Arrows indicate continuity of vaginal wall beneath muscle. (Modified from Oelrich TM. The striated urogenital sphincter muscle in the female. Anat Rec 1983;205:223-232; with permission.)

with the same layer of the anterior abdominal wall) of superficial fascia

- Membranous layer of superficial fascia, named Colles' fascia in the perineum (continuous with Scarpa's fascia of the abdominal wall)
- Superficial perineal cleft, a potential space between Colles' fascia and the muscular fascia (fascia of Gallaudet or external perineal fascia) of the superficial perineal compartment or superficial pouch
- Superficial perineal pouch including muscle fascia inferiorly (Gallaudet) and the perineal membrane superiorly. Three pairs of muscles, two pairs of erectile tissue bod-

ies, and, in the female, the vestibular glands
- The deep pouch or urethrogenital compartment (urogenital diaphragm)

The superficial and deep fasciae of the urogenital region are continuous with similar fascial layers on the anterior abdominal wall. The potential space between these fascial layers is separated from similar potential spaces in the thighs by the stout attachments of the fasciae to the ischiopubic rami. These separate the perineal space from the thigh. The attachment along the inguinal crease of Scarpa's membranous fascia of the abdominal wall to the fascia lata of the thigh separates the interfascial potential space of the abdominal wall from extension into the thighs.

## *Skin and Adipose Layer of Superficial Perineal Fascia (Camper's)*

The superficial adipose layer of the urogenital triangle is called Camper's fascia, as is the similar layer in the anterior abdominal wall. This layer of tissue continues into the anal triangle of the perineum posteriorly. Camper's fascia of the urogenital triangle provides the bulk of tissue occupying the ischioanal fossae on either side of the midline raphe and anus.

## *Membranous Layer of Superficial Perineal Fascia (Colles')*

The irregularly membranous, often laminated layer of tissue deep to Camper's fascia is called Colles' fascia. It is the counterpart of Scarpa's fascia of the abdominal wall. The membranous tissue is stoutly attached to the ischiopubic rami laterally and to the posterior edge of the urogenital musculature posteriorly. This provides an anatomic barrier between the urogenital spaces anteriorly and the ischioanal fossae posteriorly.

One should realize that a singular, well defined layer of membranous fascia is seen infrequently in the lower part of the anterior abdominal wall. A similar deterrent to simplicity and ease of understanding is seen also in the urogenital region. Simply put, one can encounter more than one layer of structurally membranous tissue in the perineum with a variable quantity of fatty tissue separating it from a subjacent layer of membranous tissue. This also occurs in the lower abdominal wall.

Tobin and Benjamin[52] took a very clear and well defended position in disputing the existence of separate adipose and membranous layers of fascia on the anterior abdominal wall or in the perineum. Current interpretations of the original work of Colles, Scarpa, and Camper are not accurate expressions of their stated observations.

## *Superficial Perineal Cleft*

### Boundaries of the Superficial Perineal Cleft
Following are the boundaries of the superficial perineal cleft:
- Inferior (below): Colles' fascia
- Superior: muscle fascia of Gallaudet (inferior or external perineal fascia)
- Lateral: Colles' fascia, attached to the ischiopubic rami
- Posterolateral: closed by the union of Colles' fascia and muscle fascia

- Anterior: communicates freely with the potential space between Scarpa's fascia and the anterior abdominal wall, laterally and superiorly

### Nature of the Superficial Perineal Cleft
Irrespective of the diversity in appearance of laminae of membranous tissues in the superficial fascia of the urogenital triangle, in every dissection we have performed on embalmed or unembalmed cadaveric specimens, we have been able to find a clearly demonstrable cleft, or potential space, between the superficial fascia and the fascia that covers the muscles of the superficial perineal compartment (Fig. 28-50).

Perhaps in any given individual there is a plane of least resistance within the superficial fascia where the fat and laminae of connective tissue can be separated with relative ease. Perhaps, too, this particular plane may depend greatly upon the exact point of entry or perforation. For all practical purposes, the superficial perineal cleft may be at one and the same time both artifactual and real upon interruption of the most readily dissectible line of separation. Although maintaining the existence of both adipose and membranous layers of superficial fascia in the perineum, Stormont et al.[53] acknowledged that the "membranous layer" is probably fenestrated.

The superficial perineal cleft can be probed with the fingertips without sharp dissection. After entering this space, blunt dissection upward ventrally from the region anterior to the perineal body, lateral to the scrotum, or deep to the subcutaneous tissues of the mons veneris reaches a continuing potential space of the lower abdominal wall. Likewise, defining the interval between superficial and deep fasciae of the abdominal wall allows tracing out the potential space inferiorly into the perineum. Extravasation of blood and/or urine into this space takes place in perineal injuries of the urethra external to the perineal membrane.

It is important to recognize and remember the difference between the superficial cleft and the superficial pouch or compartment. The superficial perineal cleft is a potential space between the membranous layer of superficial fascia and the fascia of Gallaudet. Perhaps, for easy understanding, it can be thought of as existing between Colles' fascia and the deep perineal fascia that covers the superficial perineal muscles.

The adipose and membranous layers of superficial fascia blend as they approach the external genitalia. The fatty element is essentially lost. The superficial tissue is richly infiltrated with smooth muscle fibers, forming the dartos tunic of the scrotum and the superficial fascial covering of the penis/clitoris. Near the midline of the anterior abdominal wall, this superficial fascial blending is considerably thicker and forms the fundiform ligament of the penis or clitoris.

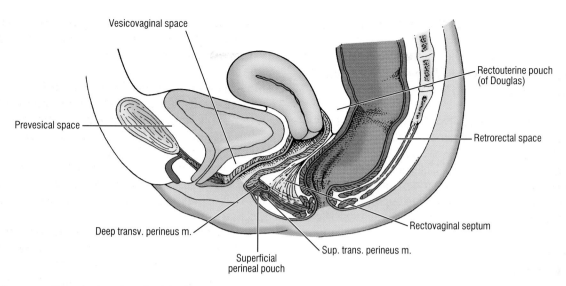

**FIG. 28-50.** Diagrammatic sagittal section of pelvis showing six unpaired spaces of pelvis. All are potential spaces except for rectouterine space of Douglas in female (rectovesical space in male) which is a true space lined with peritoneum. (Modified from Skandalakis LJ, Gadacz TR, Mansberger AR Jr, Mitchell WE Jr, Colborn GL, Skandalakis JE. Modern Hernia Repair. Pearl River NY: Parthenon, 1996; with permission.)

## *Superficial Perineal Pouch*

The superficial perineal pouch (Fig. 28-51) includes the space between the fascia of Gallaudet and the perineal membrane. It is composed of the following structures (from external to internal), which are discussed below:
- External perineal fascia or muscle fascia of Gallaudet
- Paired muscles of the superficial compartment (Fig. 28-45A)
  - Ischiocavernosus
  - Bulbospongiosus
  - Superficial transverse perineus

- Paired erectile tissue elements
  - Corpora cavernosa penis or clitoris
  - Corpora spongiosa (penile bulb or vestibular bulbs)
- Right and left vestibular (Bartholin) glands in the female (Fig. 28-45B)
- Perineal membrane
- Vasculature
- Nerves

### **External Perineal Fascia of Gallaudet**
The most superficial element in the superficial pouch is the external muscle fascia of Gallaudet. It covers the mus-

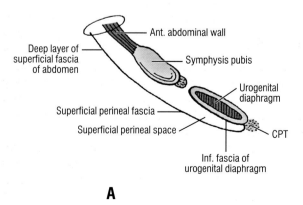

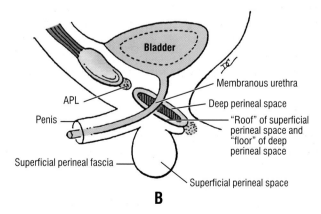

**FIG. 28-51.** Schematic of midline sections showing urogenital diaphragm and perineal spaces (pouches). Shows superficial perineal fascia (Colles' fascia) as continuation of deep or membranous layer (Scarpa's fascia) of superficial fascia of abdomen. CPT, Central perineal tendon (perineal body). APL, Arcuate pubic ligament. (Modified from Moore KL. Clinically Oriented Anatomy (2nd ed). Baltimore: Williams & Wilkins, 1985; with permission.)

cles and, between the erectile tissues, joins the deeper-lying perineal membrane. The fascia of Gallaudet covers the external abdominal oblique muscle (the so-called innominate fascia) and the deep fascia (Buck's fascia) of the penis or clitoris. However, some anatomists believe that the fascia of Buck is not related to the fascia of Gallaudet.

REMEMBER: The membranous fascia of Scarpa of the anterior abdominal wall is renamed Colles' in the perineum. Colles' is superficial fascia. Gallaudet is deep fascia. The fascia of Colles and the fascia of Gallaudet bound the superficial perineal cleft (or space); the (deep) fascia of Gallaudet and the perineal membrane bound the superficial pouch, or superficial perineal compartment. To emphasize: Colles' fascia is superficial fascia in the perineum; Gallaudet is deep, muscular fascia in the perineum.

The suspensory ligament of the penis or clitoris originates from the deep fascia just above and ventral to the symphysis pubis. The suspensory ligament is on the same deep plane as Buck's fascia and the fascia of Gallaudet. The dorsal arteries, nerves, and superficial veins lie deep to Buck's (deep) fascia on the penis or clitoris. The deep dorsal vein is invested by the fascia.

### Muscles of the Superficial Compartment

The following paragraphs discuss the paired muscles of the superficial compartment (Fig. 28-52).

ISCHIOCAVERNOSUS. The paired ischiocavernosus muscles

have an extensive bony origin that begins posteriorly at the anterior part of the ischial tuberosities and continues forward on the ischiopubic ramus. Some fibers arise from the underlying perineal membrane. The ischiocavernosus muscles embrace the crus of each of the corpora cavernosa penis or clitoris at their attachments proximally to the ischiopubic rami. The ischiocavernosus muscles insert upon the tunica albuginea of the proximal parts of the shafts of the corpora, the crus penis or crus clitoris.

The more medially situated muscle fibers of the ischiocavernosus are often difficult to separate from bundles of the bulbospongiosus muscles without artifactual division. Contraction of the ischiocavernosus results in some restriction of venous flow from the corpora cavernosa penis and clitoris that contributes to erection of these elements.

BULBOSPONGIOSUS. The bulbospongiosus muscles (Fig. 28-52) arise from the perineal body and membrane. They are invested externally by the muscle fascia of Gallaudet. They join in the midline of the male penile bulb by fusing along the midline raphe. In the female, they are separated by the pudendal cleft and cover the vestibular bulbs. The insertions of the bulbospongiosus are upon the proximal part of the corpus spongiosum in the male and the ventral extensions of the vestibular bulbs in the female.

In the male, the bulbospongiosus assists in urethral compression, "stripping" it in micturition and ejaculation. Its contraction assists also in restricting venous flow from

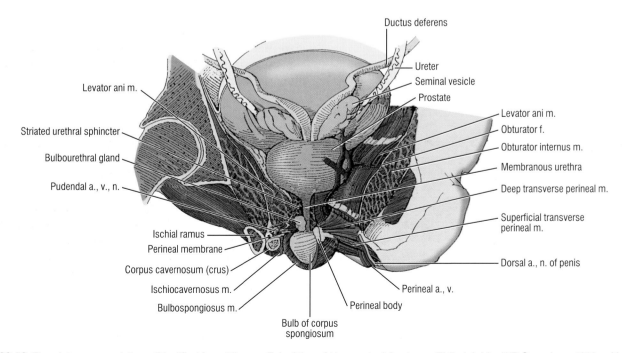

FIG. 28-52. Ejaculatory musculature. (Modified from Hinman F Jr. Atlas of Urosurgical Anatomy. Philadelphia: WB Saunders, 1993; with permission.)

the corpus spongiosum, contributing to the process of erection. In the female, the bulbospongiosus muscles provide an external sphincter for the vaginal introitus.

SUPERFICIAL TRANSVERSE PERINEUS MUSCLES. The superficial transverse perineus muscles (Fig. 28-45A, Fig. 28-52) arise bilaterally from the ischial tuberosities and insert anteromedially into the centrally located perineal body. They thereby interconnect the perineal body and the ischium in a nearly transverse way.

The superficial transverse perineus is occasionally absent. More often, it is simply difficult to define in older individuals, wherein it may be replaced by fibrous tissue. It is more difficult to find in the older female than in the older male. Some of the difficulty in finding this muscle may be due partly to atrophy with the passage of many years. Another contributing cause is that the perineal branches of the pudendal nerve and internal pudendal vessels frequently pass through the muscle, separating it into poorly defined fasciculi of muscle bundles. Tracing the neurovascular elements often destroys these bundles.

The muscle acts to fix the central fibromuscular point of the perineum, presumably assisting in the maintenance of urinary and fecal continence. Its central insertion is perpendicular to that of the external anal sphincter, and can be seen during perineal excision of the anal canal. Its motor supply, like that of other muscles of the superficial pouch, is derived from the perineal branch of the pudendal nerve from S2, S3, and S4.

### Erectile Tissues and Glandular Elements

Because the penis is suspended from the anterior abdominal wall in lower animals, the surface of the human penis which faces forward when in the flaccid state is not truly the ventral surface; it is the dorsal surface, for it becomes dorsal in position when erect.

The corpora of the penis is composed of three bodies of cavernous, erectile tissue.
- Paired corpora cavernosa penis on either side
- Corpus spongiosum medially

CORPORA CAVERNOSA OF THE PENIS AND CLITORIS. The crura (proximal or posterior parts of the corpora cavernosa) of the clitoris and penis arise from the ischial tuberosities and the rami of the ischia. Near the symphysis, the two crura are attached to the pubic bone by deep fascial connections and then bend ventrally, becoming the corpora cavernosa. Thereafter, joined by a midline fibrous septum and surrounded by a common fibrous investment, they form the body of the clitoris in the female. In the male, a ventral groove between the two corpora is occupied by the corpus spongiosum and the contained urethra.

Each corpus cavernosum of the penis or clitoris is surrounded by a tough fibrous tunica albuginea intermingled with a network of elastic fibers. The superficial layer of this tunic is composed of longitudinally oriented fibers, providing a singular tubelike covering for the two corpora. Each corpus has a separate investment of deep, circularly arranged fibers that join at the median septum. This septum completely separates the two crura proximally. Because the septum is perforated distally, the cavernous tissues of the crura communicate very freely here.

Within the corpora, a trabecular meshwork of smooth muscle bundles and a collagenous extracellular matrix receive arterial supply by the helicine branches of the right and left cavernous branches of the internal pudendal arteries (Fig. 28-53). The helicine arteries enter a complex vascular network of sinuses or lacunae lined with endothelial cells. Venules beneath the tunica albuginea provide the venous drainage for the corpora. The venules coalesce to form emissary veins. These pierce the tunic and drain to the deep dorsal vein of the penis or clitoris.[54]

In the flaccid state, the smooth muscle is tonically contracted under sympathetic stimulation and very little arterial flow enters the corpora (4 ml/min/100 g of tissue). Appropriate stimuli and parasympathetic outflow result in vasodilation of the arteries and relaxation of the smooth muscle, with concomitant compression of the peripheral venules against the tunica albuginea. This action provides the basis for erection. Sympathetic stimulation and the release of norepinephrine and other agents cause contraction of the smooth muscle, release of the venous compression, and the return to detumescence and flaccidity. The role played by the so-called polsters or cushions in the vessels of the corpora (described by McConnell et al.[55] and Conti et al.[56]) remains unresolved.

CORPUS SPONGIOSUM. The midline corpus spongiosum of the male (corpus cavernosum urethrae) ends as the expanded glans penis and transmits the penile urethra. The acorn-shaped glans penis forms a cap for the two corpora cavernosa. Its free margin is called the corona of the glans.

The corpus spongiosum, like the corpora cavernosa, is surrounded by a dense fibroelastic, unexpandable covering, the tunica albuginea. This relative inelasticity allows it to become firm when its vascular spaces are perfused with arterial blood at a rate that exceeds the rate of venous drainage. The tunica albuginea of the corpus spongiosum is thinner than that of the corpora cavernosa. The tunica and glans penis are therefore less rigid during erection than the corpora cavernosa. This allows the ejaculate to pass.

MacBride and Blight[57] estimate the tunica albuginea of

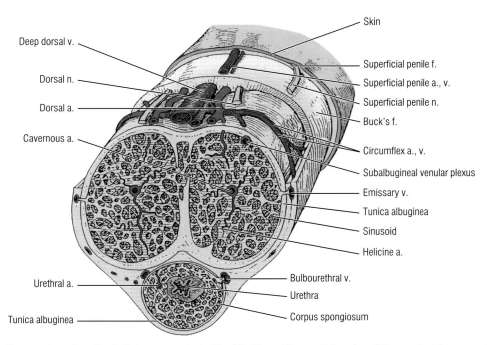

Skin
Superficial penile f.
Superficial penile a., v.
Superficial penile n.
Buck's f.
Circumflex a., v.
Subalbugineal venular plexus
Emissary v.
Tunica albuginea
Sinusoid
Helicine a.
Bulbourethral v.
Urethra
Corpus spongiosum

Deep dorsal v.
Dorsal n.
Dorsal a.
Cavernous a.
Urethral a.
Tunica albuginea

FIG. 28-53. Vasculature and innervation of penile shaft (cross-section). (Modified from Hinman F Jr. Atlas of Urosurgical Anatomy. Philadelphia: WB Saunders, 1993; with permission.)

the corpus cavernosum penis to be about 1.4 mm thick in unembalmed and embalmed cadavers, decreasing in thickness with advancing age unless fibrosis is present. The tunica of the corpus spongiosum, in contrast, is typically only about 0.3 mm thick and exhibits relatively little variation in thickness attributable to aging.

The male corpus spongiosum begins as the expanded penile bulb, formed by the fusion of two anlagen within the superficial perineal pouch. The urethra passes into the penile bulb after traversing the urethral sphincter and perineal membrane (urogenital diaphragm). After a distance of about 2.5 cm, the urethra receives the ducts of the two bulbourethral glands (of Cowper) which reside within the urogenital sphincter muscle. Here, the urethra is also characterized by the presence of the mucosal urethral glands (of Littre). At the distal end of the pendulous portion of the penis, the urethral lumen expands within the glans penis as the fossa navicularis.

The penile urethra is represented by the vestibule of the vagina, retaining the embryologic condition of the urethral groove. The unfused urethral folds on either side of the urethral groove develop into the labia minora. The original embryologic genital swellings of the female are represented by the labia majora. In the male, they form the definitive scrotum. The external meatus of the female urethra opens just above the superior aspect of the vaginal introitus (opening). On either side of the urethral meatus are the openings for the paraurethral (Skene's) glands, the female counterpart of the prostate.

### Vestibular (Bartholin) Glands

In the female, the two anlagen that fuse to form the penile bulb are represented by the two vestibular bulbs. These bulbs fuse anteriorly to form the threadlike commissure of the clitoris and expand distally as the glans clitoris. The greater vestibular glands lie within the superficial pouch, deep to the proximal ends of the vestibular bulbs and on either side of the vaginal introitus (Fig. 28-45B). The greater vestibular glands are better known as Bartholin's glands. They are small, somewhat ovoid glands whose secretory products include both lubricating and endocrine elements. According to Fettisoff et al.[58] (as cited in Gray's Anatomy[59]), the endocrine elements secreted by the glands include serotonin, calcitonin, bombesin, hCG, and katacalcin. The ducts of these mucous secreting glands open at about the 5 o'clock and 7 o'clock positions relative to the vaginal introitus, between the hymen and the labia minora.

The penile bulb and vestibular bulbs are covered by the bulbospongiosus muscle. In the female, the medial fascicles of the bilateral muscles attach to the deep fascia of the dorsum of the clitoris. The lateral fascicles attach to the perineal membrane.

## Perineal Membrane

The perineal membrane (Fig. 28-51) provides a "roof" for the superficial pouch and a "floor" for the deep pouch (urogenital diaphragm). For all practical purposes, the perineal membrane is the inferior fascia of the urogenital diaphragm. We agree with Last,[8] however, that in most cases the portion of the perineal membrane that is related to the under surface of the pelvic diaphragm (levator ani muscles) is actually areolar tissue, and that "no definitely formed membrane exists" there. Therefore a rigid description of the geographic territory of the deep perineal pouch and its contents is difficult. For a better understanding of this complicated area of the human body and for better knowledge of the contents of the deep perineal pouch we consider the perineal membrane to be present on the under surface of the levator ani muscles, thus forming a complete envelope together with its inferior layer.

## Vasculature

The vasculature of the superficial perineal pouch consists of the following:
- Posterior scrotal/labial branches of the perineal branch of the internal pudendal vessels
- Transverse perineal branch of the perineal branch of the internal pudendal artery (supplying the superficial transverse perineus muscle and tissue between the bulb and the anus)
- Also, the following arteries which enter the superficial pouch by piercing the perineal membrane, after arising from the internal pudendal artery in the deep pouch:
  – Artery of the bulb
  – Artery of the urethra
  – Deep artery of the penis or clitoris

## Nerves

The following are the nerves of the superficial perineal pouch:
- Perineal branches of the pudendal nerves:
  – Cutaneous branches (posterior scrotal/labial nerves)
  – Muscular branches (transverse perineal nerves)
- Perineal branches of the posterior femoral cutaneous nerve of the thigh

## *Urogenital Diaphragm (Deep Pouch or Compartment)*

The urogenital diaphragm is a fibromuscular layer between the pelvic floor (levator ani muscles) limited inferiorly by the perineal membrane.

## Support Function of the Deep Pouch

The ventral position of the structures within the urogenital diaphragm (Fig. 28-35) participates also in the separation of the perineum from the pelvis. This position provides an anterior support for the viscera located above the defect of the pelvic diaphragm (urogenital hiatus) between the right and left pubococcygeus muscles of the pelvic floor (Fig. 28-54). Thus, the pelvic viscera are protected and supported both by internal structures (endopelvic fascia, visceral ligaments, and levator ani and its fasciae) and external structures (urogenital diaphragm and elements of the superficial perineal compartment).

## Urogenital Diaphragm Reexamined

The term "urogenital diaphragm" is sometimes used as a synonym for the perineal membrane or triangular ligament. Most anatomic and clinical sources state that the urogenital diaphragm is composed of two connective tissue layers, the superior and inferior fasciae.

The superior layer of fascia and inferior layer of fascia (the perineal membrane, Fig. 28-45C) enclose the deep perineal compartment or pouch containing two muscles and, in the male, bulbourethral (Cowper's) glands (Fig. 28-45D). The "sandwich" formed by these two layers of fascia and the contents of the deep space (pouch) comprises the urogenital diaphragm (Fig. 28-45C, D).

Superficial (membranous layer) and deep perineal fascia attach to the ischiopubic ramus and to the posterior margin of the urogenital diaphragm and enclose the superficial perineal compartment (pouch). This area is a complex mixture of striated and smooth muscle structures arranged between the two roughly horizontal fascial laminae.

The superior and inferior fascial layers ostensibly join each other posteriorly. They provide a transversely oriented "touchdown" line for merging with the muscle fascia of Gallaudet of the superficial pouch and with the fascia of Colles. This effectively closes the superficial perineal pouch and superficial perineal cleft simultaneously.

Anteriorly, the perineal membrane and the superior layer of the diaphragm fuse into a flat, tough band of tissue, the transverse perineal ligament. The superior fascial layer, according to most contemporary sources, separates the prostate gland from the sphincter urethrae muscle and fuses medially with the inferior fascial layer of the pelvic diaphragm.

Convincing studies by Oelrich[41,50,51] cast doubt upon the existence of a superior layer of fascia of the urogenital diaphragm, at least as typically described. According to Oelrich, in the male the sphincter urethrae muscle continues superiorly through and around the substance of the prostate gland to the urinary bladder. Likewise, the same basic muscle in females continues upward from a common urethrovaginal sphincter to the sphincter urethrae and then to the bladder (Fig. 28-49C).

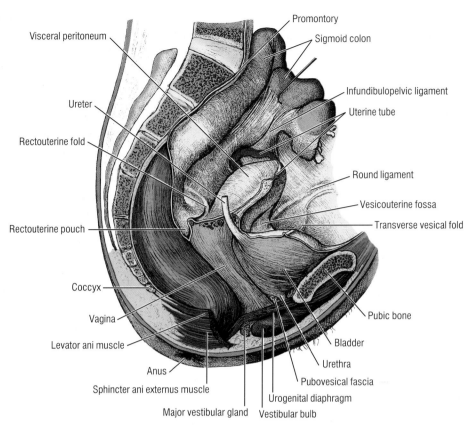

Visceral peritoneum

Ureter

Rectouterine fold

Rectouterine pouch

Coccyx

Vagina

Levator ani muscle

Anus

Sphincter ani externus muscle

Major vestibular gland

Promontory

Sigmoid colon

Infundibulopelvic ligament

Uterine tube

Round ligament

Vesicouterine fossa

Transverse vesical fold

Pubic bone

Bladder

Urethra

Pubovesical fascia

Urogenital diaphragm

Vestibular bulb

**FIG. 28-54.** Pelvic supporting structures. The urogenital diaphragm, together with endopelvic fascia and the levator ani, provides anterior support for urogenital organs. (Modified from Toldt C, Hochstetter F. Anatomischer Atlas. Munich: Urban & Schwarzenberg, 1976; with permission.)

Because the pubococcygeus muscle of the levator ani inserts in part into the lateral walls of the vagina and also into the perineal body, the urogenital hiatus of the female seals laterally. Therefore, the hiatus principally transmits endopelvic fascia, the urethra, and its sphincter. These structures also attach ventrally to the lower part of the pubic bone by the pubovesical and pubourethral ligaments, thereby assisting in closure of the urogenital hiatus.

According to Oelrich, the superior fascia of the pelvic diaphragm is the fascial layer passing through the hiatus and blending with the perineal membrane.[50] The term "urethrovaginal compartment," as he suggests, might be a more accurate name than urogenital diaphragm in the female.[51] Unfortunately, he did not offer an alternative name for the male. Perhaps "urethrogenital compartment" might be more accurate for both genders. Without adding further to the confusion of nomenclature, we will hereafter use this name or "deep compartment" or "deep pouch" to designate this rather irregularly shaped complex of muscle and connective tissue.

The findings of Strasser et al.[60] appear to agree essentially with Oelrich.[50] They observe that the sphincter urethrae muscle of the male extends inferiorly from the bladder to the penile bulb without interruption. As the sphincter urethrae continues inferiorly from the bladder it surrounds the prostate gland, contributing to the prostatic sheath. The prostate develops within the sphincter urethrae embryologycally, and its enlargement thereafter thins the surrounding portion of the sphincter urethrae.

Strasser et al.[60] further noted that the fibers of the most inferior part of the sphincter urethrae muscles are arranged omegalike about the anterior and lateral aspects of the urethra, inserting posteriorly into the perineal body. Like Oelrich,[50] they asserted that the "urogenital diaphragm," as usually described, does not exist.

### Urethral Sphincter Complex

Delancey[61] agreed with Oelrich[50,51] that the most proximal part of the striated urethral sphincter is circularly oriented and surrounds the smooth muscle of the wall of the urethra. Distally, these striated fibers lie within the deep pouch. Some encircle the urethra and vagina together, forming a combined urethral and vaginal sphincter. Others exit laterally and attach at the pubic rami and also, presumably, to the perineal membrane, as the compressor urethrae. Near the vesical neck, fibrous tissue and smooth muscle fibers from the vagina and urethra run anteriorly to attach to the pelvic wall, forming the pubourethral ligament.

A second group of connective tissue and smooth muscle fibers (known as the fibers of Luschka) connect the paraurethral sulci of the vaginal wall to the pubococcygeus muscle. Delancey called this the vaginolevator attachment.[61] Above this, the vaginal wall is attached to the levator by means of the arcus tendineus fascia pelvis.

### Fasciae

**SUPERIOR FASCIA OF THE UROGENITAL DIAPHRAGM.** In the male, the periprostatic sheath covers the prostatic capsule and its venous plexus (Fig. 28-55). Krongrad and Droller[62] report that the periprostatic sheath is composed of a coalescence of pelvic fascia and aponeurotic tissue. This tissue anchors the prostate to the sheath of the bladder above, the urogenital diaphragm inferiorly, the levator ani laterally, and the rectovesical fascia posteriorly. Further, it attaches to the pubis anteriorly by the puboprostatic ligaments.

Analyzing the pertinent literature and comparing it with our own observations, we agree with Oelrich[50,51] that the fascial complex in the male forms the superior and circumferential border of the deep pouch, a rather conical musculofascial compartment. The connective tissue attaches to the perineal membrane inferiorly. This construct is very dissimilar to the concept of a simple, flat, horizontal, roughly triangular "urogenital diaphragm." According to Krongrad and Droller,[62] the anterior periprostatic fascia (puboprostatic fascia of Denonvilliers, fascia of Zuckerkandl or Delbet) extends to the lower border of the pubic bone, where it covers the venous plexus of Santorini.

The superior fascia of the deep pouch, or urethrogenital

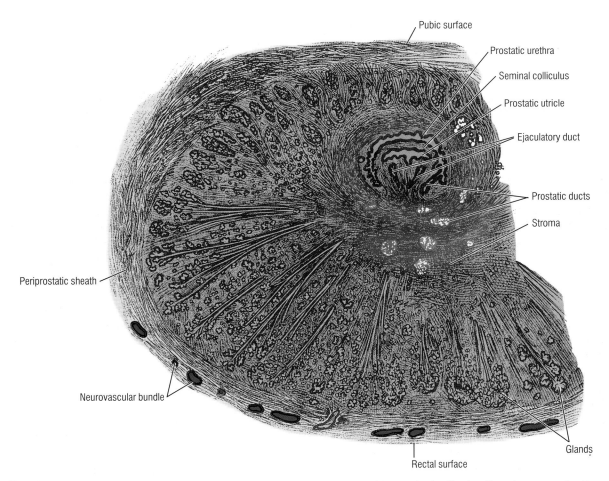

**FIG. 28-55.** Transverse section of the prostate gland and urethra, at the level of the seminal colliculus. Note the connective tissue capsule of the gland. (Modified from Toldt C, Hochstetter F. Anatomischer Atlas. Munich: Urban & Schwarzenberg, 1976; with permission.)

compartment, is difficult to demonstrate. There is great complexity in its interrelationships and coalescence with the superior and inferior fasciae of the pelvic diaphragm, pubovesical and vaginal fascia, and the prostatic fascial capsule. In the male, the superior fascia of the deep pouch clearly does not form a complete barrier between the musculature of the deep pouch and the muscle fibers of the prostate gland and prostatic urethra, as commonly supposed.

The superior layer of fascia of the pelvic diaphragm and the perineal membrane fuse together anteriorly without the intervention of muscle fibers. They form a tough fibrous band called the transverse perineal ligament. This effectively closes the deep pouch a short distance beneath the pubic arch and pubic arcuate ligament.

The dorsal nerves and arteries of the penis (clitoris) pierce the transverse perineal ligament as they leave the deep pouch to reach the dorsum of the penis (clitoris). The deep dorsal penile or clitoral vein passes between the transverse perineal ligament and the pubic arcuate ligament to enter the pelvic venous plexus. This space transmits a single or bilateral accessory pudendal artery in about 10%[11] of individuals, a vessel which may provide the dorsal artery and/or deep artery of the penis (clitoris).

**INFERIOR FASCIA OF THE DEEP POUCH.** The inferior fascia of the deep pouch is more highly organized and distinct than the superior layer. It is located between the two sides of the pubic arch and is known as the perineal membrane. Some refer to this tough layer of connective tissue as the urogenital diaphragm. It is also called the "triangular ligament," although its configuration is more trapezoidal than triangular. In light of the foregoing discussion, we might accept the term "urogenital diaphragm" as an alternative name for the perineal membrane.

The deep fascia on the inferior or superficial surface of the urogenital diaphragm is thickened to form the dense perineal membrane. It is continuous with the deep layer of fascia anteriorly and posteriorly. The perineal membrane is pierced by the urethra; in the female, the vagina also pierces this membrane.

The perineal membrane provides a "roof" for the superficial perineal pouch and a substructural basis for attachment of erectile tissue elements and muscles of that pouch. In addition, the perineal membrane acts as the "floor" for the deep pouch and its musculature.

## Muscles of the Deep Compartment

The muscles contributing to the urogenital diaphragm, as described in former years, included only two rather simply described muscles. These were the paired deep transversus perineus muscles and the sphincter urethrae. The terminology and form of these muscles were assiduously memorized by generations of obstetricians/ gynecologists, surgeons, and anatomists and many, many medical students. All pretended to see, or imagined that they saw, the structures depicted in the simple two-dimensional diagrams copied from one book to the next.

Studies including those by Krantz,[63] Oelrich,[50,51] and Tichy[42] introduced additional terminology and important concepts regarding structure and function in describing the musculature of the "urogenital diaphragm."

The muscles of the diaphragm or deep pouch are listed here and discussed below. The descriptions of muscles of the deep pouch in the female (Fig. 28-49) are drawn from the work of Oelrich.[51]

- Deep transversus perineus
- Sphincter urethrae
- Compressor urethrae (female)
- Sphincter urethrovaginalis (female)
- Transversus vaginalis (female)

**DEEP TRANSVERSUS PERINEUS MUSCLE.** Behind or dorsal to the distal part of the sphincter urethrae is the deep transversus perineus muscle of the perineum. This muscle's fibers arise from the fascia of the pudendal canal. The fibers intermingle with those of the sphincter urethrae, external anal sphincter, and smooth muscle of the rectourethral muscle at the site of the perineal body in the midline.[50]

**SPHINCTER URETHRAE.** Inferior to the prostate in the urogenital hiatus, the fibers of the sphincter urethrae are more or less circumferential (omegalike). Below the pelvic diaphragm, the sphincter expands to fill the interval between the pudendal canals. Laterally and ventrally the sphincter is associated with the rich, prostatic venous plexus and bears a resemblance to cavernous tissue. Thus, the distinctive form of the muscle is lost.

**COMPRESSOR URETHRAE.** The compressor urethrae muscle arises laterally as a slender tendon near the anterior border of the ischial tuberosity. It expands as a band about 6 mm wide as it reaches the urethra and becomes continuous with the muscle of the opposite side. Its most ventral and superior edge lies within the urogenital hiatus, where it is continuous with the lower fibers of the urethral sphincter behind the pubic symphysis. Some of its deeper fibers attach to the lateral aspect of the urethra.

**SPHINCTER URETHROVAGINALIS.** The sphincter urethrovaginalis is a thin, flat muscle about 5 mm wide that surrounds both the vagina and the urethra. Its fibers are continuous across the midline behind the vagina and continuous with the compressor urethrae ventrally. None of its fibers pass between the urethra and vagina.

**TRANSVERSUS VAGINALIS.** Some striated fibers pass medially as a fan-shaped muscle from the vicinity of the compressor urethrae to insert into the anterior half of the lateral wall of the vagina, superior to the level of the urethrovaginalis. The more posterior of these fibers could perhaps represent the deep transversus perineus muscle, although Oelrich[51] denies the presence of this muscle in the female.

### Membranous Urethra

By "membranous urethra" we mean that part of the urethra just superior to the perineal membrane or passing through it. Why have we called this 1 cm long, thin walled part of the urethra "membranous?" It is surrounded by muscle. This name is even more questionable in light of our foregoing observations about the superior fascial layer. For the part that traverses the corpus spongiosum, we use the term "spongy." The part that traverses the prostate gland, we term "prostatic." However, for the part within the deep compartment or urethrogenital diaphragm, we use the term "membranous." Logically, it should be called the "muscular" part as proposed by Waldeyer and reported by Mermigas.[64] We do not want to muddy the water further and, therefore, will continue to refer to this area as "membranous." (See the section on the male urethra in the chapter on the male genital system; and see the section on the female urethra in the chapter on the female genital system.)

The fibers of the sphincter urethrae form a sphincter for the membranous portion of the urethra in the urogenital hiatus, inferior to the prostate. The sphincter urethrae muscle provides no covering where the urethra penetrates the perineal membrane and angulates ventrally. This portion of the urethra is termed the "bare area"[65] or "pars nuda."

The bare area is incompletely supported by the corpus spongiosum.[66] Therefore, one should be cautious when using rigid urethral instruments in this area as the urethra is easily injured here.

### Internal Pudendal Vessels

The internal pudendal artery arises from the anterior division of the internal iliac artery (Fig. 28-8), either within the pelvis or after the anterior division passes through the greater sciatic foramen. Thereafter the internal iliac artery also provides origin for the inferior gluteal artery.

The course of the internal pudendal artery and its vein(s) (Fig. 28-10) after entering the pudendal canal is essentially identical to that of the pudendal nerve. The differences between the nerve and vessels occur chiefly within the urethrogenital compartment. Here, the internal puden-

dal artery sends bulbar, urethral, and deep crural branches before ending as the dorsal artery of the clitoris/penis.

The perineal membrane, visceral fascia, and the fascia of the levator ani collectively form the envelope of the "urogenital diaphragm," or urethrogenital compartment of the pelvic floor.

### Pudendal Nerve

The pudendal nerve is formed from contributions from the ventral primary rami of S2, S3, and S4 (Fig. 28-22). The nerve or its contributors leave the greater sciatic foramen in a position medial to the internal pudendal artery and vein. They then cross the sacrospinous ligament near the tip of the spine of the ischium, and pass through the lesser sciatic foramen. The pudendal nerve may receive a contribution from S4 as it passes through the coccygeus muscle (the perineal branch of the nerve to the levator ani). Passing between the underlying sacrospinous ligament and the overlying sacrotuberous ligament and gluteus maximus muscle, the nerve enters the pudendal canal of Alcock (Fig. 28-3) in the lateral wall of the ischioanal fossa.

The walls of the pudendal canal begin as extensions of ligamentous and other connective tissue from the anterolateral edge of the sacrotuberous ligament as it passes to attach on the ischial tuberosity (Fig. 28-56). The fibers from the sacrotuberous ligament that attach to the inner surface of the ischial ramus and contribute to the canal are called the falciform ligament. Thereafter, the fascial investment from the muscle fascia of the obturator internus muscle covers the nerve and accompanying internal pudendal vessels.

The pudendal nerve has three major branches: the inferior rectal nerve, the perineal nerve, and the dorsal nerve of the penis or clitoris. These branches are discussed below. NOTE: The branches may have already separated prior to entrance into the pudendal canal.

The first branch of the pudendal nerve, the inferior rectal nerve(s), originates as the pudendal nerve enters the pudendal canal. The inferior rectal nerve passes anteromedially through the fat of the ischioanal fossa. Here it reaches and supplies the levator ani (in part), the lining of the distal part of the anal canal, the external anal sphincter musculature, and the overlying subcutaneous tissue and skin.

Branches of the inferior rectal nerve are interconnected with the perineal branch of the posterior femoral cutaneous and posterior scrotal/labial nerves. The perineal branch of the ventral primary ramus of S4 may pierce the coccygeus and supply the skin between the anus and the coccyx. Somewhat further forward, the pudendal nerve divides into a perineal branch and the dorsal nerve of the penis or clitoris.

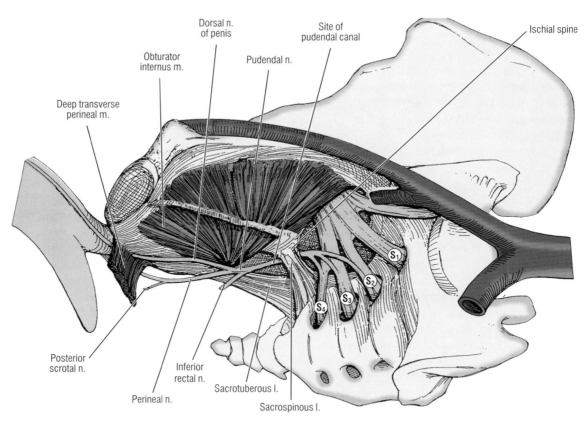

FIG. 28-56. Site of pudendal canal. (Modified from Hinman F Jr. Atlas of Urosurgical Anatomy. Philadelphia: WB Saunders, 1993; with permission.)

NOTE: In some individuals, the perineal branch of the posterior femoral cutaneous nerve figures prominently in the sensory supply of the perineum and requires selective treatment to gain adequate anesthesia of the perineum.

The perineal branch of the pudendal nerve pierces the obturator fascial wall of the pudendal canal somewhat posterior to the urogenital triangle. It frequently passes through the perineal membrane, and then the substance of the superficial transverse perineus muscle (or the cutaneous and transverse branches may pass through it separately).

The medial and lateral cutaneous branches of the perineal nerve are named either posterior labial or posterior scrotal. These branches pass through the superficial perineal cleft and Colles' membranous fascia to reach the skin.

The transverse motor branch of the perineal nerve divides into several rami to supply the musculature of the superficial and deep pouches and assist in supplying the external anal sphincter and levator ani. The branch of the perineal nerve supplying the bulbospongiosus also provides a branch to the bulb of the urethra, supplying the corpus spongiosum and urethral mucosa.[59]

The dorsal nerve of the penis or clitoris, the terminal portion of the pudendal nerve, continues forward in the pudendal canal. Its course follows the lateral aspect of the urethrogenital compartment (urogenital diaphragm) in a channel characterized by trabeculated connective tissues and muscle fibers and intermingled with highly vascular tissue.

The dorsal nerve emerges from the anterior edge of the urethrogenital compartment by piercing the transverse perineal ligament. This is the tough band of tissue formed by the coalescence of the perineal membrane inferiorly and the fascia associated with the sphincter urethrae muscle superiorly. Initially, the nerve lies deep to the suspensory ligamentous tissue of the clitoris or penis and then extends to the deep fascia of the penis or clitoris. Twigs penetrate the deep fascia to supply the superficial fascia and skin (Fig. 28-57).

### Contents of Deep Compartment Summarized

- Two bulbourethral glands (of Cowper). These pea-sized glands are located on each side of the urethra within the male urogenital diaphragm. They drain into the spongy urethra.

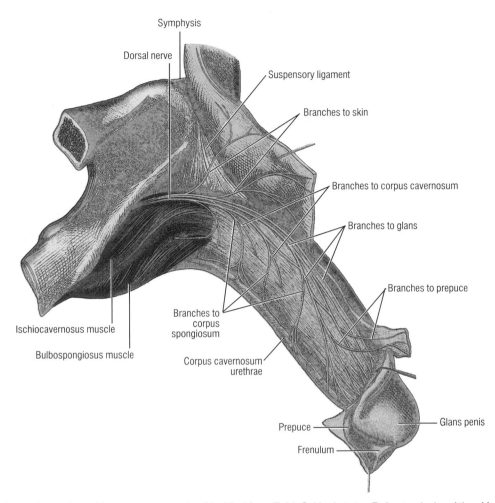

FIG. 28-57. Nerve distribution to the penis and its component parts. (Modified from Toldt C, Hochstetter F. Anatomischer Atlas. Munich: Urban & Schwarzenberg, 1976; with permission.)

- Blood vessels, ducts, and nerves (bilateral):
  - Internal pudendal artery and vein
  - Artery of the urethral bulb
  - Nerves of urethral bulb and urethra
  - Deep artery of the crus
  - Dorsal artery of the penis or clitoris
  - Deep dorsal vein of penis or clitoris (singular, midline)
  - Plexus of veins
  - Duct of bulbourethral gland
  - Dorsal nerve of penis or clitoris
- In the female, the inferior vertical portion of the vagina is considered to be contained within the urogenital diaphragm (urethrogenital compartment).

  NOTE: The main artery of the deep pouch is the continuation of the internal pudendal artery. Within the diaphragm, the internal pudendal artery gives origin to the artery of the bulb and the artery of the urethra. It then terminates by dividing into the deep artery and dorsal artery

of the penis or clitoris. The deep (motor or transverse) branch of the perineal nerve is the source of the nerve supply of the musculature within the urethrogenital pouch.

## Anal Triangle

The structure and function of the anal canal and the external anal sphincteric musculature are described in the chapter on the anorectum.

### Boundaries

The base of the anal triangle is bounded anteriorly by the transverse line through the two ischial tuberosities. In a more practical sense, the superficial transverse perineus muscle, the posterior edge of the deep compartment, and the anterior extremity of the perineal body delineate the anal triangle from the urogenital triangle. Posterolaterally, the sacrotuberous ligaments and the inferior borders of the gluteus maximus muscle provide the sides of the triangle. The coccyx creates the apex of the triangle.

### Ischioanal (Ischiorectal) Fossae

The midline raphe and anus divide the anal triangle into two smaller triangles that form the bases of the two ischioanal fossae (formerly, ischiorectal fossae). Each ischioanal fossa is pyramid-shaped. The apex points superiorly between the levator ani and obturator internus muscles (Fig. 28-3). The base of the pyramid faces inferiorly and is formed by fibrofatty tissue and overlying skin. Each fossa is filled with fat. The inferior rectal nerves and vessels pass through this fat toward the midline structures, including the superficial and deep parts of the external anal sphincter.

When tensed, the overlying gluteus maximus muscles push against the fatty tissue, compressing the fat of the ischioanal fossae and performing a role in maintaining fecal continence. When the muscles are relaxed, the softness of the adipose tissue allows dilation of the anal canal during defecation.

The two ischioanal fossae continue behind the anus, between the levator ani (levator plate and puborectalis) and the anococcygeal ligament (Fig. 28-37B). The anococcygeal ligament is an indistinct band of fibrofatty tissue. It contains mingled extensions of the superficial portion of the external sphincter ani as it passes from the circumanal region to the lower parts of the coccyx.

Each ischioanal fossa has an anterior extension beneath the posterior part of the deep compartment of the urogenital triangle, called the anterior recess, into which infections can spread. Similar posterior recesses extend posterolaterally beneath the sacrotuberous ligaments and the anococcygeal ligament. Abscesses in the ischioanal fossa can become quite large and extend from one fossa to the contralateral side, forming the so-called "horseshoe" abscess beneath the anococcygeus muscle and ligament.

### Blood Supply of the Anal Triangle

The inferior rectal artery is a branch of the internal pudendal artery (Fig. 28-16). The inferior rectal veins are tributaries to the internal pudendal vein.

### Innervation of the Anal Triangle

The anal triangle (see Fig. 28-28A&B) receives its neural and vascular supply by way of the inferior rectal nerves and vessels. The inferior rectal nerve arises from the pudendal nerve in the pudendal canal. After piercing the fascia of the obturator internus, the nerve passes anteromedially through the fatty tissue of the ischioanal fossa. Its path reaches the external anal sphincter and levator ani muscles and the mucosa of the lower part of the anal canal below the mucocutaneous junction. Cutaneous branches pass more superficially to reach the anal skin. Loss of the external sphincter following pudendal nerve injury will cause some degree of fecal incontinence.

## SURGICAL CONSIDERATIONS

- Grant and Basmajian[67] stated that the only nerve serving the perineal area is the pudendal nerve and the only artery is the internal pudendal artery. The urinary bladder and anorectum have a common nerve supply, the hypogastric plexus and pelvic splanchnic nerves. Some writers speculate that the latter fact is the reason that, after transurethral prostatectomy, many men have bladder spasms that they perceive as an urge to move their bowels.

- Pudendal nerve compression is a clinical entity that may result in chronic pain, physical disability, and severe emotional distress to the affected patient. Compression of the nerve, presumably in its perineal course, can result in pain variously localized in the perineal region; pain that can be exacerbated by standing, sexual activity, and defecation, in particular. Various invasive surgical procedures have been attempted to relieve suspected compression of, or tension upon, the nerve. These include division of the sacrospinous ligament (and, in some cases, the sacrotuberous ligament also) and dissecting the nerve free from presumably restricting tissues in its passage through the pudendal canal. Thus far, such procedures have met with limited success and debatable results in most cases.

- Based on cadaveric studies, O'Bichere et al.[68] recommend a surgical approach to the pudendal nerve that combines review of surface landmarks for anomalies with exposure of the gluteus maximus muscle, sacrotuberous ligament, and pudendal neurovascular bundle.

- The glands of the anal canal are prone to infection. This can result in the formation of fistulous tracts to the skin or localized abscesses in the ischioanal fossae.

- The rich anastomoses between the portal venous system and the systemic system can increase portal pressure. A reversal of flow within the superior rectal vein can cause dilation of submucosal tributaries to the middle rectal and inferior rectal veins and lead to hemorrhoidal varices.

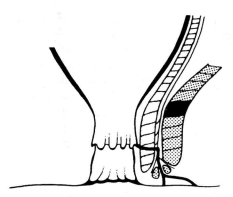

FIG. 28-58. Intersphincteric fistula. (From Parks AG, Thomson JPS. Abscess and fistula. In: Thompson JPS, Nicholls RJ, Williams CR (eds). Colorectal Disease. New York: Appleton-Century-Croft, 1981; with permission.)

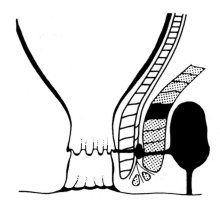

FIG. 28-60. Transsphincteric fistula. (From Parks AG, Thomson JPS. Abscess and fistula. In: Thompson JPS, Nicholls RJ, Williams CR (eds). Colorectal Disease. New York: Appleton-Century-Croft, 1981; with permission.)

- Hemorrhoids above the pectinate line are called internal hemorrhoids. Because sensory fibers from this region are carried by pelvic splanchnic nerves, and because most of the sensory receptors are sensitive only to pressure, sensation from internal hemorrhoids is poorly perceived and poorly localized. Thus, such hemorrhoids can be large and dangerous, resulting even in anemia from loss of blood.
- Hemorrhoids below the pectinate line are called external hemorrhoids. External hemorrhoids produce pain and other disagreeable sensations which are perceived acutely and localized with considerable precision.
- There are four anatomic types of rectal fistulas: inter-sphincteric, transsphincteric, suprasphincteric, and extra-sphincteric.[69]
    - Intersphincteric fistulas are the most common (70%).

The usual pathway is to the anal margin (Fig. 28-58); a subcutaneous tract is possible. Occasionally, the pathway is upward into the rectal wall and into the rectal ampulla (Fig. 28-59).
- Transsphincteric fistulas account for approximately 25 percent of rectal fistulas (Fig. 28-60). This fistula extends through the external sphincter to the ischioanal fossa and the skin.
- Suprasphincteric fistulas comprise about 4 percent of all rectal fistulas (Fig. 28-61). Their pathway is peculiarly convoluted upward into the intersphincteric space, over the puborectalis muscle, and downward into the ischioanal fossa to the skin.
- Extrasphincteric fistulas (Fig. 28-62) constitute only 1 percent of rectal fistulas. The pathway is from the perineal skin to the ischioanal fossa, through the levator

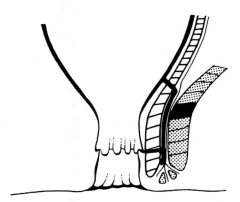

FIG. 28-59. Intersphincteric fistula with opening into rectum. (From Parks AG, Thomson JPS. Abscess and fistula. In: Thompson JPS, Nicholls RJ, Williams CR (eds). Colorectal Disease. New York: Appleton-Century-Croft, 1981; with permission.)

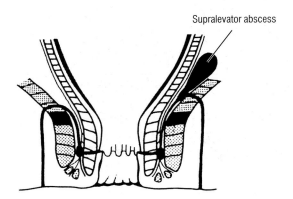

Supralevator abscess

FIG. 28-61. Suprasphincteric fistula. (From Parks AG, Thomson JPS. Abscess and fistula. In: Thompson JPS, Nicholls RJ, Williams CR (eds). Colorectal Disease. New York: Appleton-Century-Croft, 1981; with permission.)

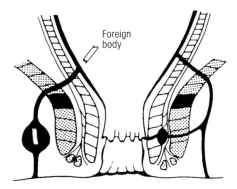

**FIG. 28-62.** Extrasphincteric fistulas. *Left,* Follows perforation of rectum due to foreign body. *Right,* Follows upward extension into rectum from ischioanal (ischiorectal) fossa, perhaps a result of injudicious use of fistula probe. (From Parks AG, Thomson JPS. Abscess and fistula. In: Thompson JPS, Nicholls RJ, Williams CR (eds). Colorectal Disease. New York: Appleton-Century-Croft, 1981; with permission.)

ani, and to the rectal wall.

- Rectal fistulas may also be divided into the following two types:
  - Anorectal, involving only the perianal tissues
  - Ischioanal, passing through the ischioanal space, often in a complicated course
- Goodsall-Salmon's rule of fistulas[70] (Fig. 28-63), which relates the internal location of the fistula to its external opening, must be learned:
  - If the external opening of the fistula is anterior to an imaginary transverse line across the anus, most likely the tract of the fistula is a straight line terminating into the anal canal.

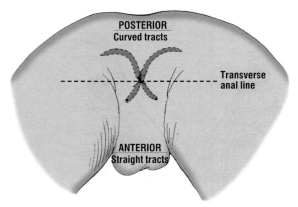

**FIG. 28-63.** Rectal fistulas. Tracts illustrate Goodsall-Salmon's rule (see text). (Modified from Imbembo AL, Zuidema GD. Anal canal and rectum. In: Nardi GL, Zuidema GD (eds). Surgery: Essentials of Clinical Practice (4th ed). Boston: Little, Brown, 1982, pp. 579-580; with permission.)

- If this external opening is located more than 3 cm anterior to the line, the tract may curve posteriorly, terminating in the posterior midline.
- In an opening posterior to the transverse line, the tract will most likely curve, terminating into the posterior wall of the anal canal.
- The subcutaneous and the superficial external sphincters of the anal canal can be divided with impunity. One must exercise care when exploring the deep external sphincter and the puborectalis.
- If fistulas requiring excision develop, they will be near the anal verge. If a fistula is deep, the seton procedure is the treatment of choice. If the fistula is simple and not deep, the fistulous tract can be completely excised, leaving the wound open.
- Most fistulas in ano are midline posterior.
- Episiotomy can be accomplished by a posterior midline incision. Incise the posterior vaginal wall, skin of the perineum, perineal body, and superficial external ani sphincter. According to Signorello et al.,[71] midline episiotomy is not effective in protecting the perineum and sphincters during childbirth and may impair anal continence. A posterolateral incision will incise the vaginal wall, skin of the ischioanal fossa, bulbospongiosus muscle, vestibular bulb, superficial transverse perineus muscle, posterior edge of the urogenital diaphragm, and perhaps the pubococcygeus muscle. If careful repair of all anatomic entities involved is not carried out, then a degree of relaxation of the perineal floor and rectocele or cystocele, or both, may develop.

## ANATOMIC COMPLICATIONS

The anatomic complications of the perineum are the complications of surgery of the several anatomic entities that are related to the perineum.

## REFERENCES

1. Galen. On the Usefulness of the Parts of the Body, Vol. II (May MT, translator). New York: Cornell University Press, 1996, p. 649.
2. Stromberg MW, Williams DJ. The misrepresentation of the human pelvis. J Biocommun 1993;20:14-28.
3. Whorwell PJ, Lupton EW, Erduran D, Wilson K. Bladder smooth muscle dysfunction in patients with irritable bowel syndrome. Gut 1986;27:1014-1017.
4. Wall LL, DeLancey JOL. The politics of prolapse: a revisionist approach to disorders of the pelvic floor in women. Perspect Biol Med 1991;34:486-496.

5. Uhlenhuth E, Day EC, Smith RD, Middleton EB. The visceral endopelvic fascia and the hypogastric sheath. Surg Gynecol Obstet 1948;86:9-28.

6. Sugaya K, Miyazato T, Koyama Y, Hatano T, Ogawa Y. Pelvic congestion syndrome caused by inferior vena cava reflux. Int J Urol 2000;7:157-159.

7. Wohlgemuth WA, Weber H, Loeprecht H, Tietze W, Bohndorf K. PTA and stenting of benign venous stenoses in the pelvis: long-term results. Cardiovasc Intervent Radiol 2000;23:9-16.

8. Last RJ. Anatomy: Regional and Applied (5th ed). Baltimore: Williams & Wilkins, 1972.

9. Gilroy AM, Hermey DC, DiBenedetto LM, Marks SC Jr, Page DW, Lei QF. Variability of the obturator vessels. Clin Anat 10(5):328-332, 1997.

10. Colborn GL, Skandalakis JE. Laparoscopic cadaveric anatomy of the inguinal area. Probl Gen Surg 1995;12:13-20.

11. Lipshutz B. A composite study of the hypogastric artery and its branches. Ann Surg 67:584-608, 1918.

12. Killackey MA. Avoidance of female genital tract complications in relation to pelvic surgery for cancer. Semin Surg Oncol 2000;18:229-234.

13. Last RJ. Anatomy: Regional and Applied (7th ed). Edinburgh: Churchill Livingstone, 1984.

14. Muntean V. The surgical anatomy of the fasciae and the fascial spaces related to the rectum. Surg Radiol Anat 21:319-324, 1999.

15. Davies WD. Abdominal and pelvic fascias with surgical applications. Surg Gynecol Obstet 1935;54:495-504.

16. McGregor AL, DuPlessis DJ. A Synopsis of Surgical Anatomy (10th ed). Baltimore: Williams & Wilkins, 1969.

17. Foshager MC, Walsh JW. CT anatomy of the female pelvis: a second look. Radiographics 1994;14:51-64; discussion 64-66.

18. Pozzi MR, Shariat RI. Anatomic characteristics of pelvic fascia and ligaments in computerized tomography [Italian]. Radiol Med 1994;88:458-464.

19. Pozzi MR, Shariat RI. Pelvic fascia, ligaments, and spaces in neoplastic disease in computerized tomography [Italian]. Radiol Med 1994;88:465-471.

20. Fritsch H, Hötzinger H. Tomographical anatomy of the pelvis, visceral pelvic connective tissue, and its compartments. Clin Anat 1995;8:17-24.

21. Havenga K, Maas CP, DeRuiter MC, Welvaart K, Trimbos JB. Avoiding long-term disturbance to bladder and sexual function in pelvic surgery, particularly with rectal cancer. Semin Surg Oncol 2000;18:235-243.

22. Church JM, Raudkivi PJ, Hill GL. The surgical anatomy of the rectum: A review with particular relevance to the hazards of rectal mobilization. Int J Colorect Dis 1987;2:158-166.

23. Pearl RK, Monsen H, Abcarian H. Surgical anatomy of the pelvic autonomic nerves: A practical approach. Am Surg 1986;52:236-237.

24. Mundy AR. An anatomical explanation for bladder dysfunction following rectal and uterine surgery. Br J Urol 1982;54:501-504.

25. Chen FP. Laparoscopic presacral neurectomy for chronic pelvic pain. Chang-Keng i Hsueh Tsa Chih 2000;23:1-7.

26. Pellegrino MJ, Johnson EW. Bilateral obturator nerve injuries during urologic surgery. Arch Phys Med Rehabil 69(1):46-7, 1988.

27. Ali HS. Ectopic pregnancy presenting with obturator nerve pain. J Accid Emerg Med 15(3):192-3, 1998.

28. Robert R, Prat-Pradal D, Labat JJ, Bensignor M, Raoul S, Rebai R, Leborgne J. Anatomic basis of chronic perineal pain: role of the pu-

dendal nerve. Surg Radiol Anat 20:93-8, 1998.

29. Klutke CG, Siegel CL. Functional female pelvic anatomy. Urol Clin North Am 1995;22:487-498.

30. Qinyao W, Weijin S, Youren Z, Wenqing Z, Zhengrui H. New concepts in severe presacral hemorrhage during proctectomy. Arch Surg 1985;120:1013-1020.

31. Nakano KK. Sciatic nerve entrapment: the piriformis syndrome. J Musculoskel Med 1987;4:33-37.

32. Brunschwig A, Walsh TS. Resection of great veins on lateral pelvic wall. Surg Gynecol Obstet 1949;88:498-500.

33. Batson OV. The vertebral vein system. Caldwell lecture, 1956. Am J Roentgenol 1957;78:195-212.

34. Heald FJ, Ryall RDH. Recurrence and survival after total mesorectal excision for rectal cancer. Lancet 1:1479-1482, 1986.

35. Enker WE. Sphincter-preserving operations for rectal cancer. Oncology 10(11):1673-1684, 1996.

36. Wagner JR, Russo P. Urologic complications of major pelvic surgery. Semin Surg Oncol 2000;18:216-228.

37. Power RMH. The unstriated muscle fiber of the female pelvis. Am J Obstet Gynecol 1939;38:27-39.

38. Shafik A. A new concept of the anatomy of the anal sphincter mechanism and the physiology of defecation: III. The longitudinal anal muscle: anatomy and role in anal sphincter mechanism. Invest Urol 1976;13:271-277.

39. Delancey JO, Starr RA. Histology of the connections between the vagina and levator ani muscles. Implications for urinary tract function. J Reprod Med 1990;35:765-771.

40. Mostwin JL. Current concepts of female pelvic anatomy and physiology. Urol Clin North Am 1991;18:175-195.

41. Oelrich TM. Pelvic and perineal anatomy of the male gorilla: Selected observations. Anat Rec 1978;191:433-445.

42. Tichy M. The morphogenesis of the human sphincter urethrae muscle. Anat Embryol 1989;180:577-582.

43. Cherry DA, Rothenberger DA. Pelvic floor physiology. Surg Clin North Am 1988;68:1217-1230.

44. de Leval J, Chantraine A, Penders L. The striated sphincter of the urethra. 1: Recall of knowledge on the striated sphincter of the urethra. J Urol (Paris) 1984;90:439-454.

45. Abitol MM. Evolution of the ischial spine and of the pelvic floor in hominoidea. Am J Phys Anthropol 1988;75:53-67.

46. Levi AC, Borghi F, Garavoglia M. Development of the anal canal muscles. Dis Colon Rectum 1991;34:262-266.

47. Jurado M, Bazan A, Elejabeitia J, Paloma V, Martinez-Monge R, Alcazar JL. Primary vaginal and pelvic floor reconstruction at the time of pelvic exenteration: a study of morbidity. Gynecol Oncol 2000;77:293-297.

48. Small T, Friedman DJ, Sultan M. Reconstructive surgery of the pelvis after surgery for rectal cancer. Semin Surg Oncol 2000;18:259-264.

49. Rufus of Ephesus. Cited in Mermigas K. Topographic Anatomy [Greek]. Athens: PG Makris, 1926, p. 10.

50. Oelrich TM. The urethral sphincter muscle in the male. Am J Anat 1980;158:229-246.

51. Oelrich TM. The striated urogenital sphincter muscle in the female. Anat Rec 1983;205:223-232.

52. Tobin CE, Benjamin JA. Anatomic and clinical reevaluation of Camper's, Scarpa's, and Colles' fasciae. Surg Gynecol Obstet 1949;88:545-559.

53. Stormont TJ, Cahill DR, King BF, Myers RP. Fascias of the male

external genitalia and perineum. Clin Anat 1994;7:115-124.

54. Lerner SE, Melman A, Christ GJ. A review of erectile dysfunction: new insights and more questions. J Urol 1993;149:1246-1255.

55. McConnell J, Benson GS, Schmidt WA. The vasculature of the human penis: a reexamination of the morphological basis for the polster theory of erection. Anat Rec 1982;203:475-484.

56. Conti G, Virag R, von Niederhausern W. The morphological basis for the polster theory of penile vascular regulation. Acta Anat 1988;133:209-212.

57. MacBride RG, Blight EM. Age-related thickness of the penile tunica albuginea. Clin Anat 1992;5:50-56.

58. Fetissof F, Arbeille B, Bellet D, Barre I, Lansac J. Endocrine cells in human Bartholin's glands. An immunohistochemical and ultrastructural analysis. Virchows Archiv B-Cell Pathol Mol Biol 1989; 57: 117-121.

59. Williams PL (ed). Gray's Anatomy (38th ed). New York: Churchill Livingstone, 1995, p. 1877.

60. Strasser H, Klima G, Poisel S, Horninger W, Bartsch G. Anatomy and innervation of the rhabdosphincter of the male urethra. Prostate 1996;28:24-31.

61. Delancey JOL. Correlative study of paraurethral anatomy. Obstet Gynecol 1986;68:91-97.

62. Krongrad A, Droller MJ. Anatomy of the prostate and its investing fascial layers. In: Paulson DF (ed). Prostatic Disorders. Philadelphia: Lea & Febiger, 1989, pp. 3-27.

63. Krantz KE. The anatomy of the urethra and anterior vaginal wall. Am J Obstet Gynecol 1951;62:374-386.

64. Mermigas K. Topographic Anatomy [Greek]. Athens: PG Makris, 1926, p. 230.

65. Khan SA, Fleagle JJ, Washecka R, Wasnick RJ, Kandel LB, D'Agostino JA, Siddharth P. The 'bare area' of the male urethra. A new anatomical concept. Urol Int 1991;46:58-60.

66. Stannard MW, Currarino G. Radiographic appearance of the pars nuda urethrae in the voiding urethrogram. Abdom Imaging 1993;18:393-395.

67. Grant JCB, Basmajian JV. Grant's Method of Anatomy (7th ed). Baltimore: Williams & Wilkins, 1965.

68. O'Bichere A, Green C, Phillips RC. New, simple approach for maximal pudendal nerve exposure: anomalies and prospects for functional reconstruction. Dis Colon Rectum 2000;43:956-960.

69. Thomson JPS. The rectum and anal canal. In: Sabiston DC Jr (ed). Textbook of Surgery (13th ed). Philadelphia: WB Saunders, 1986, pp. 1035-1052.

70. Imbembo AL, Zuidema GD. Anal canal and rectum. In: Nardi GL, Zuidema GD (eds). Surgery: Essentials of Clinical Practice (4th ed). Boston: Little, Brown, 1982, pp. 579-580.

71. Signorello LB, Harlow BL, Chekos AK, Repke JT. Midline episiotomy and anal incontinence: retrospective cohort study. BMJ 2000;320:86-90.

# Chapter 29

# Lymphatic System

John E. Skandalakis, Gene L. Colborn, Thomas A. Weidman,
Andrew N. Kingsnorth, George F. Hatch III, Kathryn F. Hatch,
Petros Mirilas, Richard C. Lauer, Lee J. Skandalakis

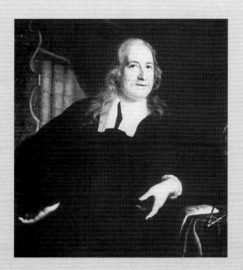

**Olof Rudbeck (1630-1702),** who may have been first to describe the lymphatic system in toto, and especially that of the liver.

*Photo:* Bokförlaget Naturoch Kultur, Stockholm, Sweden.

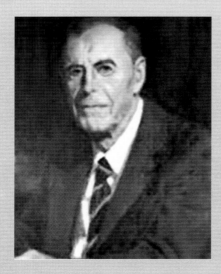

**Cushman Davis Haagensen (1900-1990),** author of the classic work *The Lymphatics in Cancer.*

*If we mistake not, in a proper time it [the lymphatics] will allow to be the greatest discovery both in physiology and pathology that anatomy has suggested, since the discovery of the circulation.*

*William Hunter*[1]

# HISTORY

The anatomic and surgical history of the lymphatic system is shown in Table 29-1.

# EMBRYOGENESIS

## Normal Development

In spite of the important role that the lymphatic system plays in human physiology and disease, much concerning its genesis remains an enigma. During the 5th week of gestation, two paired and two unpaired endothelial sacs arise as outgrowths from the venous channels. These sacs form the primordia of the lymphatic system.

The first primordial lymph sacs to appear are the paired jugular sacs in the neck. They are located bilaterally at the junction of the subclavian and internal jugular (precardinal) veins. Soon thereafter, extensions from these sacs are visible in the upper limbs. The next sac to appear is unpaired and located at the mesenteric root in the retroperitoneal space. Later the unpaired cisterna chyli develops dorsal to the mesenteric sac. The final paired sacs, two posterior (iliac) sacs, appear at the junction of the sciatic and femoral veins. In short, it may be said that embryologically the lymph system originates and terminates in the venous system.

By the end of the ninth week, these six lymphatic sacs are linked together by multiple endothelial channels to form a complicated network of lymphatic vessels (Fig. 29-1). During early fetal development mesenchymal cells invade these sacs, converting them into groups of lymph nodes. True lymph nodes, however, do not appear until the system of vessels is well established.

The earliest nodes appear in the places occupied by the primary sacs and confluences of capillary plexuses. At first, the nodes are represented by unencapsulated lymphoid tissue located within the meshwork of lymphatic channels. Later, the lymphoid mass separates into smaller portions allowing the inward growth of blood vessels and the lymphatic network. Each mass, together with portions of the surrounding network, becomes enclosed by a capsule of connective tissue. Original lymphoid tissue transforms into the medullary cords and cortical nodules of the node; the enclosed lymphatic capillaries form the peripheral lymph sinus. Cervical lymph nodes appear around the 9th week. Later, several other groups of lymph nodes are formed in various areas of the body.

The right and left thoracic ducts are channels connecting the right and left jugular lymph sacs with the cisterna chyli. The cisterna chyli also connects to the lower intercostal trunks, intestinal trunk, and lumbar trunks. The adult thoracic duct forms between weeks 6 and 8. It develops from the anastomosis of the right and left thoracic ducts at the level of the 4th to 6th thoracic segments, the distal (caudal) part of the right thoracic duct, and the proximal (cranial) part of the left thoracic duct. The right thoracic (lymphatic) duct is formed from the proximal part of the right thoracic duct. It must be noted, however, that the development presented here is speculative. The reader will find more detailed information in *Embryology for Surgeons.*[2]

Embryologically, lymphocytes are derived from the primitive stem cells in the mesenchyme of the yolk sac. From a functional standpoint, there are two types of lymphocytes: T cells and B cells. The progeny of the lymphopoietic stem cells found in the bone marrow that are destined to become T cells exit the marrow and settle in the thymus where their differentiation is completed. Ultimately T cells enter the circulation as the long-lived small lymphocytes. B cells originate in marrow, gut-associated lymphatic tissue, and the spleen. T cells are re-

**TABLE 29-1. Anatomic and Surgical History of the Lymphatic System**

| | | |
|---|---|---|
| Hippocrates (ca. 460-ca. 360 B.C.) | | Described axillary lymph nodes and "white blood" in the nodes |
| Aristotle (384-322 B.C.) | | Described "fibers which take position between blood vessels and nerves and which contain colorless liquid" |
| Herophilus of Chalcedon | 300 B.C. | Probably knew about the "milk-bearing vessels" of the mesentery |
| Erasistratus (310-250 B.C.) | | Described lymphatics of small bowel |
| Marinus (fl. A.D. 50) | | Described mesenteric lymph nodes |
| Galen (A.D. 129-199) | | Described mesenteric lymph nodes and lacteal veins |
| Paul of Aegina (A.D. 607-690) | | Most likely described infected lymph nodes at the lower neck (scrofulae) |
| Nicola Massa | 1532 | By dissecting human cadavers, saw renal lymphatic vessels |
| Gabriello Falloppio (1523-1562) | | Described mesenteric "vein" containing yellow matter in dissection on human cadavers |
| Bartholomeus Eustachius | 1563 | From dissecting a horse, described thoracic duct ("vena alba thoracica") |
| Marco Aurelio Severino (1580-1656) | | Performed radical mastectomy with axillary dissections |
| Nicolas Claude Fabrice de Peirsc (1580-1637) | | Saw chyliferous vessels in dissection of a criminal fed a rich meal before execution |
| Gaspare Aselli | 1622 | Based on vivisection of well-fed dog and dissection of mammals, described white cords (the lacteals) containing milky-appearing liquid |
| Francis Glisson (1597-1677) | | Theory of absorbent function of lymphatics |
| Johann Vesling | 1634 | Based on cadaver studies, produced earliest illustrations of human lymphatics; described thoracic duct |
| Thomas Bartholin | 1643 | First to use the word "lymphatics" |
| George Joliff (ca. 1618-1658) | | Recognized that lymphatic vessels are throughout the body carrying "aqueous humor" |
| Jean Pecquet | 1647 | Based on human and animal dissection, and injection studies, described thoracic duct and cisterna chyli |
| Johannes van Horne of Leyden | 1651 | During autopsy, accidentally discovered the thoracic duct in man without knowing the work of others |
| Marcello Malpighi (1628-1694) | | Described conglobate glands along course of lymphatics |
| Olof Rudbeck | 1651-1652 | Based on human and animal dissection, described course of lymphatics from liver and other organs to thoracic duct and venous system |
| Jan Swammerdam (1637-1680) | | Using suet and wax injections, discovered valves of the lymphatics |
| Frederick Ruysch | 1665 | Based on intravascular (intra-lymphatic?) injections, described morphology and function of lymphatic valves |
| Niels Stensen (1638-1686) | | Discovered right lymphatic duct |
| Anton Nuck | 1692 | Based on mercury injection, described fine lymphatic vessels |
| Johann Conrad Peyer (1653-1712) | | Described areas of lymph nodules in mucous membrane of small intestine (Peyer's patches) |

**TABLE 29-1 *(cont'd)*. Anatomic and Surgical History of the Lymphatic System**

| | | |
|---|---|---|
| Antonio Pacchioni | 1705 | "Glandulae" (glands) secrete lymph |
| Jean Louis Petit (1674-1760) | | First to show the spread of mammary cancer to axillary lymph nodes; advocated radical removal of the breast muscle and lymph nodes but not the nipple |
| Henri Francois LeDran (1685-1770) | | First description of spread of cancer along lymphatics |
| Johann Nathanael Lieberkuhn | 1745 | Using microscopic injections and corrosion preparations, demonstrated origin of lymphatics in intestinal villi |
| Angelo Nannoni (1715-1790) | | Removed malignant breast tumors by excision of wide margin, underlying fascia, large muscle, and nearby lymph nodes |
| William Hunter | 1746 | Based on dissection of birds, fish, and amphibians, and using mercury injection, stated that the lymphatic vessels "constitute one great and general system" |
| Johann Friedrich Meckel | 1772 | Described lymphovenous connections |
| John Hunter (1728-1793) | | Discovered lymphatics in the neck of the swan and in the crocodile. Theorized cancer spread via lymphatic route: "The red veins do not absorb in the human body" (experimental studies of intestinal veins in dogs). |
| Alexander Monro the Second (1733-1817) | | Based on injection with quicksilver, described lymph nodes |
| William Hewson (1739-1774) | | Complete account of mercury-injected lymphatic system in the human subject, and description of lacteals and lymphatic vessels in other species. Divided the lymphatic system into deep and superficial lymphatics. Noted the occurrence of lymphocytes in lymph. Performed controlled experiments with blood and lymph to study coagulation. Lymphatics involved in absorption of poisonous substances and progress of wound inflammation and cancer. Published, in 1774, important treatise, *The Lymphatic System in the Human Subject and in Other Animals.* |
| William C. Cruikshank (1745-1800) | | Via clinical observation and injection of mercury into the subdermal lymphatic channels through very thin glass catheters, traced lymph vessels from the periosteum to the cortex of the bone. Continued classification of lymphatics, regional lymph drainage, and lymphatic topography. Stated that lymphatics is involved in defense against infection and the formation of edema. |
| Benjamin Bell (1749-1806) | | First in England to advise radical mastectomy |
| Thomas Pole (1754-1829) | | Described techniques (injection and corrosion studies) for lymphatic system dissection |
| Paolo Mascagni | 1787 | Based on mercury injection, said all the lymphatics pass through one or more lymph nodes during their course; published elegant atlas with detailed anatomy of the lymphatics in human body, as well as copper engravings |
| Guillaume Dupuytren (1777-1835) | | First to identify fibrin in chyle |
| Vincenz Fohmann | 1821 | Comparative anatomic study of direct communications between lymphatics and peripheral veins |
| Gabriel Andral | 1824 or 1829 | First report of lymphangitis carcinomatosa (based on autopsy results) |
| Astley Paston Cooper | 1825 | Using mercury injection, investigated lymphatics of the breast |
| Thomas Hodgkin | 1832 | Described diseases of the lymph nodes and spleen; Hodgkin's lymphoma was one of his discoveries |
| Johannes Peter Müller (1801-1858) | | By microscopic analysis and experimentation, studied chemical and physical properties of blood, lymph, and chyle |
| Karl Langer | 1868 | Based on observations of tadpoles, suggested that the endothelium of the lymphatics is of venous origin |
| Marie Philibert, Constant Sappey | 1870s | Based on mercury injection of cutaneous and deeper lymphatic trunks, described valves, counted up to 80 valves along the length of the human arm; very accurate drawings |
| Carl F. Ludwig (1816-1895) | | Isolated and cannulated lymphatics in animals; analyzed lymph and believed it was formed by a process of filtration |

**TABLE 29-1 (cont'd). Anatomic and Surgical History of the Lymphatic System**

| | | |
|---|---|---|
| Albert von Koelliker (1817-1905) | | Studied capillary lymphatics, comparing amphibians, mammals, and humans |
| Charles Phillippe Robin (1821-1885) | | Described small spaces in the external coat of arteries communicating with lymphatics |
| Rudolf Virchow (1821-1902) | | "Barrier theory" of defensive role of lymph glands |
| Friedrich Daniel von Recklinghausen (1833-1910) | | Using silver nitrate to stain black the epithelium of the lymphatics, identified fine lymphatic vessels within their surrounding tissue |
| Dimitru Gerota | 1896 | Injected Prussian blue in turpentine and ether to visualize lymphatics; contributed to understanding of collecting lymph vessels; described the lymphatic route from the mammary glands to the liver or subdiaphragmatic nodes by which cancer of the breast may be spread |
| Louis Antoine Ranvier | 1897 | Based on microscopic studies of lymphocyte histology, hypothesized that terminal lymphatics are closed |
| Joseph Coats (1846-1899) | | Studied lymphatic and extralymphatic cancer metastasis |
| Berkeley George Andrew Moynihan | 1904 | Emphasized that the glands must be sought and removed in gastric resections for cancer |
| Ernest H. Starling (1866-1927) | | Discovered that colloid osmotic pressure of protein in plasma acts to retain fluid in the blood stream and balances the hydrostatic pressure in the capillaries. Capillaries are impermeable to protein; lymphatics absorb protein molecules and return them to the circulation. |
| Florence Rena Sabin | 1911 | Based on vertebrate embryos, said lymphatic sacs have venous origin and lymphatic vessels spring from sacs; emphasized that lymphatic and blood capillaries have the same relationship to tissue space |
| Karl Sternberg (1872-1935) Dorothy Reed (1874-1964) | | Based on pathology studies, identified multinuclear giant cells in lymph nodes and spleen in Hodgkin's disease (Reed-Sternberg cells) |
| James Bumgardner Murphy (1884-1950) | | First experimental proof that lymphocytes are involved in immunity to grafted tissue, tuberculosis, and cancer (based on grafting tumor fragments onto bird embryos) |
| Cecil K. Drinker, Joseph Mendel Yoffey, Frederick Colin Courtice | 1940s | Demonstrated that the principal function of the lymphatic system is the absorption of protein from the interstitial tissues |
| Marceau Servelle J. Deysson | 1943 | By injecting thorium dioxide (Thorotrast), visualized lymphatics in patients with elephantiasis |
| J.A. Weinberg | 1951 | Performed vital staining of lymphatics of the lung; mapped lymph nodes to minimize unnecessary dissection |
| John Bernard Kinmonth | 1952 | Developed a clinically applicable lymphangiogram |
| Denis Parsons Burkitt | 1958 | Noted that a tumor of the jaw followed unrecognized lymphoma |
| Peter Carey Nowell | 1960 | Noted mitotic activity of mononuclear leukocytes from human peripheral blood 48 to 72 hours after stimulation with a red kidney bean extract |
| R.J.V. Pulvertaft | 1964 | Described characteristics of cells from Burkitt lymphoma tumor. Later identified the morphology of the Burkitt lymphoma cell with the phytohemagglutinin-transformed lymphocyte. |
| Michael Antony Epstein (1921-?) Yvonne M. Barr (?-?) | | Studied microscopic biopsy specimens and grew cells from Burkitt tumor |
| Sayegh et al. | 1966 | Used term "sentinel node" to mean the node first visualized following injection of dye (lymphangiography) |

**TABLE 29-1 *(cont'd)*. Anatomic and Surgical History of the Lymphatic System**

| R.M. Cabanas | 1977 | Stated sentinel node concept; demonstrated that sentinel node biopsy could precede lymphadenectomy |
| Alex & Krag | 1993 | Reported on ability of radioactive tracers to identify sentinel node |

*Source:* History table adapted from Skandalakis JE. I wish I had been there: highlights in the history of lymphatics. Am Surg 61(9):799-808, 1995; with permission.

**References:**
Alex JC, Krag DN. Gamma-probe guided localization of lymph nodes. Surg Oncol 1993;2:137-143.
Cabanas RM. An approach for the treatment of penile carcinoma. Cancer 1977;39:456-466.
DePalma RG. Disorders of the lymphatic system. In: Sabiston DC Jr. (ed). Textbook of Surgery, 14th Ed. Philadelphia: WB Sauders, 1991.
Gans H. On the discovery of the lymphatic circulation. Angiology 13:530-536, 1962.
Kanter MA. The lymphatic system: an historical perspective. Plast Reconstr Surg 79(1):131-139, 1987.
Knight B. Discovering the Human Body. New York: Lippincott & Crowell, 1980.
Leeds SE. Three centuries of history of the lymphatic system. Surg Gynecol Obstet 144:927-934, 1977.
McGrew RE. Encyclopedia of Medical History. New York: McGraw-Hill, 1985.
Mayerson HS. The lymphatic system with particular reference to the kidney. Surg Gynecol Obstet 116(3):259-272.
Sayegh E, Brooks J, Sacher E, Busch F. Lymphangiography of the retroperitoneal lymph nodes through the inguinal route. J Urol 1966;95:102-107.
Schmidt JE. Medical Discoveries: Who and When. Springfield IL: CC Thomas, 1959.
Weinberg JA. Identification of regional lymph nodes in the treatment of bronchiogenic carcinoma. J Thorac Surg 1951;22:517-526.

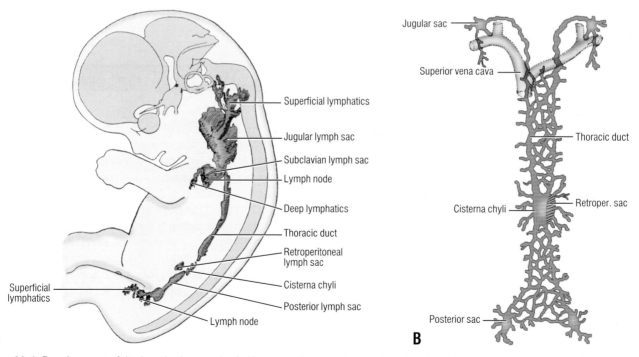

**A**                    **B**

Fɪɢ. **29-1.** Development of the lymphatic vessels. **A.** Human embryo at nine weeks, showing the primitive lymph sacs and the developing vessels. **B.** Ventral view of the formation of the single thoracic duct from the primitive paired lymphatic plexus. (Modified from Arey LB. Developmental Anatomy. Rev. 7th Ed. Philadelphia: WB Saunders, 1974. *A,* after Sabin FR. The development of the lymphatic system. In: Keibel F, Mall FP, eds. Manual of Human Embryology, vol. 2. Philadelphia: JP Lippincott, 1912. Used with permission.)

**TABLE 29-2. Anomalies of the Lymphatic System**

| Anomaly | Prenatal Age at Onset | First Appearance (or Other Diagnostic Clues) | Sex Chiefly Affected | Relative Frequency | Remarks |
|---|---|---|---|---|---|
| Variations in the course of the thoracic duct | 2nd month | No pathologic structures | Equal | Common | |
| Cystic hygroma (cystic lymphangioma) | 6th to 9th weeks? | At birth or in infancy | Equal (neck); male (groin) | Uncommon | Invasive growth; may be a neoplasm |
| Primary lymphedema: Milroy's disease | 3rd month? | At birth | Equal? | Rare | Familial tendency |
| Lymphedema precox | 3rd month? | At any age | Equal? | Rare | |
| Mesenteric, omental and retroperitoneal lymphatic cysts | ? | In infancy to middle age | Male (children); female (adults) | Uncommon | |

*Source:* Skandalakis JE, Gray SW. Embryology for Surgeons, 2nd Ed. Baltimore: Williams & Wilkins, 1994; with permission.

sponsible for cellular immunity; B cells are responsible for the synthesis of antibodies.

# Congenital Anomalies

It is not within the scope of this chapter to discuss lymphatic anomalies in detail. Table 29-2 presents an overview of some of the more common variations.

Congenital anomalies of the lymphatic system are relatively rare. One condition is seen as diffuse swelling of some portion(s) of the body called "congenital lymphedema." Whether this is due to congenital hypoplasia of the lymphatic vessels or from dilatation of the primitive lymphatic vessels is still to be established. Less commonly, there are cases of diffuse cystic dilations of the lymph vessels which exist widely throughout the body.

We quote from Musone et al.[3]:

> Cystic hygroma is a malformation of the lymphatic system that is diagnosed by ultrasound very well from the first quarter of pregnancy. It is frequently associated with chromosomal and non-chromosomal abnormalities. The presence of septae in it and amniotic fluid alpha-fetoprotein levels are prognostic indicators.

Hygromas (cystic lymphangiomas) develop as large swellings in the lower neck. Hygromas are large cavities filled with fluid which may appear at birth and frequently grow and make their presence known in the infant. Riquet et al.[4] distinguish between tissular lymphangiomas of the neck and mediastinum found in childhood through young adulthood, and the purely liquid cysts of the posterior or middle mediastinum of older adults. The former are congenital, the latter suggest an acquired origin. Hygromas,

according to Moore and Persaud,[5] apparently are derived from abnormalities in the jugular lymph sacs. Hygromas may be pinched off parts of the lymph sacs or may be lymphatic spaces which never established connections with lymph channels.

Pulmonary lymphangiectasia, a rare disease characterized by abnormal pulmonary lymphatics, was studied by Bouchard et al.[6] They reported that although it is fatal in the neonatal period, survival is possible and symptomatology decreases with age.

# SURGICAL ANATOMY

The various elements of the lymphatic system, such as the ring of Waldeyer (tonsillar ring), thymus gland, spleen, bone marrow, and lymphatic follicles of the respiratory, genitourinary, and alimentary systems are discussed in other chapters. In addition, the lymphatic drainage of each organ and region of the trunk is discussed in chapters pertinent to them. The primary purpose of this chapter is to present anatomic information which is related to surgery, rather than describing the lymphatic system in toto.

The lymphatic system can be divided into two broad categories: the lymphatic network at large and the lymphatic organs.

The lymphatic network at large includes:
- The complicated network of irregular capillaries, consisting of minute lymph vessels that drain the lymph of the body (with the exception of hyaline cartilages, epidermis, and the eye's cornea)
- Larger lymph vessels which drain the capillaries

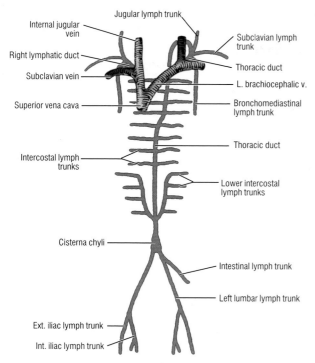

**FIG. 29-2.** The general plan of the lymphatic system. (Modified from Woodburne RT, Burkel WE. Essentials of Human Anatomy (9th ed). New York: Oxford University Press, 1994; used with permission.)

- Lymph glands which accept lymph from the lymph vessels and filter the lymph
- Large lymph vessels which are responsible for draining the lymph into the veins

The lymphatic entities to be studied in this chapter are:
- Cisterna chyli
- Thoracic duct
- Right lymphatic duct

## Cisterna Chyli

Is the cisterna chyli a typical and constant anatomic entity? Anatomists disagree. An illustration in *Gray's Anatomy*[7] designates the cisterna chyli as "atypical" and "unusual." Woodburne and Burkel,[8] quoting Nelson, indicate that the cisterna chyli is present in 25 percent of individuals as a dilatation of the thoracic duct. In only 35 percent of Rouvière's[9] dissections was a true cisterna chyli demonstrated. *Lee McGregor's Synopsis of Surgical Anatomy*[10] describes it as being present in 50 percent of cases. The authors of this chapter will designate as "cisterna chyli" a dilatation of the proximal thoracic duct or perhaps con-

fluence of lymphatic trunks that may form a sac.

The cisterna chyli is an elongated and sometimes dilated sac about 5 cm in length. It is located in the shadow of the right side of the aorta and behind the right diaphragmatic crus at the surface of L2 (variably, T12-L2). It receives the right and left lumbar trunks, the intestinal trunk, and the lowest intercostal vessels (Figs. 29-2 and 29-3).

Multiple sacculations may be present as a result of the contributing vessels. However, sacculations are not present after the convergence of the contributing vessels with the cisterna chyli. Alternatively, the meeting place of the principal vessels may be thoracic rather than abdominal. Because of the relative infrequency of a distinctly dilated cisterna, the term should be understood to be of topographic convenience but not necessarily related to the degree of distension. To diagnose such a giant cisterna chyli, MRI with gadolinium-DTPA enhancement has been used.[11]

The right and left lumbar trunks transmit lymph from the abdominal wall below the level of the navel, pelvis, kidneys, and adrenal glands. The intestinal trunk, which receives the lymph and chyle from the parts of the gastrointestinal tract supplied by the celiac and superior mesenteric arteries, occasionally empties directly into the so-called cisterna chyli. However, in most cases, the intestinal trunk is a tributary of the left lumbar trunk. The intercostal trunks enter the upper part of the cisterna chyli or empty into the beginning of the thoracic duct.

## Thoracic Duct

The thoracic duct is approximately 45 cm long and 2-5 mm in diameter. The lower end of the duct receives descending, paired, posterior intercostal lymph vessels that

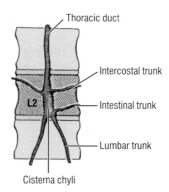

**FIG. 29-3.** Formation of the cisterna chyli by several trunks and proximal thoracic duct. (Modified from Brantigan OC. Clinical Anatomy. New York: McGraw-Hill Book Co., 1963; used with permission.)

drain the lower six or seven intercostal spaces. As it ascends, the duct receives additional tributaries from posterior mediastinal nodes and the upper intercostal spaces. Its terminal tributaries are the left jugular, subclavian, and bronchomediastinal trunks.

The duct can be subdivided into three parts: abdominal, thoracic, and cervical. The abdominal part of the thoracic duct originates from the cranial part of the cisterna chyli. With the aorta on its left and the azygos vein on its right, the thoracic duct passes through the "aortic hiatus" of the diaphragm to form the thoracic part. It maintains this relationship as it passes through the posterior mediastinum. During its ascent, the thoracic vertebrae, right intercostal arteries, and terminal portions of the hemiazygos and accessory hemiazygos veins are posterior to the thoracic duct; the esophagus, diaphragm and pericardium are anterior to it.

At the level of T7 (Fig. 29-4), the thoracic duct travels obliquely behind the esophagus to the level of the fifth thoracic vertebra. At T5, it reappears from behind the esophagus to continue its upward journey on the left of the esophagus and medial to the pleura. In the base of the neck, the thoracic duct passes posterior to the common carotid artery, internal jugular vein, vagus nerve, left anterior scalene muscle, and left phrenic nerve. It passes anterior to the vertebral artery and vein and the sympathetic trunk. The duct proceeds upward to the level of C7, whereupon it descends across the subclavian artery. It ends in the junction of the left subclavian vein and left internal jugular vein, thus forming the cervical part of the thoracic duct. A rare large thoracic duct cyst that expanded into the anterior cervico-thoracic junction has been reported by Karajiannis et al.[12]

The thoracic duct is the largest lymphatic channel in the body. It collects lymph from the entire body except the right hemithorax (thoracic wall, right lung, right side of the heart, part of the diaphragmatic surface of the liver, lower area of the right lower lobe of the liver), right head and neck, and right upper extremity. The volume of flow through the thoracic duct is between 60 and 190 cc/hr; consequently, large quantities of plasma proteins can be lost quickly from the blood in the event of trauma to the duct or in association with malignant tumors. Simple ligation of the vessel is followed by gradual restoration of normal levels of blood fat over a period of about two weeks, as collateral channels reroute the flow.[13]

Regurgitation of blood from the jugulosubclavian confluence into the thoracic duct is not possible in life because the opening of the thoracic duct into the subclavian vein is protected by valves. In cadaveric specimens, backflow of blood into the thoracic duct from the jugulosubclavian venous junction is often apparent,

causing the duct to resemble a vein.

There are several variations in the termination of the thoracic duct (Figs. 29-5 and 29-6). In 1959 Jdanov[14] reported termination in the following sites:
- Internal jugular vein                                         48%
- Subclavian vein                                               9%
- At the junction of the internal jugular

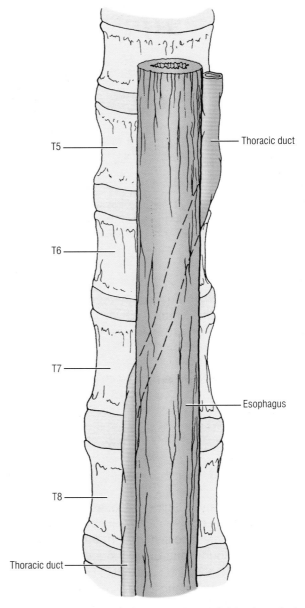

FIG. 29-4. The oblique thoracic course of the definitive thoracic duct, resulting from the anastomosis of the right and left thoracic ducts. The definitive duct represents the retention of the proximal part of the right thoracic duct and the distal segment of the left thoracic duct.

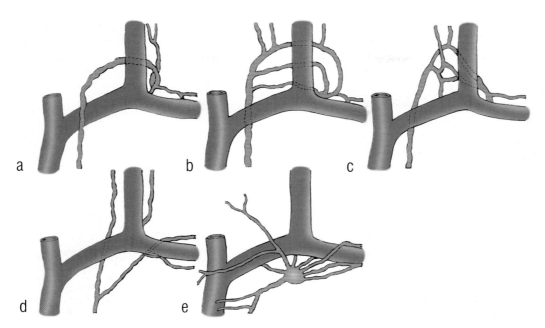

FIG. 29-5. Variations of the entry of the thoracic duct into the venous system. **a.** A single thoracic duct and a simple junction. **b.** Plexiform ramification of the final segment of a thoracic duct, but with a simple junction. **c.** Delta-like entry of the thoracic duct. **d.** Duplication of the final segment of the thoracic duct and two separate junctions. **e.** Ampullary enlargement of the thoracic duct with multiple terminal branches. (From Heberer G, van Dongen RJAM (eds). Vascular Surgery. Berlin, Heidelberg: Springer-Verlag, 1989; used with permission.)

| and subclavian veins | 35% |
|---|---|
| • Left brachiocephalic (innominate) vein | 8% |

Kinnaert[15] dissected 49 cadavers and collected 480 additional cases. He reported the termination of the thoracic duct as follows:

| • No evidence of left thoracic duct | 0-4.5% |
|---|---|
| • Multiple terminal openings: | |
|   In others' cases | 10-40% |
|   In his cases | 21% |
| • Termination into the internal jugular vein | 36% |
| • Termination into the subclavian vein | 17% |
| • Termination into the junction of internal jugular and subclavian veins | 34% |

Shimada and Sato[16] found that only 38% of Japanese had thoracic ducts that terminate in the jugulosubclavian angle. In comparison, previous studies by Kihara and Adachi[17] found this occurrence in 78.2% of Japanese and in 33% of European subjects. Shimada and Sato noted the following sites and frequencies of termination of the trunk of the thoracic duct (Fig. 29-6), each major type also possessing subtypes not discussed here:

| • Venous angle | 38% |
|---|---|
| • Internal jugular vein | 27% |
| • External jugular vein | 28% |

| • Other, complex configurations | 7% |
|---|---|

Shimada and Sato[16] noted that while the multiple complex configuration occurred only 7% of the time, this termination was highly correlated with an increased risk of metastasis in cervical or mediastinal lymph node dissections. Also, there was a high risk of injury to the terminations of the duct during radical neck dissection.

In *Clinical Anatomy and Pathology of the Thoracic Duct: An Investigation of 122 Cases,*[18] Jacobsson presented a very useful summary of the thoracic duct which we reprint here with gratitude.

*An anatomical study was made of the thoracic duct in 100 autopsy cases. A thoracic duct was found in every case and always started below the diaphragm, passed the posterior mediastinum in the thorax and discharged into the confluence of the veins in the left of the neck. In 4% of the cases a branch left the thoracic part of the thoracic duct at the aortic arch and emptied into the veins in the right side of the neck.*

*The beginning of the thoracic duct conformed to one of four types, depending on how the lumbar and intestinal trunks combined into the abdominal part. In 20% the thoracic duct arose from the confluence of the lumbar and intestinal trunks and in 55% it was formed after the intestinal trunk, branched or un-*

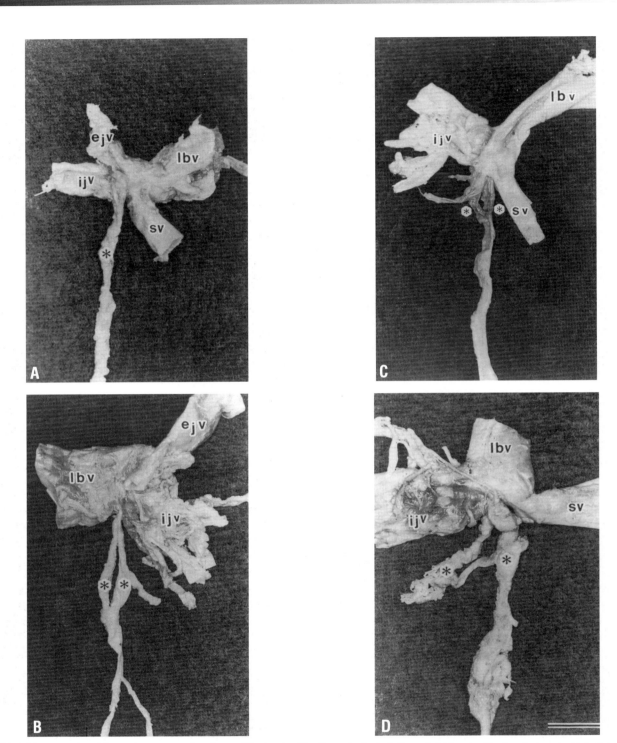

FIG. 29-6. Photographs of the various types of endings of the trunk of the thoracic duct. **A.** Type A-1. The duct is directly inserted into the venous angle. **B.** Type A-2. The duct separates into two trunks before and after running below the left brachiocephalic vein. **C.** Type A-3. The duct has two trunks, one extending to the beginning of the subclavian vein and the other to the venous angle. **D.** Type B-1. The duct with two trunks runs directly to the internal jugular vein. **E.** Type B-2. The duct separates into three trunks after running below the left brachiocephalic vein; one trunk runs to the internal jugular vein, and the others (two branches) to the subclavian vein. **F.** Type C-1. One trunk is inserted into the external jugular vein and the other into the subclavian vein. **G.** Type C-2. One trunk is inserted into the external jugular vein and the other into the internal jugular vein. **H.** Type D. There are four trunks and they are inserted into the beginning of the internal and external jugular veins, and into the subclavian vein. ejv, external jugular vein; ijv, internal jugular vein; lbv, left brachiocephalic vein; sv, subclavian vein. (From Shimada K, Sato I. Morphological and histological analysis of the thoracic duct at the jugulo-subclavian junction in Japanese cadavers. Clin Anat 1997;10:163-172; used with permission.)

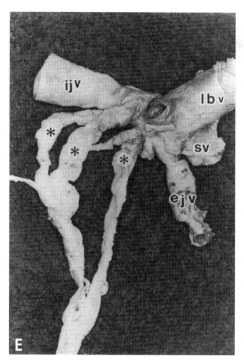

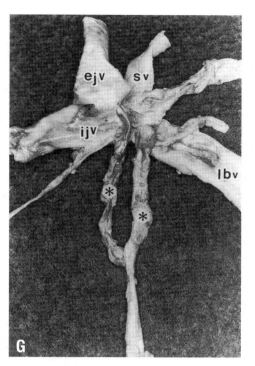

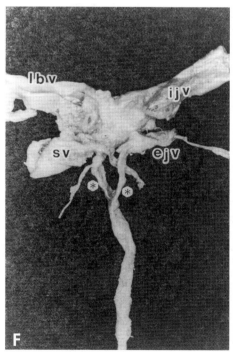

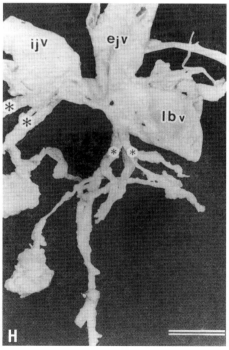

branched, had joined either the thoracic duct or one or both lumbar trunks. In 24% the thoracic duct ascended from a plexus formed by the lumbar and intestinal trunks. In 1% the thoracic duct had a plexiform structure throughout its course.

A cisterna chyli was found in 52% of the cases, with a roughly uniform distribution by sex. Its diameter averaged 6.7 mm but varied between 4 and 14 mm. In the thoracic part, insulae and plexus formations of the thoracic duct were found in 32%. The cervical part of the thoracic duct corresponded to one of 9 types, A, B and C having a single trunk with one (36%), two (13%) and three (3%) openings respectively into the venous system, D, E and F one or several insulae and one (18%), two (3%) and three (1%) openings respectively into the venous system, and G, H and I one or several plexuses and one (14%), two (9%) and three (3%) openings respectively, into the venous system on the left side of the neck. A total of 139 openings into the left veins in the neck were found in the l00 specimens of the thoracic duct. The most common site was the left subclavian vein (64), followed by the left venous angle (51), the left internal jugular vein (22) and the left external jugular vein (2).

Small lymph vessels emptied into the thoracic duct along its entire length and close connections were found with lymph nodes. Left jugular and subclavian trunks were often detected in the cervical part, emptying into the thoracic duct or independently into the cervical veins.

The thoracic duct was found to be irregular and its diameter was not constant, usually being greatest in the cervical part (excluding the cisterna chyli) and smallest in the lower thoracic part. Measurements at five levels gave the following average cross-sectional areas: (1) 14.7 sq. mm one centimeter from the opening into the venous system, (2) 11.5 sq. mm one-third of the way from the termination to the aortic arch, (3) 6.4 sq. mm at the aortic arch, (4) 4.5 sq. mm midway between the aortic arch and the diaphragm, and (5) 7.0 sq. mm one centimeter below the diaphragm. The largest and smallest external diameters measured in the cervical part were 8 mm and 1.5 mm.

Constrictions were observed along the thoracic duct, usually corresponding to the location of bicuspid valves in the vessel. The valves became more numerous as one approached the opening into the venous system, averaging 4.6 below the diaphragm, 5.9 between the diaphragm and the aortic arch, and 11.1 between the aortic arch and the termination of the thoracic duct. A terminal valve at the opening into the left cervical veins was found in 82 instances, no valve at all in the vicinity of this junction in 2 instances and a valve 1-6 mm from the opening in 55 instances.

## Right Lymphatic Duct

The right lymphatic duct "typically" begins with the union of three lymphatic trunks: right jugular, right subclavian, and right bronchomediastinal (Figs. 29-7 and 29-8).

The right bronchomediastinal trunk is regarded as the vestigial portion of the terminal (cranial) segment of the embryologic right thoracic duct. It receives lymphatic drainage from the right lung, lower left lung, right diaphragm, most of the drainage from the heart, and some drainage from the right lobe of the liver.

The right lymphatic duct is approximately 2 cm long. It is very closely related to the anterior scalene muscle. In the majority of cases, the right lymphatic duct empties into the junction of the right subclavian and right internal jugular veins. However, as demonstrated in Figures 29-7 and 29-8, its termination also has numerous variations.

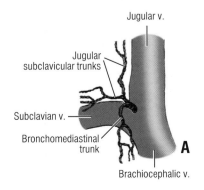
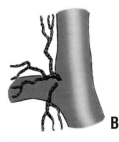
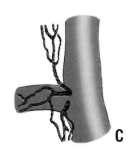

Jugular v.

Jugular subclavicular trunks

Subclavian v.

Bronchomediastinal trunk

Brachiocephalic v.

**A**   **B**   **C**

FIG. 29-7. Variations of the lymphatic junctions at the right venous angle. **A.** Entry of the tributaries into the right lymphatic duct. **B.** Partial entry into the right lymphatic duct. **C.** Separate entry of the tributaries near the right venous angle. (From Heberer G, van Dongen RJAM (eds). Vascular Surgery. Berlin, Heidelberg: Springer-Verlag, 1989; used with permission.)

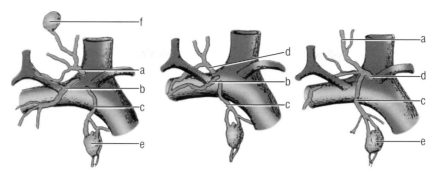

FIG. 29-8. Variations in the terminal lymph trunks of the right side. a = jugular trunk; b = subclavian trunk; c = bronchomediastinal trunk; d = right lymphatic duct; e = lymph node of parasternal chain; f = lymph node of deep cervical chain. (Modified from Williams PL (ed). Gray's Anatomy (38th ed). After Poirier & Charpy. New York: Churchill Livingstone, 1995; used with permission.)

## HISTOLOGY AND PHYSIOLOGY

Lymph capillaries are very thin. They unite to form lymphatic vessels. Lymph capillaries are lined by endothelium and are slightly larger than blood capillaries. They are unique, however, in that they lack a continuous basal lamina and are permeable only in one direction. The edges of adjacent endothelial cells overlap significantly, providing an intercellular cleft with one or two tiny points of closer apposition and adherence.

Extracellular bundles of filaments extend outward from the endothelium between collagen bundles of the surrounding connective tissues. These bundles are believed to play a role in keeping the lumen of the vessel open. Furthermore, it is presumed that as interstitial fluid increases around the lymphatic capillary, the "anchoring" filaments open the clefts, allowing the inward flow of intercellular fluid and even large molecules. As a result, relatively large products of metabolism can enter the lymph vessel, thereafter being pushed by the contraction of surrounding muscles and interstitial pressures.

The pathway of lymph starts in interstitial tissue spaces where lymph accumulates, perhaps secondary to the slight predominance of capillary filtration and reabsorption. Lymph passes from lymph capillaries to lymphatic vessels by propulsion and contraction. The lymphatic vessels carry the fluid to the lymph nodes by way of the nodal sinuses. Efferent vessels carry the lymph to the next node in the chain, and eventually the fluid flows to lymph trunks. The trunks pass the lymph into the thoracic and right lymphatic duct, where it reaches the venous circulation.

If some lymph vessels are damaged or blocked, new vessels form readily. The system drains broadly into the venous system. It is well understood that the thoracic duct and the right lymphatic duct open into their respective brachiocephalic veins, but those who have studied these vessels report openings of lymph vessels into the inferior vena cava, renal, suprarenal, azygos, and iliac veins.

Lymph capillaries and lymphatic vessels have one-way valves which open upon contraction of the vascular wall. These valves permit the passage and circulation of lymph fluid (3 to 5 liters daily) into larger vessels and, ultimately, to the thoracic ducts. The valves are bicuspid and prevent backflow.

Lymphatic vessels always follow minute arteries and veins. They resemble veins in structure but have thinner walls, more valves, and contain lymph nodes at various intervals along their length.

The exact number of lymph nodes in the body is not known and estimates vary greatly. According to Gray's Anatomy,[7] a normal young adult body contains some 400-450 lymph nodes, distributed approximately as follows: head and neck, 60-70; thorax, 100; abdomen and pelvis, 230; arm and thoracoabdominal wall (supraumbilical area), 30; leg and lower abdominal wall and superficial buttocks and perineum, 20. Conversely, Bailey and Love's Short Practice of Surgery[19] reported a total of 800 lymph nodes, 300 of which are located in the neck.

Lymph nodes are responsible for filtering lymph and producing antibodies by responding to antigens. Nodes vary greatly in size, ranging from 1-2 mm to 3-4 cm in diameter.[20] Each node (Fig. 29-9) is covered by a capsule of dense connective tissue which sends trabecular extensions to the center of the lymph node. The nodal parenchyma is divided into two regions: cortex and medulla.

The cortex is the outer and more densely staining part of the lymph node. The cortex contains lymph nodules or follicles (aggregations of lymphocytes) which contain lighter staining germinal centers. According to Roth and Reith,[21] the germinal center is a "morphological indication of lymphatic tissue response which ultimately leads to lym-

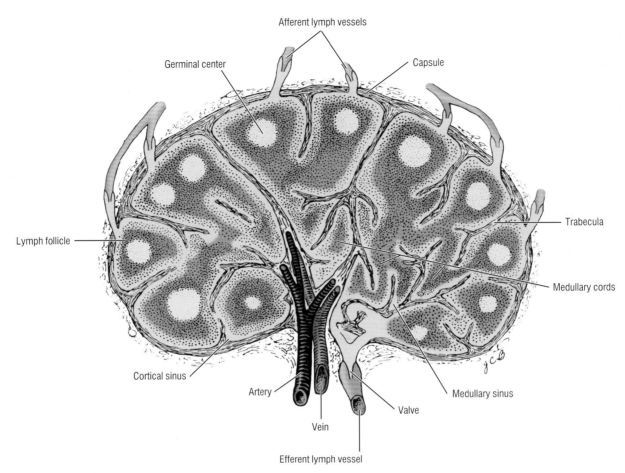

Afferent lymph vessels

Germinal center

Capsule

Lymph follicle

Trabecula

Medullary cords

Cortical sinus

Artery

Medullary sinus

Valve

Vein

Efferent lymph vessel

**FIG. 29-9.** A semi-schematic frontal section of a lymph node. (Modified from Woodburne RT, Burkel WE. Essentials of Human Anatomy, 9th Ed. New York: Oxford University Press, 1994; with permission.)

phocyte, plasma cell, and antibody formation." The germinal center may be the site of genesis of the immune system.

The innermost part of the lymph node is the medulla. The lymphoid tissue of the medulla is organized into medullary cords and medullary sinuses. The medullary cords consist of reticular fibers and cells that develop around tiny blood vessels. Accordingly, small lymphocytes, macrophages, and mature plasma cells can be found in association with medullary cords. The medullary sinuses converge in the vicinity of efferent lymphatic vessels and serve to drain the lymph node. Stellate cells found within the sinuses form a weblike series of microscopic baffles, allowing interaction with macrophages in the wall of the sinus. This interaction may create a trap for cells passing through the lumen of the sinus.

The lymphatic and blood vascular systems are fellow travelers, with multiple interactions in health and disease. There are two principal pathways by which malignant cells

spread via the lymphatic system:

- Permeation of minute lymphatic vessels, which ultimately leads to growth and spread to regional lymph nodes
- Lymphatic metastasis by tumor cell emboli, which may bypass a lymph node or become entrapped in the lymph node

The lymph nodes may act as temporary filters, in which metastatic malignant cells are trapped, propelled into vessels, or destroyed.

It is known that lymph nodes can effectively arrest the passage of particulate matter and blood cells, and entrap and destroy bacteria. Some viruses, however, can proliferate rapidly within the lymph node and thereafter easily disseminate throughout the body. Similarly, lymph nodes may fail to entrap other kinds of cells carried in the lymph. For example, a large percentage of cancer cells may transit in lymphatic vessels without being arrested at the node.

When malignant cells are entrapped within the node they may proliferate rapidly, greatly increasing the size of

## Editorial Comment

*There has been a resurgence of surgical interest in the concept of the sentinel lymph node (or primary draining lymph node). Radical cancer surgery has traditionally removed the draining nodes in the region or basin associated with the organ containing the malignancy. Using dyes or radiolabeled colloids injected adjacent to the cancer it is usually possible to identify the first node or nodes (sentinel nodes) in a basin that drain from the cancer site. In general if the sentinel node does not contain a metastasis, the other lymph nodes in that basin will also be free of metastases. In addition, it is possible to use labor intensive studies (serial sections, immunohistochemical stains, and/or polymerase chain reaction studies) to identify micrometastaes in some sentinel nodes. These studies are generally considered to be too labor intensive to apply to all the nodes in a draining basin, but may be appropriate for one or two nodes. At this writing, the sentinel node concept is under the most intensive investigation in melanoma and breast cancer, but it is also being investigated for multiple other malignancies. (RSF Jr)*

the node. Non-tender, hard, compacted masses of nodes usually contain metastatic carcinoma or very aggressive intrinsic neoplasms. The particular location of the lymph gland enlargement often provides very definite clues as to the location and nature of the primary lesion.

REMEMBER:
- Interstitial fluid from the brain and spinal cord, especially the gray matter, drains through perivascular spaces and paravascular compartments of the subarachnoid space to reach the regional lymph nodes. For example, cervical lymph nodes receive interstitial fluid drainage from the brain, while lumbar lymph nodes receive interstitial fluid drainage from the spinal cord.
- Lymphatic capillaries are present along the peripheral nerves. Lymphatics are scanty, but present, in the periosteum of bone and in tendons.
- Many anomalies and variations occur within the origin, distribution, and termination of the thoracic duct.
- When the thoracic duct itself enters the venous system on the right, there is frequently an anomalous retroesophageal right subclavian artery.
- All the lymphoid tissue of the human body forms approximately 1% of the body weight (about ½ the weight of the liver).
- The cisterna chyli and the right lymphatic duct and thoracic duct can be ligated with impunity.
- Lymphocytes and lymph always circulate within the nodal parenchyma.
- On its pathway to the neck, the thoracic duct is not interrupted by lymph nodes; therefore, lymph which is already filtered by several groups of lymph nodes is drained directly into the veins.
- Since the valves do not work after death, blood can regurgitate into the ducts, causing the involved segments to resemble veins.
- After injury or ligation of a lymphatic vessel, the lumen of the vessel becomes solid, and later the endothelium recanalizes.
- Acquired cutaneous lymphangiectasia, with areas of skin affected by obstruction and destruction of lymphatic drainage, was reported by Garcia-Doval et al.,[22] who stated that this was the first case associated with altered lymph flow in cirrhosis and ascites.
- We quote from Gidvani et al.,[23] who stressed the need to include Castleman's disease in the differential diagnosis of pediatric lymphoproliferative disorders:

    *Castleman's disease (also known as angiofollicular lymph node hyperplasia, angiomatous lymphoid hamartoma, and giant lymph node hyperplasia) is an uncommon lymphoproliferative disorder that most frequently is seen as an asymptomatic mass in the mediastinum. Little is known about the cause of this disorder, but the bulk of the evidence points toward faulty immunoregulation, which results in the excessive proliferation of B lymphocytes and plasma cells in lymphoid organs.*

- Rarely, the cisterna chyli may suffer isolated injury in blunt abdominal trauma.[24]

## SURGERY

In this book, surgery of the lymphatic system (lymphadenectomy) is presented in the chapters of the concerned organs.

Though it is not within the scope of this chapter to cover lymphedema, the senior author of this chapter (JES) asks the reader's indulgence to reminisce about a well known professor, Dr. Emmanuel Kondoleon (1879-1939), with whom he studied as a second-year medical student. The senior author watched him perform the Kondoleon operation for elephantiasis on a patient's lower extremity. From the incision to the closing, the thrill of observing "the master" remains with him today, with fond and proud memories.

## ANATOMIC COMPLICATIONS

Iatrogenic injury during surgery, or penetrating injuries of the neck, thorax, and upper abdomen may injure the thoracic duct and lead to chylorrhea. The thoracic duct may be injured at its beginning, middle, or terminal portion during a number of surgical procedures, including but not limited to:

- Hiatal hernia repair
- Distal esophageal surgery
- Surgery of aortic aneurysm
- Esophageal resection
- Thoracic aortic aneurysm surgery
- Scalene biopsy
- Left radical neck surgery

According to Woodburne and Burkel,[8] injuries to the thoracic duct can produce 75-200 cc of chylous drainage per hour. This is enough fluid to soak the patient's pillow and upper bed if it drains out, to collapse the lung (chylothorax), or to produce an enlarged abdomen (chyloperitoneum).

Chylous draining may occur during neck surgery or with penetrating injuries. It may be persistent or temporary. If the draining is persistent, ligation is essential.

Nussenbaum and colleagues[25] performed a patient trial of conservative treatment of chyle fistula, including nutritional modification, pressure dressings, and closed drainage. This medical management failed in 20%. They support early operative intervention if the peak 24-hour drainage is greater than 1000 mL: "Persistent low-output drainage after 10 days is associated with a prolonged management course and treatment-related complications. Optimal treatment of these patients is unclear."

We quote from Gregor[26] on the management of chyle fistula:

*Total parenteral nutrition allows for control of the fluid and protein loss while avoiding flow of chyle, and in most cases it results in resolution. In those cases that do not resolve, fibrin glue with some type of mesh and muscle flaps usually succeed in closure.*

If the thoracic duct is injured within the thorax, chylothorax with secondary collapse of the left lung can result. If repeated aspiration is unsuccessful, ligation is needed not only to avoid restriction of the lung but also to avoid chylous ascites and decreased nutrition.

Thoracoscopic ligation of the thoracic duct has been used to treat chylothorax following esophagectomy.[27] For the same condition, Merigliano et al.[28] advocate early thoracic duct ligation, with re-operation performed immediately after diagnosis. Sakata et al.[29] treated primary chylopericardium by thoracoscopic thoracic duct ligation and partial pericardiectomy.

Chylous ascites can occur secondary to injury of the cisterna chyli or the proximal subdiaphragmatic part of the thoracic duct. With chylous ascites, the abdominal cavity becomes tremendously enlarged due to accumulation of fluid. Again, ligation is necessary.

Beghetti et al.[30] studied the etiology and management of pediatric chylothorax:

*Prevention, early recognition, and treatment of potential complications, such as superior vena cava thrombosis or obstruction, may further improve success of conservative treatment. Congenital chylothorax seems different and may require a specific approach.*

It is well known that radiation treatment, as well as some surgical procedures, produces dilatation of the lymphatic vessels, the so-called acquired lymphangiectasis. Celis et al.[31] treat this complication with $CO_2$ laser ablation with good results.

## REFERENCES

1. Giordano JM, Trout HH, DePalma RG. The Basic Science of Vascular Surgery. Mount Kisco, NY: Futura Publishing, 1988:32.
2. Skandalakis JE, Gray SW. Embryology for Surgeons, 2nd Ed. Baltimore: Williams & Wilkins, 1994.
3. Musone E, Bonafiglia R, Menditto A, Paccone M, Cassese E, Russo G, Balbi C. Fetuses with cystic hygroma. A retrospective study. Panminerva Med 2000;42:39-43.
4. Riquet M, Briere J, Le Pimpec-Barthes F, Bely N, Dujon A, Velly JF, Brichon PY, Faillon JM, Mouroux J, Jancovici R, Dahan M. [Cystic lymphangioma of the neck and mediastinum: are there acquired forms? Report of 37 cases]. Rev Mal Resp 1999;16:71-79.

5. Moore KL, Persaud TVN. The Developing Human, 6th Ed. Philadelphia: WB Saunders, 1997.

6. Bouchard S, Di Lorenzo M, Youssef S, Simard P, Lapierre JG. Pulmonary lymphangiectasia revisited. J Pediatr Surg 2000;35:796-800.

7. Williams PL (ed). Gray's Anatomy (38th ed). New York: Churchill Livingstone, 1995, pp. 1608-1609.

8. Woodburne RT, Burkel WE. Essentials of Human Anatomy, 9th Ed. New York: Oxford University Press, 1994, p. 501.

9. As cited in Slanetz CA Jr, Herter FP. The large intestine. In: Haagensen CD, Feind CR, Herter FP, Slanetz CA Jr, Weinberg JA. The Lymphatics in Cancer. Philadelphia: WB Saunders, 1972, p. 496.

10. Decker GAG, du Plessis DJ (eds). Lee McGregor's Synopsis of Surgical Anatomy, 12th Ed. Bristol: Wright, 1986, p. 268.

11. Lee KC, Cassar-Pullicino VN. Giant cisterna chyli: MRI depiction with Gadolinium-DTPA enhancement. Clin Radiol 2000;55:51-55.

12. Karajiannis A, Krueger T, Stauffer E, Ris H. Large thoracic duct cyst - a case report and review of the literature. Eur J Cardio Thorac Surg 2000;17:754-756.

13. Ehrenhaft JL, Meyers R. Blood fat levels following supradiaphragmatic ligation of the thoracic duct. Ann Surg 1948;128:38.

14. Jdanov DA. Anatomie du canal thoracique et des principaux collecteurs lymphatiques du tronc chez l'homme. Acta Anat 1959;37: 20-47.

15. Kinnaert P. Anatomical variations of the cervical part of the thoracic duct in man. J Anat 1973;115:45-52.

16. Shimada K, Sato I. Morphological and histological analysis of the thoracic duct at the jugulo-subclavian junction in Japanese cadavers. Clin Anat 1997;10:163-172.

17. Kihara T, Adachi B. Der Ductus Thoracicus der Japaner. In: Kihara T, Adachi B. Das Lymphgefäßsystem der Japaner. Kyoto: Kenkyusha, 1953, pp. 44-49.

18. Jacobsson SI. Clinical Anatomy and Pathology of the Thoracic Duct: An Investigation of 122 Cases. Stockholm: Almqvist & Wiksell, 1972.

19. Russell RCG, Williams NS, Bulstrode CJK (eds). Bailey & Love's Short Practice of Surgery (23rd ed). London: Arnold, 2000, p. 704.

20. Haagensen CD. General anatomy of the lymphatic system. In: Haagensen CD, Feind CR, Herter FP, Slanetz CA Jr, Weinberg JA. The Lymphatics in Cancer. Philadelphia: WB Saunders, 1972, p. 30.

21. Roth MH, Reith EJ. Histology: A Text and Atlas. New York: Harper & Row/JB Lippincott, 1985, p. 309.

22. Garcia-Doval I, de la Torre C, Losada A, Ocampo C, Rodriguez T, Cruces MJ. Acquired cutaneous lymphangiectasia associated with cirrhotic ascites. J Eur Acad Dermatol Venereol 1999; 13:109-112.

23. Gidvani V, Tyree MM, Bhowmick SK. Castleman's disease: atypical manifestation in an 11-year-old girl. South Med J 2001;94:250-253.

24. Calkins CM, Moore EE, Huerd S, Patten R. Isolated rupture of the cisterna chyli after blunt trauma. J Pediatr Surg 2000;35:638-640.

25. Nussenbaum B, Liu JH, Sinard RJ. Systematic management of chyle fistula: the Southwestern experience and review of the literature. Otolaryngol Head Neck 2000;122:31-38.

26. Gregor RT. Management of chyle fistulization in association with neck dissection. Otolaryngol Head Neck Surg 2000;122:434-439.

27. Takemura M, Osugi H, Tokuhara T, Kinoshita H, Higashino M. Chylothorax after thoracoscopic esophagectomy. Jpn J Thorac Cardiovasc Surg 2000;48:238-241.

28. Merigliano S, Molena D, Ruol A, Zaninotto G, Cagol M, Scappin S, Ancona E. Chylothorax complicating esophagectomy for cancer: a plea for early thoracic duct ligation. J Thorac Cardiovasc Surg 2000;119:453-457.

29. Sakata S, Yoshida I, Otani Y, Ishikawa S, Morishita Y. Thoracoscopic treatment of primary chylopericardium. Ann Thorac Surg 2000;69:1581-1582.

30. Beghetti M, La Scala G, Belli D, Bugmann P, Kalangos A, Le Coultre C. Etiology and management of pediatric chylothorax. J Pediatr 2000;136:653-658.

31. Celis AV, Gaughf CN, Sangueza OP, Gourdin FW. Acquired lymphangiectasis. South Med J 1999;92:69-72.

# *Index*